Concise Colour

Medical Dictionary

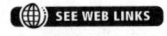 **SEE WEB LINKS**

Many entries in this dictionary have recommended web
links. When you see the above symbol at the end of an entry
go to the dictionary's web page at http://www.oup.com/
uk/reference/resources/medical, click on **Web links** in the
Resources section and locate the entry in the alphabetical
list, then click straight through to the relevant websites.

Oxford Paperback Reference

The most authoritative and up-to-date reference books for both students and the general reader.

Concise Colour

Medical Dictionary

FIFTH EDITION

OXFORD
UNIVERSITY PRESS

OXFORD
UNIVERSITY PRESS

Great Clarendon Street, Oxford OX2 6DP

Oxford University Press is a department of the University of Oxford.
It furthers the University's objective of excellence in research, scholarship,
and education by publishing worldwide in

Oxford New York

Auckland Cape Town Dar es Salaam Hong Kong Karachi
Kuala Lumpur Madrid Melbourne Mexico City Nairobi
New Delhi Shanghai Taipei Toronto

With offices in

Argentina Austria Brazil Chile Czech Republic France Greece
Guatemala Hungary Italy Japan Poland Portugal Singapore
South Korea Switzerland Thailand Turkey Ukraine Vietnam

Oxford is a registered trade mark of Oxford University Press
in the UK and in certain other countries

Published in the United States
by Oxford University Press Inc., New York

This colour edition first published as an
Oxford University Press paperback 1996.
Second edition 1998
Third edition 2002
Fourth edition, which uses the text of the seventh edition
of the Concise Medical Dictionary, 2007
Fifth edition, which uses the text of the eighth edition
of the Concise Medical Dictionary, 2010

British Library Cataloguing in Publication Data
Data available

Library of Congress Cataloging in Publication Data
Data available

Typeset by Market House Books Ltd.
Printed in China by C&C Offset Printing Co., Ltd.

ISBN 978–0–19–955715–8

10 9 8 7 6 5 4 3 2 1

Contents

Preface

The fifth edition of this dictionary provides full coverage of all the important terms and concepts used in medicine today. Written by a distinguished team of practising specialists and medical writers, it is intended primarily for workers in the paramedical fields: pharmacists, physiotherapists, speech therapists, social workers, hospital secretaries, administrators, technicians, and so on. It will also be invaluable for medical students and provides a useful reference for practising doctors. Each entry contains a basic definition, followed – where appropriate – by a more detailed explanation or description. A feature of the dictionary is that the articles are written in clear and concise English without the use of unnecessary medical jargon. For this reason the book will also be of both interest and value to the general reader who needs a home medical dictionary.

The dictionary defines terms in anatomy, physiology, biochemistry, and genetics, as well as in all the major medical and surgical specialties. Entries for medicinal drugs are given under their recommended International Non-proprietary Names (rINNs); where these differ from the names commonly used in Britain, the latter are included both as synonyms for the rINNs and as cross-reference entries (see below). Coverage of psychology and psychiatry, public health medicine, endocrinology, and dentistry is unusually comprehensive, and this edition includes over 500 new entries covering the latest developments in cardiology, oncology, and medical genetics, as well as the other medical and surgical specialties. Coverage of obstetrics and gynaecology, paediatrics, nephrology, and medical ethics has been considerably increased, and new tables and pathways have been added to the illustrations. Another feature of this edition is the addition of extra Appendices, which now include (among others) paediatric reference values, baby milk formulas, and medical certificates, and the Abbreviations section of the Appendices has been expanded.

To avoid cluttering the entry list with derivative words (e.g. adjectival forms of nouns that are defined), these words are listed at the end of the definitions of the words from which they are derived. Where necessary, articles are supplemented by clear and fully labelled line drawings. An asterisk against a word used in a definition indicates that this term has its own entry in the dictionary and that additional information can be found there. Cross-reference entries simply refer the reader to another entry, indicating either that they are synonyms or abbreviations or that they – together with related terms – are most conveniently explained in one of the dictionary's longer articles. Synonyms and abbreviations are shown in brackets after the defined term.

E.A.M.
2009

Credits

Editor

Elizabeth A. Martin MA (Oxon)

Contributors for the fifth edition

Dr Sandeep Bajwa MRCP
Dr Deborah Bowman MA, PhD
Dr Mark Donnelly FRCP
P. J. T. Drew MD, FRCP
Peter Glennon MD, FRCP
Pamela A. Hall BM, DPH, MFPHM
T. Q. Howes MA, MB, BS, MD, MRCP(I)
Dr J. Craig Jobling MA, MB, BChir, FRCS, FRCR
Nikhil Kaushik FRCOphth

Matthew Kurien MRCP
Dr Peter Lepping MD, MRCPsych, MSc
H. Manji MA, MD, FRCP
D. J. McFerran MA, FRCS
Dr Alpa N. Patel MB, BS, MRCGP, DRCOG
Amin Rahemtulla PhD, FRCP
Dr Alexandra Taylor MRCP, FRCR, MD
Jonathan White BSc (Hons), MRCP(UK)
Clare Willocks MBChB, BSc (Hons), MRCOG

Contributors and advisers for previous editions

Rajesh Aggarwal BM, MRCP, FRCS, FRCOphth
David Ahearne MB, ChB
W. Leslie Alexander FRCS, FRCOphth
J. A. D. Anderson MA, MD, FRCP, FFPHM,
    FFOM, FRCGP
J. H. Angel MD, FRCP
Dr Andrea Atherton MA, MSc, MRCP(UK)
John R. Bennett MD, FRCP
Stuart Anthony Bentley MB, BS
Dr J. N. Bowles BSc, MRCP, FRCR
Dr Peter Bradbury FRCP
Bruce M. Bryant MB, ChB, MRCP
Dr Julian L. Burton MBChB (Hons), MEd, ILTM
Philip Chan MA, MChir, FRCS
Mr Sohail Choksy MD, FRCS
Robert E. Coleman
Patrick Collins MD, MRCP
J. A. Cullen BSc, MSc
W. J. Dinning FRCS, MRCP
Ivan T. Draper MB, ChB, FRCPEd
Dr Sarah J. L. Edwards BSc, MA, PhD
John A. Gallagher MB, BS, FRACS(Orth)
J. C. Gingell MB, BCh, FRCSEd, FRCS
John M. Goldman DM, FRCP, FRCPath

Dr Helen K. Gordon FRCOG, MFFP
W. J. Gordon MD, FRCS(G), FRCOG
Michael Klaber MA, MB, FRCP
Marc E. Laniado MD, FRCS(Urol)
Alexander J. Lewis BSc, MB, BS, MRCPsych
Gordon Macpherson MB, BS
Charles V. Mann MA, MCh, FRCS
J. E. Nicholl MA, FRCS(Orth)
D. L. Phillips FRCR, FRCOG
Helen Phillips MB, BS, MRCGP, DCH, DRCOG
Heather E. Pitt Ford FDS
T. R. Pitt Ford PhD, BDS, FDS
Dr John R. Sewell MA, MB, MRCP
A. Shafiq FRCOphth, MRCP(Paeds), BM & BCh
    (Oxon)
Dr Mary Sibellas MD, FFPHM, DTM&H
B. F. Sizer BSc, MB, ChB, FRACR
Dr Tony Smith MA, BM, BCh
Dr Steve Stanaway BSc (Hons), MB, ChB, MRCP
Eric Taylor MA, MB, MRCP, MRCPsych
William F. Whimster MRCP, MRCPath
Paul Watson MA, MB, BChir, DSH, MPH, FFPHM
Robert M. Youngson MB, ChB, DRM&H, DO,
    FRCOphthal

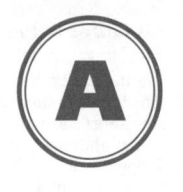

a- (an-) *prefix denoting* absence of; lacking; not. Examples: **amastia** (absence of breasts); **amorphic** (lacking definite form); **atoxic** (not poisonous).

AA *see* ALCOHOLICS ANONYMOUS.

A and E medicine accident and emergency medicine: an important specialty dealing with the immediate problems of the acutely ill and injured. *See also* ED.

ab- *prefix denoting* away from. Example: **abembryonic** (away from or opposite the embryo).

abarticulation *n.* **1.** the dislocation of a joint. **2.** a synovial joint (*see* DIARTHROSIS).

abasia *n.* an inability to walk for which no physical cause can be identified. *See also* ASTASIA.

abbreviated injury scale a quick method for determining the severity of a case of serious trauma. It can be used for purposes of *triage and *clinical audit.

abciximab *n.* an *antiplatelet drug (a *monoclonal antibody) that is used as an adjunct to lessen the chance of a heart attack during surgery to open blocked arteries of the heart (*see* CORONARY ANGIOPLASTY). It is administered by intravenous infusion; side-effects include bleeding, nausea, chest and back pain, and headache. Trade name: **ReoPro**.

abdomen *n.* the part of the body cavity below the chest (*see* THORAX), from which it is separated by the *diaphragm. The abdomen contains the organs of digestion – stomach, liver, intestines, etc. – and excretion – kidneys, bladder, etc.; in women it also contains the ovaries and uterus. The regions and quadrants of the abdomen are shown in the illustration: the four quadrants, demarcated by broken lines, are the right upper (RUQ), right lower (RLQ), left upper (LUQ), and left lower (LLQ). Terms in brackets are those used in anatomy textbooks (rather than in day-to-day medical practice) to designate the regions. —**abdominal** *adj.*

abdomin- (abdomino-) *combining form denoting* the abdomen. Examples: **abdominalgia** (pain in the abdomen); **abdominothoracic** (relating to the abdomen and thorax).

abdominal dehiscence *see* BURST ABDOMEN.

abdominal thrusts (Heimlich manoeuvre) a manoeuvre for the treatment of choking in which the patient is held firmly

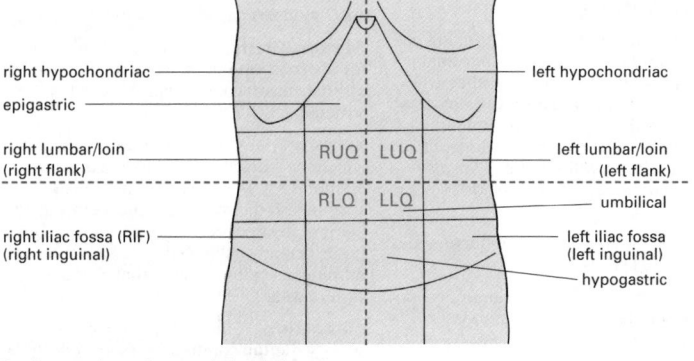

Regions and quadrants of the abdomen.

around the midriff just under the ribcage. The hands of the rescuer are held as a fist and short sharp thrusts into the patient's upper abdomen are made in order to dislodge the obstructing article from the airway. This manoeuvre should not be performed on children under the age of one year.

abducens nerve the sixth *cranial nerve (VI), which supplies the lateral rectus muscle of each eyeball, responsible for turning the eye outwards.

abduct *vb.* to move a limb or any other part away from the midline of the body. —**abduction** *n.*

abductor *n.* any muscle that moves one part of the body away from another or from the midline of the body.

aberrant *adj.* abnormal: usually applied to a blood vessel or nerve that does not follow its normal course.

aberration *n.* (in optics) a defect in the image formed by an optical device (e.g. a lens). In **chromatic aberration** the image has coloured fringes as a result of the different extent to which light of different colours is refracted. In **spherical aberration**, the image is blurred because rays from the object come to a focus in slightly different positions: the rays passing through more peripherally are bent more than those passing through centrally. This occurs even with monochromatic light.

abiotrophy *n.* degeneration or loss of function without apparent cause; for example, **retinal abiotrophy** is progressive degeneration of the retina leading to impaired vision, occurring in genetic disorders such as *retinitis pigmentosa.

ablation *n.* the removal or destruction of tissue, a part of the body, or an abnormal growth by surgery, hormonal or other drugs, or heat. For example, **ablation therapy** is an alternative to surgery for the treatment of breast cancer; it allows accurate targeting of tumours guided by MR scanning. *See also* ENDOMETRIAL ABLATION, RADIOFREQUENCY ABLATION.

ablepharia *n.* absence of or reduction in the size of the eyelids.

abortifacient *n.* a drug that induces abortion or miscarriage. *See* MIFEPRISTONE, PROSTAGLANDIN.

abortion *n.* **1.** (induced abortion, termi-

nation of pregnancy) the removal of an embryo or fetus from the uterus at a stage of pregnancy when it is deemed incapable of independent survival (i.e. at any time between conception and the 24th week of pregnancy). One of the most commonly performed gynaecological procedures in the UK, it must be carried out within the terms of the Abortion Act 1967, as amended, and the subsequent Abortion Regulations 1991. The legislation does not apply to Northern Ireland. The Department of Health keeps statistics of terminations performed in the United Kingdom, which are published annually. Two doctors must agree that termination of pregnancy is necessary for one of the reasons specified in the Regulations, which sometimes allow termination beyond the legal age of viability (24 weeks) in special circumstances (e.g. substantial risk of disability in the child if born). The majority of terminations are conducted in the first trimester. The procedure must be carried out in an approved hospital or clinic. Drugs used for medically induced abortion include *mifepristone and prostaglandin analogues (e.g. *misoprostol). Surgical methods of termination of pregnancy include vacuum aspiration of the products of conception through an intrauterine cannula, *dilatation and curettage, and uterine evacuation by ovum forceps. Termination carries little risk early in pregnancy, but complications (e.g. bleeding, infection) are more likely to occur after the 13th week of pregnancy. **2.** (spontaneous abortion) *see* MISCARRIAGE.

abortus *n.* a fetus, weighing less than 500 g, that is expelled from the uterus either dead or incapable of surviving.

ABO system *see* BLOOD GROUP.

Abrams-Griffiths number (bladder outlet obstruction index, BOOI) a scale used to estimate the degree of bladder outlet obstruction (*BOO).

abrasion *n.* **1.** a graze: a minor wound in which the surface of the skin or a mucous membrane is worn away by rubbing or scraping. **2.** the wearing of the teeth, particularly at the necks by overvigorous brushing. It is frequently enhanced by *erosion. **3.** any rubbing or scraping action that produces surface wear.

abreaction *n.* the therapeutic release of strong emotion commonly associated with a buried memory. The therapist may help the patient to retrieve the memory (sometimes through hypnosis), which is accompanied by the release and discharge of tension and anxiety associated with it; this rids the memory of its power. *See* REPRESSION.

abruptio (ablatio) *n.* separation.

abruptio placentae (placental abruption) bleeding from a normally situated placenta causing its complete or partial detachment from the uterine wall after the 24th week of gestation. There may be varying degrees of shock; *disseminated intravascular coagulation is a further complication. Abruptio placentae is often associated with hypertension and pre-eclampsia.

abscess *n.* a localized collection of pus and necrotic tissue anywhere in the body, surrounded and walled off by damaged and inflamed tissues. A *boil is an example of an abscess within the skin. The usual cause is local bacterial infection, often by staphylococci, that the body's defences have failed to overcome. In a **cold abscess**, due to tubercle bacilli, there is swelling, but little pain or inflammation (as in acute abscesses). Antibiotics, aided by surgical incision to release pus where necessary, are the usual forms of treatment.

The brain and its meninges have a low resistance to infection and a **cerebral abscess** is liable to follow any penetration of these by microorganisms. The condition is fatal unless relieved by aspiration or surgical drainage.

absence *n.* (in neurology) *see* EPILEPSY.

Absidia *n.* a genus of fungi that sometimes cause disease in humans (*see* PHYCOMYCOSIS).

absorption *n.* (in physiology) the uptake of fluids or other substances by the tissues of the body. Digested food is absorbed into the blood and lymph from the alimentary canal. Most absorption of food occurs in the small intestine – in the jejunum and ileum – although alcohol is readily absorbed from the stomach. The small intestine is lined with minute finger-like processes (*see* VILLUS), which greatly increase its surface area and therefore the speed at which absorption can take place. *See also* ASSIMILATION, DIGESTION.

abutment *n.* (in dentistry) a component of a dental *bridge or *implant.

acalculia *n.* an acquired inability to make simple mathematical calculations. It is a

symptom of disease in the dominant *parietal lobe of the brain. *See* GERSTMANN'S SYNDROME.

acamprosate calcium a drug used, in conjunction with counselling, for the maintenance of sobriety. Patients must already be abstinent at the beginning of treatment. It is administered orally; the most common side-effect is diarrhoea. Trade name: **Campral**.

acantha *n.* **1.** a spine projecting from a *vertebra. **2.** the *backbone.

Acanthamoeba *n.* a genus of amoebae commonly found in dust, soil, and fresh water. Several species can cause serious infection of the cornea, usually resulting from the use of improperly sterilized contact lenses (which may have been cleaned with tap water, for example).

acanthion *n.* the tip of the spine formed where projecting processes of the upper jaw bones (maxillae) meet at the front of the face.

acanthosis *n.* an increase in the number of *prickle cells in the innermost layer of the epidermis, leading to thickening of the epidermis. **Acanthosis nigricans** is associated with *insulin resistance; it is characterized by papillomatous growths, mainly in the armpits, giving the skin a pigmented appearance and a velvety texture. It may be benign or malignant. **Pseudoacanthosis nigricans** is more common and is associated with obesity and insulin resistance.

acapnia (hypocapnia) *n.* a condition in which there is an abnormally low concentration of carbon dioxide in the blood. This may be caused by breathing that is exceptionally deep in relation to the physical activity of the individual.

acarbose *n. see* ALPHA-GLUCOSIDASE INHIBITOR.

acardia *n.* congenital absence of the heart. The condition may occur in conjoined twins; the twin with the heart controls the circulation for both.

acariasis *n.* an infestation of mites and ticks and the symptoms, for example allergy and dermatitis, that their presence may provoke.

acaricide *n.* any chemical agent used for destroying mites and ticks.

acarid *n.* a *mite or *tick.

Acarina *n.* the group of arthropods that includes the *mites and *ticks.

Acarus (Tyroglyphus) *n.* a genus of mites. The flour mite, *A. siro* (*T. farinae*), is nonparasitic, but its presence in flour can cause a severe allergic dermatitis in flour-mill workers.

acatalasia *n.* a rare inborn lack of the enzyme *catalase, leading to recurrent infections of the gums (gingivitis) and mouth. There are two variants: Japanese (**Takahara disease**) and Swiss (asymptomatic).

acceptor *n.* (in biochemistry) a substance that helps to bring about oxidation of a reduced *substrate by accepting hydrogen ions.

accessory muscles muscles of the shoulder girdle and chest wall that (in addition to the intercostal muscles and the diaphragm) are utilized during *respiratory distress to help the flow of air in and out of the lungs. Use of these muscles can be a sign of the degree of difficulty that the patient is in, for example in cases of asthma or *airway obstruction.

accessory nerve (spinal accessory nerve) the eleventh *cranial nerve (XI), which arises from two roots, cranial and spinal. Fibres from the cranial root travel with the nerve for only a short distance before branching to join the vagus and then forming the recurrent laryngeal nerve, which supplies the internal laryngeal muscles. Fibres from the spinal root supply the sternomastoid and trapezius muscles, in the neck region (front and back).

accessory pathway an extra electrical conduction pathway between the atria and ventricles of the heart that predisposes to *re-entry tachycardia. The pathway may be contained within the atrioventricular node or may be anatomically separate, giving rise to a delta wave characteristic of the *Wolff-Parkinson-White syndrome.

accident *n.* a traumatic incident involving any part of the body. **Accident and emergency (A and E) medicine** is a specialized area of patient care dealing with acute illness.

accommodation *n.* adjustment of the shape of the lens to change the focus of the eye. When the ciliary muscle (*see* CILIARY BODY) is relaxed, suspensory ligaments attached to the ciliary body and holding the lens in position are stretched, which causes the lens to be flattened. The eye is then able to focus on distant objects. To focus the eye on near objects the ciliary muscles contract and the tension in the ligaments is thus lowered, allowing the lens to become rounder. Adjustments in *convergence also contribute to accommodation.

accommodation reflex (convergence reflex) a reflex that occurs when an individual focuses on a near object, in which the crystalline lens becomes more convex, the pupils constrict, and the eyes turn inwards.

accommodative insufficiency a weakness of accommodation as a part of the ageing process or as a result of injury, disease, or the effect of medication.

accouchement *n.* delivery of a baby.

acebutolol *n.* a *beta blocker drug used to treat high blood pressure, angina pectoris, and irregular heart rhythms. It is administered by mouth. Possible side-effects include breathing difficulty, especially in asthmatics, and cold hands and feet. Trade name: **Sectral**.

ACE inhibitor angiotensin-converting enzyme inhibitor: any one of a group of drugs used in the treatment of raised blood pressure and heart failure. ACE inhibitors act by interfering with the action of the enzyme that converts the inactive *angiotensin I to the powerful artery constrictor angiotensin II. The absence of this substance allows arteries to widen and the blood pressure to drop. ACE inhibitors are administered by mouth; they include *captopril, *enalapril, **perindopril** (Coversyl Arginine), and **ramipril** (Tritace). Possible side-effects include weakness, dizziness, loss of appetite, and skin rashes.

acentric *n.* (in genetics) a chromosome or fragment of a chromosome that has no *centromere. Since acentrics cannot attach to the *spindle they are usually lost during cell division. They are often found in cells damaged by radiation. —**acentric** *adj.*

acephalus *n.* a fetus without a head.

acervulus cerebri a collection of granules of calcium-containing material that is sometimes found within the *pineal gland as its calcification proceeds (normally after the 17th year): 'brain sand'.

acetabulum (cotyloid cavity) *n.* either of

the two deep sockets, one on each side of the *hip bone, into which the head of the thigh bone (femur) fits at the *hip joint.

acetaminophen *n. see* PARACETAMOL.

acetazolamide *n.* a *carbonic anhydrase inhibitor used mainly in the treatment of glaucoma to reduce the pressure inside the eyeball and also as a preventative for epileptic seizures and altitude sickness. It is administered by mouth or intravenous injection; side-effects include drowsiness and numbness and tingling of the hands and feet. Trade name: **Diamox**.

acetoacetic acid an organic acid produced in large amounts by the liver under metabolic conditions associated with a high rate of fatty acid oxidation (for example, in starvation). The acetoacetic acid thus formed is subsequently converted to acetone and excreted. *See also* KETONE.

acetone *n.* an organic compound that is an intermediate in many bacterial fermentations and is produced by fatty acid oxidation. In certain abnormal conditions (for example, starvation) acetone and other *ketones may accumulate in the blood (*see* KETOSIS). Acetone is a volatile liquid that is miscible with both fats and water and therefore of great value as a solvent. It is used in chromatography and in the preparation of tissues for enzyme extraction.

acetone body (ketone body) *see* KETONE.

acetonuria *n. see* KETONURIA.

acetylcholine *n.* the acetic acid ester of the organic base choline: the *neurotransmitter released at the synapses of parasympathetic nerves and at *neuromuscular junctions. After relaying a nerve impulse, acetylcholine is rapidly broken down by the enzyme *cholinesterase. *Antimuscarinic drugs block the action of acetylcholine at receptor sites; *anticholinesterases and *acetylcholinesterase inhibitors prolong the activity of acetylcholine by blocking cholinesterase.

A pharmaceutical preparation of acetylcholine is instilled into the anterior chamber of the eye as a *miotic during intraocular surgery. Trade name: **Miochol-E**.

acetylcholinesterase *n. see* CHOLINESTERASE.

acetylcholinesterase inhibitor any one of a class of drugs that block the action of acetylcholinesterase (*see* CHOLINESTERASE), an enzyme that quickly breaks down the neurotransmitter acetylcholine. This neurotransmitter is central to the functional interconnection between nerve cells in the outer layer (cortex) of the brain; the early impairment of cognitive function found in Alzheimer's disease is associated with a reduction in acetylcholine levels. By inhibiting acetylcholine breakdown, acetylcholinesterase inhibitors have been found helpful in slowing down the rate of cognitive decline in mild to moderate dementia; they do not halt the progress of the disease. The group includes **donepezil** (Aricept), **galantamine** (Reminyl), and **rivastigmine** (Exelon); these drugs are given by mouth.

acetylcysteine *n.* a drug administered as eye drops to break down mucus filaments in the eyes in the treatment of dry eyes (for example, in *Sjögren's syndrome). It is also given, by intravenous infusion, to prevent liver damage in paracetamol overdosage. Trade name: **Ilube**.

acetylsalicylic acid *see* ASPIRIN.

achalasia a condition in which the normal muscular activity of the oesophagus (gullet) is disturbed (absent or uncoordinated) due to failure or incomplete relaxation of the tight sphincter at the lower end of the oesophagus (lower oesophageal sphincter, LOS), which leads to delay in the passage of swallowed material into the stomach. It may occur at any age and affects both sexes equally: symptoms include difficulty in swallowing liquids and solids, slowly increasing over years; often regurgitation of undigested food; and occasionally severe chest pain caused by spasm of the oesophagus. Diagnosis is by a *barium swallow X-ray examination, endoscopy, and oesophageal manometric and pH studies (*see* MANOMETRY). Treatment is by forceful stretching of the LOS by surgical splitting of the muscular ring in that area (**cardiomyotomy** or **Heller's operation**), or by injecting *botulinum toxin into the sphincter.

Achilles tendon the tendon of the muscles of the calf of the leg (the *gastrocnemius and soleus muscles), situated at the back of the ankle and attached to the calcaneus (heel bone).

achlorhydria *n.* absence of hydrochloric acid in the stomach. Achlorhydria that persists despite large doses of histamine is assoa

ciated with atrophy of the lining (mucosa) of the stomach. In this condition there is usually an absence of secretion of *intrinsic factor, which will lead to *pernicious anaemia. In some people, however, achlorhydria is not associated with any disease, produces no ill-effects, and needs no treatment.

acholia *n.* absence or deficiency of bile secretion or failure of the bile to enter the alimentary canal (for example, because of an obstructed bile duct).

acholuria *n.* absence of the *bile pigments from the urine, which occurs in some forms of jaundice (**acholuric jaundice**). —**acholuric** *adj.*

achondroplasia *n.* a disorder, inherited as a *dominant characteristic, in which the bones of the arms and legs fail to grow to normal size due to a defect in both cartilage and bone. It results in a type of *dwarfism characterized by short limbs, a normal-sized head and body, and normal intelligence. —**achondroplastic** *adj.*

achromatic *adj.* without colour.

achromatic lenses lenses that are specially designed to give clear images, eliminating the coloured fringes that are produced with ordinary lenses (caused by splitting of the light into different wavelengths and hence its component colours). Such lenses are useful in scientific instruments, such as the eyepieces of microscopes.

achromatopsia *n.* the inability to differentiate different shades of colour. Such complete *colour blindness is very rare and is usually associated with poor *visual acuity, nystagmus, and sensitivity to bright light. It is usually determined by hereditary factors.

aciclovir (acyclovir) *n.* an antiviral drug that inhibits DNA synthesis in cells infected by *herpesviruses. Administered topically, by mouth, or intravenously, it is used in the treatment of herpes simplex, herpes zoster, herpetic eye disease, and herpes encephalitis and also in patients whose immune systems are compromised. Trade name: **Zovirax**.

acidaemia *n.* abnormally high blood acidity. This condition may result from an increase in the concentration of acidic substances and/or a decrease in the level of alkaline substances in the blood. *See also* ACIDOSIS. *Compare* ALKALAEMIA.

acid-base balance the balance between

the amount of carbonic acid and bicarbonate in the blood, which must be maintained at a constant ratio of 1:20 in order to keep the hydrogen ion concentration of the plasma at a constant value (pH 7.4). Any alteration in this ratio will disturb the acid-base balance of the blood and tissues and cause either *acidosis or *alkalosis. The lungs and the kidneys play an important role in the regulation of the acid-base balance.

acid-etch technique a technique for bonding resin-based materials to the enamel of teeth; it is used to retain and seal the margins of *fillings, to retain brackets of fixed *orthodontic appliances, and to retain resin-based *fissure sealants and adhesive bridges. A porous surface is created by applying phosphoric acid for one minute or less.

acid-fast *adj.* **1.** describing bacteria that have been stained and continue to hold the stain after treatment with an acidic solution. For example, tuberculosis bacteria are acid-fast when stained with a *carbol fuchsin preparation. **2.** describing a stain that is not removed from a specimen by washing with an acidic solution.

acidophil (acidophilic) *adj.* **1.** (in histology) describing tissues, cells, or parts of cells that stain with acid dyes (such as eosin). *See also* ADENOMA. **2.** (in bacteriology) describing bacteria that grow well in acid media.

acidosis *n.* a condition in which the acidity of body fluids and tissues is abnormally high. This arises because of a failure of the mechanisms responsible for maintaining a balance between acids and alkalis in the blood (*see* ACID-BASE BALANCE). In **gaseous acidosis** more than the normal amount of carbon dioxide is retained in the body, as in drowning. Patients with diabetes mellitus suffer from *diabetic ketoacidosis, in which sodium, potassium, and *ketone bodies are lost in the urine. *See also* LACTIC ACIDOSIS, RENAL TUBULAR ACIDOSIS.

acinus *n.* (*pl.* **acini**) **1.** a small sac or cavity surrounded by the secretory cells of a gland. Some authorities regard the term as synonymous with *alveolus, but others distinguish an acinus by the possession of a narrow passage (lumen) leading from the sac. **2.** (in the lung) the tissue supplied with air by one terminal *bronchiole. *Emphysema is classified by the part of the acinus involved (i.e. **centriacinar**, **panacinar**, or **periacinar**). —**acinous** *adj.*

acitretin *n. see* RETINOID.

aclasia (aclasis) *n. see* EXOSTOSIS.

acne (acne vulgaris) *n.* a common inflammatory disorder of the sebaceous glands. These grease-producing glands are under androgen control, but the cause of acne is unknown. It typically involves the face, back, and chest and is characterized by the presence of blackheads with papules, pustules, and – in more severe cases – cysts and scars. Acne is readily treatable. Mild cases respond to topical therapy with *benzoyl peroxide, while more refractory conditions require treatment with long-term antibiotics or (for treating women only) the oral contraceptive pill; severe or cystic acne can be treated with oral *isotretinoin.

aconite *n.* the dried roots of the herbaceous plant *Aconitum napellus* (monkshood or wolfbane), containing three *analgesic substances: **aconine**, **aconitine**, and **picraconitine**. Aconite was formerly used to prepare liniments for muscular pains and a tincture for toothache, but is regarded as too toxic for use today.

acoria *n.* absence of the pupil.

acoustic *adj.* of or relating to sound or the sense of hearing.

acoustic incident a sudden unexpected noise transmitted through a telephone handset or headset with the potential of triggering *acoustic shock.

acoustic nerve *see* COCHLEAR NERVE.

acoustic neuroma *see* VESTIBULAR SCHWANNOMA.

acoustic shock an adverse reaction to a sudden unexpected noise (an *acoustic incident). The condition is characterized by symptoms that may include pain, dizziness, tinnitus, anxiety, and depression. It is not associated with permanent reduction of hearing, in comparison to noise-induced hearing loss (*see* DEAFNESS).

acquired *adj.* describing a condition or disorder contracted after birth and not attributable to hereditary causes. *Compare* CONGENITAL.

acquired immune deficiency syndrome *see* AIDS.

acrania *n.* congenital absence of the skull, either partial or complete, due to a developmental defect.

acro- *combining form denoting* 1. extremity; tip. Example: **acrohypothermy** (abnormal coldness of the extremities (hands and feet)). 2. height; promontory. Example: **acrophobia** (morbid dread of heights). 3. extreme; intense. Example: **acromania** (an extreme degree of mania).

acrocentric *n.* a chromosome in which the *centromere is situated at or very near one end. —**acrocentric** *adj.*

acrocephalosyndactyly *n.* any one of a group of related inherited disorders, including *Apert syndrome, resulting in abnormalities of the skull (*craniosynostosis), face, and hands and feet (*syndactyly).

acrocyanosis *n.* bluish-purple discoloration of the hands and feet due to slow circulation of the blood through the small vessels in the skin.

acrodermatitis *n.* inflammation of the skin of the feet or hands. A diffuse chronic variety produces swelling and reddening of the affected areas, followed by atrophy. It is a manifestation of *Lyme disease. **Acrodermatitis enteropathica** is an inherited (autosomal *recessive) inability to absorb sufficient *zinc, which causes patchy sparse hair; patches of dry scaly eczematous skin on the hands, feet, scalp, and around the mouth and anogenital region; and chronic diarrhoea. Management consists of zinc supplements.

acrodynia *n. see* PINK DISEASE.

acromegaly *n.* a condition caused by excessive secretion of *growth hormone, usually by a benign tumour of the anterior pituitary gland. Overgrowth of soft tissues and bones characteristically results in large spadelike hands and feet, prominent brow ridges, broadening of the bridge of the nose, *prognathism, widely spaced teeth, enlargement of the tongue, and excessive skin tags. The condition can be associated with an increased risk of cardiovascular disease and bowel cancer. Treatment is by surgical removal of the tumour (adenomectomy) and/or radiotherapy, with or without hormone therapy.

acromion *n.* an oblong process at the top of the spine of the *scapula, part of which articulates with the clavicle (collar bone) to form the **acromioclavicular joint**. —**acromial** *adj.*

acropachy *n. see* THYROID ACROPACHY.

acroparaesthesia *n.* a tingling sensation in the hands and feet. *See* PARAESTHESIA.

acrosclerosis *n.* a skin disease thought to be a type of generalized *scleroderma. It also has features of *Raynaud's disease, with the hands, face, and feet being mainly affected.

acrosome *n.* the caplike structure on the front end of a spermatozoon. It breaks down just before fertilization (the **acrosome reaction**), releasing a number of enzymes that assist penetration between the follicle cells that still surround the ovum. Failure of the acrosome reaction is a cause of male infertility (*see also* ANDROLOGY).

acrylic resin one of a group of polymeric materials used for making denture teeth, denture bases, and orthodontic appliances and formerly as a dental filling material.

ACTH (adrenocorticotrophic hormone, adrenocorticotrophin, corticotrophin) a hormone synthesized and stored in the anterior pituitary gland, large amounts of which are released in response to any form of stress. Its release is stimulated by *corticotrophin-releasing hormone. ACTH controls the secretion of *corticosteroid hormones from the adrenal gland. An analogue of ACTH, **tetracosactide**, is administered by injection to test adrenal function (*see* SHORT SYNACTHEN TEST).

actin *n.* a protein, found in muscle, that plays an important role in the process of contraction. *See* STRIATED MUSCLE.

Actinobacillus *n.* a genus of Gram-negative nonmotile aerobic bacteria that are characteristically spherical or rodlike in shape but occasionally grow into branching filaments. Actinobacilli cause disease in animals that can be transmitted to humans.

Actinomyces *n.* a genus of Gram-positive nonmotile fungus-like bacteria that cause disease in animals and humans. The species *A. israelii* is the causative organism of human *actinomycosis.

actinomycin D *see* DACTINOMYCIN.

actinomycosis *n.* a noncontagious disease caused by the bacterium *Actinomyces israelii*, which most commonly affects the jaw but may also affect the lungs, brain, or intestines. The bacterium is normally present in the mouth but it may become pathogenic following an *apical abscess or extraction of a tooth. It is characterized by

multiple sinus tracts that open onto the skin. Treatment is by drainage of pus and a prolonged course of antibiotics.

actinotherapy *n.* the treatment of disorders with *infrared or *ultraviolet radiation.

action potential the change in voltage that occurs across the membrane of a nerve or muscle cell when a *nerve impulse is triggered. It is due to the passage of charged particles across the membrane (*see* DEPOLARIZATION) and is an observable manifestation of the passage of an impulse.

active transport (in biochemistry) an energy-dependent process in which certain substances (including ions, some drugs, and amino acids) are able to cross cell membranes against a concentration gradient. The process is inhibited by substances that interfere with cellular metabolism (e.g. high doses of digitalis).

actomyosin *n.* a protein complex formed in muscle between actin and myosin during the process of contraction. *See* STRIATED MUSCLE.

acuity *n. see* VISUAL ACUITY.

acupuncture *n.* a complementary therapy in which fine sterile needles are inserted into the skin at specific points on the body. It was developed by Eastern physicians, who recognize pathways (**meridians**) and flows of energy (called **qi**) within the body. It may work by allowing the body to release its own natural painkillers (*endorphins). Acupuncture is used to relieve the symptoms of many physical and psychological conditions, including chronic pain.

acute *adj.* **1.** describing a disease of rapid onset, severe symptoms, and brief duration. *Compare* CHRONIC. **2.** describing any intense symptom, such as severe pain.

acute abdomen an emergency surgical condition caused by damage to one or more abdominal organs following injury or disease. The patient is in severe pain and often in shock. Perforation of a peptic ulcer or a severely infected appendix, or rupture of the liver or spleen following a crushing injury, all produce an acute abdomen requiring urgent treatment.

acute coronary syndrome a combination of angina (unstable or stable), non-S–T elevation *myocardial infarction (NSTEMI), and S–T elevation myocardial infarction

(STEMI). It implies the presence of coronary artery disease.

acute fatty liver of pregnancy a rare and serious complication of pregnancy that usually presents in the third trimester with symptoms of nausea, vomiting, malaise, and abdominal pain. Liver function tests are abnormal and the features of *pre-eclampsia and often *HELLP syndrome are present. It is associated with a high maternal and fetal mortality. *Hepatic encephalopathy, *disseminated intravascular coagulation, and renal failure may develop.

acute generalized exanthematous pustulosis (toxic pustuloderma) a reaction to a medication, resulting in the appearance of fine sterile *pustules on inflamed skin; the pustules may easily be overlooked. Common causes include penicillins, and pustular psoriasis must be excluded from the diagnosis.

acute kidney injury *see* AKI.

acute renal failure acute kidney injury (*see* AKI).

acute respiratory distress syndrome *see* ADULT RESPIRATORY DISTRESS SYNDROME.

acute respiratory failure (ARF) a primary disorder of gaseous exchange (as distinct from failure of the mechanical process of breathing). The prototype of ARF is *adult respiratory distress syndrome, but the term sometimes also refers to disruption of any other part of the respiratory system, including the respiratory control centre in the brain with its *efferent and *afferent pathways.

acute retinal necrosis (ARN) severe inflammation and necrosis of the retina associated with inflammation and blockage of retinal blood vessels, haemorrhage and death of retinal tissue, and retinal detachment. It may affect both eyes (**bilateral acute retinal necrosis, BARN**), and visual prognosis is poor. ARN is thought to be due to viral infection.

acute rheumatism *see* RHEUMATIC FEVER.

acute tubular necrosis (ATN) a condition caused by acute renal injury from either ischaemia or toxins and associated with tubular damage that is usually reversible. The earliest feature is *isosthenuria, which may occur while there is still a high urine flow rate. This is followed by a reduction in

*glomerular filtration rate. *Oliguria is common and dialysis often needed for survival. If the cause of the initial damage can be removed, recovery of renal function within 6 weeks can be expected in most cases.

acyclovir *n. see* ACICLOVIR.

ad- *prefix denoting* towards or near. Examples: **adaxial** (towards the main axis); **adoral** (towards or near the mouth).

ADA deficiency *see* ADENOSINE DEAMINASE DEFICIENCY.

adalimumab *n. see* CYTOKINE INHIBITOR.

Adam's apple (laryngeal prominence) a projection, lying just under the skin, of the thyroid cartilage of the *larynx.

Adams-Stokes syndrome *see* STOKES-ADAMS SYNDROME.

ADAMTS13 *a d*isintegrin *a*nd *m*etalloproteinase with a *t*hrombo*s*pondin type *1* motif, member *13*, also known as **von Willebrand factor-cleaving protease**: an enzyme that cleaves and degrades large von Willebrand factor multimers and decreases their activity, thereby disrupting *platelet activation. Most cases of *thrombotic thrombocytopenic purpura are as a result of inhibition or deficiency of ADAMTS13.

adaptation *n.* **1.** the phenomenon in which a sense organ shows a gradually diminishing response to continuous or repetitive stimulation. The nose, for example, may become adapted to the stimulus of an odour that is continuously present so that in time it ceases to report its presence. Similarly, the adaptation of touch receptors in the skin means that the presence of clothes can be forgotten a few minutes after they have been put on. **2.** a process of change to enable adjustment to a condition or environment.

addiction *n.* a state of *dependence produced either by the habitual taking of drugs or by regularly engaging in certain activities (e.g. gambling). People can develop physical and psychological symptoms of *dependence, which include a strong desire to take the substance or exercise the behaviour, impaired capacity to control such behaviour or substance taking, a physical or psychological *withdrawal state, evidence of *tolerance development, social and mental preoccupation with substance use or the given behaviour, and persistent use despite harmful consequences. Treatment is directed to gradual withdrawal of the drug or behaviour with the aim of partial or total abstinence. *See also* AL-COHOLISM, TOLERANCE.

Addisonian crisis an acute medical emergency due to a lack of corticosteroid production by the body, caused by disease of the adrenal glands or long-term suppression of production by steroid medication. It manifests as low blood pressure and collapse, biochemical abnormalities, hypoglycaemia, and (if untreated) coma and death. Treatment is with steroids, administered initially intravenously in high doses and later orally. In patients with poor adrenal function an Addisonian crisis is usually brought on by an acute illness, such as an infection. [T. Addison (1793–1860), British physician]

Addison's disease a syndrome resulting from inadequate secretion of corticosteroid hormones due to the progressive destruction of the adrenal cortex. It is characterized by progressive deterioration with hypotension and collapse due to severe dehydration, salt loss, and *hypoglycaemia; dark pigmentation of the skin may occur. Formerly tuberculosis was a common cause, but the condition is now more likely to be due to autoimmune destruction of the adrenal cortices (*see* AUTOIMMUNE DISEASE). Treatment is with *hydrocortisone and *fludrocortisone. [T. Addison]

adduct *vb.* to move a limb or any other part towards the midline of the body. —**adduction** *n.*

adductor *n.* any muscle that moves one part of the body towards another or towards the midline of the body.

adefovir dipivoxil a drug used to treat chronic hepatitis B in patients who have not responded to or cannot tolerate interferon alfa or peginterferon alfa. It is administered by mouth; side-effects include gastrointestinal disturbances and headache. Trade name: **Hepsera**.

aden- (adeno-) *combining form denoting* a gland or glands. Examples: **adenalgia** (pain in); **adenogenesis** (development of); **adenopathy** (disease of).

adenine *n.* one of the nitrogen-containing bases (*see* PURINE) that occurs in the nucleic acids DNA and RNA. *See also* ATP.

adenitis *n.* inflammation of a gland or group of glands (or glandlike structures). For example, **mesenteric adenitis** affects the

lymph nodes (formerly called lymph glands) in the membranous support of the intestines (the mesentery); **cervical adenitis** affects the lymph nodes in the neck.

adenocarcinoma *n.* a malignant epithelial tumour arising from glandular structures, which are constituent parts of most organs of the body. The term is also applied to tumours showing a glandular growth pattern. These tumours may be subclassified according to the substances that they produce, for example **mucinous** and **serous adenocarcinomas**, or to the microscopic arrangement of their cells into patterns, for example **papillary** and **follicular adenocarcinomas** (*see also* CLEAR-CELL CARCINOMA). They may be solid or cystic (**cystadenocarcinomas**).

adenohypophysis *n.* the anterior lobe of the *pituitary gland.

adenoidectomy *n.* surgical removal of the *adenoids in patients who suffer from either *glue ear or difficulty in breathing through the nose.

adenoids (nasopharyngeal tonsil) *n.* a collection of lymphatic tissue in the *nasopharynx. Enlargement of the adenoids can cause obstruction to breathing through the nose and can block the *Eustachian tubes, causing *glue ear.

adenolymphoma *n. see* WARTHIN'S TUMOUR.

adenoma *n.* a benign tumour of epithelial origin that is derived from glandular tissue or exhibits clearly defined glandular structures. Adenomas may undergo malignant change (*see* ADENOCARCINOMA). Some show recognizable tissue elements, such as fibrous tissue (**fibroadenomas**), while others, such as some bronchial adenomas, may produce active compounds giving rise to clinical syndromes (*see* CARCINOID). Tumours in certain organs, including the pituitary gland, are often classified by their histological staining affinities, for example **eosinophil**, **basophil**, and **chromophobe adenomas**.

adenomyosis *n. see* ENDOMETRIOSIS.

adenosine *n.* a *nucleoside that contains adenine and the sugar ribose and occurs in *ATP. It is also used as an *anti-arrhythmic drug to stop *supraventricular tachycardias and restore a normal heart rhythm. As such, it needs to be injected quickly, which may fleetingly make the patient feel faint and develop chest pain. Trade name: **Adenocor.**

adenosine deaminase deficiency (**ADA deficiency**) a genetic disorder affecting about one baby in 25,000 and characterized by a defect in **adenosine deaminase** (**ADA**), an enzyme that is involved in purine metabolism. Deficiency of this enzyme results in selective damage to the antibody-producing lymphocytes; this in turn leads to a condition known as *severe combined immune deficiency (SCID), in which the affected baby has no resistance to infection and must be entirely isolated from birth. Such children have only about a 50% chance of surviving for six months. *See also* GENE THERAPY.

adenosine diphosphate *see* ADP.

adenosine monophosphate *see* AMP.

adenosine triphosphate *see* ATP.

adenosis *n.* (*pl.* **adenoses**) **1.** excessive growth or development of glands. **2.** any disease of a gland or glandlike structure, especially of a lymph node.

adenovirus *n.* one of a group of DNA-containing viruses causing infections of the upper respiratory tract that produce symptoms resembling those of the common cold.

ADEPT *n. a*ntibody-*d*irected *e*nzyme *pro*-drug therapy: a method under development for the treatment of cancer. It involves the patient being injected first with an antibody-enzyme complex that binds specifically to tumour cells, and later with a *prodrug that is inactive until it comes into contact with the antibody-enzyme complex. The enzyme converts the prodrug into a cytotoxic form, which is concentrated around the tumour and can therefore destroy the cancer cells without damaging normal tissue.

ADH antidiuretic hormone (*see* VASOPRESSIN).

ADHD *see* ATTENTION-DEFICIT/HYPERACTIVITY DISORDER.

adherence *n.* the degree to which a patient follows medical advice. **Medicines adherence** refers specifically to taking medication (drug **compliance**) but adherence may also be applied to physiotherapy exercises or attending appointments for courses of therapy. **Nonadherence** falls into two broad categories: **intentional nonadherence** involves the patient making a decision not to follow medical advice; in **unintentional nonadherence** the patient forgets or misunderstands the advice.

adhesion *n.* **1.** the union of two normally separate surfaces, such as the moving surfaces of joints, by fibrous connective tissue developing in an inflamed or damaged region. (The fibrous tissue itself is also called an adhesion.) Adhesions between loops of intestine often occur following abdominal surgery but only rarely cause symptoms, such as intestinal obstruction. If the pericardial sac is affected by adhesion, the movements of the heart may be restricted. **2.** a healing process in which the edges of a wound fit together. In **primary adhesion** there is very little *granulation tissue; in **secondary adhesion** the two edges are joined together by granulation tissue.

adhesion molecules *cell-surface molecules that are important for binding cells to neighbouring cells (**intercellular adhesion molecules**, **ICAM**) and tissues. Absence or weakening of intercellular binding facilitates the local spread of cancer.

adhesive capsulitis *see* FROZEN SHOULDER.

Adie's pupil *see* TONIC PUPIL. [W. J. Adie (1886–1935), British physician]

Adie's syndrome (**Holmes-Adie syndrome**) an abnormality of the pupils of the eyes, often affecting only one eye. The affected pupil is dilated and reacts slowly to light; the response on convergence *accommodation of the eyes is also slow (*see* TONIC PUPIL). Tendon reflexes may be absent. The condition is almost entirely restricted to women. [W. J. Adie; Sir G. M. Holmes (1876–1965), British neurologist]

adipocere *n.* a waxlike substance, consisting mainly of fatty acids, into which the soft tissues of the body can be converted after death. This usually occurs when the body is buried in damp earth or is submerged in water. Adipocere delays post-mortem decomposition and is a spontaneous form of preservation without mummification.

adipocyte *n. see* ADIPOSE TISSUE.

adipose tissue fibrous *connective tissue packed with masses of fat cells (**adipocytes**). In human adults it consists mostly of **white fat** (*see also* BROWN FAT). It forms a thick layer under the skin and occurs around the kidneys and in the buttocks. It serves both as an insulating layer and an energy store; food in excess of requirements is converted into fats and stored within these cells.

adiposis (liposis) *n.* the presence of abnormally large accumulations of fat in the body. The condition may arise from overeating, hormone irregularities, or a metabolic disorder. In **adiposis dolorosa**, a condition affecting women more commonly than men, painful fatty swellings are associated with defects in the nervous system. *See also* OBESITY.

adipsia *n. see* HYPODIPSIA.

aditus *n.* an anatomical opening or passage; for example, the opening of the tympanic cavity (middle ear) to the air spaces of the mastoid process.

adjunct *n.* a subsidiary drug used in treating a disorder, which provides additional benefits to the main drug used in treatment. For example, the *dopamine receptor agonist cabergoline is used as an adjunct to levodopa in the treatment of Parkinson's disease. —**adjunctive** *adj.*

adjuvant *n.* any substance used in conjunction with another to enhance its activity. Aluminium salts are used as adjuvants in the preparation of vaccines from the toxins of diphtheria and tetanus: by keeping the toxins in precipitated form, the salts increase the efficacy of the toxins as antigens.

adjuvant therapy treatment given to patients after the primary therapy, which is usually surgical removal of the tumour, when there is a high risk of future recurrence based on tumour stage and histology. Adjuvant therapy is aimed at destroying these microscopic tumour cells either locally (e.g. adjuvant breast irradiation after breast-conserving surgery) or systemically (e.g. adjuvant chemotherapy may be recommended for patients with breast cancer, colorectal cancer, and other types of cancer). *Compare* NEOADJUVANT CHEMOTHERAPY.

admission rate the number of people from a specified population with a specified disease or condition admitted to hospitals in a given geographical area over a specified time period.

adnexa *pl. n.* adjoining parts. For example, the **uterine adnexa** are the Fallopian tubes and ovaries (which adjoin the uterus).

adolescence *n.* the stage of development between childhood and adulthood. It begins with the start of *puberty, which in girls is usually at the age of 12–13 years and in boys about 14 years, and usually lasts until 19 years of age.

ADP (adenosine diphosphate) a compound containing adenine, ribose, and two phosphate groups. ADP occurs in cells and is involved in processes requiring the transfer of energy (*see* ATP).

adrenalectomy *n.* the surgical removal of an *adrenal gland, usually performed because of neoplastic disease.

adrenal glands (suprarenal glands) two triangular *endocrine glands, each of which covers the superior surface of a kidney. Each gland has two parts, the **medulla** and **cortex**. The medulla forms the grey core of the gland; it consists mainly of *chromaffin tissue and is stimulated by the sympathetic nervous system to produce *adrenaline and *noradrenaline. The cortex is a yellowish tissue surrounding the medulla. It is derived embryologically from mesoderm and is stimulated by pituitary hormones (principally *ACTH) to produce three kinds of *corticosteroid hormones, which affect carbohydrate metabolism (e.g. *cortisol), electrolyte metabolism (e.g. *aldosterone), and the sex glands (oestrogens and androgens).

adrenaline (epinephrine) *n.* an important hormone secreted by the medulla of the adrenal gland. It has the function of preparing the body for 'fright, flight, or fight' and has widespread effects on circulation, the muscles, and sugar metabolism. The action of the heart is increased, the rate and depth of breathing are increased, and the metabolic rate is raised; the force of muscular contraction improves and the onset of muscular fatigue is delayed. At the same time the blood supply to the bladder and intestines is reduced, their muscular walls relax, and the sphincters contract. Sympathetic nerves were originally thought to act by releasing adrenaline at their endings, and were therefore called **adrenergic** nerves. In fact the main substance released is the related substance *noradrenaline, which also forms a portion of the adrenal secretion.

Adrenaline given by injection is used in the emergency treatment of anaphylaxis and cardiac arrest. It is also included in some local anaesthetic solutions, particularly those used in dentistry, to prolong anaesthesia, and is used as eye drops for treating glaucoma.

adrenarche *n.* the start of secretion of *androgens by the adrenal glands, occurring at around 6–7 years of age in girls and 7–8 in boys. It is usually determined by the measurement of urinary 17-ketosteroids rather than direct assay of the androgens themselves. Adrenal androgens are *dehydroepiandrosterone (DHEA), DHEA sulphate, and androstenedione. The age of adrenarche is unrelated to the age of *gonadarche. Premature adrenarche is usually manifested as the early appearance of pubic hair due to levels of the adrenal androgens equivalent to those found in puberty. It does not proceed to full puberty as the gonads do not become active.

adrenergic *adj.* **1.** describing nerve fibres that release noradrenaline or adrenaline as a neurotransmitter. **2.** describing receptors that are stimulated by noradrenaline or adrenaline. See ADRENOCEPTOR.

adrenoceptor (adrenoreceptor, adrenergic receptor) any cell *receptor that binds with the catecholamines adrenaline or noradrenaline, the neurotransmitters of the *sympathetic nervous system. There are two principal types of adrenoceptor, alpha (α) and beta (β), with various subtypes of each. **Alpha adrenoceptors** have a slightly higher affinity for adrenaline than for noradrenaline; they can be divided into subtypes α_1 and α_2. α_1-adrenoceptors mediate contraction of smooth muscle; in the walls of arteries, for example, their stimulation causes constriction of arteries and a rise in blood pressure. α_2-adrenoceptors occur in the presynaptic membranes of neurons in the sympathetic nervous system, where they restrict the release of catecholamines from these neurons. **Beta adrenoceptors** also have two subtypes. β_1-adrenoceptors have an equal affinity for adrenaline and noradrenaline and are found mainly in cardiac muscle; their stimulation causes an increase in heart rate. β_2-adrenoceptors have a slightly higher affinity for adrenaline. They mediate relaxation of smooth muscle in the blood vessels, bronchi, bladder, uterus, and other organs and thus cause widening of the airways and *vasodilatation.

Drugs that stimulate these receptors (alpha agonists and beta agonists) are described as *sympathomimetic. Drugs that block their effects are the *alpha blockers and *beta blockers.

adrenocorticotrophic hormone (adrenocorticotrophin) *see* ACTH.

adrenogenital syndrome a hormonal disorder resulting from abnormal steroid production by the adrenal cortex, due to a genetic fault. It may cause masculinization in girls, precocious puberty in boys, and adrenocortical failure (*see* ADDISON'S DISEASE) in both sexes. Treatment is by life-long steroid replacement.

adrenoleukodystrophy *n.* a genetically determined condition of neurological degeneration with childhood and adult forms. Inherited as an X-linked (*see* SEX-LINKED) trait resulting in *demyelination, it is characterized by progressive *spastic paralysis of the legs, sensory loss, and cognitive impairment, associated with adrenal gland insufficiency and small gonads. The demonstration of a genetic defect in the metabolism of very long chain fatty acids aids diagnosis and has implications for future possible drug therapies. Prenatal diagnosis is possible.

adrenolytic *adj.* inhibiting the activity of *adrenergic nerves. Adrenolytic activity is opposite to that of *noradrenaline.

adult respiratory distress syndrome (acute respiratory distress syndrome, ARDS) a form of *acute respiratory failure that occurs after a precipitating event, such as trauma, aspiration, or inhalation of a toxic substance; it is particularly associated with septic shock. Lung injury is characterized by reduced oxygen in the arteries, reduced lung volume, and decreased lung compliance, and diffuse infiltrates are seen on a chest X-ray. Treatment is correction of the original cause, volume replacement, diuretics, oxygen, and mechanical ventilation.

advance decision or directive *see* ADVANCE STATEMENT, DECISION, OR DIRECTIVE.

advanced glycation end-products damaged proteins that result from the *glycation of a large number of body proteins, which can accumulate and cause permanent damage to tissues. This damage is more prevalent in diabetics due to chronic exposure to blood with high concentrations of glucose. It is believed to be partly responsible for the damage to the kidneys, eyes, and blood vessels that characterizes long-standing diabetes.

advanced life-support course an educational course to teach a structured and al-

a

gorithm-driven method of life support for use in the severest of medical emergencies, especially cardiac arrest.

advanced paediatric life-support course an educational course to teach a structured and algorithm-driven method of life support for use in severe medical emergencies in children.

advanced trauma life support *see* ATLS.

advanced trauma life-support course an educational course to teach the fundamentals of care for the victims of trauma.

advancement *n.* the detachment by surgery of a muscle, musculocutaneous flap, or tendon from its normal attachment site and its reattachment at a more advanced (anterior) point while preserving its previous nerve and blood supply. The technique is used, for example, in the treatment of squint and extensively in plastic surgery to cover large defects (*see also* PEDICLE).

advance statement, decision, or directive a legally recognized decision or statement made by an adult with *capacity that identifies any specific or general treatments the patient does not want in the event that he or she loses capacity. **Advance decisions** are very specific, should be informed, made voluntarily, and must be shown to be valid and applicable to the medical situation that arises. Such a decision could enable a critically ill patient to refuse potentially life-saving treatment (a decision known colloquially as a **living will**). The formal term for a living will is an **advance di-rective**. An **advance statement** is more general and simply indicates the sort of treatment the patient may or may not wish to undergo. Under the Mental Capacity Act 2005 statements are less binding than decisions. Advance decisions and statements cannot be used to demand treatment but only to refuse treatment and/or express preferences. Advance directives do not apply to basic care, such as nutrition, hydration, and cleanliness.

adventitia (tunica adventitia) *n.* 1. the outer coat of the wall of a *vein or *artery. It consists of loose connective tissue and networks of small blood vessels, which nourish the walls. 2. the outer covering of various other organs or parts.

adventitious *adj.* 1. occurring in a place

other than the usual one. 2. relating to the adventitia.

advocacy *n.* a role that involves acting as a proxy or speaking on behalf of a patient because the patient lacks *capacity. Under the Mental Capacity Act 2005, capacitous adults may legally nominate a proxy or an **advocate** to make health-care decisions on their behalf in the event of losing capacity. For patients without family or legally appointed advocates, an *Independent Mental Capacity Advocate should be appointed for making significant medical decisions. Health-care professionals may see their role as including advocacy for patients, e.g. in accessing services. In addition, there are many organized advocacy groups to support patients with specific conditions, such as Alzheimer's disease. Finally, every NHS trust has a *Patient Advice and Liaison Service (PALS), which can take on the role of supporting patients. *See also* PROXY DECISION, SUBSTITUTED JUDGMENT.

AECOPD *a*cute *e*xacerbation of *COPD* (*see* CHRONIC OBSTRUCTIVE PULMONARY DISEASE).

AED *see* AUTOMATED EXTERNAL DEFIBRILLATOR.

Aëdes *n.* a genus of widely distributed mosquitoes occurring throughout the tropics and subtropics. Most species are black with distinct white or silvery-yellow markings on the legs and thorax. *Aëdes* species are not only important as vectors of *dengue, *yellow fever, *filariasis, and Group B viruses causing encephalitis but also constitute a serious biting nuisance. *A. aegypti* is the principal vector of dengue and yellow fever.

aegophony *n. see* VOCAL RESONANCE.

-aemia *combining form denoting* a specified biochemical condition of the blood. Example: **hyperglycaemia** (excess sugar in the blood).

aer- (aero-) *combining form denoting* air or gas. Examples: **aerogastria** (gas in the stomach); **aerogenesis** (production of gas).

aerobe *n.* any organism, especially a microbe, that requires the presence of free oxygen for life and growth. *See also* ANAEROBE, MICROAEROPHILIC.

aerobic *adj.* 1. of or relating to aerobes: requiring free oxygen for life and growth.

2. describing a type of cellular *respiration in which foodstuffs (carbohydrates) are completely oxidized by atmospheric oxygen, with the production of maximum chemical energy from the foodstuffs.

aerobic exercises *see* EXERCISE.

aerodontalgia *n.* pain in the teeth due to change in atmospheric pressure during air travel or the ascent of a mountain.

aeroneurosis *n.* a syndrome of anxiety, agitation, and insomnia found in pilots flying unpressurized aircraft and attributed to *anoxia.

aerophagy *n.* the swallowing of air. This may be done voluntarily to stimulate belching, accidentally during rapid eating or drinking, or unconsciously as a habit. Voluntary aerophagy is used to permit oesophageal speech after surgical removal of the larynx (usually for cancer).

aerosol *n.* a suspension of extremely small liquid or solid particles (about 0.001 mm diameter) in a gas. Drugs for inhalation are in aerosol form.

aetiology (etiology) *n.* **1.** the study or science of the causes of disease. **2.** the cause of a specific disease.

afebrile *adj.* without, or not showing any signs of, a fever.

affect *n.* (in psychiatry) **1.** the predominant emotion in a person's mental state at a particular moment. **Blunted affect** is a diminished intensity of emotional response; it is a feature of some forms of chronic schizophrenia and depression. **Incongruent affect** describes an inappropriate emotional response to a situation (e.g. laughing at a funeral) and may be seen in psychotic illnesses. **2.** the emotion associated with a particular idea. —**affective** *adj.*

affective disorder (mood disorder) any psychiatric disorder featuring abnormalities of mood or emotion (*affect). The most serious of these are *depression and *mania. Other affective disorders include *SAD (seasonal affective disorder).

afferent *adj.* **1.** designating nerves or neurons that convey impulses from sense organs and other receptors to the brain or spinal cord, i.e. any sensory nerve or neuron. **2.** designating blood vessels that feed a capillary network in an organ or part. **3.** desig-

nating lymphatic vessels that enter a lymph node. *Compare* EFFERENT.

afibrinogenaemia *n.* complete absence of the coagulation factor *fibrinogen in the blood. *Compare* HYPOFIBRINOGENAEMIA.

aflatoxin *n.* a poisonous substance produced in the spores of the fungus *Aspergillus flavus*, which infects peanuts. The toxin is known to produce cancer in certain animals and is suspected of being the cause of liver cancers in human beings living in warm and humid regions of the world, where stored nuts and cereals may be contaminated by the fungus.

AFP *see* ALPHA-FETOPROTEIN.

afterbirth *n.* the placenta, umbilical cord, and ruptured membranes associated with the fetus, which normally become detached from the uterus and expelled within a few hours of birth.

aftercare *n.* long-term surveillance or rehabilitation as an adjunct or supplement to formal medical treatment of those who are chronically sick or disabled, including those with mental illness or learning disability. Aftercare includes the provision of special aids and the adaptation of homes to improve daily living.

after-image *n.* an impression of an image that is registered by the brain for a brief moment after an object is removed from in front of the eye, or after the eye is closed. A **positive afterimage**, which lasts a few seconds, retains the colour and brightness of the original image; the more common **negative afterimage** lasts longer and has colours and brightness that are complementary to the original.

afterpains *pl. n.* pains caused by uterine contractions after childbirth, especially during breast feeding, due to release of the hormone *oxytocin. The contractions help restore the uterus to its nonpregnant size and are more common in women who have given birth twice or more.

agammaglobulinaemia *n.* a total deficiency of the plasma protein *gammaglobulin. *Compare* HYPOGAMMAGLOBULINAEMIA.

agar *n.* an extract of certain seaweeds that forms a gel suitable for the solidification of liquid bacteriological *culture media. **Blood agar** is nutrient agar containing 5–10% horse blood, used for the cultivation of certain bacteria or for detecting haemolytic (blood-destroying) activity.

Age Concern (in Britain) a voluntary agency with particular interest in the well-being of older people.

(⊕) SEE WEB LINKS

• Website of Age Concern: includes advice on health issues affecting older people

agenesis *n*. absence of an organ, usually due to total failure of its development in the embryo.

age-related macular degeneration (AMD, ARMD) *see* MACULAR DEGENERATION.

agglutination (clumping) *n*. the sticking together, by serum antibodies called **agglutinins**, of such microscopic antigenic particles as red blood cells or bacteria so that they form visible clumps. Any substance that stimulates the body to produce an agglutinin is called an **agglutinogen**. Agglutination is a specific reaction; in the laboratory, sera containing different known agglutinins provide an invaluable means of identifying unknown bacteria. When blood of different groups is mixed, agglutination occurs because serum contains natural antibodies (**isoagglutinins**) that attack red cells of a foreign group, whether previously encountered or not. This is not the same process as occurs in *blood coagulation.

agglutinin *n*. an antibody that brings about the *agglutination of bacteria, blood cells, or other antigenic particles.

agglutinogen *n*. any antigen that provokes formation of an agglutinin in the serum and is therefore likely to be involved in *agglutination.

aglossia *n*. congenital absence of the tongue.

agnathia *n*. congenital absence of the lower jaw, either partial or complete.

agnosia *n*. a disorder of the brain whereby the patient cannot interpret sensations correctly although the sense organs and nerves conducting sensation to the brain are functioning normally. It is due to a disorder of the *association areas in the parietal lobes. In **auditory agnosia** the patient can hear but cannot interpret sounds (including speech). A patient with **tactile agnosia** (**astereognosis**) retains normal sensation in his hands but cannot recognize three-dimensional objects by touch alone. In **visual agnosia** the

patient can see but cannot interpret symbols, including letters (*see* ALEXIA).

agonal *adj*. describing or relating to the phenomena, such as cessation of breathing or change in the ECG or EEG, that are associated with the moment of death. For example, an **agonal rhythm** describes the ECG of a dying patient, characterized by slow, irregular, and wide ventricular complexes that eventually stop (*see* ELECTROCARDIOGRAM). It is often seen in the terminal stages of a failed attempt at cardiac resuscitation.

agonist *n*. 1. (prime mover) a muscle whose active contraction causes movement of a part of the body. Contraction of an agonist is associated with relaxation of its *antagonist. 2. a drug or other substance that acts at a cell-receptor site to produce an effect that is the same as, or similar to, that of the body's normal chemical messenger. *Sympathomimetic drugs (alpha agonists and beta agonists) are examples.

agoraphobia *n*. a morbid fear of public places and/or of open spaces. *Compare* CLAUSTROPHOBIA. *See also* PHOBIA.

agranulocytosis *n*. a disorder in which there is a severe acute deficiency of certain blood cells (*neutrophils) as a result of damage to the bone marrow by toxic drugs or chemicals. It is characterized by fever, with ulceration of the mouth and throat, and may lead rapidly to prostration and death. Treatment is by the administration of antibiotics in large quantities. When feasible, transfusion of white blood cells may be life-saving.

agraphia (dysgraphia) *n*. an acquired inability to write, although the strength and coordination of the hand remain normal. It is related to the disorders of language and it is caused by disease in the dominant *parietal lobe of the brain. *See* GERSTMANN'S SYNDROME.

ague *n*. *see* MALARIA.

Aicardi syndrome a syndrome caused by abnormal development of the brain in which the two halves of the brain do not connect. The *corpus callosum is absent. Affected individuals suffer from mental retardation and seizures. They may also have associated abnormalities of the eyes and spine. [J. D. Aicardi (20th century), French neurologist]

AIDS (acquired immune deficiency syndrome) a syndrome first identified in Los Angeles in 1981; a description of the causative virus – the human immunodeficiency virus (*HIV) – was available in 1983. The virus destroys a subgroup of lymphocytes, the *helper T cells (or *CD4 lymphocytes), resulting in suppression of the body's immune response (*see* IMMUNITY). Acute (primary) infection following exposure to the virus results in the production of antibodies (seroconversion); their presence, detected by standard tests, indicates that infection has taken place. Primary infection may be accompanied by mild or severe symptoms, lasting an average of 14 days, including fever, fatigue, lymphadenopathy, headache, and rash. Chronic HIV infection, which follows primary infection, lasts an average of 10 years, during which the person may be asymptomatic; it is followed by the development of AIDS. AIDS can be defined by a CD4 level less than 200 cells/μl or by the presence of an AIDS-defining illness, such as *Kaposi's sarcoma, recurrent pneumonia (especially caused by **Pneumocystis jiroveci*), any of various lymphomas, or any of certain cytomegalovirus-related diseases.

AIDS is largely a sexually transmitted disease, either homosexually or heterosexually. The two other main routes of spread are via infected blood or blood products (as by drug users sharing contaminated needles) and by the maternofetal route. The virus may be transmitted from an infected mother to the child in the uterus or it may be acquired from maternal blood during parturition; it may also be transmitted in breast milk. HIV has been isolated from semen, cervical secretions, plasma, cerebrospinal fluid, tears, saliva, urine, and breast milk but the concentration shows wide variations. Moreover HIV is a fragile virus and does not survive well outside the body. It is therefore considered that ordinary social contact with HIV-positive subjects involves no risk of infection. However, high standards of clinical practice are required by all health workers in order to avoid inadvertent infection via blood, blood products, or body fluids from HIV-positive people. Staff who become HIV-positive are expected to declare their status and will be counselled.

Until recently, AIDS was considered to be universally fatal, although the type and length of illness preceding death varies considerably. However, with the development of *antiretroviral drugs used in dual or triple combinations, AIDS is now perceived as a chronic disease rather than a fatal one.

(((●))) SEE WEB LINKS
• Website of the Terence Higgins Trust: includes information on HIV, AIDS, and sexual health

AIH *see* ARTIFICIAL INSEMINATION.

ainhum *n.* loss of one or more toes due to slow growth of a fibrous band around the toe that eventually causes a spontaneous amputation. The condition is rare, found mainly in Africa and associated with going barefoot.

air bed a bed with a mattress whose upper surface is perforated with thousands of holes, through which air is forced under pressure. The patient is thus supported, like a hovercraft, on a cushion of air. This type of bed is invaluable for the treatment of patients with large areas of burns.

air embolism an air bubble that obstructs the outflow of blood from the right ventricle of the heart through the lungs. Air may gain access to the circulation as a result of surgery, injury, or intravenous infusions. The patient experiences breathlessness and chest discomfort and develops acute heart failure. Tipping the patient head down, lying on the left side, may move the air bubble.

air sickness *see* MOTION SICKNESS.

airway *n.* 1. any of the passages of the respiratory system. 2. any device that enables the flow of air into and out of the lungs. *See* NASOPHARYNGEAL AIRWAY, OROPHARYNGEAL AIRWAY.

airway obstruction blockage of any of the passages by which air enters (and leaves) the lungs, which may be partial or complete. In partial obstruction, the patient can still move some air in and out of the lungs but often with difficulty. There may be a distinctive sound (*see* STRIDOR) on inspiration through a partly obstructed airway. Complete obstruction will rapidly lead to respiratory and then cardiac arrest and requires prompt airway clearance and support.

akathisia *n.* a pattern of involuntary movements induced by some antipsychotic drugs, such as *phenothiazines. An affected person is driven to restless overactivity, which can be confused with the agitation for which the drug was originally prescribed. Akathisia is mostly felt as restless legs (*see* RESTLESS LEGS SYNDROME) rather than generalized agitation or anxiety. *See also* EXTRA-PYRAMIDAL EFFECTS.

AKI acute kidney injury, also called acute renal failure. The diagnosis is usually based on changes in the serum creatinine concentration or the detection of *oliguria, neither of which is ideal as they tend to lag behind the phase of acute injury. New biomarkers of AKI are being sought as a top research priority.

akinesia *n.* a loss of normal muscular tonicity or responsiveness. **Akinetic rigid syndrome** is used to describe such conditions as *parkinsonism and *progressive supranuclear palsy. In **akinetic epilepsy** there is a sudden loss of muscular tonicity, making the patient fall with momentary loss of consciousness. **Akinetic mutism** is a state of complete physical unresponsiveness although the patient's eyes remain open and appear to follow movements. It is a consequence of damage to the *brainstem area of the brain. —**akinetic** *adj.*

ala *n.* (*pl.* **alae**) (in anatomy) a winglike structure; for example, either of the two lateral flared portions of the external nose or the winglike expansion of the ilium.

alactasia *n.* absence or deficiency of the enzyme lactase, which is essential for the digestion of milk sugar (lactose). All babies have lactase in their intestines, but the enzyme disappears during childhood in about 10% of northern Europeans, 40% of Greeks and Italians, and 80% of Africans and Asians. Alactasia causes symptoms only if the diet regularly includes raw milk, when the undigested lactose causes diarrhoea and abdominal pain.

Alagille syndrome (arteriohepatic dysplasia) an inherited condition in which the bile ducts, which drain the liver, become progressively smaller, causing increased *jaundice. It is associated with abnormalities of other organs, such as the heart, kidneys, eyes, and spine. [D. Alagille (1925–), French physician]

alanine *n. see* AMINO ACID.

alanine aminotransferase (ALT) an enzyme involved in the transamination of amino acids. Measurement of ALT in the serum is of use in the diagnosis and study of acute liver disease. It was formerly called **serum glutamic pyruvic transaminase** (SGPT).

ALARA principle *see* RADIATION PROTECTION.

alastrim *n.* a mild form of smallpox, causing only a sparse rash and low-grade fever. Medical name: **variola minor**.

albendazole *n.* an *anthelmintic drug used for treating *hydatid disease, *hookworm disease, *strongyloidiasis, and *creeping eruption. It is administered by mouth. Possible side-effects include headache, dizziness, fever, skin rashes, and loss of hair.

Albers-Schönberg disease *see* OSTEOPETROSIS. [H. E. Albers-Schönberg (1865–1921), German radiologist]

Alberti regime (GIK regime) a method for controlling blood-sugar levels in diabetic patients who are being fasted for whatever reason. It involves infusing a solution of glucose (G), insulin (I), and potassium (K) chloride intravenously over a standard time period. Blood sugar and potassium are measured frequently so that appropriate adjustments can be made to the mixture as necessary. [K. G. M. M. Alberti (1937–), British physician]

albinism *n.* the inherited absence of pigmentation in the skin, hair, and eyes, resulting in white hair and pink skin and eyes. The pink colour is produced by blood in underlying blood vessels, which are normally masked by pigment. Ocular signs are reduced visual acuity, sensitivity to light (*see* PHOTOPHOBIA), and involuntary side-to-side eye movements.

albino *n.* an individual lacking the normal body pigment (melanin). *See* ALBINISM.

Albright's hereditary osteodystrophy the skeletal abnormalities, collectively, of *pseudohypoparathyroidism. These include short stature, abnormally short fingers and toes (particularly involving the fourth and fifth metacarpals and metatarsals), and soft-tissue calcification. [F. Albright (1900–69), US physician]

albumin *n.* a protein that is soluble in water and coagulated by heat. An example is **serum albumin**, which is found in blood plasma and is important for the maintenance of plasma volume. Albumin is synthesized in the liver; the inability to synthesize it is a prominent feature of chronic liver disease (*cirrhosis).

albuminuria (proteinuria) *n.* the presence of serum albumin, serum globulin, or other serum proteins in the urine. This may be associated with kidney or heart disease.

Albuminuria is not always associated with disease: it may occur after strenuous exercise or after a long period of standing (**ortho-static albuminuria**).

albumose *n.* a substance, intermediate between albumin and peptones, produced during the digestion of proteins by pepsin and other endopeptidases (*see* PEPTIDASE).

alcaptonuria (alkaptonuria) *n.* the congenital absence of an enzyme, homogentisic acid oxidase, that is essential for the normal breakdown of the amino acids tyrosine and phenylalanine. Accumulation of *homogentisic acid causes dark brown discoloration of the skin and eyes (**ochronosis**) and progressive damage to the joints, especially of the spine. The gene responsible for the condition is recessive, so that a child is affected only if both parents are carriers of the defective gene.

alclometazone *n.* a *corticosteroid drug applied as a cream or ointment to treat inflammatory skin disorders. Possible side-effects include skin thinning and allergic reactions. Trade name: **Modrasone**.

alcohol *n.* any of a class of organic compounds formed when a hydroxyl group (–OH) is substituted for a hydrogen atom in a hydrocarbon. The alcohol in alcoholic drinks is **ethyl alcohol** (**ethanol**), which has the formula C_2H_5OH. It is produced by the fermentation of sugar by yeast. 'Pure' alcohol contains not less than 94.9% by volume of ethyl alcohol. It is obtained by distillation. A solution of 70% alcohol can be used as a preservative or antiseptic. When taken into the body ethyl alcohol depresses activity of the central nervous system (*see also* ALCOHOLISM). *Methyl alcohol (methanol) is extremely poisonous.

Alcoholics Anonymous (AA) an international voluntary agency of mutual support that is organized and operated locally among those with alcohol dependency. Members are expected to follow a 12-step programme, which includes admitting to their drink problems, recognizing a higher spiritual power that gives strength to overcome these problems, and helping and supporting fellow members.

SEE WEB LINKS
• Website of Alcoholics Anonymous

alcoholism *n.* the syndrome due to physical *dependence on alcohol, such that sudden deprivation may cause withdrawal symptoms – tremor, anxiety, hallucinations, and delusions (*see* DELIRIUM TREMENS). The risk of alcoholism for an individual depends on genetic and environmental factors. Its prevalence in any given society is closely linked to the price of alcohol and the availability of the substance. Usually several years' heavy drinking is needed for addiction to develop, with a wide range from one to 40 years. Alcoholism impairs intellectual function, physical skills, memory, and judgment: social skills, such as conversation, are preserved until a late stage. Heavy consumption of alcohol also causes *cardiomyopathy, *peripheral neuropathy, *cirrhosis of the liver, and enteritis. Treatment is usually provided on an out-patient basis, in specialist units for detoxication or medical wards. If there are complicating psychiatric problems detoxication may be part of psychiatric treatment. Psychological aspects of treatment include helping the patient to understand the psychological pressures that led to his or her heavy drinking, treatment of underlying anxiety, and *motivational interviewing. Drugs such as *disulfiram (Antabuse), which cause vomiting if alcohol is taken, may help in treatment.

aldesleukin *n. see* INTERLEUKIN.

aldosterone *n.* a steroid hormone (*see* CORTICOSTEROID) that is synthesized and released by the adrenal cortex and acts on the kidney to regulate salt (potassium and sodium) and water balance.

aldosteronism (hyperaldosteronism) *n.* overproduction of aldosterone, one of the hormones secreted by the adrenal cortex, usually due to a benign tumour (adenoma) in the cortex or hyperplasia of that tissue. It leads to abnormalities in the amounts of sodium, potassium, and water in the body. It is a rare cause of raised blood pressure (hypertension). *See also* CONN'S SYNDROME.

alendronic acid (sodium alendronate) a *bisphosphonate drug that is administered orally for the prevention and treatment of osteoporosis in postmenopausal women or induced by corticosteroid therapy. Side-effects may include abdominal pain, indigestion, and oesophageal irritation or pain. Trade name: **Fosamax**.

Aleppo boil *see* ORIENTAL SORE.

alerting device *see* ENVIRONMENTAL HEARING AID.

a

alexia *n.* an acquired inability to read. It is due to disease in the left (dominant) hemisphere of the brain in a right-handed person. In **agnosic alexia** (**word blindness**) the patient cannot read because he is unable to identify the letters and words, but he retains the ability to write and his speech is normal. This is a form of *agnosia. A patient with **aphasic alexia** (**visual asymbolia**) can neither read nor write and often has an accompanying disorder of speech. This is a form of *aphasia. *See also* DYSLEXIA.

alexin *n.* a former name for the serum component now called *complement.

alexithymia *n.* a lack of ability to understand and communicate one's own emotions and moods. It is common in *depression and can cause significant relationship difficulties during the person's illness.

alfacalcidol *n.* 1α-hydroxycholecalciferol: a derivative of vitamin D that is used to raise blood calcium levels for the prevention or treatment of rickets and *osteomalacia in patients with severe kidney disease. It is administered by mouth or by injection. Trade name: **One-Alpha**.

alfentanil *n.* an opioid *analgesic drug used mainly for pain relief during surgery (*see* OPIATE). It is administered by intravenous injection or infusion, usually at induction of anaesthesia. Trade name: **Rapifen**.

alfuzosin *n.* an *alpha blocker commonly used in the treatment of men with *lower urinary tract symptoms thought to be due to benign prostatic hyperplasia (*see* PROSTATE GLAND). It is administered orally. Trade name: **Xatral**.

ALG antilymphocyte globulin. *See* ANTILYMPHOCYTE SERUM.

algesimeter *n.* a piece of equipment for determining the sensitivity of the skin to various touch stimuli, especially those causing pain.

-algia *combining form denoting* pain. Example: **neuralgia** (pain in a nerve).

algid *adj.* cold: usually describing the cold clammy skin associated with certain forms of malaria.

alginates *pl. n.* derivatives of **alginic acid**, a complex carbohydrate extracted from certain brown seaweeds, that readily absorb water to form a gel. Alginates are included in many *antacid preparations (e.g. **Gastrocote**, **Gaviscon**) for the relief of heartburn caused by *gastro-oesophageal reflux because they form a layer on the stomach contents that protects the oesophagus from acid reflux. As they are hightly absorbent, alginates are also used in dressings for exuding wounds.

algodystrophy *n.* a specific post-traumatic syndrome after nerve injury, in which a limb remains exquisitely sensitive to any stimulus and later develops disuse *atrophy. *See* REFLEX SYMPATHETIC DYSTROPHY.

algorithm *n.* a sequential set of instructions used in calculations or problem solving. A **reconstruction algorithm** is a complex mathematical formula used by a computer to construct images from the data acquired by CT, MRI, or other scanners. A **diagnostic algorithm** or a **therapeutic algorithm** consists of a stepwise series of instructions with branching pathways to be followed to assist a physician in coming to a diagnosis or deciding on a treatment strategy, respectively.

alienation *n.* (in psychiatry) *see* THOUGHT ALIENATION.

alimemazine (**trimeprazine**) *n.* an *antihistamine drug (a *phenothiazine derivative) that also possesses sedative properties. Given by mouth, it is mainly used in the treatment of pruritus (itching) and urticaria (nettle rash), but also for premedication. Common side-effects include drowsiness, dizziness, dryness of mouth, muscular tremor and incoordination, and confusion. Trade name: **Vallergan**.

alimentary canal the long passage through which food passes to be digested and absorbed (see illustration). It extends from the mouth to the anus and each region is specialized for a different stage in the processing of food, from mechanical breakdown in the mouth to chemical *digestion and *absorption in the stomach and small intestine and finally to faeces formation and water absorption in the colon and rectum.

alitretinoin *n. see* RETINOID.

alizarin (**alizarin carmine**) *n.* an orange-red dye derived from coal tar and originally isolated from the plant madder (*Rubia tinctorum*). Alizarin is insoluble in water but dissolves in alkalis, alcohol, and ether. It is used as a pH indicator and as a histochemical reagent for calcium, thallium, titanium, and zirconium.

ALK *see* AUTOMATED LAMELLAR KERATECT-OMY.

alkalaemia *n.* abnormally high blood alkalinity. This may be caused by an increase in the concentration of alkaline substances and/or a decrease in that of acidic substances in the blood. *See also* ALKALOSIS. *Compare* ACIDAEMIA.

alkaloid *n.* one of a diverse group of nitrogen-containing substances that are produced by plants and have potent effects on body function. Many alkaloids are important drugs, including *morphine, *quinine, *atropine, and *codeine.

alkalosis *n.* a condition in which the alkalinity of body fluids and tissues is abnormally high. This arises because of a failure of the mechanisms that usually maintain a balance between alkalis and acids in the arterial blood (*see* ACID-BASE BALANCE). Alkalosis may be associated with loss of acid through vom-

iting or with excessive sodium bicarbonate intake. Breathing that is abnormally deep in relation to the amount of physical exercise may lead to **respiratory alkalosis**. Alkalosis may produce symptoms of muscular weakness or cramp.

alkaptonuria *n. see* ALCAPTONURIA.

alkylating agents a class of chemotherapy drugs that includes *cyclophosphamide, *ifosfamide, and *melphalan. These drugs bind to DNA and prevent complete separation of the two DNA chains during cell division. Side-effects are those of other *cytotoxic drugs; in addition, alkylating agents interfere with *gametogenesis and may cause sterility in men.

allantois *n.* the membranous sac that develops as an outgrowth of the embryonic hindgut. Its outer (mesodermal) layer carries blood vessels to the *placenta and so forms part of the *umbilical cord. Its cavity is small and becomes reduced further in size during fetal development (*see* URACHUS). —**allantoic** *adj.*

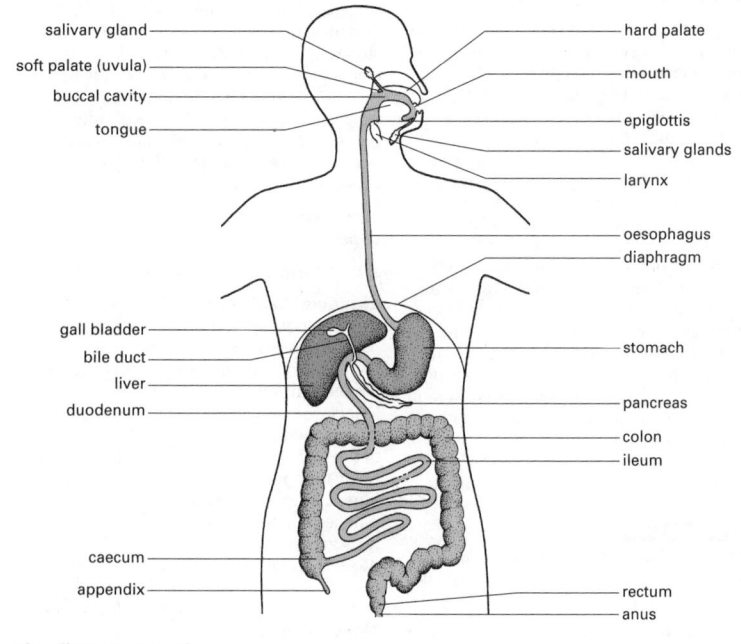

The alimentary canal.

salivary gland — hard palate
soft palate (uvula) — mouth
buccal cavity — epiglottis
tongue — salivary glands
— larynx
— oesophagus
— diaphragm
gall bladder — stomach
bile duct —
liver — pancreas
duodenum — colon
— ileum
caecum —
appendix — rectum
— anus

allele (allelomorph) *n.* one of two or more alternative forms of a *gene, only one of which can be present in a chromosome. Two alleles of a particular gene occupy the same relative positions on a pair of *homologous chromosomes. If the two alleles are the same, the individual is *homozygous for the gene; if they are different he is *heterozygous. *See also* DOMINANT, RECESSIVE. —**allelic** *adj.*

allelomorph *n. see* ALLELE.

allergen *n.* any *antigen that causes *allergy in a hypersensitive person. Allergens are diverse and affect different tissues and organs. Pollens, fur, feathers, mould, and dust may cause hay fever; house-dust mites (*see* DERMATOPHAGOIDES) have been implicated in some forms of asthma; drugs, dyes, cosmetics, and a host of other chemicals can cause rashes and dermatitis; some food allergies may cause diarrhoea or constipation or simulate acute bacterial food poisoning. When a patient's allergen has been identified (*see* PATCH TEST), it may be possible to attempt *desensitization to alleviate or prevent allergic attacks. —**allergenic** *adj.*

allergy *n.* a disorder in which the body becomes hypersensitive to particular antigens (called *allergens), which provoke characteristic symptoms whenever they are subsequently inhaled, ingested, injected, or otherwise contacted. Normally antibodies in the bloodstream and tissues react with and destroy specific antigens without further trouble. In an allergic person, however, the allergens provoke the release of a class of antibodies (IgE) that become bound to *mast cells in the body's tissues. The subsequent reaction of allergen with tissue-bound antibody (*see* REAGIN) also leads, as a side-effect, to cell damage, release of *histamine and *serotonin (5-hydroxytryptamine), inflammation, and all the symptoms of the particular allergy. Different allergies afflict different tissues and may have either local or general effects, varying from asthma and hay fever to severe dermatitis or gastroenteritis or extremely serious shock (*see* ANAPHYLAXIS). —**allergic** *adj.*

(⊕) SEE WEB LINKS
• Website of Allergy UK: provides information on a wide range of allergies together with their diagnosis and treatment

allied health professional a health-care professional with expert knowledge and experience in certain fields but without a medical or nursing qualification. Allied health professionals include speech and language therapists, radiographers, physiotherapists, occupational therapists, and dietitians.

allogeneic *adj.* describing grafted tissue derived from a donor of the same species as the recipient.

allograft (homograft) *n.* a living tissue or organ graft between two members of the same species; for example, a heart transplant from one person to another. Such grafts will not survive unless the recipient is treated to suppress his body's *immune response to the foreign tissue or the grafted organ is from an identical twin. *See also* TRANSPLANTATION.

alloisoleucine *n.* one of the isomers of the amino acid isoleucine.

allopathy *n.* (in homeopathic medicine) the orthodox system of medicine, in which the use of drugs is directed to producing effects in the body that will directly oppose and so alleviate the symptoms of a disease. *Compare* HOMEOPATHY.

allopurinol *n.* a drug used for the prevention of acute attacks of *gout and of kidney stones. It acts by reducing the level of uric acid in tissues and blood. It is administered by mouth; side-effects include nausea, vomiting, diarrhoea, headache, fever, stomach pains, and skin rashes. Occasionally, nerve damage and enlargement of the liver may occur. Trade name: **Zyloric**.

almoner *n.* a former name for a *hospital social worker.

almotriptan *n. see* 5HT$_1$ AGONIST.

alopecia (baldness) *n.* absence of hair from areas where it normally grows. **Nonscarring alopecias** include male-pattern balding, which is familial, and **androgenetic alopecia** in women, in which the hair loss is associated with increasing age. Acute hair fall (**telogen effluvium**), in which much or all of the hair is shed but may start to regrow at once, may occur after pregnancy or a serious illness. **Alopecia areata** consists of bald patches that may regrow; it is an example of an organ-specific *autoimmune disease. **Alopecia totalis** is loss of all the scalp hair, due to an autoimmune condition; in some 70% of cases it regrows within a few years. **Alopecia universalis** is loss of all body hair. In **scarring** (or **cicatricial**) **alopecias** the hair does not regrow; examples include *lichen planus and discoid *lupus erythematosus.

alpha agonist *see* SYMPATHOMIMETIC.

alpha-1 antitrypsin deficiency a rare inherited disorder associated with lung and liver diseases. It is caused by a deficiency of α_1-antitrypsin, a plasma globulin whose role is to inhibit the action of various protease enzymes (including trypsin), which protect the lungs against the action of the enzyme neutrophil elastase. This results in degradation of the *elastin of alveolar walls as well as structural proteins in other tissues, including the liver. Although many patients present in childhood, the disorder can occur in adults as well.

alpha blocker (alpha-adrenergic blocker) a drug that prevents the stimulation of alpha *adrenoceptors at the nerve endings of the sympathetic nervous system by noradrenaline and adrenaline: it therefore causes relaxation of smooth muscle, including widening of arteries (vasodilatation) and a drop in blood pressure. Alpha blockers include *doxazosin, *phentolamine, *phenoxybenzamine, *indoramin, *prazosin, *alfuzosin, and *tamsulosin. Overdosage causes a severe drop in blood pressure, a rapid pulse, nausea and vomiting, diarrhoea, a dry mouth, flushed skin, convulsions, drowsiness, and coma.

alpha-fetoprotein (AFP) *n.* a protein that is formed in the liver and yolk sac of the fetus and is present in the fetal serum and secondarily in maternal blood. Maternal AFP is used as a marker in *prenatal screening tests, which can be performed between the 15th and 20th weeks of pregnancy. Levels are elevated in open *neural tube defects (e.g. spina bifida), open abdominal wall defects (e.g. *gastroschisis), fetal death, and multiple pregnancy. Levels of AFP are decreased in *Down's syndrome. However, AFP levels are affected by the length of gestation and the mother's weight, and these factors must be considered when interpreting the results. When levels are unexpectedly high or low, further investigations (for example detailed *ultrasonography) are indicated.

Alpha-fetoprotein is also produced by certain malignant *teratomas and primary liver tumours (*hepatomas). *See* TUMOUR MARKER.

alpha-glucosidase inhibitor any member of a group of *oral hypoglycaemic drugs, including **acarbose** (Glucobay), used for treating type 2 *diabetes mellitus. They reduce the breakdown and absorption of carbohydrates in the intestine by blocking the action of an important enzyme (α-glucosidase) in this process. Side-effects include flatulence and diarrhoea.

alphavirus *n.* any member of a genus of *arboviruses transmitted by mosquitoes. Many alphaviruses can cause disease in humans and animals, including *O'nyong nyong fever and *Ross River fever.

Alport's syndrome a hereditary disease that causes *nephritis accompanied by deafness and, less commonly, ocular defects, such as cataracts. Affected males usually develop end-stage renal failure and, unless treated with a kidney transplant, die before the age of 40. Females have a better prognosis. [A. C. Alport (1880–1959), South African physician]

alprazolam *n.* a *benzodiazepine used for the short-term relief of anxiety. It is administered by mouth; side-effects include drowsiness and lightheadedness. Trade name: **Xanax**.

alprostadil *n.* a *prostaglandin drug (PGE$_1$) administered by infusion to improve lung blood flow in newborn babies with congenital heart defects who are awaiting surgery; it acts by preventing the closure of the blood vessel connecting the aorta to the pulmonary artery (*see* DUCTUS ARTERIOSUS). Possible side-effects include diminished respiratory efforts. Alprostadil is also administered by injection into the *corpora cavernosa of the penis or by application into the urethra to treat *erectile dysfunction in men; it acts by relaxing smooth muscle and dilating the cavernosal arteries, so that blood is trapped when the venules become compressed against the *tunica albuginea. Side-effects may include dizziness and headache. Trade names: **Caverject**, **MUSE**, **Prostin VR**, **Viridal Duo**.

ALS 1. *see* ANTILYMPHOCYTE SERUM. 2. amyotrophic lateral sclerosis. *See* MOTOR NEURON DISEASE.

ALT 1. *see* ALANINE AMINOTRANSFERASE. 2. argon laser *trabeculoplasty.

alteplase *n.* a *tissue-type plasminogen activator made by recombinant DNA technology (genetic engineering). Alteplase is used to dissolve blood clots (*see* FIBRINOLYTIC) in the treatment of ischaemic stroke, myocardial infarction, and pulmonary embolism. It is administered by injection. Possible side-effects include local bleeding, cerebral haemorrhage, nausea, and vomiting. Trade name: **Actilyse**.

alternative medicine *see* COMPLEMENTARY MEDICINE.

altitude sickness (mountain sickness) the condition that results from unaccustomed exposure to a high altitude (4500 m or more above sea level). Reduced atmospheric pressure and shortage of oxygen cause deep rapid breathing (*hyperventilation), which lowers the concentration of carbon dioxide in the blood (*see* ALKALOSIS). Symptoms include nausea, exhaustion, and anxiety. In severe cases there may be acute shortness of breath due to fluid collecting in the lungs (pulmonary *oedema), which requires treatment by diuretics and return to a lower altitude.

aluminium chloride hexahydrate a powerful antiperspirant used in the treatment of conditions associated with excessive sweating (*see* HYPERHIDROSIS). It is applied to the skin in the form of a solution and may cause local irritation. Trade names: **Anhydrol Forte**, **Driclor**.

aluminium hydroxide a safe slow-acting antacid. It is administered by mouth, alone or in combination with magnesium hydroxide (as **co-magaldrox**; Maalox, Mucogel), in the treatment of indigestion, gastric and duodenal ulcers, and reflux *oesophagitis. Trade name: **Alu-Cap**.

alveolitis *n.* inflammation of an *alveolus or alveoli. Chronic inflammation of the walls of the alveoli of the lungs is usually caused by inhaled organic dusts (**extrinsic allergic alveolitis**; *see* BIRD-FANCIER'S LUNG, FARMER'S LUNG) but may occur spontaneously (**cryptogenic fibrosing alveolitis, CFA**). CFA may be associated with connective-tissue diseases, such as rheumatoid arthritis or systemic sclerosis, and some experts would omit the word 'cryptogenic' if there is an association with a rheumatic disorder (*see* FARA, FASS). In addition, CFA is now commonly referred to as **idiopathic pulmonary fibrosis (IPF)**, since inflammation is not now believed to play a major role, and pathologists use the term *interstitial pneumonitis when classifying CFA. Both types of alveolitis (extrinsic and cryptogenic) may progress slowly to a state of fibrosis, and both types usually respond to corticosteroid and immunosuppressant therapy if the fibrosis is not severe.

alveolus *n.* (*pl.* **alveoli**) **1.** (in the *lung) a blind-ended air sac of microscopic size. About 30 alveoli open out of each **alveolar duct**, which leads from a respiratory *bronchiole. The **alveolar walls**, which separate alveoli, contain capillaries. The alveoli are lined by a single layer of *pneumocytes, which thus form a very thin layer between air and blood so that exchange of oxygen and carbon dioxide is normally rapid and complete. Children are born with about 20 million alveoli. The adult number of about 300 million is reached around the age of eight. **2.** the part of the upper or lower jawbone that supports the roots of the teeth (*see also* MANDIBLE, MAXILLA). After tooth extraction it is largely absorbed. **3.** the sac of a *racemose gland (*see also* ACINUS). **4.** any other small cavity, depression, or sac. —**alveolar** *adj.*

alverine citrate a bulking agent and *antispasmodic drug used to treat irritable bowel syndrome and diverticular disease. It is administered by mouth. Side-effects include occasional mild distension of the bowel. Trade name: **Spasmonal**.

alveus *n.* a cavity, groove, or canal. The **alveus hippocampi** is the bundle of nerve fibres in the brain forming a depression in which the hippocampus lies.

Alzheimer's disease the most common form of *dementia, occurring in middle age or later. It is characterized by memory impairment and, as the disease progresses, language difficulties, *apraxia, and visuospatial problems. At post mortem there are excess deposits of *amyloid protein and *neurofibrillary tangles in the brain. In cases of familial Alzheimer's, mutations in three genes have so far been detected; patients with these genes usually have early-onset (<65 years) disease. Mutations in four other genes have been implicated in the more common late-onset form of the disease. The demonstration of damage to the cholinergic pathways has led to the development of *acetylcholinesterase inhibitors, which have been shown to slow disease progression. [A. Alzheimer (1864–1915), German physician]

(())) SEE WEB LINKS

- Website of the Alzheimer's Disease Society: includes resources for health and care professionals

amalgam *n.* any of a group of alloys containing mercury. In dentistry amalgam fillings are made by mixing a silver-tin alloy with mercury in a machine known as an **amalgamator**.

Amanita *n.* a genus of fungi that contains several species of poisonous toadstools, including *A. phalloides* (death cap), *A. pantherina* (panther cap), and *A. muscaria* (fly agaric). They produce toxins that cause abdominal pain, violent vomiting, and continuous diarrhoea. In the absence of treatment death occurs in approximately 50% of cases, due to severe liver damage.

amantadine *n.* an antiviral drug that increases the activity of *dopamine in the brain and is used mainly to treat Parkinson's disease. Common side-effects include nervousness, loss of muscular coordination, and insomnia. Trade name: **Symmetrel**.

amaurosis *n.* partial or complete blindness. For example, **amaurosis fugax** is a condition in which loss of vision is transient. *See also* LEBER'S CONGENITAL AMAUROSIS. —**amaurotic** *adj.*

ambivalence *n.* (in psychology) the condition of holding opposite feelings (such as love and hate) for the same person or object. This can cause relationship difficulties and pathological grief reactions.

Amblyomma *n.* a genus of hard *ticks, several species of which are responsible for transmitting tick *typhus. The bite of this tick can also give rise to a serious and sometimes fatal paralysis.

amblyopia *n.* poor sight, not due to any detectable disease of the eyeball or visual system, known colloquially as **lazy eye**. In practice this strict definition is not always obeyed. For example, in **toxic amblyopia**, caused by tobacco, alcohol, certain other drugs, and vitamin deficiency, there is a disorder of the *optic nerve. The commonest type is **amblyopia ex anopsia**, in which factors such as squint (*see* STRABISMUS), cataract, and other abnormalities of the optics of the eye (*see* REFRACTION) impair its normal use in early childhood by preventing the formation of a clear image on the retina. This in turn leads to a cortical visual impairment.

amblyoscope (orthoptoscope, synoptophore) *n.* an instrument for measuring the angle of a squint and assessing the degree to which a person uses both eyes together. It consists of two L-shaped tubes, the short arms of which are joined by a hinge so that the long arms point away from each other. The subject looks into the short end and each eye sees, via a system of mirrors and lenses, a different picture, which is placed at the other end of each tube. If a squint is present, the tubes may be adjusted so that the short arms line up with the direction of each eye.

ambrisentan *n. see* ENDOTHELIN.

AMD age-related *macular degeneration.

amelia *n.* congenital total absence of the arms or legs due to a developmental defect. It is one of the fetal abnormalities induced by the drug *thalidomide taken early in pregnancy. *See also* PHOCOMELIA.

ameloblast *n.* a cell that forms the enamel of a tooth and disappears before tooth eruption.

ameloblastoma *n.* a locally invasive tumour in the jaw. It is considered to develop from ameloblasts although it does not contain enamel.

amelogenesis *n.* the formation of enamel by *ameloblasts, a process that is completed before tooth eruption. **Amelogenesis imperfecta** is a hereditary condition in which enamel formation is disturbed. The teeth have an unusual surface but may not be more prone to decay.

amenorrhoea *n.* the absence or stopping of the menstrual periods. It is normal for the periods to be absent before puberty, during pregnancy and milk secretion, and after the end of the reproductive period (*see* MENOPAUSE). In **primary amenorrhoea** the menstrual periods fail to appear at puberty, due to absence of the uterus or ovaries, a genetic disorder (e.g. *Turner's syndrome), or hormonal imbalance. It is diagnosed when *menarche has not occurred by the age of 16½ years but there is normal development of secondary sexual characteristics or by the age of 14 years if secondary sexual characteristics are absent. In **secondary amenorrhoea** the menstrual periods stop after establishment at puberty for a minimum of six months. Causes include disorders of the hypothalamus (a part of the brain), deficiency of ovarian, pituitary, or thyroid hormones, mental disturbance, depression, anorexia nervosa, or a major change of surroundings or circumstances.

amethocaine *n. see* TETRACAINE.

ametropia *n.* any abnormality of *refraction of the eye, resulting in blurring of the image formed on the retina. *See* ASTIGMATISM, HYPERMETROPIA, MYOPIA. *Compare* EMMETROPIA.

amfebutamone *n. see* BUPROPION.

amiloride *n.* a potassium-sparing *diuretic that causes the increased excretion of sodium and chloride; it is often combined with a thiazide or loop diuretic (e.g. hydrochlorothiazide as **co-amilozide**) to reduce the potassium loss that occurs with these drugs. Amiloride may produce dizziness and weakness and its continued use may lead to an excessive concentration of potassium in the blood.

amino acid an organic compound containing an amino group ($-NH_2$) and a carboxyl group ($-COOH$). Amino acids are fundamental constituents of all *proteins. Breakdown of proteins found in the body yields the following amino acids: alanine, arginine, asparagine, aspartic acid, cysteine, cystine, glutamic acid, glutamine, glycine, histidine, isoleucine, leucine, lysine, methionine, phenylalanine, proline, serine, threonine, tryptophan, tyrosine, and valine. Some of these amino acids can be synthesized by the body; others, the *essential amino acids, must be obtained from protein in the diet. Certain amino acids present in the body are not found in proteins; these include *citrulline, *ornithine, *taurine, and *gamma-aminobutyric acid.

aminoacidopathy *n. see* MAPLE SYRUP URINE DISEASE, METHYLMALONIC ACIDURIA.

aminoglycosides *pl. n.* a group of antibiotics active against a wide range of bacteria. It includes *gentamicin, *neomycin, and *streptomycin. Because of their toxicity (side-effects include ear and kidney damage), these drugs are used only when less toxic antibacterials are ineffective or contraindicated. They are usually administered by injection.

aminopeptidase *n.* any one of several enzymes in the intestine that cause the breakdown of a *peptide, removing an amino acid.

aminophylline *n.* a drug that relaxes smooth muscle and stimulates respiration. It is widely used to dilate the air passages in the treatment of severe asthma and some cases of chronic obstructive pulmonary disease. Administered by mouth or injection, it may cause nausea, vomiting, dizziness, and fast heart rate. *See also* THEOPHYLLINE. Trade name: **Phyllocontin Continus**.

aminosalicylates *pl. n.* drugs containing 5-aminosalicylic acid, used to treat ulcerative colitis (and to maintain patients in remission from it) and Crohn's disease affecting the colon. They include *sulfasalazine, *olsalazine, and **mesalazine** (Asacol, Ipocol, Mesren MR, Mezavant XL, Pentasa, Salofalk), which are administered orally or rectally.

amiodarone *n.* an *anti-arrhythmic drug used to control a variety of abnormal heart rhythms, including atrial *fibrillation and abnormally rapid heartbeat. It is administered by mouth or intravenous infusion. Side-effects can include harmless deposits in the cornea, photosensitivity, and peripheral neuropathy. Trade name: **Cordarone X**.

amisulpride *n. see* ANTIPSYCHOTIC.

amitosis *n.* division of the nucleus of a cell by a process, not involving *mitosis, in which the nucleus is constricted into two.

amitriptyline *n.* a tricyclic *antidepressant drug that has a mild tranquillizing action. Side-effects can include abnormal heart rhythms, which may be fatal following overdosage, and the drug is now rarely used for depression; it may be used to treat bedwetting in children and chronic pain.

amlodipine *n.* a *calcium-channel blocker used to treat hypertension and prevent angina pectoris. It is administered by mouth. Possible side-effects include headache, dizziness, fatigue, nausea, and fluid retention. Trade name: **Istin**.

amnesia *n.* total or partial loss of memory following physical injury, disease, drugs, or psychological trauma (*see* CONFABULATION, FUGUE, REPRESSION). **Anterograde amnesia** is loss of memory for the events following some trauma; **retrograde amnesia** is loss of memory for events preceding the trauma. Some patients experience both types.

amnihook *n.* a small plastic hooked instrument for performing *amniotomy. The hook is introduced through the cervix.

amniocentesis *n.* withdrawal of a sample

of the fluid (*amniotic fluid) surrounding a fetus in the uterus by piercing the amniotic sac through the abdominal wall, under direct ultrasound guidance. As the amniotic fluid contains cells from the fetus (mostly shed from the skin), cell cultures enable chromosome patterns to be studied so that *prenatal diagnosis of chromosomal abnormalities (such as *Down's syndrome) can be made. Certain metabolic errors and other abnormalities, such as *spina bifida, can also be diagnosed prenatally from analysis of the cells or of the fluid. Amniocentesis is usually performed at any time from the 15th completed week of gestation; it carries a 1–2% risk of miscarriage.

amnion *n.* the membrane that forms initially over the dorsal part of the embryo but soon expands to enclose it completely within the *amniotic cavity; it is connected to the embryo at the umbilical cord. It expands outwards and fuses with the chorion, obliterating virtually all the intervening cavity. The double membrane (**amniochorion**) normally ruptures at birth. —**amniotic** *adj.*

amnioreduction *n.* the removal of amniotic fluid in greater amounts than required for amniocentesis for therapeutic reasons (e.g. *twin-to-twin transfusion syndrome, *polyhydramnios).

amniotic cavity the fluid-filled cavity between the embryo and the *amnion. It forms initially within the inner cell mass of the *blastocyst and later expands over the back of the embryo, eventually enclosing it completely. *See also* AMNIOTIC FLUID.

amniotic fluid the fluid contained within the *amniotic cavity. It surrounds the growing fetus, protecting it from external pressure. The fluid is initially secreted from the *amnion and is later supplemented by urine from the fetal kidneys. Some of the fluid is swallowed by the fetus and absorbed through its intestine. The volume of amniotic fluid varies according to the stage of gestation: approximate normal values are 500 ml at 18 weeks, rising to a maximum of 800 ml at 34 weeks and falling to 600 ml at term. *See also* ANHYDRAMNIOS, OLIGOHYDRAMNIOS, POLYHYDRAMNIOS.

amniotic fluid embolism a condition in which amniotic fluid enters the maternal circulation causing a complex cascade similar to that seen in anaphylactic and septic *shock. It is a rare event (1 in 50,000–100,000 deliveries), with a 60–80% maternal mortality. The sudden onset of cardiopulmonary collapse, together with coma or seizures, in labour or shortly after delivery, should prompt the diagnosis. Most of the women who survive have permanent neurological damage.

amniotomy (artificial rupture of membranes, ARM) *n.* a method of surgically inducing labour by puncturing the *amnion surrounding the baby in the uterus using an *amnihook or similar instrument.

amobarbital (amylobarbitone) *n.* an intermediate-acting *barbiturate used to treat severe insomnia in patients already taking barbiturates. Trade name: **Sodium Amytal**.

amoeba *n.* (*pl.* **amoebae**) any protozoan of jelly-like consistency and irregular and constantly changing shape. Found in water, soil and other damp environments, they move and feed by means of flowing extensions of the body (*see* PSEUDOPODIUM). Some amoebae cause disease in humans (*see* ACANTHAMOEBA, ENTAMOEBA). —**amoebic** *adj.*

amoebiasis *n. see* DYSENTERY.

amoebocyte *n.* a cell that moves by sending out processes of its protoplasm in the same way as an amoeba.

amoeboma *n.* a rare manifestation of longstanding or partially treated infection due to *Entamoeba histolytica*, leading to development of a nonmalignant tumour-like (pseudotumorous) inflammatory mass. It can occur in the caecum, appendix, and *rectosigmoid area in descending order of frequency. These pseudotumours may ulcerate and become infected with pus-forming (pyogenic) bacteria, causing severe inflammation of the bowel wall. They can cause symptoms of *intestinal obstruction, weight loss, and low-grade fever. Colonic amoeboma with multiple amoebic liver abscesses can masquerade as colorectal carcinoma and liver metastases; imaging with ultrasound and CT scan is used to differentiate between these.

amok *n.* a sudden outburst of furious and murderous aggression, directed indiscriminately at everybody in the vicinity.

amorolfine *n.* an antifungal drug used to treat fungal infections of the skin and nails. It is applied externally as a cream or nail lacquer; possible side-effects include itching and a transient burning sensation. Trade name: **Loceryl**.

amoxicillin *n.* a semisynthetic *penicillin used to treat infections caused by a wide range of bacteria and other microorganisms (*see also* BETA-LACTAM ANTIBIOTIC). It is administered by mouth or injection. Side-effects include nausea, vomiting, diarrhoea, rashes, and anaemia. Sensitivity to penicillin prohibits its use. Trade names: **Amoxil, Galenamox, Rimoxallin**.

AMP (adenosine monophosphate) a compound containing adenine, ribose, and one phosphate group. AMP occurs in cells and is involved in processes requiring the transfer of energy (*see* ATP).

ampere *n.* the basic *SI unit of electric current. It is equal to the current flowing through a conductor of resistance 1 ohm when a potential difference of 1 volt is applied between its ends. The formal definition of the ampere is the current that when passed through two parallel conductors of infinite length and negligible cross section, placed 1 metre apart in a vacuum, produces a force of 2×10^{-7} newton per metre between them. Symbol: A.

amphetamines *pl. n.* a group of *sympathomimetic drugs that have a marked *stimulant action on the central nervous system, alleviating fatigue and producing a feeling of mental alertness and wellbeing. **Dexamfetamine** (**dexamphetamine**; Dexedrine) is used in the treatment of *narcolepsy and in selected cases of *attention-deficit/hyperactivity disorder in children. It is administered by mouth; side-effects include insomnia and restlessness. *Tolerance to amphetamines develops rapidly, and prolonged use may lead to *dependence; these drugs should not be used to treat depressive illness or obesity.

amphiarthrosis *n.* a slightly movable joint in which the bony surfaces are separated by fibrocartilage (*see* SYMPHYSIS) or hyaline cartilage (*see* SYNCHONDROSIS).

amphoric breath sounds *see* BREATH SOUNDS.

amphotericin *n.* an *antifungal drug that is used to treat deep-seated fungal infections. It can be administered by mouth, but is usually given by intravenous infusion. Common side-effects include headache, fever, muscle pains, and diarrhoea; more severe side-effects, such as kidney damage, can be reduced if the drug is administered in a lipid preparation (*see* LIPOSOME). Trade names: **Abelcet, AmBisome, Amphocil, Fungizone**.

ampicillin *n.* a semisynthetic *penicillin used to treat a variety of infections, including those of the urinary, respiratory, biliary, and intestinal tracts. It is inactivated by *penicillinase and therefore cannot be used against organisms producing this enzyme. It is given by mouth or injection; side-effects include nausea, vomiting, and diarrhoea, and some allergic reactions may occur. Trade names: **Penbritin, Rimacillin**.

ampoule (ampule) *n.* a sealed glass or plastic capsule containing one dose of a drug in the form of a sterile solution for injection.

ampulla *n.* (*pl.* **ampullae**) an enlarged or dilated ending of a tube or canal. The semicircular canals of the inner ear are expanded into ampullae at the point where they join the vestibule. The **ampulla of Vater** is the dilated part of the common bile duct where it is joined by the pancreatic duct.

amputation *n.* the removal of a limb, part of a limb, or any other portion of the body (such as a breast or the rectum). The term is customarily modified by an adjective showing the particular type of amputation. Examples include above-knee, through-knee, and below-knee amputations of the lower limb. Once a common operation in surgery, it is now performed mostly in elderly people, when circulation to a lower limb is inadequate and gangrene develops. It is also performed in cases of severe injury to limbs. In planning an amputation the surgeon takes account of the blood supply, the patient's mobility, and the type of artificial part (prosthesis) that will be fitted.

amsacrine *n.* a *cytotoxic drug administered by intravenous injection to treat acute myeloid leukaemia. Possible side-effects include nausea, vomiting, hair loss, and interference with bone marrow blood-cell production. Trade name: **Amsidine**.

Amsler grid a chart usually consisting of a grid of black lines on a white background. It is used to detect and monitor problems of central vision affecting the retina; for example, in early macular disease, the square edges of the grid may appear distorted. [M. Amsler (1891–1968), Swiss ophthalmologist]

amygdala (amygdaloid nucleus) *n.* one

of the *basal ganglia and part of the *limbic system: a roughly almond-shaped mass of grey matter deep inside each cerebral hemisphere. It has extensive connections with the olfactory system and sends nerve fibres to the hypothalamus; its functions are concerned with perception of threat, fear, learning, emotion, and memory.

amylase *n.* an enzyme that occurs in saliva and pancreatic juice and aids the digestion of starch, which it breaks down into glucose, maltose, and dextrins. Amylase will also hydrolyse *glycogen to yield glucose, maltose, and dextrins.

amylobarbitone *n. see* AMOBARBITAL.

amyloid *n.* a *glycoprotein, resembling starch, that is deposited in the internal organs in amyloidosis. β-amyloid protein has been found in the brains of Alzheimer's patients but the significance of this is unclear.

amyloidosis *n.* infiltration of the liver, kidneys, spleen, and other tissues with amyloid, a starchlike substance. In **primary amyloidosis** the disorder arises without any apparent cause; **secondary amyloidosis** occurs as a late complication of such chronic infections as tuberculosis or leprosy and also in *Hodgkin's disease. Amyloidosis is also very common in the genetic disease familial Mediterranean fever (*see* POLYSEROSITIS).

amylopectin *n. see* STARCH.

amylose *n. see* STARCH.

amyotonia congenita (floppy baby syndrome) a former diagnosis for various conditions, present at birth, in which the baby's muscles are weak and floppy (i.e. hypotonic). The term is becoming obsolete as more specific diagnoses are discovered to explain the cause of floppiness in babies.

amyotrophy *n.* a progressive loss of muscle bulk (wasting) associated with weakness of these muscles. It is caused by disease of the motor nerve that activates the affected muscle. Amyotrophy is a feature of any chronic *neuropathy and it may be found in some diabetic patients (*see* DIABETIC AMYOTROPHY). A combination of amyotrophy and spasticity may be found in the different forms of *motor neuron disease.

an- *prefix. see* A-.

anabolic *adj.* promoting tissue growth by increasing the metabolic processes involved in protein synthesis. Anabolic steroids are synthetic forms of male sex hormones (*see* ANDROGEN); they include *nandrolone. They were formerly used to help weight gain in underweight patients, such as the elderly and those with serious illnesses, but are now used mainly to stimulate the production of blood cells by the bone marrow in some forms of aplastic anaemia. Some anabolic steroids cause virilization in women and liver damage.

anabolism *n.* the synthesis of complex molecules, such as proteins and fats, from simpler ones by living things. *See also* ANABOLIC, METABOLISM.

anacidity *n.* a deficiency or abnormal absence of acid in the body fluids.

anacrotism *n.* the condition in which there is an abnormal curve in the ascending line of a pulse tracing. It may be seen in cases of aortic stenosis. —**anacrotic** *adj.*

anaemia *n.* a reduction in the quantity of the oxygen-carrying pigment *haemoglobin in the blood. The main symptoms are excessive tiredness and fatigability, breathlessness on exertion, pallor, and poor resistance to infection.

There are many causes of anaemia. It may be due to loss of blood (**haemorrhagic anaemia**), resulting from an accident, operation, etc., or from chronic bleeding, as from an ulcer or haemorrhoids. **Iron-deficiency anaemia** results from lack of iron, which is necessary for the production of haemoglobin (*see* SIDEROPENIA). **Haemolytic anaemias** result from the increased destruction of red blood cells (which contain the pigment). This can be caused by toxic chemicals; *autoimmunity; the action of parasites, especially in *malaria; or conditions such as *thalassaemia and *sickle-cell disease, associated with abnormal forms of haemoglobin, or *spherocytosis, which is associated with abnormal red blood cells. (*See also* HAEMOLYTIC DISEASE OF THE NEWBORN.) Anaemia can also be caused by the impaired production of red blood cells, as in *leukaemia (when red-cell production in the bone marrow is suppressed) or *pernicious anaemia. **Aplastic anaemia** is characterized by a failure of blood cell production resulting in *pancytopenia and reduced bone marrow cellularity.

Anaemias can be classified on the basis of the size of the red cells, which may be large (**macrocytic anaemias**), small (**microcytic anaemias**), or normal-sized (**normocytic**

anaemias). (*See also* MACROCYTOSIS, MICRO-CYTOSIS.) The treatment of anaemia depends on the cause. —**anaemic** *adj.*

anaerobe *n.* any organism, especially a microbe, that is able to live and grow in the absence of free oxygen. A **facultative anaerobe** is a microorganism that grows best in the presence of oxygen but is capable of some growth in its absence. An **obligate anaerobe** can grow only in the absence of free oxygen. *Compare* AEROBE, MICROAEROPHILIC.

anaerobic *adj.* **1.** of or relating to anaerobes. **2.** describing a type of cellular respiration in which foodstuffs (usually carbohydrates) are never completely oxidized because molecular oxygen is not used. *Fermentation is an example of anaerobic respiration.

anaesthesia *n.* loss of feeling or sensation in a part or all of the body. Anaesthesia of a part of the body may occur as a result of injury to or disease of a nerve; for example in leprosy. The term is usually applied, however, to the technique of reducing or abolishing an individual's sensation of pain to enable surgery to be performed. This is effected by administering drugs (*see* ANAESTHETIC) or by the use of other methods, such as *acupuncture or hypnosis.

General anaesthesia is total unconsciousness, usually achieved by administering a combination of injections and gases (the latter are inhaled through a mask). **Local anaesthesia** abolishes pain in a limited area of the body and is used for minor operations, particularly many dental procedures. It may be achieved by injections of substances such as lidocaine (commonly used in dentistry) close to a local nerve, which deadens the tissues supplied by that nerve. Local anaesthesia may be combined with intravenous sedation. An appropriate injection into the spinal column produces *spinal anaesthesia or *epidural anaesthesia in the lower limbs or abdomen. **Regional anaesthesia**, usually of a limb, is achieved by encircling local anaesthetic solutions or direct application of anaesthetic to one or more peripheral nerves.

anaesthetic **1.** *n.* an agent that reduces or abolishes sensation, affecting either the whole body (**general anaesthetic**) or a particular area or region (**local anaesthetic**). General anaesthetics, used for surgical procedures, depress activity of the central nervous system, producing loss of consciousness. *Anaesthesia is induced by intravenous anaesthetics, such as *thiopental, **etomidate**, or **propofol**, and maintained by inhalation anaesthetics (such as *sevoflurane). Local anaesthetics inhibit conduction of impulses in sensory nerves in the region where they are injected or applied; they include *tetracaine, *bupivacaine, and *lidocaine. **2.** *adj.* reducing or abolishing sensation.

anaesthetist *n.* a medically qualified doctor who administers an anaesthetic to induce unconsciousness in a patient before a surgical operation.

anagen *n.* the growth phase of a hair follicle, lasting two to three years. It is followed by a transitional stage, called **catagen**, which lasts for about two weeks, and then a resting phase, **telogen**. On average about 85% of hairs are in anagen and hence growing actively. There are about 100,000 hairs on the human scalp and up to 100 may be shed each day.

anákhré *n. see* GOUNDOU.

anal *adj.* of, relating to, or affecting the anus; for example an anal *fissure or an anal *fistula.

anal canal the terminal portion of the large intestine, which is surrounded by the muscles of defecation (**anal sphincters**). The canal ends on the surface at the anal orifice (*see* ANUS).

analeptic (respiratory stimulant) *n.* a drug that acts on the central nervous system to stimulate the muscles involved in breathing. Analeptics, such as *doxapram, are used to treat respiratory depression and respiratory failure.

anal fissure a break in the skin lining the anal canal, usually causing pain during bowel movements and sometimes bleeding. Anal fissures occur as a consequence of constipation or sometimes of diarrhoea. The commonest site is midline posteriorly, followed by midline anteriorly. Medical treatment involves using stool softeners along with the application of soothing ointments and smooth muscle relaxants locally (e.g. 0.4% glyceryl trinitrate or 2% diltiazem). Surgical treatment includes the operation of **lateral sphincterotomy** (cutting the muscle of the anal sphincter) if the condition is severe and not responding to medical management.

analgesia *n.* reduced sensibility to pain, without loss of consciousness and without the sense of touch necessarily being affected. The condition may arise accidentally, if nerves are diseased or damaged, or be induced deliberately by the use of pain-killing drugs (*see* ANALGESIC). Strictly speaking, local *anaesthesia should be called **local analgesia**. *See also* RELATIVE ANALGESIA.

analgesic 1. *n.* a drug that relieves pain. **Nonopioid analgesics**, such as *aspirin and *paracetamol, are used for the relief of headache, toothache, and mild rheumatic pain. More potent **opioid analgesics**, such as *morphine, *pethidine, *alfentanil, and *buprenorphine, are used to relieve moderate or severe pain; these drugs may produce *dependence and *tolerance (*see* OPIATE). Some analgesics, including aspirin and *indometacin, also reduce fever and inflammation and are used in rheumatic and other inflammatory conditions (*see* NSAID). **2.** *adj.* relieving pain.

analgesic nephropathy disease of the *tubulointerstitium of the kidney associated with chronic use of mixed analgesic preparations. Phenacetin, paracetamol, and salicylates have all been implicated. The condition is progressive and results in bilateral atrophy of the kidneys and chronic renal failure. In the early stages the condition is asymptomatic. The earliest clinical manifestations relate to disordered tubular function with impaired concentration and acidification of the urine.

anal incontinence *see* INCONTINENCE.

analogous *adj.* describing organs or parts that have similar functions in different organisms although they do not have the same evolutionary origin or development. *Compare* HOMOLOGOUS.

analogue *n.* a drug that differs in minor ways in molecular structure from its parent compound. Examples are *calcipotriol (an analogue of vitamin D), *betahistine (an analogue of histamine), and the *gonadorelin analogues. Useful analogues of existing drugs are either more potent or cause fewer side-effects. *Carboplatin and *oxaliplatin, for example, are less toxic analogues of *cisplatin.

analogue image a traditional X-ray image on film that is in shades that range smoothly from black to white with no appreciable steps from one shade of grey to the next (*see* GREY SCALE). Analogue images can be converted to digital format (*see* DIGITIZATION) for manipulation and storage by computers and other electronic devices.

anal sphincter tears *see* PERINEAL TEAR, OBSTETRIC ANAL SPHINCTER INJURY (OASIS).

analysis *n.* (in psychology) any means of understanding complex mental processes or experiences. There are several systems of analysis used by different schools of psychology; for example, *psychoanalysis; **transactional analysis**, in which people's relationships are explained in psychoanalytic terms; and **functional analysis**, in which a particular kind of behaviour is thoroughly described with reference to its frequency, its antecedents, and its consequences.

anamnesis *n.* a medical, psychiatric, or dental history before the onset of the condition being investigated, based on the patient's personal account.

anankastic *adj.* describing a collection of longstanding personality traits in ICD-10 (*see* INTERNATIONAL CLASSIFICATION OF DISEASES), including stubbornness, meanness, an over-meticulous concern to be accurate in small details, a disposition to check things unnecessarily, severe feelings of insecurity about personal worth, and an excessive tendency to doubt evident facts. *See* PERSONALITY DISORDER.

anaphase *n.* the third stage of *mitosis and of each division of *meiosis. In mitosis and anaphase II of meiosis the chromatids separate, becoming daughter chromosomes, and move apart along the spindle fibres towards opposite ends of the cell. In anaphase I of meiosis the pairs of homologous chromosomes separate from each other. *See* DISJUNCTION.

anaphylaxis *n.* an emergency condition resulting from an abnormal and immediate allergic response to a substance to which the body has become intensely sensitized. It results in flushing, itching, nausea and vomiting, swelling of the mouth and tongue and airway enough to often cause obstruction, wheezing, a sudden drop in blood pressure, and even sudden death. In this extreme form it is called **anaphylactic shock**. Common causes are peanuts, latex, and wasp or bee stings. Treatment, which must be given immediately, consists of adrenaline (epinephrine) injection, oxygen with possible advanced support of the airway, intravenous fluids, intravenous corticosteroids, and antihistamines. —**anaphylactic** adj.

anaplasia n. a loss of normal cell characteristics or differentiation, which may be to such a degree that it is impossible to define the origin of the cells. Anaplasia is typical of rapidly growing malignant tumours, which are described as **anaplastic**.

anasarca n. massive swelling of the legs, trunk, and genitalia due to retention of fluid (*oedema): found in congestive heart failure and some forms of renal failure.

anastomosis n. **1.** (in anatomy) a communication between two blood vessels without any intervening capillary network. See ARTERIOVENOUS ANASTOMOSIS. **2.** (in surgery) an artificial connection between two tubular organs or parts, especially between two normally separate parts of the intestine or two blood vessels. See also SHUNT.

anastrazole n. see AROMATASE INHIBITOR.

anatomical position the internationally accepted body position for anatomical descriptions, such that any part of the body can be related to any other part of it. A person in the anatomical position stands erect, the arms hanging by the sides with the palms facing frontwards and the legs and feet together with the toes pointing forwards (see illustration).

anatomical snuffbox the triangular area on the most radial and distal aspect of the wrist overlying the *scaphoid bone and bounded by the extensor tendons of the thumb. It is often tender in injuries to the scaphoid (see SCAPHOID FRACTURE).

anatomy n. the study of the structure of living organisms. In medicine it refers to the study of the form and gross structure of the various parts of the human body. The term **morphology** is sometimes used synonymously with anatomy but it is usually used for **comparative anatomy**: the study of differences in form between species. See also CYTOLOGY, HISTOLOGY, PHYSIOLOGY. —**anatomical** adj. —**anatomist** n.

anatoxin n. a former name for *toxoid.

ANCA antineutrophil cytoplasmic antibodies: autoantibodies associated with various vasculitic syndromes, including *Wegener's granulomatosis, microscopic polyangiitis, and Churg-Strauss syndrome.

ANCA have long been suspected of having a pathogenic role.

anconeus n. a muscle behind the elbow that assists in extending the forearm.

Ancylostoma (Ankylostoma) n. a genus of small parasitic nematodes (see HOOKWORM) that inhabit the small intestine and are widely distributed in Europe, America, Asia, and Africa. The worms suck blood from the gut wall, to which they are attached by means of cutting teeth. Humans are the principal and optimum hosts for A. duodenale.

The anatomical position.

ancylostomiasis n. an infestation of the small intestine by the parasitic hookworm Ancylostoma duodenale. See HOOKWORM DISEASE.

Anderson-Fabry disease see FABRY DISEASE.

ANDI an acronym for abnormal development and *i*nvolution, used to tabulate benign disorders of the breast.

andr- (andro-) *combining form denoting* men or the male sex. Example: **androphobia** (morbid fear of).

androblastoma (arrhenoblastoma) *n.* a rare tumour of the ovary, composed of Sertoli cells, Leydig cells, or both. It can produce male or female hormones and may give rise to *masculinization; in children it may cause precocious puberty. Up to 30% of these tumours are malignant, but probably as many as 85% of all cases are cured by surgery alone.

androgen *n.* one of a group of steroid hormones, including *testosterone and *dihydrotestosterone, that stimulate the development of male sex organs and male secondary sexual characteristics (e.g. beard growth, deepening of the voice, and muscle development). The principal source of these hormones is the testis (production being stimulated by *luteinizing hormone) but they are also secreted by the adrenal cortex (*see* DEHYDROEPIANDROSTERONE) and ovaries in small amounts. In women excessive production of androgens gives rise to *masculinization.

Naturally occurring and synthetic androgens are used in replacement therapy (to treat such conditions as delayed puberty in adolescent boys, *hypogonadism, and impotence due to testicular insufficiency) and as *anabolic agents. Side-effects include salt and water retention, increased bone growth, and masculinization in women. Androgens should not be used in patients with cancer of the prostate gland or in pregnant women. —**androgenic** *adj.*

androgen insensitivity syndrome (AIS) an X-linked (*see* SEX-LINKED) disorder in which the body does not react to androgens because of structural abnormalities in androgen receptors. In its most extreme form, **complete AIS** (formerly known as **testicular feminization syndrome**), there is a fully female body appearance with breast development and a short vagina (but no uterus; testes are present internally). Psychosexuality is female orientated. **Partial AIS** is also known as *Reifenstein's syndrome.

androgenization *n.* the final effects of the exposure of sensitive tissues to androgens, i.e. the development of secondary male sexual characteristics. Androgenization can also

occur abnormally in females, who may develop excessive body hair, male-pattern baldness, and *clitoromegaly.

andrology *n.* **1.** the study of male infertility and erectile dysfunction. *Seminal analysis reveals the presence of gross abnormalities in the shape and motility of spermatozoa, as well as their concentration in the semen, but further procedures are required to diagnose the underlying causes of the sperm dysfunction. These include the diagnosis of abnormalities in the genital tract (e.g. varicocele, obstruction of the vas deferens), which may be corrected surgically, and testing for the presence of antisperm antibodies in the semen and for the ability of the sperm to penetrate the cervical mucus, as well as for the presence of hormonal disorders. More sophisticated techniques include computer-assisted quantitative motility measurements, which monitor the precise speed and motility patterns of individual sperm; biochemical tests for the production of free oxygen radicals, which cause damage to developing sperm; and *acrosome-reaction assays, which reveal the ability of the sperm to penetrate the barriers surrounding the ovum. The development of all these techniques has enabled the identification of several previously undiagnosed causes of infertility and the selection of treatments most likely to succeed in remedying them. **2.** the study of androgen production and the relationship of plasma androgen to androgen action. This study is necessary to understand *hirsutism and other conditions caused by abnormal androgen production.

andropause *n.* the decline in production of testosterone that occurs with age in men. Unlike the female menopause, there is no circumscribed time at which testosterone production irreversibly ceases. Instead it tends to undergo a steady reduction from the third decade onwards.

androstenedione *n. see* ADRENARCHE, DEHYDROEPIANDROSTERONE, TESTOSTERONE.

androsterone *n.* a steroid that is formed in the liver as a metabolite of testosterone. *See also* ANDROGEN.

anencephaly *n.* partial or complete absence of the bones of the rear of the skull, the meninges, and the cerebral hemispheres of the brain. It occurs as a developmental defect, and most affected infants are stillborn;

if born live they do not survive for more than a few hours. Anencephaly is often associated with other defects of the nervous system, such as *spina bifida. Prenatal screening tests for anencephaly include detection of alpha-fetoprotein levels and ultrasound scanning.

anergy *n.* **1.** lack of response to a specific antigen or allergen. **2.** lack of energy. —**anergic** *adj.*

aneuploidy *n.* the condition in which the chromosome number of a cell is not an exact multiple of the normal basic (haploid) number. *See* MONOSOMY, TRISOMY; *compare* EUPLOIDY. —**aneuploid** *adj., n.*

aneurine *n. see* VITAMIN B₁.

aneurysm *n.* an abnormal balloon-like swelling in the wall of an artery. This may be due to degenerative disease or infection, which damages the muscular coats of the vessel, or it may be the result of congenital deficiency in the muscular wall. An **aortic aneurysm** most frequently occurs in the abdominal aorta, below the level of the renal arteries. Beyond a certain size it is prone to rupture, presenting as an acute surgical emergency with abdominal and back pain and haemorrhagic shock. A **dissecting aneurysm** usually affects the first part of the aorta and results from a degenerative condition of its muscular coat. This weakness predisposes to a tear in the lining of the aorta, which allows blood to enter the wall and track along (dissect) the muscular coat. A dissecting aneurysm may rupture or it may compress the blood vessels arising from the aorta and produce infarction (localized necrosis) in the organs they supply. The patient complains of severe chest pain that has a tearing quality and often spreads to the back or abdomen. Surgical repair may help in some cases. A **ventricular aneurysm** may develop in the wall of the left ventricle after myocardial infarction. A segment of myocardium becomes replaced by scar tissue, which expands to form an aneurysmal sac. Heart failure may result or thrombosis within the aneurysm may act as a source of *embolism. *See also* ARTERIOVENOUS ANEURYSM.

Most aneurysms within the brain are congenital: there is a risk that they may burst, causing a *subarachnoid haemorrhage. **Berry aneurysms** are small saccular aneurysms most commonly occurring in the branches of the *circle of Willis. Usually as-

sociated with congenital weakness of the vessels, these aneurysms are a cause of fatal intracranial haemorrhage in young adults. **Charcot-Bouchard aneurysms** are small aneurysms found on tiny arteries within the brain of elderly and hypertensive subjects. These aneurysms may rupture, causing cerebral haemorrhage. Options for treatment of cerebral aneurysms include surgical clipping of the aneurysm and placing metallic coils within the aneurysm to establish a clot within it (*endovascular coiling).

In a **pseudoaneurysm** (or **false aneurysm**) the swelling of the artery is contained by clotted blood rather than the wall of the artery. —**aneurysmal** *adj.*

Angelman syndrome a neurogenetic disorder characterized by severe developmental delay, absence of speech, seizures, a jerky puppet-like gait (*see* ATAXIA), and paroxysmal laughter (giving it the alternative name **happy puppet syndrome**). Affected children commonly have cranial and facial abnormalities, such as a small or flattened head. Angelman syndrome is a prototype of genomic *imprinting: a deletion on maternal chromosome 15 is the cause in a majority of cases. [H. Angelman (1915–96), British paediatrician]

angi- (angio-) *combining form denoting* blood or lymph vessels. Examples: **angiectasis** (abnormal dilation of); **angiopathy** (disease of); **angiotomy** (cutting of).

angiitis *n. see* VASCULITIS.

angina *n.* a sense of suffocation or suffocating pain. *See* ANGINA PECTORIS, LUDWIG'S ANGINA.

angina pectoris pain in the centre of the chest, which is induced by exercise and relieved by rest and may spread to the jaws and arms. Angina pectoris occurs when the demand for blood by the heart exceeds the supply of the coronary arteries and it usually results from coronary artery *atheroma. It may be prevented or relieved by such drugs as *glyceryl trinitrate and *beta blockers. If drug treatment proves ineffective, *coronary angioplasty or *coronary artery bypass grafts may be required, the former being less invasive than the latter.

angiodysplasia *n.* an abnormal collection of small blood vessels usually in the lining (mucosal surface) of the gastrointestinal tract, which can bleed. These are common in the large and small intestine, but can also be found in the lining of stomach and mouth. The condition is diagnosed by gastroscopy, *colonoscopy, *video capsule endoscopy, enteroscopy (*see* ENTEROSCOPE), or mesenteric *angiography. Treatment options include endoscopic coagulation with *diathermy, *argon plasma, or laser application, and surgical removal in cases not responding to endoscopic treatments.

angiogenesis *n.* the formation of new blood vessels, which occurs during wound healing and is promoted by growth factors (*see* VASCULAR ENDOTHELIAL GROWTH FACTOR). This process is also seen in many malignant tumours and has become a target for anticancer therapy (*see* ANGIOGENESIS INHIBITOR).

angiogenesis inhibitor an agent that prevents the development of new blood vessels (*angiogenesis) by inhibiting the action of *vascular endothelial growth factor (it is also known as **anti-VEGF**). Angiogenesis inhibitors are now used as anticancer drugs, since growing cancers have a greater need for blood supply than normal tissue and must develop new blood vessels before progressing beyond a very small size. They include *bevacizumab and *thalidomide.

angiography *n.* X-ray imaging of blood vessels (*see also* CORONARY ANGIOGRAPHY, LYMPHANGIOGRAPHY) after injection of *radiopaque contrast medium. *Digital subtraction increases the visibility of the vessels. **Magnetic resonance angiography** (MRA) can be performed either by injection of a magnetic resonance contrast agent (*see* CONTRAST MEDIUM), which gives an increased signal from the blood, or by relying on the movement of blood to give a lack of signal in the plane being examined. These images can be reconstructed in two or three dimensions. **Computerized tomographic angiography** (CTA) uses a radiographic contrast agent, usually injected into a vein, to enhance the density of the blood. This can then be clearly seen on either two- or three-dimensional images, with other surrounding tissues hidden by the computer. **Fluorescein angiography** is a common method of investigation in ophthalmology. *Fluorescein sodium is injected into a vein in the arm, from which it circulates throughout the body. Light of an appropriate wavelength is shone into the eye, causing the dye in the retinal blood vessels to fluoresce. This allows the circulation through the retinal blood vessels to be observed and photographed. **Indocyanine**

green (ICG) angiography uses indocyanine green dye, which fluoresces in infrared light. It is valuable in assessing circulation in the deeper layers of the *fundus.

angioid streaks reddish to dark-brown irregular streaks radiating outwards from the optic disc underneath the retina. They represent irregular linear cracks in *Bruch's membrane and can be the site for the development of new vessels from the choroid. They are seen in such systemic conditions as pseudoxanthoma elasticum, Paget's disease, and sickle-cell anaemia.

angiokeratoma *n.* a localized collection of thin-walled blood vessels covered by a cap of warty material. It is most often seen as an isolated malformation in the genital skin of the elderly or on the hands and feet of children. It is not malignant and its cause is unknown. Angiokeratomas may be removed surgically. *See also* FABRY DISEASE.

angioma *n.* a benign tumour composed of blood vessels or lymph vessels. **Cherry angiomas** (or **Campbell de Morgan spots**) are small red spots on the trunk in middle-aged or elderly people. They are completely harmless and consist of a minor vascular malformation. An **arteriovenous angioma** (or **malformation**) is a knot of distended blood vessels overlying and compressing the surface of the brain. It may cause epilepsy, or one of the vessels may burst, causing a *subarachnoid haemorrhage or a haemorrhage within the brain (intracerebral haemorrhage). This type of angioma may be suitable for surgical removal or stereotactic radiotherapy (*see* STEREOTACTIC LOCALIZATION). It may be associated with a purple birthmark on the face: this is called the **Sturge-Weber syndrome**. Arteriovenous malformations may occur in many other parts of the body, where they are often asymptomatic. *See also* HAEMANGIOMA, LYMPHANGIOMA.

angio-oedema (angioneurotic oedema) *n. see* URTICARIA.

angioplasty *n.* repair or reconstruction of a narrowed or completely obstructed blood vessel. Traditionally, this was performed during open surgery, but in modern practice angioplasty commonly refers to **percutaneous transluminal angioplasty** (**PTA; balloon angioplasty**), in which an inflatable balloon, mounted on the tip of a flexible catheter, is placed within the lumen of the affected vessel at the site of the narrowing/

blockage, under X-ray control. On inflation of the balloon the lumen is reopened. In an artery this disrupts the *intima (which reduces the chances of the stenosis recurring). This procedure may be performed before introducing a vascular *stent. Common sites for PTA are coronary, carotid, renal, and leg arteries. *See also* CORONARY ANGIOPLASTY.

angioscope *n.* **1.** a modified microscope used to study capillaries. **2.** a narrow flexible endoscope used to examine the interior of blood vessels.

angiospasm *n. see* RAYNAUD'S DISEASE.

angiotensin *n.* either of two peptides: **angiotensin I** or **angiotensin II**. Angiotensin I is derived, by the action of the enzyme *renin, from a protein (alpha globulin) secreted by the liver into the bloodstream. As blood passes through the lungs, another enzyme, **angiotensin-converting enzyme** (**ACE**), acts on angiotensin I to form angiotensin II. This peptide causes constriction of blood vessels and stimulates the release of the hormones *vasopressin and *aldosterone, which increase blood pressure. *See also* ACE INHIBITOR, ANGIOTENSIN II ANTAGONIST.

angiotensin II antagonist any one of a class of drugs that block the action of the hormone *angiotensin II, which constricts blood vessels; they are therefore useful in treating *hypertension. These drugs include **candesartan** (Amias), **irbesartan** (Aprovel), **losartan** (Cozaar), **telmisartan** (Micardis), and **valsartan** (Diovan). They are taken by mouth and side-effects are usually mild.

angle *n.* **1.** (in anatomy) a corner. For example, the **angle of the eye** is the outer or inner corner of the eye; the **angle of the mouth** is the site where the upper and lower lips join on either side. **2.** the degree of divergence of two lines or planes that meet each other; the space between two such lines. The **carrying angle** is the obtuse angle formed between the forearm and the upper arm when the forearm is fully extended and the hand is supinated.

angstrom *n.* a unit of length equal to one ten millionth of a millimetre (10^{-10} m). It is not a recommended *SI unit but is sometimes used to express wavelengths and interatomic distances: the *nanometre (1 nm = 10 Å) is now the preferred unit. Symbol Å.

anhedonia *n.* a reduction in or the total loss of the feeling of pleasure in acts that normally give pleasure.

anhidrosis *n.* the absence of sweating in the presence of an appropriate stimulus for sweating, such as heat. A reduction in sweating is known as **hypohidrosis**. Anhidrosis and hypohidrosis may accompany disease or occur as a congenital defect.

anhidrotic **1.** *n.* any drug that inhibits sweating, such as an *antimuscarinic drug. **2.** *adj.* inhibiting sweating.

anhydraemia *n.* a decrease in the proportion of water, and therefore plasma, in the blood.

anhydramnios *n.* absence of amniotic fluid (liquor) surrounding the fetus. This can be associated with premature rupture of membranes, placental insufficiency, intrautering growth restriction, and certain fetal renal abnormalities (e.g. *Potter syndrome).

anhydrase *n.* an enzyme that catalyses the removal of water from a compound.

anima *n.* (in Jungian psychology) an *archetype that is the feminine component of a male's personality.

animus *n.* the *archetype that is the masculine component of a female's personality.

anion *n.* an ion of negative charge, such as a bicarbonate ion (HCO_3^-) or a chloride ion (Cl^-) (*see also* ELECTROLYTE). The **anion gap** is the difference between the concentrations of cations (positively charged ions) and anions, calculated from the formula:

$$(Na^+ + K^+) - (HCO_3^- + Cl^-)$$

It is used to estimate the unaccounted-for anions in the blood in cases of metabolic disturbance. The normal anion gap is 12–16 mmol/l.

aniridia *n.* congenital absence of the iris (of the eye). This may be a hereditary condition, associated with macular dysplasia, sensory nystagmus, and congenital cataract. *See also* WAGR SYNDROME.

aniseikonia *n.* a condition in which the image of an object differs markedly in size or shape between the two eyes.

anisocoria *n.* inequality in the size of the pupils of the two eyes, usually a difference of more than 1 mm in diameter. For diagnosis, it is important to establish which of the pupils is behaving abnormally.

anisocytosis *n.* an excessive variation in size between individual red blood cells. Anisocytosis is measured by some automatic analysers; these automated instruments calculate the red cell distribution width (RDW), which reflects anisocytosis. Anisocytosis may be a feature of almost any disease affecting the blood.

anisomelia *n.* a difference in size or shape between the arms or the legs.

anisometropia *n.* the condition in which the power of *refraction in one eye differs significantly from that in the other.

ankle *n.* **1.** the hinge joint between the leg and the foot. It consists of the *talus (ankle bone), which projects into a socket formed by the lower ends of the *tibia and *fibula. **2.** the whole region of the ankle joint, including the *tarsus and the ends of the tibia and fibula.

ankle jerk a deep tendon reflex elicited when the Achilles tendon is stretched and then struck with a tendon hammer. The normal response is reflex contraction of the calf muscles and plantar flexion of the ankle. The ankle jerk may be increased if the spinal cord is compressed above the level of the first sacral spinal nerve (which arises at the level of the second lumbar vertebra). If the nerve itself is cut or compressed the reflex is reduced or absent.

ankyloblepharon *n.* an abnormal fusion (partial or complete) of the upper and lower eyelid margins.

ankylosing spondylitis *see* SPONDYLITIS.

ankylosis *n.* pathological fusion of two bones across a joint space resulting from prolonged joint inflammation or infection. In **bony ankylosis** the joint space is obliterated by bony tissue as a result of chronic inflammatory conditions, such as ankylosing *spondylitis or *septic arthritis. **Fibrous ankylosis**, in which there is a shortening of the connecting fibrous tissue, results from healing with fibrosis and is commonly associated with chronic arthritis due to tuberculous infection.

Ankylostoma *n. see* ANCYLOSTOMA.

annulus *n.* (in anatomy) a circular opening or ring-shaped structure. —**annular** *adj.*

anodontia *n.* absence of the teeth because they have failed to develop. It is more common for only a few teeth to fail to develop (*see* HYPODONTIA).

anodyne *n.* any treatment or drug that soothes and eases pain.

anogenital warts *see* CONDYLOMA, WART.

anomaloscope *n.* an instrument for testing colour discrimination. By adjusting the controls the subject has to produce a mixture of red and green light to match a yellow light. The matching is done on a brightly illuminated disc viewed down a telescope.

anomalous pulmonary venous drainage a congenital abnormality in which the pulmonary veins enter the right atrium or vena cava instead of draining into the left atrium. The clinical features are those of an *atrial septal defect.

anomaly *n.* any deviation from the normal, especially a congenital or developmental defect.

anomia *n.* a form of *aphasia in which the patient is unable to give the names of objects, although retaining an understanding of their use and the ability to put words together into speech.

anonychia *n.* congenital absence of one or more nails.

Anopheles *n.* a genus of widely distributed mosquitoes, occurring in tropical and temperate regions, with some 350 species. The malarial parasite (*see* PLASMODIUM) is transmitted to humans solely through the bite of female *Anopheles* mosquitoes. Some species of *Anopheles* may transmit the parasites of bancroftian *filariasis.

anophthalmos *n.* congenital absence of the eye.

anoplasty *n.* a surgical technique used to repair a weak or injured anal sphincter.

anorchism *n.* congenital absence of one or both testes.

anorexia *n.* weight loss.

anorexia nervosa a psychiatric illness in which the patients starve themselves or use other techniques, such as vomiting or taking laxatives, to induce weight loss. To fulfil ICD-10 criteria for anorexia nervosa patients must have a distorted body image (thinking they are overweight when they are not), a defined weight loss or *body mass index reduction, amenorrhoea, and vomiting or purging. The illness is most common in female adolescents, but about 10% of sufferers are male. There is a significant mortality associated with anorexia nervosa because of the medical consequences of weight loss. The causes of the illness are not well understood: problems within the family, rejection of adult sexuality, self-harming behaviour in the context of a borderline-type *emotionally unstable personality disorder, and performance pressure are hypothesized as factors involved. Patients must be persuaded to eat enough to maintain a normal body weight and their emotional disturbance is usually treated with *psychotherapy supported by a dietitian and possibly the *community mental health team. *See also* BULIMIA.

anosmia *n.* absence of the sense of smell. This can be temporary, as with a cold or other forms of *rhinitis, or it can be permanent, following certain viral infections, head injuries, and tumours affecting the *olfactory nerve. If loss of the sense of smell is partial rather than total, the condition is called **hyposmia**.

anovulation *n.* failure of the ovary to develop and release a female germ cell (ovum). **Anovular menstruation** is uterine bleeding in the absence of ovulation.

anoxaemia *n.* a condition in which there is less than the normal concentration of oxygen in the blood. *See also* ANOXIA, HYPOXAEMIA.

anoxia *n.* a condition in which the tissues of the body receive inadequate amounts of oxygen. This may result from low atmospheric pressure at high altitudes; a shortage of circulating blood, red blood cells, or haemoglobin; or disordered blood flow, such as occurs in heart failure. It can also result from insufficient oxygen reaching the blood in the lungs due to poor breathing movements or because disease, such as pneumonia, is reducing the effective surface area of lung tissue. *See also* HYPOXIA. —**anoxic** *adj.*

ANP atrial *natriuretic peptide.

ansa *n.* (in anatomy) a loop; for example, the **ansa hypoglossi** is the loop formed by the descending branch of the hypoglossal nerve.

ansiform *adj.* (in anatomy) shaped like a loop. The term is applied to certain lobules of the cerebellum.

ant- (**anti-**) *prefix denoting* opposed to; counteracting; relieving. Examples: **antarthritic** (relieving arthritis); **antibacterial** (destroying or stopping the growth of bacteria).

Antabuse *n. see* DISULFIRAM.

antacid *n.* a drug that neutralizes the hydrochloric acid secreted in the digestive juices of the stomach. Antacids, which include aluminium and magnesium compounds, are used to relieve pain and discomfort in disorders of the digestive system, including peptic ulcer.

antagonist *n.* **1.** a muscle whose action (contraction) opposes that of another muscle (called the **agonist** or **prime mover**). Antagonists relax to allow the agonists to effect movement. **2.** a drug or other substance with opposite action to that of another drug or natural body chemical, which it inhibits. Examples are the *antimetabolites. —**antagonism** *n.*

antazoline *n.* a short-acting *antihistamine drug, applied topically in combination with the sympathomimetic drug *xylometazoline (as **Otrivine-Antistin**) to treat allergic conjunctivitis.

ante- *prefix denoting* before. Examples: **antenatal** (before birth); **anteprandial** (before meals).

anteflexion *n.* the bending forward of an organ. A mild degree of anteflexion of the uterus is considered to be normal.

ante mortem before death. *Compare* POST MORTEM.

antenatal diagnosis *see* PRENATAL DIAGNOSIS.

antepartum *adj.* occurring before the onset of labour.

antepartum haemorrhage bleeding from the genital tract after the 20th week of pregnancy until the birth of the baby. Dangerous causes include *abruptio placentae and *placenta praevia.

anterior *adj.* **1.** describing or relating to the front (ventral) portion of the body or limbs. **2.** describing the front part of any organ. For example, the **anterior chamber** of the eye is that part of the eye between the cornea and the lens, which is filled with aqueous humour.

anteroposterior (AP) *adj.* from the front

to the back. In radiography, AP denotes a radiograph in the *coronal plane taken when the X-ray beam is directed from the front to the back of the patient. *Portable chest radiographs are usually AP. *Compare* DE-CUBITUS, POSTEROANTERIOR.

anteversion *n.* the forward inclination of an organ, especially the normal forward inclination of the uterus.

anthelmintic 1. *n.* any drug or chemical agent used to destroy parasitic worms (helminths), e.g. tapeworms, roundworms, and flukes, and/or remove them from the body. Anthelmintics include *albendazole, *mebendazole, *niclosamide, *piperazine, and *praziquantel. 2. *adj.* having the power to destroy or eliminate helminths.

anthracosis *n. see* COAL-WORKER'S PNEU-MOCONIOSIS.

anthracycline *n.* any of 500 or so antibiotics synthesized or isolated from species of *Streptomyces.* *Doxorubicin is the most important member of this group of compounds, which have wide activity, particularly against breast cancer and lymphoma; others include *daunorubicin and **epirubicin** (Pharmorubicin). *See* CYTOTOXIC DRUG.

anthrax *n.* an acute infectious disease of farm animals caused by the bacterium *Bacillus anthracis*, which can be transmitted to humans by contact with animal hair, hides, or excrement. In humans the disease attacks either the lungs, causing pneumonia, or the skin, producing severe ulceration (known as **malignant pustule**). **Woolsorter's disease** is a serious infection of the skin or lungs by *B. anthracis*, affecting those handling wool or pelts (*see* OCCUPATIONAL DISEASE). Untreated anthrax can be fatal but administration of large doses of penicillin or tetracycline is usually effective.

anthrop- (**anthropo-**) *combining form denoting* the human race. Examples: **anthropogenesis** or **anthropogeny** (origin and development of); **anthropoid** (resembling); **anthropology** (science of).

anthropometry *n.* the taking of measurements of the human body or its parts. Comparisons can then be made between individuals of different sexes, ages, and races to determine the difference between normal and abnormal development. —**anthropometric** *adj.*

anthropozoonosis *n.* a disease that is transmissible from an animal to a human, or vice versa, under natural conditions. Diseases that are found primarily in animals and sometimes affect humans include *leptospirosis, *anthrax, and *rabies.

anti-androgen *n.* any one of a group of drugs that block the cellular uptake of testosterone by the prostate gland and are therefore used in the treatment of prostate cancer, which is an androgen-dependent tumour. Anti-androgens include *bicalutamide, *cyproterone, *finasteride, and *flutamide.

anti-arrhythmic *adj.* describing a group of drugs used to correct irregularities in the heartbeat (*see* ARRHYTHMIA). They include *adenosine, *amiodarone, *verapamil, *disopyramide, *flecainide, and *lidocaine.

antibacterial *adj.* describing an antibiotic that is active against bacteria.

antibiotic *n.* a substance, produced by or derived from a microorganism, that destroys or inhibits the growth of other microorganisms. Antibiotics are used to treat infections caused by organisms that are sensitive to them, usually bacteria or fungi. They may alter the normal microbial content of the body (e.g. in the intestine, lungs, bladder) by destroying one or more groups of harmless or beneficial organisms, which may result in infections (such as thrush in women) due to overgrowth of resistant organisms. These side-effects are most likely to occur with **broad-spectrum antibiotics** (those active against a wide variety of organisms). Resistance may also develop in the microorganisms being treated; for example, through incorrect dosage or overprescription (*see also* SUPERINFECTION). Antibiotics should not be used to treat minor infections, which will clear up unaided. Some antibiotics may cause allergic reactions. *See also* AMINOGLY-COSIDES, ANTIFUNGAL, ANTIVIRAL DRUG, CEPHALOSPORIN, PENICILLIN, QUINOLONE, TETRACYCLINES.

antibody *n.* a special kind of blood protein that is synthesized in lymphoid tissue in response to the presence of a particular *antigen and circulates in the plasma to attack the antigen and render it harmless. The production of specific antibodies against antigens as diverse as invading bacteria, inhaled pollen grains, and foreign red blood cells is the basis of both *immunity and *allergy.

Chemically, antibodies are proteins of the globulin type; they are classified according to their structure and function (*see* IMMUNO-GLOBULIN).

anticholinergic *adj. see* ANTIMUSCARINIC.

anticholinesterase *n.* any substance that inhibits the action of *cholinesterase, the enzyme that is responsible for the breakdown of the neurotransmitter acetylcholine, and therefore allows acetylcholine to continue transmitting nerve impulses. Drugs with anticholinesterase activity include *neostigmine, *pyridostigmine, and *edrophonium; their uses include the diagnosis and treatment of *myasthenia gravis. *See also* PARASYMPATHOMIMETIC.

anticoagulant *n.* an agent that prevents the clotting of blood. The natural anticoagulant *heparin directly interferes with blood clotting and is active both within the body and against a sample of blood in a test tube. Synthetic drugs, such as *warfarin, are effective only within the body, since they act by affecting blood coagulation factors (*see* BLOOD COAGULATION). They take longer to act than heparin. Anticoagulants are used to prevent the formation of blood clots or to break up blood vessels in such conditions as thrombosis and embolism. Incorrect dosage may result in haemorrhage. *See also* FIBRINOLYTIC.

anticonvulsant *n.* a drug that prevents or reduces the severity and frequency of seizures in various types of epilepsy; the term **antiepileptic drug** is now preferred since not all epileptic seizures involve convulsions. The choice of drug is dictated by the type of seizure and the patient's response, and the dosage must be adjusted carefully as individuals vary in their response to these drugs and side-effects may be troublesome. Commonly used antiepileptic drugs include *carbamazepine, *lamotrigine, *phenytoin, *sodium valproate, **topiramate** (Topamax), *gabapentin, **pregabalin** (Lyrica), **vigabatrin** (Sabril), and **oxcarbazepine** (Trileptal). Phenobarbital is no longer commonly prescribed.

Certain anticonvulsants have shown efficacy in treating bipolar disorder, and some are used in the treatment of chronic pain, as in postherpetic neuralgia.

antidepressant *n.* a drug designed to alleviate the symptoms of depression. Antidepressants act by altering the availability of

serotonin and noradrenaline in the brain; they are also likely to influence synaptic transmission regulation and postsynaptic conduction. There are four main classes of antidepressants. The **selective serotonin re-uptake inhibitors**, such as fluoxetine and citalopram (*see* SSRI), are recommended as first-line treatment for depression and anxiety by current NICE guidelines. Their mode of action is entirely on serotonin. Side-effects include gastrointestinal problems and nausea. **Tricyclic antidepressants**, such as *imipramine, *doxepin, *lofepramine, *clomipramine, *amitriptyline, and **dosulepin** (Prothiaden), are also widely used. They act on noradrenaline as well as serotonin, although most of them primarily have a noradrenergic action. They are also used in chronic pain management. Their side-effect profile varies from that of SSRIs; on the whole they have more *antimuscarinic effects and are more sedative and more dangerous in overdose. **Serotonin and nora-drenaline reuptake inhibitors**), such as venlafaxine and duloxetine (*see* SNRI), are a common second-line choice in the treatment of depression and anxiety.
Monoamine oxidase inhibitors (MAOs), such as the reversible moclobemide and the irreversible phenelzine (*see* MAO INHIBITOR), are older antidepressants now less used because of significant side-effects and interactions with other drugs. The irreversible MAOIs also require certain dietary restrictions. Antidepressants are not addictive, but depending on their half-life they show a varying prevalence of *discontinuation syndrome. Their usefulness in mild depression is debated, but they are part of the gold-standard treatment for moderate and severe depression.

antidiabetic drugs drugs used to control *diabetes mellitus. Type 1 diabetes is treated with the wide range of formulations of *insulin. Type 2 diabetes is treated mainly with *oral hypoglycaemic drugs but in some cases insulin may be required.

anti-D immunoglobulin (anti-D Ig) a preparation of anti-D, a *rhesus factor antibody formed by Rh-negative individuals following exposure to Rh-positive blood (usually by exchange between fetal and maternal blood in Rh-negative women who carry a Rh-positive fetus). Anti-D Ig is administered (by intramuscular injection) to Rh-negative women within 72 hours of giving birth to a Rh-positive child (or following miscarriage or abortion) to prevent the risk of *haemolytic disease of the newborn in a subsequent child. It rapidly destroys any remaining Rh-positive cells, which could otherwise stimulate antibody production affecting the next pregnancy. Anti-D is also available as antenatal prophylaxis to all Rh-negative pregnant women.

antidiuretic hormone (ADH) see VASO-PRESSIN.

antidote n. a drug that counteracts the effects of a poison or of overdosage by another drug. For example, *dimercaprol is an antidote to arsenic, mercury, and other heavy metals.

antidromic adj. describing impulses travelling 'the wrong way' in a nerve fibre. This is rare but may happen in shingles, when the irritation caused by the virus in the spinal canal initiates impulses that travel outwards in normally afferent nerves. The area of skin that the sensory nerves supply (usually a strip on the trunk) becomes painfully blistered. Antidromic impulses cannot pass *synapses, which work in one direction only.

antiemetic n. a drug that prevents vomiting. Various drugs have this effect, including some *antihistamines (e.g. cyclizine, promethazine) and *antimuscarinic drugs. They are used for such conditions as motion sickness and vertigo; drugs used to counteract nausea and vomiting due to other causes (e.g. cytotoxic drugs) include *domperidone, *metoclopramide, and *ondansetron.

antiepileptic drug see ANTICONVULSANT.

antifibrinolytic adj. describing an agent that inhibits the dissolution of blood clots (see FIBRINOLYSIS). Antifibrinolytic drugs include *tranexamic acid.

antifungal (antimycotic) adj. describing a drug that kills or inactivates fungi and is used to treat fungal (including yeast) infections. Antifungal drugs include *amphotericin, *griseofulvin, the *imidazoles, *itraconazole, *nystatin, and *terbinafine.

antigen n. any substance that may be specifically bound by an *antibody molecule. In order to generate antibodies specific for small molecules, the latter are attached to a larger molecule before immunization. The small molecule is called a **hapten**; the larger molecule is called a **carrier**. —**antigenic** adj.

antigen-presenting cell (APC) a cell,

such as a *dendritic cell or a *macrophage, that processes antigen for presentation to a T lymphocytes (see HELPER T CELL).

antihelix (anthelix) n. the curved inner ridge of the *pinna of the ear.

antihistamine n. a drug that inhibits the action of *histamine in the body by blocking either of two types of receptors for histamine, H_1 or H_2. Antihistamines that block H_1 receptors (**H_1-receptor antagonists**) are used for symptomatic relief of allergic conditions, such as hay fever, pruritus (itching), and urticaria (nettle rash). Many H_1-receptor antagonists, e.g. *cyclizine and *promethazine, also have a strong *antiemetic activity and are used to prevent motion sickness. The most common side-effect of these drugs, especially the older antihistamines (e.g. *alimemazine, promethazine), is drowsiness and because of this they are sometimes used for sedation. Newer antihistamines, e.g. **cetirizine**, **loratidine**, **mizolastine** (Mizollen), are less sedating. Other side-effects include dizziness, blurred vision, tremors, digestive upsets, and lack of muscular coordination.

H_2 receptors are mainly found in the stomach, where stimulation by histamine causes secretion of acid gastric juice. **H_2-receptor antagonists** (e.g. *cimetidine, *nizatidine, *ranitidine, and *famotidine) block these receptors and reduce gastric acid secretion; they are used in the treatment of functional dyspepsia, *peptic ulcers, and *gastro-oesophageal reflux disease.

antihypertensive drugs drugs used in treating high blood pressure (see HYPERTEN-SION).

anti-inflammatory 1. adj. describing a drug that reduces *inflammation. The various groups of anti-inflammatory drugs act against one or more of the mediators that initiate or maintain inflammation. Some groups suppress only certain aspects of the inflammatory response. The main groups of anti-inflammatory drugs are the *antihistamines, the glucocorticoids (see CORTICO-STEROID), and the nonsteroidal anti-inflammatory drugs (see NSAID). 2. n. an anti-inflammatory drug.

antiketogenic n. an agent that prevents formation of *ketones in the body.

antilymphocyte serum (antilympho-cyte globulin, ALS, ALG) an *antiserum, containing antibodies that suppress lymphocytic activity, prepared by injecting an animal with lymphocytes. ALS may be given to a patient to prevent the immune reaction that causes tissue rejection following transplantation of such organs as kidneys or of bone marrow. Administration naturally also impairs other immunity mechanisms, making infection a serious hazard.

antimetabolite *n.* any one of a group of drugs that interfere with the normal metabolic processes within cells by combining with the enzymes responsible for them. Some drugs used in the treatment of cancer, e.g. *cytarabine *fluorouracil, *methotrexate, and *mercaptopurine, are antimetabolites that prevent cell growth by interfering with enzyme reactions essential for nucleic acid synthesis. For example, fluorouracil inhibits the enzyme thymidylate synthetase. Side-effects of antimetabolites can be severe, involving blood cell disorders and digestive disturbances. *See also* CHEMOTHERAPY, CYTO-TOXIC DRUG.

antimitotic *n.* any one of a group of drugs that inhibit cell division and growth, e.g. *doxorubicin. The drugs used to treat cancer are mainly antimitotics. *See also* ANTIME-TABOLITE, CYTOTOXIC DRUG.

anti-Müllerian hormone *see* MÜLLERIAN DUCT.

antimuscarinic (**anticholinergic**) *adj.* inhibiting the action of *acetylcholine, the neurotransmitter that conveys information in the parasympathetic nervous system. Antimuscarinic drugs block the effects of certain (muscarinic) receptors (hence their name). The actions of these drugs include relaxation of smooth muscle, decreased secretion of saliva, sweat, and digestive juices, and dilation of the pupil of the eye. *Atropine and similar drugs have these effects; they are used in the treatment of gut spasms (e.g. *propantheline) and of parkinsonism (e.g. *trihexyphenidyl) as bronchodilators (e.g. *ipratropium), and as *mydriatics. Characteristic side-effects include dry mouth, thirst, blurred vision, dry skin, increased heart rate, and difficulty in urination.

antimutagen *n.* a substance that can either reduce the spontaneous production of mutations or prevent or reverse the action of a *mutagen.

antimycotic *adj. see* ANTIFUNGAL.

anti-oestrogen (**oestrogen-receptor an-** tagonist) *n.* one of a group of drugs that oppose the action of oestrogen by binding to *oestrogen receptors in the body's tissues. The most important of these drugs is currently *tamoxifen, which is used in the treatment of breast cancers dependent on oestrogen. Because they stimulate the production of pituitary *gonadotrophins, some anti-oestrogens (e.g. *clomifene, tamoxifen) are used to induce or stimulate ovulation in infertility treatment. Side-effects of anti-oestrogens include hot flushes, itching of the vulva, nausea, vomiting, fluid retention, and sometimes vaginal bleeding.

antioxidant *n.* a substance capable of neutralizing oxygen free radicals, the highly active and damaging atoms and chemical groups produced by various disease processes and by poisons, radiation, smoking, and other agencies. Antioxidants occur naturally in the body and in certain foods and beverages; they may also be ingested in the form of supplements. They include *vitamin C (ascorbic acid), *vitamin E (tocopherols), and β-*carotene.

antiphospholipid antibody syndrome (**APS**, **Hughes syndrome**) an autoimmune disease in which the presence of antibodies against phospholipid is associated with a tendency to arterial or venous thrombosis and – in women of childbearing age – recurrent miscarriage. APS may be primary or occur in association with systemic lupus erythematosus (SLE) or other connective-tissue diseases. Treatment is by low-dose aspirin or heparin.

antiplatelet drug any one of a class of drugs that reduce platelet aggregation (*see* PLATELET ACTIVATION) and therefore the formation of clot (*see* THROMBOSIS). Examples are *abciximab, *aspirin, and *clopidogrel.

antipruritic *n.* an agent that relieves itching (*pruritus). Examples are *doxepin and *crotamiton, applied in creams or lotions, and some *antihistamine drugs (e.g. *alimemazine), used if the itching is due to an allergy.

antipsychotic *adj.* describing a group of drugs used to treat severe mental disorders (psychoses), including schizophrenia and mania; some are administered in small doses to relieve anxiety and tic disorders and to treat impulsivity in emotionally unstable personality disorder. Formerly called **major tranquillizers**, they are now known as first-

and second-generation antipsychotics. The **first-generation** (or **typical**) **antipsychotics** include the *phenothiazines (e.g. *chlorpromazine), *butyrophenones (e.g. *haloperidol), and **thioxanthenes** (e.g. *flupentixol). Side-effects of antipsychotic drugs can include *extrapyramidal effects, sedation, *antimuscarinic effects, weight gain, and *long QT syndrome. The **second-generation** (or **atypical**) **antipsychotics** are a group of more recently developed drugs that are in theory associated with fewer extrapyramidal effects than first-generation antipsychotics: they include *clozapine, *risperidone, **amisulpride** (Solian), **aripiprazole** (Abilify), **olanzapine** (Zyprexa), **quetiapine** (Seroquel), and **zotepine** (Zoleptil). Recent research results have suggested that there are significant differences among the second-generation antipsychotics regarding their efficacy and side-effect profiles. Antipsychotics act on various neurotransmitter receptors in the brain, including dopamine, histamine, serotonin, and cholinergic receptors. Most of them block neurotransmitter activity, but some have partially agonistic effects.

antipyretic   *n.* a drug that reduces fever by lowering the body temperature. Several analgesic drugs have antipyretic activity, including *aspirin and *paracetamol.

antiretroviral drug (ARV) any of a group of drugs that inhibit or slow the growth of *retroviruses, specifically HIV, and are used in the treatment of HIV infection and *AIDS. They include the *reverse transcriptase inhibitors and the *protease inhibitors (*see also* MARAVIROC, RALTEGRAVIR). Treatment with a combination of antiretrovirals is known as **highly active antiretroviral therapy (HAART)**.

antisecretory drug any drug that reduces the normal rate of secretion of a body fluid, usually one that reduces acid secretion into the stomach. Such drugs include *antimuscarinic drugs, H_2-receptor antagonists (*see* ANTIHISTAMINE), and *proton-pump inhibitors.

antisepsis   *n.* the elimination of bacteria, fungi, viruses, and other microorganisms that cause disease by the use of chemical or physical methods.

antiseptic   *n.* a chemical that destroys or inhibits the growth of disease-causing bacteria and other microorganisms and is sufficiently nontoxic to be applied to the skin or

mucous membranes to cleanse wounds and prevent infections or to be used internally to treat infections of the intestine and bladder. Examples are *cetrimide, *chlorhexidine, and povidone-*iodine.

antiserum   *n.* (*pl.* **antisera**) a serum that contains antibodies against antigens of a particular kind; it may be injected to treat, or give temporary protection (passive *immunity) against, specific diseases. Antisera are prepared in large quantities in such animals as horses. In the laboratory, they are used to identify unknown organisms responsible for infection (*see* AGGLUTINATION).

antisocial personality disorder a *personality disorder characterized by callous unconcern for others, irresponsibility, violence, disregard for social rules, and an incapacity for maintaining enduring relationships. It is also known as **dyssocial personality** in ICD-10, **psychopathy**, and **sociopathy**.

antispasmodic   *n.* a drug that relieves spasm of smooth muscle in the gut. Antispasmodics, which include *alverine citrate, *dicycloverine, and **mebeverine** (Colofac), are used to treat irritable bowel syndrome and diverticular disease. *Compare* ANTISPASTIC.

antispastic   *n.* a drug that relieves spasm of skeletal muscle. *See also* MUSCLE RELAXANT. *Compare* ANTISPASMODIC.

antitachycardia pacing termination of a *tachycardia by temporarily pacing the heart at a faster rate.

antithyroid drugs drugs that are used to counteract the excessive production and release of thyroid hormones in thyrotoxic states. The main agents are *carbimazole and *propylthiouracil. *See also* THIONAMIDES.

anti-TNF drugs   *see* CYTOKINE INHIBITOR.

antitoxin   *n.* an antibody produced by the body to counteract a toxin formed by invading bacteria or from any other source.

antitragus   *n.* a small projection of cartilage above the lobe of the ear, opposite the tragus. *See* PINNA.

antitussive (cough suppressant)   *n.* a drug, such as *pholcodine (a weak opioid), that suppresses coughing, possibly by reducing the activity of the cough centre in the brain and by depressing respiration. Some opioid analgesics also have antitussive activity, e.g. *codeine, *diamorphine, and *methadone.

anti-VEGF an agent that inhibits the action of *vascular endothelial growth factor (VEGF). *See* ANGIOGENESIS INHIBITOR.

antivenene (antivenin) *n.* an *antiserum containing antibodies against specific poisons in the venom of such an animal as a snake, spider, or scorpion.

antiviral drug a drug effective against viruses that cause disease. Antiviral drugs include *DNA polymerase inhibitors (e.g. *aciclovir, *foscarnet, *ganciclovir), *ribavirin, and *oseltamivir; they are used for treating herpes, cytomegalovirus and respiratory syncytial virus infections, and influenza. Antiviral drugs are also used for treating HIV infection and AIDS (*see* ANTIRETROVIRAL DRUG).

antrectomy *n.* **1.** surgical removal of the bony walls of an *antrum. *See* ANTROSTOMY. **2.** a surgical operation in which a part of the stomach (the antrum) is removed. Most secretions of acid, pepsin, and the hormone gastrin occur in the antrum and the operation may be required (usually combined with *vagotomy) in the treatment of peptic ulcers that have recurred after vagotomy and are resistant to such drugs as *proton-pump inhibitors and H_2-blocking drugs (*see* ANTIHISTAMINE).

antroscopy *n.* inspection of the inside of the maxillary sinus (*see* PARANASAL SINUSES) using an *endoscope (called an **antroscope**).

antrostomy *n.* a surgical operation to produce a permanent or semipermanent artificial opening on an *antrum in a bone, so providing drainage for any fluid. The operation is sometimes carried out to treat infection of the *paranasal sinuses.

antrum *n.* **1.** a cavity, especially a cavity in a bone. The **mastoid** (or **tympanic**) **antrum** is the space connecting the air cells of the *mastoid process with the chamber of the inner ear. **2.** the part of the *stomach adjoining the pylorus (**pyloric** or **gastric antrum**).

anuria *n.* failure of the kidneys to produce urine. This can occur in a variety of conditions that produce a sustained drop in blood pressure. Urgent assessment is required to differentiate lack of production of urine from an obstruction to the flow of urine from the kidneys, which can readily be relieved. Anuria is associated with increasing *uraemia and may require *haemodialysis.

anus *n.* the opening at the lower end of the alimentary canal, through which the faeces are discharged. It opens out from the *anal canal and is guarded by two sphincters. The anus is closed except during defecation. —**anal** *adj.*

anvil *n.* (in anatomy) *see* INCUS.

anxiety *n.* generalized pervasive *fear. **Anxiety disorders** are conditions in which anxiety dominates the patient's life or is experienced in particular situations; they include *panic disorder, *post-traumatic stress disorder, and *generalized anxiety disorder. Treatment usually includes antidepressants, cognitive behavioural therapy, and anxiety management techniques.

anxiolytic *adj.* describing a group of drugs used for the short-term treatment of anxiety of various causes. Formerly known as **minor tranquillizers**, they include the *benzodiazepines and *buspirone. Common side-effects of these drugs are drowsiness and dizziness, and prolonged use may result in *dependence.

A-O Association for Osteosynthesis: denoting a widely used system for treating fractures by metal inserts.

aorta *n.* (*pl.* **aortae** or **aortas**) the main artery of the body, from which all others derive. It arises from the left ventricle (**ascending aorta**), arches over the top of the heart (*see* AORTIC ARCH) and descends in front of the backbone (**descending aorta**), giving off large and small branches and finally dividing to form the right and left *iliac arteries. The part of the descending aorta from the aortic arch to the diaphragm is called the **thoracic aorta**; the part below the diaphragm is the **abdominal aorta**. —**aortic** *adj.*

aortic aneurysm *see* ANEURYSM.

aortic arch that part of the aorta that extends from the ascending aorta, upward over the heart and then backward and down as far as the fourth thoracic vertebra. *Stretch receptors in its outer wall monitor blood pressure and form part of the system maintaining this at a constant level.

aortic regurgitation a leak of the aortic valve resulting in reflux of blood from the aorta into the left ventricle during diastole. Aortic regurgitation is most commonly due to degenerative 'wear and tear' of the aortic valve. Other causes include dilatation of the aortic root with secondary dilatation of the aortic valve, scarring of the aortic valve as a result of previous acute rheumatic fever, or dissecting aortic aneurysm. Mild cases are symptom-free, but patients more severely affected develop breathlessness, angina pectoris, and enlargement of the heart; all have a diastolic murmur. A badly affected valve may be replaced surgically with a prosthesis.

aortic replacement a surgical technique used to replace a diseased length of aorta, most often the abdominal aorta. It usually involves inserting into the aorta a flexible tube of artificial material, which functions as a substitute for the diseased section.

aortic stenosis narrowing of the opening of the aortic valve due to fusion of the cusps that comprise the valve. It may result from previous rheumatic fever, or from calcification and scarring in a valve that has two *cusps instead of the normal three, or it may be congenital. Aortic stenosis obstructs the flow of blood from the left ventricle to the aorta during systole. Breathlessness on effort, angina pectoris, and fainting may follow. The patient has a systolic *murmur. When symptoms develop the valve should be replaced surgically with a mechanical or biological prosthesis.

aortic valve a valve in the heart, lying between the left ventricle and the aorta. It is a *semilunar valve that prevents blood returning to the ventricle from the aorta.

aortitis *n.* inflammation of the aorta, which was previously common as a late complication of syphilis but is more often now associated with a variety of poorly understood autoimmune conditions (such as *Behçet's syndrome and *Takayasu's disease). Inflammation of the aortic wall may result in the formation of an aneurysm or vascular stenosis, obstructing blood flow to target organs. Chest pain may occur from pressure on surrounding structures or from the reduced blood supply to the heart. *Aortic regurgitation may be found. Surgical repair to the aortic aneurysm or valve may be needed.

aortocaval compression (supine hypotension) compression of the aorta and inferior vena cava by a pelvic mass, such as the pregnant uterus, causing maternal hypotension when the woman adopts the supine position. The blood pressure usually returns to normal when the woman is turned onto a left lateral tilt.

aortography *n.* X-ray examination of the aorta, in which a series of images is taken during the injection of a *radiopaque contrast medium (*see* ANGIOGRAPHY). This technique has been largely replaced as a primary investigation by other *cross-sectional imaging methods.

AP *see* ANTEROPOSTERIOR.

apareunia *n.* inability to have penetrative intercourse due to physical discomfort, *vaginismus, or an underlying psychological problem. *See* DYSPAREUNIA.

apathetic hyperthyroidism a condition seen in older patients with *thyrotoxicosis, characterized by weight loss, slow atrial fibrillation, and severe depressive illness, rather than the usual florid symptoms. They have small goitres on examination and the blood tests confirm thyrotoxicosis, which is treated in the standard manner.

APC *see* ANTIGEN-PRESENTING CELL.

APD 1. *see* AUDITORY PROCESSING DISORDER. 2. automated *peritoneal dialysis.

aperient *n.* a mild *laxative.

Apert syndrome a hereditary disorder characterized by *craniosynostosis, underdevelopment of the midfacial tissues resulting in a sunken facial appearance, and *syndactyly (fusion) of 2–5 digits ('mitten glove'). Variable mental deficits and cleft palate may result. The condition may be associated with *Crouzon syndrome, in which case the fusion of the digits is less marked. *See also* ACROCEPHALOSYNDACTYLY. [E. Apert (1868–1940), French physician]

apex *n.* the tip or summit of an organ; for example the heart or lung. The apex of a *tooth is the tip of the root, where there is a small hole (the **apical foramen**) through which vessels and nerves pass from the pulp to the periapical tissues. —**apical** *adj.*

apex beat the impact of the heart against the chest wall during *systole. It can be felt or heard to the left of the breastbone, in the space between the fifth and sixth ribs.

apexification *n.* a procedure to allow the end of the root of an immature tooth to form a hard tissue barrier following traumatic injury that has caused the pulp to die.

apexogenesis *n.* a procedure that allows the root tip to continue forming when an im-

Apgar score	0	1	2
Appearance	Blue	Acrocyanotic	Pink
Pulse rate (bpm)	Absent	<100	>100
Reflex irritability	No response	Grimace	Vigorous cough/sneeze
Muscle tone	Limp	Some flexion of extremities	Active movement
Respiratory effort	Absent	Slow/irregular breaths	Good respiratory effort and cry

Apgar score.

mature tooth has sustained limited injury following trauma.

Apgar score a method of rapidly assessing the general state of a baby immediately after birth. A score of 0, 1, or 2 points is given for each sign, usually measured at one minute and five minutes after delivery (see table). Thus an infant scoring a total of 10 points would be in optimum condition. When the score is low, the test is repeated at intervals as a guide to short-term progress. [V. Apgar (1909–74), US anaesthetist]

aphakia *n.* absence of the lens of the eye: the state of the eye after a cataract has been removed when no intraocular lens has been inserted. —**aphakic** *adj.*

aphakic spectacles eyeglasses prescribed after cataract surgery when no intraocular lens is inserted into the eye (not common practice now). Usually these are thick convex lenses.

aphasia (dysphasia) *n.* a disorder of language affecting the generation and content of speech and its understanding (it is not a disorder of articulation: *see* DYSARTHRIA). It is caused by damage to the language-dominant half of the brain, which is usually the left hemisphere in a right-handed person. In **expressive aphasia** there is difficulty in producing language; in **receptive aphasia** there is difficulty with the comprehension of the spoken word. Aphasia is commonly accompanied by difficulties in reading and writing. —**aphasic** *adj.*

aphonia *n.* absence or loss of the voice caused by disease of the larynx or mouth or by disease of the nerves and muscles involved in the generation and articulation of speech. If loss of speech is due to a language

defect in the cerebral hemispheres, the disorder is *aphasia.

aphrodisiac *n.* an agent that stimulates sexual excitement.

aphthous ulcer a small ulcer, occurring singly or in groups in the mouth as white or red spots; their cause is unknown. Treatment is with topical tetracycline or topical corticosteroids.

apical abscess an abscess in the bone around the apex of a tooth. An acute abscess is extremely painful, causing swelling of the jaw and sometimes also the face. A chronic abscess may cause no pain or swelling. An abscess invariably results from damage to and infection of the pulp of the tooth. Treatment is drainage and *root canal treatment or extraction of the tooth; antibiotics may give temporary relief.

apicectomy *n.* (in dentistry) surgical removal of the apex of the root of a tooth, now often referred to as **root end resection**. It is usually accompanied by placement of a filling in a cavity prepared in the root end. It is carried out when *root canal treatment has failed and cannot be redone.

aplasia *n.* total or partial failure of development of an organ or tissue. *See also* AGENESIS. —**aplastic** *adj.*

aplasia cutis congenita the congenital absence of skin on the scalp, usually in one or more small patches. It may result from an infection in the uterus or from a developmental abnormality.

aplastic anaemia *see* ANAEMIA.

APMPPE acute posterior multifocal placoid *pigment epitheliopathy.

apneusis *n.* a state in which prolonged inhalation occurs. It occurs when the appropriate inhibitory influences are prevented from reaching the inspiratory centre of the brain.

apnoea *n.* temporary cessation of breathing from any cause, formally defined as a reduction in nasal airflow to less than 30% of normal for more than 10 seconds. The presence of more than five episodes of apnoea per hour of sleep is indicative of *obstructive sleep apnoea. Attacks of apnoea are common in newborn babies and should be taken seriously although they do not necessarily indicate serious illness. *See also* SLEEP APNOEA. —**apnoeic** *adj.*

apnoea index the number of *apnoea episodes per hour of sleep.

apnoea monitor an electronic alarm that is activated by a sensor that responds to a baby's respiratory movements. It can be used at home to monitor babies thought to be at risk of *sudden infant death syndrome.

apocrine *adj.* **1.** describing sweat glands that occur only in hairy parts of the body, especially the armpit and groin. These glands develop in the hair follicles and appear after puberty has been reached. The strong odours associated with sweating result from the action of bacteria on the sweat produced by apocrine glands. *Compare* ECCRINE. **2.** describing a type of gland that loses part of its protoplasm when secreting. *See* SECRETION.

apolipoprotein *n.* any one of a family of proteins that form the protein components of *lipoproteins, which transport hydrophobic lipid molecules in the plasma. Individual members of the family are designated by the abbreviation 'Apo' followed by a capital letter. Apolipoproteins have a range of molecular weights and perform a variety of functions during the life cycle of the lipoproteins in which they are found. These include acting as ligands for the binding of enzymes (ApoB) and as cofactors for the action of other enzymes (ApoA and ApoC).

apomorphine *n.* a *dopamine receptor agonist used in the treatment of Parkinson's disease that is poorly controlled by *levodopa. It is given by subcutaneous injection or infusion; side-effects include involuntary movements and instability of posture. Apomorphine is also given by mouth for the treatment of erectile dysfunction. Trade name: **APO-go**.

aponeurosis *n.* a thin but strong fibrous sheet of tissue that replaces a *tendon in muscles that are flat and sheetlike and have a wide area of attachment (e.g. to bones). —**aponeurotic** *adj.*

apophysis *n.* **1.** a protuberance of bone to which a tendon is attached. It ossifies separately from the rest of the bone and fuses with it at maturity. **2.** a projection of any other part, e.g. of the brain (**apophysis cerebri**: the *pineal gland).

apophysitis *n.* inflammation of an unfused *apophysis resulting from excessive traction from a large tendon attachment. It most commonly occurs around the knee (*see* OSGOOD-SCHLATTER DISEASE) and the heel (*see* SEVER'S DISEASE). *See also* OSTEOCHONDRITIS.

apoplexy *n. see* STROKE.

apoptosis *n.* programmed cell death, which results in the ordered removal of cells and occurs naturally as part of the normal development, maintenance, and renewal of cells, tissues, and organs. During embryonic development, for example, the fingers are 'sculpted' from the embryonic spadelike hand by apoptosis of the cells between them. Defects in apoptosis, for example if it is absent or blocked, have been implicated in the uncontrolled division of malignant cells that occurs in cancer. Abnormal apoptosis, due to failure of the mechanisms that control it, may be a causative factor in autoimmune disease.

appendectomy *n.* the usual US term for *appendicectomy.

appendicectomy *n.* surgical removal of the vermiform appendix. *See also* APPENDICITIS.

appendicitis *n.* inflammation of the vermiform *appendix. **Acute appendicitis**, which became common in the 20th century, usually affects young people. The chief symptom is abdominal pain, first central and later (with tenderness) in the right lower abdomen, over the appendix (*see* MCBURNEY'S POINT). Unusual positions of the appendix may cause pain in different sites, leading to difficulty in diagnosis. Vomiting and diarrhoea sometimes occur, but fever is slight. If not treated by surgical removal (appendicectomy) the condition usually progresses to cause an abscess or generalized *peritonitis. Conditions that mimic appendicitis include mesenteric *lymphadenitis, terminal ileitis (see CROHN'S DISEASE), right-sided ectopic pregnancy, a right-sided kidney stone, *pyelonephritis, and (rarely) right-sided pneumonia. **Chronic appendicitis** was a term used 20–50 years ago to explain recurrent pains in the lower abdomen; it is no longer used.

appendicular *adj.* **1.** relating to or affecting the vermiform appendix. **2.** relating to the limbs: the **appendicular skeleton** comprises the bones of the limbs.

appendix (vermiform appendix) *n.* the short thin blind-ended tube, 7–10 cm long, that is attached to the end of the caecum (a pouch at the start of the large intestine). It has no known function in humans and is liable to become infected and inflamed, especially in young adults (see APPENDICITIS).

apperception *n.* (in psychology) the process by which the qualities of an object, situation, etc., perceived by an individual are correlated with his/her preexisting knowledge.

appestat *n.* a region in the brain that controls the amount of food intake. Appetite suppressants probably decrease hunger by changing the chemical characteristics of this centre.

applanation *n.* a method of flattening the cornea that is used to determine the intraocular pressure in applanation tonometry (see TONOMETER).

apple-core *adj.* describing the characteristic radiographic appearance of a *stricture of the bowel resulting from the presence of a malignant tumour. The bowel is narrow with an irregular outline and the ends of the stricture are 'shouldered' – the angle between the normal wall and the start of the narrow area approaches 90° on both sides. This contrasts with smooth tapering strictures, which are commonly benign.

applicator *n.* any device used to apply medication or treatment to a particular part of the body.

apposition *n.* the state of two structures, such as parts of the body, being in close contact. For example, the fingers are brought into apposition when the fist is clenched, and the eyelids when the eyes are closed.

appraisal *n.* formal review of a health-care professional's performance, carried out on an annual basis by a trained appraiser in order to provide feedback on past performance, chart continuing progress, and identify needs for development. For doctors, the content of the appraisal is based on the General Medical Council's document *Good Medical Practice. See also* CLINICAL GOVERNANCE.

apraclonidine *n.* an alpha agonist (see SYMPATHOMIMETIC) administered in the form of eye drops to reduce or prevent raised intraocular pressure, mostly used after laser surgery. Trade name: **Iopidine**.

apraxia (dyspraxia) *n.* an inability to make skilled movements with accuracy. This is a disorder of the *cerebral cortex resulting in the patient's inability to organize the movements rather than clumsiness due to weakness, sensory loss, or disease of the *cerebellum. It is most often caused by disease of the dominant *parietal lobe of the brain and sometimes by disease of the frontal lobe, causing, for example, difficulty in walking (**gait apraxia**).

aproctia *n.* congenital absence of the anus or its opening. *See* IMPERFORATE ANUS.

apronectomy *n.* the surgical removal of excessive redundant skin and subcutaneous tissue from the front of the abdomen, usually after massive weight loss in morbidly obese patients.

aprosexia *n.* inability to fix the attention on any subject, due to poor eyesight, defective hearing, or mental weakness.

APTT activated partial thromboplastin time (see PTTK).

APUD cells cells that share the metabolic property of *a*mine-*p*recursor *u*ptake and *de*carboxylation. They have a wide distribution, especially in the mucosa of the gastrointestinal tract and pancreas, and are able to form a large variety of peptide hormonal substances; they are often known as the **diffuse endocrine system**.

apudoma *n.* a tumour that contains *APUD cells and may give rise to symptoms caused by excessive production of the hormones and other peptides that these cells produce. *Carcinoids are a good example of this group of tumours, but there are many others (e.g. *gastrinomas, *somatostatinomas, and *VIPomas).

apyrexia *n.* the absence of fever.

aquaporin *n.* any of a class of proteins

that function as transmembrane water channels. Genetic mutations of aquaporin 2 (*AQP-2*) are responsible for some distinct forms of *nephrogenic diabetes insipidus.

aqueduct *n.* (in anatomy) a canal containing fluid. An example is the *cerebral aqueduct.

aqueous humour the watery fluid that fills the chamber of the *eye immediately behind the cornea and in front of the lens. It is continually being formed – chiefly by capillaries of the ciliary processes – and it drains away into Schlemm's canal, at the junction of the cornea and sclera.

arachidonic acid *see* ESSENTIAL FATTY ACID.

arachnidism *n.* poisoning from the bite of a spider. Toxins from the less venomous species of spider cause only local pain, redness, and swelling. Toxins from more venomous species, such as the black widow (*Lactrodectus mactans*), cause muscular pains, convulsions, nausea, and paralysis.

arachnodactyly *n.* abnormally long and slender fingers: usually associated with excessive height and congenital defects of the heart and eyes in *Marfan's syndrome.

arachnoid (arachnoid mater) *n.* the middle of the three membranes covering the brain and spinal cord (*see* MENINGES), which has a fine, almost cobweb-like, texture. Between it and the pia mater within lies the subarachnoid space, containing cerebrospinal fluid and large blood vessels; the membrane itself has no blood supply.

arachnoiditis *n.* an inflammatory process causing thickening and scarring (fibrosis) of the membranous linings (*meninges) of the spinal canal. The resulting entrapment of nerve roots may result in weakness, pain, and numbness in the affected area. The condition may result from infection or inflammation of the meninges, surgery, or as a response to the oil-based dyes previously used in *myelography. The reaction to myelography is prevented by the current use of water-soluble dyes.

arachnoid villus one of the thin-walled projections outwards of the arachnoid membrane into the blood-filled sinuses of the dura, acting as a one-way valve for the flow of cerebrospinal fluid from the subarachnoid space into the bloodstream. Large villi, known as **arachnoid granulations** (or **Pac-**

chionian bodies), are found in the region of the superior sagittal sinus. They may be so distended as to cause pitting of the adjacent bone.

arbor *n.* (in anatomy) a treelike structure. **Arbor vitae** is the treelike outline of white matter seen in sections of the cerebellum; it also refers to the treelike appearance of the inner folds of the cervix (neck) of the uterus.

arbovirus *n.* one of a group of RNA-containing viruses that are transmitted from animals to humans by insects (i.e. arthropods; hence *ar*thropod-*bor*ne viruses) and cause diseases resulting in encephalitis or serious fever, such as dengue and yellow fever.

ARC AIDS-related complex.

arc-eye *n.* a painful condition of the eyes caused by damage to the surface of the cornea by ultraviolet light from arc welding. It usually resolves if the eyes are padded for 24 hours. It is similar to *snow blindness and the condition caused by overexposure of the eye to sun-tanning lamps.

arch- (**arche-, archi-, archo-**) *combining form denoting* first; primitive; ancestral. Example: **archinephron** (first-formed embryonic kidney).

archenteron *n.* a cavity that forms in the very early embryo as the result of gastrulation (*see* GASTRULA). In humans it forms a tubular cavity, the **archenteric canal**, which connects the amniotic cavity with the yolk sac. —**archenteric** *adj.*

archetype *n.* (in Jungian psychology) an inherited idea or mode of thought supposed to be present in the *unconscious mind and to derive from the experience of the whole human race (the collective unconscious), not from the life experience of the individual.

archipallium *n.* the *hippocampal formation of the cerebrum. The term is seldom used.

arcuate keratotomy a curved incision made in the periphery of the cornea. It is usually performed in the region of greatest curvature of the cornea in order to flatten it and hence reduce *astigmatism.

arcus *n.* an arch; for example the **arcus aortae** (*aortic arch) or an **arcus senilis** or **arcus juvenilis** (*see* CORNEAL ARCUS).

ARDS *see* ADULT RESPIRATORY DISTRESS SYNDROME.

areola *n.* 1. the brownish or pink ring of tissue surrounding the nipple of the breast. 2. the part of the iris that surrounds the pupil of the eye. 3. a small space in a tissue. —**areolar** *adj.*

areolar tissue loose *connective tissue consisting of a meshwork of collagen, elastic tissue, and reticular fibres interspersed with numerous connective tissue cells. It binds the skin to underlying muscles and forms a link between organs while allowing a high degree of relative movement.

ARF *see* ACUTE RESPIRATORY FAILURE.

Argasidae *n. see* TICK.

argentaffin cells cells that stain readily with silver salts. Such cells occur, for example, in the crypts of Lieberkühn in the intestine.

argentaffinoma *n. see* CARCINOID.

arginine *n.* an *amino acid that plays an important role in the formation of *urea by the liver.

argon laser a type of *laser that utilizes argon gas to produce a beam of intense light, used especially in eye surgery to treat disease of the retina (e.g. diabetic retinopathy) or glaucoma (as in argon laser *trabeculoplasty). *See also* PHOTOCOAGULATION.

argon plasma coagulation an endoscopic procedure used predominantly to control active bleeding in the gastrointestinal tract. A monopolar electrosurgical current is delivered to tissue via an ionized argon gas stream (argon plasma) leading to coagulation. Other uses of this procedure include debulking of tumours not amenable to surgical intervention.

Argyll Robertson pupil a disorder of the eyes in which the *pupillary (light) reflex is absent. Although the pupils contract normally for near vision (the accommodation reflex), they fail to contract in bright light. It may occur, for example, as a result of syphilis or diabetes. [D. Argyll Robertson (1837–1909), Scottish ophthalmologist]

argyria (argyrosis) *n.* the deposition of silver in the skin and other tissues, either resulting from industrial exposure or following ingestion or long-term administration of silver salts. A slate-grey pigmentation develops slowly; this is accentuated in areas exposed to light. Deposition of silver in the conjunctiva, corneal epithelium, stroma, and Descemet's membrane is usually due to chronic exposure to silver compounds or instillation of eye drops containing silver.

ariboflavinosis *n.* the group of symptoms caused by deficiency of riboflavin (vitamin B_2). These symptoms include inflammation of the tongue and lips and sores in the corners of the mouth.

Arimidex *n. see* AROMATASE INHIBITOR.

aripiprazole *n. see* ANTIPSYCHOTIC.

Aristolochia *n.* a genus of plants containing aristolochic acid, a nephrotoxin associated with progressive renal failure and a tendency to urothelial tumours. Species are associated with *Balkan nephropathy (*A. clematis*) and *Chinese herb nephropathy (*A. fangchi*).

ARMD age-related *macular degeneration.

ARN *see* ACUTE RETINAL NECROSIS.

Arnold-Chiari malformation a congenital disorder in which there is distortion of the base of the skull with protrusion of the lower brainstem and parts of the cerebellum through the opening for the spinal cord at the base of the skull (*see* BANANA AND LEMON SIGNS). It is associated commonly with *neural tube defects, *hydrocephalus, and a *syringomyelia. [J. Arnold (1835–1915) and H. Chiari (1851–1916), German pathologists]

Aromasin *n. see* AROMATASE INHIBITOR.

aromatase inhibitor any one of a class of drugs used in the treatment of early and advanced oestrogen-dependent breast cancer in postmenopausal women. These drugs act by inhibiting the action of aromatase, an enzyme that promotes the conversion of testosterone to oestradiol. They therefore reduce oestrogen levels, which can be helpful in the control of oestrogen-dependent tumours. Aromatase inhibitors include **anastrozole** (Arimidex), **exemestane** (Aromasin), and **letrozole** (Femara), which are taken by mouth; side-effects include symptoms of oestrogen deficiency (e.g. hot flushes), nausea and vomiting, and headache.

aromatherapy *n.* a form of complementary medicine that utilizes fragrant essential oils to improve physical, psychological, and emotional wellbeing. The oils can be massaged into the skin or their fragrances can be inhaled via an infusion.

arousal *n.* **1.** a state of alertness and of high responsiveness to stimuli. It is produced by strong motivation, by anxiety, and by a stimulating environment. **2.** physiological activation of the *cerebral cortex by centres lower in the brain, such as the *reticular activating system, resulting in wakefulness and alertness. It is hypothesized that unduly high or low degrees of arousal lead to neuropsychiatric problems, such as *narcolepsy and *mania.

arrhenoblastoma *n.* *see* ANDROBLASTOMA.

arrhythmia *n.* any deviation from the normal rhythm (sinus rhythm) of the heart. The natural pacemaker of the heart (the sinoatrial node), which lies in the wall of the right atrium, controls the rate and rhythm of the whole heart under the influence of the autonomic nervous system. It generates electrical impulses that spread to the atria and ventricles, via specialized conducting tissues, and cause them to contract normally. Arrhythmias result from a disturbance of the generation or the conduction of these impulses and may be intermittent or continuous. Arrhythmias are subdivided into **tachyarrhythmias** (fast rate) and **bradyarrhythmias** (slow rate). They include *ectopic beats (extrasystoles), ectopic tachycardias (*see* SUPRAVENTRICULAR TACHYCARDIA, VENTRICULAR TACHYCARDIA), atrial and ventricular *fibrillation, and *heart block (which is often associated with slow heart rates). Symptoms include palpitations, breathlessness, and chest pain. In more serious arrhythmias the *Stokes-Adams syndrome or *cardiac arrest may occur. Arrhythmias may result from most heart diseases but they also occur without apparent cause.

arsenic *n.* a poisonous greyish metallic element producing the symptoms of nausea, vomiting, diarrhoea, cramps, convulsions, and coma when ingested in large doses. Drugs used as antidotes to arsenic poisoning include *dimercaprol. Arsenic was formerly readily available in the form of rat poison and in fly-papers and was the poisoner's first choice during the 19th century, its presence in a body being then difficult to detect. Today detection is relatively simple. Arsenic was formerly used in medicine, the most important arsenical drugs being **arsphenamine** (Salvarsan) and **neoarsphenamine**, used in the treatment of syphilis and dangerous parasitic diseases. Symbol: As.

artefact *n.* *see* ARTIFACT.

artemisinin *n.* the active ingredient of qinghaosu, a Chinese herbal medicine prepared from a species of wormwood (*Artemisia annua*) and long used for treating malaria. Derivatives of artemisinin (including artesunate and artemether) have been developed for the treatment of malignant (falciparum) malaria; they act by killing the asexual stages of the parasite (*see* PLASMODIUM) and are used in combination with other antimalarial drugs. In the UK, for example, artemether is available in combination with lumefantrine (as **Riamet**).

arter- (arteri-, arterio-) *combining form denoting* an artery. Examples: **arteriopathy** (disease of); **arteriorrhaphy** (suture of); **arteriovenous** (relating to arteries and veins).

arterial ulcer a localized area of damage and breakdown of the skin due to inadequate arterial blood supply (*ischaemia). Usually it is seen on the feet of patients with severe atheromatous narrowings of the arteries supplying the legs.

arteriectomy *n.* surgical excision of an artery or part of an artery. This may be performed as a diagnostic procedure (for example, to take an arterial biopsy in the diagnosis of arteritis) or during reconstruction of a blocked artery when the blocked segment is replaced by a synthetic graft.

arteriogenesis *n.* the enlargement of pre-existing collateral channels to form collateral arteries in order to bypass an occluded primary artery (*see* COLLATERAL CIRCULATION). This is an active process involving remodelling of the vessel wall mediated by cellular and chemical signals.

arteriography *n.* imaging of arteries (*see* ANGIOGRAPHY). The major roles of arteriography are to demonstrate the site and extent of atheroma, especially in the coronary arteries (*see* CORONARY ANGIOGRAPHY) and leg arteries (**peripheral arteriography**), and to demonstrate the anatomy of aneurysms within the skull (**carotid** and **vertebral arteriography**).

arteriole *n.* a small branch of an *artery, leading into many smaller vessels – the *capillaries. By their constriction and dilation, under the regulation of the sympathetic nervous system, arterioles are the principal controllers of blood flow and pressure.

arteriolitis *n.* inflammation of the arterioles (the smallest arteries), which may complicate severe hypertension. This produces **necrotizing arteriolitis**, which may result in kidney failure. A similar condition may affect the lung in pulmonary hypertension.

arteriolosclerosis *n. see* NEPHROSCLEROSIS.

arterioplasty *n.* surgical reconstruction of an artery; for example, in the treatment of *aneurysms.

arteriosclerosis *n.* an imprecise term used for any of several conditions affecting the arteries. The term is often used as a synonym for atherosclerosis (*see* ATHEROMA).

arteriotomy *n.* an incision into, or a needle puncture of, the wall of an artery. This is most often performed as a diagnostic procedure in the course of *arteriography or cardiac *catheterization. It may also be required to remove an embolus (*see* EMBOLECTOMY).

arteriovenous anastomosis a thick-walled blood vessel that connects an arteriole directly with a venule, thus bypassing the capillaries. Arteriovenous anastomoses are commonly found in the skin of the lips, nose, ears, hands and feet; their muscular walls can constrict to reduce blood flow or dilate to allow blood through to these areas.

arteriovenous aneurysm a direct communication between an artery and vein, without an intervening capillary bed. It can occur as a congenital abnormality or it may be acquired following injury or surgery. It may affect the limbs, lungs, or viscera and may be single or multiple. If the connection is large, the short-circuiting of blood may produce heart failure. Large isolated arteriovenous aneurysms may be closed surgically.

arteriovenous malformation *see* ANGIOMA.

arteritis *n.* an inflammatory disease that affects the muscular walls of the arteries. It may be part of a *connective-tissue disease or it may be due to an infection, such as syphilis. The affected vessels are swollen and tender and may become blocked. **Temporal** (or **giant-cell**) **arteritis** occurs in the elderly and most commonly affects the arteries of the scalp. The patient complains of severe headache, and double vision or scalp tenderness may be present; blindness may result

from thrombosis of the arteries to the eyes. Treatment with cortisone derivatives is rapidly effective.

artery *n.* a blood vessel carrying blood away from the heart. All arteries except the *pulmonary artery carry oxygenated blood. The walls of arteries contain smooth muscle fibres, which contract or relax under the control of the sympathetic nervous system. See illustrations. *See also* AORTA, ARTERIOLE.

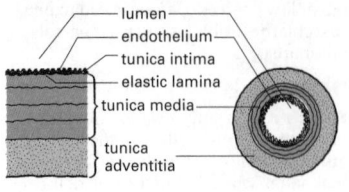

Transverse section through an artery.

arthr- (arthro-) *combining form denoting* a joint. Examples: **arthrology** (science of); **arthrosclerosis** (stiffening or hardening of).

arthralgia (arthrodynia) *n.* severe pain in a joint, without swelling or other signs of arthritis. *Compare* ARTHRITIS.

arthrectomy *n.* surgical excision of a joint. It is usually performed on a painful joint that has ceased to function, as may result from intractable infection, or after a failed joint replacement. *See also* (EXCISION) ARTHROPLASTY.

arthritis *n.* inflammation of one or more joints, characterized by pain, swelling, warmth, redness of the overlying skin, and diminished range of joint motion. There are four basic subgroups of arthritis: **noninflammatory arthritis**, including *osteoarthritis, *neuropathic arthritis, and *osteochondritis dissecans; **inflammatory arthritis**, including *rheumatoid arthritis, *gout, *psoriatic arthritis, and *juvenile chronic arthritis; **infectious arthritis**, including *septic arthritis; and **haemorrhagic arthritis**, including haemophilic arthritis (which occurs in patients with haemophilia). Arthritis may be **monoarticular** (involving one joint), **pauciarticular** (involving four or fewer joints), or **polyarticular** (involving five or more joints, either simultaneously or in sequence). Diagnosis is based on clinical and laboratory findings, including X-rays, blood tests, and where necessary analysis of synovial fluid obtained by *arthrocentesis. Treatment is

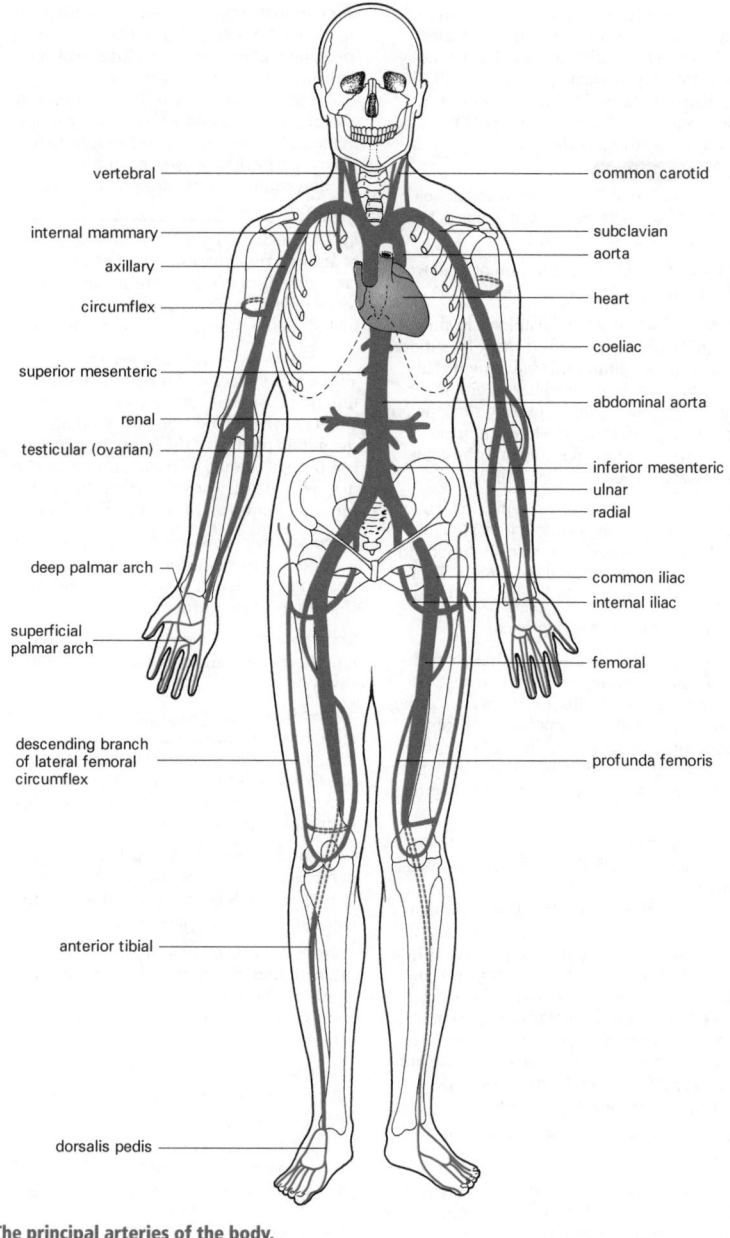

The principal arteries of the body.

specific for each subgroup and may include any combination of supportive measures with activity modification, analgesics, anti-inflammatory medications (e.g. *NSAIDs), corticosteroids, and surgical procedures, such as joint replacement (*see* ARTHRO-PLASTY). —**arthritic** *adj.*

((()) SEE WEB LINKS

• Website of Arthritis Care: includes advice on living with arthritis together with resources for health and care professionals

arthrocentesis *n.* aspiration of fluid from a joint through a puncture needle.

arthrodesis *n.* artificial ankylosis: the fusion of bones across a joint space by surgical means, which eliminates movement. This operation is performed when a joint is very painful, highly unstable, grossly deformed or chronically infected, or when an *arthroplasty would be inadvisable or impossible. *See also* CHARNLEY CLAMPS.

arthrodic joint (gliding joint) a form of *diarthrosis (freely movable joint) in which the bony surfaces slide over each other without angular or rotational movement. Examples are the joints of the carpus and tarsus.

arthrodynia *n. see* ARTHRALGIA.

arthrography *n.* an X-ray imaging technique for examining joints. A contrast medium (either *radiolucent gas or a *radio-paque material) is injected into the joint space, outlining its contents and extent accurately. Arthrography has now largely been replaced by *magnetic resonance imaging (MRI).

arthrogryposis *n.* congenital limitation of joint movement due to *contractures affecting two or more joints. This is accompanied by joint stiffness, cylindrical limbs, and absence of skin creases. The most common of such syndromes is **arthrogryposis multiplex congenita**, a congenital condition of multiple contractures in which muscles are replaced by fibrous tissue, resulting in narrow limbs. Treatment, which begins soon after birth, consists initially of manipulation and splintage of deformed joints followed by contracture release and osteotomies.

arthropathy *n.* any disease or disorder involving a joint.

arthroplasty *n.* surgical refashioning of a diseased joint to relieve pain and to maintain or regain movement. An **excision** (or **re-**section) **arthroplasty** involves the excision of enough bone to create a gap at which movement can occur. In an **interposition arthroplasty** a biological or artificial barrier is placed between the two bony surfaces. In a **total arthroplasty** both joint surfaces are replaced by *prostheses; in a **hemiarthroplasty**, performed for some fractures of the hip and shoulder, only one end of a joint is replaced.

arthropod *n.* any member of a large group of animals that possess a hard external skeleton and jointed legs and other appendages. Many arthropods are of medical importance, including the *mites, *ticks, and *insects.

arthroscope *n.* a rigid telescope fitted with a lens system and fibreoptic illumination that is inserted into a joint through a small ('keyhole') incision and generates a magnified picture of the joint interior that can be viewed on a television monitor. The diameter of arthroscopes ranges from 2 mm for small joints to 5 mm for larger joints.

arthroscopy *n.* inspection of a joint cavity with an *arthroscope, enabling percutaneous surgery (such as *meniscectomy) and *biopsy to be performed.

arthrostomy *n.* a procedure to enable a temporary opening to be made into a joint cavity.

arthrotomy *n.* the surgical opening of any joint. It is performed to allow joint inspection, removal of a loose body, drainage of pus (from an infected joint) or of a haematoma, synovectomy, joint reconstruction, or joint replacement.

articaine *n.* a local *anaesthetic used in dentistry. It is available in combination with adrenaline (as **Septanest**) to achieve better and longer lasting anaesthesia.

articular *adj.* relating to a joint. For example, **articular cartilage** is the layer of cartilage at the ends of adjoining bones at a joint. *See also* EXTRA-ARTICULAR, INTRA-ARTICULAR, PERIARTICULAR.

articulation *n.* (in anatomy) the point or type of contact between two bones. *See* JOINT.

articulator *n.* (in dentistry) an apparatus for relating the upper and lower models of a patient's dentition in a fixed position, usually with maximum tooth contact. Some articulators can reproduce jaw movements.

They are used in the construction of crowns, bridges, and dentures.

artifact (artefact) *n.* **1.** (in radiography) an appearance on an image reflecting a problem with the radiographic technique rather than representing the true appearance of the patient. For example, a movement artifact is blurring of the image due to movement of the patient or organ during the exposure. All imaging techniques are susceptible to a range of artifacts. *See also* PARTIAL VOLUME ARTIFACT. **2.** (in microscopy) a structure seen in a tissue under a microscope that is not present in the living tissue. Artifacts, which are produced by faulty *fixation or staining of the tissue, may give a false impression that disease or abnormality is present in the tissue when it is not.

artificial heart a titanium pump that is implanted into the body to take over the function of a failing left ventricle in patients with heart disease. This allows the diseased ventricle time to recover its function. The pump is powered by an external battery, strapped to the patient's body, to which it is connected by wires passed through the patient's skin. Originally pumps were implanted into the abdomen, but the most recent devices are small enough to fit into the heart itself.

artificial insemination instrumental introduction of semen into the vagina in order that a woman may conceive. Insemination is timed to coincide with the day on which the woman is expected to ovulate (*see* MENSTRUAL CYCLE). The semen specimen may be provided by the husband (**AIH – artificial insemination husband**), for example in cases of erectile dysfunction, or by an anonymous donor (**DI – donor insemination**), usually in cases where the husband is sterile.

artificial nutrition and hydration the use of enteral feeding tubes or cannulas to provide nutrients and prevent a patient becoming dehydrated. Such interventions may be considered to be either active treatment or merely supportive, leading to debate about withdrawal from insentient patients who have no prospect of meaningful recovery. Commonly, when other intensive treatments are judged *futile, artificial nutrition and hydration are considered *extraordinary means of prolonging life. It is permissible to withdraw such treatment when it is no longer in the patient's interests and when the primary intention is not to kill the patient, although death is foreseen (*see* DOCTRINE OF DOUBLE EFFECT). In cases of patients in a *persistent vegetative state, the matter must be referred to the courts following the case of Tony Bland. Where food and water are withdrawn it is still considered important to moisten the patient's lips and to keep him or her comfortable until death.

artificial respiration (artificial ventilation) an emergency procedure for maintaining a flow of air into and out of a patient's lungs when the natural breathing reflexes are absent or insufficient. This may occur after drowning, poisoning, etc., or during a surgical operation on the thorax or abdomen when muscle-relaxing drugs are administered. The simplest and most efficient method is *mouth-to-mouth resuscitation. In hospital the breathing cycle is maintained by means of a *ventilator.

artificial rupture of membranes (ARM) *see* AMNIOTOMY.

artificial sphincter an apparatus designed to replace or support a *sphincter that is either absent or ineffective. *See also* NEOSPHINCTER.

ARV *see* ANTIRETROVIRAL DRUG.

arytenoid cartilage either of the two pyramid-shaped cartilages that lie at the back of the *larynx next to the upper edges of the cricoid cartilage.

arytenoidectomy *n.* surgical excision of the arytenoid cartilage of the larynx in the treatment of paralysis of the vocal folds.

asbestosis *n.* a lung disease – a form of *pneumoconiosis – caused by fibres of asbestos inhaled by those who are exposed to the mineral. The incidence of lung cancer is high in such patients, particularly if they smoke cigarettes (*see also* MESOTHELIOMA). Asbestosis does not include *asbestos-related pleural disease. This is important because patients with asbestosis due to occupational exposure can often claim compensation, whereas this is only rarely possible for those with asbestos-related pleural disease.

asbestos-related pleural disease any one of a variety of conditions involving the *pleura, but not the lungs (*see* ASBESTOSIS), in subjects exposed to asbestos. These include the formation of pleural plaques, diffuse pleural thickening, and pleural effusions (*see* OEDEMA).

A-scan *n.* examination of ocular tissue, including measurement of the length of the eye (axial length), by means of a high-frequency ultrasound machine. *See also* B-SCAN.

ascariasis *n.* a disease caused by an infestation with the parasitic worm *Ascaris lumbricoides*. Adult worms in the intestine can cause abdominal pain, vomiting, constipation, diarrhoea, appendicitis, and peritonitis; in large numbers they may cause obstruction of the intestine. The presence of the migrating larvae in the lungs can provoke pneumonia. Ascariasis occurs principally in areas of poor sanitation; it is treated with *levamisole.

Ascaris *n.* a genus of parasitic nematode worms. *A. lumbricoides*, widely distributed throughout the world, is the largest of the human intestinal nematodes – an adult female measures up to 35 cm in length. Eggs, passed out in the stools, may be transmitted to a new host in contaminated food or drink. Larvae hatch out in the intestine and then undergo a complicated migration, via the hepatic portal vein, liver, heart, lungs, windpipe, and pharynx, before returning to the intestine where they later develop into adult worms (*see also* ASCARIASIS).

ascites (hydroperitoneum) *n.* the accumulation of fluid in the peritoneal cavity, causing abdominal swelling. Causes include infections (such as tuberculosis), heart failure, *portal hypertension, *cirrhosis, and various cancers (particularly of the ovary and liver): the presence of malignant cells in the fluid, revealed by cytological examination, is usually evidence of secondary spread. Obstruction to the drainage of lymph from the abdomen results in **chylous ascites** (*see* CHYLE). **Pancreatic ascites**, due to direct communication between the pancreatic duct and the peritoneal cavity, usually following trauma or severe pancreatitis, is diagnosed by very high amylase levels in aspirated ascitic fluid. *See also* OEDEMA.

ascorbic acid *see* VITAMIN C.

ASD *see* ATRIAL SEPTAL DEFECT.

-ase *suffix denoting* an enzyme. Examples: **lactase; dehydrogenase**.

asepsis *n.* the complete absence of bacteria, fungi, viruses, or other microorganisms that could cause disease. Asepsis is the ideal state for the performance of surgical operations and is achieved by using *sterilization techniques. —**aseptic** *adj.*

Asherman syndrome a condition in which *amenorrhoea and infertility follow a major haemorrhage in pregnancy. It may result from overvigorous curettage of the uterus in an attempt to control the bleeding. This removes the lining, the walls adhere, and the cavity is obliterated to a greater or lesser degree. Some 50% of such patients are subsequently infertile, and of those who become pregnant, only a minority achieve an uncomplicated delivery. *Compare* SHEEHAN'S SYNDROME. [J. G. Asherman (20th century), Czechoslovakian gynaecologist]

Askanazy cells *see* HÜRTHLE CELL TUMOUR.

asparaginase *n.* an enzyme that inhibits the growth of certain tumours. **Crisantaspase**, the form produced by the bacterium *Erwinia chrysanthemi*, is used in the treatment of acute lymphoblastic leukaemia. Administered by injection, it may cause allergic reactions and *anaphylaxis. Trade name: **Erwinase**.

asparagine *n. see* AMINO ACID.

aspartate aminotransferase (AST) an enzyme involved in the transamination of amino acids. Measurement of AST in the serum may be used in the diagnosis of acute myocardial infarction and acute liver disease. It was formerly called **serum glutamic oxaloacetic transaminase** (**SGOT**).

aspartic acid (aspartate) *see* AMINO ACID.

Asperger's syndrome a condition, often considered to be a mild form of *autism, characterized by social aloofness, lack of interest in other people, stilted and pedantic styles of speech, and an excessive preoccupation with a very specialized interest (such as timetables). Intelligence can be normal or enhanced, but is more commonly in the lower average range. [H. Asperger (1906–80), Austrian paediatrician]

aspergillosis *n.* a group of conditions caused by fungi of the genus *Aspergillus*, usually *Aspergillus fumigatus*. These conditions nearly always arise in patients with pre-existing lung disease and fall into three categories. The allergic form most commonly affects asthmatic patients and may cause collapse of segments or lobes of a lung. The colonizing form leads to formation of a fungus ball (**aspergilloma**), usually within a pre-existing cavity in the lung (such as an emphysematous *bulla or a healed tuberculous cavity). Similar fungus balls may be found in other cavities, such as the eye or the sinuses around the nose. The third form of aspergillosis, in which the fungus spreads throughout the lungs and may even disseminate throughout the body, is rare but potentially fatal. It is usually associated with deficiency in the patient's immunity.

Aspergillus *n.* a genus of fungi, including many common moulds, some of which cause infections of the respiratory system in humans. The species *A. fumigatus* causes *aspergillosis. *A. niger* is commonly found in the external ear and can become pathogenic.

aspermia *n.* strictly, a lack or failure of formation of semen. More usually, however, the term is used to mean the total absence of sperm from the semen (*see* AZOOSPERMIA).

asphyxia *n.* suffocation: a life-threatening condition in which oxygen is prevented from reaching the tissues by obstruction of or damage to any part of the respiratory system. Drowning, choking, and breathing poisonous gas all lead to asphyxia. Unless the condition is remedied by removing the obstruction (when present) and by artificial respiration if necessary, there is progressive *cyanosis leading to death. Brain cells cannot live for more than about four minutes without oxygen.

aspiration *n.* the withdrawal of fluid from the body by means of suction using an instrument called an **aspirator**. There are various types of aspirator: some employ hollow needles for removing fluid from cysts, inflamed joint cavities, etc.; another kind is used to suck debris and water from the patient's mouth during dental treatment.

aspiration cytology the *aspiration of specimens of cells from tumours or cysts through a hollow needle, using a syringe, and their subsequent examination under the microscope after suitable preparation (by staining, etc.). The technique is now used widely, especially for superficial cysts or tumours, and has become a specialized branch of diagnostic pathology. *See also* FINE-NEEDLE ASPIRATION CYTOLOGY.

aspirin (acetylsalicylic acid) *n.* a drug that relieves pain and also reduces inflammation and fever. Largely superseded by modern anti-inflammatory agents (*see* NSAID), aspirin is now most commonly taken regularly in low doses as an *antiplatelet drug. In this role it reduces the risk of vascular thrombosis that may lead to events such as heart attack or stroke. Aspirin works by inhibiting the production of *prostaglandins; it may irritate the lining of the stomach, causing nausea, vomiting, pain, and bleeding. Tablets should not be held on the gum adjacent to a painful tooth as ulceration may occur. High doses cause dizziness, disturbed hearing, mental confusion, and overbreathing (*see* SALICYLISM). Aspirin has been implicated as a cause of *Reye's syndrome and should therefore not be given to children below the age of 16 years unless specifically indicated by a physician. *See also* ANALGESIC.

assay *n.* a test or trial to determine the strength of a solution, the proportion of a compound in a mixture, the potency of a drug, or the purity of a preparation. *See also* BIOASSAY.

assent *n.* agreement to undergo medical treatment obtained from an adult or child who lacks capacity to *consent. Assent has ethical but not legal force. The practice of involving noncapacitous individuals in decisions regarding their health care wherever possible is becoming increasingly common and is often considered to be 'best practice'. In research, it is particularly difficult to justify proceeding without assent, since research is not principally and inevitably in patients' *best interests.

assertive outreach team (AOT) a multidisciplinary psychiatric team specialized in the treatment of patients with severe mental illness who are difficult to engage. Most AOTs will only see patients who have had a number of recent hospital admissions ('revolving door' patients).

assimilation *n.* the process by which food substances are taken into the cells of the body after they have been digested and absorbed.

assisted suicide the act of helping a patient to commit suicide by giving him or her the means (e.g. drugs) to do so. Aiding and abetting a suicide is a criminal offence in England and Wales by virtue of the Suicide Act 1961, section 2. However, a number of high-profile cases involving those who assist terminally ill patients in suicide – e.g. by accompanying people to jurisdictions where euthanasia is lawful, such as Switzerland – have not been prosecuted. There is an important ethicolegal distinction between acts and omissions such that respecting a capacitous patient's choice to refuse life-saving or life-preserving treatment is not legally regarded as assisted suicide (*see* ADVANCE STATEMENT, DECISION, OR DIRECTIVE). *See also* EUTHANASIA.

assistive listening device a device for helping people with hearing difficulties. An assistive listening device can be a stand-alone device or can work in conjunction with a *hearing aid or *cochlear implant. Assistive listening devices include *induction loop systems, amplifiers for telephones, and radio headphones to wear when listening to the radio or television. Such devices increase the loudness of the desired sound without increasing the level of any background noise; i.e. they improve the signal-to-noise ratio. *See also* ENVIRONMENTAL HEARING AID.

association area an area of *cerebral cortex that lies away from the main areas that are concerned with the reception of sensory impulses and the start of motor impulses but is linked to them by many neurons known as **association fibres**. The areas of association are thought to be responsible for the elaboration of the information received by the primary sensory areas and its correlation with the information fed in from memory and from other brain areas. They are thus responsible for the maintenance of many higher mental activities. *See also* BODY IMAGE.

association of ideas (in psychology) linkage of one idea to another in a regular way according to their meaning. In **free association** the linkage of ideas arising in dreams or fantasy may be used to discover the underlying motives of the individual. In **word association tests** stimulus words are produced to which the subject has to respond as quickly as possible.
   Loosening of associations is a form of *formal thought disorder in which the linkage of the person's train of thoughts gets lost or disrupted.

ASSR *see* AUDITORY STEADY STATE RESPONSE.

AST *see* ASPARTATE AMINOTRANSFERASE.

astasia *n.* an inability to stand for which no physical cause can be found. **Astasia-abasia** is an inability to stand or walk in the absence of any recognizable physical illness. The patient's attempts are bizarre and careful examination reveals contradictory features. It is most commonly an expression of *conversion disorder.

aster *n.* a star-shaped object in a cell that surrounds the *centrosome during mitosis and meiosis and is concerned with the formation of the *spindle.

astereognosis *n. see* AGNOSIA.

asteroid hyalosis 1. a degenerative condition, formerly known as **asteroid hyalitis**, in which tiny deposits of calcium are suspended in the vitreous humour. They are more commonly seen in the elderly and usually cause no decrease in vision. 2. *see* SYNCHYSIS SCINTILLANS.

asthenia *n.* weakness or loss of strength.

asthenic *adj.* describing a personality characterized by low energy, susceptibility to physical and emotional stress, and a diminished capacity for pleasure. It was first published by the German psychiatrist Emil Kraepelin (1856–1926), who described asthenic, pyknic, and hypoplastic personality types. These descriptions are now largely obsolete.

asthenopia *n. see* EYESTRAIN.

asthenospermia *n. see* OLIGOSPERMIA.

asthma *n.* the condition of subjects with widespread narrowing of the bronchial airways, which changes in severity over short periods of time (either spontaneously or under treatment) and leads to cough, wheezing, and difficulty in breathing. **Bronchial asthma** may be precipitated by exposure to one or more of a wide range of stimuli, including *allergens, drugs (such as aspirin and other NSAIDs and beta blockers), exertion, emotion, infections, and air pollution. The onset of asthma is usually early in life and in atopic subjects (*see* ATOPY) may be accompanied by other manifestations of hypersensitivity, such as hay fever and dermatitis; however, the onset may be delayed into adulthood or even middle or old age. Treatment is with *bronchodilators, with or without corticosteroids, usually administered via aerosol or dry-powder inhalers, or – if the condition is more severe – via a nebulizer. Oral corticosteroids are reserved for those patients who fail to respond adequately to these measures. Severe asthmatic attacks may need large doses of oral corticosteroids (*see* STATUS ASTHMATICUS). Selection of treatment for individual cases is made using stepped guidelines issued by respiratory organizations, e.g. the British and American Thoracic Societies and the European Respiratory Society. A new group of drug treatments, using *monoclonal antibodies to target components in the allergic response, have recently become available (*see* OMALIZUMAB). Avoidance of known allergens, especially the house dust mite, allergens arising from domestic pets, and food additives, will help to reduce the frequency of attacks, as will the discouragement of smoking.

Cardiac asthma occurs in left ventricular heart failure and must be distinguished from bronchial asthma, as the treatment is quite different. —**asthmatic** *adj.*

SEE WEB LINKS
• Website of Asthma UK

astigmatism *n.* a defect of vision in which the image of an object is distorted because not all the light rays come to a focus on the retina. Some parts of the object may be in focus but light from other parts may be focused in front of or behind the retina. This is usually due to irregular curvature of the cornea and/or lens (*see* REFRACTION), whose surface resembles part of the surface of an egg (rather than a sphere). The defect can be corrected by wearing **cylindrical lenses**, which produce exactly the opposite degree of distortion and thus cancel out the distortion caused by the eye itself. —**astigmatic** *adj.*

astragalus *n. see* TALUS.

astringent *n.* a drug that causes cells to shrink by precipitating proteins from their surfaces. Astringents are used in lotions to harden and protect the skin and to reduce bleeding from minor abrasions. They are also used in mouth washes, throat lozenges, eye drops, etc., and in antiperspirants.

astrocyte (astroglial cell) *n.* a type of cell with numerous sheet-like processes extending from its cell body, found throughout the central nervous system. It is one of the several different types of cell that make up the *glia. The cells have been ascribed the function of providing nutrients for neurons and possibly of taking part in information storage processes.

astrocytoma *n.* a brain tumour derived from non-nervous cells (*glia), which – unlike the neurons – retain the ability to reproduce themselves by mitosis. All grades of malignancy occur, from slow-growing tumours whose histological structure resembles normal glial cells, to rapidly growing highly invasive tumours whose cell structure is poorly differentiated (including **anaplastic astrocytoma** and *glioblastoma). In adults astrocytomas are usually found in the cerebral hemispheres but in children they also occur in the cerebellum.

asymbolia *n. see* ALEXIA.

asymmetric septal hypertrophy (ASH) *see* HYPERTROPHIC CARDIOMYOPATHY.

asymmetric tonic neck reflex a primitive reflex that is present from birth but should disappear by six months of age. If the infant is lying on its back and the head is turned to one side, the arm and leg on the side to which the head is turned should straighten, and the arm and leg on the opposite side should bend (the 'fencer' position). Persistence of the reflex beyond six months is suggestive of *cerebral palsy.

asymptomatic *adj.* not showing any symptoms of disease, whether disease is present or not.

asynclitism *n.* tilting of the fetal skull towards one or other shoulder causing the top of the skull to be either nearer to the sacrum (**anterior asynclitism** or **Naegele's obliquity**) or nearer to the pubis (**posterior asynclitism** or **Litzmann's obliquity**). These mechanisms enable the fetal head to pass more easily through the maternal pelvis.

asystole *n.* a condition in which the heart no longer beats, accompanied by the absence of complexes in the *electrocardiogram. The clinical features, causes, and treatment are those of *cardiac arrest.

atavism *n.* the phenomenon in which an individual has a character or disease known to have occurred in a remote ancestor but not in his parents.

ataxia *n.* the shaky movements and unsteady gait that result from the brain's failure to regulate the body's posture and the strength and direction of limb movements. In **cerebellar ataxia**, due to disease of the *cerebellum, there is clumsiness of willed movements. The patient staggers when walking; he cannot pronounce words properly and may have *nystagmus. The common causes are alcohol, drugs (e.g. phenytoin), multiple sclerosis, hereditary degenerative conditions, and *paraneoplastic syndromes. **Friedreich's ataxia** is an inherited disorder appearing first in adolescence. It has the features of cerebellar ataxia, together with spasticity of the limbs. The unsteady movements of **sensory ataxia**, caused by disease of the sensory nerves, are exaggerated when the patient closes his eyes (*see* ROMBERG'S SIGN). *See also* ATAXIA TELANGIECTASIA, TABES DORSALIS (LOCOMOTOR ATAXIA). —**ataxic** *adj*.

ataxia telangiectasia an inherited (autosomal *recessive) neurological disorder. *Ataxia is usually noted early in life, and a key feature is the presence of dilated blood vessels visible in the sclerae of the eyes and on the cheeks and ears. Other symptoms may include slow slurred speech, abnormal eye movements, skin lesions, and immune deficiency. Affected individuals may develop malignant disease. A raised level of *alpha-fetoprotein is found in the blood.

atel- (**atelo-**) *combining form denoting* imperfect or incomplete development. Examples: **atelencephaly** (of the brain); **atelocardia** (of the heart).

atelectasis *n*. failure of part of the lung to expand. This occurs when the cells lining the air sacs (alveoli) are too immature, as in premature babies, and unable to produce the wetting agent (surfactant) with which the surface tension between the alveolar walls is overcome. It also occurs when the larger bronchial tubes are blocked from within by retained secretions, inhaled foreign bodies, or bronchial cancers, or from without by enlarged lymph nodes, such as are found in patients with tuberculosis and lung cancers. The lung can usually be helped to expand by physiotherapy and removal of the internal block (if present) via a *bronchoscope, but prolonged atelectasis becomes irreversible.

ateleiosis *n*. failure of sexual development owing to lack of pituitary hormones. *See* INFANTILISM, DWARFISM.

atenolol *n*. a cardioselective *beta blocker used to treat angina, high blood pressure, and irregular heart rhythms. It is administered by mouth or by intravenous injection or infusion and the commonest side-effects are fatigue, depression, and digestive upsets. Trade name: **Tenormin**.

atherectomy *n*. excision or destruction of *atheroma within an artery using equipment introduced by *catheter. **Directional atherectomy** involves the use of a device with an incising blade that can be directed to one side of the artery at a time. **Rotational**

atherectomy (**rotablation**) is achieved with a diamond-tipped drill (burr) that rotates at up to 185,000 times per minute.

atheroembolic renal disease a disease associated with diffuse atherosclerosis and sloughing of atheromatous plaques in the aorta and main renal arteries. This results in occlusion of smaller arteries and arterioles downstream within the kidney, with ischaemic and inflammatory reactions. This leads to the onset of renal impairment. Precipitating factors include invasive procedures with aortic cannulae, vascular surgery, and therapy with thrombolytics or anticoagulants. Less commonly the condition can occur spontaneously.

atheroma *n*. degeneration of the walls of the arteries due to the formation in them of fatty plaques and scar tissue. This limits blood circulation and predisposes to thrombosis. It is common in adults in Western countries. A diet rich in animal fats (*see* CHOLESTEROL) and refined sugar, cigarette smoking, obesity, and inactivity are the principal causes. Individuals with diabetes, hypertension, or a family history of early atheroma are particularly predisposed to the condition. It may be symptomless but often causes complications from arterial obstruction in middle and late life (such as angina pectoris, heart attack, stroke, and gangrene). Treatment is by prevention, but some symptoms may be ameliorated by drug therapy (e.g. angina by glyceryl trinitrate), by surgical bypass of the arterial obstruction, or by *atherectomy. —**atheromatous** *adj*.

atherosclerosis *n*. a disease of the arteries in which fatty plaques develop on their inner walls, with eventual obstruction of blood flow. *See* ATHEROMA. —**atherosclerotic** *adj*.

athetosis *n*. a writhing involuntary movement especially affecting the hands, face, and tongue. It is usually a form of *cerebral palsy. It impairs the child's ability to speak or use his hands; intelligence is often unaffected. Such movements may also be caused by drugs used to treat *parkinsonism or by the phenothiazines (*see also* DYSKINESIA). —**athetotic** *adj*.

athlete's foot a fungal infection of the skin between the toes: a type of *ringworm. Medical name: **tinea pedis**.

athyreosis *n*. absence of or lack of function of the thyroid gland, causing *cretinism in infancy and *myxoedema in adult life.

atlas *n.* the first *cervical vertebra, by means of which the skull is articulated to the backbone.

ATLS advanced trauma life support, which comprises the treatment programmes for patients who have been subjected to major trauma (e.g. serious road traffic accidents, missile injuries). Doctors, nurses, and para-medical personnel involved in ATLS receive special training for dealing with such emergencies.

ATN *see* ACUTE TUBULAR NECROSIS.

atomoxetine *n.* a CNS *stimulant used for the treatment of attention-deficit/hyperactivity disorder in children and adolescents. It is taken by mouth; side-effects include anorexia, dry mouth, gastrointestinal upsets, palpitation, and sleep disturbance, and there is a small risk of suicidal thoughts and behaviour. Trade name: **Strattera**.

atony *n.* a state in which muscles are floppy, lacking their normal elasticity. —**atonic** *adj.*

atopen *n.* any substance responsible for *atopy.

atopy *n.* a form of *allergy in which there is a hereditary or constitutional tendency to develop hypersensitivity reactions (e.g. hay fever, allergic asthma, atopic *eczema) in response to allergens (**atopens**). Individuals with this predisposition – and the conditions provoked in them by contact with allergens – are described as **atopic**.

atorvastatin *n.* a drug used to reduce abnormally high levels of cholesterol and other lipids in the blood (*see* STATIN). It is administered by mouth; side-effects include insomnia, abdominal pain, flatulence, diarrhoea, and nausea. Trade name: **Lipitor**.

atosiban *n. see* TOCOLYTIC.

ATP (adenosine triphosphate) a compound that contains adenine, ribose, and three phosphate groups and occurs in cells. The chemical bonds of the phosphate groups store energy needed by the cell, for muscle contraction; this energy is released when ATP is split into ADP or AMP. ATP is formed from ADP or AMP using energy produced by the breakdown of carbohydrates or other food substances. *See also* MITOCHONDRION.

atracurium besilate a nondepolarizing *muscle relaxant administered by injection during anaesthesia or intensive care. Side-effects including flushing and an increase in heart rate. Trade name: **Tracrium**.

atresia *n.* **1.** congenital absence or abnormal narrowing of a body opening. *See* BILI-ARY ATRESIA, DUODENAL ATRESIA, TRICUSPID ATRESIA. **2.** the degenerative process that affects the majority of ovarian follicles. Usually only one Graafian follicle will ovulate in each menstrual cycle. —**atretic** *adj.*

atri- (atrio-) *combining form denoting* an atrium, especially the atrium of the heart. Example: **atrioventricular** (relating to the atria and ventricles of the heart).

atrial fibrillation *see* FIBRILLATION.

atrial natriuretic peptide (ANP) *see* NATRIURETIC PEPTIDE.

atrial septal defect (ASD) a congenital defect of the heart in which there is a hole in the partition (septum) separating the two atria (*see* SEPTAL DEFECT). There are two kinds of ASD – **ostium primum** and **ostium secundum**. Ostium primum defects are rarer but more serious as the defect lies low down near the valves of the heart. Affected children often have heart failure, although in some a heart murmur detected at routine medical examinations is the only indication of the defect. Ostium secundum defects lie away from the valves and most children have no symptoms; the defect is most commonly indicated by the detection of a heart murmur, and may not be apparent until adulthood. Small defects may close spontaneously. Most persisting ostium secundum defects can now be treated with an umbrella-shaped closure device passed to the heart through the venous system under X-ray and ultrasound control. Ostium primum defects still require surgical closure.

Intrauterine surgical techniques now enable a fetus in which an ASD has been detected to proceed to full term by using the placental circulation as a substitute for the *extracorporeal circulation that would otherwise be required.

atrioventricular bundle (AV bundle, bundle of His) a bundle of modified heart muscle fibres (**Purkinje fibres**) passing from the *atrioventricular (AV) node forward to the septum between the ventricles, where it divides into right and left bundles, one for each ventricle. The fibres transmit contraction waves from the atria, via the AV node, to the ventricles.

a

atrioventricular node (AV node) a mass of modified heart muscle situated in the lower middle part of the right atrium. It receives the impulse to contract from the *sinoatrial node, via the atria, and transmits it through the *atrioventricular bundle to the ventricles.

at-risk register *see* CHILD PROTECTION REGISTER.

atrium *n.* (*pl.* **atria**) **1.** either of the two upper chambers of the *heart. Their muscular walls are thinner than those of the ventricles; the left atrium receives oxygenated blood from the lungs via the pulmonary vein; the right atrium receives deoxygenated blood from the venae cavae. *See also* AURICLE. **2.** any of various anatomical chambers into which one or more cavities open. —**atrial** *adj.*

atrophic vaginitis *see* VAGINITIS.

atrophy *n.* the wasting away of a normally developed organ or tissue due to degeneration of cells. This may be physiological or pathological. Physiological atrophy occurs during embryonic life and the neonatal period (web spaces, notochord, umbilical vessels), in adolescence (the thymus), in adult life (the *corpus luteum during the menstrual cycle), and in a variety of organs and tissues in old age. Pathological atrophy may occur through starvation, disuse, denervation, abnormal hormonal stimulation, lack of hormonal stimulation, or ischaemia. **Muscular atrophy** is associated with various diseases, such as poliomyelitis.

atropine *n.* an *antimuscarinic drug that occurs in deadly nightshade (*see* BELLADONNA). Because it dilates the pupil and paralyses the ciliary muscle (*see* CYCLOPLEGIA, MYDRIATIC), atropine is used in eye examinations and the treatment of anterior *uveitis. It is also administered by injection to treat a slow heart rate (*bradycardia) associated with arrhythmias or, with *neostigmine, to reverse the action of muscle relaxants used during surgery. It is occasionally used to treat gut spasms and for *premedication. Common side-effects include dryness of the throat, thirst, impaired vision, and increased heart rate. Trade names: **Minims Atropine Sulphate**, **Minijet Atropine**.

attachment *n.* **1.** (in psychology) the process of developing the first close selective relationship of a child's life, most commonly with the mother. The relationship acts to reduce anxiety in strange settings and forms a base from which children develop further relationships. Seriously disturbed attachment is hypothesized to lead to personality disorders, depression, or anxiety in later life. **2.** (in the National Health Service) working arrangements by which workers employed by public bodies (such as *district nurses and social workers) are engaged in association with specific general practitioners, caring for their registered patients rather than working solely on a geographical or district basis. **3. (clinical attachment)** (in the NHS) a person shadowing a clinical professional, often in order to gain experience in that professional's field or in the UK in general.

attachment disorder a psychiatric disorder in infants and young children resulting from *institutionalization, emotional neglect, or *child abuse. Affected children are either withdrawn, aggressive, and fearful or attention-seeking and indiscriminately friendly. Treatment requires the provision of stable caring adults as parents over a long period of time.

attendance allowance *see* DISABILITY LIVING ALLOWANCE.

attention-deficit/hyperactivity disorder (ADHD, attention deficit disorder, hyperkinetic disorder) a mental disorder, usually of children, characterized by a grossly excessive level of activity and a marked impairment of the ability to attend. The behaviour may be predominantly hyperactive-impulsive, predominantly inattentive, or combined. It is hypothesized that the majority of patients have a higher than normal number of dopamine transporter complexes, reducing the amount of freely available dopamine in the synaptic cleft. This leads to cognitive problems, including an inability to keep attention, to focus attention, and to perform organizational planning. Learning is impaired as a result, and behaviour can be disruptive and may be defiant or aggressive. ADHD is highly genetic. Untreated, many children develop later conduct problems or even personality disorders. Treatment usually involves drugs (such as amphetamines and *methylphenidate) and behaviour therapy; the family needs advice and practical help. The illness can carry on into adult life, but more commonly improves as the affected children mature.

attenuation *n.* reduction of the disease-producing ability (virulence) of a bacterium or virus by chemical treatment, heating, drying, by growing under adverse conditions, or by passing through another organism. Treated (**attenuated**) bacteria or viruses are used for many *immunizations.

atticotomy *n.* a surgical operation to remove *cholesteatoma from the ear. It is a form of limited *mastoidectomy.

attrition *n.* (in dentistry) the wearing of tooth surfaces by the action of opposing teeth. A small amount of attrition occurs with age but accelerated wear may occur in *bruxism and with certain diets.

atypical antipsychotics *see* ANTIPSYCHOTIC.

atypical facial pain *see* PERSISTENT IDIOPATHIC FACIAL PAIN.

atypical mole syndrome (dysplastic naevus syndrome) a condition in which patients have numerous moles, some of which are relatively large and irregular in shape or pigmentation. There may be a family history of this syndrome or of malignant *melanoma.

atypical pneumonia any one of a group of community-acquired *pneumonias that do not respond to penicillin but do respond to such antibiotics as tetracycline and erythromycin. They include infection with *Mycoplasma pneumoniae, Chlamydia psittaci* (*see* PSITTACOSIS), and *Coxiella burnetii* (*see* Q FEVER).

audi- (audio-) *combining form denoting* hearing or sound.

audiogram *n.* the graphic record of a test of hearing carried out on an audiometer. The term is also commonly used to refer to types of hearing test. A **pure tone audiogram** (**PTA**) is a test that uses tones of a single frequency, played to the test subject through headphones. A **free field audiogram** uses sounds presented to the patient through loudspeakers. A **speech audiogram** uses lists of words played to the patient through headphones.

audiology *n.* the study of disorders of hearing.

audiometer *n.* an apparatus for testing hearing at different sound frequencies, so helping in the diagnosis of deafness. —**audiometry** *n.*

audit *n. see* CLINICAL AUDIT.

auditory *adj.* relating to the ear or to the sense of hearing.

auditory brainstem response audiometry (ABR audiometry, brainstem evoked response audiometry, BSER) an objective test of hearing that measures the electrical activity in the auditory nerve and *brainstem following sound stimulation using repeated clicks.

auditory canal (auditory meatus) the canal leading from the pinna to the eardrum.

auditory nerve *see* COCHLEAR NERVE.

auditory processing disorder (APD, central auditory processing disorder, CAPD) difficulty in hearing and processing auditory information, especially in poor acoustic environments, despite normal or near-normal ear function. It may be due to genetic factors, maturational delay in the central nervous system, or focal abnormalities of the central nervous system (such as tumours). Treatments include *hearing therapy, *auditory skills training, educational support, use of *assistive listening devices, and training with computerized therapy tools.

auditory skills training a method of teaching people to use their hearing to its best potential, undertaken in the treatment of *auditory processing disorder.

auditory steady state response (ASSR) an objective test of hearing that measures the electrical activity in the auditory nerve and *brainstem following sound stimulation using repeated tones.

auditory verbal therapy (AVT) a technique for teaching deaf children to communicate that focuses on speech and residual hearing rather than sign language.

Auerbach's plexus (myenteric plexus) a collection of nerve fibres – fine branches of the *vagus nerve – within the walls of the intestine. It supplies the muscle layers and controls the movements of *peristalsis. [L. Auerbach (1828–97), German anatomist]

AUR acute urinary retention (*see* RETENTION).

aura *n.* the forewarning of an epileptic or migrainous attack. An **epileptic aura** may take many forms, such as an odd smell or taste. The **migrainous aura** may affect the patient's eyesight with brilliant flickering lights or blurring of vision, but it may also result in pins and needles, weakness of the limbs, or *aphasia.

aural *adj.* relating to the ear.

auranofin *n.* a *gold preparation administered by mouth to treat rheumatoid arthritis. The most common side-effect is diarrhoea. Trade name: **Ridaura**.

auricle *n.* **1.** a small pouch in the wall of each *atrium of the heart: the term is also used incorrectly as a synonym for *atrium. **2.** *see* PINNA.

auriscope (auroscope, otoscope) *n.* an apparatus for examining the eardrum and the passage leading to it from the ear (external meatus). It consists of a funnel (speculum), a light, and lenses (see illustration).

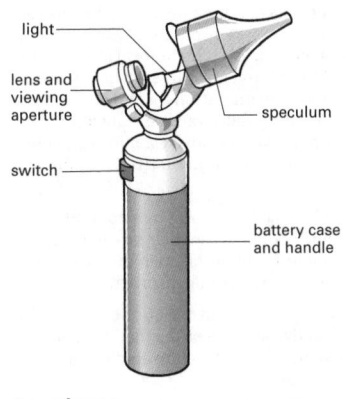

light
lens and viewing aperture
switch
speculum
battery case and handle

An auriscope.

auscultation *n.* the process of listening, usually with the aid of a *stethoscope, to sounds produced by movement of gas or liquid within the body. Auscultation is an aid to diagnosis of abnormalities of the heart, lungs, intestines, and other organs according to the characteristic changes in sound pattern caused by different disease processes. —**auscultatory** *adj.*

auscultatory gap a silent period in the knocking sounds heard with a stethoscope over an artery, between the systolic and diastolic blood pressures, when the blood pressure is measured with a *sphygmomanometer.

Austin Flint murmur a heart *murmur that is loudest in diastole and associated with a third heart sound. It is a sign of *aortic regurgitation, which allows retrograde filling and rapid rise in left intraventricular pressure. This prevents the mitral valve from opening fully, giving rise to the murmur, which is best heard in the mitral area (apex) rather than the aortic area (where the problem lies). [Austin Flint (1812–86), US physician]

Australia antigen another name for the *hepatitis B antigen, which was first discovered in the blood of an Australian aborigine. This disease is caused by a virus of which the Australia antigen forms part.

aut- (auto-) *combining form denoting* self. Example: **autokinesis** (voluntary movement).

autism *n.* **1.** (Kanner's syndrome, infantile autism) a psychiatric disorder of childhood, with an onset before the age of 2½ years. It is marked by severe difficulties in communicating and forming relationships with other people, in developing language, and in using abstract concepts; repetitive and limited patterns of behaviour (*see* STEREOTYPY); and obsessive resistance to tiny changes in familiar surroundings. Autistic children find it hard to understand how other people feel, and so tend to remain isolated even into adult life. About 50% have learning disabilities, but some are very intelligent and may even be gifted in specific areas. The cause is unknown, but genetic factors and brain damage may be important. The condition often progresses into adulthood, and independent living is uncommon. Treatment is not specific, but lengthy specialized education is usually necessary. Behaviour problems and anxiety can be controlled with behaviour therapy and drugs (such as *antipsychotics). Autism and similar developmental disorders, including *Asperger's syndrome and *Rett's syndrome, are known as **autistic spectrum disorders**. **2.** the condition of retreating from realistic thinking to self-centred fantasy thinking: a symptom of personality disorder and schizophrenia. —**autistic** *adj.*

((⊕)) SEE WEB LINKS

• Website of the National Autistic Society: links to a database for researchers and professionals and to the UK's Autism Services Directory

autoagglutination *n.* the clumping together of the body's own red blood cells by antibodies produced against them, which occurs in acquired haemolytic anaemia (an *autoimmune disease).

autoantibody *n.* an antibody formed against one of the body's own components in an *autoimmune disease.

autochthonous *adj.* 1. remaining at the site of formation. A blood clot that has not been carried in the bloodstream from its point of origin is described as autochthonous. 2. originating in an organ without external stimulus, like the beating of the heart.

autoclave 1. *n.* a piece of equipment for sterilizing surgical instruments, dressings, etc. It consists of a chamber, similar to a domestic pressure cooker, in which the articles are placed and treated with steam at high pressure. 2. *vb.* to sterilize in an autoclave.

autocrine *adj.* describing the production by a cell of substances, such as hormones or *growth factors, that can influence the growth of the cell that produces them.

autofluorescence *n.* *fluorescence of structures in the absence of fluorescein dye. Structures such as optic disc *drusen fluoresce when stimulated by cobalt blue light.

autogenous *adj.* originating within the body of the patient. For example, an autogenous vein graft, to bypass a blocked artery, is made from material derived from the body of the patient receiving the graft.

autograft *n.* a tissue graft taken from one part of the body and transferred to another part of the same individual. The repair of burns is often done by grafting on strips of skin taken from elsewhere on the body, usually the upper arm or thigh. Unlike *allografts, autografts are not rejected by the body's immunity defences. *See also* SKIN GRAFT, TRANSPLANTATION.

autoimmune disease one of a number of otherwise unrelated disorders caused by inflammation and destruction of tissues by the body's own *immune response. These disorders include acquired haemolytic anaemia, pernicious anaemia, rheumatic fever, rheumatoid arthritis, glomerulonephritis, systemic lupus erythematosus, myasthenia gravis, Sjögren's syndrome, and several forms of thyroid dysfunction, including Hashimoto's disease. It is not known why the body should lose the ability to distin-

guish between substances that are 'self' and those that are 'non-self'.

autoimmunity *n.* a disorder of the body's defence mechanisms in which an *immune response is generated against components or products of its own tissues, treating them as foreign material and attacking them. *See* AUTOIMMUNE DISEASE, IMMUNITY.

autoinoculation *n.* the accidental transfer of inoculated material from one site in the body to another. Following vaccination against smallpox, for example, satellite lesions may occur around the site of inoculation. Sometimes the conjunctiva is affected.

autointoxication *n.* poisoning by a toxin formed within the body.

autologous *adj.* denoting a graft that is derived from the recipient of the graft.

autolysis *n.* the destruction of tissues or cells brought about by the actions of their own enzymes. *See* LYSOSOME.

automated external defibrillator (AED) a type of external *defibrillator that can analyse the heart rhythm it detects and advise via voice prompts on therapy to be given according to the latest guidelines. In cases of ventricular fibrillation, some defibrillators will make decisions on delivering electric shocks and do so after issuing appropriate warnings to the attending health-care professionals.

automated lamellar keratectomy (ALK) excision of the outer layers of the cornea using an automated *keratome. It is usually used as part of a surgical procedure, to alter the shape of the cornea to correct errors of refraction.

automated perimeter *see* PERIMETER.

automatism *n.* behaviour that may be associated with *epilepsy, in which the patient performs well-organized movements or tasks while unaware of doing so. The movements may be simple and repetitive, such as hand clapping and lip smacking, or they may be so complex as to mimic a person's normal conscious activities.

autonomic nervous system the part of the *peripheral nervous system responsible for the control of involuntary muscles (e.g. the heart, bladder, bowels) and hence those bodily functions that are not consciously directed, including regular beating of the heart, intestinal movements, sweating, salivation, etc. The autonomic system is subdivided into **sympathetic** and **parasympathetic nervous systems**. Sympathetic nerves lead from the middle section of the spinal cord and parasympathetic nerves from the brain and lower spinal cord. The heart, smooth muscles, and most glands receive fibres of both kinds: the interplay of sympathetic and parasympathetic reflex activity (the actions are often antagonistic) governs their working. For example, the parasympathetic system is responsible for slowing the heart rate and constricting the pupillary muscles; the sympathetic system increases the heart rate and dilates the pupil. Sympathetic nerve endings liberate *noradrenaline as a neurotransmitter; parasympathetic nerve endings release *acetylcholine.

autonomy *n.* the right to self-determination (literally, 'self-rule'), which all people with *capacity have. Respect for, and fostering of, the autonomy of the patient is one of the *four principles of medical ethics and is sometimes said to be pre-eminent in that all ethical practice flows from facilitating and respecting autonomous choices. Respect for autonomy finds its legal translation in the concept of valid *consent. In practice therefore, respecting a patient's autonomy usually takes the form of listening to concerns, sharing sufficient information, and seeking consent for any proposed treatment or research. Autonomy is not unlimited in its scope, e.g. the law constrains an autonomous wish for assisted suicide and, as a general principle, patients can request but not demand treatment. Professional autonomy involves *reflective practice and attempting to follow one's own principles consistently and confidently. —**autonomous** *adj.*

autophony *n.* abnormal awareness of one's own voice or other internally generated sounds. It occurs in some cases of conductive *deafness and *superior canal dehiscence syndrome.

autoploidy *n.* the normal condition in cells or individuals, in which each cell has a chromosome set consisting of *homologous pairs, enabling cells to divide normally. —**autoploid** *adj., n.*

autopsy (necropsy, post mortem) *n.* a review of the clinical history of a deceased person followed by external examination of the body, evisceration and dissection of the internal organs, and ancillary investigations (such as histopathology, microbiology, or

toxicology) to determine the cause of death. Autopsies may be performed on the instruction of a medicolegal authority or at the request of clinicians (with consent of the family). In addition to determining the cause of death, autopsies have a role in research, audit, clinical governance, and medical education.

autoradiography (radioautography) *n.* a technique for examining the distribution of a radioactive *tracer in the tissues of an experimental animal. The tracer is injected into the animal, which is killed after a certain period. Thin sections of its organs are placed in close contact with a radiation-sensitive material, such as a photographic emulsion, and observed under a microscope. Blackening of the film indicates a high concentration of radioactive material.

autorefractor *n.* a machine that automatically determines the spectacle prescription for the eye. *See also* OPTOMETER.

autoscopy *n.* the experience of seeing one's whole body as though from a vantage point some distance away. It can be a symptom in *epilepsy. *See also* OUT-OF-BODY EXPERIENCE.

autosomal dominant *see* DOMINANT.

autosomal recessive *see* RECESSIVE.

autosome *n.* any chromosome that is not a *sex chromosome and occurs in pairs in diploid cells. —**autosomal** *adj.*

autosuggestion *n.* self-suggestion or self-conditioning that involves repeating ideas to oneself in order to change psychological or physiological states. Autosuggestion is used primarily in **autogenic training**, a technique used to help patients control their anxiety or their habits. *See* SUGGESTION.

autotransfusion *n.* reintroduction into a patient of his or her own blood. This may be blood previously drawn and stored in the blood bank or blood that has been lost from the patient's circulation during surgical operation. The blood is collected by suction during the operation, filtered to remove bubbles and small blood clots, and returned into one of the patient's veins through a drip. *See also* CELL SAVER.

autotrophic (lithotrophic) *adj.* describing organisms (known as **autotrophs**) that synthesize their organic materials from carbon dioxide and nitrates or ammonium compounds, using an external source of energy. **Photoautotrophic** organisms, including green plants and some bacteria, derive their energy from sunlight; **chemoautotrophic** (or **chemosynthetic**) organisms obtain energy from inorganic chemical reactions. All autotrophic bacteria are nonparasitic. *Compare* HETEROTROPHIC.

aux- (auxo-) *combining form denoting* increase; growth. Example: **auxocardia** (enlargement of the heart).

auxotroph *n.* a strain of a microorganism, derived by mutation, that requires one or more specific factors for growth not needed by the parent organism.

avascular *adj.* lacking blood vessels or having a poor blood supply. The term is usually used with reference to cartilage.

avascular necrosis *see* OSTEONECROSIS.

Avastin *n. see* BEVACIZUMAB.

aversion therapy a form of *behaviour therapy that is used to reduce the occurrence of undesirable behaviour, such as sexual deviations or drug addiction. *Conditioning is used, with repeated pairing of some unpleasant stimulus with a stimulus related to the undesirable behaviour. An example is the use of *disulfiram in the treatment of alcoholism. Aversion therapy is little used nowadays. *See also* SENSITIZATION.

avian influenza a disease of poultry and other birds caused by strains of *influenza A virus. The severity of the disease depends on the strain of virus involved: H5N1 is particularly deadly (causing fowl plague (or pest), with a mortality approaching 100%) and very contagious, being spread between domestic flocks by wild birds. This virus is not easily transmissible to humans, requiring close contact with infected birds or their faeces. The first human cases of H5N1 infection ('bird flu') were reported in 1997 and restricted to Hong Kong: 18 people were infected, six of whom died. Since then half of the people infected with H5N1 in Asia, Europe, the Near East, and Africa have died. Most cases of avian influenza in humans have resulted from contact with infected poultry; human-to-human transmission has been extremely rare. However, if H5N1 should develop this ability, a serious pandemic could occur. *See also* SWINE INFLUENZA.

avitaminosis *n.* the condition caused by

lack of a vitamin. *See also* DEFICIENCY DISEASE.

AVM arteriovenous malformation (*see* ANGIOMA).

avoidant *adj.* describing a personality type characterized by self-consciousness, hypersensitivity to rejection and criticism from others, avoidance of normal situations because of their potential risk, high levels of tension and anxiety, and consequently a restricted life.

AVPU a system for assessing the depth of unconsciousness: A = alert; V = voice responses present; P = pain responses present; U = unresponsive. It is useful for judging the severity of head injury and the need for specialized neurosurgical assistance before proceeding to formal evaluation by the *Glasgow Coma Scale.

AVT *see* AUDITORY VERBAL THERAPY.

avulsion *n.* 1. the tearing or forcible separation of part of a structure. For example, a tendon may be torn from the bone to which it attaches or the skin of the scalp may be torn from the underlying tissue and bone. 2. (in dentistry) the knocking out of a tooth by trauma. The tooth may be replanted (*see* REPLANTATION).

axial *adj.* at right angles to the long *axis of the body, i.e. denoting a horizontal plane through a standing patient at 90° to the *coronal and *sagittal planes. This is the usual plane for the primary images obtained at *computerized tomography. *See also* MULTIPLANAR RECONSTRUCTION.

axilla *n.* (*pl.* **axillae**) the armpit. —**axillary** *adj.*

axis *n.* 1. a real or imaginary line through the centre of the body or one of its parts or a line about which the body or a part rotates. 2. the second *cervical vertebra, which articulates with the atlas vertebra above and allows rotational movement of the head.

axolemma *n.* the fine cell membrane, visible only under the electron microscope, that encloses the protoplasm of an *axon.

axon *n.* a nerve fibre: a single process extending from the cell body of a *neuron and carrying nerve impulses away from it. An axon may be over a metre in length in certain neurons. In large nerves the axon has a sheath (**neurilemma**) made of *myelin; this is interrupted at intervals by gaps called

nodes of Ranvier, at which branches of the axon leave. An axon ends by dividing into several branches called **telodendria**, which make contact with other nerves or with muscle or gland membranes.

axonotmesis *n.* rupture of nerve fibres (axons) within an intact nerve sheath. This may result from prolonged pressure or crushing and it is followed by degeneration of the nerve beyond the point of rupture. The prognosis for *nerve regeneration is good. *Compare* NEURAPRAXIA, NEUROTMESIS.

axoplasm *n.* the semifluid material of which the *axon of a nerve cell is composed. It flows slowly outwards from the cell body.

azathioprine *n.* an *immunosuppressant drug, used mainly to aid the survival of organ or tissue transplants. It may also be used in the treatment of rheumatoid arthritis (*see* DISEASE-MODIFYING ANTIRHEUMATIC DRUG) and myasthenia gravis. It is administered by mouth. Azathioprine may damage bone marrow, causing blood disorders; other possible side-effects include nausea and vomiting, malaise, muscle pain, and skin rashes. Trade name: **Imuran**.

azelaic acid an antibacterial drug applied externally as a cream in the treatment of acne and rosacea. Possible side-effects include local irritation and light sensitivity. Trade name: **Skinoren**.

azelastine *n.* an *antihistamine drug administered as a metered-dose nasal spray for the treatment of hay fever and as eye drops to treat allergic conjunctivitis. Possible side-effects include nasal irritation and disturbances of taste sensation. Trade names: **Optilast**, **Rhinolast**.

azithromycin *n.* an antibiotic used to treat respiratory, skin, soft-tissue, and other infections, including genital infections caused by *Chlamydia trachomatis*. It is administered by mouth. Possible side-effects include allergic reactions, nausea, and vomiting. Trade name: **Zithromax**.

azo- (azoto-) *combining form denoting* a nitrogenous compound, such as urea. Example: **azothermia** (raised temperature due to nitrogenous substances in the blood).

azoospermia (aspermia) *n.* the complete absence of sperm from the seminal fluid. This is due either to profound impairment of sperm formation (*spermatogenesis) due to damage to the testes (e.g. caused by *cryptorchidism, mumps *orchitis, or radio- or chemotherapy) or – more commonly – to obstruction of the genital tract (e.g. resulting from vasectomy, gonorrhoea, or *Chlamydia* infection). A biopsy of the testis is necessary in order to differentiate these two causes of azoospermia; if a blockage is present it may be possible to relieve it surgically (*see* EPIDIDYMOVASOSTOMY).

azotaemia *n.* a former name for *uraemia.

azoturia *n.* the presence in the urine of an abnormally high concentration of nitrogen-containing compounds, especially urea.

aztreonam *n.* an antibiotic administered by injection used to treat infections of the lungs, bones, skin, and soft tissues caused by Gram-negative organisms (*see* GRAM'S STAIN), including lung infections in patients with cystic fibrosis. Possible side-effects include skin rashes, diarrhoea, and vomiting. Trade name: **Azactam**.

azygos vein an unpaired vein that arises from the inferior vena cava and drains into the superior vena cava, returning blood from the thorax and abdominal cavities.

Babinski reflex *see* PLANTAR REFLEX. [J. F. F. Babinski (1857–1932), French neurologist]

baby blues (postpartum blues) a colloquial name for the brief episodes of misery, tearfulness, poor sleep, and irritability that affect about half of all women during the first week after delivery. Reassurance and support are the mainstay of management. *Compare* POSTNATAL DEPRESSION, PUERPERAL PSYCHOSIS.

bacillaemia *n.* the presence of bacilli in the blood, resulting from infection.

bacille Calmette-Guérin *see* BCG. [A. L. C. Calmette (1863–1933) and C. Guérin (1872–1961), French bacteriologists]

bacilluria *n.* the presence of bacilli in the urine, resulting from a bladder or kidney infection. *See* CYSTITIS.

bacillus *n.* (*pl.* **bacilli**) any rod-shaped bacterium. *See also* BACILLUS, LACTOBACILLUS, STREPTOBACILLUS.

Bacillus *n.* a large genus of Gram-positive spore-bearing rodlike bacteria. They are widely distributed in soil and air (usually as spores). Most feed on dead organic material and are responsible for food spoilage. The species *B. anthracis*, which is nonmotile, causes *anthrax, a disease of farm animals transmissible to humans. *B. polymyxa*, commonly found in soil, is the source of the polymyxin group of antibiotics. *B. subtilis* may cause conjunctivitis in humans; it is also a source of the antibiotic *bacitracin zinc.

bacitracin zinc an antibiotic effective against a number of microorganisms. Combined with polymyxin B, it is applied externally to treat infections of the skin and eyes.

backbone (spinal column, spine, vertebral column) *n.* a flexible bony column extending from the base of the skull to the small of the back. It encloses and protects the spinal cord, articulates with the skull (at the atlas), ribs (at the thoracic vertebrae), and hip girdle (at the sacrum), and provides attachment for the muscles of the back. It is made up of individual bones (*see* VERTEBRA) connected by discs of fibrocartilage (*see* INTERVERTEBRAL DISC) and bound together by ligaments. The backbone of a newborn baby contains 33 vertebrae: seven cervical (neck), 12 thoracic (chest), five lumbar (lower back), five sacral (hip), and four coccygeal. In the adult the sacral and coccygeal vertebrae become fused into two single bones (sacrum and coccyx, respectively); the adult vertebral column therefore contains 26 bones (see illustration). Anatomical name: **rachis**.

back slaps a manoeuvre for the treatment of a choking patient. Firm slaps are given to the patient's back in an attempt to dislodge the obstructing article from the upper airway.

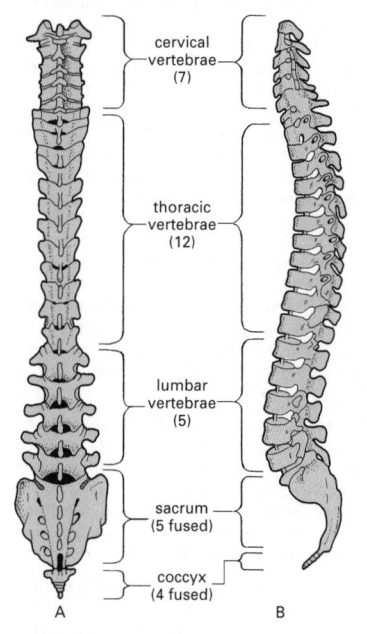

cervical vertebrae (7)

thoracic vertebrae (12)

lumbar vertebrae (5)

sacrum (5 fused)

coccyx (4 fused)

A   B

The backbone. Seen from the back (A) and left side (B).

baclofen *n.* a skeletal *muscle relaxant drug administered orally or by *intrathecal injection to relieve spasm resulting from injury or disease of the brain or spinal cord, including cerebral palsy and multiple sclerosis. Side-effects include dizziness, drowsiness, and nausea. Trade name: **Lioresal**.

bacteraemia *n.* the presence of bacteria in the blood: a sign of infection.

bacteri- (bacterio-) *combining form denoting* bacteria. Example: **bacteriolysis** (dissolution of).

bacteria *pl. n.* (*sing.* **bacterium**) a group of microorganisms all of which lack a distinct nuclear membrane (and hence are considered more primitive than animal and plant cells) and most of which have a cell wall of unique composition (many antibiotics act by destroying the bacterial cell wall). Most bacteria are unicellular; the cells may be spherical (*coccus), rod-shaped (*bacillus), spiral (*Spirillum), comma-shaped (*Vibrio) or corkscrew-shaped (*spirochaete). Generally, they range in size between 0.5 and 5 μm. Motile species bear one or more fine hairs (flagella) arising from their surface. Many possess an outer slimy *capsule, and some have the ability to produce an encysted or resting form (*endospore). Bacteria reproduce asexually by simple division of cells; incomplete separation of daughter cells leads to the formation of *colonies consisting of different numbers and arrangements of cells. Some colonies are filamentous in shape, resembling those of fungi. Transfer of DNA from one bacterium to another takes place in the process of *conjugation.

Bacteria are very widely distributed. Some live in soil, water, or air; others are parasites of humans, animals, and plants. Many parasitic bacteria do not harm their hosts; some cause diseases by producing poisons (*see* ENDOTOXIN, EXOTOXIN).

bacterial vaginosis a condition caused by overgrowth of certain species of the bacteria that are normally present in the vagina (e.g. *Bacteroides*, *Gardnerella vaginalis*). One of the most common vaginal infections, it is marked by a greyish watery vaginal discharge with a characteristic fishy odour.

bactericidal *adj.* being capable of killing bacteria. Substances with this property include antibiotics, antiseptics, and disinfectants; they are known as **bactericides**. *Compare* BACTERIOSTATIC.

bacteriology *n.* the science concerned with the study of bacteria. It is a branch of *microbiology. —**bacteriological** *adj.* —**bacteriologist** *n.*

bacteriolysin *n. see* LYSIN.

bacteriophage (phage) *n.* a virus that attacks bacteria. In general, a phage consists of a head, tail, and tail fibres, all composed of protein molecules, and a core of DNA. The tail and tail fibres are responsible for attachment to the bacterial surface and for injection of the DNA core into the host cell. The phage grows and replicates in the bacterial cell, which is eventually destroyed with the release of new phages. Each phage acts specifically against a particular species of bacterium. This is utilized in **phage typing**, a technique of identifying bacteria by the action of known phages on them. *See also* LYSOGENY.

bacteriostatic *adj.* capable of inhibiting or retarding the growth and multiplication of bacteria. Erythromycin is bacteriostatic. *Compare* BACTERICIDAL.

bacterium *n. see* BACTERIA.

Bacteroides *n.* a genus of Gram-negative, mostly nonmotile, anaerobic rodlike bacteria. They are normally present in the alimentary and urinogenital tracts of mammals and are found in the mouth, particularly in dental plaque associated with periodontal disease. Some species have now been classified into the genera *Porphyromonas* and *Prevotella*.

bagassosis *n.* a form of external allergic *alveolitis caused by exposure to the dust of mouldy bagasse, the residue of sugar cane after the sugar has been extracted, which is used in the production of hardboard and other thermal boards. Symptoms usually appear in the evening after exposure during the day and include fever, malaise, irritant cough, and respiratory distress.

Baghdad boil *see* ORIENTAL SORE.

Bagolini lens a lens with fine parallel lines (almost invisible striations) across its width, used in various vision tests; for example, to test suppression and abnormal retinal correspondence. [20th-century Italian ophthalmologist]

BAHA *see* BONE-ANCHORED HEARING AID.

Baker's cyst a cyst behind the knee resulting from rupture or herniation of the synovial membrane from a knee joint affected by osteoarthritis. [W. M. Baker (1839–96), British surgeon]

BAL 1. see BRONCHOALVEOLAR LAVAGE.
2. British Anti-Lewisite (see DIMERCAPROL).

balanced salt solution (BSS) a solution containing physiological concentrations of sodium chloride, potassium chloride, calcium chloride, magnesium chloride, sodium acetate, and sodium citrate. Such fluids are isotonic to eye tissue; they are used during intraocular surgery and to replace intraocular fluids.

balanitis n. inflammation of the glans penis, usually associated with tightness of the foreskin (*phimosis). It is more common in childhood than in adult life. An acute attack is associated with redness and swelling of the glans. Treatment is by antibiotics, and further attacks are prevented by *circumcision. In **Zoon's plasma cell balanitis** persistent shiny red patches develop on the glans; the cause is unknown. **Balanitis xerotica obliterans** (**BXO**) is an autoimmune condition characterized by ivory-white patches on the glans.

balanoposthitis n. inflammation of the foreskin and the surface of the underlying glans penis. It usually occurs as a consequence of *phimosis and represents a more extensive local reaction than simple *balanitis. The affected areas become red and swollen, which further narrows the opening of the foreskin and makes passing urine difficult and painful. Treatment of an acute attack is by administration of antibiotics, and further attacks are prevented by *circumcision.

balantidiasis n. an infestation of the large intestine with the parasitic protozoan *Balantidium coli*. Humans usually become infected by ingesting food or drink contaminated with cysts from the faeces of a pig. The parasite invades and destroys the intestinal wall, causing ulceration and *necrosis, and the patient may experience diarrhoea and dysentery. Balantidiasis is a rare cause of dysentery, mainly affecting farm workers; it is treated with various antibiotics.

Balantidium n. a genus of one of the largest parasitic *protozoans affecting humans (70 μm or more in length). The oval body is covered with threadlike cilia (for locomotion). *B. coli*, normally living in the gut

of pigs as a harmless *commensal, occasionally infects humans (see BALANTIDIASIS).

baldness n. see ALOPECIA.

Balkan nephropathy a severe and progressive form of tubulointerstitial renal disease (see TUBULOINTERSTITIUM), first described in 1956 and endemic to certain rural areas along the tributaries of the Danube in Bosnia, Bulgaria, Croatia, Romania, and Serbia. The natural course of the disease is progression to end-stage kidney failure and frequent development of tumours in the upper urinary tract. It seems likely that an environmental factor is responsible for the disease, and evidence supports the theory that long-term consumption of food contaminated with seeds from plants of *Aristolochia* spp. underlies the pathogenesis.

ball-and-cage valve a form of mechanical prosthesis commonly used in the past for replacing damaged heart valves. Currently, most mechanical valve replacements are of the tilting-disc variety.

ball-and-socket joint see ENARTHROSIS.

Ballantyne syndrome (maternal mirror syndrome) a condition that occurs in cases of *hydrops fetalis when the maternal condition begins to mirror the state of the fetus. The maternal signs and symptoms are similar to those of *pre-eclampsia, including vomiting, hypertension, oedema, and proteinuria.

balloon n. an inflatable plastic cylinder of variable size that is mounted on a thin tube and used for dilating narrow areas in blood vessels (see CORONARY ANGIOPLASTY), in the alimentary tract (*strictures), or in the urinary tract (see ENDOPYELOTOMY).

ballottement n. the technique of examining a fluid-filled part of the body to detect a floating object. During pregnancy, a sharp tap with the fingers, applied to the uterus through the abdominal wall or the vagina, causes the fetus to move away and then return to impart an answering tap to the examiner's hand as it floats back to its original position. This confirms that swelling of the uterus is due to a fetus rather than a tumour or other abnormality.

balneotherapy n. the treatment of disease by bathing, usually in the mineral-containing waters of hot springs. The once fashionable 'water cures', taken at spas, certainly had a more psychological than physical effect. Today, specialized remedial treatment in baths, under the supervision of physiotherapists, is used to alleviate pain and improve blood circulation and limb mobility in arthritis and in nerve and muscle disorders.

bamboo spine an X-ray appearance of the spine in which there is squaring of the vertebrae and vertical *syndesmophytes that span adjacent vertebrae, so that the spine resembles a stick of bamboo. It is seen in ankylosing *spondylitis.

banana and lemon signs ultrasound features of the *Arnold-Chiari malformation in fetuses with open neural tube defects. The **banana sign** refers to the shape of the cerebellum owing to caudal displacement; the **lemon sign** refers to the lemon-shaped head resulting from scalloping of the frontal bones. See illustration.

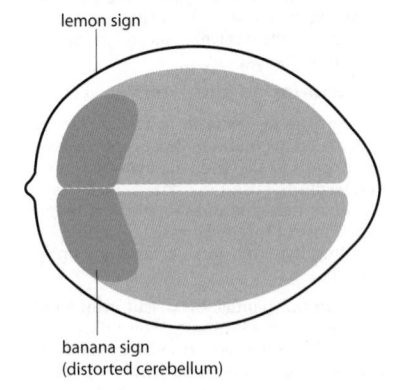

lemon sign

banana sign
(distorted cerebellum)

Banana and lemon signs.

bandage *n.* a piece of material, in the form of a pad or strip, applied to a wound or used to bind around an injured or diseased part of the body.

bandage lens a soft contact lens that can be useful in managing certain external eye disorders, including tiny perforations.

band keratopathy the deposition of calcium in the superficial layers of the cornea, usually as a horizontal band starting peripherally and moving centrally. It is associated with chronic eye disease, e.g. chronic *uveitis, particularly juvenile chronic uveitis.

Bandl's ring *see* RETRACTION RING. [L. Bandl (1842–92), German obstetrician]

Banti's syndrome a disorder in which enlargement and overactivity of the spleen occurs as a result of increased pressure within the splenic vein (*see* HYPERSPLENISM, SPLENOMEGALY). It arises primarily in children and occurs with *cirrhosis of the liver. [G. Banti (1852–1925), Italian pathologist]

barbiturate *n.* any of a group of drugs, derived from barbituric acid, that depress activity of the central nervous system and were formerly widely used as sedatives and hypnotics. They are classified into three groups according to their duration of action – short, intermediate, and long. Because they produce *tolerance and psychological and physical *dependence, have serious toxic side-effects (*see* BARBITURISM), and can be fatal following large overdosage, barbiturates have been largely replaced in clinical use by safer drugs. The main exception is the very short-acting drug *thiopental, which is used to induce anaesthesia. *See also* AMOBARBITAL, BUTOBARBITAL, PHENOBARBITAL.

barbiturism *n.* addiction to drugs of the barbiturate group. Signs of intoxication include confusion, slurring of speech, yawning, sleepiness, loss of memory, loss of balance, and reduction in muscular reflexes. Withdrawal of the drugs must be undertaken slowly, over 1–3 weeks, to avoid the withdrawal symptoms of tremors and convulsions, which can prove fatal.

barefoot doctor *see* MEDICAL ASSISTANT.

bariatric surgery surgery performed for the purpose of weight loss in obese patients. Most procedures are restrictive, being designed to promote feelings of fullness and satiety after meals (*see* GASTRIC BANDING, STOMACH STAPLING). *See also* GASTRIC BYPASS SURGERY, JAW WIRING.

baritosis *n.* a lung disease – a form of *pneumoconiosis – caused by inhaling barium dust. It gives dramatic shadows on chest X-rays but no respiratory disability.

barium enema an imaging technique for examination of the large bowel. Prior bowel cleansing is usually required with a colonic cleansing preparation; intravenous *hyoscine butylbromide (Buscopan) or glucagon is usually given to reduce colonic spasm. A tube is then inserted into the rectum through the anus, and barium sulphate

is run into the bowel to the caecum. For
*double contrast, air is then pumped
through the tube to distend the colon. A series of radiographs is then taken, usually on
a tilting table with the patient lying and
standing. Barium enema is used mainly to
identify cancers, polyps, and diverticular disease in the colon. Its role has been largely
taken over by colonoscopy as this latter technique enables mucosal sampling and therapeutic interventions.

barium follow-through *see* SMALL-
BOWEL MEAL.

barium sulphate a barium salt, extremely
insoluble in water, that is opaque to X-rays
and is used as a *contrast medium in radiography of the gastrointestinal tract (*see* BAR-
IUM ENEMA, BARIUM SWALLOW AND MEAL).

barium swallow and meal a technique
for examining the oesophagus, stomach, and
duodenum. The patient swallows barium
sulphate to coat the lining of the organs.
Granules that produce gas to distend the
stomach may be given to produce a *double-
contrast effect. A series of X-rays is taken.
This can be used to diagnose disorders of
oesophageal motor function, tumours, gastric and duodenal ulcers, hiatus *hernia, and
*gastro-oesophageal reflux disease. Many in-
dications for this examination have been replaced by the use of gastroscopy.

Barlow manoeuvre a test for *congenital
dislocation of the hip that detects whether or
not a hip can be readily dislocated. With the
baby lying supine and the pelvis steadied
with one hand, the hip being tested is gently
adducted and backward pressure is applied
to the head of the femur. If the hip is dislo-
catable, a clunk will be felt and sometimes
heard (**Von Rosen's sign**). If the hip is gently
abducted, it will usually relocate. [T. Barlow
(1845–1945), British physician]

BARN bilateral *acute retinal necrosis.

baroreceptor (baroceptor) *n.* a collection
of sensory nerve endings specialized to monitor changes in blood pressure. The main receptors lie in the *carotid sinuses and the
*aortic arch; others are found in the walls of
other large arteries and veins and some
within the walls of the heart. Impulses from
the receptors reach centres in the medulla;
from here autonomic activity is directed so
that the heart rate and resistance of the peripheral blood vessels can be adjusted appropriately.

barotitis *n.* disease of the ear caused by
changing air pressure, as experienced during
air travel.

barotrauma *n.* damage to the ear, *Eustachian tube, or paranasal sinuses caused
by changes in ambient pressure, as experienced during air flight or deep-sea diving.

Barr body *see* SEX CHROMATIN. [M. L. Barr
(1908–95), Canadian anatomist]

**Barrett's oesophagus (columnar-lined
oesophagus, CLO)** a condition in which the
normal squamous *epithelium lining the
oesophagus is replaced by columnar epithelium of the type normally lining the intestine ('intestinal metaplasia') because of
damage caused by *gastro-oesophageal
reflux or (occasionally) corrosive *oesophagitis. The condition may be associated with
an ulcer (**Barrett's ulcer**), and the epithelium has an abnormally high likelihood of
undergoing malignant change. [N. R. Barrett
(1903–79), British thoracic surgeon]

barrier cream a preparation used to protect the skin against water-soluble irritants
(e.g. detergents, breakdown products of
urine). Usually applied in the form of a
cream or ointment and often containing a
silicone (such as *dimeticone), barrier
creams are useful in the alleviation of various skin disorders, including napkin rash
and pressure sores.

Barron's banding apparatus an apparatus for treating haemorrhoids in which a
tight elastic band is applied across their base
to cause ischaemic necrosis leading to
sloughing off within a few days.

bartholinitis *n.* inflammation of
*Bartholin's glands. In **chronic bartholinitis**
cysts may form in the glands as a result of
blockage of their ducts. In **acute bartholinitis** abscess formation may occur (**Bartholin's
abscess**).

**Bartholin's glands (greater vestibular
glands)** a pair of glands that open at the
junction of the vagina and the external genitalia (vulva). Their secretions lubricate the
vulva and so assist penetration by the penis
during coitus. The **lesser vestibular glands**,
around the vaginal opening, perform the
same function. [C. Bartholin (1655–1738),
Danish anatomist]

Bartonella (Haemobartonella) *n.* a genus
of Gram-negative bacteria that are facultative intracellular parasites. They occur in the

red blood cells and cells of the lymphatic system, spleen, liver, and kidneys and cause several infections in humans (*see* BARTONELLOSIS).

bartonellosis *n.* an infectious disease, largely confined to high river valleys in Peru, Ecuador, and Colombia, caused by the bacterium *Bartonella bacilliformis*. The parasite, present in red blood cells and cells of the lymphatic system, is transmitted to humans by sandflies. There are two clinical types of the disease: **Oroya fever** (**Carrion's disease**), whose symptoms include fever, anaemia, and enlargement of the liver, spleen, and lymph nodes; and **verruga peruana**, characterized by wartlike eruptions on the skin that can bleed easily and ulcerate. Oroya fever accounts for nearly all fatalities. Bartonellosis can be treated successfully with penicillin and other antibiotics and blood transfusions may be given to relieve the anaemia.

Other species of *Bartonella* cause *cat-scratch disease and *trench fever.

Bartter syndrome an inherited condition of the kidney, which causes abnormalities in the excretion and reabsorption of salts from the blood. This results in lowered levels of potassium and chloride and an increased level of calcium. The baby fails to grow properly and becomes progressively weaker and dehydrated. Treatment consists of correcting the salt imbalance with appropriate supplements. [F. C. Bartter (1914–83), US physician]

basal cell carcinoma (BCC) the commonest form of skin cancer. Although classified as a malignant tumour, it grows very slowly. BCC usually occurs on the central area of the face, especially in fair-skinned people; the prevalence increases greatly with episodes of sunburn. The initial sign is a spot or lump that fails to heal, which slowly enlarges. Treatment depends on subtype and is usually straightforward, e.g. topical chemotherapy agents (such as 5-fluorouracil), *curettage and cautery, surgical excision, *cryotherapy, or *radiotherapy. High-risk BCCs around the eyes or nose may be treated with *Mohs' micrographic surgery to ensure low rates of recurrence and maximal tissue conservation. Only if neglected for decades does a BCC eventually become a so-called **rodent ulcer** and destroy the surrounding tissue. However, the term 'rodent ulcer' is still sometimes used to mean any basal cell carcinoma.

basal ganglia several large masses of grey matter embedded deep within the white matter of the *cerebrum (see illustration). They include the **caudate** and **lenticular nuclei** (together known as the **corpus striatum**) and the **amygdaloid nucleus**. The lenticular nucleus consists of the **putamen** and **globus pallidus**. The basal ganglia have complex neural connections with both the cerebral cortex and thalamus: they are involved with the regulation of voluntary movements at a subconscious level.

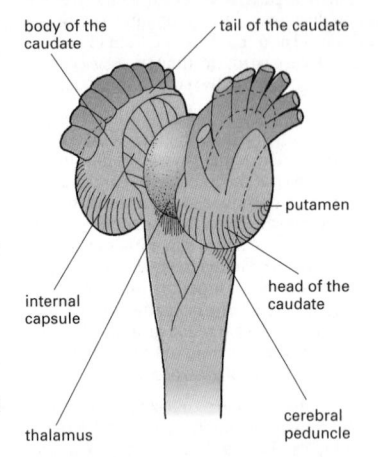

The basal ganglia. Showing its position in relation to neighbouring parts (seen from the front).

basal metabolism the minimum amount of energy expended by the body to maintain vital processes, e.g. respiration, circulation, and digestion. It is expressed in terms of heat production per unit of body surface area per day (**basal metabolic rate – BMR**), and for an average man the BMR is 1.7 Calories (7.115 kilojoules) per day. BMR may be determined by the direct method, in which the subject is placed in a respiratory chamber and the amount of heat evolved is measured, or (more normally) by the indirect method, based on the *respiratory quotient. Measurements are best taken during a period of least activity, i.e. during sleep and 12–18 hours after a meal, under controlled temperature conditions. Various factors, such as age, sex, and particularly thyroid activity, influence the value of the BMR.

basement membrane   the thin delicate membrane that lies at the base of an *epithelium. It is composed of mucopolysaccharide and fibres of protein.

base pairing   the linking of the two strands of a DNA molecule by means of hydrogen bonds between the bases of the nucleotides. Adenine always pairs with thymine and cytosine with guanine. *See* DNA.

basic life support   the provision of treatment designed to maintain adequate circulation and ventilation to a patient in *cardiac arrest, without the use of drugs or specialist equipment.

basilar artery   an artery in the base of the brain, formed by the union of the two vertebral arteries. It extends from the lower to the upper border of the pons Varolii and then divides to form the two posterior cerebral arteries.

basilar membrane   a membrane in the *cochlea of the ear that separates two of the three channels (scalae) that run the length of the spiral cochlea. The organ of Corti is situated on the basilar membrane, inside the scala media.

basilic vein   a large vein in the arm, extending from the hand along the back of the forearm, then passing forward to the inner side of the arm at the elbow.

basion   *n.* the midpoint of the anterior border of the large hole (foramen magnum) at the base of the *skull.

basophil   1. *n.* a variety of white blood cell distinguished by a lobed nucleus and the presence in its cytoplasm of coarse granules that stain purple-black with *Romanowsky stains. Basophils are capable of ingesting foreign particles and contain *histamine and *heparin. There are normally $30–150 \times 10^6$ basophils per litre of blood. *See also* POLYMORPH. 2. (basophilic) *adj.* describing any cell that stains well with basic dyes. For example, certain cells in the anterior pituitary gland are basophilic.

basophilia   *n.* 1. a property of a microscopic structure whereby it shows an affinity for basic dyes. 2. an increase in the number of certain white blood cells (*basophils) in the blood, which may occur in a variety of blood diseases.

basophilic   *adj. see* BASOPHIL.

bat ears   protuberent external ears as a result of the absence of the antihelical fold in the *pinna. It is a normal variant but can be surgically corrected if desired using an *otoplasty operation.

bathyaesthesia   *n.* sensation experienced in the deeper parts of the body, such as the joints and muscles.

Batten's disease   one of a group of rare hereditary disorders (known as the **neuronal ceroid lipofuscinoses**) that also includes *Tay-Sachs disease. Fatty substances accumulate in the cells of the nervous system, causing progressive dementia, epilepsy, spasticity, and visual failure. The condition starts in late infancy or childhood. There is no treatment. [F. E. Batten (1865–1918), British neurologist]

battered baby syndrome   *see* NONACCIDENTAL INJURY.

battery   *n.* (in law) the wrongful touching of another person, which may be a criminal offence or a tort in civil law (the latter is known as **trespass against the person**). Any intentional touching of another is a potential battery unless it occurs with the *consent of the person involved. Consent therefore provides a defence against a charge of battery brought in relation to medical treatment.

Bazin's disease   a rare disease of young women in which tender nodules develop under the skin in the calves. The condition is a *tuberculide; the nodules may break down and ulcerate though they may clear up spontaneously. Medical name: **erythema induratum**. [A. P. E. Bazin (1807–78), French dermatologist]

BCC   *see* BASAL CELL CARCINOMA.

B cell   *n. see* LYMPHOCYTE.

BCG (bacille Calmette-Guérin)   a strain of tubercle bacillus that has lost the power to cause *tuberculosis but retains its antigenic activity; it is therefore used to prepare a vaccine against the disease.

BCI   bladder contractility index: a scale used to grade how strongly the urinary bladder can contract.

bear tracks   (in ophthalmology) areas of hypertrophy of retinal pigment epithelium (*see* RETINA) that clinically resemble the prints of bears' paws.

Beau's lines transverse depressions on the nails appearing some weeks or months after a severe illness or chemotherapy. [J. H. S. Beau (1806–65), French physician]

Becker muscular dystrophy a *sex-linked (X-linked) disorder in which affected males develop an increase in muscle size followed by weakness and wasting. It usually starts between the ages of 5 and 15, and 25 years after onset most patients are wheelchair-bound. Although most men become severely disabled, life expectancy is close to normal. The disorder is similar to Duchenne *muscular dystrophy but less severe. [P. E. Becker (20th century), German geneticist]

Beck's triad *see* CARDIAC TAMPONADE. [C. S. Beck (1894–1971), US surgeon]

beclometasone *n.* a *corticosteroid drug that is administered by mouth to treat ulcerative colitis, by nasal spray to treat hay fever, and by inhaler for the prevention of asthma. For the latter it may be combined with formoterol (as **Fostair**). Possible side-effects include nasal irritation and hoarseness. Trade names: **Becodisks**, **Beconase**, **Clenil Modulite**, **Clipper**, **Qvar**, etc.

becquerel *n.* the *SI unit of activity of a radioactive source, being the activity of a radionuclide decaying at a rate of one spontaneous nuclear transition per second. It has replaced the curie. Symbol: Bq.

bed bug a bloodsucking insect of the genus *Cimex*. *C. hemipterus* of the tropics and *C. lectularius* of temperate regions have reddish flattened bodies and vestigial wings. They live and lay their eggs in the crevices of walls and furniture and emerge at night to suck blood; although bed bugs are not known vectors of disease their bites leave a route for bacterial infection. Premises can be disinfested with appropriate insecticides.

bed occupancy the number of hospital beds occupied by patients expressed as a percentage of the total beds available in the ward, specialty, hospital, area, or region. It may be recorded in relation to a defined point in time or more usefully for a period, when the calculation is based on bed-days. It is used with other indices (such as *admission rate) to assess the demands for hospital beds in relation to diseases, specialties, or populations and hence to gauge an appropriate balance between demand for health care and number of beds.

bedsore *n. see* PRESSURE SORE.

bedwetting *n. see* ENURESIS.

behaviourism *n.* an approach to psychology postulating that only observable behaviour need be studied, thus denying any importance to unconscious processes. Behaviourists are concerned with the laws regulating the occurrence of behaviour (*see* CONDITIONING). —**behaviourist** *n.*

behaviour modification the use of the methods of behaviourist psychology (*see* BEHAVIOURISM) – especially operant *conditioning – to alter people's behaviour. Behaviour modification has wider applications than *behaviour therapy, since it is also used in situations in which the client is not ill; for example, in education. *See also* CHAINING, PROMPTING.

behaviour therapy treatment based on the belief that certain psychological problems are the products of faulty learning. Treatment is directed at the problem or target behaviour and is designed for the particular patient, not for the particular underlying diagnosis the patient may have. *See also* AVERSION THERAPY, CONDITIONING, DESENSITIZATION, EXPOSURE, RESPONSE PREVENTION.

Behçet's syndrome an idiopathic disease of the immune system characterized by *aphthous ulcers in the mouth, genital ulcers, skin lesions, and severe inflammation of the uveal tract of the eye (*see* UVEITIS). It may also involve the joints and nervous system and cause inflammation of the veins. The condition occurs more often in men than women. Treatment is aimed at controlling the immune system. [H. Behçet (1889–1948), Turkish dermatologist]

bejel (endemic syphilis) *n.* a long-lasting nonvenereal form of *syphilis that occurs in the Balkans, Turkey, eastern Mediterranean countries, and the dry savannah regions of North Africa; it is particularly prevalent where standards of personal hygiene are low. The disease is spread among children and adults by direct body contact. Early skin lesions are obvious in the moist areas of the body (mouth, armpits, and groin) and later there may be considerable destruction of the tissues of the skin, nasopharynx, and long bones. Wartlike eruptions in the anal and genital regions are common. Bejel, which is rarely fatal, is treated with penicillin.

bel *n. see* DECIBEL.

belladonna *n.* the deadly nightshade plant (*Atropa belladonna*) or the mixture of alkaloids derived from it, which include *atropine and *hyoscine.

bell and pad a psychological method of treating bed-wetting in children and adults. When the subject starts to pass urine it is detected by a pad (or by sheets of metallic mesh) and this sets off a bell (or loud buzzer). The modern form of the apparatus has a small electronic sensor worn under the underclothes and produces a loud bleep. The purpose of the alarm is to waken the subject, who then empties the bladder fully. A process of conditioning leads to the subject learning to be dry. It is effective in about 80% of cases.

belle indifference a symptom of *conversion disorder in which an apparently grave physical affliction or disability (which has no physical cause) is accepted in a smiling and calm fashion.

Bell's palsy paralysis of the *facial nerve causing weakness of the muscles of one side of the face and an inability to close the eye. In some patients hearing may be affected so that sounds seem abnormally loud, and a loss of taste sensation may occur. The cause of this condition is usually a viral infection, and recovery normally occurs spontaneously. [Sir C. Bell (1774–1842), Scottish physiologist]

Bell's phenomenon the normal outward and upward rotation of the eyes that occurs when the lids are closed, but not during blinking. [Sir C. Bell]

belly *n.* **1.** the *abdomen or abdominal cavity. **2.** the central fleshy portion of a muscle.

bemiparin sodium *see* LOW-MOLECULAR-WEIGHT HEPARIN.

Bence-Jones protein a protein of low molecular weight found in the urine of patients with multiple *myeloma and rarely in patients with *lymphoma, *leukaemia, and *Hodgkin's disease. [H. Bence-Jones (1814–73), British physician]

bendroflumethiazide (bendrofluazide) *n.* a potent thiazide *diuretic used in the treatment of conditions involving retention of fluid, such as congestive heart failure, hypertension, and *oedema. Side-effects include a fall in blood pressure on standing up,

dizziness, lethargy, and muscle cramps. Trade names: **Aprinox, Neo-NaClex**.

bends *n. see* COMPRESSED AIR ILLNESS.

Benedict's test a test for the presence of sugar in urine or other liquids. A few drops of the test solution are added to **Benedict's solution**, prepared from sodium or potassium citrate, sodium carbonate, and copper sulphate. The mixture is boiled and shaken for about two minutes, then left to cool. The presence of up to 2% glucose is indicated by the formation of a reddish, yellowish, or greenish precipitate, the highest levels corresponding to the red coloration, the lowest (about 0.05%) to the green. [S. R. Benedict (1884–1936), US surgeon]

beneficence *n.* doing good: one of the *four principles of medical ethics. The obligation to act in patients' *best interests at all times is recognized in ancient and modern codes of professional conduct, e.g. the *Hippocratic oath. Benefits in health care, and therefore beneficence, must commonly be balanced against risks or harms (i.e. *nonmaleficence). The courts have been clear that beneficence extends beyond medical interests. Respect for *autonomy requires that professionals determine what the patient considers to be doing good in any given situation.

benign *adj.* **1.** describing a tumour that does not invade and destroy the tissue in which it originates or spread to distant sites in the body, i.e. a tumour that is not cancerous. Benign tumours may nonetheless cause serious morbidity or mortality by compressing or obstructing vital structures. **2.** describing any disorder or condition that does not produce harmful effects. *Compare* MALIGNANT.

benign intracranial hypertension (idiopathic intracranial hypertension, pseudotumour cerebri) a syndrome of raised pressure within the skull caused by impaired reabsorption of cerebrospinal fluid. The symptoms include headache, vomiting, double vision, and *papilloedema. The diagnosis is made by finding a high opening pressure at *lumbar puncture. It normally subsides spontaneously but drug therapy or neurosurgical treatment may be required to protect the patient's vision.

benign paroxysmal positional vertigo (BPPV) a common cause of vertigo in which the patient complains of brief episodes of rotatory vertigo precipitated by sudden head movements. It is thought to be due to microscopic debris derived from the *otoliths of the utricle and displaced into one of the semicircular canals, most commonly the posterior semicircular canal. The debris is most commonly thought to be free in the canal (canalithiasis; *see* CANALITH) but can be attached to the *cupula (cupulolithiasis; *see* CUPULOLITH). Diagnosis is by performing a *Dix-Hallpike test. Treatment is with a predetermined set of head movements to move the debris from the semicircular canal (*see* EPLEY PARTICLE REPOSITIONING MANOEUVRE, SEMONT LIBERATORY MANOEUVRE, BRANDT-DAROFF EXERCISES). Surgery is occasionally used to occlude the relevant semicircular canal, cut the *singular nerve or vestibular nerves, or perform a *labyrinthectomy. Drugs are generally ineffective in the treatment of this condition.

benign prostatic hyperplasia (BPH) *see* PROSTATE GLAND.

benperidol *n.* a *butyrophenone antipsychotic drug used mainly to treat deviant and antisocial sexual behaviour. It is administered by mouth. Trade name: **Anquil**.

benserazide *n. see* LEVODOPA.

benzalkonium *n.* an antiseptic used in preparations for treating infections of the mouth and throat and various skin conditions.

benzhexol *n. see* TRIHEXYPHENIDYL.

benzodiazepines *pl. n.* a group of pharmacologically active compounds used as *anxiolytics and hypnotics. The group includes *chlordiazepoxide, *diazepam, *oxazepam, and *temazepam.

benzoic acid an antiseptic, active against fungi and bacteria, used as a preservative in foods and pharmaceutical preparations and, combined with salicylic acid, in the form of an ointment (Whitfield's ointment) for the treatment of ringworm.

benzoyl peroxide a preparation used in the treatment of acne. It acts by removing the surface layers of the epidermis and unblocking skin pores and has an antiseptic effect on skin bacteria. It is administered as a cream or gel, alone or in combination with an antibiotic. Side-effects may include skin irritation. Trade names: **Acnecide**, **Brevoxyl**, **PanOxyl**.

benzydamine hydrochloride an anti-inflammatory drug (*see* NSAID) administered as a mouthwash or spray for the relief of inflammatory ulcerative conditions of the mouth and throat. Trade name: **Difflam**.

benzyl benzoate an oily aromatic liquid that is applied to the body – in the form of an emulsion – for the treatment of scabies. It causes skin irritation and should not be used to treat children. Trade name: **Ascabiol**.

benzylpenicillin *n. see* PENICILLIN.

Berger's nephropathy (IgA nephropathy) an abnormality of the kidney in which there is a focal area of inflammation (*glomerulonephritis). This causes microscopic amounts of blood in the urine. A quarter of the patients with this condition may develop kidney failure. [J. Berger (20th century), French nephrologist]

beriberi *n.* a nutritional disorder due to deficiency of vitamin B_1 (thiamine). It is widespread in rice-eating communities in which the diet is based on polished rice, from which the seed coat (which is rich in thiamine) has been removed. Beriberi takes two forms: **wet beriberi**, in which there is an accumulation of tissue fluid (*oedema), and **dry beriberi**, in which there is extreme emaciation. There is nervous degeneration in both forms of the disease and death from heart failure is often the outcome.

berry aneurysm *see* ANEURYSM.

berylliosis *n.* poisoning by beryllium or its compounds, either by inhalation or by skin contamination. Inhalation of fumes from molten beryllium causes an acute *alveolitis and is usually fatal. Subacute and chronic forms can result from extremely low levels of exposure to the powder and can produce granulomata in the skin or lungs very similar to those seen in *sarcoidosis. In the lungs, these lead to fibrosis, which can, however, be prevented by prompt use of oral corticosteroids. Although the incidence of berylliosis has been greatly reduced since the use of beryllium compounds in the manufacture of fluorescent light tubes was discontinued in Britain in 1948, new cases are still occurring.

best interests a legal and moral standard often invoked in questions of medical ethics. A doctor has both an ethical and a legal obligation to maximize a patient's welfare or wellbeing. When cases have gone to court, the judiciary has been clear that the concept of best interests extends beyond the purely medical. The principle of *autonomy requires that a capacitous patient is in the best position to determine what is in his or her best interests. Where a patient lacks capacity, health-care professionals must act in his or her best interests. Under the Mental Capacity Act 2005, a doctor must take account of the patient's wishes and try to determine what he or she would have wanted, possibly with reference to an advance directive (*see* ADVANCE STATEMENT, DECISION, OR DIRECTIVE), an appointed proxy, or an *Independent Mental Capacity Advocate. The interests of children are especially important, and doctors must be particularly vigilant where there is a potential conflict of interests, as when reporting cases of suspected child abuse or recruiting for paediatric research.

Best's disease *see* VITELLIFORM DEGENERATION. [F. Best (20th century), German physician]

beta agonist *see* SYMPATHOMIMETIC.

beta blocker (beta-adrenergic blocker) a drug that prevents stimulation of the beta *adrenoceptors at the nerve endings of the sympathetic nervous system. Blockade of β_1 receptors causes a decrease in heart rate and force; blockade of β_2 receptors causes constriction of the airways and the arteries. Beta blockers include *acebutolol, *atenolol, *bisoprolol, *oxprenolol, *propranolol, and *sotalol; they are used to control abnormal heart rhythms, to treat angina, and to reduce high blood pressure (although they are no longer regarded by some experts as the first choice of drug for treating hypertension in the absence of heart disease, being less effective than newer antihypertensive drugs). Beta blockers that block both β_1 and β_2 receptor sites cause constriction of air passages in the lungs, and these drugs should not be used in patients with asthma and bronchospasm. Other beta blockers are relatively selective for the heart (cardioselective) and are less likely to constrict the airways. Some beta blockers (e.g. *carteolol, *levobunolol, and *timolol) reduce the production of aqueous humour and therefore the pressure inside the eye; they are taken as eye drops in the treatment of *glaucoma.

beta cells *see* ISLETS OF LANGERHANS.

betahistine *n.* a drug that is an *analogue of *histamine and increases blood flow through the inner ear. It is administered by mouth to treat *Ménière's disease. Side-effects are uncommon but include gastric upset. Trade name: **Serc**.

beta-lactam antibiotic one of a group of drugs that includes the *penicillins and the *cephalosporins. All have a four-membered **beta-lactam** ring as part of their molecular structure. Beta-lactam antibiotics function by interfering with the growth of the cell walls of multiplying bacteria. Bacteria become resistant to these antibiotics by producing **beta-lactamases**, enzymes (such as *penicillinase) that disrupt the beta-lactam ring. To counteract this, **beta-lactamase inhibitors** (e.g. *clavulanic acid) may be added to beta-lactam antibiotics. For example, **co-amoxiclav** (Augmentin) is a mixture of *amoxicillin and clavulanic acid.

betamethasone *n.* a synthetic corticosteroid used to treat inflammatory and allergic conditions and congenital adrenal hyperplasia. It is administered by mouth or injection; as drops for the ear, eye, or nose; or as a cream or ointment. The side-effects are those of *cortisone. Trade names: **Betnelan**, **Betnesol**, **Betnovate**, **Vistamethasone**.

betaxolol *n.* a *beta blocker administered as eye drops to treat chronic simple *glaucoma. Possible side-effects are local stinging and burning. Trade name: **Betoptic**.

bethanechol *n.* a cholinergic drug (*see* PARASYMPATHOMIMETIC) that acts mainly on the bowel and bladder, stimulating these organs to empty. Administered by mouth, it may be used to relieve urinary retention. Possible side-effects include nausea, vomiting, and abdominal cramps. Trade name: **Myotonine**.

bevacizumab *n.* a *monoclonal antibody that interferes with the growth of new blood vessels (*see* ANGIOGENESIS) by inhibiting the action of *vascular endothelial growth factor. Administered by intravenous infusion, it is licensed for the treatment of metastatic colorectal cancer, breast cancer, renal cell carcinoma, and non-small-cell lung cancer. Side-effects include hypertension, bowel perforation, and bleeding. Trade name: **Avastin**.

bezafibrate *n.* a drug that is used to treat hyperlipidaemia that fails to respond to diet (*see* FIBRATES). It is administered by mouth. Possible side-effects include skin rashes, nausea and vomiting, and muscle pain. Trade name: **Bezalip**.

bezoar *n.* a mass of swallowed indigestible material within the stomach. The material, which is usually swallowed by psychiatrically disturbed patients, accumulates and ultimately causes gastric obstruction. Its removal often requires a surgical operation. *See also* TRICHOBEZOAR.

bi- *combining form denoting* two; double. Examples: **biciliate** (having two cilia); **binucleate** (having two nuclei).

bicalutamide *n.* an *anti-androgen commonly used to treat locally advanced and advanced prostate cancer because in men it blocks androgen receptors without reducing levels of testosterone in the blood, preserving libido and general energy levels. It is taken by mouth; side-effects include breast enlargement, tenderness, and pain. Trade name: **Casodex**.

biceps *n.* a muscle with two heads. The **biceps brachii** extends from the shoulder joint to the elbow (see illustration). It flexes the arm and forearm and supinates the forearm and hand. The **biceps femoris** is situated at the back of the thigh and is responsible for flexing the knee, extending the thigh, and rotating the leg outwards.

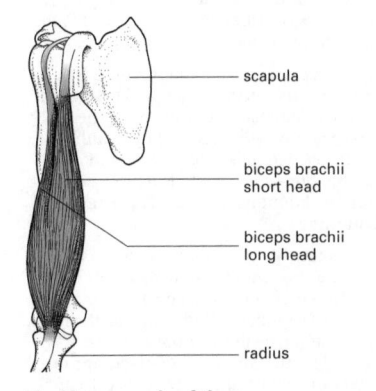

scapula

biceps brachii
short head

biceps brachii
long head

radius

The biceps muscle of the arm.

biceps jerk a deep tendon reflex mediated by the fifth cervical *spinal nerve (C5). The examiner's thumb or index finger is placed over the patient's biceps tendon in the elbow crease and struck sharply with a tendon hammer; the normal response is a reflex contraction of the biceps and flexion of the elbow. The jerk is exaggerated in upper *motor neuron lesions, such as a stroke, and reduced or absent in lower motor neuron lesions, such as a disc herniation, peripheral nerve injury, or peripheral neuropathy (e.g. diabetes, alcoholism).

biconcave *adj.* having a hollowed surface on both sides. Biconcave lenses are used to correct short-sightedness. *Compare* BICONVEX.

biconvex *adj.* having a surface on each side that curves outwards. Biconvex lenses are used to correct long-sightedness. *Compare* BICONCAVE.

bicornuate *adj.* having two hornlike processes or projections. The term is applied to an abnormal uterus that is divided into two separate halves at the upper end.

bicuspid 1. *adj.* having two *cusps, as in the premolar teeth and the mitral valve of the heart. 2. *n.* (in the USA) a premolar tooth.

bicuspid valve *see* MITRAL VALVE.

Bielschowsky head tilt an orthoptic eye test used mainly to differentiate between a weakness of the superior oblique muscle and a weakness of the contralateral superior rectus muscle (*see* EXTRINSIC MUSCLE). [A. Bielschowsky (1871–1940), German ophthalmologist]

bifid *adj.* split or cleft into two parts.

bifocal lens a lens with two principal focal lengths: usually the upper part of the lens gives a sharp image of distant objects and the lower part gives a sharp image of near objects. Examples are bifocal spectacles, bifocal contact lenses, and bifocal intraocular lenses. *See also* TRIFOCAL LENSES, MULTIFOCAL LENSES.

bifurcation *n.* (in anatomy) the point at which division into two branches occurs; for example in blood vessels or in the trachea.

bigeminal body one of the two swellings that develop in the roof of the midbrain during its development in the embryo.

bigeminy *n.* the condition in which alternate *ectopic beats of the heart are transmitted to the pulse and felt as a double pulse beat (**pulsus bigeminus**). It is a common manifestation of digitalis poisoning.

biguanide *n.* one of the group of drugs including *metformin, which is used to treat noninsulin-dependent (type 2) diabetes mellitus. Biguanides are *oral hypoglycaemic drugs: they act by reducing the release of glucose from the liver and increasing glucose uptake by muscles.

bilateral *adj.* (in anatomy) relating to or affecting both sides of the body or of a tissue or organ or both of a pair of organs (e.g. the eyes, breasts, or ovaries).

bile *n.* a thick alkaline fluid that is secreted by the *liver and stored in the *gall bladder, from which it is ejected intermittently into the duodenum via the common *bile duct. Bile may be yellow, green, or brown, according to the proportions of the *bile pigments (excretory products) present; other constituents are lecithin, cholesterol, and *bile salts. The bile salts help to emulsify fats in the duodenum so that they can be more easily digested by pancreatic *lipase into fatty acids and glycerol. Bile salts also form compounds with fatty acids, which can then be transported into the *lacteals. Bile also helps to stimulate *peristalsis in the duodenum.

bile acids the organic acids in bile; mostly occurring as bile salts (sodium glycocholate and sodium taurocholate). They are cholic acid, deoxycholic acid, glycocholic acid, and taurocholic acid.

bile-acid sequestrant a drug that binds to bile acids, forming a complex that is excreted in the faeces. Bile acids are formed in the liver from *cholesterol and the effect of loss of bile acids is a reduction in total body cholesterol and a decrease in *low-density lipoprotein serum levels. These drugs, which include *colestyramine and *colestipol, are used to treat patients with abnormally high blood cholesterol levels who are liable to develop coronary heart disease.

bile duct any of the ducts that convey bile from the liver. Bile is drained from the liver cells by many small ducts into the right and left hepatic ducts, which unite to form the main bile duct of the liver, the **common hepatic duct**. This joins the **cystic duct**, which leads from the *gall bladder, to form the **common bile duct**, which drains into the duodenum.

bile pigments coloured compounds – breakdown products of the blood pigment *haemoglobin – that are excreted in *bile. The two most important bile pigments are **bilirubin**, which is orange or yellow, and its

oxidized form **biliverdin**, which is green. Mixed with the intestinal contents, they give the brown colour to the faeces (*see* URO-BILINOGEN).

bile salts sodium glycocholate and sodium taurocholate – the alkaline salts of *bile – necessary for the emulsification of fats. After they have been absorbed from the intestine they are transported to the liver for reuse.

bi-level positive airways pressure *see* BiPAP.

Bilharzia *n. see* SCHISTOSOMA.

bilharziasis *n. see* SCHISTOSOMIASIS.

bili- *combining form denoting* bile.

biliary *adj.* relating to or affecting the bile duct or bile. *See also* FISTULA.

biliary atresia a congenital or acquired condition in which there is obstruction of bile flow due to destruction or absence of the bile ducts. Babies usually present within the first few weeks of life with jaundice that does not improve with time. Some forms of biliary atresia can be corrected surgically, but if diagnosis has been delayed the condition may lead to irreversible liver damage requiring liver transplantation.

biliary colic pain resulting from obstruction of the gall bladder or common bile duct, usually by a stone. The pain, which is very severe, is usually felt in the upper abdomen (in the midline or to the right) but can also be poorly localized due to its visceral nature. It often occurs about an hour after a meal (particularly if fatty), may last several hours, and is usually steady in severity (unlike other forms of *colic). Vomiting often occurs simultaneously.

bilious *adj.* **1.** containing bile; for example **bilious vomiting** is the vomiting of bile-containing fluid. **2.** a lay term used to describe attacks of nausea or vomiting.

bilirubin *n. see* BILE PIGMENTS.

biliuria (choluria) *n.* the presence of bile in the urine: a feature of certain forms of jaundice.

biliverdin *n. see* BILE PIGMENTS.

Billings method a method of planning pregnancy involving the daily examination of cervical mucus, which varies in consistency and colour throughout the menstrual cycle. Use of a **Billings mucus observation chart** to help identify the type of mucus enables the woman to have six days' warning of impending ovulation. [J. and E. Billings (20th century), Australian physicians]

bimanual *adj.* using two hands to perform an activity, such as a gynaecological examination.

binaural *adj.* relating to or involving the use of both ears.

binder *n.* a bandage that is wound around a part of the body, usually the abdomen, to apply pressure or to give support or protection.

binge–purge syndrome *see* BULIMIA.

binocular *adj.* relating to or involving the use of both eyes.

binocular vision the ability to focus both eyes on an object at the same time, so that a person sees one image of the object he is looking at. It is not inborn, but acquired during the first few months of life. Binocular vision enables judgment of distance and perception of depth. *See also* STEREOSCOPIC VISION.

bio- *combining form denoting* life or living organisms. Example: **biosynthesis** (formation of a compound within a living organism).

bioassay *n.* estimation of the activity or potency of a drug or other substance by comparing its effects on living organisms with effects of a preparation of known strength. Bioassay is used to determine the strength of preparations of hormones or other material of biological origin when other physical or chemical methods are not available.

bioavailability *n.* the proportion of a drug that is delivered to its site of action in the body. This is usually the amount entering the circulation and may be low when the drugs are given by mouth.

biochemistry *n.* the study of the chemical processes and substances occurring in living things. —**biochemical** *adj.* —**biochemist** *n.*

biocompatibility *n.* the ability of a material or device to be tolerated by tissue. This is important for materials embedded in the body. —**biocompatible** *adj.*

bioengineering *n.* the application of biological and engineering principles to the development and manufacture of equipment and devices for use in biological systems. Examples of such products include orthopaedic prostheses and heart pacemakers.

bioethics *n.* an area of applied *ethics relating to moral decisions and behaviour in the life sciences and incorporating but not limited to *medical ethics, which is commonly considered to be a subspecialty of bioethics (**biomedical ethics**).

biofeedback *n.* the giving of immediate information to a subject about his or her bodily processes (such as heart rate), which are usually unconscious, by means of monitoring devices. This may enable some voluntary control over such processes. These processes can then be subject to operant *conditioning. This is an experimental treatment for disturbances of bodily regulation, such as hypertension.

biofilm *n.* an organized layer of microorganisms that forms on a surface. Biofilm may be implicated in several disease processes, including dental infections (*see* PLAQUE), *endocarditis, infections of surgical implants, lung infections in people with *cystic fibrosis, and *glue ear. Its organized structure makes the biofilm resistant to attack.

biological response modifier a therapeutic agent, such as *interferon or *interleukin, that influences the body's defence mechanisms to act against a cancer cell. These substances are normally produced in small amounts by the body; relatively large doses are being studied for cancer treatment, especially in melanoma and renal cancer.

biology *n.* the study of living organisms – plants, animals, and microorganisms – including their structure and function and their relationships with one another and with the inanimate world. —**biological** *adj.*

biometry *n.* the measurement of living things and the processes associated with life, including the application of mathematics, particularly statistics, to problems in biology.

bionics *n.* the science of mechanical or electronic systems that function in the same way as, or have characteristics of, living systems. *Compare* CYBERNETICS. —**bionic** *adj.*

bionomics *n. see* ECOLOGY.

biophysical profile a physiological assessment of fetal wellbeing, based on scores for each of the following: fetal breathing, fetal movement, fetal tone, and *amniotic fluid volume (as observed on ultrasound) and fetal heart rate (measured by *cardiotocography). The maximum score is 10 (with 2 points for each component).

biopsy *n.* the removal of a small piece of living tissue from an organ or part of the body for microscopic examination. Biopsy is an important means of diagnosing cancer from examination of a fragment of tumour. It is often carried out with a special hollow needle, inserted into the liver, kidney, or other organ, with relatively little discomfort to the patient.

biostatistics *n.* statistical information and techniques used with special reference to studies of health and social problems. It embraces, overlaps, and is to some extent synonymous with the fields of **vital statistics** (e.g. *fertility and *mortality rates) and *demography.

biotechnology *n.* the development of techniques for the application of biological processes to the production of materials of use in medicine and industry. For example, the production of many antibiotics relies on the activity of various fungi and bacteria. Recent techniques of *genetic engineering, in which human genes are cloned in bacterial cells, have enabled the large-scale production of hormones (notably insulin), vaccines, interferon, and other useful products.

biotin *n.* a vitamin of the B complex that is essential for the metabolism of fat, being involved in fatty acid synthesis and *gluconeogenesis. A biotin deficiency is extremely rare in humans; it can be induced by eating large quantities of raw egg white, which contains a protein – avidin – that combines with biotin, making it unavailable to the body. Rich sources of the vitamin are egg yolk and liver.

BiPAP (bi-level positive airways pressure) trade name for a device that provides ventilation for patients by delivering air to the lungs at two levels of pressure, either cyclically in an anaesthetized patient or triggered by the patient's attempts at breathing when awake. The higher pressure inflates the lungs to whatever volume can safely be achieved, while the lower pressure enables controlled exhalation against a resistance: this minimizes *atelectasis, a risk with conventional positive-pressure ventilators, which allow exhalation against zero resistance (by open-

ing a valve in the device). Although BiPAP is a trade name, it is now widely used generically for this type of ventilation (or ventilator). There are also other devices that utilize the same principle, for example **vPAP** (variable positive airways pressure).

biparietal diameter the ultrasound measurement used to assess gestational age of a fetus between 13 and 22 weeks. It is the distance between the upper edge of the proximal parietal bone and the upper edge of the distal one, i.e. the greatest transverse diameter of the fetal skull.

biphasic defibrillator *see* DEFIBRILLATOR.

bipolar *adj.* (in neurology) describing a neuron (nerve cell) that has two processes extending in different directions from its cell body.

bipolar affective disorder (BPAD) a severe mental illness causing repeated episodes of *depression, *mania, and/or *mixed affective state. **Type I BPAD** consists equally of depressive and manic episodes, whereas **Type II BPAD** consists primarily of depressive episodes with occasional phases of *hypomania. Treatment is that of the individual episode; mood stabilizers (e.g. *lithium) are used to prevent or lessen future episodes. Combinations of mood stabilizers with *antidepressant or *antipsychotic medication may be used in more severe cases. Certain types of *psychotherapy can be used to prevent relapse as well as to treat the individual episode. 50% of BPAD patients have substance abuse problems, and many suffer from minor mood symptoms between episodes.

bird-fancier's lung a form of extrinsic allergic *alveolitis caused by the inhalation of avian proteins present in the droppings and feathers of certain birds, especially pigeons and caged birds (such as budgerigars). As in *farmer's lung, there is an acute and a chronic form.

bird flu *see* AVIAN INFLUENZA.

birefringence *n.* the property possessed by some naturally occurring substances (such as cell membranes) of doubly refracting a beam of light, i.e. of bending it in two different directions. —**birefringent** *adj.*

birth *n.* (in obstetrics) *see* LABOUR.

birth asphyxia *see* HYPOXIC-ISCHAEMIC ENCEPHALOPATHY.

birth control the use of *contraception or *sterilization (male or female) to prevent unwanted pregnancies.

birthing chair a chair specially adapted to allow childbirth to take place in a sitting position. Its introduction in the Western world followed the increasing demand by women for greater mobility during labour. The chair is electronically powered and can be tilted back quickly and easily should the need arise.

birthmark *n.* a skin blemish or mark present at birth. The cause is unknown but most birthmarks grow before the baby is born. *See* NAEVUS.

birth rate the number of live births occurring in a year per 1000 total population (the **crude birth rate**). *See* FERTILITY RATE.

bisacodyl *n.* a stimulant *laxative that acts on the large intestine to cause reflex movement and bowel evacuation. Bisacodyl is administered by mouth or in a suppository. The commonest side-effect is the development of abdominal cramps. Trade name: **Dulco-lax**.

bisexual *adj.* 1. describing an individual who is sexually attracted to both men and women. 2. describing an individual who possesses the qualities of both sexes.

Bishop score a scoring system to assess the state of the maternal cervix and position of the fetal head to determine the ease or difficulty with which labour may be induced.

Bismarck brown a basic aniline dye used for staining and counterstaining histological and bacterial specimens. [O. von Bismarck (1815–98), German statesman]

bisoprolol *n.* a cardioselective *beta blocker used to treat angina pectoris, hypertension, and heart failure. It is administered by mouth. Possible side-effects include breathing difficulty, fatigue, cold extremities, and sleep disturbances. Trade names: **Cardicor**, **Emcor**.

bisphosphonates *pl. n.* a class of drugs that inhibit the resorption of bone by blocking the action of *osteoclasts. This property makes them useful for treating certain bone disorders, such as Paget's disease and osteoporosis, as well as malignant disease – both in terms of pain relief and in treating hypercalcaemia due to cancer. Bisphosphonates include *alendronic acid, **etidronate** (di-

sodium etidronate; Didronel), *pamidronate, **risedronate** (Actonel), **clodronate** (sodium clodronate; Bonefos, Clasteon, Loron), and *zoledronic acid.

bistoury *n.* a narrow surgical knife, with a straight or curved blade.

bite-raiser *n.* an appliance to prevent normal closure of the teeth in orthodontic treatment and in the treatment of the *temporomandibular joint syndrome.

bite-wing *n.* a dental X-ray film that provides a view of the crowns of the teeth in part of both upper and lower jaws. This view is used in the diagnosis of caries and periodontal disease.

Bitot's spots cheesy foamy greyish spots that form on the surface of dry patches of conjunctiva at the sides of the eyes. They consist of fragments of keratinized epithelium. A common cause is vitamin A deficiency. [P. A. Bitot (1822–88), French physician]

bivalent *n.* (in genetics) a structure consisting of homologous chromosomes attached to each other by *chiasmata during the first division of *meiosis. —**bivalent** *adj.*

bivalirudin *n. see* HIRUDIN.

blackdamp (chokedamp) *n.* (in mining) the poisonous gas containing carbon dioxide, carbon monoxide, or other suffocating material, sometimes found in pockets in underground workings. *Compare* FIREDAMP.

Black Death *see* PLAGUE.

black eye bruising of the eyelids.

black fly a small widely distributed bloodsucking insect of the genus *Simulium*. Black flies are also known as buffalo gnats from their humpbacked appearance. Female flies can inflict painful bites and constitute a serious pest at certain times of the year. *S. damnosum* in Africa and *S. ochraceum* in Central America and Venezuela transmit the parasites causing *onchocerciasis.

blackhead *n.* a plug formed of fatty material (sebum and keratin) in the outlet of a *sebaceous gland in the skin; the black colour is due to *melanin. *See also* ACNE. Medical name: **comedo**.

black heel a black area, sometimes called a 'talon noir', resulting from the rupture of capillaries in the skin in those who play basketball, squash, etc. It may be mistaken for malignant melanoma.

blackwater fever a rare and serious complication of malignant (falciparum) *malaria in which there is massive destruction of the red blood cells, leading to the presence of the blood pigment haemoglobin in the urine. The condition is probably brought on by inadequate treatment with *quinine; it is marked by fever, bloody urine, jaundice, vomiting, enlarged liver and spleen, anaemia, exhaustion, and – in fatal cases – a reduced flow of urine resulting from a blockage of the kidney tubules. Treatment involves rest, administration of alkaline fluids and intravenous glucose, and blood transfusions.

bladder *n.* 1. (urinary bladder) a sac-shaped organ that has a wall of smooth muscle and stores the urine produced by the kidneys. Urine passes into the bladder through the *ureters; the release of urine from the bladder is controlled by a sphincter at its junction with the *urethra. The **bladder neck** is the outlet of the bladder where it joins the urethra and in males it is in contact with the *prostate gland; it is under the control of the autonomic nerves of the pelvis. The neck of the bladder is the commonest site for *retention of urine, usually by an enlarged prostate or a urethral *stricture. *See also* DETRUSOR. 2. any of several other hollow organs containing fluid, such as the *gall bladder.

bladder augmentation (bladder enhancement) a surgical method of increasing the capacity of the bladder. This is usually achieved by ileocystoplasty or ileocaecocystoplasty (*see* CYSTOPLASTY).

bladder neck incision an operation that involves an incision through the bladder neck and prostate to relieve *lower urinary tract symptoms. This is usually performed under a general or spinal anaesthetic through a cystoscope and is smaller than a transurethral resection of the prostate.

bladder pressure study a combined X-ray and manometry examination of the bladder to look for abnormal function. The bladder is filled slowly with contrast medium using a small urinary catheter and the pressure is monitored during filling and voiding (micturition). X-ray images of the bladder and urethra (*see* URETHROGRAPHY) are taken. The test is used to differentiate between ob-

struction to bladder outflow and abnormal contractions of the muscle in the bladder wall.

bladder replacement *see* CYSTECTOMY.

bladderworm *n. see* CYSTICERCUS.

blast *n.* an important cause of serious soft-tissue injury that is associated with explosions or high-velocity missiles. The eardrums, lungs, and gastrointestinal tract are especially vulnerable to the indirect effects of the blast wave.

-blast *combining form denoting* a formative cell. Example: **osteoblast** (formative bone cell).

blastema *n.* any zone of embryonic tissue that is still differentiating and growing into a particular organ. The term is usually applied to the tissue that develops into the kidneys and gonads.

blasto- *combining form denoting* a germ cell or embryo. Example: **blastogenesis** (early development of an embryo).

blastocoele *n.* the fluid-filled cavity that develops within the *blastocyst. The cavity increases the surface area of the embryo and thus improves its ability to absorb nutrients and oxygen.

blastocyst *n.* an early stage of embryonic development that consists of a hollow ball of cells with a localized thickening (the **inner cell mass**) that will develop into the actual embryo; the remainder of the blastocyst is composed of *trophoblast (see illustration). At first the blastocyst is unattached, but it

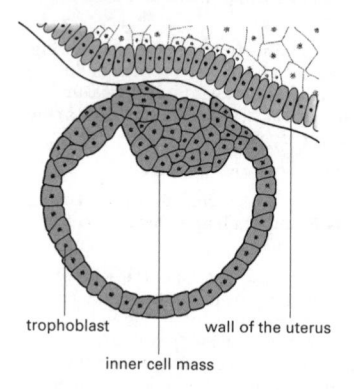

trophoblast   wall of the uterus

inner cell mass

Section through a blastocyst.

soon implants in the wall of the uterus. *See also* IMPLANTATION.

blastomere *n.* any of the cells produced by *cleavage of the zygote, comprising the earliest stages of embryonic development until the formation of the *blastocyst. Blastomeres divide repeatedly without growth and so decrease in size.

blastomycosis *n.* any disease caused by parasitic fungi of the genus *Blastomyces*, which may affect the skin (forming wartlike ulcers and tumours on the face, neck, hands, arms, feet, and legs) or involve various internal tissues, such as the lungs, bones, liver, spleen, and lymphatics. There are two principal forms of the disease: **North American blastomycosis** (**Gilchrist's disease**), caused by *B. dermatitidis*; and **South American blastomycosis**, caused by *B. brasiliensis*. Both diseases are treated with antifungal drugs (such as amphotericin).

blastopore *n.* the opening that forms as a result of invagination of the surface layer of the early embryo (*gastrula). It is very much reduced in humans, in which it gives rise to the archenteric canal (*see* ARCHENTERON).

blastula *n.* an early stage of the embryonic development of many animals. The equivalent stage in mammals (including humans) is the *blastocyst.

bleaching *n.* (in dentistry) a procedure to lighten the colour of teeth. Internal bleaching involves placing chemicals within an existing cavity in a discoloured tooth that has had *root canal treatment. External bleaching involves placing chemicals on the tooth surface.

bleb *n.* a blister or large vesicle. A **filtering bleb** is a blister-like cyst underneath the conjunctiva resulting from a surgical procedure such as *trabeculectomy, used in the treatment of glaucoma.

bleeding *n. see* HAEMORRHAGE.

blenn- (blenno-) *combining form denoting* mucus. Example: **blennorrhagia** (excessive production of).

blennorrhagia *n.* a copious discharge of mucus, particularly from the urethra. This usually accompanies *urethritis and sometimes occurs with acute *prostatitis. Treatment is directed to clearing the underlying causative organism by antibiotic administration.

blennorrhoea *n.* a profuse watery discharge from the urethra. This, like *blennorrhagia, is associated with either prostatitis or urethritis, and is cleared by the usual measures undertaken in the treatment of these conditions.

bleomycin *n.* an antibiotic with action against cancer cells (*see* CYTOTOXIC DRUG), used in the treatment of Hodgkin's lymphoma and testicular cancer. It can be inserted into the pleural cavity to create a chemical *pleurodesis for treatment of a pleural effusion. It is administered by injection and can cause toxic side-effects in the skin and lungs.

blephar- (blepharo-) *combining form denoting* the eyelid. Example: **blepharotomy** (incision into).

blepharitis *n.* inflammation of the eyelids. In **squamous blepharitis**, often associated with dandruff of the scalp, white scales accumulate among the eyelashes. **Chronic ulcerative blepharitis** is characterized by yellow crusts overlying ulcers of the lid margins. The lashes become matted together and tend to fall out or become distorted. **Allergic blepharitis** may occur in response to drugs or cosmetics put in the eye or on the eyelids.

blepharochalasis *n.* excessive eyelid skin resulting from recurrent episodes of oedema and inflammation of the eyelid. It occurs in young people, causing drooping of the lid. *Compare* DERMATOCHALASIS.

blepharoconjunctivitis *n.* inflammation involving the eyelid margins and conjunctiva.

blepharon *n. see* EYELID.

blepharophimosis *n.* a small aperture between the eyelids. It is usually congenital.

blepharoplasty (tarsoplasty) *n.* any operation to repair or reconstruct the eyelid. It involves either rearrangement of the tissues of the lid or the use of tissue from other sites (e.g. skin or mucous membrane).

blepharoptosis *n. see* PTOSIS.

blepharospasm *n.* involuntary tight contraction of the eyelids, either in response to painful conditions of the eye or as a form of *dystonia.

blind loop syndrome (stagnant loop syndrome) a condition of stasis of the small intestine allowing the overgrowth of bacteria, which causes *malabsorption and the passage of fatty stools (*see* STEATORRHOEA). It is usually a result of chronic obstruction (resulting, for example, from *Crohn's disease, a *stricture, or intestinal tuberculosis), or surgical bypass operations producing a stagnant length of bowel, or conditions (e.g. a jejunal *diverticulum) in which a segment of intestine is out of continuity with the rest.

blindness *n.* the inability to see. Lack of all light perception constitutes total blindness but there are degrees of visual impairment far less severe than this that may be classed as blindness for administrative or statutory purposes. For example, marked reduction in the *visual field is classified as blindness, even if objects are still seen sharply. The commonest causes of blindness worldwide are *trachoma, *onchocerciasis, and vitamin A deficiency (*see* NIGHT BLINDNESS) but there is wide geographic variation. In Great Britain the commonest causes are age-related *macular degeneration, *glaucoma, *cataract, myopic retinal degeneration, and diabetic *retinopathy.

(⊕) SEE WEB LINKS
• Website of the Royal National Institute of Blind People

blind and partially sighted register (in Britain) a list of persons who are technically blind or partially sighted due to reduced visual acuity, or who have severely restricted fields of vision (*see* BLINDNESS). Such people may be entitled to special education and to financial and other social benefits. The list is maintained by local authorities (England and Wales), regional or island councils (in Scotland), or the Health and Social Care Board (Northern Ireland).

blind spot the small area of the *retina of the eye where the nerve fibres from the light-sensitive cells (*see* CONE, ROD) lead into the optic nerve. There are no rods or cones in this area and hence it does not register light. Anatomical name: **punctum caecum**.

blind trial *see* INTERVENTION STUDY.

blinking *n.* the action of closing and opening the eyelids, which wipes the front of the eyeball and helps to spread the *tears. Reflex blinking may be caused by suddenly bringing an object near to the eye: the eyelids close involuntarily in order to protect the eye.

blister *n.* a swelling containing watery

fluid (serum) and sometimes also blood (**blood blister**) or pus, within or just beneath the skin. Blisters commonly develop as a result of unaccustomed friction on the hands or feet or at the site of a burn but are also a feature of certain skin diseases. Blisters may be treated with antiseptics and dressings. An unduly painful blister may be punctured with a sterile needle so that the fluid is released.

block *n.* any interruption of physiological or mental function, brought about intentionally (as part of a therapeutic procedure) or by disease. *See also* HEART BLOCK, NERVE BLOCK.

blocking *n.* (in psychiatry) **1.** a sudden halting of the flow of thought or speech. Thought block is a common symptom in severe mental illness. Blocking of speech may be a consequence of thought block or a result of a mechanical impediment in speech, such as *stammering. **2.** the failure to recall a specific event, or to explore a specific train of thought, because of its unpleasant associations.

blood *n.* a fluid that circulates throughout the body, via the arteries and veins, providing a vehicle by which an immense variety of different substances are transported between the various organs and tissues. It is composed of *blood cells, which are suspended in a liquid medium, the *plasma. An average individual has approximately 70 ml of blood per kilogram body weight (about 5 litres in an average adult male).

blood bank a department within a hospital or blood transfusion centre in which blood collected from donors is stored prior to transfusion. Blood must be kept at a temperature of 4°C and may be used up to four weeks after collection.

blood-brain barrier the mechanism that controls the passage of molecules from the blood into the cerebrospinal fluid and the tissue spaces surrounding the cells of the brain. The endothelial cells lining the walls of the brain capillaries are more tightly joined together at their edges than those lining capillaries supplying other parts of the body. This allows the passage of solutions and fat-soluble compounds but excludes particles and large molecules. The importance of the blood-brain barrier is that it protects the brain from the effect of many substances harmful to it. A disadvantage, however, is that many useful drugs pass only in small amounts into the brain, and much larger doses may have to be given than normal. Brain cancer, for example, is relatively insensitive to chemotherapy, although drugs such as diazepam, alcohol, and fat-soluble general anaesthetics pass readily and quickly to the brain cells.

blood cell (blood corpuscle) any of the cells that are present in the blood in health or disease. The cells may be subclassified into three major categories, namely red cells (*erythrocytes); white cells (*leucocytes), which include granulocytes, lymphocytes, and monocytes; and *platelets (see illustration). The blood cells account for approximately 40% of the total volume of the blood in health; red cells comprise the vast majority.

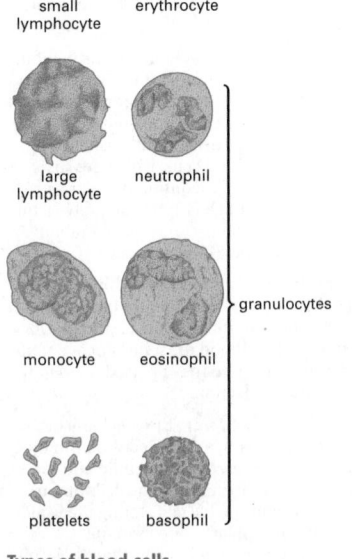

small lymphocyte   erythrocyte

large lymphocyte   neutrophil

monocyte   eosinophil

⎫
⎬ granulocytes
⎭

platelets   basophil

Types of blood cells.

blood clot a solid or semisolid mass formed as the result of *blood coagulation, either within the blood vessels and heart after death or elsewhere in the body during life (a mass of coagulated blood formed in the cardiovascular system during life is

called a thrombus: *see* THROMBOSIS). A blood clot consists of a meshwork of the protein *fibrin in which various blood cells are trapped.

blood clotting *see* BLOOD COAGULATION.

blood coagulation (blood clotting) the process whereby blood is converted from a liquid to a solid state. The process may be initiated by contact of blood with a foreign surface (**intrinsic system**) or with damaged tissue (**extrinsic system**). These systems involve the interaction of a variety of substances (*coagulation factors) and lead to the production of the enzyme thrombin, which converts the soluble blood protein *fibrinogen to the insoluble protein *fibrin, forming the blood clot. Finally, fibrin is broken down by the action of *plasmin. Anticoagulants and tissue-type plasminogen activators act by inhibiting or activating various pathways in this cascade (see illustration). Blood coagulation is an essential mechanism for the arrest of bleeding (*haemostasis). *See also* PLATELET ACTIVATION.

blood corpuscle *see* BLOOD CELL.

blood count the numbers of different blood cells in a known volume of blood, usually expressed as the number of cells per litre. A sample of blood at known dilution is passed through a narrow opening in an electronic counting device. Blood-count investigations are important in the diagnosis of blood diseases. *See also* DIFFERENTIAL LEUCOCYTE COUNT.

blood donor a person who gives blood for storage in a *blood bank. The blood can then be used for *transfusion into another patient. In Britain collection is organized by the National Blood Transfusion Services, but the armed forces have their own services. *See also* BLOOD GROUP.

blood group any one of the many types into which a person's blood may be classified, based on the presence or absence of certain inherited antigens on the surface of the red blood cells. Blood of one group contains antibodies in the serum that react against the cells of other groups.

There are more than 30 blood group systems, one of the most important of which is the **ABO system**. This system is based on the presence or absence of antigens A and B: blood of groups A and B contains antigens A and B, respectively; group AB contains both antigens and group O neither. Blood of

Blood coagulation. The clotting cascade showing sites of action of anticoagulants and tissue-type plasminogen activators.

group A contains antibodies to antigen B; group B blood contains anti-A antibodies or *isoagglutinins; group AB has neither antibody and group O has both. A person whose blood contains either (or both) of these antibodies cannot receive a transfusion of blood containing the corresponding antigens. The table below illustrates which blood groups can be used in transfusion for each of the four groups.

blood plasma see PLASMA.

blood poisoning the presence of either bacterial toxins or large numbers of bacteria in the bloodstream causing serious illness. See PYAEMIA, SEPTICAEMIA, TOXAEMIA.

blood pressure the pressure of blood against the walls of the main arteries. Pressure is highest during *systole, when the ventricles are contracting (**systolic pressure**), and lowest during *diastole, when the ventricles are relaxing and refilling (**diastolic pressure**). Blood pressure is measured – in millimetres of mercury (mmHg) – by means of a *sphygmomanometer at the brachial artery of the arm, where the pressure is most similar to that of blood leaving the heart. The normal range varies with age, but a young adult would be expected to have a systolic pressure of around 120 mmHg and a diastolic pressure of 80 mmHg at rest. These are recorded as 120/80 mmHg.

Individual variations are common. Muscular exertion and emotional factors, such as fear, stress, and excitement, all raise systolic blood pressure (see HYPERTENSION). Systolic

Donor's blood group	Blood group of people donor can receive blood from	Blood group of people donor can give blood to
A	A, O	A, AB
B	B, O	B, AB
AB	A, B, AB, O	AB
O	O	A, B, AB, O

Blood group.

b

blood pressure is normally at its lowest during sleep. Severe shock may lead to an abnormally low blood pressure and possible circulatory failure (*see* HYPOTENSION). Blood pressure is adjusted to its normal level by the *sympathetic nervous system and hormonal controls.

blood serum *see* SERUM.

blood sugar the concentration of glucose in the blood, normally expressed in millimoles per litre. The normal range is 3.5–5.5 mmol/l. Blood-sugar estimation is an important investigation in a variety of diseases, most notably in diabetes mellitus. *See also* HYPERGLYCAEMIA, HYPOGLYCAEMIA.

blood test any test designed to discover abnormalities in a sample of a person's blood, such as the presence of alcohol, drugs, or bacteria, or to determine the *blood group.

blood transfusion *see* TRANSFUSION.

blood vessel a tube carrying blood away from or towards the heart. Blood vessels are the means by which blood circulates throughout the body. *See* ARTERY, ARTERIOLE, VEIN, VENULE, CAPILLARY.

Bloom's syndrome a specific abnormality of chromosome 15 in which the individual suffers from recurrent infections, blisters on the hands and lips, and poor growth. Such children have a much higher than normal risk of developing cancer. [D. Bloom (20th century), US dermatologist]

Blount disease a condition causing *bow-legs as a result of abnormal growth at the *epiphysis at the top of the tibia (shin bone). It is more common in Africans and is most noticeable in childhood. The condition may affect one or both legs, and affected children are often obese. Treatment depends upon the severity and the age of the child but usually involves surgery. [W. P. Blount (1900–92), US orthopaedic surgeon]

blue baby a colloquial name, becoming obsolete, for an infant suffering from congenital cyanotic heart disease, the commonest forms of which are *tetralogy of Fallot and *transposition of the great vessels, in which the circulation is misdirected. Both of these conditions result in the presence of partially deoxygenated blood (which is blue in colour) in the peripheral circulation, which gives the skin and lips a characteristic purple colour. Surgical correction is often possible at an early stage. If untreated, infants may survive months or years with persistent *cyanosis.

blue bloater the characteristic appearance of a patient suffering from heart failure as a result of *chronic obstructive pulmonary disease, marked by *cyanosis, oedema, and breathlessness at rest. The left ventricle of the heart is enlarged (*see* COR PULMONALE).

B lymphocyte *n. see* LYMPHOCYTE.

B-Lynch brace suture a technique in which a compression suture is applied to the uterus, which can be used in cases of severe *postpartum haemorrhage as an alternative to an emergency hysterectomy. A pair of vertical sutures are inserted around the uterus to appose the anterior and posterior walls and to apply continuous compression, which stems the bleeding. [C. Balogun-Lynch (21st century), British obstetrician and gynaecologist]

BMA *see* BRITISH MEDICAL ASSOCIATION.

BMI *see* BODY MASS INDEX.

BNF *see* BRITISH NATIONAL FORMULARY.

BNP brain *natriuretic peptide.

Boari flap an operation in which a tube of bladder tissue is constructed to replace the lower third of the ureter when this has been destroyed, damaged, or surgically removed because of the presence of a tumour. *See also* URETEROPLASTY. [A. Boari (19th century), Italian surgeon]

Boas's sign excessive sensitivity in the region of the wing of the right scapula, associated with acute *cholecystitis. [I. I. Boas (1858–1938), German gastroenterologist]

body *n.* 1. an entire animal organism. 2. the trunk of an individual, excluding the limbs. 3. the main or largest part of an organ (such as the stomach or uterus). 4. a solid discrete mass of tissue; e.g. the carotid body. *See also* CORPUS.

body dysmorphic disorder *see* DYSMORPHOPHOBIA.

body image (body schema) the individual's concept of the disposition of his limbs and the identity of the different parts of his body. It is a function of the *association areas of the brain. *See also* GERSTMANN'S SYNDROME.

body mass index (BMI) the weight of a

person (in kilograms) divided by the square of the height of that person (in metres): used as an indicator of whether or not a person is over- or underweight. For example, a person who is 1.7 m tall and weighs 65 kg has a BMI of $65/1.7^2 = 22.5$. A BMI of between 20 and 25 is considered normal, between 25 and 30 is overweight, and greater than 30 indicates clinical *obesity. A BMI of less than 20 is considered underweight. A limitation of the BMI is that it cannot distinguish whether the weight is due to muscle or fat.

body temperature the temperature of the body, as measured by a thermometer. Body temperature is accurately controlled by a small area at the base of the brain (the *hypothalamus); in normal individuals it is maintained at about 37°C (98.4°F). Heat production by the body arises as the result of vital activities (e.g. respiration, heartbeat, circulation, secretion) and from the muscular effort of exercise and shivering. A rise in body temperature occurs in fever.

body type (somatotype) the characteristic anatomical appearance of an individual, based on the predominance of the structures derived from the three germ layers (ectoderm, mesoderm, endoderm). The three types are described as *ectomorphic, *mesomorphic, and *endomorphic.

Boeck's disease *see* SARCOIDOSIS. [C. P. M. Boeck (1845–1913), Norwegian dermatologist]

Boerhaave's syndrome spontaneous rupture (*see* PERFORATION) of the gullet (oesophagus), especially following forceful retching and vomiting. Usual symptoms are chest pain, fever, and shortness of breath. Surgical *emphysema is often present on the front of the chest and base of the neck. Diagnosis is usually made with CT scanning. Surgery is required in most of the cases, along with broad-spectrum antibiotics and parenteral *nutrition. [H. Boerhaave (1668–1738), Dutch physician]

boil *n.* a tender inflamed area of the skin containing pus. The infection is usually caused by the bacterium *Staphylococcus aureus* entering through a hair follicle or a break in the skin, and local injury or lowered constitutional resistance may encourage the development of boils. Boils usually heal when the pus is released or with antibiotic treatment, though occasionally they may

cause more widespread infection. Medical name: **furuncle**.

Bolam test where clinical *negligence is claimed, a test used to determine the standard of care owed by professionals to those whom they serve, e.g. the standards of care provided to patients by doctors. The case *Bolam v Friern Hospital Management Committee* (1957) 1 WLR 583 established that if a doctor acts in accordance with a responsible body of medical opinion, he or she will not be negligent. Subsequently, this standard of care test was amended – the *Bolitho amendment – to include the requirement that the doctor should also have behaved in a way that 'withstands logical analysis' regardless of the body of medical opinion. The determination of whether a professional's actions or omissions withstand logical analysis is the responsibility of the court.

Bolitho amendment an addition to the *Bolam test of the legal standard of care required in *negligence actions, which states that a professional's acts or omissions be assessed to see if (i) they accord with a reasonable body of opinion and (ii) they withstand the logical analysis of the court.

bolus *n.* 1. a soft mass of chewed food. 2. a large dose of a drug administered by rapid injection, as opposed to infusion.

bonding *n.* 1. (in psychology) the development of a close and selective relationship, such as that of *attachment. **Mother–child bonding** is the supposed process that starts with physical contact between mother and child in the child's first hours of life and continues throughout childhood. It promotes the mother's loving and caring for her baby as well as the child's sense of security. 2. (in dentistry) the attachment of dental restorations, sealants, and orthodontic brackets to teeth. Bonding may be mechanical (*see* ACID-ETCH TECHNIQUE) or chemical, by the use of adhesive *cements or resins. Dentine bonding agents are increasingly used to attach dental fillings to dentine as well as to enamel. In certain artificial *crowns porcelain is bonded to a metal substructure to produce a bonded porcelain crown.

bone *n.* the hard extremely dense connective tissue that forms the skeleton of the body. It is composed of a matrix of collagen fibres impregnated with bone salts (chiefly calcium carbonate and calcium phosphate; *see* HYDROXYAPATITE), in which are embed-

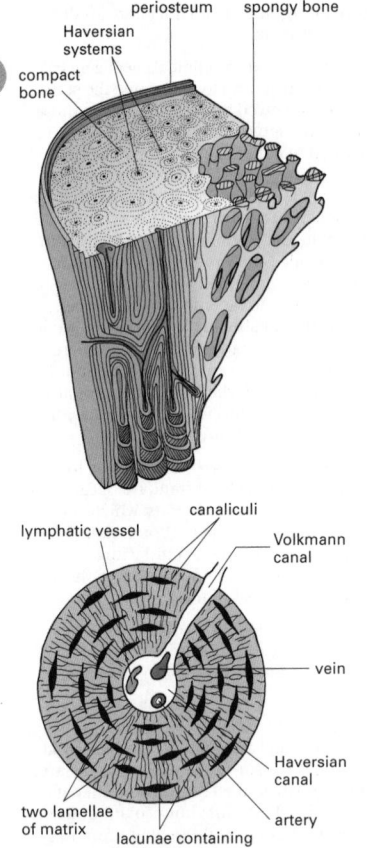

Bone. Section of the shaft of a long bone (above) with detail of single Haversian system (below).

ded bone cells (*see* OSTEOCYTE). **Compact** (or **cortical**) **bone** forms the outer shell of bones; it consists of a hard virtually solid mass made up of bony tissue arranged in concentric layers (**Haversian systems**). **Spongy** (or **cancellous**) **bone**, found beneath compact bone, consists of a meshwork of bony bars (**trabeculae**) with many interconnecting spaces containing marrow. (See illustration.)

Individual bones may be classed as long, short, flat, or irregular. The outer layer of a bone is called the *periosteum. The **medullary cavity** is lined with *endosteum and contains the marrow. Bones not only form the skeleton but also act as stores for mineral salts and play an important part in the formation of blood cells.

bone-anchored hearing aid (BAHA) a specialized form of *hearing aid for patients with certain forms of conductive *deafness. A small titanium screw is surgically fixed into the bone of the skull behind the external ear using a process called *osseointegration. Sound energy is passed from a miniature microphone and amplifier to the screw, through the bone, to the *cochlea.

bone graft the use of bone or a bonelike synthetic substance to fill a bony defect or to augment bone formation. Bone grafts are usually *autografts or *allografts, but synthetic bone grafts, using calcium compounds and hydroxyapatite, are increasingly being used. Hard cortical bone can be used to replace structural defects, softer cancellous bone is used to fill voids or to encourage bony union, and synthetic bone grafts act as a scaffold through which normal bony healing can occur.

bone growth factors a group of *growth factors that promote new bone formation. **Bone morphogenic protein** (BMP), a naturally occurring substance that induces *osteoblast formation, has been genetically synthesized to form **bone morphogenetic protein**, which stimulates new bone formation and assists with fracture healing. Other bone growth factors include a type of transforming growth factor (TGFβ) and insulin-like growth factor II (IGF-II), which encourage collagen formation.

bone marrow (marrow) the tissue contained within the internal cavities of the bones. At birth, these cavities are filled entirely with blood-forming **myeloid tissue** (**red marrow**) but in later life the marrow in the limb bones is replaced by fat (**yellow marrow**). Samples of bone marrow may be obtained for examination by *aspiration through a stout needle or by *trephine biopsy. *See also* HAEMOPOIESIS.

bone scan an imaging investigation of the musculoskeletal system using radioactive *tracers. *Technetium-99m phosphate is injected intravenously and absorbed into the hydroxyapatite crystals of bone. It concentrates in areas of increased blood flow and metabolism, such as areas of infection, trauma, and *neoplasia, before giving off radiation that can be detected by a *gamma camera, which produces a map or scan of activity in the target area. A bone scan is particularly useful in the diagnosis of subtle fractures (including stress fractures), avascular necrosis (*see* OSTEONECROSIS), osteomyelitis, and loosening of orthopaedic implants.

bony labyrinth *see* LABYRINTH.

BOO bladder outlet obstruction, usually by an enlarged *prostate gland but also by a high bladder neck or uncoordinated contraction of the urinary sphincters and detrusor muscle of the bladder.

BOOI bladder outlet obstruction index: *see* ABRAMS-GRIFFITHS NUMBER.

BOOP *see* BRONCHIOLITIS OBLITERANS ORGANIZING PNEUMONIA.

borborygmus *n.* (*pl.* **borborygmi**) an abdominal gurgle due to movement of fluid and gas in the intestine. Excessive borborygmi can occur when intestinal movement is increased, for example in the *irritable bowel syndrome and in intestinal obstruction, or when there is more intestinal gas than normal.

borderline *adj.* 1. denoting a type of *emotionally unstable personality disorder. 2. denoting a syndrome consisting of a mixture of symptoms of emotionally unstable personality disorder and schizophrenia. Borderline syndrome was first defined by Tölle in the 1980s.

Bordetella *n.* a genus of tiny Gram-negative aerobic bacteria. *B. pertussis* causes *whooping cough, and all the other species are able to break down red blood cells and cause diseases resembling whooping cough.

borneol *n.* an essential oil used, in preparations with other essential oils, such as camphene, cineole, and pinene, to disperse gallstones and kidney stones. It is administered by mouth. Trade names: **Rowachol**, **Rowatinex**.

Bornholm disease (devil's grip, epidemic myalgia, epidemic pleurodynia) a disease caused by *Coxsackie viruses, named after the Danish island where the first documented cases occurred. It is spread by contact and epidemics usually occur during warm weather in temperate regions and at any time in the tropics. Symptoms include fever, headache, and attacks of severe pain in the lower chest. The illness lasts about a week and is rarely fatal. There is no specific treatment.

Borrelia *n.* a genus of large parasitic *spirochaete bacteria. Various species, transmitted by lice or ticks, cause *relapsing fever; the species *B. burgdorferi*, transmitted by ticks, causes *Lyme disease.

bortezomib *n.* a *cytotoxic drug that works by inhibiting *proteasomes and causing death of malignant cells. It is administered intravenously in the treatment of relapsed myeloma. Side-effects include *peripheral neuropathy, *thrombocytopenia, and nausea. Trade name: **Velcade**.

bosentan *n. see* ENDOTHELIN.

bottom shuffling a normal variant of crawling in which babies sit upright and move on their bottoms, usually by pulling forward on their heels. Babies who bottom-shuffle tend to walk slightly later. There is often a family history of bottom shuffling.

botulinum toxin a powerful nerve toxin, produced by the bacterium *Clostridium botulinum*, that has proved effective, in minute dosage, for the treatment of various conditions of muscle dysfunction, such as dystonic conditions (*see* DYSTONIA), including *torticollis and spasm of the orbicularis muscle in patients with *blepharospasm, and spastic paralysis associated with cerebral palsy and stroke. It is also used for the treatment of severe *hyperhidrosis and wrinkles between the eyebrows. It is administered by injection. The toxin may also be used to treat *achalasia, being injected through an endoscope into the gastro-oesophageal sphincter, and is used in the bladder to treat urinary incontinence due to *detrusor overactivity (as in multiple sclerosis) that is resistant to other treatments. Side-effects include prolonged local muscle paralysis. Trade names: **Botox**, **Dysport**, **NeuroBloc**, **Vistabel**, **Xeomin**.

botulism *n.* a serious form of *food poisoning from foods containing the toxins produced by the bacterium *Clostridium botulinum*. The toxins selectively affect the central nervous system, causing symmetric descending paralysis; in fatal cases, death is often caused by respiratory failure due to muscular paralysis. The bacterium thrives in improperly preserved foods, typically canned raw meats. The toxins are unstable to heat and therefore invariably destroyed in cooking.

Bouchard's node a bony thickening arising at the proximal interphalangeal joint of a finger in osteoarthritis. It is often found together with *Heberden's nodes. [J. C. Bouchard (1837–1915), French physician]

bougie *n.* a hollow or solid cylindrical instrument, usually flexible, that is inserted into tubular passages, such as the oesophagus (gullet), rectum, or urethra. Bougies are used in diagnosis and treatment, particularly by enlarging *strictures (for example, in the urethra).

Bourneville's disease *see* TUBEROUS SCLEROSIS. [D.-M. Bourneville (1840–1909), French neurologist]

boutonnière deformity (buttonhole deformity) a deformity seen in a finger when the central strand of the tendon of the extensor muscle of the digits is ruptured. This results in marked flexion of the middle phalanx across the proximal interphalangeal joint and hyperextension of the distal phalanx.

bovine spongiform encephalopathy (BSE) *see* SPONGIFORM ENCEPHALOPATHY.

bowel *n. see* INTESTINE.

Bowen's disease a type of in-situ carcinoma of the squamous epidermal cells of the skin that does not spread to the basal layers. [J. T. Bowen (1857–1941), US dermatologist]

bow-legs *pl. n.* abnormal out-curving of the legs, resulting in a gap between the knees on standing. A certain degree of bowing is normal in small children, but persistence into adult life, or later development of this deformity, results from abnormal growth of the *epiphysis or arthritis. The condition can be corrected by *osteotomy. Medical name: **genu varum**.

Bowman's capsule the cup-shaped end of a *nephron, which encloses a knot of blood capillaries (**glomerulus**). It is the site of primary filtration of the blood into the kidney tubule. [Sir W. P. Bowman (1816–92), British physician]

BPAD *see* BIPOLAR AFFECTIVE DISORDER.

BPH benign prostatic hyperplasia. *See* PROSTATE GLAND.

BPPV *see* BENIGN PAROXYSMAL POSITIONAL VERTIGO.

brachi- (brachio-) *combining form denoting* the arm. Example: **brachialgia** (pain in).

brachial *adj.* relating to or affecting the arm.

brachial artery an artery that extends from the axillary artery, at the armpit, down the side and inner surface of the upper arm to the elbow, where it divides into the radial and ulnar arteries.

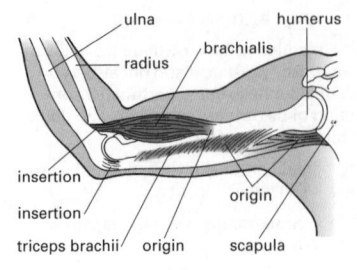

Brachialis and triceps muscles.

brachialis *n.* a muscle that is situated at the front of the upper arm and contracts to flex the forearm (see illustration). It works against the triceps brachii.

brachial plexus a network of nerves, arising from the spine at the base of the neck, from which arise the nerves supplying the

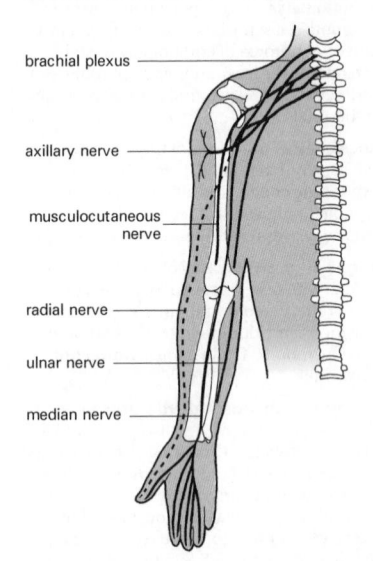

The brachial plexus.

arm, forearm and hand, and parts of the shoulder girdle (see illustration). *See also* RADIAL NERVE.

brachiocephalic artery *see* INNOMINATE ARTERY.

brachium *n.* (*pl.* **brachia**) the arm, especially the part of the arm between the shoulder and the elbow.

brachy- *combining form denoting* shortness. Example: **brachydactylia** (shortness of the fingers or toes).

brachycephaly *n.* shortness of the skull, with a *cephalic index of about 80. —**brachycephalic** *adj.*

brachytherapy *n.* radiotherapy administered by implanting a radioactive source into or close to a tumour. This technique is used in the treatment of many accessible tumours (e.g. gynaecological cancers) and is increasingly used in the treatment of localized prostate cancer. **Intravascular brachytherapy** has been used to prevent *restenosis in stented coronary arteries but this technique has been obviated by the introduction of drug-eluting *stents.

bracket *n.* (in dentistry) the component of a fixed *orthodontic appliance that is bonded to the tooth.

brady- *combining form denoting* slowness. Example: **bradylalia** (abnormally slow speech).

bradyarrhythmia *n. see* ARRHYTHMIA.

bradycardia *n.* slowing of the heart rate to less than 50 beats per minute. **Sinus bradycardia** is often found in healthy individuals, especially athletes, but it is also seen in some patients with reduced thyroid activity, jaundice, hypothermia, or *vasovagal attacks. Bradycardia may also result from *arrhythmias, especially complete *heart block, when the slowing is often extreme and often causes loss of consciousness.

bradykinesia *n.* a symptom of *parkinsonism comprising a difficulty in initiating movements and slowness in executing movements.

bradykinin *n.* a naturally occurring polypeptide consisting of nine amino acids. Bradykinin is a very powerful vasodilator and causes contraction of smooth muscle; it is formed in the blood under certain conditions and is thought to play an important role as a mediator of inflammation. *See* KININ.

braille *n.* an alphabet, developed by Louis Braille (1809–1852) in 1837, in which the letters are represented by patterns of raised dots, which are read by feeling with the finger tips. It is the main method of reading used by the blind.

brain *n.* the enlarged and highly developed mass of nervous tissue that forms the upper end of the *central nervous system (see illus-

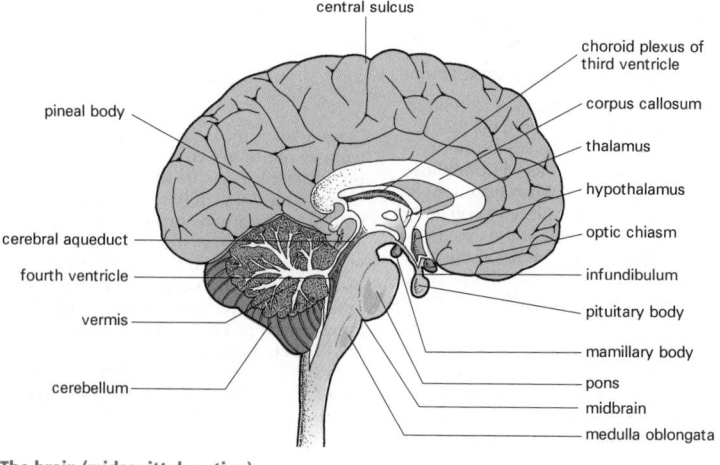

central sulcus

choroid plexus of third ventricle

corpus callosum

thalamus

hypothalamus

pineal body

optic chiasm

cerebral aqueduct

infundibulum

fourth ventricle

pituitary body

vermis

mamillary body

cerebellum

pons

midbrain

medulla oblongata

The brain (midsagittal section).

tration). The average adult human brain weighs about 1400 g (approximately 2% of total body weight) and is continuous below with the spinal cord. It is invested by three connective tissue membranes, the *meninges, and floats in *cerebrospinal fluid within the rigid casing formed by the bones of the skull. The brain is divided into the hindbrain (rhombencephalon), consisting of the *medulla oblongata, *pons, and *cerebellum; the *midbrain (mesencephalon); and the forebrain (prosencephalon), subdivided into the *cerebrum and the *diencephalon (including the *thalamus and *hypothalamus). Anatomical name: **encephalon**.

brain death *see* DEATH.

brain natriuretic peptide (BNP) *see* NATRIURETIC PEPTIDE.

brainstem *n.* the enlarged extension upwards within the skull of the spinal cord, consisting of the medulla oblongata, the pons, and the midbrain. The pons and medulla are together known as the **bulb**, or **bulbar area**. Attached to the midbrain are the two cerebral hemispheres. *See* BRAIN.

brainstem evoked response audiometry *see* AUDITORY BRAINSTEM RESPONSE AUDIOMETRY.

brain tumour *see* CEREBRAL TUMOUR.

branchial arch *see* PHARYNGEAL ARCH.

branchial cleft *see* PHARYNGEAL CLEFT.

branchial cyst a cyst that arises at the site of an embryonic *pharyngeal pouch and is due to a developmental anomaly.

branchial pouch *see* PHARYNGEAL POUCH.

Brandt Andrews method a technique for expelling the placenta from the uterus. Upward pressure is applied to the uterus through the abdominal wall while holding the umbilical cord taut. When the uterus is elevated in this way, the placenta will be in the cervix or upper vagina and is then expelled by applying pressure below the base of the uterus. [T. Brandt (1819–95), Swedish obstetrician; H. R. Andrews (1872–1942), British gynaecologist]

Brandt-Daroff exercises a sequence of exercises used in the treatment of *benign paroxysmal positional vertigo. Patients are taught how to perform the exercises and then continue the programme at home.

Braxton Hicks contractions irregular

painless contractions of the uterus that occur during pregnancy and may become stronger towards term. [J. Braxton Hicks (1825–97), British obstetrician]

BRCA1 and BRCA2 genes associated with susceptibility to breast and ovarian cancer. Women with mutations in either of these genes have a 56–85% risk of developing breast cancer, and this form of the cancer tends to develop at a relatively young age. The risk of ovarian cancer is 36–66% in women with *BRCA1* mutations and 10–20% with *BRCA2*. Targeted therapy specific to these mutations using a *PARP inhibitor is undergoing investigation.

breakbone fever *see* DENGUE.

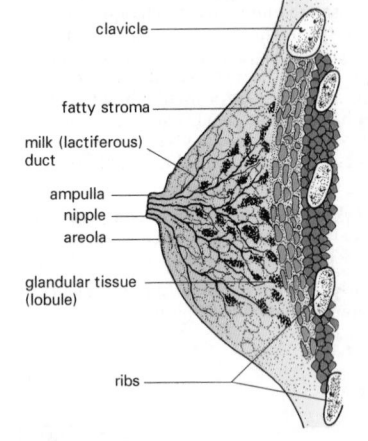

Breast (longitudinal section).

clavicle

fatty stroma

milk (lactiferous) duct

ampulla

nipple

areola

glandular tissue (lobule)

ribs

breast *n.* 1. the mammary gland of a woman: one of two compound glands that produce milk. Each breast consists of glandular lobules – the milk-secreting areas – embedded in fatty tissue (see illustration). The milk passes from the lobules into ducts, which join up to form 15–20 **lactiferous ducts**. Near the front of the breast the lactiferous ducts are dilated into **ampullae**, which act as reservoirs for the milk. Each lactiferous duct discharges through a separate orifice in the nipple. The dark area around the nipple is called the **areola**. *See also* LACTATION. Anatomical name: **mamma**. 2. the front part of the chest (thorax).

breastbone *n. see* STERNUM.

breast cancer a malignant tumour of the breast, usually a *carcinoma, rarely a *sarcoma. It is unusual in men but is the most common form of cancer in women, in some cases involving both breasts. Cumulative exposure to higher oestrogen levels is implicated as a causal factor: breast cancer is most strongly associated with early menarche and late menopause, childlessness, and late age at the birth of the first child, and hence with an increase in the total number of menstrual cycles in a woman's life. Approximately 5% of cases are due to the *BRCA1 and BRCA2 gene mutations.

The classic sign is a lump in the breast, usually painless; bleeding or discharge from the nipple may occur infrequently. Sometimes the first thing to be noticed is a lump in the axilla (armpit), which is caused by spread of the cancer to the drainage lymph nodes. The tumour may also spread to the bones, lungs, and liver. Current treatment of a localized tumour is usually by surgery (*see* LUMPECTOMY, MASTECTOMY), with or without radiotherapy; cytotoxic drugs and hormone therapy are used as *adjuvant therapy and *neoadjuvant chemotherapy and for widespread (metastatic) disease. Anti-oestrogenic agents used include *tamoxifen and (more recently) *aromatase inhibitors and *trastuzumab (Herceptin).

(SEE WEB LINKS)

• Website of Breast Cancer Care: information on screening, diagnosis, and treatment

breast implant a prosthesis to replace breast tissue that has been removed surgically during a simple *mastectomy in the treatment of breast cancer. The type of implant in current use is a silicone sac filled with silicone gel; it has recently been found that coating the sac with polyurethane to give a textured surface reduces the incidence of fibrosis around the implant and consequent hardening of breast tissue. Alternatively, an implant with a soya-oil filling may be used. The implant is inserted subcutaneously at the time of operation (the skin and nipple are retained), and follow-up radiotherapy is not normally required. Implants are also used to augment existing breast tissue.

breast-milk jaundice prolonged jaundice lasting several weeks after birth in breast-fed babies for which no other cause can be found. It improves with time and is not an indication to stop breast-feeding.

breath-holding attacks episodes in which a child (usually aged between one and five) cries, holds its breath, and goes blue. Such attacks are usually precipitated by temper and may cause loss of consciousness. Drug treatment is not necessary and the attacks cease spontaneously.

breathing *n.* the alternation of active **inhalation** (or **inspiration**) of air into the lungs through the mouth or nose with the passive **exhalation** (or **expiration**) of the air. During inhalation the *diaphragm and *intercostal muscles contract, which enlarges the chest cavity and draws air into the lungs. Relax-

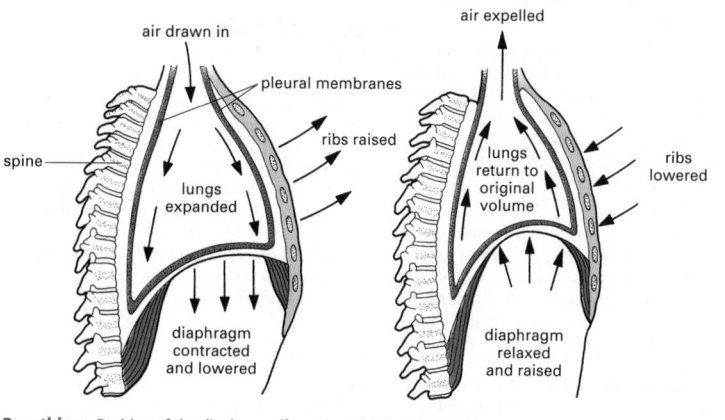

Breathing. Position of the diaphragm (from the side) during breathing.

ation of these muscles forces air out of the lungs at exhalation. (See illustration.) Breathing is part of *respiration and is sometimes called external respiration. There are many types of breathing in which the rhythm, rate, or character is abnormal. *See also* APNOEA, BRONCHOSPASM, CHEYNE-STOKES RESPIRATION, DYSPNOEA, STRIDOR.

breathlessness *n. see* DYSPNOEA.

breath sounds the sounds heard through a stethoscope placed over the lungs during breathing. Normal breath sounds are soft and called **vesicular** – they may be increased or decreased in disease states. The sounds heard over the larger bronchi are louder and harsher. Breath sounds transmitted through consolidated lungs in pneumonia are louder and harsher; they are similar to the sounds heard normally over the larger bronchi and are termed **bronchial breath sounds**. *Crepitations and *rhonchi are sounds added to the breath sounds in abnormal states of the lung. **Amphoric** or **cavernous** sounds have a hollow quality and are heard over cavities in the lung; the amphoric quality may also be heard in voice sounds and on percussion.

breech presentation the position of a baby in the uterus such that it will be delivered buttocks first (instead of the normal head-first delivery). This type of delivery increases the risk of damage to the baby. *See also* CEPHALIC VERSION, LØVSET'S MANOEUVRE, MAURICEAU-SMELLIE-VIET MANOEUVRE.

bregma *n.* the point on the top of the skull at which the coronal and sagittal *sutures meet. In a young infant this is an opening, the anterior *fontanelle.

Breslow thickness the distance (in millimetres) between the surface and the deepest extent of a malignant *melanoma. The measurement the best prognostic indicator in melanoma; tumours that are less than 0.76 mm thick have a 5-year survival in well over 90% of patients. [A. Breslow (1928–80), US pathologist]

bridge *n.* (in dentistry) a fixed replacement for missing teeth. The artificial tooth is attached to one or more natural teeth, usually by a crown. Bridges may also be fitted on dental *implants. The supporting teeth (or implants) are referred to as **abutments**, and the artificial teeth that fit over them are referred to as **retainers**. The replacements of missing teeth are known as **pontics**. **Adhesive bridges** are attached to one or more ad-

jacent teeth by a metal plate that adheres to the enamel on the tooth surface prepared by the *acid-etch technique; these bridges require minimal tooth preparation compared with conventional types of bridges.

Bright's disease *see* NEPHRITIS. [R. Bright (1789–1858), British physician]

brimonidine *n.* an alpha agonist (*see* SYMPATHOMIMETIC) used in the form of eye drops in the treatment of *glaucoma and ocular hypertension. The drug reduces the production of aqueous humour and increases its outflow from the eye; it may be used when betablocker eye drops are medically undesirable or are ineffective in controlling the glaucoma. Trade name: **Alphagan**.

brinzolamide *n.* a *carbonic anhydrase inhibitor used to reduce intraocular pressure in the treatment of *glaucoma when beta blockers are not effective or appropriate: it decreases the production of aqueous humour. Administered as eye drops, it may cause local irritation and taste disturbance. Trade name: **Azopt**.

British Medical Association (BMA) a professional body for doctors and also an independent trade union dedicated to protecting individual members and the collective interests of doctors. It has a complex structure that allows representation both by geographical area of work and through various committees, including the General Practice Committee (GPC), Central Consultants and Specialists Committee, Junior Doctors Committee, and the Medical Students Committee.

(⊕) SEE WEB LINKS
• Website of the BMA

British National Formulary (BNF) a reference source published by the Royal Pharmaceutical Society of Great Britain and the British Medical Journal (BMJ) Group twice a year (in March and September). It contains comprehensive information on medications from various sources, including the manufacturer as well as regulatory and professional bodies, resulting in information that is relevant to practice and takes into account national guidelines.

British Sign Language (BSL) *see* SIGN LANGUAGE.

British thermal unit a unit of heat equal to the quantity of heat required to raise the temperature of 1 pound of water by 1°

Fahrenheit. 1 British thermal unit = 1055 joules. Abbrev.: Btu.

brittle diabetes type 1 *diabetes mellitus that constantly causes disruption of lifestyle due to recurrent attacks of hypo- or hyperglycaemia from whatever cause. The most common reasons are therapeutic errors, emotional disorders, intercurrent illnesses, and self- or carer-induced episodes.

Broca's area the area of cerebral motor cortex responsible for the initiation and control of speech. It is situated in the left frontal lobe in most (but not all) right-handed people, in the region of *Brodmann areas 44 and 45. [P. P. Broca (1824–80), French surgeon]

Brodie's abscess a chronic abscess of bone that develops from acute bacterial *osteomyelitis. The classic appearance on X-ray is a small walled-off cavity in the bone with little or no periosteal reaction. Treatment is by surgical drainage and antibiotics. [Sir B. C. Brodie (1783–1862), British surgeon]

Brodmann areas the numbered areas (1–47) into which a map of the *cerebral cortex may conveniently be divided for descriptive purposes, based upon the arrangement of neurons seen in stained sections under the microscope. On the map area 4, for example, corresponds to primary motor cortex, while the primary visual cortex comes into area 17. [K. Brodmann (1868–1918), German neurologist]

bromism *n.* a group of symptoms caused by excessive intake of bromides, formerly widely used as sedatives. Overuse for long periods leads to mental dullness, weakness, drowsiness, loss of sensation, slurred speech, and sometimes coma. A form of acne may also develop.

bromocriptine *n.* a *dopamine receptor agonist, derived from ergot, that is used in the treatment of *parkinsonism. It is also used to treat disorders associated with excessive secretion of *prolactin (such as *prolactinoma and galactorrhoea), since it inhibits the secretion of this hormone by the pituitary gland, and to treat *acromegaly, as it suppresses the release of growth hormone. The drug is administered by mouth. Side-effects may include nausea, constipation, drowsiness, and dizziness. Trade name: **Parlodel**.

Brompton cocktail a mixture of alcohol, morphine, and cocaine sometimes given to control severe pain in terminally ill people, especially those dying of cancer. The mixture was first tried at the Brompton Hospital, London.

bromsulphthalein *n.* a blue dye used in tests of liver function. A small quantity of the dye is injected into the bloodstream, and its concentration in the blood is measured after 5 and then 45 minutes. The presence of more than 10% of the dose in the circulation after 45 minutes indicates that the liver is not functioning normally.

bronch- (**broncho-**) *combining form denoting* the bronchial tree. Examples: **bronchoalveolar** (relating to the bronchi and alveoli); **bronchopulmonary** (relating to the bronchi and lungs).

bronchial carcinoma cancer of the bronchus, one of the commonest causes of death in smokers. *See also* LUNG CANCER; SMALL-CELL LUNG CANCER.

bronchial tree a branching system of tubes conducting air from the trachea (windpipe) to the lungs: includes the bronchi (*see* BRONCHUS) and their subdivisions and the *bronchioles.

bronchiectasis *n.* widening of the bronchi or their branches. It may be congenital or it may result from infection (especially whooping cough or measles in childhood) or from obstruction, either by an inhaled foreign body or by a growth (including cancer). Pus may form in the widened bronchus so that the patient coughs up purulent sputum, which may contain blood. Diagnosis is on the clinical symptoms and by X-ray and CT scan. Treatment consists of antibiotic drugs to control the infection and physiotherapy to drain the sputum. Surgery may be used if only a few segments of the bronchi are affected.

bronchiole *n.* a subdivision of the bronchial tree that does not contain cartilage or mucous glands in its wall. Bronchioles open from the fifth or sixth generation of bronchi and extend for up to 20 more generations before reaching the **terminal bronchioles**. Each terminal bronchiole divides into a number of **respiratory bronchioles**, from which the *alveoli open. Each terminal bronchiole conducts air to an acinus in the *lung. —**bronchiolar** *adj.*

bronchiolitis *n.* inflammation of the small airways in the lungs (the *bronchioles) due to viral infection, usually the *respiratory syncytial virus. Bronchiolitis occurs in epidemics and is commonest in infants of less than one year. The bronchioles become swollen, the lining cells die, and the tubes become blocked with debris and mucopus. This prevents air reaching the alveoli and the child becomes short of oxygen (hypoxic) and breathless. In mild cases no treatment is necessary; more severe cases require supportive treatment – administration of oxygen and feeding via a nasogastric tube. Antibiotics are indicated only if there is evidence of a secondary infection. If the child is particularly vulnerable, specific treatment with *ribavirin or artificial ventilation may be beneficial. Recurrent attacks of bronchiolitis may herald the onset of *asthma.

bronchiolitis obliterans organizing pneumonia (BOOP) a disease entity characterized clinically by a flulike illness with cough, fever, shortness of breath, and late inspiratory crackles; there are specific histological features and patchy infiltrates on X-ray. It is sometimes the result of a viral infection, but may follow medication with certain drugs or be associated with connective-tissue disease, such as rheumatoid arthritis. The condition usually responds to oral corticosteroids; however, if a drug is implicated, it must be withdrawn.

bronchitis *n.* inflammation of the bronchi (*see* BRONCHUS). **Acute bronchitis** is caused by viruses or bacteria and is characterized by coughing, the production of mucopurulent sputum, and narrowing of the bronchi due to spasmodic contraction (*see* BRONCHOSPASM). In **chronic bronchitis** the patient coughs up excessive mucus secreted by enlarged bronchial mucous glands on most days for at least three consecutive months in at least two consecutive years; the bronchospasm cannot always be relieved by bronchodilator drugs. It is not primarily an inflammatory condition, although it is frequently complicated by acute infections. The disease is particularly prevalent in Britain in association with cigarette smoking, air pollution, and *emphysema. The combination of chronic bronchitis and emphysema is often referred to as *chronic obstructive pulmonary disease (COPD).

bronchoalveolar lavage (BAL) a method of obtaining cellular material from the lungs that is used particularly in the investigation and monitoring of interstitial lung disease and in the investigation of pulmonary infiltrates in immunosuppressed patients. A saline solution is infused into the lung, via a bronchoscope, and immediately removed. Examination of the cells in the lavage fluid may help to identify the cause of interstitial lung disease. The combination of cytological and microbiological examination can lead to a very high rate of diagnostic accuracy in such conditions as *Pneumocystis jiroveci* pneumonia.

bronchoconstrictor *n.* a drug that causes narrowing of the air passages by producing spasm of bronchial smooth muscle.

bronchodilator *n.* an agent that causes widening of the air passages by relaxing bronchial smooth muscle. *Sympathomimetic drugs that stimulate β_2 adrenoceptors, such as *formoterol, *salbutamol, and *terbutaline, are potent bronchodilators and are used for relief of bronchial asthma and chronic obstructive pulmonary disease. These drugs are often administered as aerosols, giving rapid relief, but at high doses they may stimulate the heart. Some antimuscarinic drugs (e.g. *ipratropium and *theophylline) are also used as bronchodilators.

bronchography *n.* X-ray examination of the bronchial tree after it has been made visible by the injection of *radiopaque dye or contrast medium. It was used particularly in the diagnosis of *bronchiectasis, but has now been largely superseded by CT scanning.

bronchophony *n. see* VOCAL RESONANCE.

bronchopneumonia *n. see* PNEUMONIA.

bronchopulmonary dysplasia a condition, seen usually in premature babies as a result of *respiratory distress syndrome, requiring prolonged treatment with oxygen beyond the age of 28 days. The babies have overexpanded lungs, which on X-rays show characteristic changes. Management consists of oxygen support and treating infections. Recovery is slow, sometimes over several years, but most babies do recover.

bronchoscope *n.* an instrument used to look into the trachea and bronchi. In addition to the rigid tubular metal type, used for many years, there is now a narrower flexible *fibreoptic instrument with which previously inaccessible bronchi can be inspected. With either instrument the bronchial tree can be washed out (*see* BRONCHOALVEOLAR LAVAGE) and samples of tissue and foreign bodies can be removed with long forceps. —**bronchoscopy** *n.*

bronchospasm *n.* narrowing of bronchi by muscular contraction in response to some stimulus, as in *asthma and *bronchitis. The patient can usually inhale air into the lungs, but exhalation may require visible muscular effort and is accompanied by expiratory noises that are clearly audible (*see* WHEEZE) or detectable with a stethoscope. The condition in which bronchospasm can usually be relieved by bronchodilator drugs is known as **reversible obstructive airways disease** and includes asthma; that in which bronchodilator drugs usually have no effect is **irreversible obstructive airways disease** and includes chronic bronchitis.

bronchus *n.* (*pl.* **bronchi**) any of the air passages beyond the *trachea (windpipe) that has cartilage and mucous glands in its wall (see illustration). The trachea divides into two main bronchi, which divide successively into five **lobar bronchi**, 20 **segmental bronchi**, and two or three more divisions. *See also* BRONCHIOLE. —**bronchial** *adj.*

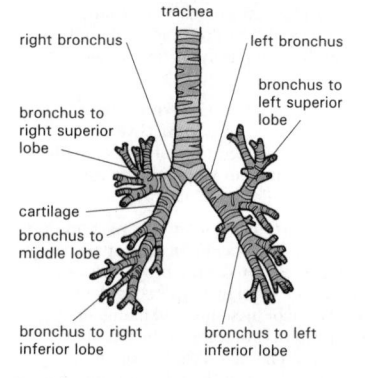

Bronchus. The bronchi and their principal (lobar) branches.

bronze diabetes *see* HAEMOCHROMATOSIS.

brown fat a form of fat in adipose tissue that is a rich source of energy and can be converted rapidly to heat. It accounts for 5% of body weight in human infants; adults have little or no brown fat. The main form of adipose tissue in adults, **white fat** (accounting for 20–25% body weight), stores energy; infants have little or no white fat. Some forms of obesity may be linked to lack of – or inability to synthesize – brown fat.

Brown-Séquard syndrome the neurological condition resulting when the spinal cord has been damaged. In those parts of the body supplied by the damaged segment there is a flaccid weakness and loss of feeling in the skin. Below the lesion there is a spastic paralysis on the same side and a loss of pain and temperature sensation on the opposite side. The causes include trauma and multiple sclerosis. [C. E. Brown-Séquard (1818–94), French physiologist]

Brown's syndrome a condition, usually congenital, in which the tendon sheath of the superior oblique muscle of the *eye does not relax, thus limiting the elevation of the eye, especially in adduction. [H. W. Brown (20th century), US ophthalmologist]

Brucella *n.* a genus of Gram-negative aerobic spherical or rodlike parasitic bacteria responsible for *brucellosis (undulant fever) in humans and contagious abortion in cattle, pigs, sheep, and goats. The principal species are *B. abortus* and *B. melitensis*. **Brucella ring test** is a diagnostic test for brucellosis involving the clumping together of a standard *Brucella* strain by antibodies in an infected person's serum.

brucellosis (Malta fever, Mediterranean fever, undulant fever) *n.* a chronic disease of farm animals caused by bacteria of the genus *Brucella, which can be transmitted to humans either by contact with an infected animal or by drinking nonpasteurized contaminated milk. Symptoms include headache, fever, aches and pains, sickness, loss of appetite, and weakness; occasionally a chronic form develops, with recurrent symptoms. Untreated the disease may last for years but prolonged administration of tetracycline antibiotics or streptomycin is effective.

Bruch's membrane the transparent innermost layer of the *choroid, which is in contact with the retinal pigment epithelium (*see* RETINA). [K. W. L. Bruch (1819–84), German anatomist]

Brudzinski sign a sign present when there is irritation of the meninges (the membranes covering the brain); it is present in meningitis. As the neck is pulled forward, the hips and knees bend involuntarily. [J. von Brudzinski (1874–1917), Polish physician]

Brufen *n. see* IBUPROFEN.

Brugia *n.* a genus of threadlike parasitic worms (*see* FILARIA). *B. malayi* infects humans throughout southeast Asia, causing *filariasis and *elephantiasis (especially of the feet and legs). *B. pahangi*, a parasite of wild cats and domestic animals, produces an allergic condition in humans, with coughing, breathing difficulty, and an increase in the number of *eosinophils in the blood. *Brugia* undergoes part of its development in mosquitoes of the genera *Anopheles* and *Mansonia*, which transmit the parasite from host to host.

bruise (contusion) *n.* an area of skin discoloration caused by the escape of blood from ruptured underlying vessels following injury. Initially red or pink, a bruise gradually becomes bluish, and then greenish yellow, as the haemoglobin in the tissues breaks down chemically and is absorbed. It may be necessary to draw off blood from very severe bruises through a needle, to aid healing.

bruit *n.* a sharp or harsh systolic sound, heard on *auscultation, that is due to turbulent blood flow in a peripheral artery, usually the carotid or iliofemoral artery. Bruits can also be heard over arteriovenous *fistulae or malformations.

Brunner's glands compound glands of the small intestine, found in the *duodenum and the upper part of the jejunum. They are embedded in the submucosa and secrete mucus. [J. C. Brunner (1856–1927), Swiss anatomist]

brush border *see* MICROVILLUS.

Brushfield spots greyish-brown spots seen in the iris of the eye. They can be found in normal individuals but are usually associated with *Down's syndrome. [T. Brushfield (1858–1937), British physician]

bruxism *n.* a habit in which an individual grinds his or her teeth, which may lead to excessive wear. This usually occurs during sleep.

B-scan examination of the tissues of the eye in cross section by means of a high-frequency ultrasound machine. It is useful in the diagnosis of eye disease, especially in the posterior segment of the eye when direct viewing is obscured (e.g. by dense cataracts). *See also* A-SCAN.

BSE bovine *spongiform encephalopathy. *See also* CREUTZFELDT-JAKOB DISEASE.

BSER brainstem evoked response audiometry. *See* AUDITORY BRAINSTEM RESPONSE AUDIOMETRY.

BSS *see* BALANCED SALT SOLUTION.

bubo *n.* a swollen inflamed lymph node in the armpit or groin, commonly developing in some sexually transmitted diseases (e.g. soft sore), bubonic plague, and leishmaniasis.

bubonic plague *see* PLAGUE.

buccal *adj.* 1. relating to the mouth or the hollow part of the cheek. 2. describing the surface of a tooth adjacent to the cheek.

buccal cavity the cavity of the mouth, which contains the tongue and teeth and leads to the pharynx. Here food is tasted, chewed, and mixed with saliva, which begins the process of digestion.

buccal glands small glands in the mucous membrane lining the mouth. They secrete material that mixes with saliva.

buccinator *n.* a muscle of the cheek that has its origin in the maxilla and mandible (jaw bones). It is responsible for compressing the cheek and is important in mastication.

buclizine *n.* an *antihistamine with marked sedative properties. Given by mouth, it is used (combined with codeine and paracetamol in **Migraleve**) to treat migraine; side-effects include drowsiness.

Budd-Chiari syndrome a rare condition that follows obstruction of the hepatic veins by a blood clot. In the majority of cases the cause is unknown but hypercoagulable states, local or disseminated malignancy, and infections are some of the possible causes. It is characterized by abdominal pain, hepatomegaly, jaundice, ascites, and rapid decline in liver function. [G. Budd (1808–82), British physician; H. Chiari (1851–1916), German pathologist]

budesonide *n.* a *corticosteroid drug used in a nasal spray to treat hay fever or as an inhalant for asthma (for which it may be combined with *formoterol as **Symbicort**). It is also administered by mouth or enema for the treatment of Crohn's disease and ulcerative colitis. Trade names: **Budenofalk**, **Entocort**, **Novolizer**, **Pulmicort**, **Rhinocort Aqua**.

Buerger's disease an inflammatory condition of the arteries, especially in the legs, that predominantly affects young male cigarette smokers. Intermittent *claudication (pain due to reduced blood supply) and gangrene of the limbs may develop. Coronary thrombosis may occur and venous thrombosis is common. The treatment is similar to that of *atheroma but cessation of smoking is essential to prevent progression of the disease. Medical name: **thromboangiitis obliterans**. [L. Buerger (1879–1943), US physician]

buffalo hump excessive subcutaneous adipose tissue forming a hump on the back over the lower cervical (neck) and upper thoracic regions of the spine. It is seen classically in *Cushing's syndrome but also in patients who are obese. *Compare* DOWAGER'S HUMP.

buffer *n.* a solution whose hydrogen ion concentration (pH) remains virtually unchanged by dilution or by the addition of acid or alkali. The chief buffer of the blood and extracellular body fluids is the bicarbonate (H_2CO_3/HCO_3^-) system. *See also* ACID-BASE BALANCE.

bulb *n.* (in anatomy) any rounded structure or a rounded expansion at the end of an organ or part.

bulbar *adj.* **1.** relating to or affecting the medulla oblongata. **2.** relating to a bulb. **3.** relating to the eyeball.

bulbourethral glands *see* COWPER'S GLANDS.

bulimia *n.* insatiable overeating. This symptom may be psychogenic, occurring, for example, as a phase of *anorexia nervosa (**bulimia nervosa** or the **binge–purge syndrome**); or it may be due to neurological causes, such as a lesion of the *hypothalamus.

bulla *n.* (*pl.* **bullae**) **1.** a large blister, containing serous fluid. **2.** (in anatomy) a rounded bony prominence. **3.** a thin-walled air-filled space within the lung, arising congenitally or in *emphysema. It may cause trouble by rupturing into the pleural space (*see* PNEUMOTHORAX), by adding to the air that does not contribute to gas exchange, and/or by compressing the surrounding lung and making it inefficient. —**bullous** *adj.*

bullous keratopathy a pathological con-

dition of the cornea of the eye due to failure in the functioning of its endothelium. It results in corneal oedema, seen as small blisters in the cornea that cause blurring of vision. *See* FUCHS' ENDOTHELIAL DYSTROPHY.

bullous pemphigoid *see* PEMPHIGOID.

bull's-eye maculopathy *see* MACULOPATHY.

bumetanide *n.* a quick-acting loop *diuretic used to relieve the fluid retention (oedema) occurring in heart failure, kidney disease, or cirrhosis of the liver. It is administered by mouth, intravenously, or by intramuscular injection. A possible side-effect is dizziness. Trade name: **Burinex**.

BUN blood urea nitrogen: a measurement of nitrogen in the form of urea in the blood, usually reported as mg/dl, in common usage in the USA (each molecule of urea has two nitrogen atoms, each of molar mass 14 g/mol). Elsewhere, the concentration of urea in the serum is reported as mmol/L:

serum urea (in mmol/L) = BUN (in mg/dl of nitrogen)/2.8

BUN or serum urea is used as a measure of kidney function but is less precise than the serum creatinine or estimates of glomerular filtration rate based on the serum creatinine (*see* EGFR). A disproportionate rise in blood urea nitrogen (or serum urea) compared with creatinine may be seen with volume depletion, cardiac failure, high protein diets, gastrointestinal bleeding, loss of muscle (the classic example is the bilateral amputee), and catabolic states associated with severe burns and fevers.

bundle *n.* a group of muscle or nerve fibres situated close together and running in the same direction; e.g. the *atrioventricular bundle.

bundle branch block a defect in the specialized conducting tissue of the heart (*see* ARRHYTHMIA) that is identified on an *electrocardiogram. Right bundle branch block is a normal variant in children and young adults, but may reflect chronic lung disease or ischaemic heart disease in older adults. Left bundle branch block may occur with ischaemic heart disease, hypertension, or cardiomyopathy.

bundle of His *see* ATRIOVENTRICULAR BUNDLE. [W. His (1863–1934), Swiss anatomist]

bunion *n.* an area of thickened tissue overlying the joint at the base of the big toe. It arises when a protective *bursa develops around the joint in response to friction and pressure from ill-fitting footwear. The condition is most commonly associated with *hallux valgus. Treatment may range from modified footwear to surgery.

buphthalmos (hydrophthalmos) *n.* infantile or congenital glaucoma: increased pressure within the eye due to a defect in the development of the tissues through which fluid drains from the eye (the *trabecular meshwork). Since the outer coat (sclera) of the eyeball of children is distensible, the eye enlarges as the inflow of fluid continues. It usually affects both eyes and may accompany congenital abnormalities in other parts of the body. Treatment is by surgical operation, e.g. *goniotomy, to improve drainage of fluid from the eye. Spontaneous arrest of buphthalmos may occur before vision is completely lost.

bupivacaine *n.* a potent local anaesthetic, used mainly for regional *nerve block. It is significantly longer acting than many other local anaesthetics. It has been used in childbirth, but may cause slowing of the baby's heart, with a risk of death. Trade name: **Marcain**.

buprenorphine *n.* a powerful opioid analgesic (*see* OPIATE) used for the relief of moderate to severe pain. It acts for 6–8 hours and is administered by mouth, injection, or transdermal (skin) patches. Side-effects include drowsiness, nausea and vomiting, and constipation. Trade names: **BuTrans**, **Temgesic**, **Transtec**.

bupropion (amfebutamone) *n.* a drug used to help people stop smoking. It is taken by mouth; side-effects include insomnia, headaches, dizziness, depression, and rashes. Bupropion should not be taken by those with a history of epilepsy or eating disorders. Trade name: **Zyban**.

bur *n.* **1.** a cutting instrument that fits in a dental handpiece (*see* DRILL). It may be made from hardened steel, stainless steel, or tungsten carbide or be coated with diamond particles. Burs are mainly used for cutting cavities in teeth, removing old restorations, and preparing teeth to receive artificial crowns. **2. (burr)** a surgical drill for cutting through bone or other tissue.

bur hole (burr hole) a circular hole drilled through the skull to release intracranial tension (due to blood, pus, or cerebrospinal fluid) or to facilitate such procedures as needle aspiration or biopsy.

Burkitt's lymphoma a malignant tumour of the lymphatic system, most commonly affecting children and largely confined to tropical Africa in a zone 15° north and south of the equator. It is the most rapidly growing malignancy, with a tumour doubling time of about five days. It can arise at various sites, most commonly the facial structures, such as the jaw, and in the abdomen. The *Epstein-Barr virus plays a role in the origin and growth of the tumour. Complications affecting the nervous system occur in up to 50% of cases. Non-African Burkitt's lymphoma is increasingly being recognized. All forms are very sensitive to cytotoxic drug therapy but cure is uncommon. [D. P. Burkitt (1911–93), Irish surgeon]

burn *n.* tissue damage caused by such agents as heat, cold, chemicals, electricity, ultraviolet light, or nuclear radiation. A **first-degree burn** affects only the outer layer (epidermis) of the skin. In a **second-degree burn** both the epidermis and the underlying dermis are damaged. A **third-degree burn** involves damage or destruction of the skin to its full depth and damage to the tissues beneath. Burns cause swelling and blistering, due to loss of plasma from damaged blood vessels. In serious burns, affecting 15% or more of the body surface in adults (10% or more in children), this loss of plasma results in severe *shock and requires immediate transfusion of blood or saline solution. Burns may also lead to bacterial infection, which can be prevented by administration of antibiotics. Third-degree burns may require skin grafting.

burr *n. see* BUR.

bursa *n.* (*pl.* **bursae**) a small sac of fibrous tissue that is lined with *synovial membrane and filled with fluid (synovia). Bursae occur where parts move over one another; they help to reduce friction. They are normally formed round joints and in places where ligaments and tendons pass over bones. However, they may be formed in other places in response to unusual pressure or friction.

bursitis *n.* inflammation of a *bursa, resulting from repetitive slight injury, pressure, or friction or from infection or inflammatory conditions. Commonly affecting the shoulder, elbow, hip, knee, or heel, it produces pain and tenderness and sometimes restricts joint movement. Treatment of bursitis not due to infection includes rest, *NSAIDs, and possibly local anaesthetic and corticosteroid injections. *See also* HOUSEMAID'S KNEE.

burst abdomen (abdominal dehiscence) spontaneous opening of the wound after an abdominal operation.

Busacca nodule a type of nodule seen on the anterior surface of the iris in granulomatous *uveitis. [A. Busacca (20th century) Italian physician]

buserelin *n.* a *gonadorelin analogue that is administered as a nasal spray or by subcutaneous injection for the treatment of endometriosis, to help in the management of advanced prostate cancer, and in the treatment of infertility by in vitro fertilization. Possible side-effects include hot flushes, headache, emotional upset, and loss of libido. Trade names: **Suprecur**, **Suprefact**.

buspirone *n.* a drug used for the short-term relief of the symptoms of anxiety (*see* ANXIOLYTIC). It is administered by mouth; common side-effects are headache, nausea, dizziness, and nervousness. Trade name: **Buspar**.

busulfan (busulphan) *n.* an *alkylating agent that destroys cancer cells by acting on the bone marrow. It is administered by mouth or intravenous infusion, mainly in the treatment of chronic myeloid leukaemia. It

may cause blood disorders producing bleeding. Trade names: **Busilvex**, **Myleran**.

butobarbital (butobarbitone) *n.* an intermediate-acting *barbiturate, taken by mouth for the treatment of severe insomnia that has not responded to other drugs. Prolonged administration may lead to *dependence and its use with alcohol should be avoided; overdosage has serious effects (*see* BARBITURISM). Trade name: **Soneryl**.

butterfly rash *see* LUPUS ERYTHEMATOSUS.

buttonhole deformity *see* BOUTONNIÈRE DEFORMITY.

butyrophenone *n.* one of a group of chemically related *antipsychotic drugs that includes *haloperidol and *benperidol. Butyrophenones inhibit the effects of *dopamine by occupying dopamine receptor sites in the body.

bypass *n.* a surgical procedure to divert the flow of blood or other fluid from one anatomical structure to another; a *shunt. A bypass can be temporary or permanent and is commonly performed in the treatment of cardiac and gastrointestinal disorders. *See also* CARDIOPULMONARY BYPASS, CORONARY ARTERY BYPASS GRAFT.

byssinosis *n.* an industrial disease of the lungs caused by inhalation of dusts of cotton, flax, hemp, or sisal. The patient characteristically has chest tightness and *wheeze after the weekend break, which wears off during the working week.

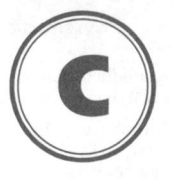

CA125 *n.* a *tumour marker that can be detected by a simple blood test and is particularly useful in the diagnosis of ovarian cancer and also for subsequently monitoring its response to treatment. In a patient being evaluated for a pelvic mass, a CA125 level greater than 65 is associated with malignancy in approximately 90% of cases (*see* RISK OF MALIGNANCY INDEX). A number of benign conditions, including benign ovarian tumours, can also cause elevations of the CA125 level, as can cancers other than ovarian cancer, including malignancies of the endometrium, lung, breast, and gastrointestinal tract.

CA19-9 *n.* a substance whose presence in the bloodstream can be increased in certain cancers, such as pancreatic cancers, and is increasingly used as a *tumour marker in blood tests.

cabergoline *n.* a dopamine receptor agonist (*see* DOPAMINE) that is used alone or as an adjunct to *levodopa combined with benserazide or carbidopa to treat Parkinson's disease. It has other uses and effects similar to those of *bromocriptine. Trade name: **Dostinex**.

CABG *see* CORONARY ARTERY BYPASS GRAFT.

cac- (**caco-**) *combining form denoting* disease or deformity. Example: **cacosmia** (unpleasant odour).

cachet *n.* a flat capsule containing a drug that has an unpleasant taste. The cachet is swallowed intact by the patient.

cachexia *n.* a condition of abnormally low weight, weakness, and general bodily decline associated with chronic disease. It occurs in such conditions as cancer, pulmonary tuberculosis, and malaria.

cacosmia *n.* a disorder of the sense of smell in which scents that are inoffensive to most people are objectionable to the sufferer or in which a bad smell seems to be perpetually present. The disorder is usually due to damage to pathways within the brain rather than in the nose or olfactory nerve.

CAD *see* CORONARY ARTERY DISEASE.

cadmium *n.* a silvery metallic element that can cause serious lung irritation if the fumes of the molten metal are inhaled. Long-term exposure may also cause kidney damage. Symbol: Cd.

caecostomy *n.* an operation in which the caecum is brought through the abdominal wall and opened in order to drain or decompress the intestine, usually when the colon is obstructed or injured. This may be performed surgically or endoscopically (**percutaneous endoscopic caecostomy, PEC**).

caecum *n.* a blind-ended pouch at the junction of the small and large intestines, situated below the *ileocaecal valve. The upper end is continuous with the colon and the lower end bears the vermiform appendix. *See* ALIMENTARY CANAL.

caeruloplasmin *n.* a copper-containing protein present in blood plasma. Congenital deficiency of caeruloplasmin leads to abnormalities of the brain and liver (*see* WILSON'S DISEASE).

Caesarean section a surgical operation for delivering a baby through the abdominal wall. The operation most commonly performed is **lower uterine segment Caesarean section** (**LUSCS**), carried out through a transverse incision in the lower portion of the uterus (*see* LOWER UTERINE SEGMENT). **Classical Caesarean section**, in which the upper segment of the uterus is incised vertically, is now rarely performed. In addition to its use in cases of obstructed labour, *malpresentation (breech, brow, and shoulder), and in severe *antepartum haemorrhage, Caesarean section is being performed increasingly when the baby is at risk and is exhibiting signs of distress. Because of improved techniques in perinatal care, particularly of the preterm baby, the operation may be performed, if necessary, as soon as the child is viable.

caesium-137 *n.* an artificial radioactive isotope of the metallic element caesium. The radiation given off by caesium-137 can be employed in the technique of *radiotherapy, but is now rarely used. Symbol: Cs-137. *See also* TELETHERAPY.

café au lait spots well-defined pale-brown patches on the skin. They are present in up to 20% of the normal population, but the presence of six or more in an individual is strongly suggestive of *neurofibromatosis type 1.

caffeine *n.* an alkaloid drug, present in coffee and tea, that has a stimulant action, particularly on the central nervous system. It is used to promote wakefulness and increase mental activity; it also possesses diuretic properties, and large doses may cause headache. Caffeine is often included with aspirin or codeine in analgesic preparations.

Caffey's disease *see* HYPEROSTOSIS. [J. Caffey (1895–1966), US paediatrician]

caisson disease *see* COMPRESSED AIR ILLNESS.

calamine *n.* a preparation of zinc carbonate used as a mild astringent on the skin in the form of a lotion, cream, or ointment. It is also included in a *coal tar preparation for the treatment of psoriasis.

calc- (calci-, calco-) *combining form denoting* calcium or calcium salts.

calcaneus (heel bone) *n.* the large bone in the *tarsus of the foot that forms the projection of the heel behind the foot. It articulates with the cuboid bone in front and with the talus above.

calcar *n.* a spurlike projection. The **calcar avis** is the projection in the medial wall of the lateral ventricle of the brain.

calcicosis *n.* *pneumoconiosis due to breathing marble dust. The term is not in current use.

calciferol *n.* *see* VITAMIN D.

calcification *n.* the deposition of calcium salts in tissue. This occurs as part of the normal process of bone formation (*see* OSSIFICATION). *Compare* DYSTROPHIC CALCIFICATION, METASTATIC CALCIFICATION.

calcineurin inhibitors drugs that act by inhibiting the calcium-dependent protein *phosphatase calcineurin, an enzyme that initiates a sequence of events that bring about activation of T *lymphocytes. The group includes *ciclosporin and *tacrolimus, which are major maintenance immunosup-

pressants used in transplantation. Topical calcineurin inhibitors (e.g. tacrolimus, **pimecrolimus** [Elidel]) are used in the treatment of eczema when topical steroids have failed or are contraindicated. Stinging is a common transient side-effect, and reactivation of infections may occur.

calcinosis *n.* the abnormal deposition of calcium salts in the tissues. This may occur only in the fat layer beneath the skin or it may be more widespread. *See also* METASTATIC CALCIFICATION.

calciphylaxis *n.* calcific uraemic arteriolopathy: a rare and often fatal complication of end-stage renal failure associated with small vessel calcification, intractable skin ulceration, and a high risk of septic complications.

calcipotriol *n.* a vitamin D analogue administered as an ointment, cream, or scalp lotion for the treatment of psoriasis. Possible side-effects include skin irritation and facial dermatitis. Trade name: **Dovonex**.

calcitonin (thyrocalcitonin) *n.* a hormone, produced by *C cells in the thyroid gland, that lowers the levels of calcium and phosphate in the blood. A recombinant form of calcitonin, **salcatonin** (Miacalcic), is given by injection or nasal spray to treat malignant hypercalcaemia, Paget's disease of the bone, and postmenopausal osteoporosis. *Compare* PARATHYROID HORMONE.

calcitriol *n.* 1,25-dihydroxycholecalciferol: the final and most metabolically active form of vitamin D_3. It is formed in the kidney by the addition of two hydroxy (–OH) groups to the basic vitamin D molecule, which itself is produced in the skin from 7-dehydrocholesterol or ingested in certain foods. Calcitriol is given by mouth or intravenous injection to raise blood calcium levels in patients with severe kidney disease and to treat postmenopausal osteoporosis. It is also used as an ointment to treat psoriasis. Trade names: **Calcijex, Rocaltrol, Silkis**.

calcium *n.* a metallic element essential for the normal development and functioning of the body. Calcium is an important constituent of bones and teeth: the matrix of *bone, consisting principally of calcium phosphate, accounts for about 99% of the body's calcium. It is present in the blood at a concentration of about 10 mg/100 ml, being maintained at this level by hormones (*see* CALCITONIN, PARATHYROID HORMONE). It is essential for many metabolic processes, including nerve function, muscle contraction, and blood clotting.

The normal dietary requirement of calcium is about 1 g per day: dairy products (milk and cheese) are the principal sources. Its uptake by the body is facilitated by *vitamin D; a deficiency of this vitamin may therefore result in such conditions as *rickets, *osteoporosis, and *osteomalacia. A deficiency of calcium in the blood may lead to *tetany. Excess calcium may be deposited in the body as *calculi (stones). Symbol: Ca.

calcium-channel blocker (calcium antagonist) a drug that inhibits the influx of calcium ions into cardiac and smooth-muscle cells; it therefore reduces the strength of heart-muscle contraction, reduces conduction of impulses in the heart, and causes *vasodilatation. Calcium-channel blockers, which include *amlodipine, *diltiazem, *nicardipine, *nifedipine, and *verapamil, are used to treat angina and high blood pressure.

calculosis *n.* the presence of multiple calculi (stones) in the body. *See* CALCULUS.

calculus *n.* (*pl.* **calculi**) 1. a stone: a hard pebble-like mass formed within the body, particularly in the gall bladder (*see* GALL-STONE) or anywhere in the urinary tract (*see* CYSTOLITHIASIS, NEPHROLITHIASIS, STAGHORN CALCULUS). Calculi in the urinary tract are commonly composed of calcium oxalate and are usually visible on X-ray examination. Some of these stones cause pain if they cause obstruction and prevent urine flow in the ureter or kidney, or by direct irritation of the bladder. Stones passing down a duct (such as the ureter) cause severe colicky pain. Most stones pass spontaneously, but some need to be broken into smaller pieces, usually by extracorporeal *lithotripsy, and the remainder by endosurgical techniques (*see* LITHOLAPAXY) or rarely by open surgery. Calculi may also occur in the ducts of the salivary glands. 2. a calcified deposit that forms on the surface of a tooth as it is covered with dental *plaque. **Supragingival calculus** forms above the *gingivae (gums), principally in relation to the openings of the salivary gland ducts. **Subgingival calculus** forms beneath the crest of the gingivae. Calculus hinders the cleaning of teeth and its presence contributes to *gingivitis and *periodontal disease.

Caldicott guardian an individual appointed by an NHS trust or health authority board with overall responsibility for ensuring that the confidentiality and security of patient information is maintained.

calibrator *n.* 1. an instrument used for measuring the size of a tube or opening. 2. an instrument used for dilating a tubular part, such as the gullet.

caliectasis (hydrocalycosis) *n.* dilatation or distension of the calyces of the kidney, which is mainly associated with *hydronephrosis and usually demonstrated by ultrasound or intravenous urography.

calliper (caliper) *n.* 1. an instrument with two prongs or jaws, used for measuring diameters: used particularly in obstetrics for measuring the diameter of the pelvis. 2. (calliper splint) a surgical appliance (*see* ORTHOSIS) that is used to correct or control deformity of a joint in the leg. It consists of a metal bar that is fixed to the shoe and held to the leg by means of straps.

callosity (callus) *n.* a hard thick area of skin occurring in parts of the body subject to pressure or friction. The soles of the feet and palms of the hands are common sites, and if much hard dead skin develops, a callosity can become painful. A *corn is a type of callosity.

callotasis *n.* the process of stretching the callus that forms between the ends of a bone that has been divided. It is achieved by means of an external fixator attached to the bone in the procedure for *limb lengthening. The elongated callus consolidates to form new bone.

callus *n.* 1. the composite mass of tissue that forms between bone ends when a fracture is healing. It initially consists of blood clot and *granulation tissue, which develops into cartilage and then calcifies to form bone. Callus formation is an essential part of the process of healthy union in a fractured bone. 2. *see* CALLOSITY.

calor *n.* heat: one of the classical signs of inflammation in a tissue, the other three being *rubor (redness), *dolor (pain), and *tumor (swelling). An inflamed region has a higher temperature than normal because of the distended blood vessels, which allow an increased flow of blood.

calorie *n.* a unit of heat equal to the amount of heat required to raise the temperature of 1 gram of water from 14.5°C to

15.5°C (the 15° calorie). One Calorie (also known as the **kilocalorie** or **kilogram calorie**) is equal to 1000 calories; this unit is used to indicate the energy value of foods. Except in this context, the calorie has largely been replaced by the *joule (1 calorie = 4.1855 joules).

calorimeter *n.* any apparatus used to measure the heat lost or gained during various chemical and physical changes. For example, calorimeters may be used to determine the total energy value of different foods in terms of calories. —**calorimetry** *n.*

calvaria *n.* the vault of the *skull.

calyx *n.* (*pl.* **calyces**) a cup-shaped part, especially any of the divisions of the pelvis of the *kidney. Each calyx receives urine from the urine-collecting tubes in one sector of the kidney.

Cameron's ulcer linear *erosion found on the lining of the stomach at or near the level of the diaphragm in patients with hiatus *hernia. The cause is unclear but interruption in the blood supply (*ischaemia) is one of the likely explanations. Treatment involves *antisecretory drugs and treatment of anaemia, which is often present.

Campbell de Morgan spots *see* AN-GIOMA. [C. G. de Morgan (1811–76), British physician]

camphor *n.* a crystalline aromatic substance obtained from the tree *Cinnamomum camphora*. It is used in creams, liniments, and sprays as a counterirritant and antipruritic.

camptodactyly *n.* congenital and permanent flexion of a finger, most commonly the little finger; it can occur at one or both interphalangeal joints. It often affects both hands and is first noticed at the age of about ten; no treatment is needed.

Campylobacter *n.* a genus of spiral motile Gram-negative bacteria. Species of *Campylobacter* are a common cause of food poisoning, producing headache, nausea, diarrhoea, and vomiting lasting for 3–5 days. *See also* HELICOBACTER.

canal *n.* a tubular channel or passage; e.g. the *alimentary canal and the auditory canal of the ear.

canaliculitis *n.* inflammation of a canaliculus, especially a lacrimal canaliculus (*see* LACRIMAL APPARATUS).

canaliculus *n.* (*pl.* **canaliculi**) a small channel or canal. Canaliculi occur, for example, in compact bone, linking lacunae containing bone cells. **Bile canaliculi** are minute channels within the liver that transport bile to the bile duct. **Lacrimal canaliculi** drain tears into the lacrimal sac (*see* LACRIMAL APPARATUS).

canalith *n.* a particle derived from *otoliths in the *utricle of the inner ear, displaced from its normal site and located within the canal portion of one of the semicircular canals. Canaliths are implicated in *benign paroxysmal positional vertigo.

cancellous *adj.* lattice-like: applied to the porous spongy network of flattened sheets of *bone, interconnected like a honeycomb, that forms the interior of bones and has a lower density than the surrounding cortical bone. *See also* LAMELLAR BONE.

cancer *n.* any *malignant tumour, including *carcinoma, *lymphoma, *leukaemia, and *sarcoma. It arises from the abnormal, purposeless, and uncontrolled division of cells that then invade and destroy the surrounding tissues. Spread of cancer cells (*metastasis) may occur via the bloodstream or the lymphatic channels or across body cavities such as the pleural and peritoneal spaces (*see* TRANSCOELOMIC SPREAD), thus setting up secondary tumours (metastases) at sites distant from the original tumour. Each individual primary tumour has its own pattern of local behaviour and spread; for example, bone metastasis is very common in cancers of the breast, bronchus, thyroid, kidney, and prostate but less common in other tumours.

There are many causative factors, some of which are known; for example, cigarette smoking is associated with lung cancer, radiation with some sarcomas and leukaemia, and several viruses are implicated (*see* ONCOGENIC). A genetic element is implicated in the development of many cancers. In many cancers a gene called *p53 is deleted or impaired: its normal function is to prevent the uncontrolled division of cells (*see* TUMOUR NECROSIS FACTOR). Whatever the initiating cause, cancer always results ultimately from DNA mutations.

Treatment of cancer depends on the type of tumour, the site of the primary tumour, and the extent of spread.

((🌐)) SEE WEB LINKS

• Cancerbackup website: information on all aspects of cancer provided by Macmillan Cancer Support

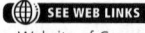

• Website of Cancer Research UK: includes information for patients

cancer phobia a disorder of the phobic type in which minor symptoms are interpreted as signs of cancer and panic attacks may occur. As with any other phobic disorder, cancer phobia cannot be treated by appeals to reason. Some success has been achieved by various forms of *behaviour therapy and *SSRIs.

candela *n.* the *SI unit of luminous intensity, equal to the intensity in a given direction of a source that emits monochromatic radiation of frequency 540×10^{12} Hz and has a radiant intensity in that direction of 1/683 watt per steradian. Symbol: cd.

candesartan *n. see* ANGIOTENSIN II ANTAGONIST.

Candida *n.* a genus of *yeasts (formerly called *Monilia*) that inhabit the vagina and alimentary tract and can – under certain conditions – cause *candidiasis. The species *C. albicans*, a small oval budding fungus, is primarily responsible for candidiasis.

candidiasis (candidosis) *n.* a common *yeast infection of moist areas of the body, usually caused by *Candida albicans*. It is especially common in the vagina, where it is known as **thrush**, but is also found in the mouth and skin folds. On the skin, the lesions are bright red with small satellite pustules, while in the mouth candidiasis appears as white patches on the tongue or inside the cheeks. In the vagina it produces itching and sometimes a thick white discharge. Candidiasis may develop in patients receiving broad-spectrum antibiotics as well as in those who are *immunocompromised. Topical, intravaginal, or oral therapy with *imidazoles is effective; oral *nystatin helps to reduce candidal infection of the bowel.

canine *n.* the third tooth from the midline of each jaw. There are thus four canines, two in each jaw, in both the permanent and primary (deciduous) *dentitions. It is known colloquially as the **eye tooth**.

cannabis *n.* a recreational drug prepared from the Indian hemp plant (*Cannabis sativa*), also known as **pot**, **marijuana**, **hashish**, and **bhang**. Smoked or swallowed, it produces euphoria and affects perception and awareness, particularly of time; high doses may cause hallucinations. The nonmedical use of cannabis is illegal; its principal psychoactive ingredient, *tetrahydrocannabinol, has a limited therapeutic value in the treatment of cancer and AIDS. Cannabis is currently classified as a class B drug under the *Misuse of Drugs Act 1971 (as amended).

cannula *n.* a hollow tube designed for insertion into a body cavity, such as the bladder, or a blood vessel. The tube contains a sharp pointed solid core (**trocar**), which facilitates its insertion and is withdrawn when the cannula is in place.

cantharidin *n.* the active principle of **cantharides**, or **Spanish fly** (the dried bodies of a blister beetle, *Lytta vesicatoria*). A toxic and irritant chemical, cantharidin causes blistering of the skin and was formerly used in veterinary medicine as a counterirritant and vesicant. If swallowed it causes nausea, vomiting, and inflammation of the urinary tract, the latter giving rise to its reputation as an aphrodisiac. It is very dangerous and may cause death.

cantholysis *n.* surgical division of the attachment of the *canthus (corner of the eye) from its underlying bone and tendon. It is performed as part of some eye operations.

canthoplasty *n.* a surgical procedure to reconstruct the *canthus (corner of the eye).

canthus *n.* either corner of the eye; the angle at which the upper and lower eyelids meet. —**canthal** *adj.*

cap *n.* a covering or a cover-like part. The **duodenal cap** is the superior part of the duodenum as seen on X-ray after a barium swallow and meal.

capacity *n.* the state of being able to make decisions about one's medical care, i.e. to consent to or to refuse treatment. The law, by virtue of the *Mental Capacity Act 2005, requires that to assess capacity doctors should evaluate whether a patient can comprehend, retain, and weigh up information in the balance such as to make a considered decision that can be communicated. The patient must understand the nature, purpose, and possible consequences of having and not having investigations or treatments. The term **competence** is often used as a synonym, but since the Mental Capacity Act 2005 came into force capacity is the preferred term. *See also* INCOMPETENCE. — **ca-pacitous** *adj.*

CAPD 1. chronic (or continuous) ambulatory *peritoneal dialysis: a method of treating renal failure on an out-patient basis. **2.** central *auditory processing disorder.

capecitabine *n.* a drug of the *fluoro-pyrimidine class that is used in treatment of advanced or metastatic colorectal cancer and breast cancer. Taken by mouth, it is converted to *fluorouracil in the body; side-effects may include blood disorders (*see* MYELOSUPPRESSION) and mouth ulcers. Trade name: **Xeloda**.

Capgras' syndrome (illusion of doubles) the delusion that a person closely involved with the patient has been replaced by an identical-looking impostor. It is often, but not necessarily, a symptom of paranoid *schizophrenia. [J. M. J. Capgras (1873–1950), French psychiatrist]

capillary *n.* an extremely narrow blood vessel, approximately 5–20 μm in diameter.

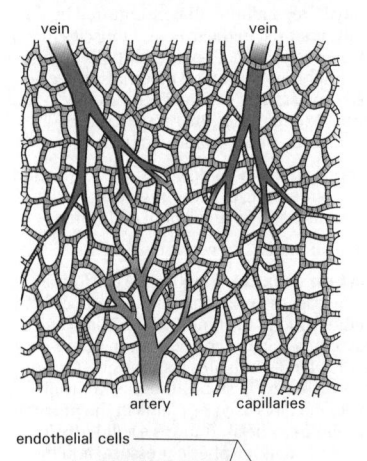

Capillary. A network of capillaries (above); a single capillary (below).

Capillaries form networks in most tissues; they are supplied with blood by arterioles and drained by venules. The vessel wall is only one cell thick, which enables exchange of oxygen, carbon dioxide, water, salts, etc., between the blood and the tissues (see illustrations).

capillary refill time a quickly performed test to assess the adequacy of circulation in an individual with poor cardiac output. An area of skin is pressed firmly by (say) a fingertip until it loses its colour; the number of seconds for the area to return to its original colour indicates capillary refill time. Normal capillary refill takes around 2 seconds. Slow capillary refill may occur globally in an individual with poor circulation or in a small area (e.g. a toe) in which local circulation is compromised (due, for example, to peripheral vascular disease). This test may not be very useful in people with dark skin.

capitate *adj.* head-shaped; having a rounded extremity.

capitate bone the largest bone of the wrist (*see* CARPUS). It articulates with the scaphoid and lunate bones behind, with the second, third, and fourth metacarpal bones in front, and with the trapezoid and hamate laterally.

capitellum *n. see* CAPITULUM.

capitulum *n.* the small rounded end of a bone that articulates with another bone. For example, the **capitulum humeri** (or **capitellum**) is the round prominence at the elbow end of the humerus that articulates with the radius.

capping *n.* (in dentistry) **1.** a colloquial term for crowning: the technique of fitting a tooth with an artificial *crown. **2.** *see* PULP CAPPING.

capreomycin *n.* an antibiotic, derived from the bacterium *Streptomyces capreolus*, that is used in the treatment of tuberculosis. It is given with other antituberculosis drugs to reduce the development of resistance by the infective bacteria. Capreomycin is poorly absorbed from the gastrointestinal tract and therefore must be administered by intramuscular injection. The more serious side-effects include ear and kidney damage. Trade name: **Capastat**.

capsule *n.* **1.** a membrane, sheath, or other structure that encloses a tissue or organ. For example, the kidney, adrenal gland, and lens of the eye are enclosed within capsules. A **joint capsule** is the fibrous tissue, including the synovial membrane, that surrounds a freely movable joint. **2.** a soluble case, usually made of gelatin, in which certain drugs are administered. **3.** the slimy substance that forms a protective layer around certain bacteria, hindering their ingestion by phagocytes. It is usually made of *polysaccharide.

capsulitis *n.* inflammation of the capsule surrounding a joint. *See also* FROZEN SHOULDER.

capsulorrhexis *n.* a continuous tear made in the lens capsule of the eye. In **anterior capsulorrhexis**, performed during cataract surgery, the tear is made in the anterior surface of the capsule. It has the advantage over a *capsulotomy in making the residual capsule much more resilient to being torn during surgery.

capsulotomy *n.* an incision made in the capsule of the lens. In **posterior capsulotomy** a hole is made in the centre of the posterior capsule using a *YAG laser, thus providing a clear path for light rays to reach the retina. The laser light is aimed using a modified slit-lamp microscope from outside the eye.

captopril *n.* a drug used in the treatment of heart failure, hypertension, and diabetic nephropathy; it acts by inhibiting the action of angiotensin (*see* ACE INHIBITOR). Side-effects include rash, *neutropenia or *agranulocytosis, hypotension, and loss of taste. Trade names: **Acepril**, **Capoten**.

caput succedaneum a temporary swelling of the soft parts of the head of a newly born infant that occurs during labour, due to compression by the muscles of the cervix (neck) of the uterus, and resolves after delivery.

carbamazepine *n.* an *anticonvulsant drug used in the treatment of epileptic tonic–clonic seizures, the prophylaxis of bipolar affective disorder, and to relieve the pain of trigeminal neuralgia. It is given by mouth or as rectal suppositories. Common side-effects include drowsiness, dizziness, and muscular incoordination; abnormalities of liver and bone marrow may occur with long-term treatment. Trade names: **Carbagen SR**, **Tegretol**.

carbidopa *n. see* LEVODOPA.

carbimazole *n.* a *thionamide used to reduce the production of thyroid hormone in cases of overactivity of the gland (thyrotoxicosis); it is the most commonly used antithyroid drug in the UK. A prodrug, it is administered by mouth and converted to its biologically active metabolite, **methimazole**, within the body. Gastrointestinal upsets, rashes, and itching may occur; more rarely, carbimazole may cause *myelosuppression. Trade name: **Neo-Mercazole**.

carbocisteine *n. see* MUCOLYTIC.

carbohydrate *n.* any one of a large group of compounds, including the *sugars and *starch, that contain carbon, hydrogen, and oxygen and have the general formula $C_x(H_2O)_y$. Carbohydrates are important as a source of energy: they are manufactured by plants and obtained by animals from the diet, being one of the three main constituents of food (*see also* FAT, PROTEIN). All carbohydrates are eventually broken down in the body to the simple sugar *glucose, which can then take part in energy-producing metabolic processes. Excess carbohydrate, not immediately required by the body, is stored in the liver and muscles in the form of *glycogen. In plants carbohydrates are important structural materials (e.g. cellulose) and storage products (commonly in the form of starch). *See also* DISACCHARIDE, MONOSACCHARIDE, POLYSACCHARIDE.

carbol fuchsin a red stain for bacteria and fungi, consisting of carbolic acid and *fuchsin dissolved in alcohol and water.

carbolic acid *see* PHENOL.

carbon dioxide a colourless gas formed in the tissues during metabolism and carried in the blood to the lungs, where it is exhaled (an increase in the concentration of this gas in the blood stimulates respiration). Carbon dioxide occurs in small amounts in the atmosphere; it is used by plants in the process of *photosynthesis. It forms a solid (dry ice) at $-75°C$ (at atmospheric pressure) and in this form is used as a refrigerant. Formula: CO_2.

carbonic anhydrase inhibitor any one of a class of drugs that act by blocking the action of the enzyme carbonic anhydrase. This enzyme greatly speeds up the reaction between carbon dioxide and water to form carbonic acid, a compound needed for the production of many of the body's secretions. Carbonic anhydrase is present in high concentrations in the eye, kidneys, stomach lining, and pancreas. Carbonic anhydrase inhibitors reduce the production of aqueous humour in the eye and are used mainly in treating *glaucoma. They include *acetazolamide, *brinzolamide, and *dorzolamide.

carbon monoxide a colourless almost odourless gas that is very poisonous. When breathed in it combines with haemoglobin in the red blood cells to form *carboxyhaemoglobin, which is bright red in colour. This compound is chemically stable and thus the haemoglobin can no longer combine with oxygen. Carbon monoxide is present in coal gas and motor exhaust fumes. Formula: CO.

carbon tetrachloride a pungent volatile fluid used as a dry-cleaner. When inhaled or swallowed it may severely damage the heart, liver, and kidneys, causing cirrhosis and nephrosis, and it can also affect the optic nerve and other nerves. Treatment is by administration of oxygen. Formula: CCl_4.

carboplatin *n.* a derivative of platinum that is used in the treatment of advanced ovarian and lung cancers. Given intravenously, it is similar to *cisplatin but has fewer side-effects; in particular, it causes less nausea and nephrotoxicity but more myelosuppression.

carboprost *n.* a synthetic *prostaglandin used to control severe postpartum haemorrhage that has not responded to ergometrine and oxytocin. It is administered by deep intramuscular injection; side-effects include nausea and vomiting, diarrhoea, and flushing. Trade name: **Hemabate**.

carboxyhaemoglobin *n.* a substance formed when carbon monoxide combines with the pigment *haemoglobin in the blood. Carboxyhaemoglobin is incapable of transporting oxygen to the tissues and this is the cause of death in carbon monoxide poisoning. Large quantities of carboxyhaemoglobin are formed in carbon monoxide poisoning, and low levels are always present in the blood of smokers and city dwellers.

carboxylase *n.* an enzyme that catalyses the addition of carbon dioxide to a substance.

carbuncle *n.* a collection of *boils with multiple drainage channels. The infection is usually caused by *Staphylococcus aureus* and may result in an extensive slough of skin.

Treatment is with antibiotics and sometimes also by surgery.

carcin- (carcino-) *combining form denoting* cancer or carcinoma. Example: **carcinogenesis** (development of).

carcino-embryonic antigen (CEA) a protein produced in the fetus but not in normal adult life. It may be produced by carcinomas, particularly of the colon, and is a rather insensitive marker of malignancy. It is an example of an *oncofetal antigen that is used as a *tumour marker, particularly in the follow-up of colorectal cancer.

carcinogen *n.* any substance that, when exposed to living tissue, may cause the production of cancer. Known carcinogens include ionizing radiation and many chemicals, e.g. those found in cigarette smoke and those produced in certain industries. They cause damage to the DNA of cells that may persist if the cell divides before the damage is repaired. Damaged cells may subsequently develop into a *cancer (*see also* CARCINOGENESIS). An inherent susceptibility to cancer may be necessary for a carcinogen to promote the development of cancer. *See also* ONCOGENIC. —**carcinogenic** *adj.*

carcinogenesis *n.* the evolution of an invasive cancer cell from a normal cell. This is a multistep process characterized by successive genetic mutations caused by carcinogens. Intermediate stages, sometimes called **premalignant**, **preinvasive**, or **noninvasive**, may be recognizable, but the interchangeable use of these terms can be confusing, and they have been replaced by *carcinoma in situ.

carcinoid (argentaffinoma) *n.* a tumour of the *argentaffin cells in the glands of the intestine (*see* APUDOMA). Carcinoids typically occur in the tip of the appendix and are among the commonest tumours of the small intestine. They may also occur in the rectum and other parts of the digestive tract and in the bronchial tree (**bronchial carcinoid adenoma**). Carcinoids sometimes produce 5-hydroxytryptamine (serotonin), prostaglandins, and other physiologically active substances, which are inactivated in the liver. If a gastrointestinal tumour has spread to the liver, excess amounts of these substances are released into the systemic circulation and the **carcinoid syndrome** results – flushing, headache, diarrhoea, bronchial constriction causing asthma-like attacks, and in some cases damage to the right side of the heart associated with fibrosis of the tricuspid valve. Bronchial carcinoids can give rise to the syndrome without metastasizing.

carcinoma *n.* *cancer that arises in epithelium, the tissue that lines the skin and internal organs of the body. It may occur in any tissue containing epithelial cells. In many cases the site of origin of the tumour may be identified by the nature of the cells it contains. Organs may exhibit more than one type of carcinoma; for example, an adenocarcinoma and a squamous carcinoma may be found in the cervix (but not usually concurrently). Treatment depends on the nature of the primary tumour, different types responding to different drug combinations. —**carcinomatous** *adj.*

carcinoma in situ (CIS) the earliest stage of cancer spread, in which the neoplasm is confined by the basement membrane of the epithelium. Surgical removal of the growth should lead to cure. *See also* CERVICAL CANCER, CERVICAL INTRAEPITHELIAL NEOPLASIA, DUCTAL CARCINOMA IN SITU.

carcinomatosis *n.* carcinoma that has spread widely throughout the body. Spread of the cancer cells occurs via the lymphatic channels and bloodstream and across body cavities, for example the peritoneal cavity.

carcinosarcoma *n.* a malignant tumour of the cervix, uterus, or vagina containing a mixture of *adenocarcinoma, sarcoma cells, and stroma, previously called **malignant mixed Müllerian tumours** (**MMMT**). Sarcomatoid differentiation of epithelial cancers often indicates a poor prognosis.

cardi- (**cardio-**) *combining form denoting* the heart. Examples: **cardiomegaly** (enlargement of); **cardiopathy** (disease of).

cardia *n.* **1.** the opening at the upper end of the *stomach that connects with the oesophagus (gullet). **2.** the heart.

cardiac *adj.* **1.** of, relating to, or affecting the heart. **2.** of or relating to the upper part of the stomach (*see* CARDIA).

cardiac arrest the cessation of effective pumping action of the heart. This may be because the heart stops beating altogether (*asystole), because there is normal electrical activity without mechanical pumping activity (*pulseless electrical activity), or because there is rapid, chaotic, ineffective electrical

and mechanical activity of the heart (ventricular *fibrillation or *ventricular tachycardia). There is abrupt loss of consciousness, absence of the pulse, and breathing stops. Unless treated promptly, irreversible brain damage and death follow within minutes. Some patients may be resuscitated by airway clearance and support, artificial ventilation, massage of the heart, and (if ventricular fibrillation or tachycardia is present) *defibrillation.

cardiac arrest simulation a form of education in resuscitation skills using a *resuscitation mannikin wired up to a heart rhythm simulator that can mimic all common cardiac arrest situations. Candidates may be expected to perform basic life support as well as advanced life support and display skills in airway maintenance and team leadership. This form of teaching and assessment is widely used in advanced life support courses.

cardiac-arrest team a designated team of doctors in a hospital who attend *cardiac arrests as they occur and administer protocol-driven treatment according to the latest guidelines. *See also* MEDICAL EMERGENCY TEAM.

cardiac cycle the sequence of events between one heartbeat and the next, normally occupying less than a second. The atria contract simultaneously and force blood into the relaxed ventricles. The ventricles then contract very strongly and pump blood out through the aorta and pulmonary artery. During ventricular contraction, the atria relax and fill up again with blood. *See* DIASTOLE, SYSTOLE.

cardiac glycosides *see* GLYCOSIDE, DIGOXIN.

cardiac muscle the specialized muscle of which the walls of the *heart are composed. It is composed of a network of branching elongated cells (fibres) whose junctions with neighbouring cells are marked by irregular transverse bands known as **intercalated discs**.

cardiac reflex reflex control of the heart rate. Sensory fibres in the walls of the heart are stimulated when the heart rate increases above normal. Impulses are sent to the cardiac centre in the brain, stimulating the vagus nerve and leading to slowing of the heart rate.

cardiac rehabilitation a programme of staged exercises and lifestyle classes designed for people recovering from a heart attack and run through the local hospital by dedicated health care professionals, who may include specialist nurses, occupational therapists, and physiotherapists.

cardiac resynchronization therapy (CRT) a treatment for heart failure that involves ventricular pacing with multiple *leads. The aim is to restore coordinated ventricular contraction and hence improve cardiac function.

cardiac tamponade a dangerous situation in which there is a build-up of fluid around the heart within the pericardial sac. This causes compression of the heart, which is therefore unable to fill with blood adequately in order to pump effectively. Cardiac tamponade can result in heart failure, a drop in blood pressure, or cardiac arrest. It requires treatment by drainage of the fluid. The classical diagnostic features, known as **Beck's triad**, consist of dilated neck veins, a fall in blood pressure, and muffled heart sounds.

cardinal veins two pairs of veins in the embryo that carry blood from the head (**anterior cardinal veins**) and trunk (**posterior cardinal veins**); they unite to form the **common cardinal vein**, which drains into the sinus venosus of the heart.

cardiogenic shock see HEART FAILURE, SHOCK.

cardiology n. the science concerned with the study of the structure, function, and diseases of the heart. See also NUCLEAR CARDIOLOGY. —**cardiologist** n.

cardiomyopathy n. any chronic disorder affecting the muscle of the heart. It may be inherited but can be caused by various conditions, including virus infections, alcohol abuse, beriberi (vitamin B_1 deficiency), and amyloidosis. The cause is often unknown. It may result in enlargement of the heart, *heart failure, *arrhythmias, and *thromboembolism. Modern drug treatment improves symptoms and prognosis. See also HYPERTROPHIC CARDIOMYOPATHY.

cardiomyoplasty n. a surgical technique to replace or reinforce damaged cardiac muscle with skeletal muscle. It is now rarely performed.

cardiomyotomy n. see ACHALASIA, MYOTOMY.

cardioplegia n. a technique in which the heart is stopped by injecting it with a solution of salts, by hypothermia, or by an electrical stimulus. This has enabled complex cardiac surgery and transplants to be performed safely.

cardiopulmonary bypass a method by which the circulation to the body is maintained while the heart is deliberately stopped during heart surgery. The function of the heart and lungs is carried out by a pump-oxygenator (see HEART-LUNG MACHINE) until the natural circulation is restored.

cardiopulmonary resuscitation (CPR) an emergency procedure for life support, consisting of artificial respiration and manual external cardiac massage. It is used in cases of cardiac arrest or apparent sudden death resulting from electric shock, drowning, respiratory arrest, or other causes, to establish effective circulation and ventilation in order to prevent irreversible brain damage. External cardiac massage compresses the heart, forcing blood into the systemic and pulmonary circulation; venous blood refills the heart when the compression is released. *Mouth-to-mouth resuscitation or a mechanical form of ventilation oxygenates the blood being pumped through the circulatory system.

cardiotocograph n. the instrument used in *cardiotocography to produce a **cardiotocogram**, the graphic printout of the measurements obtained.

cardiotocography n. the electronic monitoring of the fetal heart rate and the frequency of uterine contractions. The former is detected by an external transducer or a fetal scalp electrode, and the latter by a second external transducer.

cardiotomy syndrome (postcardiotomy syndrome) a condition that may develop weeks or months after heart surgery and is characterized by fever and *pericarditis. Pneumonia and pleurisy may form part of the syndrome. It is thought to be an *autoimmune disease and may be recurrent. A similar syndrome (**Dressler's syndrome**) may follow myocardial infarction. It may respond to anti-inflammatory drugs.

cardiovascular system (circulatory system) the heart together with two networks

C

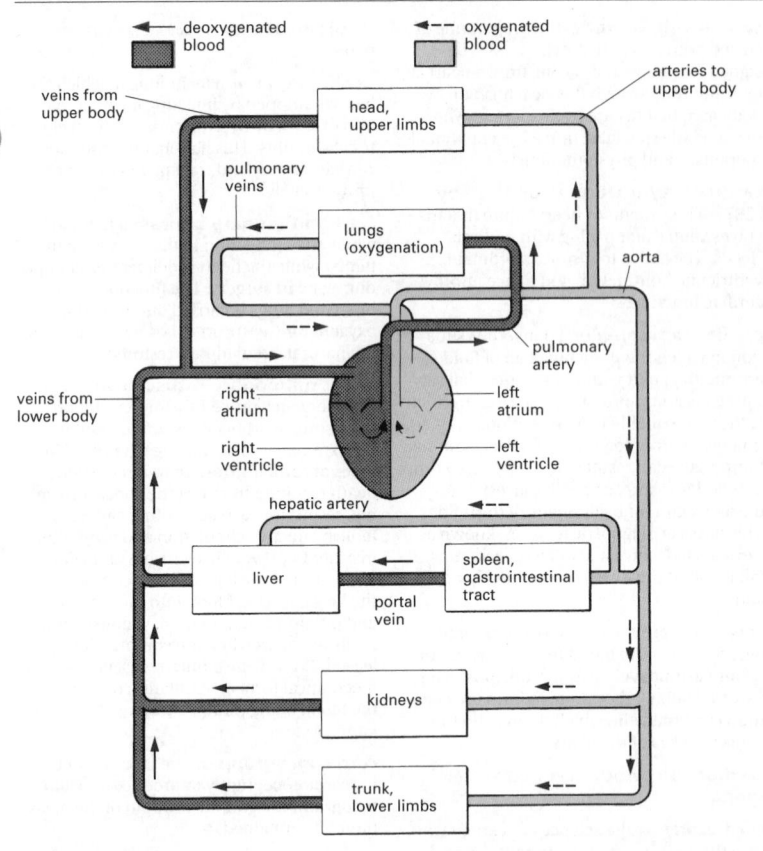

deoxygenated blood
oxygenated blood

veins from upper body

head, upper limbs

arteries to upper body

pulmonary veins

lungs (oxygenation)

aorta

pulmonary artery

veins from lower body

right atrium

left atrium

right ventricle

left ventricle

hepatic artery

liver

spleen, gastrointestinal tract

portal vein

kidneys

trunk, lower limbs

Cardiovascular system.

of blood vessels – the *systemic circulation and the *pulmonary circulation (see illustration). The cardiovascular system effects the circulation of blood around the body, which brings about transport of nutrients and oxygen to the tissues and the removal of waste products.

cardioversion (countershock) *n.* restoration of normal heart rhythm in patients with tachyarrhythmia (*see* ARRHYTHMIA). Electrical (synchronized) cardioversion involves the application of a controlled shock, synchronized with the R wave of the *electrocardiogram, through electrodes placed on the chest wall of the anaesthetized patient. The apparatus is called a **cardiovertor** and is a

modified *defibrillator. It is synchronized (usually by pressing a specific button on the control panel) because inadvertent delivery of the shock at the peak of the T wave can trigger ventricular fibrillation. Pharmacological cardioversion is achieved through oral, or more commonly intravenous, drug administration.

care assistant a person who helps with the general care of a patient, usually assisting a nurse or social worker with care of the vulnerable elderly in the community. Care assistants include home helps.

Care Quality Commission (CQC) an independent organization established in 2009 and responsible for regulation of health and social care in England; it replaced the *Healthcare Commission, the *Commission for Social Care Inspection, and the *Mental Health Act Commission. The responsibilities of the commission include publication of national health-care standards; annual assessment of the performance of NHS and social-care organizations; reviewing other (i.e. private and voluntary) health- and social-care organizations; reviewing complaints about the services when it has not been possible to resolve them locally; and investigating serious service failures.

(())) SEE WEB LINKS

- Website of the Care Quality Commission: includes guidance for health and social care professionals

care trust an organization similar to a *primary care trust but with additional responsibilities for social care services in partnership with local authorities.

caries n. decay and crumbling of the substance of a tooth (see DENTAL CARIES) or a bone. —**carious** adj.

carina n. a keel-like structure, such as the keel-shaped cartilage at the bifurcation of the trachea into the two main bronchi.

cariogenic adj. causing caries, particularly dental caries: refers especially to the sugar in food and drinks.

cariology n. the branch of dentistry concerned with the study of tooth decay (see DENTAL CARIES).

carminative n. a drug that relieves flatulence, used to treat gastric discomfort and colic.

carmustine n. a drug (an *alkylating agent) used in the treatment of myeloma, non-Hodgkin lymphomas, and certain brain tumours (gliomas and glioblastoma). Administered intravenously or (for brain tumours) as implants, it may cause kidney damage. Trade name: **Gliadel**.

carneous mole a fleshy mass in the uterus consisting of pieces of placenta and products of conception that have not been expelled after miscarriage.

Caroli's disease an inherited condition in which the bile ducts, which drain the liver, are widened, causing an increased risk of infection or cancer in the gall bladder. Compare CAROLI'S SYNDROME. [J. Caroli (20th century), French physician]

Caroli's syndrome an inherited condition in which the bile ducts, which drain the liver, are widened and there are fibrous changes in the liver and cysts within the kidneys. Compare CAROLI'S DISEASE. [J. Caroli]

carotenaemia n. see XANTHAEMIA.

carotene n. a yellow or orange plant pigment – one of the carotenoids – that occurs in four forms: alpha (α), beta (β), gamma (γ), and delta (δ). The most important form is β-carotene, which is an *antioxidant and can be converted in the body to retinol (vitamin A). Foods containing β-carotene (for example, milk and some vegetables) are therefore a source of the vitamin.

carotenoid n. any one of a group of about 100 naturally occurring yellow to red pigments found mostly in plants. The group includes the *carotenes.

carotid artery either of the two main arteries in the neck whose branches supply the head and neck. The **common carotid artery** arises on the left side directly from the aortic arch and on the right from the innominate artery. They ascend the neck on either side as far as the thyroid cartilage (Adam's apple), where they each divide into two branches, the **internal carotid**, supplying the cerebrum, forehead, nose, eye, and middle ear, and the **external carotid**, sending branches to the face, scalp, and neck.

carotid artery stenosis (carotid stenosis) narrowing of the carotid artery, which reduces the supply of blood to the brain and is a cause of strokes. Many cases can be treated by surgical excision or bypass of the narrowed segment (see also ENDARTEREC- TOMY), but inserting a *stent into the carotid artery is becoming more common.

carotid body a small mass of tissue in the carotid sinus containing *chemoreceptors that monitor levels of oxygen, carbon dioxide, and hydrogen ions in the blood. If the oxygen level falls, the chemoreceptors send impulses to the cardiac and respiratory centres in the brain, which promote increases in heart and respiration rates. It can give rise to carotid body tumours, which are a form of *paraganglioma.

carotid sinus a pocket in the wall of the carotid artery, at its division in the neck, containing receptors that monitor blood pressure (see BARORECEPTOR). When blood pressure is raised, impulses travel from the receptors to the vasomotor centre in the brain, which initiates a reflex *vasodilatation and slowing of heart rate to lower the blood pressure to normal.

carp- (carpo-) *combining form denoting* the wrist (carpus).

carpal 1. *adj.* relating to the wrist. 2. *n.* any of the bones forming the carpus.

carpal tunnel the space between the carpal bones of the wrist and the connective tissue (retinaculum) over the flexor tendons. It contains the flexor tendons and the median nerve.

carpal tunnel syndrome a combination of *paraesthesia (pins and needles), numbness, and pain in the hand, usually affecting the thumb, index, and middle fingers. The symptoms are usually worse at night, and in longstanding cases there may be weakness of grip due to wasting of the *thenar eminence of the thumb. It is caused by pressure on the median nerve as it passes through the wrist (*see* CARPAL TUNNEL), which may result from any continuous repetitive movements of the hand, such as typing, or any condition causing local swelling. It is common in rheumatoid arthritis, myxoedema, pregnancy, and at the menopause. Treatment is by splinting of the wrist, injection of a steroid, or – in severe cases – by surgical release of the nerve under local anaesthesia.

carphology *n. see* FLOCCILLATION.

carpopedal spasm *see* SPASM.

carpus *n.* the eight bones of the wrist (see illustration). The carpus articulates with the metacarpals distally and with the ulna and radius proximally.

carrier *n.* 1. a person who harbours the microorganisms causing a particular disease without experiencing signs or symptoms of infection and who can transmit the disease to others. 2. (in genetics) a person who bears a gene for an abnormal trait without showing any signs of the disorder; the carrier is usually *heterozygous for the gene concerned, which is *recessive. 3. an animal, usually an insect, that passively transmits infectious organisms from one animal to another or from an infected animal to a human being. *See also* VECTOR.

carteolol *n.* a *beta blocker used as eye drops in the treatment of *glaucoma; side-

effects may include local stinging and burning. Trade name: **Teoptic.**

cartilage *n.* a dense connective tissue composed of a matrix produced by cells called **chondroblasts**, which become embedded in the matrix as **chondrocytes**. It is a semiopaque grey or white substance, consisting chiefly of *chondroitin sulphate, that is capable of withstanding considerable pressure. There are three types: *hyaline cartilage, *elastic cartilage, and *fibrocartilage (see illustration). In the fetus and infant cartilage occurs in many parts of the body, but most of this cartilage disappears during development. In the adult, hyaline cartilage is found in the costal cartilages, larynx, trachea, bronchi, nose, and covering the surface of bones at joints, where wear and damage results in *osteoarthritis. Elastic cartilage occurs in the external ear, and fibrocartilage in the intervertebral discs and tendons. Cartilage is the precursor of bone following a fracture (*see* CALLUS).

caruncle *n.* a small red fleshy swelling. The **lacrimal caruncle** is the red prominence at the inner angle of the eye. **Hymenal caruncles** occur around the mucous membrane lining the vaginal opening.

caseation *n.* the breakdown of diseased tissue into a dry cheeselike mass: a type of *necrosis associated with tubercular lesions.

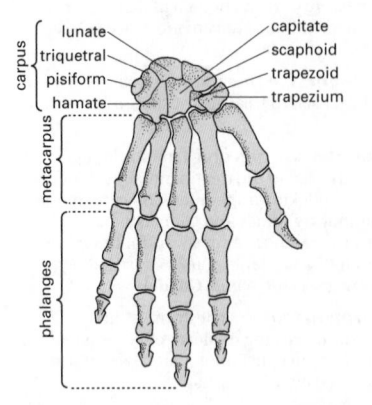

Carpus. Bones of the left wrist and hand (from the front).

case control study comparison of a group of people with a disease or condition and a control group of people free from that

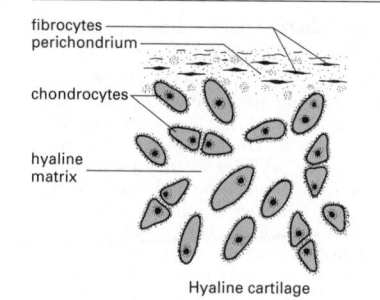

fibrocytes
perichondrium
chondrocytes
hyaline
matrix

Hyaline cartilage

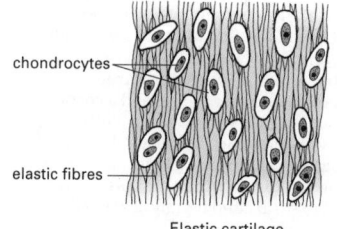

chondrocytes

elastic fibres

Elastic cartilage

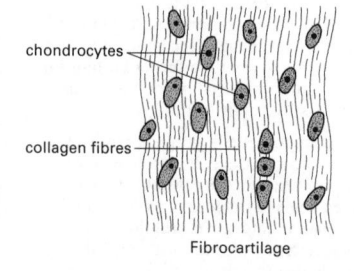

chondrocytes

collagen fibres

Fibrocartilage

Types of cartilage.

disease (e.g. people diagnosed with lung cancer and people without lung cancer). The groups are compared in terms of the frequency of *variables in their backgrounds (e.g. cigarette smoking). This method can be used to investigate risk factors for diseases. In the more precise **matched pair study** each individual with the disease is paired with a control matched on the basis of (say) age, sex, and occupation in order to account for some of the main risk factors for the disease. This places greater emphasis on the factors for which the pairs have not been matched.

Compare COHORT STUDY, CROSS-SECTIONAL STUDY.

case fatality rate the number of fatalities from a specified disease in a given period per 100 diagnosed cases of the disease arising in the same period. Unless deaths occur very rapidly after the onset of the disease (e.g. cholera), they may be the outcome of episodes that started in an earlier period. It is possible for more people to die from a condition than to develop it during the time period under investigation. Different time periods will be appropriate depending on the disease of interest. Comparison of the annual number of admissions and fatalities in a given hospital in respect of a specific disease is known as the **hospital fatality rate**.

casein *n.* a milk protein. Casein is precipitated out of milk in acid solution or by the action of rennin: it is the principal protein of cheese. Casein is very easily prepared and is useful as a protein supplement, particularly in the treatment of malnutrition.

case work *see* SOCIAL SERVICES.

Casodex *n. see* BICALUTAMIDE.

cassette *n.* (in radiography) a thin light-proof box in which a piece of photographic film is placed. It usually contains special screens, which fluoresce on exposure to X-rays, intensifying the image formed on photographic film when a radiographic exposure is taken. In *computerized radiography the cassette may contain an electrically charged plate.

cast *n.* **1.** a rigid casing for a limb or other part of the body, made of plaster of Paris, fibreglass, or plastic, that is designed to protect a broken bone and prevent movement of the aligned bone ends until healing has progressed sufficiently. **2.** a mass of dead cellular, fatty, and other material that forms within a body cavity and takes its shape. It may then be released and appear elsewhere. For example, *granular casts appearing in the urine indicate kidney disease.

cast nephropathy (myeloma kidney) a complication of multiple myeloma seen in approximately half of those who have renal disease. The casts typically involve the distal convoluted and collecting tubules and often have a fractured or crystalline appearance. They are frequently surrounded by multinucleate giant cells. Deposition of the casts is associated with progressive renal failure.

castration *n.* removal of the sex glands (the testes or the ovaries). Castration in childhood causes failure of sexual development but when done in adult life (usually as part of hormonal treatment for cancer) it produces less marked physical changes in both sexes. Castration inevitably causes sterility but it need not cause impotence or loss of sexual desire.

casuistry *n.* **1.** an approach to ethical analysis that is based on cases as distinct from principle-dependent or rule-based methods of evaluating moral problems. **2.** an excessively subtle or opaque form of reasoning often presented with the intention to mislead.

CAT computerized axial tomography, now referred to as *computerized tomography (CT).

cata- *prefix denoting* downward or against.

catabolism *n.* the chemical decomposition of complex substances by the body to form simpler ones, accompanied by the release of energy. The substances broken down include nutrients in food (carbohydrates, proteins, etc.) as well as the body's storage products (such as glycogen). *See also* METABOLISM. —**catabolic** *adj.*

catagen *n. see* ANAGEN.

catalase *n.* an enzyme, present in many cells (including red blood cells and liver cells), that catalyses the breakdown of hydrogen peroxide.

catalepsy *n.* the abnormal maintenance of postures, occurring in *catatonia. These may have arisen spontaneously or they may be induced by the examiner.

catalyst *n.* a substance that alters the rate of a chemical reaction but is itself unchanged at the end of the reaction. The catalysts of biochemical reactions are the *enzymes.

cataphoresis *n.* the introduction into the tissues of positively charged ionized substances (cations) by the use of a direct electric current. *See* IONTOPHORESIS.

cataplasia *n.* degeneration of tissues to an earlier developmental form.

cataplexy *n.* a sudden onset of muscle weakness that may be precipitated by excitement or emotion. There may be total loss of muscle tone, resulting in collapse, or simply jaw dropping or head nodding. It occurs in 60–90% of patients with *narcolepsy.

cataract *n.* an opacity in the lens of the eye that may result in blurred vision. Minor degrees of cataract do not necessarily impair vision seriously. Cataracts may be congenital or acquired. The latter are most commonly a result of age (**senile cataract**); metabolic disease (such as diabetes), injury to the eye, or exposure of the eye to infrared rays (e.g. **glass-blowers' cataract**) or ionizing radiation can also cause a cataract. A type commonly related to ageing is **nuclear sclerotic cataract**, which results from increasing density and yellowing of the centre of the lens. A **posterior subcapsular cataract** (at the rear surface of the lens within the lens capsule) is also related to ageing but may occur with prolonged use of steroids and chronic ocular inflammation. **Brunescent cataracts** are dark brown and very dense, and a **cortical cataract** is one in which the opacity occurs in the soft outer part (cortex) of the lens. A **Morgagnian cataract** is a longstanding very opaque cataract in which the cortex has started to shrink and liquefy, leaving a central shrunken nucleus.

Cataract is treated by removal of the affected lens (*see* CATARACT EXTRACTION, PHACOEMULSIFICATION); patients may wear appropriate spectacles or a contact lens to compensate for the missing lens but in modern practice a synthetic **intraocular lens implant** is routinely placed inside the eye as a part of the surgical procedure.

cataract extraction surgical removal of a cataract from the eye. In **extracapsular cataract extraction** the cataract alone is removed, leaving the lens capsule behind. **Intracapsular cataract extraction** is the removal of the whole lens, including the capsule that surrounds it.

catarrh *n.* the excessive secretion of thick phlegm or mucus by the mucous membrane of the nose, nasal sinuses, nasopharynx, or air passages. The term is not used in any precise or scientific sense.

catatonia *n.* a state in which a person becomes mute or stuporous or adopts bizarre postures. The features include **flexibilitas cerea**, in which the limbs may be moved passively by another person into positions that are then retained for hours on end. Catatonia was once a noted feature of *schizophrenia but is now hardly ever seen in developed countries. It remains common in developing countries. Treatment includes high-dose *benzodiazepines and *electro-convulsive therapy. —**catatonic** *adj.*

CATCH-22 *see* DI GEORGE SYNDROME.

catchment area the geographic area from which a hospital can expect to receive patients and on which (in Britain) the designated population of the hospital is based. There is no statutory requirement for patients to use the hospital(s) of their area, but a code of zoning practice exists for some specialties (e.g. mental illness). A hospital may have a smaller catchment area for common specialties than for rarer ones, which may be shared between several districts (**regional specialty**) or regions (**supraregional specialty**).

catecholamines *pl. n.* a group of physiologically important substances, including *adrenaline, *noradrenaline, and *dopamine, having various different roles (mainly as *neurotransmitters) in the functioning of the sympathetic and central nervous systems. Chemically, all contain a benzene ring with adjacent hydroxyl groups (catechol) and an amine group on a side chain. Catecholamines act at both alpha (α) and beta (β) *adrenoceptors. Some tumours (e.g. *phaeochromocytoma) secrete excess catecholamines.

categorical imperative *see* IMPERATIVE.

catgut *n.* a natural fibrous material prepared from the tissues of animals, usually from the walls of sheep intestines, twisted into strands of different thicknesses and formerly widely used to sew up wounds (*see* SUTURE) and tie off blood vessels during surgery. The catgut gradually dissolves and is absorbed by the tissues, so that the stitches do not have to be removed later. This also minimizes the possibility of long-term irritation at the site of operation. Some catgut is treated with chromic acid during manufacture (**chromic catgut**). This gives catguts that last for longer periods before absorption is complete.

catharsis *n.* 1. purging or cleansing out of the bowels by giving the patient a *laxative (cathartic) to stimulate intestinal activity. 2. the release of strong pent-up emotions. *See* ABREACTION.

cathartic *n. see* LAXATIVE.

cathepsin *n.* one of a group of enzymes

found in animal tissues, particularly the spleen, that digest proteins.

catheter *n.* a flexible tube for insertion into a narrow opening so that fluids may be introduced or removed (see illustration). **Urinary catheters** are passed into the bladder through the urethra to allow drainage of urine in certain disorders and to empty the bladder before abdominal operations.

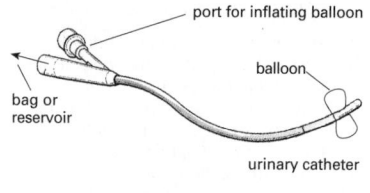

urinary catheter

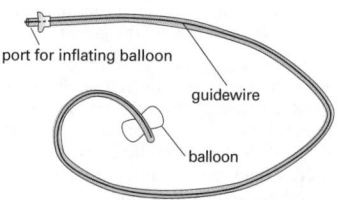

embolectomy catheter (Fogarty)

Catheters.

catheterization *n.* the introduction of a *catheter into a hollow organ or vessel. In **urethral catheterization** a catheter is introduced into the bladder to relieve obstruction to the outflow of urine (*see also* INTERMITTENT SELF-CATHETERIZATION). Catheters can also be passed above the pubis through the abdominal wall (**suprapubic catheterization**) directly into an enlarged bladder if urethral catheterization is not possible. **Cardiac catheterization** entails the introduction of special catheters, usually via the femoral blood vessels in the groin, into the chambers of the heart. This allows the measurement of pressures in the chambers and pressure gradients across the heart valves, as well as the injection of contrast medium for visualization of structures using X-rays (*see* CORONARY ANGIOGRAPHY). **Vascular catheterization** enables the introduction into the arteries or veins of: (1) contrast medium for radiography; (2) drugs to constrict or expand vessels or to dissolve a thrombus (*see* THROMBOLYSIS); (3) metal coils or other solid materials to block bleeding vessels or to thrombose *aneurysms (*see* EMBOLIZATION); (4) devices for monitoring pressures within important vessels (e.g. *Swan-Ganz catheters for monitoring pulmonary artery pressure in critically ill patients); or (5) balloons and *stents to relieve obstruction.

cation *n.* an ion of positive charge, such as a sodium ion (Na⁺). *Compare* ANION. *See* ELECTROLYTE.

cation-exchange resins complex insoluble chemical compounds that may be administered with the diet to alter the *electrolyte balance of the body in the treatment of heart, kidney, and metabolic disorders. For example, in patients on a strict low-sodium diet such resins combine with sodium in the food so that it cannot be absorbed and passes out in the faeces.

cat-scratch disease an infectious disease caused by the bacterium *Bartonella henselae*, which infects cats and is transmitted to humans by a cat scratch or bite. A papule or pustule develops at the site of the injury followed, a week to two months after infection, by swelling of the lymph nodes (usually those closest to the wound). Fever and malaise are common. The condition usually resolves without treatment but antibiotics may be given to prevent complications.

cauda *n.* a tail-like structure. The **cauda equina** is a bundle of nerve roots from the lumbar, sacral, and coccygeal spinal nerves that descend nearly vertically from the spinal cord until they reach their respective openings in the vertebral column.

caudal *adj.* relating to the lower part or tail end of the body.

caul *n.* **1.** (in obstetrics) the *amnion, either as a piece of membrane that covers an infant's head at birth or the entire unruptured sac that encloses the fetus during pregnancy. **2.** (in anatomy) *see* OMENTUM.

causal agent a factor associated with the definitive onset of an illness (or other response, including an accident). Examples are bacteria and trauma. The relationship is more direct than in the case of a *risk factor; in general, the ill health only occurs if the agent is a precursor.

causalgia *n.* an intensely unpleasant burning pain felt in a limb where there has

been partial damage to the sympathetic and somatic sensory nerves.

caustic *n.* an agent, such as silver nitrate, that destroys tissue. Caustic agents may be used to remove dead skin, warts, etc., but care must be taken not to damage the surrounding area.

caustic soda *see* SODIUM HYDROXIDE.

cauterize *vb.* to destroy tissues by direct application of a heated instrument (known as a **cautery**): used for the removal of small warts or other growths (*see also* CURETTAGE) and also to stop bleeding from small vessels. —**cautery** *n.*

Caverject *n. see* ALPROSTADIL.

cavernitis *n.* inflammation of the corpora cavernosa of the *penis or the corpus cavernosum of the clitoris.

cavernosography *n.* a radiological examination of the erectile tissue of the penis (*see* CORPUS CAVERNOSUM) that entails the infusion of *radiopaque contrast medium into the corpora cavernosa via a small butterfly needle. The contrast medium flow rate needed to maintain erection can be measured, and radiographs taken during the procedure give information regarding the veins draining the penis.

cavernosometry *n.* the measurement of pressure within the corpora cavernosa of the penis during infusion. The flow rate required to produce an erection is recorded and also the flow necessary to maintain the induced erection. The examination is important in the investigation of erectile dysfunction.

cavernous breathing *see* BREATH SOUNDS.

cavernous sinus one of the paired cavities within the *sphenoid bone, at the base of the skull behind the eye sockets, into which blood drains from the brain, eye, nose, and upper cheek before leaving the skull through connections with the internal jugular and facial veins. Through the sinus, in its walls, pass the internal carotid artery and the abducens, oculomotor, trochlear, ophthalmic, and maxillary nerves.

cavity *n.* **1.** (in anatomy) a hollow enclosed area; for example, the abdominal cavity or the buccal cavity (mouth). **2.** (in dentistry) **a.** the hole in a tooth caused by *caries or abrasion. **b.** the hole shaped in a tooth by a dentist to retain a filling.

cavity varnish (in dentistry) a solution of natural or synthetic resin in an organic solvent. It is used as a sealer for amalgam fillings or as a coating over newly inserted cement fillings.

CBT *see* COGNITIVE BEHAVIOURAL THERAPY.

CBW (chemical and biological warfare) the use of poisonous gases and other chemicals, bacteria, viruses, and toxins during war.

CCDC *see* CONSULTANT IN COMMUNICABLE DISEASE CONTROL.

C cells parafollicular cells of the thyroid gland, which are derived from neural crest tissue. They produce *calcitonin. *Medullary carcinoma of the thyroid has its origin in the C cells.

CCF congestive cardiac failure (*see* HEART FAILURE).

CCST Certification of Completion of Specialist Training. *See* CONSULTANT.

CCU *see* CORONARY CARE UNIT.

CD cluster of differentiation: a numerical system for classifying antigens expressed on the surface of lymphocytes. *See also* CD4.

CD4 a surface antigen on *helper T cells that is particularly important for immune resistance to viruses. It is also a receptor for the human immunodeficiency virus (HIV); progressive reduction of CD4-bearing T cells reflects the progression of *AIDS.

CDH 1. *see* CONGENITAL DIAPHRAGMATIC HERNIA. 2. *see* CONGENITAL DISLOCATION OF THE HIP.

C. diff *Clostridium difficile. See* CLOSTRIDIUM.

cefaclor *n.* a second-generation *cephalosporin antibiotic used in the treatment of otitis media, upper and lower respiratory-tract infections, urinary-tract infections, and skin infections. It is administered by mouth; side-effects include diarrhoea and skin eruptions. Trade name: **Distaclor**.

cefadroxil *n.* a first-generation *cephalosporin antibiotic used in the treatment of urinary-tract infections, skin infections, pharyngitis, and tonsillitis. It is administered by mouth; side-effects include skin rash and generalized itching. Trade name: **Baxan**.

cefalexin *n.* a first-generation *cephalo-

sporin antibiotic used in the treatment of respiratory-tract, genitourinary-tract, and skin infections and otitis media. It is administered by mouth; diarrhoea is the most common side-effect. Trade names: **Ceporex, Keflex**.

cefotaxime *n. see* CEPHALOSPORIN.

ceftazidime *n.* a third-generation *cephalosporin antibiotic that has good activity against Gram-negative bacteria (including *Pseudomonas*). It is administered by intravenous or intramuscular injection for the treatment of urinary and respiratory tract infections, cellulitis, meningitis, and septicaemia. Side-effects include reaction at the site of injection, diarrhoea, and hypersensitivity reactions. Trade names: **Fortum, Kefadim**.

cefuroxime *n.* a second-generation *cephalosporin antibiotic that is less susceptible to beta-lactamase enzymes than the older members of the group. It is used in the treatment of infections of the urinary and lower respiratory tracts and the skin, Lyme disease, gonorrhoea, epiglottitis, meningitis, and otitis media. It is usually administered by injection. Side-effects include nausea, diarrhoea, and rash. Trade names: **Zinacef, Zinnat**.

-cele (-coele) *combining form denoting* swelling, hernia, or tumour. Example: **gastrocele** (hernia of the stomach).

celecoxib *n.* an anti-inflammatory drug (*see* NSAID) that selectively inhibits cyclooxygenase 2 (*see* COX-2 INHIBITOR). It is taken by mouth in the treatment of osteoarthritis, rheumatoid arthritis, and ankylosing spondylitis. Trade name: **Celebrex**.

cell *n.* the basic unit of all living organisms, which can reproduce itself exactly (*see* MITOSIS). Each cell is bounded by a **cell membrane** of lipids and protein, which controls the passage of substances into and out of the cell. Cells contain *cytoplasm, in which are suspended a *nucleus and other structures (*organelles) specialized to carry out particular activities in the cell (see illustration).

Complex organisms are built up of millions of cells that are specially adapted to carry out particular functions. The process of cell differentiation begins early on in the development of the embryo and cells of a particular type (e.g. blood cells, liver cells) always give rise to cells of the same type. Each cell has a particular number of *chro-

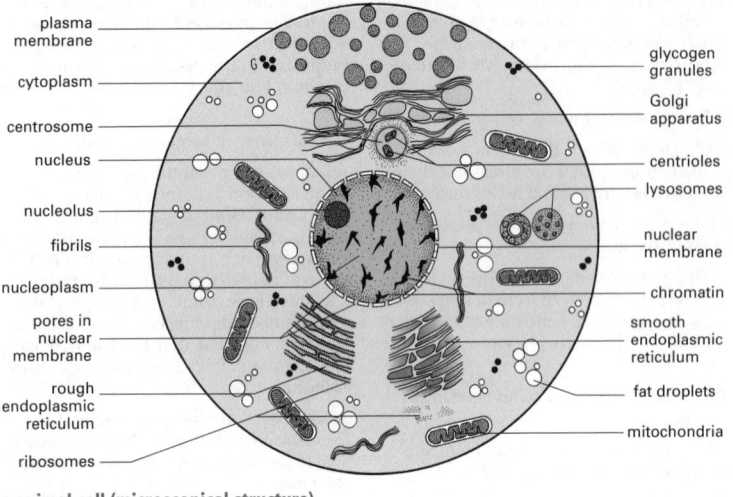

plasma membrane

cytoplasm

centrosome

nucleus

nucleolus

fibrils

nucleoplasm

pores in nuclear membrane

rough endoplasmic reticulum

ribosomes

glycogen granules

Golgi apparatus

centrioles

lysosomes

nuclear membrane

chromatin

smooth endoplasmic reticulum

fat droplets

mitochondria

An animal cell (microscopical structure).

mosomes in its nucleus. The sex cells (sperm and ova) always contain half the number of chromosomes of all the other cells of the body (*see* MEIOSIS); at fertilization a sperm and ovum combine to form a cell with a complete set of chromosomes that will develop into the embryo.

cell body (perikaryon) the enlarged portion of a *neuron (nerve cell), containing the nucleus. It is concerned more with the nutrition of the cell than with propagation of nerve impulses.

cell division reproduction of cells by division first of the chromosomes (karyokinesis) and then of the cytoplasm (cytokinesis). Cell division to produce more body (somatic) cells is by *mitosis; cell division during the formation of gametes is by *meiosis.

cellophane maculopathy *see* EPIRETINAL MEMBRANE.

cell saver (intraoperative cell salvage device) a machine that aspirates blood lost during surgery and spins, washes, and filters it for retransfusion back into the patient's body (*see* AUTOTRANSFUSION). The device is used in surgery that has significant blood loss, such as orthopaedic and vascular surgery, and avoids the costs and risks of *allogeneic transfusion.

cell-surface molecules molecules on the surface of cell membranes that are responsible for most cellular functions directly related to their immediate environment. Many have very precise functions of adhesion (*see* ADHESION MOLECULES), metabolic exchange, hormone reception, respiration, and immune reactions. Cell-to-cell exchanges involve specialized surface structures (junctions), which form a communicating nexus.

cellulitis *n.* an infection of the deep layers of the skin and subcutaneous tissue by staphylococci, streptococci, or other bacteria. The patient is systemically unwell and feverish. It is most common on the lower legs and there may be associated *lymphangitis and *lymphadenitis. It is otherwise similar to *erysipelas, but the margins are less clearly defined because the infection is deeper. Intravenous antibiotics are often required.

cellulose *n.* a carbohydrate consisting of linked glucose units. It is an important constituent of plant cell walls. Cellulose cannot be digested by humans and is a component of *dietary fibre (roughage).

Celsius temperature (centigrade temperature) temperature expressed on a scale in which the melting point of ice is assigned a temperature of 0° and the boiling point of water a temperature of 100°. For many medical purposes this scale has superseded the Fahrenheit scale (*see* FAHRENHEIT TEMPERATURE). The formula for converting from Celsius (C) to Fahrenheit (F) is: $F = 9/5C + 32$. [A. Celsius (1701–44), Swedish astronomer]

CEMACH Confidential Enquiry into Maternal Deaths and Child Health. *See* CONFIDENTIAL ENQUIRIES.

cement *n.* **1.** any of a group of materials used in dentistry either as fillings or as *lutes for crowns. *Glass ionomer cements are used for filling, and zinc phosphate, zinc polycarboxylate, and glass ionomer cements are used for luting. Zinc oxide–eugenol cements are widely used as temporary fillings or as an impression material. **2.** a fast-setting material used to fix prostheses (e.g. artificial hips) in place. **3.** *see* CEMENTUM.

cementocyte *n.* a cell found in cementum.

cementoma *n.* a benign overgrowth of cementum.

cementum (cement) *n.* a thin layer of hard tissue on the surface of the root of a *tooth. It attaches the fibres of the *periodontal membrane to the tooth.

censor *n.* (in psychology) the mechanism, postulated by Freud, that suppresses or modifies desires that are inappropriate or feared. The censor is usually regarded as being located in the *superego but was also described by Freud as being in the *ego itself.

census *n.* a ten-yearly enumeration of the population based on the actual presence of individuals in a house or institution on a designated night (known as a **de facto census**). This contrasts with the approach in the USA, where enumeration is based on official address (**de jure census**).

-centesis *combining form denoting* puncture or perforation. Example: **amniocentesis** (surgical puncture of the amnion).

centi- *prefix denoting* one hundredth or a hundred.

centigrade temperature *see* CELSIUS TEMPERATURE.

centile chart a graph with lines showing average measurements of height, weight, and head circumference compared with age and sex, against which the physical development of a child or fetus can be assessed. The lines of growth on the graph are called **centiles**, and the number of a centile predicts the percentage of individuals who are below that measurement for a given age; for example, the 10th centile means that 10% of the age- and sex-matched population will be smaller and 90% will be bigger. A child or fetus will normally follow a particular centile, but if growth crosses centiles or lies outside the 97th or 3rd centiles, further investigation may be warranted.

central auditory processing disorder
see AUDITORY PROCESSING DISORDER.

central island an area of significant irregular astigmatism seen on *corneal topography after laser refractive surgery. It may affect the postoperative outcome.

central nervous system (CNS) the *brain and the *spinal cord, as opposed to the cranial and spinal nerves and the *autonomic nervous system, which together form the peripheral nervous system. The CNS is responsible for the *integration of all nervous activities.

central serous chorioretinopathy
shallow *retinal detachment in the area of the macula due to a localized leakage through the retinal pigment epithelium (*see* RETINA) into the subretinal space. The cause is unknown. It affects young adult males, causing reduced or distorted central vision that usually settles in a few months.

central venous catheter an intravenous catheter for insertion directly into a large vein, most commonly the subclavian vein, during its passage under the clavicle, or the jugular in the neck. Such catheters can also be inserted into the femoral vein at the groin. They enable intravenous drugs and fluids to be given and intravenous pressures to be measured, which is often useful during operations or in intensive care. Central venous catheters must be inserted under strictly sterile conditions using a local anaesthetic.

central venous pressure (CVP) the pressure of blood within the right atrium. Measurement of CVP is obtained by *catheterization of the right side of the heart; the catheter is attached to a manometer. CVP measurements are used to estimate circulatory function and blood volume in cases of shock or severe haemorrhage and to monitor blood replacement. In a recumbent patient, with the zero point of the manometer level with the mid-axilla (centre of the armpit), CVP should measure between 5 and 8 cm saline under normal conditions. In clinical practice the CVP is often estimated by inspecting the *jugular venous pressure (JVP).

centre *n.* (in neurology) a collection of neurons (nerve cells) whose activities control a particular function. The **respiratory** and **cardiovascular centres**, for example, are regions in the lower brainstem that control the movements of respiration and the functioning of the circulatory system, respectively.

centrencephalic *adj.* (in electroencephalography) describing discharges that can be recorded synchronously from all parts of the brain. The source of this activity is in the *reticular formation of the midbrain. **Centrencephalic epilepsy** is associated with a congenital predisposition to seizures.

centri- *combining form denoting* centre. Example: **centrilobular** (in the centre of a lobule (especially of the liver)).

centrifugal *adj.* moving away from a centre, as from the brain to the peripheral tissues.

centrifuge *n.* a device for separating components of different densities in a liquid, using centrifugal force. The liquid is placed in special containers that are spun at high speed around a central axis.

centriole *n.* a small particle found in the cytoplasm of cells, near the nucleus. Centrioles are involved in the formation of the *spindle and aster during cell division. During interphase there are usually two centrioles in the *centrosome; when cell division occurs these separate and move to opposite sides of the nucleus, and the spindle is formed between them.

centripetal *adj.* moving towards a centre, as from the peripheral tissues to the brain.

centromere (kinetochore) *n.* the part of a chromosome that joins the two *chromatids to each other and becomes attached to the spindle during *mitosis and *meiosis. When chromosome division takes place the centromeres split longitudinally.

centrosome (centrosphere) *n.* an area of clear cytoplasm, found next to the nucleus in nondividing cells, that contains the *centrioles.

centrosphere *n.* **1.** an area of clear cytoplasm seen in dividing cells around the poles of the spindle. **2.** *see* CENTROSOME.

centrum *n.* (*pl.* **centra**) the solid rodshaped central portion of a *vertebra.

cephal- (cephalo-) *combining form denoting* the head. Example: **cephalalgia** (pain in).

cephalad *adj.* towards the head.

cephalhaematoma *n.* a swelling on the head caused by a collection of bloody fluid between one or more of the skull bones (usually the *parietal bone) and its covering membrane (periosteum). It is most commonly seen in newborn infants delivered with the aid of forceps or vacuum extraction or subjected to pressures during passage through the birth canal. No treatment is necessary and the swelling disappears in a few months. If it is extensive, the blood in the fluid may break down, releasing bilirubin into the bloodstream and causing *jaundice. A cephalhaematoma in an older baby or child is evidence of some recent injury to the head; occasionally an unsuspected fracture is revealed on X-ray. *See also* CHIGNON, SUBAPONEUROTIC HAEMORRHAGE.

cephalic *adj.* of or relating to the head.

cephalic index a measure of the shape of a skull, commonly used in *craniometry: the ratio of the greatest breadth, multiplied by 100, to the greatest length of the skull. *See also* BRACHYCEPHALY, DOLICHOCEPHALY.

cephalic version (external cephalic version) a procedure in which a fetus that is lying in the breech position is turned so that its head will enter the birth canal first. It may give rise to complications (e.g. abruptio placentae) and is therefore only carried out in selected cases.

cephalin *n.* one of a group of *phospholipids that are constituents of cell membranes and are particularly abundant in brain.

cephalocele *n. see* NEURAL TUBE DEFECTS.

cephalogram *n.* a special standardized X-ray picture that can be used to measure alterations in the growth of skull bones.

cephalometry *n.* the study of facial growth by examination of standardized lateral radiographs of the head. It is used mainly for diagnosis in *orthodontics.

cephalopelvic disproportion (CPD) the state in which the diameter of the fetal head is greater than the pelvic outlet, preventing successful vaginal delivery. This may be relative when there is *malposition of the vertex (back of the head) or absolute when the vertex is in the occipitoanterior position (*see* OC-CIPUT), and can only be considered when the cervix is fully dilated.

cephalosporin *n.* any one of a group of semisynthetic *beta-lactam antibiotics, derived from the mould *Cephalosporium*, which are effective against a wide range of microorganisms and are therefore used in a variety of infections. The older (first-generation) cephalosporins include *cefadroxil and *cefalexin; more recent (second-generation) drugs include *cefaclor, *cefuroxime, and **cefotaxime**. Third-generation cephalosporins, such as *ceftazidime, **cefotaxime**, **cefpodoxime** (Orelox), and **ceftriaxone** (Rocephin), have greater activity against Gram-negative bacteria. Cross-sensitivity with penicillin may occur and the principal side-effects are allergic reactions and irritation of the digestive tract.

CEPOD Confidential Enquiry into Peri-Operative Deaths: an influential enquiry by the Royal College of Surgeons of England that is used to monitor standards of surgical treatment. *See also* CONFIDENTIAL ENQUIRIES.

CERA *see* CORTICAL EVOKED RESPONSE AUDIOMETRY.

cercaria *n.* (*pl.* **cercariae**) the final larval stage of any parasitic trematode (*see* FLUKE). The cercariae, which have tails but otherwise resemble the adults, are released into water from the snail host in which the parasite undergoes part of its development. Several thousand cercariae may emerge from a single snail in a day.

cerebellum *n.* the largest part of the hindbrain, bulging back behind the pons and the medulla oblongata and overhung by the occipital lobes of the cerebrum. Like the cerebrum, it has an outer grey cortex and a core of white matter. Three broad bands of nerve fibres – the inferior, middle, and superior cerebellar peduncles – connect it to the medulla, the pons, and the midbrain respectively. It has two hemispheres, one on each side of the central region (the **vermis**), and its surface is thrown into thin folds called

The cerebellum (anterior view).

folia (see illustration). Within lie four pairs of nuclei.

The cerebellum is essential for the maintenance of muscle tone, balance, and the synchronization of activity in groups of muscles under voluntary control, converting muscular contractions into smooth coordinated movement. It does not, however, initiate movement and plays no part in the perception of conscious sensations or in intelligence. —**cerebellar** *adj.*

cerebr- (**cerebri-**, **cerebro-**) *combining form denoting* the cerebrum or brain.

cerebral abscess *see* ABSCESS.

cerebral aqueduct (aqueduct of Sylvius) the narrow channel, containing cerebrospinal fluid, that connects the third and fourth *ventricles of the brain.

cerebral cortex the intricately folded outer layer of the *cerebrum, making up some 40% of the brain by weight and composed of an estimated 15 thousand million neurons (*see* GREY MATTER). This is the part of the brain most directly responsible for consciousness, with essential roles in perception, memory, thought, mental ability, and intellect, and it is responsible for initiating voluntary activity. It has connections, direct or indirect, with all parts of the body. The folding of the cortex provides a large surface area, the greater part lying in the clefts (**sulci**), which divide the upraised convolutions (**gyri**). On the basis of its microscopic appearance in section, the cortex is mapped into *Brodmann areas; it is also divided into functional regions; including *motor cortex, *sensory cortex, and *association areas.

Within, and continuous with it, lies the *white matter, through which connection is made with the rest of the nervous system.

cerebral haemorrhage bleeding from a cerebral blood vessel into the tissue of the brain. It is commonly caused by degenerative disease of the arteries and high blood pressure but it may result from bleeding from congenital abnormalities of blood vessels. The extent and severity of the symptoms depend upon the site and volume of the haemorrhage; they vary from a transient weakness or numbness to profound coma and death. *See also* ATHEROMA, HYPERTENSION, STROKE.

cerebral hemisphere one of the two paired halves of the *cerebrum.

cerebral palsy a disorder of movement and/or posture as a result of nonprogressive but permanent damage to the developing brain. This damage may occur before, during, or immediately after delivery and has many causes, including an inadequate supply of oxygen to the brain, low levels of glucose in the blood (*hypoglycaemia), and infection. It is often associated with other problems, such as learning difficulties, hearing difficulties, poor speech, poor balance, and epilepsy. There are three main types of cerebral palsy: **spastic**, in which the limbs are difficult to control and which may affect the whole body (quadriplegic), one side of the body (hemiplegic), or both legs (diplegic); **ataxic hypotonic**, in which the main problem is poor balance and uncoordinated movements; and **dyskinetic**, in which there is involuntary movement of the limbs. Management requires a multidisciplinary approach, the main components of which are physiotherapy, speech and language therapy, educational assistance, and appropriate appliances.

((⊕)) SEE WEB LINKS

- Website of Scope, the UK's leading cerebral palsy charity

cerebral tumour an abnormal multiplication of brain cells. Any tumorous swelling tends to compress or even destroy the healthy brain cells surrounding it and – because of the rigid closed nature of the skull – increases the pressure on the brain tissue. Malignant brain tumours, which are much more common in children than in adults, include *medulloblastomas and *gliomas; these grow rapidly, spreading through the otherwise normal brain tissue and causing progressive neurological disability. Benign tumours, such as *meningiomas, grow slowly and compress the brain tissue. Both benign and malignant tumours commonly cause fits. Benign tumours are often cured by total surgical resection. Malignant tumours may be treated by neurosurgery, chemotherapy, and radiotherapy, but the outcome for most patients remains poor.

cerebration *n.* 1. the functioning of the brain as a whole. 2. the unconscious activities of the brain.

cerebroside *n.* one of a group of compounds occurring in the *myelin sheaths of nerve fibres. They are *glycolipids, containing a sphingolipid bound to a sugar, usually galactose (in **galactocerebrosides**) or glucose (in **glucocerebrosides**).

cerebrospinal fever (spotted fever) *see* MENINGITIS.

cerebrospinal fluid (CSF) the clear watery fluid that surrounds the brain and spinal cord. It is contained in the *subarachnoid space and circulates in the *ventricles of the brain and in the central canal of the spinal cord. The brain floats in the fluid (its weight so being reduced from about 1400 g to less than 100 g) and is cushioned by it from contact with the skull when the head is moved vigorously. The CSF is secreted by the *choroid plexuses in the ventricles, circulates through them to reach the subarachnoid space, and is eventually absorbed into the bloodstream through the *arachnoid villi. Its normal contents are glucose, salts, enzymes, and a few white cells, but no red blood cells.

cerebrovascular disease any disorder of the blood vessels of the brain and its covering membranes (meninges). Most cases are due to atheroma and/or hypertension, clinical effects being caused by rupture of diseased blood vessels (*cerebral or *subarachnoid haemorrhage) or inadequacy of the blood supply to the brain (ischaemia), due to cerebral thrombosis or embolism. The term **cerebrovascular accident** is given to the clinical syndrome accompanying a sudden and sometimes severe attack, which leads to a *stroke.

cerebrum (telencephalon) *n.* the largest and most highly developed part of the brain, composed of the two **cerebral hemispheres**, separated from each other by the **longitudi-**

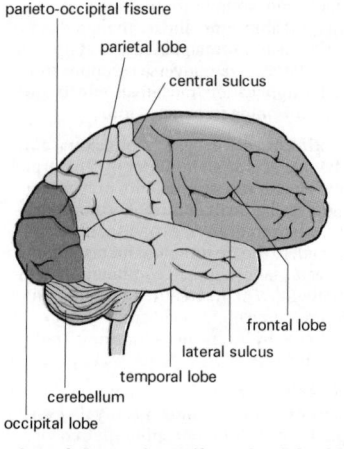

parieto-occipital fissure

parietal lobe

central sulcus

frontal lobe

lateral sulcus

temporal lobe

cerebellum

occipital lobe

Lobes of the cerebrum (from the right side).

nal fissure in the midline (see illustration). Each hemisphere has an outer layer of grey matter, the *cerebral cortex, below which lies white matter containing the *basal ganglia. Connecting the two hemispheres at the bottom of the longitudinal fissure is the **corpus callosum**, a massive bundle of nerve fibres. Within each hemisphere is a crescent-shaped fluid-filled cavity (lateral *ventricle), connected to the central third ventricle in the *diencephalon. The cerebrum is responsible for the initiation and coordination of all voluntary activity in the body and for governing the functioning of lower parts of the nervous system. The cortex is the seat of all intelligent behaviour. —**cerebral** *adj*.

cerumen (earwax) *n*. the waxy material that is secreted by the sebaceous glands in the external auditory meatus of the outer ear. Its function is to protect the delicate skin that lines the inside of the meatus.

cervic- (cervico-) *combining form denoting* **1.** the neck. Example: **cervicodynia** (pain in). **2.** the cervix, especially of the uterus. Example: **cervicectomy** (surgical removal of).

cervical *adj*. **1.** of or relating to the neck. **2.** of, relating to, or affecting the cervix (neck region) of an organ, especially the cervix of the uterus.

cervical cancer (cervical carcinoma) cancer of the neck (cervix) of the uterus. The tumour may develop from the surface epithelium of the cervix (squamous carci-

noma) or from the epithelial lining of the cervical canal (adenocarcinoma). In both cases the tumour is invasive, spreading to involve surrounding tissue and subsequently to neighbouring lymph nodes and adjacent organs, such as the bladder and rectum. Cancer of the cervix can be detected in an early stage of development (*see* CERVICAL SCREENING) and diagnosis is established by biopsy (*see* COLPOSCOPY). In carcinoma in situ (*see* CERVICAL INTRAEPITHELIAL NEOPLASIA) the tumour is confined to the epithelium: there is no invasion of surrounding tissue but, if untreated (by local ablation, *LLETZ, or surgical excision), it can become invasive. Common early features of invasive disease are abnormal vaginal bleeding and a foul-smelling blood-stained vaginal discharge. Treatment is by surgery with or without postoperative radiotherapy. *See also* HUMAN PAPILLOMAVIRUS.

cervical cerclage a procedure to help prevent *preterm delivery. It involves inserting a suture around the cervix of the uterus, either transvaginally or transabdominally, to keep it closed and reduce the possibility of preterm cervical dilatation and rupture of membranes.

cervical ectopy *see* ECTROPION.

cervical fracture a fracture of a vertebra in the neck (*see* CERVICAL VERTEBRAE). Cervical fractures range from minor, requiring no treatment, to those associated with paralysis and instant death. Treatment can be support with a collar, skull traction, an *orthosis attached to the skull, or surgery, depending on the severity of the fracture.

cervical incompetence spontaneous dilatation of the cervix of the uterus during the second trimester of pregnancy. The membranes bulge and subsequently rupture, and the fetus is expelled prematurely. It may be caused by forcible dilatation of the cervix during the operation of *dilatation and curettage or it may be related to laceration of the cervix during a previous confinement or to previous cervical surgical procedures (e.g. knife *cone biopsy).

cervical intraepithelial neoplasia (CIN) cellular changes in the cervix of the uterus preceding the invasive stages of *cervical cancer. The CIN grading system distinguishes three stages: **CIN 1** (mild dysplasia); **CIN 2** (moderate dysplasia); and **CIN 3** (severe dysplasia, *carcinoma in situ). CIN is uncommon after the menopause. Treatment may be by local ablation (e.g. cryocautery, electrodiathermy, or carbon dioxide *laser vaporization) or surgical excision (e.g. *LLETZ, *cone biopsy, or hysterectomy).

cervical screening *screening tests to detect the presence of precancerous changes in the cervix (neck) of the uterus (see CERVICAL INTRAEPITHELIAL NEOPLASIA). *Cervical smears are the standard first-line screening tools in most countries: screening programmes based on the traditional **Papanicolaou (Pap) test** have been mostly superseded by *liquid-based cytology. *Colposcopy is indicated when abnormal cells (*dyskaryosis) are detected.

cervical smear a specimen of cellular material scraped from the *transformation zone of the cervix (neck) of the uterus that is stained and examined under a microscope in order to detect cell abnormalities indicating the presence of precancerous change. *See* CERVICAL SCREENING.

cervical vertebrae the seven bones making up the neck region of the *backbone. The first cervical vertebra – the **atlas** – consists basically of a ring of bone that supports the skull by articulating with the occipital condyles (see OCCIPITAL BONE). The second vertebra – the **axis** – has an upward-pointing process (the **odontoid process** or **dens**) that forms a pivot on which the atlas can rotate, enabling the head to be turned. *See also* VERTEBRA.

cervicitis *n.* inflammation of the neck (cervix) of the uterus.

cervix *n.* a necklike part, especially the **cervix uteri** (neck of the uterus), which projects at its lower end into the vagina. The cervical canal passes through it, linking the cavity of the uterus with the vagina; the canal is lined with mucous membrane (see ENDOCERVIX) and normally contains mucus, the viscosity of which changes throughout the menstrual cycle. The cervix is capable of wide dilation during childbirth.

CESDI Confidential Enquiries into Stillbirths and Deaths in Infancy. *See* CONFIDENTIAL ENQUIRIES.

cestode *n. see* TAPEWORM.

cetirizine *n. see* ANTIHISTAMINE.

cetrimide *n.* a detergent disinfectant used alone or in combination for cleansing skin

surfaces and wounds, for treating minor burns and abrasions, and as an ingredient of *barrier creams for napkin rash and pressure sores. There are few adverse reactions from external application; most toxic effects are due to poisoning from ingestion.

cetuximab *n.* a drug (a *monoclonal antibody) that acts as an inhibitor of *epidermal growth factor receptor (EGFR), preventing tumour-cell growth. It is used, in combination with irinotecan (see TOPOISOMERASE INHIBITOR), in the treatment of metastatic colorectal cancer and, in combination with radiotherapy, in the treatment of squamous cell carcinoma of the head and neck. It is administered by intravenous infusion. Trade name: **Erbitux**.

CFS/ME/PVF a condition, known variously as **chronic fatigue syndrome**, **myalgic encephalomyelitis** (or **encephalopathy**), or **postviral fatigue syndrome**, characterized by extreme disabling fatigue that has lasted for at least six months, is made worse by physical or mental exertion, does not resolve with bed rest, and cannot be attributed to other disorders. The fatigue is accompanied by at least some of the following: muscle pain or weakness (*fibromyalgia), poor coordination, joint pain, recurrent sore throat, slight fever, painful lymph nodes in the neck and armpits, depression, cognitive impairment (especially an inability to concentrate), and general malaise. The cause is unknown, but in some cases some viral conditions (especially glandular fever) are thought to trigger the disease; however, no viral aetiology has yet been identified. Treatment is restricted to relieving the symptoms and helping sufferers to plan their lives with a minimum of energy expenditure. Graded physiotherapy may be helpful in some cases. Many psychiatrists consider CFS/ME/PVF to be a mood disorder and use behavioural and cognitive techniques as well as antidepressants to treat it.

(⊕) SEE WEB LINKS

• Website of Action for ME: includes information for health-care professionals

Chagas' disease a disease caused by the protozoan parasite *Trypanosoma cruzi*. It is transmitted to humans when the trypanosomes, present in the faeces of nocturnal bloodsucking *reduviid bugs, come into contact with wounds and scratches on the skin or the delicate internal tissues of the nose and mouth. The presence of the parasite in the heart muscles and central nervous system results in serious inflammation and lesions, which can prove fatal. The disease, limited to poor rural areas of South and Central America, is especially prevalent in children and young adults. It may be treated with nifurtimox. *See also* TRYPANOSOMIASIS. [C. Chagas (1879–1934), Brazilian physician]

chaining *n.* (in psychology) a technique of *behaviour modification in which a complex skill is taught by being broken down into its separate components, which are gradually built up into the full sequence. Usually the last component in the sequence is taught first, because it is this component that is followed by *reinforcement: this is termed **backwards chaining**.

chalazion (meibomian cyst) *n.* a swollen sebaceous (meibomian) gland in the eyelid caused by blockage of its duct. The gland becomes inflamed and converted into a jelly-like mass, producing disfigurement of the lid. It may disappear spontaneously over a period of time but treatment by application of antibiotic ointments and/or surgical incision and curettage will result in its rapid cure.

chalcosis *n.* the deposition of copper in the tissues of the eye, usually resulting from the presence of a copper foreign body within the eye.

chancre *n.* a painless ulcer that develops at the site where infection enters the body, e.g. on the lips, penis, urethra, or eyelid. It is the primary symptom of such infections as sleeping sickness and syphilis.

chancroid *n. see* SOFT SORE.

channelopathy *n.* an inherited condition predisposing to arrhythmia that is characterized by a genetic mutation affecting one of the cell membrane channels responsible for transport of ions (e.g. potassium or sodium) into or out of the cardiac cells.

CHAPS *see* CHILDREN'S AUDITORY PERFORMANCE SCALE.

Charcot-Leyden crystals fine colourless sharp-pointed crystals seen in the sputum of asthmatics. [J. M. Charcot (1825–93), French neurologist; E. V. von Leyden (1832–1910), German physician]

Charcot-Marie-Tooth disease (peroneal muscular atrophy) a group of inherited diseases of the peripheral nerves, also known as

hereditary sensorimotor neuropathy, causing a gradually progressive weakness and wasting of the muscles of the legs and the lower part of the thighs. The hands and arms are eventually affected. The genetic defect responsible for the most common form, type Ia, is a duplication on chromosome 17. The diagnosis is made by nerve conduction tests followed by genetic blood tests. [J. M. Charcot; P. Marie (1853–1940), French physician; H. H. Tooth (1856–1925), British physician]

Charcot's joint *see* NEUROPATHIC ARTHRITIS. [J. M. Charcot]

Charcot's triad the combination of pain, fever (and rigors), and jaundice that can indicate acute *cholangitis. [J. M. Charcot]

Charnley clamps an apparatus used to encourage *arthrodesis between the ends of two bones on either side of a joint. Parallel pins driven through the bone ends are connected on each side of the joint by bolts bearing wing nuts; tightening of the screw arrangements forces the surfaces of the bones together. When the two bones have joined, by growth and reshaping, the clamps can be removed. [Sir J. Charnley (1911–82), British orthopaedic surgeon]

CHART *n.* *c*ontinuous *h*yperfractionated *a*ccelerated *r*adio*t*herapy: a radiotherapy technique aimed at the rapid destruction of tumour cells when they are actively proliferating – and therefore most sensitive to radiation – by treating them several times a day over a greatly shortened total treatment time. The technique has been shown to be of benefit in the treatment of lung cancer and locally advanced head and neck cancer.

Chediak-Higashi syndrome a rare fatal hereditary (autosomal *recessive) condition causing enlargement of the liver and spleen, albinism, and abnormalities of the eye. It is thought to be due to a disorder of glycolipid metabolism. [A. Chediak (20th century), Cuban physician; O. Higashi (20th century) Japanese paediatrician]

cheil- (cheilo-) *combining form denoting* the lip(s). Example: **cheiloplasty** (plastic surgery of).

cheilectomy *n.* a surgical procedure involving the removal of *osteophytes from around a degenerate joint to regain further range of motion. It is commonly performed in degenerative arthritis of the big toe (*see* HALLUX RIGIDUS).

cheilitis *n.* inflammation of the lips. **Angular cheilitis** affects the angles of the lips and may be caused by a staphylococcal or candidal infection, though mechanical, nutritional, and immune factors may be implicated.

cheiloplasty *n. see* LABIOPLASTY.

cheiloschisis *n. see* CLEFT LIP.

cheilosis *n.* swollen cracked bright-red lips. This is a common symptom of many nutritional disorders, including ariboflavinosis (vitamin B_2 deficiency).

cheir- (cheiro-) *combining form denoting* the hand(s). Examples: **cheiralgia** (pain in); **cheiroplasty** (plastic surgery of).

cheiroarthropathy *n.* the restricted hand movement seen in long-standing diabetes. Due to chronic thickening of the skin limiting joint flexibility, it is part of the *diabetic hand syndrome.

cheiropompholyx (acute vesicular eczema of the hands) *n.* a type of blistering *eczema affecting the palms and fingers. The thickness of the skin in these areas prevents the pinhead vesicles from breaking and eventually the skin peels after a period of intense itching. *See* POMPHOLYX.

chelating agent a chemical compound that forms complexes by binding metal ions. Some chelating agents, including *desferrioxamine and *penicillamine, are drugs used to treat metal poisoning: the metal is bound to the drug and excreted safely. Chelating agents often form the active centres of enzymes.

chem- (chemo-) *combining form denoting* chemical or chemistry.

chemodectoma *n.* a former name for *paraganglioma.

chemoembolization *n.* a procedure in which the blood supply to a tumour is blocked with a synthetic embolic agent and cytotoxic drugs are then administered directly into the tumour. It is most frequently used for the treatment of liver cancer.

chemokine *n.* any one of a group of small proteins that guide leucocytes to sites of infection and are vital for immune function. They fall into two main classes, CC chemokines and CXC chemokines; receptors (denoted R) are named after the class that bind to them, and subtypes of each class are indicated by numbers (e.g. CCR5).

chemoradiotherapy *n.* the use of concurrent chemotherapy with radical irradiation in the treatment of malignant disease. Combined treatment in this way offers higher response rates, particularly in some gastrointestinal malignancies, such as rectal cancer and (particularly) anal cancer. It is also of proven benefit in locally advanced squamous cancers, such as those arising from the head and neck region or the cervix of the uterus.

chemoreceptor *n.* a cell or group of cells that responds to the presence of specific chemical compounds by initiating an impulse in a sensory nerve. Chemoreceptors are found in the taste buds and in the mucous membranes of the nose. *See also* RECEPTOR.

chemosis *n.* swelling (oedema) of the *conjunctiva. It is usually due to inflammation but may occur if the drainage of blood and lymph from around the eye is obstructed.

chemotaxis *n.* movement of a cell or organism in response to the stimulus of a gradient of chemical concentration.

chemotherapy *n.* the prevention or treatment of disease by the use of chemical substances. The term is increasingly restricted to the treatment of cancer with antimetabolites and similar drugs (*see* CYTOTOXIC DRUG) in contrast to *radiotherapy, but is also still sometimes used for antibiotic and other treatment of infectious diseases.

cherry angioma *see* ANGIOMA.

chest *n. see* THORAX.

Cheyne-Stokes respiration a striking form of breathing in which there is a cyclical variation in the rate, which becomes slower until breathing stops for several seconds before speeding up to a peak and then slowing again. It occurs when the sensitivity of the respiratory centres in the brain is impaired, particularly in states of coma. [J. Cheyne (1777–1836), Scottish physician; W. Stokes (1804–78), Irish physician]

chiasma *n.* (*pl.* **chiasmata**) (in genetics) the point at which homologous chromosomes remain in contact after they have started to separate in the first division of *meiosis. Chiasmata occur from the end of prophase to anaphase and represent the point at which mutual exchange of genetic material takes place (*see* CROSSING OVER).

chickenpox *n.* a highly infectious disease caused by a *herpesvirus (the varicella-zoster virus) that is transmitted by airborne droplets. After an incubation period of 11–18 days a mild fever develops, followed after about 24 hours by an itchy rash of red pimples that soon change to vesicles. These usually start on the trunk or scalp and spread to the face and limbs; they crust over and resolve after about 12 days. Treatment is aimed at reducing the fever and controlling the itching (e.g. by the application of calamine lotion). Complications are rare but include secondary infection and occasionally *encephalitis. The patient is infectious from the onset of symptoms until all the spots have gone. One attack usually confers life-long immunity, although the virus may reactivate at a later date and cause shingles (*see* HERPES). In adult patients who are particularly vulnerable, e.g. those with AIDS or who are otherwise immunosuppressed, chickenpox can be a serious disease, which may be treated with *aciclovir. Medical name: **varicella**.

chiclero's ulcer a form of *leishmaniasis of the skin caused by the parasite *Leishmania tropica mexicana*. The disease, occurring in Panama, Honduras, and the Amazon, primarily affects men who visit the forests to collect chicle (gum) and takes the form of an ulcerating lesion on the ear lobe. The sore usually heals spontaneously within six months.

Chief Medical Officer (CMO) the government's most senior medical adviser, who is responsible to the Secretary of State for Health for all of the *Department of Health's medical matters. There are separate CMOs for England, Scotland, Wales, and Northern Ireland.

Chief Nursing Officer the government's chief nursing adviser, who is responsible for providing an expert professional contribution and advice on nursing, midwifery, and health visiting matters to ministers and senior officials. There are separate Chief Nursing Officers for England, Scotland, Wales, and Northern Ireland.

chigger *n. see* TROMBICULA.

chignon *n.* a temporary swelling on the head seen in *newborn infants delivered with

the aid of vacuum suction. *See also* CEPHAL-HAEMATOMA, SUBAPONEUROTIC HAEMOR-RHAGE.

chigoe *n. see* TUNGA.

chikungunya fever a disease, occurring in Africa and Asia, caused by an *arbovirus and transmitted to humans by mosquitoes of the genus *Aëdes*. The disease is similar to *dengue and symptoms include fever, headache, joint and muscle pain, and an irritating rash. The patient is given drugs to relieve the pain and reduce the fever; the joint pain, which may progress to arthritis, can persist for up to 3 years after the infection.

chilblains (perniosis) *pl. n.* dusky red itchy swellings that develop on the extremities in cold weather. They usually settle in two weeks but treatment with *nifedipine is helpful in severe cases. There may be a genetic predisposition to chilblains.

child abuse the maltreatment of children. It may take the form of **sexual abuse**, when a child is involved in sexual activity with an adult; **physical abuse**, when physical injury is caused by cruelty or undue punishment (*see* NONACCIDENTAL INJURY); **neglect**, when basic physical provision for needs is lacking; and **emotional abuse**, when lack of affection and/or hostility from caregivers damage a child's emotional development (*see* ATTACHMENT DISORDER).

(( )) SEE WEB LINKS

• ChildLine website: advice on physical, emotional, and sexual abuse together with a confidential helpline

childbirth *n. see* LABOUR.

child health clinic (in Britain) a special clinic for the routine care of infants and preschool children, formerly known as a **child welfare centre**. Sometimes these clinics are staffed by doctors, *health visitors, and clinic nurses; the children attending them are drawn from the neighbourhood around the clinic. Alternatively general practitioners may run their own child health clinic on a regular basis, with health visitors and other staff in attendance; it is unusual for children not registered with the practice to attend such clinics. The service provides screening tests for such conditions as *congenital dislocation of the hip, suppressed squint (*see* COVER TEST), and impaired speech and/or hearing. The *Guthrie test may also be performed if this has not been done before the baby leaves hospital. The staff of child health clinics also educate mothers (especially those having their first child) in feeding techniques and hygiene and see that children receive the recommended immunizations against infectious diseases. They also ensure that the families of children with disabilities receive maximum support from health and social services and that such children achieve their maximum potential in the preschool period. *See also* COMMUNITY PAEDIATRICIAN.

child protection register a confidential list of children whose social circumstances render them at risk of neglect or abuse. Each local authority maintains a child protection register, and children on the register should undergo extra support and surveillance from health and/or social services.

Children's Auditory Performance Scale (CHAPS) a questionnaire designed to assess children's hearing abilities in certain situations. It is used in the diagnosis of *auditory processing disorder.

children's centre a building housing a range of services to support children up to five years of age and their families, including childcare, early education, parenting advice, and access to health advice. Children's centres are being introduced throughout the country, starting with the most deprived and disadvantaged communities. *See also* HEALTH INEQUALITIES.

Child-Turcotte-Pugh score a useful scoring system to assess the severity of liver disease using five criteria: serum bilirubin level, serum albumin level, presence of ascites, neurological disturbance, and prothrombin time.

Chinese herb nephropathy a condition that came to prominence in the 1990s when hundreds of young European women developed end-stage renal disease after receiving slimming pills containing Chinese herbs. The condition is also associated with a high incidence of urothelial tumours. It was eventually proved that the product was contaminated with aristolochic acid, a main toxic product of *Aristolochia* plant species. Its presence in the slimming regimen was the result of accidental substitution of the prescribed herb *Stephania tetrandra* (han fang-ji) by *A. fangchi* (guang fang-ji).

chir- (chiro-) *combining form denoting* the hand(s). *See also* CHEIR-.

chiropody *n. see* PODIATRY. —**chiropodist** *n.*

chiropractic *n.* a system of treating diseases by manipulation, mainly of the vertebrae of the backbone. It is based on the theory that nearly all disorders can be traced to the incorrect alignment of bones, with consequent malfunctioning of nerves and muscle throughout the body. Practitioners in the UK are required to register at the General Chiropractic Council, set up in 1997 to regulate the profession.

chi-square test (in statistics) a test to determine if the difference between two groups of observations is statistically significant (*see* SIGNIFICANCE), used in controlled trials and other studies. It measures the differences between theoretical and observed frequencies (*see* FREQUENCY DISTRIBUTION) and identifies whether or not *variables are dependent.

Chlamydia *n.* a genus of Gram-negative bacteria that are *obligate intracellular parasites in humans and other animals, in which they cause disease. *Chlamydia psittaci* causes *psittacosis, and *C. trachomatis* is the causative agent of the eye disease *trachoma. Some strains of *Chlamydia*, especially *C. trachomatis*, are a common cause of sexually transmitted infections, being responsible for nonspecific *urethritis in men, *pelvic inflammatory disease in women, and *inclusion conjunctivitis in the newborn. *C. pneumoniae* causes pneumonia. —**chlamydial** *adj.*

chloasma (melasma) *n.* ill-defined symmetrical brown patches on the cheeks or elsewhere on the face. Chloasma is a *photosensitivity reaction in women on combined oral contraceptive pills or who are pregnant; very rarely it occurs in men. It can usually be prevented by the use of sunscreens and may be treated with bleaching creams.

chlor- (chloro-) *combining form denoting* 1. chlorine or chlorides. 2. green.

chloracne *n.* an occupational acne-like skin disorder that occurs after regular contact with chlorinated hydrocarbons. These chemicals are derived from oil and tar products; 'cutting oils' used in engineering also cause the disease. The skin develops blackheads, papules, and pustules, mainly on hairy parts (such as the forearm). Warts and skin cancer may develop after many years of exposure to these chemicals.

chloral hydrate a sedative and hypnotic drug formerly widely used (as an oral solution) to induce sleep, mainly in children and the elderly; its derivative **cloral betaine** (Welldorm) is formulated as tablets. Nausea, vomiting, and other gastrointestinal side-effects limit the use of these drugs. Prolonged use may lead to *dependence.

chlorambucil *n.* an *alkylating agent used in chemotherapy, mainly in the treatment of chronic lymphocytic leukaemia and lymphomas. It is given by mouth; prolonged large doses may cause damage to the bone marrow. Trade name: **Leukeran**.

chloramphenicol *n.* an antibiotic, derived from the bacterium *Streptomyces venezuelae* and also produced synthetically, that is effective against a wide variety of microorganisms. However, due to its serious side-effects, especially damage to the bone marrow, it is usually reserved for serious infections (especially those caused by **Haemophilus influenzae*) when less toxic drugs are ineffective, being administered by mouth or intravenously. Chloramphenicol is also used in the form of eye drops to treat superficial eye infections. Trade names: **Chloromycetin**, **Kemicetine**, **Minims Chloramphenicol**.

chlordiazepoxide *n.* a *benzodiazepine drug with *muscle relaxant properties, used for the short-term relief of anxiety and to lessen the severity of symptoms in alcohol withdrawal. It is administered by mouth; side-effects include drowsiness, lightheadedness, and shaky movements. Trade names: **Librium**, **Tropium**.

chlorhexidine *n.* an antiseptic widely used as a solution to disinfect and cleanse the skin (especially before surgery), wounds, and burns. It is also used in the form of a mouthwash, gel, or spray for treating gingivitis and mouth ulcers and as a solution for washing out urinary catheters and treating some bladder infections. Skin sensitivity to chlorhexidine occurs rarely. Trade names: **Cepton**, **ChloraPrep**, **Chlorohex**, **Corsodyl**, **Hibitane Obstetric**, **Periogard**, etc.

chlorination *n.* the addition of noninjurious amounts of chlorine (often one part per million) to water supplies before human consumption to ensure that harmful microorganisms are destroyed. *See also* FLUORIDATION.

chlorine *n.* an extremely pungent gaseous element with antiseptic and bleaching properties. It is widely used to sterilize drinking water and purify swimming pools. In high concentrations it is toxic; it was used in World War I as a poison gas in the trenches. Symbol: Cl.

chlormethiazole *n. see* CLOMETHIAZOLE.

chloroform *n.* a volatile liquid formerly widely used as a general anaesthetic. Because its use as such causes liver damage and affects heart rhythm, chloroform is now used only in low concentrations as a flavouring agent and preservative, in the treatment of flatulence, and in liniments as a *rubefacient.

chlorophenothane *n. see* DDT.

chlorophyll *n.* one of a group of green pigments, found in all green plants and some bacteria, that absorb light to provide energy for the synthesis of carbohydrates from carbon dioxide and water (photosynthesis). The two major chlorophylls, a and b, consist of a porphyrin/magnesium complex.

chloropsia *n.* green vision: a rare symptom of digitalis poisoning.

chloroquine *n.* a drug used principally in the treatment and prevention of benign *malarias but also occasionally in the treatment of rheumatoid arthritis and lupus erythematosus. It is administered by mouth or injection and may cause gastrointestinal disturbance, headache, and skin rashes or itching; a side-effect of prolonged use in large doses is eye damage. Trade names: **Avloclor**, **Malarivon**, **Nivaquine**. *See also* PROGUANIL.

chlorphenamine (chlorpheniramine) *n.* a potent *antihistamine used to treat such allergies as hay fever and urticaria and in the emergency treatment of anaphylactic shock. It is administered by mouth or, to relieve severe conditions, by injection. Trade name: **Piriton**.

chlorpromazine *n.* a phenothiazine *antipsychotic drug used in the treatment of schizophrenia and mania; it is also used to control nausea and vomiting in terminal illness. Chlorpromazine is administered by mouth or injection or as a rectal suppository; common side-effects are drowsiness and dry mouth. It also causes abnormalities of movement, especially *dystonias, *tardive dyskinesia, and *parkinsonism. Trade name: **Largactil**.

chlorpropamide *n.* an oral hypogly-caemic drug (*see* SULPHONYLUREA) used in the treatment of type 2 diabetes and diabetes insipidus. Because it is very long acting, chlorpropamide has more side effects than other sulphonylureas and carries a risk of hy-poglycaemia; it is therefore not now recommended for type 2 diabetes.

chlortalidone (chlorthalidone) *n.* a thia-zide *diuretic used to treat fluid retention (oedema), *ascites due to cirrhosis, high blood pressure (hypertension), heart failure, and diabetes insipidus. It is administered by mouth and may cause a fall in blood pressure on standing up, dizziness, and reduced blood potassium levels. Trade name: **Hygroton**.

choana *n.* (*pl.* **choanae**) a funnel-shaped opening, particularly either of the two openings between the nasal cavity and the pharynx.

chokedamp *n. see* BLACKDAMP.

chol- (chole-, cholo-) *combining form denoting* bile. Example: **cholemesis** (vomiting of).

cholagogue *n.* a drug that stimulates the flow of bile from the gall bladder and bile ducts into the duodenum.

cholangiocarcinoma *n.* a rare malignant tumour of the *bile ducts. It is particularly likely to occur at the junction of the right and left hepatic ducts within the liver (in which case it is often known as a **Klatskin tumour**), causing obstructive jaundice. Primary scle-rosing *cholangitis, ulcerative *colitis, chronic infection with certain liver flukes, and exposure to the imaging contrast agent Thorotrast are some of the risk factors for development of cholangiocarcinoma. Differentiation from other causes of bile duct *stricture(s), e.g. sclerosing cholangitis, can be very difficult.

cholangiography *n.* imaging of the bile ducts in order to demonstrate anatomical abnormalities, generalized diseases of the bile ducts, the presence of stones, or the site and nature of local blockages. It may be combined with imaging of the pancreatic duct (**cholangiopancreatography**), as in **en-doscopic retrograde cholangiopancreatog-raphy** (*see* ERCP). **Magnetic resonance cholangiopancreatography** (**MRCP**) is a noninvasive *magnetic resonance imaging technique that is increasingly used as an al-

ternative to ERCP for diagnosis, but does not allow any treatment to be performed at the same examination. In **operative** (or **on-table**) **cholangiography**, a radiopaque *con-trast medium is injected into the bile ducts during *cholecystectomy, to make sure there are no stones remaining in the main ducts. **Percutaneous transhepatic cholangiogra-phy** (**PTC**) is an invasive fluoroscopic tech-nique in which a needle is passed through the skin, across the liver, and into a bile duct; contrast material can then be injected to outline the ducts. Using a *Seldinger tech-nique, drains or stents can be placed to treat infection or malignant strictures of the ducts. **T-tube cholangiography** involves the postoperative injection of radiopaque con-trast material via a drain left in the main bile duct after cholecystectomy.

cholangioma *n.* an extremely rare benign tumour originating from the bile duct.

cholangiopancreatography *n. see* CHOLANGIOGRAPHY.

cholangioscope *n.* an illuminated optical telescope using digital video technology to examine the interior of the bile ducts.

cholangitis *n.* inflammation of the bile ducts. It usually occurs when the ducts are obstructed, especially by stones or *stricture (benign or malignant), or after operations or intervention on the bile ducts. Symptoms in-clude intermittent fever, usually with *rigors; pain; and intermittent jaundice (a combina-tion known as **Charcot's triad**). Initial treat-ment is by broad-spectrum antibiotics, but relief of the obstruction is essential for per-manent cure. Liver abscess is a possible complication, and recurrent episodes of cholangitis can lead to secondary biliary *cir-rhosis. **Sclerosing cholangitis** is a disease process involving intra- or extrahepatic *bile ducts leading to progressive occlusion of the bile ducts due to ongoing inflammation and stricture formation. It is known to be associ-ated with *ulcerative colitis and certain auto-immune diseases.

cholecalciferol *n. see* VITAMIN D.

cholecyst- *combining form denoting* the gall bladder. Example: **cholecystotomy** (inci-sion of).

cholecystectomy *n.* surgical removal of the gall bladder, usually for *cholecystitis or gallstones. Formerly always performed by *laparotomy, the operation is now often done by *laparoscopy (**percutaneous laparoscopic cholecystectomy**). *See also* MINIMALLY INVASIVE SURGERY.

cholecystenterostomy *n.* a surgical procedure in which the gall bladder is joined to the small intestine. It is performed in order to allow bile to pass from the liver to the intestine when the common bile duct is obstructed by an irremovable cause.

cholecystitis *n.* inflammation of the gall bladder. **Acute cholecystitis** is a frequent complication of *gallstones but in a minority of cases can occur in the absence of gallstones (**acute acalculous cholecystitis**). It is usually treated by analgesics, intravenous fluid therapy, and broad-spectrum antibiotics, but *cholecystectomy is the usual definitive treatment of cholecystitis. **Chronic cholecystitis** was used in the past to describe recurrent episodes of biliary colic; the term should be avoided. *See also* CHOLESTEROSIS, MURPHY'S SIGN.

cholecystoduodenostomy *n.* a form of *cholecystenterostomy in which the gall bladder is joined to the duodenum.

cholecystography *n.* X-ray examination of the gall bladder. A radiopaque compound is taken by mouth, absorbed by the intestine, and excreted by the liver into the bile, which is then concentrated in the gall bladder. An X-ray image (**cholecystogram**) of the gall bladder indicates whether or not it is functioning, and gallstones may be seen as contrasting (nonopaque) areas within it. A fatty meal is often given to demonstrate the ability of the gall bladder to contract. This technique has largely been replaced by ultrasound scanning.

cholecystokinin *n.* a hormone secreted by the cells of the duodenum in response to the presence of partly digested food in the duodenum. It causes contraction of the gall bladder and expulsion of bile into the intestine and stimulates the production of digestive enzymes by the pancreas (*see also* PANCREATIC JUICE). In the brain cholecystokinin functions as a neurotransmitter, involved in the control of satiety.

cholecystotomy *n.* a surgical operation in which the gall bladder is opened, usually to remove gallstones. It is performed rarely, only when *cholecystectomy would be impracticable or dangerous.

choledoch- (choledocho-) *combining form denoting* the common bile duct. Example: **choledochoplasty** (plastic surgery of).

choledocholithiasis *n.* stones within the common bile duct. The stones usually form in the gall bladder and pass into the bile duct, but they may develop within the duct after *cholecystectomy.

choledochotomy *n.* a surgical operation in which the common bile duct is opened, to search for or to remove stones within it. It may be performed at the same time as *cholecystectomy or if stones occur in the bile duct after cholecystectomy.

cholelithiasis *n.* the formation of stones in the gall bladder (*see* GALLSTONE).

cholelithotomy *n.* removal of gallstones by *cholecystotomy.

cholera *n.* an acute infection of the small intestine by the bacterium *Vibrio cholerae*, which causes severe vomiting and diarrhoea (known as **ricewater stools**) leading to dehydration. The disease is contracted from food or drinking water contaminated with faeces from a patient. Cholera often occurs in epidemics; outbreaks are rare in good sanitary conditions. After an incubation period of 1–5 days symptoms commence suddenly; the resulting dehydration and the imbalance in the concentration of body fluids can cause death within 24 hours in severe cases if untreated. Initial treatment involves replacing the fluid loss by *oral rehydration therapy; tetracycline eradicates the bacteria and hastens recovery. The mortality rate in untreated cases is over 50%. Vaccination against cholera is effective for only 6–9 months.

choleresis *n.* the production of bile by the liver.

choleretic *n.* an agent that stimulates the secretion of bile by the liver thereby increasing the flow of bile.

cholestasis *n.* failure of normal amounts of bile to reach the intestine, resulting in obstructive *jaundice. The cause may be a mechanical blockage in the bile ducts, such as a stone (**extrahepatic biliary obstruction**), or liver disease, such as that caused by the drug *chlorpromazine in some hypersensitive individuals (**intrahepatic cholestasis**); it may also occasionally occur in pregnancy (*see* OBSTETRIC CHOLESTASIS) and is present in primary biliary *cirrhosis. The symptoms are jaundice with dark urine, pale faeces, and usually itching (pruritus).

cholesteatoma *n.* a skin-lined sac containing debris from dead skin cells that grows from the eardrum into the *mastoid bone, eroding normal structures in its path. Left untreated, it can carry infection to the brain, causing meningitis or a cerebral *abscess. Treatment is by means of *mastoidectomy. Rarely, cholesteatoma can arise congenitally in the *temporal bone or central nervous system.

cholesterol *n.* a fatlike material (a *sterol) present in the blood and most tissues, especially nervous tissue. Cholesterol and its esters are important constituents of cell membranes and are precursors of many steroid hormones and bile salts. Western dietary intake is approximately 500–1000 mg/day. Cholesterol is synthesized in the body from acetate, mainly in the liver, and blood concentration is normally 140–300 mg/100 ml (3.6–7.8 mmol/l). An elevated concentration of cholesterol in the blood (*see* HYPERCHOLESTEROLAEMIA) is often associated with *atheroma, of which cholesterol is a major component. Hypercholesterolaemia and the resulting atheroma have been linked with a high dietary intake of saturated fats and cholesterol. However, current thinking suggests that the damage to blood vessels is caused by high levels (over 4.4 mmol/l) of *low-density lipoprotein (LDL), one of the forms in which cholesterol and other lipids are transported in the bloodstream. *See also* HYPERLIPIDAEMIA, LIPOPROTEIN.

cholesterosis *n.* an uncommon form of chronic inflammation of the gall bladder in which small crystals of cholesterol are deposited on the internal wall, like the pips of a strawberry: hence its descriptive term **strawberry gall bladder**. The crystals may enlarge to become *gallstones.

cholestyramine *n. see* COLESTYRAMINE.

cholic acid (cholalic acid) *see* BILE ACIDS.

choline *n.* a basic compound important in the synthesis of phosphatidylcholine (lecithin) and other *phospholipids and of *acetylcholine. It is also involved in the transport of fat in the body. Choline is sometimes classed as a vitamin but, although it is essential for life, it can be synthesized in the body.

cholinergic *adj.* **1.** describing nerve fibres

that release *acetylcholine as a neurotransmitter. **2.** describing *receptors at which acetylcholine acts to pass on messages from cholinergic nerve fibres. **3.** describing drugs that mimic the actions of acetylcholine (*see* PARASYMPATHOMIMETIC). *Compare* ADRENERGIC.

cholinergic urticaria *see* URTICARIA.

cholinesterase *n.* an enzyme that breaks down a choline ester into its choline and acid components. The term usually refers to **acetylcholinesterase**, which breaks down the neurotransmitter *acetylcholine into choline and acetic acid. It is found in all *cholinergic nerve junctions, where it rapidly destroys the acetylcholine released during the transmission of a nerve impulse so that subsequent impulses may pass. Other cholinesterases are found in the blood and other tissues.

choluria *n.* bile in the urine, which occurs when the level of bile in the blood is raised, especially in obstructive *jaundice. The urine becomes dark brown or orange, and bile pigments and bile salts may be detected in it.

chondr- (chondro-) *combining form denoting* cartilage. Example: **chondrogenesis** (formation of).

chondrin *n.* a material that resembles gelatin, produced when cartilage is boiled.

chondriosome *n. see* MITOCHONDRION.

chondroblast *n.* a cell that produces the matrix of *cartilage.

chondroblastoma *n.* a tumour derived from *chondroblasts, having the appearance of a mass of well-differentiated cartilage.

chondrocalcinosis *n.* the appearance of calcific material in joint cartilage, most commonly an incidental finding on X-ray of the knees in elderly patients and usually causing no symptoms. It is also seen less commonly in several disorders, including Wilson's disease, pseudogout, hyperparathyroidism, hypothyroidism, and haemochromatosis.

chondroclast *n.* a cell that is concerned with the absorption of cartilage.

chondrocranium *n.* the embryonic skull, which is composed entirely of cartilage and is later replaced by bone. *See also* MENINX.

chondrocyte *n.* a *cartilage cell, found embedded in the matrix.

chondrodermatitis nodularis helicis a fairly common painful nodule on the upper part of the ear. It occurs mainly in middle-aged or elderly men and characteristically prevents the sufferer from sleeping on the affected side; it is readily treated by being cut out.

chondrodysplasia (chondro-osteodystrophy, chondrodystrophy) *n.* any of various conditions in which there is abnormal cartilage development. It affects long bones and can cause short-limb dwarfism, overgrowth of the epiphysis, or other deformities. One particular form is an autosomal *recessive syndrome most commonly found in Old Order Amish populations. *See also* ACHONDROPLASIA.

chondroitin sulphate a mucopolysaccharide that forms an important constituent of cartilage, bone, and other connective tissues. It is composed of glucuronic acid and N-acetyl-D-galactosamine units.

chondroma *n.* a relatively common benign tumour of cartilage-forming cells, which may occur at the growing end of any bone but is found most commonly in the bones of the feet and hands. It may be a chance finding on X-ray, it may expand the bone, or it may be the site of a *pathological fracture.

chondromalacia *n.* softening, inflammation, and degeneration of cartilage at a joint. **Chondromalacia patellae** is the most common kind, affecting the undersurface of the kneecap; it results in pain in the front of the knee and grating (*crepitus), which is made worse by kneeling, squatting, and climbing stairs. Treatment includes physiotherapy, anti-inflammatory drugs, weight loss, and avoidance of aggravating factors.

chondroplasty *n.* the refashioning of articular cartilage, commonly performed by shaving areas of worn and unstable cartilage with the aid of an *arthroscope.

chondrosarcoma *n.* an uncommon malignant tumour of cartilage cells occurring in a bone, most frequently in the femur, humerus, ribs, or pelvis, and most commonly affecting adults in their fifties and sixties. It has a typical 'snowstorm' appearance on X-ray. Treatment is by surgical removal; these tumours are not usually sensitive to radiotherapy or chemotherapy.

choose and book an electronic booking system introduced in the NHS from 2005 to enable patient choice. At the point of referral, it allows patients to choose which hospital they are referred to by their general practitioner and then to book a convenient date and time for the appointment.

chord- (chordo-) *combining form denoting* 1. a cord. 2. the notochord.

chorda *n.* (*pl.* **chordae**) a cord, tendon, or nerve fibre. The **chordae tendineae** are stringlike processes in the heart that attach the margins of the mitral and tricuspid valve leaflets to projections of the wall of the ventricle (**papillary muscles**). Rupture of the chordae, through injury, endocarditis, or degenerative changes, results in *mitral regurgitation.

chordee *n.* acute angulation of the penis. In *Peyronie's disease, this is due to a localized fibrous plaque in the penis, which fails to engorge on erection. As a result, the penis angulates at this point making intercourse impossible. In a child, downward chordee is an associated deformity in *hypospadias and the more severe forms are corrected surgically.

chordoma *n.* a rare tumour arising from remnants of the embryologic *notochord. The classical sites are the base of skull and the region of the sacrum.

chorea *n.* a jerky involuntary movement particularly affecting the head, face, or limbs. Each movement is sudden but the resulting posture may be prolonged for a few seconds. The symptoms are usually due to disease of the *basal ganglia but may result from drug therapy for *parkinsonism or phenothiazines. Such movements are characteristic of *Huntington's disease, in which they are associated with progressive dementia. *See also* SYDENHAM'S CHOREA.

chorioamnionitis *n.* inflammation and infection of the inner and outer fetal membranes, often after preterm premature rupture of membranes (*PPROM). This condition is associated with poor fetal outcome and can lead to maternal sepsis from *endometritis.

choriocarcinoma (chorionepithelioma) *n.* a rare malignant tumour of the placenta originating in the outer membrane (chorion) surrounding the fetus. Usually it is a complication of a *hydatidiform mole, although it may follow a miscarriage or even a normal

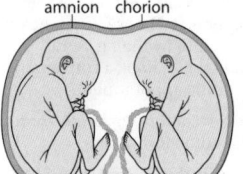
monoamniotic monochorionic
amnion chorion

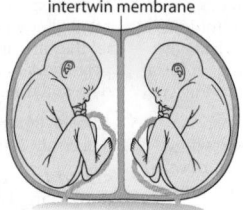
diamniotic monochorionic
intertwin membrane

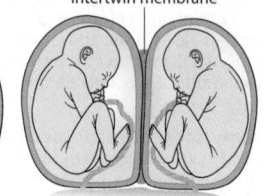
diamniotic dichorionic (fused)
intertwin membrane

single placental mass

diamniotic dichorionic (separated)

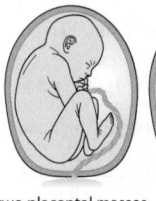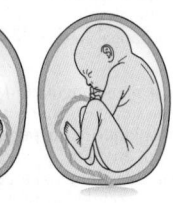

two placental masses

Chorionicity.

pregnancy. The tumour rapidly spreads to the lungs, but is relatively sensitive to chemotherapy. *See also* GESTATIONAL TROPHOBLASTIC NEOPLASIA.

chorion *n.* the embryonic membrane that totally surrounds the embryo from the time of implantation. It is formed from *trophoblast lined with mesoderm and becomes closely associated with the *allantois. The blood vessels (supplied by the allantois) are concentrated in the region of the chorion that is attached to the wall of the uterus and forms the *placenta. *See also* VILLUS. —**chorionic** *adj.*

chorionicity *n.* the number of chorionic membranes present on direct examination of the placenta and membranes following delivery of *twins. Chorionicity can be determined antenatally by ultrasound, ideally between 10 and 14 weeks gestation. Where two placental masses are identified, the pregnancy is **dichorionic**. More frequently a single placental mass exists and chorionicity can only be determined by evaluation of the intertwin membrane; the pregnancy is **monochorionic** when the fetuses share a chorion (see illustration; *see also* LAMBDA SIGN, T-SIGN). Chorionicity rather than zygosity is a better determinant of perinatal

outcome in twins. The perinatal mortality rate of monochorionic pregnancies may be up to four times that of dichorionic.

chorionic villus sampling (CVS) an invasive procedure for *prenatal diagnosis in which a sample of placental tissue (containing chorionic *villi) is aspirated through the cervix or abdomen under ultrasound visualization. It is usually performed between the 10th and 13th weeks of gestation. The cells so obtained are subjected to chromosomal analysis to determine if any abnormalities are present in the fetus. This enables the diagnosis of chromosomal abnormalities, such as Down's syndrome.

chorioretinopathy *n.* any eye disease involving both the choroid and the retina. *See* CENTRAL SEROUS CHORIORETINOPATHY.

choristoma *n.* a mass of tissue composed of tissue not normally found at the affected site. A *dermoid cyst is an example.

choroid *n.* the layer of the eyeball between the retina and the sclera (*see also* BRUCH'S MEMBRANE). It contains blood vessels and a pigment that absorbs excess light and so prevents blurring of vision. *See* EYE. —**choroidal** *adj.*

choroidal detachment the separation of the *choroid from the *sclera of the eye as a result of leakage of fluid from the vessels of the choroid. It occurs when pressure inside the eyeball is very low, usually after trauma or intraocular surgery.

choroideraemia *n.* a sex-linked hereditary condition in which the retinal pigment epithelium (*see* RETINA) and the choroid begin to degenerate in the first few months or years of life. In males this results in blindness, but in females it rarely causes any significant visual loss.

choroiditis *n.* inflammation of the choroid layer of the eye. It may be inflamed together with the iris and ciliary body (*see* UVEITIS) but often is involved alone and in patches (**focal** or **multifocal choroiditis**). Vision becomes blurred but the eye is usually pain-free.

choroid plexus a rich network of blood vessels, derived from those of the pia mater, in each of the brain's ventricles. It is responsible for the production of *cerebrospinal fluid.

Christmas disease (haemophilia B) a disorder that is identical in its effects to *haemophilia A, but is due to a deficiency of a different blood coagulation factor, the **Christmas factor** (Factor IX). [S. Christmas (20th century), in whom the factor was first identified]

chrom- (chromo-) *combining form denoting* colour or pigment.

chromaffin *n.* tissue in the medulla of the *adrenal gland consisting of modified neural cells containing granules that are stained brown by chromates. Adrenaline and noradrenaline are released from the granules when the adrenal gland is stimulated by its sympathetic nerve supply. *See also* NEUROHORMONE.

-chromasia *combining form denoting* staining or pigmentation.

chromat- (chromato-) *combining form denoting* colour or pigmentation.

chromatid *n.* one of the two threadlike strands formed by longitudinal division of a chromosome during *mitosis and *meiosis. They remain attached at the *centromere. Chromatids can be seen between early prophase and metaphase in mitosis and between diplotene and the second metaphase

of meiosis, after which they divide at the centromere to form daughter chromosomes.

chromatin *n.* the material of a cell nucleus that stains with basic dyes and consists of DNA and protein: the substance of which the chromosomes are made. *See* EUCHROMATIN, HETEROCHROMATIN.

chromatography *n.* any of several techniques for separating the components of a mixture by selective absorption. Two such techniques are quite widely used in medicine, for example to separate mixtures of amino acids. In one of these, **paper chromatography**, a sample of the mixture is placed at the edge of a sheet of filter paper. As the solvent soaks along the paper, the components are absorbed to different extents and thus move along the paper at different rates. In **column chromatography** the components separate out along a column of a powdered absorbent, such as silica or aluminium oxide.

chromatolysis *n.* the dispersal or disintegration of the microscopic structures within the nerve cells that normally produce proteins. It is part of the cell's response to injury.

chromatophore *n.* a cell containing pigment. In humans chromatophores containing *melanin are found in the skin, hair, and eyes.

chromatopsia *n.* abnormal coloured vision: a rare symptom of various conditions. Sometimes everything looks reddish to patients after removal of their cataracts; patients suffering from digitalis poisoning may see things in green or yellow. Similar disturbances of colour may be experienced by people recovering from inflammation of the optic nerve.

chromoblastomycosis (chromomycosis) *n.* a chronic fungal infection of the skin usually occurring at the site of an injury; for example, a wound from a wood splinter. It produces pigmented wartlike lumps on exposed areas that sometimes ulcerate. In the immunocompromised it may spread rapidly and even prove fatal.

chromophobe (chromophobic) *adj.* describing cells or tissues that do not stain well with either acidic or basic dyes. Chromophobic cells may be seen, for example, in the anterior pituitary gland. *See also* ADENOMA.

chromosome *n.* one of the threadlike

Chromosome. Human male chromosomes, arranged in numbered pairs according to a standard classification. The female set differs only in the sex chromosomes (XX instead of XY).

structures in a cell nucleus that carry the genetic information in the form of *genes. It is composed of a long double filament of *DNA coiled into a helix together with associated proteins, with the genes arranged in a linear manner along its length. It stains deeply with basic dyes during cell division (*see* MEIOSIS, MITOSIS). The nucleus of each human somatic cell contains 46 chromosomes, 23 of which are of maternal and 23 of paternal origin (see illustration). Each chromosome can duplicate an exact copy of itself between each cell division (*see* INTERPHASE) so that each new cell formed receives a full set of chromosomes. *See also* CHROMATID, CENTROMERE, SEX CHROMOSOME. —**chromosomal** *adj.*

chron- (chrono-) *combining form denoting* time. Example: **chronophobia** (abnormal fear of).

chronic *adj.* 1. describing a disease of long duration involving very slow changes. Such a disease is often of gradual onset. The term does not imply anything about the severity of a disease. *Compare* ACUTE. 2. describing a type of inflammation characterized by the presence of lymphocytes, plasma cells, and macrophages. —**chronicity** *n.*

chronic fatigue syndrome *see* CFS/ME/PVF.

chronic idiopathic facial pain *see* PERSISTENT IDIOPATHIC FACIAL PAIN.

chronic obstructive pulmonary disease (COPD, chronic obstructive airways disease) a disease of adults, especially those over the age of 45 with a history of smoking or inhalation of airborne pollution, characterized by airflow obstruction that is not fully reversible. The disease has features of *emphysema, chronic *bronchitis, and asthmatic bronchitis. It is now diagnosed, according to the *GOLD guidelines, at different stages:
Stage 0: the presence of risk factors and symptoms (e.g. cough and wheeze) with normal *forced expiratory volume in 1 second (FEV_1).
Stage 1: FEV_1 is normal, but the ratio of FEV_1 to forced *vital capacity (FVC) is less than 70%.
Stage 2: FEV_1 is less than 80% but more than 50% of the predicted value for the patient's age and height.
Stage 3: FEV_1 less than 50% but more than 30%.
Stage 4: FEV_1 less than 30% or the presence of chronic respiratory failure.

The guidelines for COPD recommend different treatment regimens for different stages. Although the response to inhaled corticosteriods is less for COPD than for asthma, these drugs, especially combined with inhaled long-acting beta agonists (e.g. *salmeterol), can improve quality of life and survival in stages 3 and 4. There is also a decrease in the number of acute exacerbations of COPD (**AECOPD**): increased sputum volume or purulence and/or breathlessness, with or without symptoms (e.g. cough, wheeze, chest pain, malaise, fever).

chronic pelvic pain (CPP) intermittent or constant pain in the lower abdomen or pelvis of at least six months' duration, not occurring exclusively with menstruation or intercourse and not associated with pregnancy. It may be caused by an underlying gynaecological condition, such as *endometriosis or adhesions, but bowel or bladder disorders (e.g. irritable bowel syndrome, insterstitial cystitis), visceral hypersensitivity, and psychological conditions may all contribute.

Chronic Sick and Disabled Persons Act 1970 (in Britain) an Act providing for the identification and care of those suffering from a chronic or degenerative disease for which there is no cure and which can be only partially alleviated by treatment. Such people are usually distinguished from the elderly who may also suffer from chronic diseases. It is the responsibility of local authorities to identify those with such problems and to ensure that services are available to meet their needs. Identification can be difficult because of the lack of a clear and agreed definition of what constitutes a disability of such severity as to warrant inclusion in such a register. *See* HANDICAP.

chrys- (chryso-) *combining form denoting* gold or gold salts.

chrysiasis *n.* the deposition of gold in the eye and other tissues as a result of prolonged or excessive treatment with gold salts.

Chrysops *n.* a genus of bloodsucking flies, commonly called deer flies. Female flies, found in shady wooded areas, bite humans during the day. Certain species in Africa may transmit the tropical disease *loiasis to humans. In the USA *C. discalis* is a vector of *tularaemia.

chrysotherapy *n.* the treatment of disease by the administration of *gold or its compounds.

Churg-Strauss syndrome a clinical syndrome comprising severe asthma associated with an increased *eosinophil count in the peripheral blood and eosinophilic deposits in the small vessels of the lungs. It usually responds to oral corticosteroids. Untreated, it may result in severe and widespread systemic *vasculitis. [J. Churg (1910–) and L. Strauss (1913–85), US pathologists]

Chvostek's sign twitching of the facial muscles elicited by stimulation of the facial nerve by tapping. This indicates muscular irritability, usually due to calcium depletion (*see* TETANY). [F. Chvosteck (1835–84), Austrian surgeon]

chyle *n.* an alkaline milky liquid found within the *lacteals after a period of absorption. It consists of lymph with a suspension of minute droplets of digested fats (triglycerides), which have been absorbed from the

small intestine. It is transported in the lymphatic system to the *thoracic duct. *See also* ASCITES.

chylomicron *n.* a *lipoprotein particle present in the blood after digested fat has been absorbed from the small intestine. The lipid portion consists largely of triglycerides, which are released by the action of *lipoprotein lipase.

chyluria *n.* the presence of *chyle in the urine.

chyme *n.* the semiliquid acid mass that is the form in which food passes from the stomach to the small intestine. It is produced by the action of *gastric juice and the churning movements of the stomach.

chymotrypsin *n.* a protein-digesting enzyme (*see* PEPTIDASE). It is secreted by the pancreas in an inactive form, **chymotrypsinogen**, that is converted into chymotrypsin in the duodenum by the action of *trypsin.

chymotrypsinogen *n. see* CHYMOTRYPSIN.

Cialis *n. see* SILDENAFIL.

cicatricial *adj.* associated with scarring. For example, **cicatricial alopecia** is a type of baldness associated with scarring (*see* ALOPECIA).

ciclosporin (cyclosporin) *n.* an *immunosuppressant drug used to prevent and treat rejection of a transplanted organ or bone marrow. It may also be used to treat severe rheumatoid arthritis, psoriasis, and atopic eczema. Ciclosporin is administered orally or by intravenous infusion; side-effects include nausea, gum swelling, tremor, excessive hair growth, and kidney impairment. Trade names: **Neoral**, **Sandimmun**.

-cide *combining form denoting* killer or killing. Examples: **bactericide** (of bacteria); **infanticide** (of children).

ciliary body the part of the *eye that connects the choroid with the iris. It consists of three zones: the **ciliary ring**, which adjoins the choroid; the **ciliary processes**, a series of about 70 radial ridges behind the iris to which the suspensory ligament of the lens is attached; and the **ciliary muscle**, contraction of which alters the curvature of the lens (*see* ACCOMMODATION).

cilium *n.* (*pl.* **cilia**) **1.** a hairlike process, large numbers of which are found on certain epithelial cells and on certain (ciliate) protozoa. Cilia are particularly characteristic of the epithelium that lines the upper respiratory tract, where their beating serves to remove particles of dust and other foreign material. **2.** an eyelash or eyelid. —**ciliary** *adj.*

cimetidine *n.* an H$_2$-receptor antagonist (*see* ANTIHISTAMINE) that is used to treat stomach and duodenal ulcers, reflux oesophagitis, and other digestive disorders. It is administered by mouth or injection and the most common side-effects are dizziness, diarrhoea, muscular pains, and rash. Trade name: **Tagamet**.

Cimex *n. see* BED BUG.

CIN *see* CERVICAL INTRAEPITHELIAL NEOPLASIA.

cinchocaine *n.* a local anaesthetic used in combination with corticosteroids in ointments and suppositories to relieve the pain of haemorrhoids.

cinchona *n.* the dried bark of *Cinchona* trees, formerly used in medicine to stimulate the appetite and to prevent haemorrhage and diarrhoea. Taken over prolonged periods, it may cause *cinchonism. Cinchona is the source of *quinine.

cinchonism *n.* poisoning caused by an overdose of cinchona or the alkaloids quinine, quinidine, or cinchonine derived from it. The symptoms are commonly ringing noises in the ears, dizziness, blurring of vision (and sometimes complete blindness), rashes, fever, and low blood pressure. Treatment with *diuretics increases the rate of excretion of the toxic compounds from the body.

cine- *combining form denoting* any technique of recording a rapid series of X-ray images on cine film for later analysis. Examples: **cineangiography; cinefluorography**. Cine film is now being replaced by electronic storage (digital) media. *See also* VIDEO-.

cingulectomy *n.* surgical excision of the *cingulum, the part of the brain concerned with anger and depression. The procedure has occasionally been carried out as *psychosurgery for intractable mental illness.

cingulum *n.* (*pl.* **cingula**) **1.** a curved bundle of nerve fibres in each cerebral hemisphere, nearly encircling its connection with the corpus callosum. *See* CEREBRUM. **2.** a

small protuberance on the lingual surface of the crowns of incisor and canine teeth.

ciprofibrate *n. see* FIBRATES.

ciprofloxacin *n.* a broad-spectrum *quinolone antibiotic that can be given orally or by intravenous infusion and is particularly useful against Gram-negative bacteria, such as *Pseudomonas*, that are resistant to all other oral antibiotics. Side-effects can include nausea, diarrhoea, abdominal pain, and headache. It is also applied as eye drops or ointment for eye infections and corneal ulcers. Trade names: **Ciloxan**, **Ciproxin**.

circadian *adj.* denoting a biological rhythm or cycle of approximately 24 hours. *Compare* NYCTOHEMERAL, ULTRADIAN.

circle of Willis a circle on the undersurface of the brain formed by linked branches of the arteries that supply the brain (see illustration). Most cerebral *aneurysms occur on or near the circle of Willis. [T. Willis (1621–75), English anatomist]

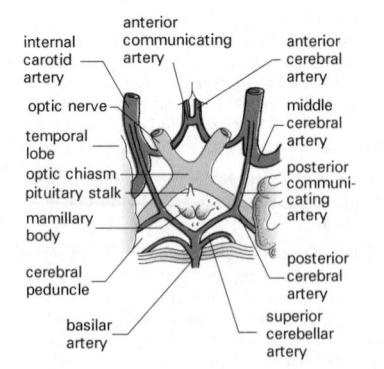

The circle of Willis (seen from below).

circulatory system *see* CARDIOVASCULAR SYSTEM.

circum- *prefix denoting* around; surrounding. Example: **circumanal** (surrounding the anus).

circumcision *n.* surgical removal of the foreskin of the penis. This operation is usually performed for religious and ethnic reasons but is sometimes required for medical conditions, mainly *phimosis and *paraphimosis. **Female circumcision** (or **female genital mutilation**) involves removal of the clitoris, labia minora, and labia majora for cultural reasons. The extent of excision varies from tribe to tribe and from country to country. The simplest and least damaging form is **clitoridectomy** (removal of the clitoris); the next form entails excision of the prepuce, clitoris, and all or part of the labia minora. The most extensive form, **infibulation**, involves excision of clitoris, labia minora, and labia majora. The vulval lips are sutured together and a piece of wood or reed is inserted to preserve a small passage for urine and menstrual fluid. In the majority of women who are circumcised, *episiotomy, often extensive, is required to allow delivery of a child. Female circumcision is prohibited under the Female Genital Mutilation Act 2003.

circumduction *n.* a circular movement, such as that made by a limb.

circumflex nerve a mixed sensory and motor nerve of the upper arm. It arises from the fifth and sixth cervical segments of the spinal cord and is distributed to the deltoid muscle of the shoulder and the overlying skin.

circumoral *adj.* situated around the mouth.

circumstantiality *n.* a disorder of thought in which thinking and speech proceed slowly and with many unnecessary trivial details. It is sometimes seen in organic *psychosis, in *schizophrenia, and in people of pedantic and obsessional personality.

cirrhosis *n.* a condition in which the liver responds to injury or death of some of its cells (*hepatocytes) by producing interlacing strands of fibrous tissue between which are nodules of regenerating cells. The liver becomes tawny and characteristically knobbly (due to the nodules). Causes include chronic *alcoholism (**alcoholic cirrhosis**), viral *hepatitis, *nonalcoholic fatty liver disease (NAFLD), chronic obstruction of the common bile duct (**secondary biliary cirrhosis**), autoimmune diseases (**chronic autoimmune hepatitis**, **primary biliary cirrhosis**), sclerosing *cholangitis, and chronic heart failure (**cardiac cirrhosis**). In a small minority of cases no cause is found (**cryptogenic cirrhosis**). Complications include *portal hypertension, *ascites, *hepatic encephalopathy, and *hepatoma. Cirrhosis cannot be cured

but its progression may be stopped if the cause can be removed or it can be treated by liver transplantation. This particularly applies in alcoholism (when all alcohol must be prohibited); in chronic autoimmune hepatitis (in which corticosteroid treatment may reduce inflammation); in viral hepatitis (treatment to eradicate or suppress viral replication helps); in secondary biliary cirrhosis (in which surgery may relieve obstruction); and in cardiac failure that can be treated. —**cirrhotic** *adj.*

cirs- (cirso-) *combining form denoting* a varicose vein. Example: **cirsectomy** (excision of).

cirsoid *adj.* describing the distended knotted appearance of a varicose vein. The term is used for a type of tumour of the scalp (**cirsoid aneurysm**), which is an arteriovenous aneurysm.

CIS *see* CARCINOMA IN SITU.

cisatracurium *n. see* MUSCLE RELAXANT.

CISC clean intermittent self-catheterization. *See* INTERMITTENT SELF-CATHETERIZATION.

cisplatin *n.* a platinum-containing compound: a *cytotoxic drug that impedes cell division by damaging DNA. Administered intravenously, it is used in the treatment of various cancers, including testicular tumours and cancers of the head and neck. It is highly toxic; side-effects include nausea, vomiting, kidney damage, peripheral neuropathy, and hearing loss. Less toxic *analogues of cisplatin are available (*see* CARBOPLATIN, OXALIPLATIN).

cisterna *n.* (*pl.* **cisternae**) **1.** one of the enlarged spaces beneath the *arachnoid that act as reservoirs for cerebrospinal fluid. The largest (**cisterna magna**) lies beneath the cerebellum and behind the medulla oblongata. **2.** a dilatation at the lower end of the thoracic duct, into which the great lymph ducts of the lower limbs drain.

cistron *n.* the section of a DNA or RNA chain that controls the amino-acid sequence of a single polypeptide chain in protein synthesis. A cistron can be regarded as the functional equivalent of a *gene.

citalopram *n.* an antidepressant drug that acts by prolonging the action of the neurotransmitter serotonin (5-hydroxytryptamine) in the brain (*see* SSRI). It is taken by mouth for the treatment of depression and panic disorder; side-effects may include dizziness, agitation, tremor, nausea, and diarrhoea. Trade name: **Cipramil**.

citric acid an organic acid found naturally in citrus fruits. Citric acid is formed in the first stage of the *Krebs cycle, the important energy-producing cycle in the body.

citric acid cycle *see* Krebs cycle.

Citrobacter *n.* a genus of Gram-negative anaerobic rod-shaped bacteria widely distributed in nature. The organisms cause infections of the intestinal and urinary tracts, gall bladder, and the meninges that are usually secondary, occurring in the elderly, newborn, debilitated, and immunocompromised.

citrullinaemia *n.* an inborn lack of one of the enzymes concerned with the chemical breakdown of proteins to urea: in consequence both the amino acid citrulline and ammonia accumulate in the blood. Affected children fail to thrive, and show signs of mental retardation.

citrulline *n.* an *amino acid produced by the liver as a by-product during the conversion of ammonia to *urea.

CJD *see* Creutzfeldt-Jakob disease.

clamp *n.* a surgical instrument designed to compress a structure, such as a blood vessel or a cut end of the intestine (see illustration). A variety of clamps have been designed for specific surgical procedures. **Blood-vessel** (**atraumatic**) **clamps** are used to stop bleeding from the cut vessels and are designed not to damage the arterial wall. **Intestinal clamps** prevent the intestinal contents from leaking into the abdominal cavity during operations on the intestines and are designed

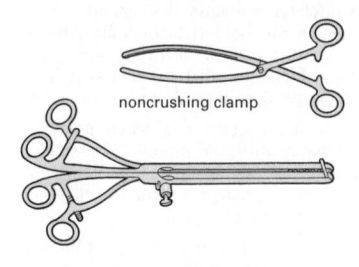

noncrushing clamp

twin gastrointestinal clamp

Intestinal clamps.

either not to damage the intestinal wall (noncrushing clamps) or to close the open end (crushing clamps) prior to suturing.

Clark's levels the five vertical levels of skin that are successively penetrated by an invading *melanoma. They are: epidermis, papillary dermis, intervening zone, reticular dermis, and subcutaneous tissue. They usually correlate with the *Breslow thickness. [W. H. Clark (1924–97), US dermatologist]

clasp *n.* (in dentistry) the part of a *denture or *orthodontic appliance that keeps it in place. It is made of flexible metal.

clasp-knife rigidity *see* spasticity.

claudication *n.* limping. **Intermittent claudication** is a cramping pain, induced by exercise and relieved by rest, that is caused by an inadequate supply of blood to the affected muscles. It is most often seen in the calf and leg muscles as a result of *atheroma of the leg arteries. The leg pulses are often absent and the feet may be cold. The treatment is that of atheroma.

claustrophobia *n.* a morbid fear of enclosed places. *Compare* agoraphobia. *See also* phobia.

claustrum *n.* a thin vertical layer of grey matter in each cerebral hemisphere, between the surface of the *insula and the lenticular nucleus (*see* basal ganglia).

clavicle *n.* the collar bone: a long slender curved bone, a pair of which form the front part of the shoulder girdle. Each clavicle articulates laterally with the *scapula and medially with the manubrium of the sternum (breastbone). Fracture of the clavicle is a common *sports injury: the majority of cases require no treatment other than supporting the weight of the arm in a sling. —**clavicular** *adj.*

clavulanic acid a drug that interferes with the *penicillinases that inactivate *beta-lactam antibiotics, such as *amoxicillin or *ticarcillin. Combined with the antibiotic, clavulanic acid can overcome drug resistance.

clavus *n.* a sharp pain in the head, as if a nail were being driven in.

claw-foot *n.* an excessively arched foot, giving an unnaturally high instep. In most cases the cause is unknown, but the deformity may sometimes be due to an imbalance between the muscles flexing the toes and the shorter muscles that extend them; this type is found in some neuromuscular diseases, such as Friedreich's *ataxia. Surgical treatment is effective in childhood but less so in adult life. Medical name: **pes cavus**.

claw-hand   n. flexion and contraction of the fingers with extension at the joints between the fingers and the hand, giving a claw-like appearance. Any kind of damage to the nerves or muscles may lead to claw-hand; causes include injuries, *syringomyelia, and leprosy. *See also* DUPUYTREN'S CONTRACTURE.

clearance (renal clearance)   n. a quantitative measure of the rate at which waste products are removed from the blood by the kidneys or through the process of dialysis. It is expressed in terms of the volume of blood that could be completely cleared of a particular substance in a particular unit of time. Clearance by the kidney is usually measured as ml/min while clearance with, say, peritoneal dialysis is usually measured in litres/week.

clear-cell carcinoma (clear-cell adenocarcinoma)   a variant of *adenocarcinoma that tends to arise from the kidneys or the female genital tract. In the latter case it is linked to intrauterine exposure to *diethylstilbestrol during the 1950s and 1960s and takes the form of a vaginal cancer, which can be treated by radical surgery followed by radiotherapy.

clearing   n. (in microscopy) the process of removing the cloudiness from microscopical specimens after *dehydration by means of a **clearing agent**. This increases the transparency of the specimens. Xylene, cedar oil, methyl benzoate plus benzol, and methyl salicylate plus benzol are commonly used as clearing agents.

cleavage   n. (in embryology) the process of repeated cell division of the fertilized egg to form a ball of cells that becomes the *blastocyst. The cells (**blastomeres**) do not grow between divisions and so they decrease in size.

cleft lip (harelip)   the congenital deformity of a cleft in the upper lip, on one or both sides of the midline. It occurs when the three blocks of embryonic tissue that go to form the upper lip fail to fuse and it is often associated with a *cleft palate. Medical name: **cheiloschisis**.

cleft palate   a fissure in the midline of the palate due to failure of the two sides to fuse in embryonic development. Only part of the palate may be affected, or the cleft may extend the full length with bilateral clefts at the front of the maxilla; it may be accompanied by a *cleft lip and disturbance of tooth formation. Cleft palates can be corrected by surgery.

cleid- (cleido-, clid-, clido-)   *combining form denoting* the clavicle (collar bone). Example: **cleidocranial** (of the clavicle and cranium).

cleidocranial dysostosis   a congenital defect of bone formation in which the skull bones ossify imperfectly and the collar bones (clavicles) are absent.

clemastine   n. an antihistamine used for the treatment of symptoms of hay fever and urticaria. It is administered by mouth; common side-effects are dizziness, sleepiness, and stomach upset. Trade name: **Tavegil**.

client-centred therapy (Rogerian therapy)   a method of psychotherapy in which the therapist refrains from directing clients in what they should do and instead concentrates on communicating understanding and acceptance. Frequently the therapist reflects the clients' own words or feelings back to them. The aim is to enable clients to solve their own problems.

climacteric   n. 1. *see* MENOPAUSE. 2. (male climacteric) declining sexual drive and fertility in men, usually occurring around or after middle age. *See* ANDROPAUSE.

clindamycin   n. an antibiotic used to treat serious bacterial infections, such as staphylococcal bone and joint infections. It is administered by mouth or injection. The most serious side-effect is pseudomembranous colitis, caused by overgrowth of *Clostridium difficile*, which limits the use of this drug; other side-effects include nausea, vomiting, and occasional hypersensitivity reactions. Trade name: **Dalacin C**.

clinic   n. 1. an establishment or department of a hospital devoted to the treatment of particular diseases or the medical care of out-patients. 2. a gathering of instructors, students, and patients, usually in a hospital ward, for the examination and treatment of the patients.

clinical audit   a quality-improvement process that seeks to improve patient care and outcomes through systematic review. Aspects of the structure, processes, and out-

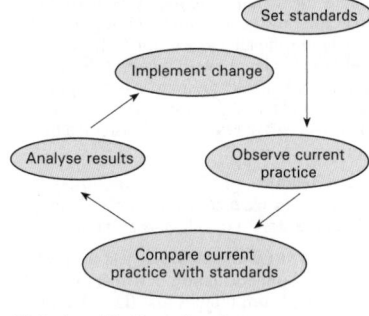

Clinical audit. The audit cycle.

comes of care are selected and systematically evaluated against explicit criteria. Where indicated, changes are implemented at an individual, team, or service level and further monitoring is used to confirm improvement in health-care delivery. The assessment, evaluation, and improvement of quality then forms a cycle of activity (audit cycle) that promotes sustained improvement (see diagram).

A distinction may be made between clinical audit, which refers to total care (involving doctors, nurses, paramedical staff, etc.), and **medical audit**, which refers to medical care specifically performed by doctors, although in practice the two terms are often used interchangeably.

clinical ethics consideration of the moral issues attendant upon, and questions arising from, clinical practice, as distinct from research. In North America, it is common for hospitals to employ a clinical ethicist or provide a formal clinical ethics consultation service. In the UK, clinical *ethics committees are increasingly common in the NHS.

clinical governance the framework through which the NHS aims to deliver high-quality services within a safe system, with continuous efforts for service improvement. Introduced in 1998, clinical governance emphasizes the concept of accountability: organizations, teams, and individuals should understand and accept their roles and responsibilities in delivering care. The range of activities undertaken under the banner of clinical governance includes ensuring clinical effectiveness of treatments, *risk management, *clinical audit, *quality assurance, patient and public involvement (see LOCAL INVOLVEMENT NETWORKS), staff education,

development, and training (see APPRAISAL, REVALIDATION), and research. There is a push in the NHS towards **integrated governance**: a cohesive approach to all governance arrangements (clinical, corporate, and financial) in organizations, with an emphasis on involving patients and external stakeholders in the development of future arrangements. See also CARE QUALITY COMMISSION, INTEGRATED CARE PATHWAY, NATIONAL INSTITUTE FOR HEALTH AND CLINICAL EXCELLENCE, NATIONAL PATIENT SAFETY AGENCY, NATIONAL SERVICE FRAMEWORKS.

clinical medical officer see COMMUNITY HEALTH.

clinical medicine the branch of medicine dealing with the study of actual patients and the diagnosis and treatment of disease at the bedside, as opposed to the study of disease by *pathology or other laboratory work.

clinical trial see INTERVENTION STUDY.

clinodactyly n. congenital deflection of one or more digits from the central axis of the hand or foot. Clinodactyly may affect both hands (or feet) but most commonly affects the fifth finger (which curves towards the fourth). It has an incidence of 9% and may be found in isolation, in association with other congenital malformations, or as part of a syndrome (e.g. Down's syndrome). No treatment is necessary.

clitoridectomy n. the surgical removal of the clitoris (see (FEMALE) CIRCUMCISION).

clitoris n. the female counterpart of the penis, which contains erectile tissue (see CORPUS CAVERNOSUM) but is unconnected with the urethra. Like the penis it becomes erect under conditions of sexual stimulation, to which it is very sensitive.

clitoromegaly n. abnormal development of the clitoris due to excessive exposure to androgens, either from abnormal endogenous production or exogenous administration.

clivus n. (in anatomy) a surface that slopes, as in part of the sphenoid bone.

CLO 1. columnar-lined oesophagus: see BARRETT'S OESOPHAGUS. 2. Campylobacter-like organism: the original (now obsolete) term for *Helicobacter pylori, still widely used as the commercial name for one of the mucosal urease biopsy test kits available (**CLO test**).

cloaca *n.* the most posterior part of the embryonic *hindgut. It becomes divided into the rectum and the urinogenital sinus, which receives the bladder together with the urinary and genital ducts.

clomethiazole (chlormethiazole) *n.* a hypnotic and sedative drug used to treat severe insomnia, agitation, and restlessness in the elderly, and alcohol withdrawal symptoms. It is administered by mouth and the most common side-effects are tingling sensations in the nose and sneezing. Trade name: **Heminevrin**.

clomifene (clomiphene) *n.* a synthetic nonsteroidal compound (*see* ANTI-OESTROGEN) that induces ovulation and subsequent menstruation in women who fail to ovulate (for example, due to polycystic ovary syndrome). It is administered by mouth; common side-effects are hot flushes and abdominal discomfort. Trade name: **Clomid**.

clomipramine *n.* a sedative tricyclic *antidepressant taken by mouth to treat depressive illness, phobias, and obsessional states. Common side-effects are dry mouth and blurred vision. Trade name: **Anafranil**.

clonazepam *n.* a benzodiazepine with *anticonvulsant properties, used to treat epilepsy (including status epilepticus). It is administered by mouth or injection; drowsiness is a common side-effect. Trade name: **Rivotril**.

clone 1. *n.* a group of cells (usually bacteria) descended from a single cell by asexual reproduction and therefore genetically identical to each other and to the parent cell. 2. *n.* an organism derived from a single cell of its parent and therefore genetically identical to it. The first cloned animal, born in 1997, was produced by fusing a somatic nucleus of the parent with a denucleated egg cell of a second animal. The resulting 'embryo' was implanted into the uterus of a third animal to complete its development. 3. *n.* (gene clone) a group of identical genes produced by *genetic engineering. The parent gene is isolated using *restriction enzymes and inserted, via a **cloning vector** (e.g. a bacteriophage), into a bacterium, in which it is replicated. *See also* VECTOR. 4. *vb.* to form a clone. *See also* CLONING.

clonic *adj.* of, relating to, or resembling clonus. The term is most commonly used to describe the rhythmical limb movements

seen as part of a generalized tonic-clonic seizure (*see* EPILEPSY).

clonidine *n.* a drug that interacts with *adrenoceptors in the brain to reduce sympathetic stimulation of the arteries (*see* CATECHOLAMINES, NORADRENALINE). It is occasionally used to treat high blood pressure; administered by mouth or injection, it commonly causes drowsiness and dry mouth, and sudden withdrawal may worsen the hypertension. Trade name: **Catapres**.

In the **clonidine suppression test**, used in the diagnosis of *phaeochromocytoma, clonidine is administered orally and plasma catecholamines sampled then and at hourly intervals for 3 hours. In normal subjects clonidine suppresses release of catecholamines and plasma levels are reduced, but in people with phaeochromocytoma plasma catecholamines remain elevated.

cloning *n.* the process of making identical copies (*clones) of genes, cells, or organisms. **Therapeutic cloning**, which is lawful if licensed by the Human Fertilization and Embryology Authority, produces human blastocysts to harvest their *stem cells. In **reproductive cloning**, whole animals are produced: *see* CLONE (sense 2); reproductive cloning of humans is currently unlawful in the UK. The moral issues relative to therapeutic and reproductive cloning are hotly debated, although for many it is the purpose of cloning that determines its moral acceptability or otherwise.

clonogenic *adj.* describing a cell capable of producing a colony of cells of a predetermined minimum size. Such a cell is known as a **colony forming unit** (**CFU**).

clonorchiasis *n.* a condition caused by the presence of the fluke *Clonorchis sinensis* in the bile ducts. The infection, common in the Far East, is acquired through eating undercooked, salted, or pickled freshwater fish harbouring the larval stage of the parasite. Symptoms include fever, abdominal pain, diarrhoea, liver enlargement, loss of appetite, emaciation and – in advanced cases – cirrhosis and jaundice. Treatment is unsatisfactory although *praziquantel has proved beneficial in some cases.

Clonorchis *n.* a genus of liver flukes, common parasites of humans and other fish-eating mammals in the Far East. The adults of *C. sinensis* cause clonorchiasis. Eggs are passed out in the stools and the larvae undergo their development in two other hosts, a snail and a fish.

clonus *n.* rhythmical contraction of a muscle in response to a suddenly applied and then sustained stretch stimulus. It is most readily obtained at the ankle when the examiner bends the foot sharply upwards and then maintains an upward pressure on the sole. It is caused by an exaggeration of the stretch reflexes and is usually a sign of disease in the brain or spinal cord.

clopidogrel *n.* an *antiplatelet drug that is administered by mouth to prevent strokes or heart attacks in those at risk. Side-effects may include gastrointestinal bleeding. Trade name: **Plavix**.

Clostridium *n.* a genus of mostly Gram-positive anaerobic spore-forming rodlike bacteria commonly found in soil and in the intestinal tract of humans and animals. Many species cause disease and produce extremely potent *exotoxins. *C. botulinum* grows freely in badly preserved canned foods, producing a toxin causing serious food poisoning (*botulism); an extremely dilute form of this toxin is now used to treat muscle spasm (*see* BOTULINUM TOXIN). *C. histolyticum*, *C. oedematiens*, and *C. septicum* all cause *gas gangrene when they infect wounds. *C. tetani* lives as a harmless *commensal in the intestine but causes *tetanus on contamination of wounds (with manured soil). The species *C. perfringens* – Welch's bacillus – causes blood poisoning, *food poisoning, and gas gangrene. Overgrowth of *Clostridium difficile* (often shortened to *C. diff*), a normal inhabitant of the human large intestine, is not uncommon as a complication of some antibiotic therapy and produces a specific condition – **pseudomembranous colitis** (*see* PSEUDOMEMBRANE) – which is life-threatening unless treated promptly and is becoming more common as a hospital-acquired infection.

clotrimazole *n.* an antifungal drug used to treat all types of fungal skin infections (including ringworm), infection in otitis externa, and vaginal candidiasis (thrush). It is applied to the infected part as a cream or solution or as vaginal pessaries and occasionally causes mild burning or irritation. Trade name: **Canesten**.

clotting factors *see* COAGULATION FACTORS.

clotting time *see* COAGULATION TIME.

clozapine *n.* an atypical *antipsychotic drug used in the treatment of schizophrenia in patients who are unresponsive to conventional antipsychotics. Administered by mouth, it is notable for the absence of tremors and repetitive movements that are associated with these drugs. Side-effects include dizziness, headache, and increased salivation, and in a few cases the drug may depress levels of white blood cells. Trade names: **Clozaril**, **Denzapine**, **Zaponex**.

clubbing *n.* thickening of the tissues at the bases of the finger and toe nails so that the normal angle between the nail and the digit is filled in. The nail becomes convex in all directions and in extreme cases the digit end becomes bulbous like a club or drumstick. Clubbing is seen in pulmonary tuberculosis, bronchiectasis, empyema, infective endocarditis, cyanotic congenital heart disease, lung cancer, and cirrhosis and as a harmless congenital abnormality.

club-foot (talipes) *n.* a congenital deformity of one or both feet in which the patient cannot stand with the sole of the foot flat on the ground. In the most common variety (**congenital talipes equinovarus**) the foot points downwards, the heel is inverted, and the forefoot twisted. It is diagnosed at birth and may be associated with other congenital abnormalities. Treatment is initially by physiotherapy and strapping or a plaster cast, but if this fails to correct the deformity surgical correction is performed. Other varieties are **talipes varus**, inward deviation of the hind foot; and **talipes valgus**, an outward deviation of the hind foot, which is much less common.

clumping *n. see* AGGLUTINATION.

cluster headache a variant of *migraine more common in men than in women (ratio 9:1). The unilateral pain around one eye is very severe and lasts between 15 minutes and three hours. The attacks commonly occur in the early hours of the morning but may occur up to eight times a day. The pain is associated with drooping of the eyelid (*ptosis), a bloodshot eye, a small pupil, and/or excessive production of tears in the eye. The acute treatment is with anti-migraine drugs (5HT$_1$ agonists) and prophylaxis is with such drugs as verapamil, lithium, or methysergide.

Clutton's joint a painless joint effusion in

a child, usually in the knee, caused by inflammation of the synovial membranes due to congenital syphilis. [H. H. Clutton (1850–1909), British surgeon]

clyster *n.* an old-fashioned term for an *enema.

CMO *see* CHIEF MEDICAL OFFICER.

CMV *see* CYTOMEGALOVIRUS.

CNS *see* CENTRAL NERVOUS SYSTEM.

coagulant *n.* any substance capable of converting blood from a liquid to a solid state. *See* BLOOD COAGULATION.

coagulase *n.* an enzyme, formed by disease-producing varieties of certain bacteria of the genus *Staphylococcus*, that causes blood plasma to coagulate. Staphylococci that are positive when tested for coagulase production are classified as belonging to the species *Staphylococcus aureus.*

coagulation *n.* the process by which a colloidal liquid changes to a jelly-like mass. *See* BLOOD COAGULATION.

coagulation factors (clotting factors) a group of substances present in blood plasma that, under certain circumstances, undergo a series of chemical reactions leading to the conversion of blood from a liquid to a solid state (*see* BLOOD COAGULATION). Although they have specific names, most coagulation factors are referred to by an agreed set of Roman numerals (e.g. *Factor VIII, *Factor IX). Lack of any of these factors in the blood results in the inability of the blood to clot. *See also* HAEMOPHILIA.

coagulation time (clotting time) the time taken for blood or blood plasma to coagulate (*see* BLOOD COAGULATION). When measured under controlled conditions and using appropriate techniques, coagulation times may be used to test the function of the various stages of the blood coagulation process.

coagulum *n.* a mass of coagulated matter, such as that formed when blood clots.

coalesce *vb.* to grow together or unite. —**coalescence** *n.*

coal tar a complex mixture of hydrocarbons obtained from the distillation of coal. It has anti-inflammatory and antiscaling activity and is used in the treatment of psoriasis, eczema, and dandruff, being applied as a cream, paste, ointment, lotion, solution, or

shampoo, alone or in combination with other ingredients. Side-effects may include local irritation and photosensitivity. Trade names: **Clinitar, Exorex, Psoriderm**, etc.

coal-worker's pneumoconiosis a lung disease caused by coal dust. It affects mainly coal miners but also other exposed workers, such as lightermen, if the lungs' capacity to accommodate and remove the particles is exceeded. *See* PNEUMOCONIOSIS.

co-amoxicla v*see* BETA-LACTAM ANTIBIOTIC.

coarctation *n.* (of the aorta) a congenital narrowing of a short segment of the aorta. The most common site of coarctation is just beyond the origin of the left subclavian artery from the aorta. This results in high blood pressure (*hypertension) in the upper part of the body and arms and low blood pressure in the legs. The defect is corrected surgically.

Coats' disease a congenital anomaly of the blood vessels of the retina, which are abnormally dilated and leaking. This results in subretinal haemorrhage and exudative *retinal detachment. [G. Coats (1876–1915), British ophthalmologist]

cobalamin *n.* see VITAMIN B_{12}.

cobalt *n.* a metallic element. The artificial radioisotope **cobalt-60**, or **radiocobalt**, is a powerful emitter of gamma radiation and is used in the radiation treatment of cancer (*see* RADIOTHERAPY, TELETHERAPY). Cobalt itself forms part of the *vitamin B_{12} molecule. Symbol: Co.

cobalt-chromium *n.* a silver-coloured nonprecious alloy of cobalt and chromium used for the metal frame of partial *dentures.

coblation *n.* a technique that uses high-frequency electric current passed through saline to generate relatively low levels of heat that can simultaneously cut through tissue and coagulate bleeding vessels by means of a device called a **coblator**. The technique can be used for several operations, most notably *tonsillectomy.

cocaine *n.* an alkaloid that is derived from the leaves of the coca plant (*Erythroxylon coca*) or prepared synthetically and is sometimes used as a local anaesthetic applied to mucous membranes in ear, nose, and throat surgery. It constricts the small blood vessels at the site of application and therefore need not be given with *adrenaline. Since it causes feelings of exhilaration and may lead to psychological *dependence, cocaine has largely been replaced by safer anaesthetics.

coccidioidomycosis *n.* an infection caused by inhaling the spores of the fungus *Coccidioides immitis*. In 60% of patients infection produces no symptoms at all. In the primary form there is an influenza-like illness that usually resolves within about eight weeks. In a few patients the disease becomes progressive and resembles tuberculosis. Severe or progressive infections are treated with intravenous injections of amphotericin. The disease is endemic in the desert areas of the Americas, especially the southwestern United States, northern Mexico, and northern Argentina.

coccobacillus *n.* a rod-shaped bacterium (bacillus) that is so small that it resembles a spherical bacterium (coccus). Examples of such bacteria are *Bacteroides* and *Brucella*.

coccus *n.* (*pl.* **cocci**) any spherical bacterium. *See also* GONOCOCCUS, MENINGOCOCCUS, MICROCOCCUS, PNEUMOCOCCUS, STAPHYLOCOCCUS, STREPTOCOCCUS.

coccy- (coccyg-, coccygo-) *combining form* denoting the coccyx. Example: **coccygectomy** (excision of).

coccygodynia (coccydynia) *n.* pain in the lowermost segment of the spine (coccyx) and the neighbouring area, usually as a result of trauma.

coccyx *n.* (*pl.* **coccyges** or **coccyxes**) the lowermost element of the *backbone: the vestigial human tail. It consists of four rudimentary **coccygeal vertebrae** fused to form a triangular bone that articulates with the sacrum. *See also* VERTEBRA. —**coccygeal** *adj.*

cochlea *n.* the spiral organ of the *labyrinth of the ear, which is concerned with the reception and analysis of sound. As vibrations pass from the middle ear through the cochlea, different frequencies cause particular regions of the basilar membrane to vibrate: high notes cause vibration in the region nearest the middle ear; low notes cause vibration in the region nearest the tip of the spiral. The **organ of Corti**, which lies within a central triangular membrane-bound canal (**scala media** or **cochlear duct**), contains sensory hair cells attached to an overlying **tectorial membrane** (see illustration). When the basilar membrane vibrates the sensory cells become distorted and send nerve im-

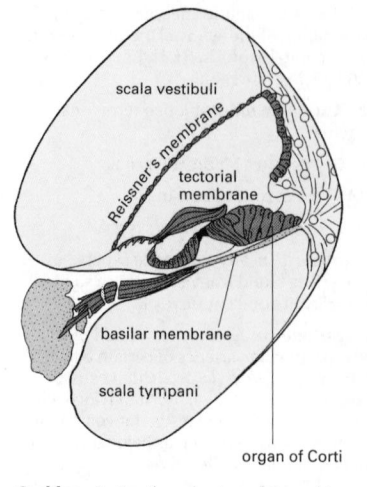

Cochlea. Section through a turn of the cochlea.

pulses to the brain via the *cochlear nerve. —**cochlear** *adj.*

cochlear duct (scala media) *see* COCHLEA.

cochlear implant a device to improve the hearing of profoundly deaf people who derive no benefit from conventional *hearing aids. It consists of an electrode that is permanently implanted into the inner ear (*cochlea). An external device with a microphone and an electronic processing unit passes information to the electrode using radio-frequency waves. The implant is powered by batteries in the external part of the device.

cochlear nerve (acoustic nerve, auditory nerve) the nerve connecting the cochlea to the brain and therefore responsible for transmitting the nerve impulses relating to hearing. It forms part of the *vestibulocochlear nerve (cranial nerve VIII).

Cockayne's syndrome a hereditary disorder (inherited as an autosomal *recessive condition) associated with *trisomy of chromosome no. 20. Clinical features include *epidermolysis bullosa, dwarfism, mental retardation, and pigmentary degeneration of the retina. [E. A. Cockayne (1880–1956), British physician]

Cockcroft-Gault formula a formula for calculating the *glomerular filtration rate based on the patient's age, body mass, and plasma creatinine level. A correction factor can be used to differentiate males from females.

co-codamol *n. see* CODEINE.

codeine *n.* an opioid analgesic derived from *morphine but less potent as a pain killer and sedative and less toxic. It is administered by mouth or intramuscular injection to relieve pain and by mouth to suppress dry coughs and treat diarrhoea. Common side-effects include constipation, nausea, vomiting, dizziness, and drowsiness, but *dependence is uncommon. Codeine may also be administered orally in combination with paracetamol (as **co-codamol**) or aspirin (as **co-codaprin**) for pain relief.

Codman's triangle a triangular area of new bone seen on X-ray at the edge of a malignant bone tumour resulting from elevation of the *periosteum by malignant tissue. It is most often seen in *osteosarcomas. [E. A. Codman (1869–1940), US surgeon]

codon *n.* the unit of the *genetic code that determines the synthesis of one particular amino acid. Each codon consists of a section of the DNA molecule, and the order of the codons along the molecule determines the order of amino acids in each protein made in the cell.

co-dydramol *n. see* DIHYDROCODEINE.

-coele *combining form denoting* 1. a body cavity. Example: **blastocoele** (cavity of blastocyst). 2. *see* -CELE.

coeli- (coelio-) *combining form denoting* the abdomen or belly. Example: **coeliectasia** (abnormal distension of).

coeliac *adj.* of or relating to the abdominal region. The **coeliac trunk** is a branch of the abdominal *aorta supplying the stomach, spleen, liver, and gall bladder.

coeliac disease a condition in which the small intestine fails to digest and absorb food. Affecting 1–2% of the population worldwide, it is due to a permanent sensitivity of the intestinal lining to the protein gliadin, which is contained in *gluten in the germ of wheat and rye and causes atrophy of the digestive and absorptive cells of the intestine. Symptoms include stunted growth, distended abdomen, and pale frothy foul-smelling stools; the disease can be diagnosed by *biopsy of the jejunum and is treated suc-

cessfully by a strict and lifelong gluten-free diet. Medical name: **gluten-sensitive enteropathy**.

(⊕) SEE WEB LINKS
• Website of Coeliac UK: provides information on coeliac disease and gluten-free living

coelioscopy *n.* the technique of introducing an *endoscope through an incision in the abdominal wall to examine the intestines and other organs within the abdominal cavity.

coelom *n.* the cavity in an embryo between the two layers of mesoderm. It develops into the body cavity.

coenzyme *n.* a nonprotein organic compound that, in the presence of an *enzyme, plays an essential role in the reaction that is catalysed by the enzyme. Coenzymes, which frequently contain the B vitamins in their molecular structure, include *coenzyme A, *FAD, and *NAD.

coenzyme A a *nucleotide containing pantothenic acid, which is an important coenzyme in the Krebs cycle and in the metabolism of fatty acids.

cofactor *n.* a nonprotein substance that must be present in suitable amounts before certain *enzymes can act. Cofactors include *coenzymes and metal ions (e.g. sodium and potassium ions).

coffee-ground vomit vomit that contains dark brown granules resembling coffee grounds. It is a sign of upper gastrointestinal bleeding.

Cogan's syndrome a disorder in which *keratitis and iridocyclitis (*see* UVEITIS) are associated with tinnitus, vertigo, and bilateral sensorineural deafness. [D. G. Cogan (1908–93), US ophthalmologist]

cognition *n.* the mental processes by which knowledge is acquired. These include perception, reasoning, acts of creativity, problem-solving, and possibly intuition.

cognitive behavioural therapy (CBT) a *cognitive therapy that is combined with behavioural elements (*see* BEHAVIOUR THERAPY). The patient is encouraged to analyse his or her specific ways of thinking around a problem. The therapist then looks at the resulting behaviour and the consequences of that thinking and tries to encourage the patient to change his or her cognition in order to avoid adverse behaviour or its consequences. CBT is successfully used to treat phobias, anxiety, and depression (it is among the recommended treatments for anxiety and depression in the NICE guidelines).

cognitive psychology the branch of psychology concerned with all human activities relating to knowledge. More specifically, cognitive psychology is concerned with how knowledge is acquired, stored, correlated, and retrieved, by studying the mental processes underlying attention, concept formation, information processing, memory, and speech. Cognitive psychology views the brain as an information-processing system operating on, and storing, the data acquired by the senses. It investigates this function by experiments designed to measure and analyse human performance in carrying out a wide range of mental tasks. The data obtained allows possible models of the underlying mental processes to be constructed. These models do not purport to represent the actual physiological activity of the brain. Nevertheless, as they are refined by testing and criticism, it is hoped that they may approach close to reality and gradually lead to a clearer understanding of how the brain operates.

cognitive therapy a form of *psychotherapy based on the belief that psychological problems are the products of faulty ways of thinking about the world. For example, a depressed patient may use wrongly negative automatic associations in everyday situations. The therapist assists the patient to identify these false ways of thinking and to avoid them. In *cognitive behavioural therapy this is combined with an analysis and retraining of unhelpful behaviours. In **cognitive analytical therapy** (CAT) there is an element of psychodynamic exploration of the patient's problems; CAT is mostly used to treat personality disorders.

cohort study (longitudinal study) a systematic study of a group of people, which may be conducted prospectively or retrospectively. A **prospective cohort study** involves a systematic follow-up for a defined period of time or until the occurrence of a specified event (e.g. onset of illness, retirement, or death) in order to observe patterns of disease and/or cause of death. A **retrospective cohort study** examines data relating to the group's history of exposure and disease experience.

coitus (sexual intercourse, copulation) *n.* sexual contact between a man and a woman during which the erect penis enters the vagina and is moved within it by pelvic thrusts until *ejaculation occurs. *See also* ORGASM. —**coital** *adj.*

coitus interruptus a contraceptive method in which the penis is removed from the vagina before ejaculation of semen (orgasm). The method is unreliable (10–20 pregnancies per 100 woman-years) and it may lead to sexual disharmony and anxiety in one or both partners.

col- (coli-, colo-) *combining form denoting* the colon. Example: **coloptosis** (prolapse of).

colchicine *n.* a drug obtained from the meadow saffron (*Colchicum autumnale*), used to relieve pain in attacks of gout and in the prevention of attacks of hereditary *polyserositis. It is administered by mouth; common side-effects are nausea, vomiting, diarrhoea, and stomach pains.

cold (common cold) *n.* a widespread infectious virus disease causing inflammation of the mucous membranes of the nose, throat, and bronchial tubes. The disease is transmitted by coughing and sneezing. Symptoms commence 1–2 days after infection and include a sore throat, stuffy or runny nose, headache, cough, and general malaise. The disease is mild and lasts only about a week but it can prove serious to young babies and to patients with a pre-existing respiratory complaint.

cold sore *see* HERPES.

colectomy *n.* surgical removal of the colon. **Total colectomy** is removal of the whole colon, usually for extensive *colitis; **partial colectomy** is removal of a segment of the colon. *See also* HEMICOLECTOMY, PROCTOCOLECTOMY.

colestipol *n.* a *bile-acid sequestrant used, in conjunction with dietary reduction of cholesterol, to lower cholesterol levels in the blood in patients with hyperlipidaemia and primary hypercholesterolaemia that have not responded to diet. It is administered by mouth; constipation is a common side-effect. Trade name: **Colestid**.

colestyramine (cholestyramine) *n.* a drug that binds with bile salts so that they are excreted (*see* BILE-ACID SEQUESTRANT). It is administered by mouth to relieve conditions due to irritant effects of bile salts (such as the itching that occurs in obstructive jaundice), to treat diarrhoea, and to lower the blood levels of cholesterol and other fats in patients with hyperlipidaemia. Common side-effects include constipation, heartburn, and nausea. Trade names: **Questran, Questran Light**.

colic *n.* severe abdominal pain, usually of fluctuating severity, with waves of pain seconds or a few minutes apart. **Infantile colic** is common among babies, due to wind in the intestine associated with feeding difficulties. **Intestinal colic** is due to partial or complete obstruction of the intestine or to constipation. Colic arising from the small intestine is felt in the upper abdomen; colic from the colon is felt in the lower abdomen. Medical name: **enteralgia**. **Renal colic** is excruciating pain caused by dilatation and spasm of the ureter when stones are present in the kidney, renal pelvis, or ureter. *See also* BILIARY COLIC.

coliform bacteria a group of Gram-negative rodlike bacteria that are normally found in the gastrointestinal tract and have the ability to ferment the sugar lactose. The group includes the genera *Enterobacter*, *Escherichia*, and *Klebsiella*.

colistin *n.* an antibiotic given by intravenous injection to treat Gram-negative infections resistant to other antimicrobials and by mouth to sterilize the bowel before surgery. Colistin is a mixture of antimicrobial substances produced by a strain of the bacterium *Bacillus polymyxa*. Its most serious side-effects are nerve and kidney damage. Trade name: **Colomycin**.

colitis *n.* inflammation of the colon. The usual symptoms are diarrhoea, often with passage of blood and mucus, and lower abdominal pain. It is diagnosed by demonstrating inflammation of the colon's lining (mucosa) by *sigmoidoscopy, *colonoscopy, or (less likely) *barium enema X-ray. Colitis may be due to infection by *Entamoeba histolytica* (**amoebic colitis**) or by bacteria (**infective colitis**); it may also occur in *Crohn's disease (**Crohn's colitis**). Partial or temporary cessation of blood supply to the colon may cause **ischaemic colitis**. **Ulcerative colitis** (**idiopathic proctocolitis**) almost always involves the rectum (*see* PROCTITIS) as well as a varying extent of the colon, which become inflamed and ulcerated. Its cause is unknown. It varies in severity, relapses being treated by drugs, including corticosteroids and *aminosalicylates (sulfasalazine,

mesalazine, and olsalazine, as tablets or enemas), and bed rest. Severe, continuous, or extensive colitis not responding to medical management requires surgery (*see* COLECTOMY, PROCTOCOLECTOMY). **Microscopic colitis** is characterized by watery diarrhoea and the presence of inflammation on microscopic examination of biopsies of the colonic mucosa (the mucosa are macroscopically normal-looking).

collagen *n.* a protein that is the principal constituent of white fibrous connective tissue (as occurs in tendons). Collagen is also found in skin, bone, cartilage, and ligaments. It is relatively inelastic but has a high tensile strength.

collagen disease an obsolete term for *connective-tissue disease.

collapsing pulse *see* CORRIGAN'S PULSE.

collar bone *see* CLAVICLE.

collateral 1. *adj.* accessory or secondary. 2. *n.* a branch (e.g. of a nerve fibre) that is at right angles to the main part.

collateral circulation 1. an alternative route provided for the blood by secondary vessels when a primary vessel becomes blocked. 2. the channels of communication between the blood vessels supplying the heart. At the apex of the heart, where the coronary arteries form *anastomoses, these are very complex.

Colles' fracture a fracture of the distal end of the *radius, which is displaced backwards and upwards to produce a 'dinner fork' deformity. *Avulsion of the ulnar styloid process (*see* ULNA) usually takes place as well. It is usually caused by a fall on the outstretched hand. The bone is restored to its normal position under anaesthesia, and a plaster cast is applied for about six weeks. Complications are residual deformity and stiffness of the wrist. [A. Colles (1773–1843), Irish surgeon]

colliculus *n.* (*pl.* **colliculi**) a small protuberance or swelling. Two pairs of colliculi, the **superior** and **inferior colliculi**, protrude from the roof of the midbrain (*see* TECTUM).

collimator *n.* a device, used in diagnostic radiology or radiotherapy, to produce a narrow beam of radiation by means of metallic slits that control the size of the beam from a radiation source. Many newer *linear accelerators use **multi-leaf collimators**, a specialized form of collimator using individual 'leaves' (1 cm or smaller) to shape the radiation *treatment field around the tumour. Collimators are also used on radiation detectors, in particular in *gamma cameras, for which the exact source of radioactivity needs to be known to produce an accurate image.

collodion *n.* a syrupy solution of nitrocellulose in a mixture of alcohol and ether. When applied to the surface of the body it evaporates to leave a thin clear transparent skin, useful for the protection of minor wounds. Flexible collodion also contains camphor and castor oil, which allow the skin to stretch a little more.

colloidian baby the distinctive appearance of a newborn baby that is covered in a shiny membrane, resembling a sausage skin. Although the baby is occasionally normal it is more likely that it will suffer from chronic skin disorders, such as *ichthyosis.

collyrium *n.* a medicated solution used to bathe the eyes.

coloboma *n.* a defect in the development of the eye causing abnormalities ranging in severity from a notch in the lower part of the iris, making the pupil pear-shaped, to defects behind the iris in the *fundus. A coloboma of the eyelid is a congenital notch in the lid margin.

colography (colonography) *n.* imaging of the colon, as an alternative to *barium enema or colonoscopy, to detect polyps, tumours, and anatomical abnormalities. **CT colography** uses *computerized tomography to obtain many *axial thin-slice images (usually less than 3 mm thick), which can be electronically reformatted in two or three dimensions (*see* MULTIPLANAR RECONSTRUCTION). It has the added advantage of imaging all the other abdominal organs, including the liver. **MR colography**, using *magnetic resonance imaging, is in development as a widely used clinical tool; it has the advantage over CT of no radiation dose for the patient.

colon *n.* the main part of the large intestine, which consists of four sections – the **ascending**, **transverse**, **descending**, and **sigmoid colons** (see illustration). The colon has no digestive function but it absorbs large amounts of water and electrolytes from the undigested food passed on from the small intestine. At intervals strong peristaltic movements move the dehydrated contents (faeces) towards the rectum. —**colonic** *adj.*

colonic irrigation washing out the contents of the large bowel by means of copious enemas, using either water, with or without soap, or a liquid medication.

colonography *n. see* COLOGRAPHY.

colonoscopy *n.* an endoscopic procedure for examining the interior of the entire colon and often the terminal ileum using a flexible steerable telescopic instrument utilizing digital video technology (**colonoscope**) introduced through the anus. Insertion may be aided by using an external *3-D magnetic imager (e.g. ScopeGuide). It is possible to obtain biopsies for microscopic examination using flexible forceps passed through the colonoscope (**diagnostic colonoscopy**) and to remove polyps using a *diathermy snare, dilate strictures with the scope balloons, or insert self-expandable metal stents (SEMS) into benign or malignant strictures (**therapeutic colonoscopy**).

colony *n.* a discrete population or mass of microorganisms, usually bacteria, all of which are considered to have developed from a single parent cell. Bacterial colonies that grow on agar plates differ in shape, size, colour, elevation, translucency, and surface texture, depending on the species. This is used as a means of identification. *See also* CULTURE.

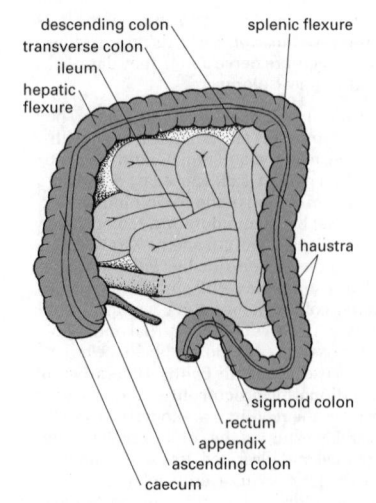

The colon.

colony-stimulating factor (CSF) one of a group of substances (haemopoietic growth factors or hormones) that are produced in the bone marrow and stimulate the production of specific blood cells. Genetically engineered granulocyte colony-stimulating factor (G-CSF) stimulates neutrophil production and also limits bone marrow toxicity from chemotherapy.

colorimeter *n.* an instrument for determining the concentration of a particular compound in a preparation by comparing the intensity of colour in it with that in a standard preparation of known concentration. The instrument is used particularly for measuring the amount of haemoglobin in the blood.

colostomy *n.* a surgical operation in which a part of the colon is brought through the abdominal wall and an artificial opening is created in order to drain or decompress the contents of colon. The part of the colon chosen depends on the site of obstruction or disease process. Depending on the indication a colostomy may be temporary, eventually being closed after months or years to restore intestinal continuity; or permanent, when the colon distal to the colostomy has been removed or is diseased. A bag is usually worn over the colostomy opening (*stoma) to collect the faeces for disposal.

(((🌐))) SEE WEB LINKS
• Website of the Colostomy Association
• Living with a Colostomy: an interactive website for ostomists and their families

colostrum *n.* the first secretion from the breast, occurring shortly after, or sometimes before, birth prior to the secretion of true milk. It is a relatively clear fluid containing serum, white blood cells, and protective antibodies.

colour blindness any of various conditions in which certain colours are confused with one another. True lack of colour appreciation is extremely rare (*see* MONOCHROMAT), but some defect of colour discrimination is present in about 8% of Caucasian males, and 0.4% of Caucasian females. The most common type of colour blindness is **Daltonism** (**protanopia**) – red-blindness – in which the person cannot distinguish between reds and greens. Occasional cases are due to acquired disease of the retina but in the vast majority it is inherited. The defect is thought to be in the functioning of the light-sensitive cells in the retina responsible for colour perception (*see* CONE). *See also* DEUTERANOPIA, TRICHROMATIC.

colour flow ultrasound imaging *see* DOPPLER ULTRASOUND.

colp- (colpo-) *combining form denoting* the vagina. Example: **colpoplasty** (plastic surgery of).

colpoperineorrhaphy *n.* an operation to repair tears in the vagina and the muscles surrounding its opening.

colporrhaphy (perineal repair) *n.* an operation designed to remove lax and redundant vaginal tissue and so reduce the diameter of the vagina in cases of prolapse of the base of the bladder (**anterior colporrhaphy**; *see* CYSTOCELE) or of the rectum (**posterior colporrhaphy**; *see* RECTOCELE).

colposcopy *n.* examination of the cervix under low-power binocular magnification and an intense light source. If abnormalities are revealed (identified as white areas after application of acetic acid, then iodine, to the cervix), a diagnostic biopsy is taken for histological assessment. Confirmation of the diagnosis is followed by appropriate treatment (*see* CERVICAL INTRAEPITHELIAL NEOPLASIA). —**colposcopic** *adj.*

colposuspension *n.* a surgical procedure for treating stress incontinence in women in which the upper part of the vaginal wall is fixed to the anterior abdominal wall by unabsorbable suture material. It may be performed through an abdominal incision (**Burch colposuspension**) or using a laparoscope (**laparoscopic colposuspension**). These techniques have now been largely replaced by other less invasive sling procedures, such as *tension-free vaginal tape.

columella *n.* (in anatomy) a part resembling a small column. For example, the **columella cochleae** (**modiolus**) is the central pillar of the cochlea, around which the spiral cochlear canal winds. The **columella nasi** is the anterior part of the nasal septum.

column *n.* (in anatomy) any pillar-shaped structure, especially any of the tracts of grey matter found in the spinal cord.

COM chronic otitis media (*see* OTITIS).

coma *n.* a state of unrousable unconsciousness. *See also* GLASGOW COMA SCALE.

co-magaldrox *n. see* ALUMINIUM HYDROX-IDE.

combined therapy therapy that combines several types of treatment in order to improve results. It is usually a combination of surgery with radiotherapy and/or chemotherapy for the treatment of malignant tumours (*see* ADJUVANT THERAPY). *See also* SANDWICH THERAPY.

Combitube *n.* trade name for an airway support device, initially designed for use by relatively untrained personnel on the battlefield, that is referred to in modern hospital resuscitation guidelines but rarely used. The device has two tubes and is introduced through the mouth blindly into the back of the throat. It may end up in either the oesophagus or the airway: ventilation is provided either through the hole in the end of the tracheal tube or via perforations in the side of the oesophageal tube.

comedo *n.* (*pl.* **comedones**) *see* BLACK-HEAD.

commando operation a major operation performed to remove a malignant tumour from the head and neck. Extensive dissection, often involving the face, is followed by reconstruction to restore function and cosmetic acceptability.

commensal *n.* an organism that lives in close association with another of a different species without either harming or benefiting it. For example, some microorganisms living in the gut obtain both food and a suitable habitat but neither harm nor benefit humans. *Compare* SYMBIOSIS. —**commensalism** *n.*

comminuted fracture a fracture in which the bone is broken into more than two pieces. A crushing force is usually responsible and there is often extensive injury to surrounding soft tissues.

Commission for Patient and Public Involvement in Health (CPPIH) a nondepartmental public body set up in 2003 to ensure that the public is involved in decisions about health-care services. The CPPIH was abolished in 2008 when *PPI forums were replaced by *local involvement networks (LINks).

Commission for Social Care Inspection (CSCI) (in England) a nondepartmental public body responsible for inspecting and reporting on social care services. The

CSCI was replaced in 2009 by the *Care Quality Commission.

commissure *n.* **1.** a bundle of nerve fibres that crosses the midline of the central nervous system, often connecting similar structures on each side. **2.** any other tissue connecting two similar structures.

commotio retinae swelling of the retina, usually resulting from blunt trauma to the eye. The swelling usually resolves over a few days.

communicable disease (contagious disease, infectious disease) any disease that can be transmitted from one person to another. This may occur by direct physical contact, by common handling of an object that has picked up infective microorganisms (*see* FOMES), through a disease *carrier, or by spread of infected droplets coughed or exhaled into the air. The most dangerous communicable diseases are on the list of *notifiable diseases. Specific legal obligations arise in respect of notifiable diseases by virtue of the Public Health (Control of Disease) Act 1984 (as amended), delegated legislation, and the Health and Social Care Act 2008.

communicable disease control the control of disease due to infectious agents or their toxic products. *See* CONSULTANT IN COMMUNICABLE DISEASE CONTROL.

communicans *adj.* communicating or connecting. The term is applied particularly to blood vessels or nerve fibres connecting two similar structures.

communitarianism *n.* an approach to ethical problems that rejects excessive emphasis on the individual and focuses instead on social cohesion and community interests, arguing that every single person is embedded within society and depends on others to flourish. As such, individual *rights and personal *autonomy may be morally less important than the collective experience and social responsibility.

community health preventive services, mainly outside the hospital, involving the surveillance of special groups of the population, such as preschool and school children, women, and the elderly, by means of routine clinical assessment and *screening tests. Routine preventive measures, such as immunization, family planning, and dietary advice, are offered in special clinics staffed by

*community nurses, **clinical medical officers**, and **senior clinical medical officers** and sometimes by *community paediatricians. When somebody is identified as having an illness, he (or she) is referred for treatment to a *general practitioner or hospital as appropriate. *See also* CHILD HEALTH CLINIC, SCHOOL HEALTH SERVICE.

community hospital *see* HOSPITAL.

community medicine *see* PUBLIC HEALTH MEDICINE.

community mental health team (CMHT) a multidisciplinary team consisting of psychiatrists, psychiatric nurses, psychologists, social workers, and occupational therapists who treat patients with severe mental illness in the community.

community midwife (domiciliary midwife) (in Britain) a registered *nurse with special training in midwifery (both hospital and domiciliary practice). The midwife must be registered with the *Nursing and Midwifery Council in order to practise; this requires regular refresher courses to supplement the basic qualification of **Registered Midwife** (RM). Community midwives are attached to general practices or hospitals, and their work includes **home deliveries** and antenatal and postnatal care in the community.

community nurses (in Britain) a generic term for *health visitors, *community midwives, and *district nurses. *See also* DOMICILIARY SERVICES.

community paediatrician a consultant in paediatrics with special responsibility for the care of children outside the hospital. *See also* COMMUNITY HEALTH.

community services *see* DOMICILIARY SERVICES.

Community Treatment Order *see* MENTAL HEALTH ACT.

comparative mortality figure *see* OCCUPATIONAL MORTALITY.

compartment *n.* (in anatomy) any one of the spaces in a limb that are bounded by bone and thick sheets of fascia and enclose the muscles and other tissues of the limb.

compartment syndrome the condition that results from swelling of the muscles in a *compartment of a limb, which raises the pressure within the compartment so that the blood supply to the muscle is cut off, causing *ischaemia and further swelling. If it persists, the muscles and nerves within the compartment die, leading to *Volkmann's contracture. Causes are trauma, damage to blood vessels, reperfusion after ischaemia, and tight casts or bandages. Treatment is to release any tight dressings and to divide the fascia surrounding the compartment to relieve the pressure (*see* FASCIOTOMY).

compatibility *n.* the degree to which the body's defence systems will tolerate the presence of intruding foreign material, such as blood when transfused or a kidney when transplanted. Complete compatibility exists between identical twins: a blood transfusion between identical twins will evoke no *antibody formation in the recipient. In severe **incompatibility**, for example between completely unrelated people, there are likely to be swift immune reactions as antibodies attack and destroy any offending antigenic material. *See also* HISTOCOMPATIBILITY, IMMUNITY. —**compatible** *adj.*

compensation *n.* **1.** the act of making up for a functional or structural deficiency. For example, compensation for the loss of a diseased kidney is brought about by an increase in size of the remaining kidney, so restoring the urine-producing capacity. **2.** monetary payment in redress for injury or loss. The amount of compensation awarded to an injured party usually corresponds to the degree of harm suffered, damages being split into general and special damages.

competence *n. see* CAPACITY.

complaints system a process that enables patients to voice concerns about the standard of care they receive within the NHS and through which they may be awarded *compensation. Strict procedural rules apply to the management of complaints. A grievance is usually resolved at a local level within the institution or trust concerned. The Independent Complaints Advocacy Service is available to provide advice and guidance to complainants. If a patient is not satisfied with the outcome of local resolution, the matter can be referred to the *Health Service Ombudsman. Legal action cannot usually proceed at the same time and only a small proportion of complaints proceed to law. Disciplinary procedures are separate from the complaints procedure although complaints may prompt or inform disciplinary action.

complement *n.* a system of functionally linked proteins that interact with one another to aid the body's defences when *antibodies combine with *antigens. Complement is involved in the breaking-up (*lysis) and *opsonization of foreign organisms. It is also involved in inflammation and clearing immune (antigen-antibody) complexes.

complementary medicine various forms of therapy that are viewed as complementary to conventional medicine. These include (but are not confined to) *osteopathy, *acupuncture, *homeopathy, *massage, *aromatherapy, *reflexology, and *reiki. Previously, complementary therapies were regarded as an alternative to conventional therapies, and the two types were considered to be mutually exclusive (hence the former names **alternative medicine** and **fringe medicine**). However, many practitioners now have dual training in conventional and complementary therapies. There is very limited provision for complementary medicine within the confines of the National Health Service.

complement fixation the binding of *complement to the complex that is formed when an antibody reacts with a specific antigen. Because complement is taken up from the serum only when such a reaction has occurred, testing for the presence of complement after mixing a suspension of a known organism with a patient's serum can give confirmation of infection with a suspected organism. The *Wassermann reaction for diagnosing syphilis is a complement-fixation test.

complex *n.* (in psychoanalysis) an emotionally charged and repressed group of ideas and beliefs that is capable of influencing an individual's behaviour. The term in this sense was originally used by Jung, but it is now widely used in a looser sense to denote an unconscious motive.

complex partial seizure *see* EPILEPSY.

complex regional pain syndrome *see* REFLEX SYMPATHETIC DYSTROPHY.

compliance *n. see* ADHERENCE.

complication *n.* a disease or condition arising during the course of or as a consequence of another disease.

compomer *n.* a dental filling material that is a hybrid of *composite resin and *glass ionomer.

composite resin a tooth-coloured filling material for teeth. It is composed of two different materials: an inorganic filler chemically held in an organic resin. Composite resins are usually hardened by polymerization initiated by intense light.

compress *n.* a pad of material soaked in hot or cold water and applied to an injured part of the body to relieve the pain of inflammation.

compressed air illness (caisson disease) a syndrome occurring in people working under high pressure in diving bells or at great depths with breathing apparatus. On return to normal atmospheric pressure nitrogen dissolved in the bloodstream expands to form bubbles, causing pain (the **bends**) and blocking the circulation in small blood vessels in the brain and elsewhere (**decompression sickness**). Pain, paralysis, and other features may be eliminated by returning the victim to a higher atmospheric pressure and reducing this gradually, so causing the bubbles to redissolve. Chronic compressed air illness may cause damage to the bones (*see* OSTEONECROSIS), heart, and lungs.

compression venography an *ultrasound technique to look for blockages in leg veins, usually deep vein *thrombosis. Pressing the vein with the ultrasound probe usually causes it to empty and flatten, which does not occur if there is thrombus in the lumen. *See also* VENOGRAPHY.

compulsion *n.* an *obsession that takes the form of a motor act, such as repetitive washing based on a fear of contamination, as seen in obsessive–compulsive disorder.

compulsory admission (involuntary admission) (in Britain) the entry and detention of a person within an institution without his consent, either because of mental illness (*see* MENTAL HEALTH ACT) or severe social deprivation and self-neglect (*see* SECTION 47 REMOVAL). *Compare* VOLUNTARY ADMISSION.

computerized radiography (CR) a system for replacing photographic film with a charged plate. Exposure to X-rays knocks charge off the plate. The resultant image can be read by a laser beam and stored digitally or printed out as required. This system is widely used in conjunction with *PACS systems.

computerized tomography (CT) a form of X-ray examination in which the X-ray source and detector (**CT scanner**) rotate around the object to be scanned and the information obtained can be used to produce cross-sectional images (*see* CROSS-SECTIONAL IMAGING) by computer (a **CT scan**). A higher radiation dose is received by the patient than with some conventional X-ray techniques, but the diagnostic information obtained is far greater and should outweigh the increased risk. CT scanning can be used for all parts of the body, but is particularly useful in the head, chest, and abdomen. The data obtained can be used to construct three-dimensional images of structures of interest. *See also* MULTIDETECTOR COMPUTERIZED TOMOGRAPHY, SPIRAL CT SCANNING.

conception *n.* 1. (in gynaecology) the start of pregnancy, when a male germ cell (sperm) fertilizes a female germ cell (ovum) in the *Fallopian tube. 2. (in psychology) an idea or mental impression.

conceptus *n.* the products of conception: the developing fetus and its enclosing membrane at all stages in the uterus.

concha *n.* (*pl.* **conchae**) (in anatomy) any part resembling a shell. For example, the **concha auriculae** is a depression on the outer surface of the pinna (auricle), which leads to the external auditory meatus of the outer ear. *See also* NASAL CONCHA.

concomitant *adj.* at the same time: describing drugs that are administered together or symptoms that occur during the same period.

concordance *n.* similarity of any physical characteristic that is found in both of a pair of twins.

concretion *n.* a stony mass formed within such an organ as the kidney, especially the coating of an internal organ (or a foreign body, such as a urinary catheter) with calcium salts. *See also* CALCULUS.

concussion *n.* a condition caused by injury to the head, characterized by headache, confusion, and amnesia. These symptoms may be prolonged and constitute a **post-concussional syndrome**. There may be no recognizable structural damage to the brain, but scans may reveal evidence of *contusion (bruising) within the brain. Repeated concussion eventually causes symptoms suggesting brain damage. *See also* PUNCH-DRUNK SYNDROME.

condenser *n.* (in microscopy) an arrangement of lenses beneath the stage of a microscope. It can be adjusted to provide correct focusing of light on the microscope slide.

conditioned reflex a reflex in which the response occurs not to the sensory stimulus that normally causes it but to a separate stimulus, which has been learnt to be associated with it. In Pavlov's classic experiments, dogs learned to associate the sound of a bell with feeding time and would salivate at the bell's sound whether food was then presented to them or not.

conditioning *n.* the establishment of new behaviour by modifying the stimulus/response associations. In **classical conditioning** a stimulus not normally associated with a particular response is presented together with the stimulus that evokes the response automatically. This is repeated until the first stimulus evokes the response by itself (*see* CONDITIONED REFLEX). In **operant conditioning** a response is rewarded (or punished) each time it occurs, so that in time it comes to occur more (or less) frequently (*see* REINFORCEMENT).

condom *n.* a sheath made of latex rubber, plastic, or silk that is fitted over the penis during sexual intercourse. Use of a condom protects both partners against sexually transmitted diseases (including AIDS) and, carefully used, it is a reasonably reliable contraceptive (between 2 and 10 pregnancies per 100 woman-years). A more recent development is the **female condom** (e.g. **Femidom**), which is fitted into the vagina. Manufactured from similar materials as male condoms, they too act as both contraceptives and as barriers to sexually transmitted diseases.

conduct disorder a repetitive and persistent pattern of aggressive or otherwise antisocial behaviour. It is usually recognized in childhood or adolescence and can lead to *antisocial personality disorder. Treatment is usually with *behaviour therapy or *family therapy.

condylarthrosis (condyloid joint) *n.* a form of *diarthrosis (freely movable joint) in which an ovoid head fits into an elliptical cavity. Examples are the knee joint and the joint between the mandible (lower jaw) and the temporal bone of the skull.

condyle *n.* a rounded protuberance that occurs at the ends of some bones, e.g. the *occipital bone, and forms an articulation with another bone.

condyloma *n.* (*pl.* **condylomata**) a raised wartlike growth. **Condylomata acuminata** (*sing.* **condyloma acuminatum**) are warts caused by *human papillomavirus and are found on the vulva, under the foreskin, or on the skin of the anal region. They may be treated with podophyllin, trichloroacetic acid, topical *imiquimod, or cryotherapy; patients should be checked for the presence of other sexually transmitted diseases. **Condylomata lata** (*sing.* **condyloma latum**) are flat plaques found in the secondary stage of syphilis, occurring in the anogenital region.

cone *n.* one of the two types of light-sensitive cells in the *retina of the eye (*compare* ROD). The human retina contains 6–7 million cones; they function best in bright light and are essential for acute vision (receiving a sharp accurate image). The area of the retina called the *fovea contains the greatest concentration of cones. Cones can also distinguish colours. It is thought that there are three types of cone, each sensitive to the wavelength of a different primary colour – red, green, or blue. Other colours are seen as combinations of these three primary colours.

cone beam CT *see* IMAGE-GUIDED RADIO-THERAPY.

cone biopsy surgical removal, by knife or laser, of a cone-shaped segment of tissue from the cervix of the uterus. It may be performed if a cervical biopsy (*see* COLPOSCOPY) reveals evidence of cervical carcinoma in situ (*cervical intraepithelial neoplasia type 3): the abnormal tissue is removed and examined microscopically for confirmation of complete removal of the abnormality.

confabulation *n.* the invention of circumstantial but fictitious detail about events supposed to have occurred in the past. Usually this is to disguise an inability to remember past events. It may be a symptom of any form of loss of memory, but typically occurs in *Korsakoff's syndrome.

confection *n.* (in pharmacy) a sweet substance that is combined with a medicinal preparation to make it suitable for administration.

confidence interval (in statistics) a range of values (interval) that contains the parameter of interest within a given probability. For example, with a 95% confidence interval the parameter value will lie in this interval 95 times out of every 100.

confidential enquiries special enquiries that seek to improve health and health care by collecting evidence on aspects of care and disseminating recommendations based on these findings. The **Confidential Enquiry into Maternal Deaths and Child Health** (**CEMACH**, now incorporating **Confidential Enquiries into Stillbirths and Deaths in Infancy, CESDI**) reports on the care of mothers and children (*see* INFANT MORTALITY RATE, MATERNAL DEATH, MATERNAL MORTALITY RATE, PERINATAL MORTALITY RATE). The **National Confidential Enquiry into Patient Outcome and Death** investigates general medical and surgical care, and the **National Confidential Inquiry into Suicide and Homicide by People with Mental Illness** covers the care of people with mental illness. The *National Patient Safety Agency manages the contracts with the confidential enquiries.

confidentiality *n.* an ethical and legal obligation that requires doctors to keep information about their patients private. It is the foundation on which trust and the therapeutic relationship is built. A doctor automatically assumes such an obligation during a patient consultation. Confidentiality is generally considered to be held within the health-care team rather than with one particular professional in order to facilitate effective care. Confidentiality is not an unlimited duty and sometimes it is permissible or even obligatory to breach a patient's confidence, e.g. for child protection or when a patient suffers from a *notifiable disease. One of the most common situations in which confidentiality can be breached is where there is a serious risk of physical harm to an identifiable individual or individuals. There is no 'duty to warn' in the UK, which means that doctors may be entitled to breach confidentiality where there is a serious risk of harm, but not obliged to do so. The GMC requires that doctors should be prepared to justify their decision whether or not they decide to breach confidentiality in cases of serious risk. *See also* DATA PROTECTION, PRIVACY. —**confidential** *adj.*

conflict *n.* (in psychology) the state produced when a stimulus produces two opposing reactions. The basic types of conflict situation are **approach–approach**, in which the individual is drawn towards two attractive – but mutually incompatible – goals; **approach–avoidance**, where the stimulus evokes reactions both to approach and to avoid; and **avoidance–avoidance**, in which the avoidance reaction to one stimulus would bring the individual closer to an equally unpleasant stimulus. Conflict has been used to explain the development of neurotic disorders, and the resolution of conflict remains an important part of psychoanalysis. *See also* CONVERSION.

conflict of interest (in medical ethics) the situation in which a health professional is subject to potential or actual pressures that may conflict with his or her obligation to promote the *best interests of the patient over and above all else. A conflict of interest arises from a particular context or situation and may threaten a doctor's integrity and undermine trust between professional and patient. For example, a drug company may encourage a doctor to prescribe a particular medicine, which may not be the treatment of choice for a patient. In medical research, there is always a potential conflict between protecting the individual and benefiting society. Particular problems of this kind occur in randomized controlled trials (*see* EQUIPOISE, INTERVENTION STUDY). Doctors will always experience competing pressures and it is important for them to be able to recognize and then, where possible, disclose, resolve, or mitigate morally problematic conflicts.

confluence *n*. a point of coalescence. The **confluence of the sinuses** is the meeting point of the superior sagittal, transverse, straight, and occipital venous sinuses in the dura mater in the occipital region of the skull.

congenital *adj*. describing a condition that is recognized at birth or that is believed to have been present since birth. Congenital malformations include all disorders present at birth whether they are inherited or caused by an environmental factor.

congenital adrenal hyperplasia a family of autosomal *recessive genetic disorders causing decreased activity of any of the enzymes involved in the synthesis of *cortisol from *cholesterol. The most commonly affected enzymes are 21-hydroxylase and 11-hydroxylase, and each enzyme deficiency

can itself be due to a variety of genetic mutations. The clinical manifestations depend on which enzyme is affected and the resultant deficiencies and build-up products produced. The most serious consequence is adrenal crisis and/or severe salt wasting due to lack of cortisol and/or aldosterone, which may prove fatal if undiagnosed. The condition is often easier to spot at birth in females, who may have indeterminate genitalia due to high levels of *testosterone in utero. Adrenal hyperplasia occurs due to excessive stimulation of the glands by *ACTH (adreno-corticotrophic hormone) in response to the resultant cortisol deficiency of these conditions.

congenital diaphragmatic hernia (CDH) herniation of the fetal abdominal organs into the fetal chest, which occurs in one in 2000–5000 live births. This leads to pulmonary *hypoplasia, which is the main cause of the associated high neonatal mortality. The risk of pulmonary hypoplasia is substantially greater where there is herniation of the liver into the thoracic cavity. CDH is commonly associated with additional structural abnormalities (cardiac, neural tube defects, and exomphalos), and the risk of chromosomal abnormality (*aneuploidy) is 10–20%. Demonstration of a fluid-filled bowel at the level of the heart on ultrasound is diagnostic.

congenital dislocation of the hip (CDH) an abnormality present at birth in which the head of the femur is displaced or easily displaceable from the acetabulum (socket) of the ilium, which is poorly developed; it frequently affects both hip joints. CDH occurs in about 1.5 per 1000 live births, being more common in first-born girls, in breech deliveries, and if there is a family history of the condition. The leg is shortened and has a reduced range of movement, and the skin creases may be asymmetrical. All babies are routinely screened for CDH at birth and at developmental check-ups by gentle manipulation of the hip causing it to be reduced and dislocated with a clunk (*see* BARLOW MANOEUVRE, ORTOLANI MANOEUVRE). The diagnosis is confirmed by X-ray or ultrasound scan. Treatment is with a special harness holding the hip in the correct position. If this is unsuccessful, the hip is reduced under anaesthetic and held with a plaster of Paris cast or the defect is corrected by surgery. Successful treatment of an infant can give a normal hip; if the dislocation is not detected, the hip does not develop normally and osteoarthritis develops at a young age.

congenitally corrected transposition
see TRANSPOSITION OF THE GREAT VESSELS.

congestion *n.* an accumulation of blood within an organ, which is the result of back pressure within its veins (for example congestion of the lungs and of the liver occurs in heart failure). Congestion may be associated with *oedema (accumulation of fluid in the tissues). It is relieved by treatment of the cause.

congestive cardiac failure (CCF, congestive heart failure) *see* HEART FAILURE.

Congo red a dark-red or reddish-brown pigment that becomes blue in acidic conditions. It is used as a histological *stain. *Amyloidosis is indicated if over 60% of the dye disappears from the blood within one hour of injection.

coniine *n.* an extremely poisonous alkaloid, found in hemlock (*Conium maculatum*), that paralyses the nerves, mainly the motor nerves. Coniine has been included in drug preparations for the treatment of asthma and whooping cough.

coning *n.* prolapse of the brainstem through the *foramen magnum as a result of raised intracranial pressure: it is usually immediately fatal. A similar emergency can occur through the hiatus of the *tentorium.

conization *n.* surgical removal of a cone of tissue. The technique is commonly used in excising a portion of the cervix (neck) of the uterus (*see* CONE BIOPSY) for the treatment of cervicitis or early cancer (carcinoma in situ).

conjoined twins identical twins that are physically joined together at birth, known colloquially as **Siamese twins**. The condition ranges from twins joined only by the umbilical blood vessels (allantoido-angiopagous twins) to those in whom conjoined heads or trunks are inseparable.

conjugate (conjugate diameter, true conjugate) *n.* the distance between the front and rear of the pelvis measured from the most prominent part of the sacrum to the back of the pubic symphysis. Since the true conjugate cannot normally be measured during life it is estimated by subtracting 1.3–1.9 cm from the **diagonal conjugate**, the distance between the lower edge of the symphysis and the sacrum (usually about 12.7 cm). If the true conjugate is less than about 10.2 cm, delivery of an infant through the natural passages may be difficult or impossible, and *Caesarean section may have to be performed.

conjugation *n.* the union of two microorganisms in which genetic material (DNA) passes from one organism to the other. In bacteria minute projections on the donor 'male' cell (**pili**) form a bridge with the recipient 'female' cell; the exact function of the pili is not known, but they are believed to have an important role in conjugation.

conjunctiva *n.* the delicate mucous membrane that covers the front of the eye and lines the inside of the eyelids. The conjunctiva lining the eyelids contains many blood vessels but that over the eyeball contains few and is transparent. —**conjunctival** *adj.*

conjunctivitis (pink eye) *n.* inflammation of the conjunctiva, which becomes red and swollen and produces a watery or pus-containing discharge. It causes discomfort rather than pain and does not usually affect vision. Conjunctivitis may be caused by infection by bacteria or viruses (in which case it usually spreads rapidly to the other eye) or physical or chemical irritation. The patient usually recovers with no after-effects in one to three weeks; bacterial infections respond to antibiotic eye drops. **Allergic** (or **vernal**) **conjunctivitis** is acute or chronic inflammation of the cornea usually due to a specific allergen, such as pollen, animal danders, or dust. It is characterized by itching, irritation, redness, watering of the eyes, and light sensitivity. *See also* INCLUSION CONJUNCTIVITIS, TRACHOMA.

connective tissue the tissue that supports, binds, or separates more specialized tissues and organs or functions as a packing tissue of the body. It consists of an amorphous **ground substance** of mucopolysaccharides in which may be embedded white (collagenous), yellow (elastic), and reticular fibres, fat cells, *fibroblasts, *mast cells, and *macrophages (see illustration). Variations in chemical composition of the ground substance and in the proportions and quantities of cells and fibres give rise to tissues of widely differing characteristics, including bone, cartilage, tendons, and ligaments as well as *adipose, *areolar, and *elastic tissues.

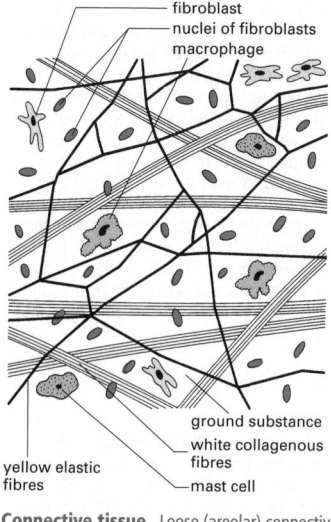

- fibroblast
- nuclei of fibroblasts
- macrophage
- ground substance
- white collagenous fibres
- yellow elastic fibres
- mast cell

Connective tissue. Loose (areolar) connective tissue.

connective-tissue disease any one of a group of diseases that are characterized by inflammatory changes in connective tissue and can affect virtually any body system. Formerly known as **collagen diseases** (connective-tissue disease has been the preferred term since 1978), they include *dermatomyositis, systemic and discoid *lupus erythematosus, *morphoea, *polyarteritis nodosa, and *rheumatoid arthritis.

Conn's syndrome the combination of muscular weakness, abnormally intense thirst (polydipsia), the production of large volumes of urine (polyuria), and hypertension, resulting from excessive production of the hormone aldosterone by the adrenal cortex (*see* ALDOSTERONISM). It is a rare cause of hypertension. [W. J. Conn (1907–94), US physician]

consanguinity *n.* relationship by blood; the sharing of a common ancestor within a few generations.

conscientious objection a refusal to behave in a socially or legally accepted way because such behaviour is counter to one's personal beliefs, principles, or values. Conscientious objection is commonly, but not always, based on religious belief. In some areas of medical practice, there is legal provision allowing for conscientious objection; for example, by virtue of the Abortion Act 1967, section 4(1), a doctor can lawfully refuse to perform an abortion on the grounds of a conscientious objection but must refer the patient to a colleague who will carry out the procedure. Adherents of some religious denominations, such as Jehovah's Witnesses, may refuse life-saving treatments, frequently those involving blood products, on the grounds of conscience and religious belief, and provided the patient has capacity, a doctor is bound to respect the wishes or *autonomy of the patient.

consent *n.* agreement to undergo any medical treatment or to participate in medical research. There are four criteria that must be met for consent to be legally valid, namely: (i) the patient must have capacity to make a choice; (ii) the patient must be provided with sufficient information (*see* INFORMED CONSENT) as to the nature of treatment, its likely consequences, and the possible effects of not having treatment; (iii) the patient must be in a position to decide voluntarily, i.e. without external pressure or influence, which may entail giving the patient time to consider the options; and (iv) the patient should be largely consistent in their views and understand that they can change their mind about treatment at any point. Valid consent usually provides a legal defence against the charge of *battery (trespass against the person). Claims of *negligence may be brought if the doctor discloses insufficient or inadequate information or fails to answer the patient's questions and address his or her concerns.

The law requires consent to be evidenced in writing only in special cases, such as recruiting a subject to a clinical trial. However, consent forms are commonly used for evidential purposes and to communicate a patient's choice within the health-care team. Valid consent is not required in an emergency or where a patient lacks capacity. It used to be that the concept of *therapeutic privilege provided a further exception to the requirement that patients should give valid consent, but such a position is contentious and considered by many commentators to be outdated and inappropriate. *See also* ASSENT, AUTONOMY.

consequentialism *n.* a theoretical approach arguing that the morality or otherwise of an action or question can be determined according to the consequences that will ensue. As such, the theory proposes that actions should be judged by their consequences and not according to their intrinsic nature or the motives or character of those performing them. Consequences may be considered according to probability and impact. According to this view, the ethical course of action is that which will maximize good outcomes and minimize bad outcomes. The best known example of consequentialism is *utilitarianism, which in general seeks to achieve maximum utility or good outcomes for the greatest possible number of people in society.

Consequentialism is a major theory within medical ethics, where the twin principles of *beneficence and *nonmaleficence can be seen as essentially consequentialist. A *cost–benefit analysis or *risk–benefit analysis on utilitarian principles is often carried out when distributing medical resources or deciding between treatments. A calculation of this kind also forms the basis of the quality-adjusted life years (QALYs) system (*see* QUALITY OF LIFE).

The main objection to strict consequentialism is that the consequences of actions cannot always be predicted or perceived. Furthermore, it depends on measuring the measurable. There are also questions as to who should be included in the calculus (e.g. should the interests of fetuses or animals be considered?). Finally, despite 'everyone' counting once and only once in the equation, it can lead to seemingly unfair, unforeseen, or unintended outcomes for certain individuals or groups. —**consequentialist** *adj.*

conservative treatment treatment aimed at preventing a condition from becoming worse, in the expectation that either natural healing will occur or progress of the disease will be so slow that no drastic treatment will be justified. *Compare* RADICAL TREATMENT.

consolidation *n.* 1. the state of the lung in which the alveoli (air sacs) are filled with fluid produced by inflamed tissue, as in *pneumonia. It is diagnosed from its dullness to *percussion, bronchial breathing (*see* BREATH SOUNDS) in the patient, and from the distribution of shadows on the chest X-ray. 2. the stage of repair of a broken bone following *callus formation, during which the callus is transformed by *osteoblasts into mature bone.

constipation *n.* a condition in which bowel evacuations occur infrequently, or in which the faeces are hard and small, or where passage of faeces causes difficulty or pain. The frequency of bowel evacuation varies considerably from person to person and the normal cannot be precisely defined. Constipation developing in a person of previously regular bowel habit may be a symptom of intestinal disease. Recurrent or longstanding constipation is treated by increasing fluid intake, *dietary fibre (roughage), *laxatives, or *enemas. **Faecal impaction**, the end-result of chronic constipation commoner in elderly and very young patients, often requires manual removal of the faecal bolus, sometimes under an anaesthetic.

constrictor *n.* any muscle that compresses an organ or causes a hollow organ or part to contract.

consultant *n.* a fully trained specialist in a branch of medicine. In Britain, consultants are responsible for the care of patients within a distinct specialty, usually in hospital wards, but they are allowed to opt for some sessions in private practice in addition to any National Health Service commitments. After registration and completion of the *Foundation Programme, doctors continuing in hospital service are appointed as **senior house officers** and then obtain a **specialist registrar** post in their chosen specialty. When a specialist registrar has successfully completed a defined college or faculty specialist training programme, he or she is awarded a **Certificate of Completion of Specialist Training** (CCST) and is eligible to apply for a consultant post. Doctors who do not complete full specialist training or doctors who are not working as consultants may work in hospitals as **specialist** and **associated specialist doctors** with a variety of titles carrying increasing responsibility, such as **clinical assistant**, **staff grade**, and **associate specialist**. *See also* DOCTOR.

Consultant in Communicable Disease Control (**CCDC**) a consultant within the *Health Protection Agency who is responsible for the surveillance, prevention, and control of communicable disease and noncommunicable environmental exposures. *See also* PUBLIC HEALTH CONSULTANT.

consumption *n.* any disease causing wasting of tissues, especially (formerly) pulmonary tuberculosis. —**consumptive** *adj.*

contact *n.* transmission of an infectious

disease by touching or handling an infected person or animal (**direct contact**) or by **indirect contact** with airborne droplets, faeces, etc., containing the infective microorganism.

contact lenses lenses worn directly against the eye, separated from it only by a film of tear fluid. **Corneal microlenses** cover only the cornea, while **haptic lenses** cover some of the surrounding sclera as well. Contact lenses are used mainly in place of spectacles, to correct errors of refraction, but also in a protective capacity (see BANDAGE LENS). Contact lenses are made of a variety of materials, such as glass, plastic, and silicone; soft gas-permeable lenses have mostly replaced hard Perspex lenses.

contact therapy a form of *radiotherapy in which a radioactive substance is brought into close contact with the part of the body being treated. Needles or capsules of the isotope may be implanted in or around a tumour so that the radiation they emit will destroy it. *Compare* TELETHERAPY.

contagious disease originally, a disease transmitted only by direct physical contact: now usually taken to mean any *communicable disease.

continent diversion see URINARY DIVERSION.

continuity of care a continuous relationship between a patient and an identified health-care professional who is the sole source of care and information for the patient. However, as a patient's health-care needs over time can rarely be met by a single professional, multiprofessional pathways of continuity exist to achieve both quality of care and patient satisfaction.

continuous positive airways pressure (CPAP) an air pressure in the range 5–30 cm H_2O (1.2–7.5 mPa). It can be applied to the upper airways using a full face mask or a nasal mask only (nCPAP). It is used in high-dependency units to optimize oxygen delivery to patients who are being weaned from ventilators and on patients at home with *obstructive sleep apnoea. It works by improving nasopharyngeal airways, reducing the work of breathing, and preventing basal *atelectasis during sleep.

continuous subcutaneous insulin infusion the administration of insulin by continuous infusion into the subcutaneous tissue via a small pump worn under the clothing and connected to the skin by a tube and a fine needle. The insulin is delivered at a precalculated background rate, but patient-activated *boluses can be administered at meal times. This method is particularly appropriate (as an alternative to regular injections) for patients with repeated or unpredictable episodes of hypoglycaemia.

contra- *prefix denoting* against or opposite. Example: **contraversion** (turning away from).

contraception *n.* the prevention of unwanted pregnancy, which can be achieved by various means. Hormonal contraceptives (combined oestrogen and progestogen or progestogen only) act by preventing ovulation. They are usually taken in regular oral doses (see ORAL CONTRACEPTIVE), but may also be administered through the skin, by means of an adhesive patch impregnated with the hormones, or by three- or two-monthly injections of a long-acting progestogen. More recently developed methods for continuous administration of the hormones include subcutaneous implants of progestogen and hormonal intra-uterine devices (see IUS). Methods that aim to prevent fertilization of the ovum include *coitus interruptus, the *condom, the *diaphragm, and surgical intervention (tubal occlusion and vasectomy: see STERILIZATION). Methods that aim to prevent implantation of a fertilized ovum in the uterus include the intrauterine contraceptive device (see IUCD); these methods can be used after intercourse but before implantation (see POST-COITAL CONTRACEPTION). Couples whose religious beliefs forbid the use of mechanical or hormonal contraceptives may use the *rhythm method, in which intercourse is limited to those days in the menstrual cycle when conception is least likely.

contraction *n.* the shortening of a muscle in response to a motor nerve impulse. This generates tension in the muscle, usually causing movement.

contracture *n.* *fibrosis of skeletal muscle or connective tissue producing shortening and resulting in deformity of a joint. *See also* DUPUYTREN'S CONTRACTURE, VOLKMANN'S CONTRACTURE.

contraindication *n.* any factor in a patient's condition that makes it unwise to pursue a certain line of treatment. For example, an attack of pneumonia in a patient would be a strong contraindication against the use of a general anaesthetic.

contralateral *adj.* on or affecting the opposite side of the body: applied particularly to paralysis (or other symptoms) occurring on the opposite side of the body from the brain lesion that caused them.

contrast *n.* **1.** short for *contrast medium, e.g. **post-contrast CT scan**. **2.** the difference in the shade of grey between different tissues on a diagnostic image, such as radiograph or CT scan (*see* GREY SCALE).

contrast medium (contrast agent) a substance administered to enhance the visibility of structures (i.e. increase the contrast) during imaging. In *radiography a positive contrast agent (e.g. *barium sulphate or a water-soluble iodine-containing compound) increases the density of a structure. Gas is a negative contrast agent. Positive and negative contrast media can be used together (e.g. barium sulphate and gas in a double-contrast *barium enema). Magnetic resonance (MR) contrast agents contain either a positive contrast atom (usually gadolinium) to increase the signal or a negative contrast atom (such as iron) to decrease it. Ultrasound contrast medium consists of tiny (1–10 μm diameter) bubbles of gas, which reflect back the sound waves strongly. They can also be made to resonate or rupture to increase the signal to the ultrasound probe.

contrast nephropathy deterioration in renal function (of more than 25%) after administration of radiocontrast material. Development of this condition is more likely when there is pre-existing renal disease (the most important factor) or diabetes, vasoconstriction, simultaneous use of NSAIDs, and large amounts of radiocontrast are used. It is thought that the radiocontrast induces vasoconstriction in the vessels supplying the medulla of the kidney and aggravates hypoxia in this part of the kidney.

contrecoup *n.* injury of a part resulting from a blow on its opposite side. This may happen, for example, if a blow on the back of the head causes the front of the brain to be pushed against the inner surface of the skull.

controlled drug *see* MISUSE OF DRUGS ACT 1971.

controlled trial *see* INTERVENTION STUDY.

contusion *n.* **1.** *see* BRUISE. **2.** any of various degrees of bruising of the brain (**cerebral contusion**), resulting from *head injury or surgery. Clinical signs range from *concussion to *coma, reflecting the severity of the trauma.

conus arteriosus the front upper portion of the right ventricle adjoining the pulmonary arteries.

conus medullaris the conical end of the spinal cord, at the level of the lower end of the first lumbar vertebra.

convergence *n.* **1.** (in neurology) the formation of nerve tracts by fibres coming together into one pathway from different regions of the brain. **2.** (in ophthalmology) the ability of the eyes to turn inwards and focus on a near point so that a single image is formed on both retinas. The closer the object, the greater the degree of convergence.

convergence insufficiency a condition in which the eyes fail to turn inwards enough to achieve fusion of separate images during near vision. In some cases, convergence exercises (*see* ORTHOPTICS) can improve the condition.

conversion *n.* (in psychiatry) the expression of *conflict as physical symptoms. Psychoanalysts believe that the repressed instinctual drive is manifested as motor or sensory loss, such as paralysis, rather than as speech or action. This is thought to be one of the ways in which *conversion disorder is produced.

conversion disorder a psychological conflict or need that manifests itself as an organic dysfunction or physical symptom. The sufferer may display symptoms of blindness, deafness, loss of sensation, gait abnormalities, false memory, or paralysis of various parts of the body. None of these can be accounted for by organic disease. Conversion disorder was formerly known as *hysteria. It is classified with *dissociative disorders (as dissociative (conversion) disorders) in ICD-10 (*see* INTERNATIONAL CLASSIFICATION OF DISEASES). It is also included under the classification of *somatoform disorders.

convolution *n.* a folding or twisting, such as one of the many that cause the fissures, sulci, and gyri of the surface of the *cerebrum.

convulsion *n.* an involuntary contraction of the muscles producing contortion of the body and limbs. Rhythmic convulsions of the limbs are a feature of major *epilepsy.

*Febrile convulsions are provoked by fever in otherwise healthy infants and young children.

Cooksey-Cawthorne exercises a series of physical exercises used in the rehabilitation of patients with certain forms of *vertigo.

Cooley's anaemia *see* THALASSAEMIA. [T. B. Cooley (1871–1945), US paediatrician]

Coombs' test a means of detecting rhesus antibodies on the surface of red blood cells that precipitate proteins (globulins) in the blood serum. The test is used in the diagnosis of haemolytic anaemia in babies with rhesus incompatibility in whom there is destruction of red blood cells (*see* HAEMOLYTIC DISEASE OF THE NEWBORN). [R. R. A. Coombs (1921–2006), British immunologist]

Copaxone *n. see* GLATIRAMER.

COPD *see* CHRONIC OBSTRUCTIVE PULMONARY DISEASE.

co-phenotrope *n.* a drug administered by mouth in the treatment of diarrhoea. It consists of a mixture of diphenoxylate hydrochloride (an opioid that reduces *peristalsis) and atropine (which relaxes the smooth muscle of the gut) in a ratio of 100 to 1. Trade name: **Lomotil**.

copr- (copro-) *combining form denoting* faeces. Example: **coprophobia** (abnormal fear of).

coprolalia *n.* the repetitive speaking of obscene words. It can be involuntary, as part of *Tourette's syndrome.

coprolith *n. see* FAECALITH.

coproporphyrin *n.* a *porphyrin compound formed during the synthesis of protoporphyrin IX, a precursor of *haem. Coproporphyrin is excreted in the faeces in **hereditary coproporphyria.**

copulation *n. see* COITUS.

cor *n.* the heart.

coracoid process a beaklike process that curves upwards and forwards from the top of the *scapula, over the shoulder joint.

cord *n.* any long flexible structure, which may be solid or tubular. Examples include the spermatic cord, spinal cord, umbilical cord, and vocal cord.

cordectomy *n.* surgical removal of a vocal cord or, more usually, a piece of the vocal cord (**partial cordectomy**).

cordocentesis *n.* the removal of a sample of fetal blood by inserting a fine hollow needle through the abdominal wall of a pregnant woman, under ultrasound guidance, into the umbilical vein. Cordocentesis is most commonly performed for confirmation of fetal *packed cell volume prior to intrauterine transfusion or for confirmation of infection in the fetus. *See also* FETAL BLOOD SAMPLING.

cordotomy *n.* a surgical procedure for the relief of severe and persistent pain in the pelvis or lower limbs. The nerve fibres that transmit the sensation of pain to consciousness pass up the spinal cord in special tracts (the **spinothalamic tracts**). In cordotomy the spinothalamic tracts are severed in the cervical (neck) region.

cord presentation the position of the umbilical cord when it lies below the presenting part of the fetus in an intact bag of membranes. *See also* CORD PROLAPSE.

cord prolapse rupture of the membranes in cases of a *cord presentation. It is an obstetric emergency: there is a severe risk of cord compression and spasm causing fetal asphyxia (*see* HYPOXIC-ISCHAEMIC ENCEPHALOPATHY). Delivery must occur as soon as possible and the presenting part displaced away from the cord.

Cordylobia *n. see* TUMBU FLY.

core-and-cluster *n.* a form of housing for handicapped people. Institutional organizations are replaced by small self-contained living units associated with a central facility providing more intensive resources.

corectopia *n.* displacement of the pupil towards one side from its normal position in the centre of the iris. When present from birth, the displacement is usually inwards towards the nose. Scarring of the iris from inflammation may also draw the pupil out of position.

co-registration *n.* in diagnostic imaging, the process of taking two images obtained by different techniques and (usually electronically) laying them on top of each other after suitable adjustment, so that the anatomical landmarks coincide. This can give increased information about any disease present. Co-registration is typically used in *PET/CT scanning.

corium *n. see* DERMIS.

corn *n.* an area of hard thickened skin on or between the toes or elsewhere on the foot: a type of *callosity produced by ill-fitting shoes. The horny skin layers form an inverted pyramid that presses down into the deeper skin layers, causing pain. A corn may be treated by applying salicylic acid or by podiatry.

cornea *n.* the transparent circular part of the front of the eyeball. It refracts the light entering the eye onto the lens, which then focuses it onto the retina. The cornea contains no blood vessels and it is extremely sensitive to pain. The innermost layer (**corneal endothelium**) consists of a single layer of cells that cannot regenerate. —**corneal** *adj.*

corneal arcus a white or greyish line in the periphery of the cornea, concentric with but separated from the edge by a clear zone. It begins above and below but may become a continuous ring. It consists of an infiltration of fatty material and is common in the elderly (**arcus senilis**). When it occurs in younger people (**arcus juvenilis**) it may indicate *hyperlipidaemia. It does not affect vision.

corneal graft *see* KERATOPLASTY.

corneal reflex reflex blinking of both eyes normally elicited by lightly touching the cornea of one eye. This reflex is lost in deep coma, during general anaesthesia, and in death; it is therefore one of the tests used to confirm brainstem death.

corneal ring a ring designed to be inserted into the peripheral tissue of the cornea in order to alter the curvature of the corneal surface. It is undergoing trials to assess its ability to correct errors of refraction. In myopia (short-sightedness), for example, the ring would be required to stretch the corneal tissue peripherally and thus flatten the central corneal curvature in order to correct the myopia.

corneal topography (videokeratography) an imaging technique used to study the shape and refractive power of the cornea in detail. An image projected onto the cornea is analysed by a computer to produce a representation of the shape and refractive power of the corneal surface. Corneal topography has an important role in the management of corneal disease and refractive surgery.

cornification *n. see* KERATINIZATION.

cornu *n.* (*pl.* **cornua**) (in anatomy) a horn-shaped structure, such as the horn-shaped processes of the hyoid bone and thyroid cartilage. *See also* HORN.

corona *n.* a crown or crownlike structure. The **corona capitis** is the crown of the head.

coronal *adj.* relating to the crown of the head or of a tooth. The **coronal plane** divides the body into dorsal and ventral parts (see illustration).

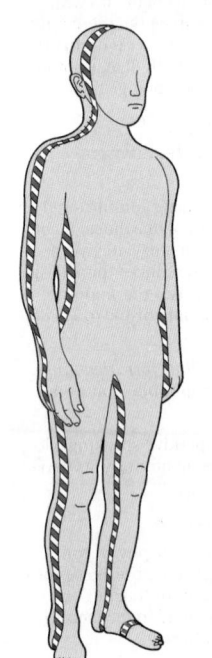

Coronal. The coronal plane of section through the body and through the left foot.

coronal suture *see* SUTURE.

corona radiata 1. a series of radiating fibres between the cerebral cortex and the internal capsule of the brain. 2. a layer of follicle cells that surrounds a freshly ovulated ovum. The cells are elongated radially to the ovum when seen in section.

coronary angiography an X-ray technique for examination of the coronary arteries, often taken to also include examination of the chambers of the heart. A catheter is introduced via the radial artery at the wrist or the femoral artery at the groin and manipulated into the heart under X-ray control. *Contrast medium is then injected to outline the ventricles and coronary arteries. Video images are recorded during contrast-medium injection, either on film or electronic media, often using *digital subtraction techniques. Coronary angiography is used to diagnose cardiac disease, specifically narrowing or blockage in the coronary arteries, and plan treatment by surgery or radiological interventional techniques (*see* CORONARY ARTERY BYPASS GRAFT, PERCUTANEOUS CORONARY INTERVENTION).

coronary angioplasty a procedure in which a segment of coronary artery narrowed by atheroma is stretched by the inflation of a balloon introduced into it by means of cardiac *catheterization under X-ray screening (*see* ANGIOPLASTY). The site of the obstruction is identified by prior *coronary angiography. Not all narrowed segments can be improved by angioplasty, but results may be improved by placement of metallic *stents. *See also* PERCUTANEOUS CORONARY INTERVENTION.

coronary arteries the arteries supplying blood to the heart. The **right** and **left coronary arteries** arise from the aorta, just above the aortic valve, and form branches encircling the heart. *See* CORONARY ANGIOPLASTY, CORONARY ARTERY BYPASS GRAFT.

coronary artery bypass graft (CABG) *coronary revascularization in which a segment of a coronary artery narrowed by atheroma is bypassed by an *autologous section of healthy saphenous vein or internal mammary artery at *thoracotomy. The improved blood flow resulting from one or more such grafts relieves *angina pectoris and reduces the risk of *myocardial infarction. Recently developed techniques of *minimally invasive surgery have enabled the operation to be performed without the need for thoracotomy.

coronary artery disease (CAD) *atherosclerosis of the coronary arteries, which may cause *angina pectoris and lead to *myocardial infarction. One of the leading causes of death in Western countries, the disease occurs most frequently in populations with diets high in cholesterol, saturated fats, and refined carbohydrates. Other risk factors include hypertension, diabetes mellitus, and smoking.

coronary care unit (CCU) a designated ward of a hospital to which the most serious cardiac cases are transferred for specialist monitoring and treatment.

coronary revascularization the restoration of blood flow to ischaemic heart muscle (*see* ISCHAEMIA) by *coronary angioplasty and *stenting or by a *coronary artery bypass graft.

coronary thrombosis the formation of a blood clot (thrombus) in the coronary artery, which obstructs the flow of blood to the heart. This is usually due to *atheroma and results in the death (infarction) of part of the heart muscle. For symptoms and treatment, *see* MYOCARDIAL INFARCTION.

coroner *n.* the official who presides at an *inquest. He or she must be either a medical practitioner or a lawyer of at least five years' standing.

coronoid process 1. a process on the upper end of the *ulna. It forms part of the notch that articulates with the humerus. 2. the process on the ramus of the *mandible to which the temporalis muscle is attached.

cor pulmonale enlargement of the right ventricle of the heart due to excessive pressure loading that results from diseases of the lungs or the pulmonary arteries. Such diseases include those affecting the structure of the lungs (e.g. emphysema) or their function (e.g. obesity) except when these changes result from congenital heart disease or diseases primarily affecting the left side of the heart.

corpus *n.* (*pl.* **corpora**) any mass of tissue that can be distinguished from its surroundings.

corpus albicans the residual body of scar tissue that remains in the ovary at the point where a *corpus luteum has regressed after its secretory activity has ceased.

corpus callosum the broad band of nervous tissue that connects the two cerebral hemispheres, containing an estimated 300 million fibres. *See* CEREBRUM.

corpus cavernosum either of a pair of cylindrical blood sinuses that form the erectile tissue of the *penis and clitoris. In the penis a third sinus, the corpus spongiosum, encloses the urethra and extends into the glans. All these sinuses have a spongelike structure that allows them to expand when filled with blood.

corpuscle *n.* any small particle, cell, or mass of tissue.

corpus luteum the glandular tissue in the ovary that forms at the site of a ruptured *Graafian follicle after ovulation. It secretes the hormone *progesterone, which prepares the uterus for implantation. If implantation fails the corpus luteum becomes inactive and degenerates. If an embryo becomes implanted the corpus luteum continues to secrete progesterone until the fourth month of pregnancy, by which time the placenta has taken over this function.

corpus spongiosum the blood sinus that surrounds the urethra of the male. Together with the corpora cavernosa, it forms the erectile tissue of the *penis. It is expanded at the base of the penis to form the urethral bulb and at the tip to form the glans penis.

corpus striatum the part of the *basal ganglia in the cerebral hemispheres of the brain consisting of the caudate nucleus and the lentiform nucleus.

correlation *n.* (in statistics) the degree of linear relationship between two or more *variables. Pairs of observations can be plotted as a series of points on a **graph**. The **correlation coefficient** measures the extent to which the points on the resulting **scatter diagram** form a straight line. The correlation coefficient varies within the range of +1 (where an increase of one variable is associated with a corresponding increase in the other, and vice versa) to –1 (where an increase of one variable is associated with a corresponding decrease of the other); a coefficient of 0 indicates no linear relationship between the two variables. The statistical technique known as **multivariate analysis** can be used to investigate the variation in several variables.

Corrigan's pulse (collapsing pulse) a type of pulse that has an exaggerated rise followed by a sudden fall. It is typical of *aortic regurgitation. [Sir D. J. Corrigan (1802–80), Irish physician]

Corrigan's sign powerful pulsation of the carotid arteries causing ear movement and/or head nodding. It is a sign of *aortic regurgitation. [Sir D. J. Corrigan]

cortex *n.* (*pl.* **cortices**) the outer part of an organ, situated immediately beneath its capsule or outer membrane; for example, the **adrenal cortex** (*see* ADRENAL GLANDS), **renal cortex** (*see* KIDNEY), or *cerebral cortex. —**cortical** *adj.*

cortical evoked response audiometry (CERA) an objective test of hearing that measures the electrical activity in the *cerebral cortex following sound stimulation.

cortical Lewy body disease a disorder characterized by a combination of *parkinsonism and *dementia, which typically fluctuates. Visual hallucinations are common, and there is exquisite sensitivity to phenothiazine drugs. Abnormal proteins called **Lewy bodies** are found within the nerve cells of the cortex and the basal ganglia. It is the second most common cause of dementia (**dementia with Lewy bodies**) after *Alzheimer's disease.

corticosteroid (corticoid) *n.* any steroid hormone synthesized by the adrenal cortex. There are two main groups of corticosteroids. The **glucocorticoids** (e.g. *cortisol, *cortisone, and corticosterone) are essential for the utilization of carbohydrate, fat, and protein by the body and for a normal response to stress. Naturally occurring and synthetic glucocorticoids have very powerful anti-inflammatory effects and are used to treat conditions that involve inflammation. The **mineralocorticoids** (e.g. *aldosterone) are necessary for the regulation of salt and water balance.

corticosterone *n.* a steroid hormone (*see* CORTICOSTEROID) synthesized and released in small amounts by the adrenal cortex.

corticotrophin *n. see* ACTH.

corticotrophin-releasing hormone (CRH) a peptide hypothalamic hormone (of 41 amino acids) stimulating the release of *ACTH (adrenocorticotrophic hormone) from the anterior pituitary. Its own release is suppressed by a *negative feedback loop involving cortisol, and its action is increased by antidiuretic hormone (*see* VASOPRESSIN) and *angiotensin II. It can be administered intravenously as part of the **CRH test**, during which blood is analysed at 15-minute intervals for one hour for the ACTH response, which is excessive in cases of primary adrenal failure and suppressed in cases of anterior *hypopituitarism.

cortisol *n.* a steroid hormone: the major glucocorticoid synthesized and released by the human adrenal cortex (*see* CORTICO-STEROID). It is important for normal carbohydrate metabolism and for the normal response to any stress. *See also* HYDROCORTISONE.

cortisone *n.* a naturally occurring *corticosteroid that is used mainly to treat deficiency of corticosteroid hormones in *Addison's disease and following surgical removal of the adrenal glands. It is administered by mouth or injection and may cause serious side-effects such as stomach ulcers and bleeding, nervous and hormone disturbances, muscle and bone damage, and eye changes.

cor triloculare a rare congenital condition in which there are three instead of four chambers of the heart due to the presence of a single common ventricle. *Cyanosis (blueness) is common. Most patients die in infancy.

Corynebacterium *n.* a genus of Gram-positive, mostly aerobic, nonmotile rodlike bacteria that frequently bear club-shaped swellings. Many species cause disease in humans, domestic animals, birds, and plants; some are found in dairy products. The species *C. diphtheriae* (**Klebs-Loeffler bacillus**) is the causative organism of *diphtheria, producing a powerful *exotoxin that is harmful to heart and nerve tissue. It occurs in one of three forms: *gravis*, *intermedius*, and *mitis*.

coryza (cold in the head) *n.* a catarrhal inflammation of the mucous membrane in the nose due to either a *cold or *hay fever. *See also* CATARRH.

COSHH (control of substances hazardous to health) (in occupational health) legislation and resulting regulations concerning the duties and responsibilities of employers and employees to ensure that **hazardous substances** used in a workplace (e.g. toxic chemicals in factories, anaesthetic gases in operating theatres) do not affect adversely the workforce or others.

cost- (costo-) *combining form denoting* the ribs. Example: **costectomy** (excision of).

costal *adj.* of or relating to the ribs.

costal cartilage a cartilage that connects a *rib to the breastbone (*sternum). The first seven ribs (true ribs) are directly connected to the sternum by individual costal cartilages. The next three ribs are indirectly connected to the sternum by three costal cartilages, each of which is connected to the one immediately above it.

costalgia *n.* pain localized to the ribs. This term is now rarely used.

cost–benefit analysis an analytical process for weighing up the possible losses (costs) and gains (benefits) of an action or policy, often in monetary or numerical form, and usually as a means of deciding between alternatives. In medicine, it is particularly associated with the setting of priorities in allocating limited health-care resources. Analysis may result in a cost–benefit ratio. *Compare* RISK–BENEFIT ANALYSIS. *See also* CONSEQUENTIALISM, QUALITY OF LIFE, RATIONING.

costochondritis *n. see* TIETZE'S SYNDROME.

cot death *see* SUDDEN INFANT DEATH SYNDROME.

co-trimoxazole *n.* an antibacterial drug consisting of **sulfamethoxazole** (a *sulphonamide) and *trimethoprim, each of which potentiates (increases) the action of the other. Since both these drugs are well absorbed and rapidly excreted, co-trimoxazole can be taken by mouth; it may also be administered by intravenous infusion. Because of the severity of its side-effects, which are those of the sulphonamides, co-trimoxazole is now usually limited to treating *Pneumocystis* pneumonia, toxoplasmosis, and nocardiasis. Trade name: **Septrin**.

cotton-wool spots soft fluffy spots in the retina resulting from accumulations of *axoplasm in the nerve-fibre layer of the retina. These may indicate diseases causing hypoxia (oxygen deficiency) in the nerve-fibre layer (e.g. diabetes, hypertension, connective-tissue disease, or AIDS).

cotyledon *n.* any of the major convex subdivisions of the mature *placenta. Each cotyledon contains a major branch of the umbilical blood vessels, which branch further into the numerous villi that make up the surface of the cotyledon.

cotyloid cavity *see* ACETABULUM.

couching *n.* an operation for cataract in which the lens is pushed out of the pupil downwards and backwards into the jelly-like vitreous humour by a small knife inserted through the edge of the cornea. It was widely employed in ancient Hindu civilizations but developments in surgery and anaesthesia leave little place for it today.

coughing *n.* a form of violent exhalation by which irritant particles in the airways can be expelled. Stimulation of the cough reflexes results in the glottis being kept closed until a high expiratory pressure has built up, which is then suddenly released. Medical name: **tussis**.

cough suppressant *see* ANTITUSSIVE.

coulomb *n.* the *SI unit of electric charge, equal to the quantity of electricity transferred by 1 ampere in 1 second. Symbol: C.

counselling *n.* 1. a method of approaching psychological difficulties in adjustment that aims to help the client work out his own problems. The counsellor listens sympathetically, attempting to identify with the client, tries to clarify current problems, and sometimes gives advice. It involves less emphasis on insight and interpretation than does psychotherapy or psychoanalytic therapy. *See also* CLIENT-CENTRED THERAPY. 2. *see* GENETIC COUNSELLING.

counterextension *n.* *traction on one part of a limb, while the remainder of the limb is held steady: used particularly in the treatment of a fractured femur (thigh bone).

counterirritant *n.* an agent, such as methyl salicylate, that causes irritation when applied to the skin and is used in order to relieve more deep-seated pain or discomfort. —**counterirritation** *n.*

countertraction *n.* the use of an opposing force to balance that being applied during *traction, when a strong continuous pull is applied, for example, to a limb so that broken bones can be kept in alignment during healing.

coupling agents items that help to improve contact between the two paddles of a manual *defibrillator and the chest wall of the patient, thus reducing the *transthoracic impedance and the risk of contact burns. The most common agents are **defibrillation gel pads**, thin pads of electrically conductive material placed between the patient's skin and the defibrillation paddles. The two pads must not touch during defibrillation or a short circuit will form between the paddles. Liquid gels can also be used, but there is a greater risk of short-circuiting as the gel can spread between the two paddles.

couvade *n.* 1. a custom in some tribes whereby a father takes to his bed during or after the birth of his child. 2. a symptom of abdominal pain experienced by a man in relation to his wife's giving birth. It may be due to *conversion disorder, anxiety, or sympathy.

couvelaire *n.* the appearance of the uterus following a massive placental abruption (*abruptio placentae) when blood has extravasated (leaked) through the *myometrium to the subserosal surface of the uterus. The uterus is hard and tender and a bruised discoloration can be seen at the time of Caesarean section.

covariate (covariable) *n.* (in statistics) a continuous *variable that is not part of the main experimental manipulation but has an effect on the dependent variable. The inclusion of covariates increases the power of the statistical test and removes the bias of confounding variables (which have effects on the dependent variable that are indistinguishable from those of the independent variable).

cover-slip *n.* an extremely thin square or circle of glass used to protect the upper surface of a preparation on a microscope slide.

cover test a test to detect a squint. The observer looks at a target object, one eye at a time being covered. If the uncovered eye deviates to focus on the target, then a squint is confirmed. The movement can be up, down, sideways, or a combination, depending on the type of squint (*see* STRABISMUS).

Cowper's glands (bulbourethral glands) a pair of small glands that open into the urethra at the base of the penis. Their secretion contributes to the seminal fluid, but less than that of the prostate gland or seminal vesicles. [W. Cowper (1660–1709), English surgeon]

cowpox *n.* a virus infection of cows' udders, transmitted to humans by direct contact, causing very mild symptoms similar to *smallpox. An attack confers immunity to smallpox. Medical name: **vaccinia**.

cox- (coxo-) *combining form denoting* the hip. Example: **coxalgia** (pain in).

coxa *n.* (*pl.* **coxae**) **1.** the hip bone. **2.** the hip joint.

Coxiella *n.* a genus of rickettsiae that cause disease in animals and humans. They are transmitted to humans by inhalation and produce disease characterized by inflammation of the lungs, without a rash (*compare* TYPHUS). The single species, *C. burnetii*, causes *Q fever.

COX-2 inhibitor any one of a group of anti-inflammatory drugs (*see* NSAID) that selectively block the action of the enzyme cyclo-oxygenase 2 (COX-2), which mediates the production of *prostaglandin at sites of inflammation, especially in joints; they are less likely to inhibit COX-1, which controls the production of prostaglandin in the stomach (where it is involved in the production of protective mucus), and therefore less likely than nonselective NSAIDs to cause peptic bleeding or ulceration. COX-2 inhibitors are used in the treatment of arthritis, acute gout, and moderate or severe pain. They include *celecoxib and **etoricoxib** (Arcoxia). However, because their use is associated with an increased incidence of heart attack and stroke, COX-2 inhibitors should be taken only by those who are not at risk of developing these conditions and who have a high risk of developing peptic ulceration. Other side-effects include fluid retention (oedema), intestinal upset, dizziness, insomnia, and sore throat.

Coxsackie virus (echovirus) one of a group of RNA-containing viruses that are able to multiply in the gastrointestinal tract (*see* ENTEROVIRUS). About 30 different types exist. **Type A Coxsackie viruses** generally cause less severe and less well-defined diseases, such as *hand, foot, and mouth disease, although some cause meningitis and severe throat infections (*see* HERPANGINA). **Type B Coxsackie viruses** cause inflammation or degeneration of heart tissue, resulting in pericarditis or myocarditis, or brain tissue, producing meningitis or encephalitis. They can also attack the muscles of the chest wall, the bronchi, pancreas, thyroid, or conjunctiva and recent evidence suggests they may be implicated in diabetes in children and in motor neuron disease. *See also* BORNHOLM DISEASE.

CPAP *see* CONTINUOUS POSITIVE AIRWAYS PRESSURE.

C-peptide *n.* a peptide (so-called because of its C shape) formed when insulin is produced from its precursor molecule, proinsulin. It is secreted in equal molar amounts to insulin. However, as it remains detectable in the plasma much longer than insulin it can be more easily assayed as a marker of the degree of insulin secretion. This can be useful to assess the ability of the pancreas to secrete insulin, for example when trying to determine whether somebody has type 1 or type 2 diabetes or to distinguish an insulin-secreting tumour (an *insulinoma) from surreptitious insulin usage in somebody presenting with unexplained hypoglycaemia.

CPPIH *see* COMMISSION FOR PATIENT AND PUBLIC INVOLVEMENT IN HEALTH.

CPR *see* CARDIOPULMONARY RESUSCITATION.

CQC *see* CARE QUALITY COMMISSION.

crab louse *see* PHTHIRUS.

cradle *n.* a framework of metal strips or other material that forms a cage over an injured part of the body of a patient lying in bed, to protect it from the pressure of the bedclothes.

cradle cap a common condition in young babies in which crusty white or yellow scales form a 'cap' on the scalp. It is treated by applying oil or using a special shampoo and usually resolves in the first year of life, although it may represent the start of seborrhoeic *eczema.

cramp *n.* prolonged painful contraction of a muscle. It is sometimes caused by an imbalance of calcium and potassium in the body, but is more often a result of fatigue, imperfect posture, or stress. Spasm in the muscles making it impossible to perform a specific task but allowing the use of these muscles for any other movement is called **occupational cramp**. It most often affects the hand muscles for writing (**writer's cramp**), a form of *dystonia.

crani- (cranio-) *combining form denoting* the skull. Example: **cranioplasty** (plastic surgery of).

cranial nerves the 12 pairs of nerves that arise directly from the brain and leave the skull through separate apertures; they are conventionally given Roman numbers, as follows: I *olfactory; II *optic; III *oculomotor; IV *trochlear; V *trigeminal; VI *abducens; VII *facial; VIII *vestibulocochlear; IX *glossopharyngeal; X *vagus; XI *accessory; XII *hypoglossal. *Compare* SPINAL NERVES.

craniometry *n.* the science of measuring the differences in size and shape of skulls.

craniopagus (dicephalus) *n.* *conjoined twins united by their heads.

craniopharyngioma *n.* a brain tumour, situated above the *sella turcica, that is derived from remnants of **Rathke's pouch**, the earliest detectable embryonic precursor of the pituitary gland. The patient may show raised intracranial pressure and *diabetes insipidus due to reduced secretion of the hormone *vasopressin. An X-ray of the skull typically shows calcification within the tumour and loss of the normal skull structure around the pituitary gland.

craniostenosis *n.* premature closing of the *sutures and fontanelles between the cranial bones during development, resulting in the skull remaining abnormally small. *Compare* CRANIOSYNOSTOSIS.

craniosynostosis *n.* premature fusion of some of the cranial bones, usually before birth, so that the skull is unable to expand in certain directions to assume its normal shape under the influence of the growing brain. Depending on which cranial *sutures fuse early, the skull may become elongated from front to back, broad and short, peaked (**oxycephaly** or **turricephaly**), or asymmetrical. Craniosynostosis is a feature of several related inherited disorders (*see* ACROCEPHALOSYNDACTYLY). *Compare* CRANIOSTENOSIS.

craniotomy *n.* **1.** surgical removal of a portion of the skull (cranium), performed to expose the brain and *meninges for inspection or biopsy or to relieve excessive intracranial pressure (as in a subdural *haematoma). **2.** surgical perforation of the skull of a dead fetus during difficult labour, so that delivery may continue.

For both operations the instrument used is called a **craniotome**.

cranium *n.* the part of the skeleton that encloses the brain. It consists of eight bones connected together by immovable joints (*see* SKULL). —**cranial** *adj.*

C-reactive protein (CRP) a protein whose plasma concentrations are raised in infections and inflammatory states and in the presence of tissue damage or necrosis.

cream *n.* a preparation for use on the skin consisting of an emulsion of oil in water, which may or may not contain medication. It rubs into the skin easily and contains preservatives, which may be allergenic. *Compare* OINTMENT.

creatinase (creatine kinase) *n.* an enzyme involved in the metabolic breakdown of creatine to creatinine.

creatine *n.* a product of protein metabolism found in muscle. Its phosphate, **creatine phosphate** (**phosphocreatine**, **phosphagen**), acts as a store of high-energy phosphate in muscle and serves to maintain adequate amounts of *ATP (the source of energy for muscular contraction).

creatine kinase an enzyme involved in the metabolic breakdown of creatine to creatinine. Isomers of creatine kinase originate from brain and thyroid (BB), skeletal muscle (MM), and cardiac muscle (MB). Any damage to these tissues causes an increase of the isomer in the serum, which can be used in diagnosis, particularly of myocardial infarction.

creatinine *n.* a substance derived from creatine and creatine phosphate in muscle. Creatinine is excreted in the urine.

creatinuria *n.* an excess of the nitrogenous compound creatine in the urine.

creeping eruption (larva migrans) a skin disease caused either by larvae of certain nematode worms (e.g. *Ancylostoma braziliense*) normally parasitic in dogs and cats or by the maggots of certain flies (*see* HYPODERMA, GASTEROPHILUS). The larvae burrow within the skin tissues, their movements marked by long thin red lines that cause the patient intense irritation. The nematode infections are treated with albendazole, ivermectin, or tiabendazole; maggots can be surgically removed.

cremasteric reflex a superficial reflex in males elicited by stroking the inner side of the upper thigh with a sharp object. If the reflex is intact the scrotum on that side is pulled upwards as the cremaster muscle contracts. Absence or reduction of both cremasteric reflexes indicates an upper *motor neuron lesion; absence of the reflex on one side suggests a lower motor neuron lesion at the level of the first lumbar spinal nerve.

crenation *n.* an abnormal appearance of red blood cells seen under a microscope, in which the normally smooth cell margins appear crinkly or irregular. Crenation may be a feature of certain blood disorders, but most commonly occurs as a result of prolonged storage of a blood specimen prior to preparation of a blood film.

crepitation (rale) *n.* a soft fine crackling sound heard in the lungs through the stethoscope. Crepitations are made either by air passages and alveoli (air sacs) opening up during inspiration or by air bubbling through fluid. They are not normally heard in healthy lungs.

crepitus *n.* 1. a crackling sound or grating feeling produced by bone rubbing on bone or roughened cartilage, detected on movement of an arthritic joint. Crepitus in the knee joint is a common sign of *chondromalacia patellae in the young and *osteoarthritis in the elderly. 2. a similar sound heard with a stethoscope over an inflamed lung when the patient breathes in.

crest *n.* a ridge or linear protuberance, particularly on a bone. Examples include the crest of fibula and the iliac crest (of the ilium).

CREST syndrome a disease characterized by the association of *calcinosis, Raynaud's phenomenon (*see* RAYNAUD'S DISEASE), (o)esophageal malfunction, sclerodactyly (tapering fingers), and telangiectasia (*see* TELANGIECTASIS). It represents a variant of *systemic sclerosis and is also called **limited cutaneous systemic sclerosis**. It may be associated with severe pulmonary hypertension.

cretinism *n.* a syndrome of *dwarfism, mental retardation, and coarseness of the skin and facial features due to lack of thyroid hormone from birth (congenital *hypothyroidism).

Creutzfeldt-Jakob disease (CJD) a rapidly progressive rare neurological disease, a form of human *spongiform encephalopathy in which dementia progresses to death after a period of 3–12 months. There is no effective treatment. The causative agent is an abnormal *prion protein that accumulates in the brain and causes widespread destruction of tissue. CJD typically affects middle-aged to elderly people. Some 15% of cases are due to a form of the disease that is inherited as an autosomal *dominant trait but most cases are sporadic, susceptibility being genetically determined. A few cases of CJD are acquired:

the agent is known to have been transmitted by tissue and organ transplantation and by human growth hormone injections, but the disease may take years to manifest itself.

Variant Creutzfeldt-Jakob disease (vCJD) is the human form of bovine spongiform encephalopathy (BSE), which is most likely acquired by the ingestion of infected beef products. Patients are younger than those affected with sporadic CJD and present with psychiatric symptoms (e.g. depression, anxiety) and hypersensitivity to touch, which are followed after months by myoclonic jerks (*see* MYOCLONUS) and dementia. [H. G. Creutzfeldt (1885–1964) and A. M. Jakob (1884–1931), German psychiatrists]

CRH *see* CORTICOTROPHIN-RELEASING HORMONE.

cribriform plate *see* ETHMOID BONE.

cricoid cartilage the cartilage, shaped like a signet ring, that forms part of the anterior and lateral walls and most of the posterior wall of the *larynx.

cricoid pressure a technique in which a trained assistant presses downwards on the *cricoid cartilage of a supine patient to aid endotracheal *intubation.

cricothyroid membrane the fibrous tissue in the anterior aspect of the neck between the lower border of the *thyroid cartilage (the 'Adam's apple') and the upper border of the *cricoid cartilage, lying immediately below it. It is the site where certain emergency airway devices can be inserted.

cricothyroidotomy *n.* a technique for obtaining an emergency airway through the *cricothyroid membrane when standard airway techniques have failed. There are two main techniques. In **needle cricothyroidotomy**, a large-bore intravenous cannula is inserted directly through the membrane. Ventilation by this technique can only be through a high-pressure system, must only be performed by trained personnel, and must only continue for a maximum of 45 minutes. Damage to the lungs can ensue. In **surgical cricothyroidotomy**, a surgical hole is made in the membrane and a cuffed tube, similar to a short endotracheal tube (*see* IN-TUBATION), is inserted directly. This affords much better airway protection.

cri-du-chat syndrome a congenital condition of severe mental retardation associated with an abnormal facial appearance, spasticity, and a characteristic catlike cry in infancy. It results from a chromosomal abnormality in which there is a loss (*deletion) of part of the short arm of chromosome no. 5.

Crigler-Najjar syndrome a genetic disease in which the liver enzyme glucuronyl transferase, responsible for dealing with bilirubin, is absent. A large amount of unconjugated bilirubin accumulates in the blood and the syndrome presents in early childhood with worsening jaundice. The only definitive treatment is a liver transplant, without which life expectancy is usually less than two years. [J. F. Crigler (1919–) and V. A. Najjar (1914–), US paediatricians]

Crimean Congo haemorrhagic fever a disease caused by bunyaviruses that has occurred in the former USSR, the Middle East, and Africa. It causes bleeding into the intestines, kidneys, genitals, and mouth with up to 50% mortality. The virus is spread by various types of tick from wild animals and birds to domestic animals (especially goats and cattle) and thus to humans.

crisantaspase *n. see* ASPARAGINASE.

crisis *n.* **1.** the turning point of a disease, after which the patient either improves or deteriorates. Since the advent of antibiotics, infections seldom reach the point of crisis. **2.** the occurrence of sudden severe pain in certain diseases. *See also* DIETL'S CRISIS.

crisis resolution and home treatment team (CRHT) (in psychiatry) a multidisciplinary team in psychiatric services specialized in the treatment of severely mentally ill patients in their home environment. An additional remit of CRHTs is to try and avoid acute hospital admissions.

crista *n.* (*pl.* **cristae**) **1.** the sensory structure within the ampulla of a *semicircular canal within the inner ear (see illustration). The cristae respond to changes in the rate of movement of the head, being activated by pressure from the fluid in the semicircular canals. **2.** one of the infoldings of the inner membrane of a *mitochondrion. **3.** any anatomical structure resembling a crest.

critical incident an event or episode that deviates from the expected or desired course and could have potentially negative effects for patient care or safety. Related terms include 'significant and adverse events'. Such episodes may inform *reflective practice.

Crohn's disease a condition in which segments of the alimentary tract become inflamed, thickened, ulcerated, and scarred. It can affect any part of the intestinal tract from mouth to anus; common areas affected are the small bowel and/or colon. It commonly affects the terminal part of the ileum, which in its acute form (acute ileitis) can mimic acute {appendicitis}. The main symptoms are abdominal pain, diarrhoea, tiredness, and loss of weight. Longstanding Crohn's disease can often cause partial obstruction of the intestine due to stricture(s) and *malabsorption. *Fistulae around the anus, between adjacent loops of intestine, or from intestine to skin, bladder, etc., are known complications of Crohn's disease. The cause is unknown, but various environmental and genetic factors are thought to be involved. Treatment includes aminosalicylates, corticosteroids, immunosuppressant drugs, monoclonal antibodies, antibiotics, dietary modification, or (in many cases) surgical correction or removal of the affected part of the intestine. Alternative names: **regional enteritis, regional ileitis**. [B. B. Crohn (1884–1983), US physician]

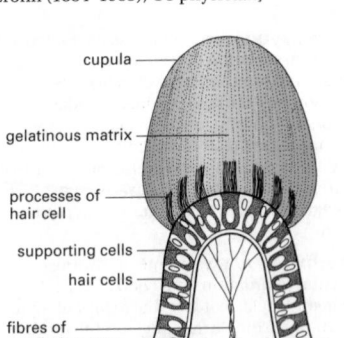

A crista.

cromoglicate (sodium cromoglicate, cromoglycate) *n.* a drug thought to prevent the release of histamine from mast cells. It is used to prevent asthma attacks and hay fever and to treat other allergic conditions, including allergic conjunctivitis and food allergies. It is administered by inhalation, as a nasal spray, or as eye drops, and may cause local irritation. Trade names: **Rynacrom, Vividrin**.

crossbite *n.* a condition in which some or

all of the lower teeth close outside the upper teeth during normal closure.

cross-dressing *n. see* TRANSVESTISM.

crossing over (in genetics) the exchange of sections of chromatids that occurs between pairs of homologous chromosomes, which results in the recombination of genetic material. It occurs during *meiosis at a *chiasma.

cross-over trial *see* INTERVENTION STUDY.

cross-sectional imaging any technique that produces an image in the form of a plane through the body with the structures cut across. The main techniques are *ultrasonography, *computerized tomography, *magnetic resonance imaging, and some *nuclear medicine techniques (*see* POSITRON EMISSION TOMOGRAPHY; SPECT SCANNING). If a series of thin-section images is stacked they can be 'cut' through to show other planes or allow reconstruction of three-dimensional images.

cross-sectional study the collection and analysis of information relating to persons in a population or group at a defined point in time (or within a defined period), with particular reference to their disease status, individual characteristics and exposure to factors thought likely to predispose to disease.

crotamiton *n.* a drug that is used to relieve itching, including that associated with scabies. It is applied to the skin as a lotion or cream and sometimes causes reddening and hypersensitivity reactions. Trade name: **Eurax**.

croup *n.* acute inflammation and obstruction of the respiratory tract, involving the larynx and the main air passages (trachea and bronchi), in young children (usually aged between six months and three years). The usual cause is a virus infection but bacterial secondary infection can occur. The symptoms are those of *laryngitis, accompanied by signs of obstruction – harsh difficult breathing (*see* STRIDOR), a characteristic barking cough, a rising pulse rate, restlessness, and *cyanosis. Treatment is by reassurance and humidification of the inspired air. In severe cases the obstruction may require treatment by steroid nebulizers, *intubation, or *tracheostomy. *See also* EPIGLOTTITIS.

Crouzon syndrome (craniofacial dysostosis) a genetic disorder characterized by premature fusion of the skull sutures, leading to distortion in the shape of the head. It is a generalized form of *craniosynostosis, with a wide skull, high forehead, widely spaced eyes (ocular *hypertelorism), and *exophthalmos. *See also* APERT SYNDROME. [O. Crouzon (1874–1938), French neurologist]

crown *n.* **1.** the part of a tooth normally visible in the mouth and usually covered by enamel. **2.** a dental *restoration that covers most or all of the natural crown. It may be made of porcelain (sometimes bonded to a metal substructure), gold, a combination of these, or less commonly other materials. Most crowns are like thimbles and are custom made to fit over a trimmed-down tooth. Preformed metal crowns may be used on primary teeth. A **post crown** is used to restore a tooth when insufficient of the natural crown remains. A post is inserted into the root and the missing centre of the tooth is built up; over it is fitted a thimble-like crown to restore the natural shape of the tooth. *Root canal treatment is required before a post crown can be made.

crowning *n.* **1.** the stage of labour when the upper part of the infant's head is encircled by, and just passing through, the vaginal opening. **2.** (in dentistry) the technique of treating and fitting a tooth with an artificial *crown.

crown–rump length (CRL) the longest measurement of the fetus from end to end. Measurement of the CRL of the embryo in the first trimester has been shown to be the most accurate parameter for assessment of gestational age; the measurement is less accurate at the end of the first trimester because of fetal flexion.

CRP *see* C-REACTIVE PROTEIN.

CRT *see* CARDIAC RESYNCHRONIZATION THERAPY.

cruciate ligaments a pair (anterior and posterior) of ligaments inside each knee joint, which help to prevent excessive anteroposterior glide. Damage to the cruciate ligaments is a common *sports injury, especially in football players.

crude rate the total number of events (e.g. cases of lung cancer) expressed as a rate per 1000 population. When factors such as age structure or sex of populations can significantly affect the rates (as in *mortality or *morbidity rates) it is more meaningful to compare age/sex specific rates using one or more age groups of a designated sex (e.g. lung cancer in males aged 55–64 years). More complex calculations, which take account of the age and sex structure of a population as a whole, can produce *standardized rates and *standardized mortality ratios (SMR).

crural *adj.* **1.** relating to the thigh or leg. **2.** relating to the crura cerebri (*see* CRUS).

crus *n.* (*pl.* **crura**) an elongated process or part of a structure. The **crus cerebri** is one of two symmetrical nerve tracts situated between the medulla oblongata and the cerebral hemispheres.

crush syndrome *see* MYOGLOBINURIC ACUTE RENAL FAILURE.

cry- (cryo-) *combining form denoting* cold.

cryaesthesia *n.* **1.** exceptional sensitivity to low temperature. **2.** a sensation of coldness.

cryoglobulin *n.* an abnormal protein – an *immunoglobulin (*see* PARAPROTEIN) – that may be present in the blood in certain diseases. Cryoglobulins become insoluble at low temperatures, leading to obstruction of small blood vessels in the fingers and toes in cold weather and producing a characteristic rash. The presence of cryoglobulins (**cryoglobulinaemia**) may be a feature of a variety of diseases, including *macroglobulinaemia, systemic *lupus erythematosus, and certain infections.

cryoprecipitate *n.* a precipitate produced by freezing and thawing under controlled conditions. An example of a cryoprecipitate is the residue obtained from fresh frozen blood plasma that has been thawed at 4°C. This residue is extremely rich in a clotting factor, Factor VIII (antihaemophilic factor), and is used in the control of bleeding in *haemophilia.

cryopreservation *n.* preservation of tissues by freezing. Cryopreservation of embryos, egg cells, or sperm may be employed as part of *in vitro fertilization procedures, for example if there are medical reasons for delaying the pregnancy. *See also* VITRIFICATION.

cryoprobe *n. see* CRYOSURGERY.

cryoretinopexy *n.* the use of extreme cold to freeze areas of weak or torn retina in order to cause scarring and seal breaks. It is used in *cryosurgery for *retinal detachment and also in certain other ischaemic conditions of the retina (e.g. diabetic retinopathy).

cryostat *n.* **1.** a chamber in which frozen tissue is sectioned with a *microtome. **2.** a device for maintaining a specific low temperature.

cryosurgery *n.* the use of extreme cold in a localized part of the body to freeze and destroy unwanted tissues. Cryosurgery is usually undertaken with an instrument called a **cryoprobe**, which has a fine tip cooled by allowing carbon dioxide or nitrous oxide gas to expand within it. Cryosurgery is commonly used for the treatment of retinal detachment (*see* CRYORETINOPEXY), the destruction of certain bone tumours, and the obliteration of skin blemishes.

cryotherapy *n.* the destruction of diseased or unwanted tissue based on freezing. For example, prostate cryotherapy involves the infusion of argon gas through the perineum to destroy prostate cancer cells, either after failed radiotherapy or as primary treatment. *See also* CYCLOCRYOTHERAPY, CRYOSURGERY, HYPOTHERMIA.

crypt *n.* a small sac, follicle, or cavity; for example, the crypts of Lieberkühn (*see* LIEBERKÜHN'S GLANDS), which are intestinal glands.

crypt- (crypto-) *combining form denoting* concealed. Example: **cryptogenic** (of unknown origin).

cryptococcosis (torulosis) *n.* a disease of worldwide distribution, but recognized mainly in the USA, caused by the fungus *Cryptococcus neoformans*. The fungus attacks the lung, resulting in a tumour-like solid mass (**toruloma**), but produces few or no symptoms referable to the lungs. It may spread to the brain, leading to meningitis; this may occur as an opportunistic infection in those suffering from AIDS. The condition responds well to treatment with *amphotericin.

Cryptococcus *n.* a genus of unicellular yeastlike fungi that cause disease in humans. They are found in soil (particularly when enriched with pigeon droppings), and they are common in pigeon roosts and nests. The species *C. neoformans* causes *cryptococcosis.

cryptomenorrhoea *n.* severe cyclical abdominal pain in association with *amen-orrhoea, usually about a year after the expected onset of menstruation and usually due to an *imperforate hymen. On parting the labia, a bulging blue membrane is seen above the hymen and a pelvic mass is felt on examination. Treatment is by incision of the membrane.

cryptophthalmos *n.* apparent absence of the eyes due to failure of normal eyelid formation during embryonic development, resulting in absence of the opening between the upper and lower eyelids.

cryptorchidism (cryptorchism) *n.* the condition in which the testes fail to descend into the scrotum and are retained within the abdomen or inguinal canal. The operation of *orchidopexy is necessary to bring the testes into the scrotum before puberty in order to allow subsequent normal development; it is thought that the higher temperature in the abdomen interferes with sperm production. —**cryptorchid** *adj., n.*

cryptosporidiosis *n.* an intestinal infection of mammals and birds caused by parasitic protozoa of the genus *Cryptosporidium*, which is usually transmitted to humans via farm animals. Ingestion of water or milk contaminated with infective oocysts results in severe diarrhoea and abdominal cramps, caused by release of a toxin. Most patients recover in 7–14 days, but the disease can persist in the immunocompromised (including AIDS patients), the elderly, and young children.

CSF 1. *see* CEREBROSPINAL FLUID. 2. *see* COLONY-STIMULATING FACTOR.

CS gas a powerful incapacitating gas used in warfare and riot control. The sufferer experiences a burning sensation in the eyes, difficulty in breathing, tightness of the chest, nausea, vomiting, and streaming from the eyes and nose. In confined spaces the gas can prove fatal.

CSOM chronic suppurative otitis media (*see* OTITIS).

CT *see* COMPUTERIZED TOMOGRAPHY.

CTPA computerized tomographic pulmonary angiography: a modification of computerized tomographic *angiography in which the computer software optimizes the view of the pulmonary arteries. Also known as **SVCT** (spiral volumetric computerized to-

mography), it has become a useful tool for the diagnosis of pulmonary embolism.

cubital *adj.* relating to the elbow or forearm; for example the **cubital fossa** is the depression at the front of the elbow.

cuboid bone the outer bone of the *tarsus, which articulates with the fourth and fifth metatarsal bones in front and with the calcaneus (heel bone) behind.

cuirass ventilator *see* VENTILATOR.

culdoplasty (McCall culdoplasty) *n.* a surgical procedure to correct a *vault prolapse after hysterectomy using sutures to suspend the vaginal vault at the origin of the uterosacral ligaments (which support the vagina) and to close off the *pouch of Douglas.

Culex *n.* a genus of mosquitoes, worldwide in distribution, of which there are some 600 species. Certain species are important as vectors of filariasis (*see also* WUCHERERIA) and viral encephalitis.

culicide *n.* an agent that destroys mosquitoes or gnats.

Cullen sign a bluish bruiselike appearance around the umbilicus due to bleeding into the peritoneum. Causes include a ruptured ectopic pregnancy and acute *pancreatitis. [T. S. Cullen (1868–1953), US gynaecologist]

culmen *n.* an area of the upper surface of the *cerebellum, anterior to the declive and posterior to the central lobule and separated from them by deep fissures.

culture 1. *n.* a population of microorganisms, usually bacteria, grown in a solid or liquid laboratory medium (**culture medium**), which is usually *agar, broth, or *gelatin. A **pure culture** consists of a single bacterial species. A **stab culture** is a bacterial culture growing in a plug of solid medium within a bottle (or tube); the medium is inoculated by 'stabbing' it with a bacteria-coated straight wire. A **stock culture** is a permanent bacterial culture, from which subcultures are made. *See also* TISSUE CULTURE. 2. *vb.* to grow bacteria or other microorganisms in cultures.

cumulative action the toxic effects of a drug produced by repeated administration of small doses at intervals that are not long enough for it to be either broken down or excreted by the body.

cumulus oophoricus a cluster of follicle cells that surround a freshly ovulated ovum. By increasing the effective size of the ovum they may assist its entrance into the end of the Fallopian tube. They are dispersed at fertilization by the contents of the *acrosome.

cuneiform bones three bones in the *tarsus – the **lateral** (external), **intermediate** (middle), and **medial** (internal) cuneiform bones – that articulate respectively with the first, second, and third metatarsal bones in front. All three bones articulate with the navicular bone behind.

cuneus *n.* a wedge-shaped area of *cerebral cortex that forms the inner surface of the occipital lobe.

Cuniculus *n.* a genus of large forest-dwelling rodents, the pacas or spotted cavies, found in South and Central America. In Brazil these animals are a natural reservoir of the parasite *Leishmania braziliensis*, which causes espundia (*see* LEISHMANIASIS).

cupola *n.* **1.** the small dome at the end of the cochlea. **2.** any of several dome-shaped anatomical structures.

cupping *n.* the traditional Chinese practice of applying a heated cup to the skin and allowing it to cool, which causes swelling of the tissues beneath and an increase in the flow of blood in the area. This is thought to draw out harmful excess blood from diseased organs nearby and so promote healing. In **wet cupping** the skin is previously cut, so that blood will flow into the cup and can be removed.

cupula *n.* a small dome-shaped structure consisting of sensory hairs embedded in gelatinous material, forming part of a *crista in the ampullae of the semicircular canals of the ear.

cupulolith *n.* a particle derived from *otoliths in the *utricle of the inner ear, displaced from its normal site and attached to the *cupula within the ampullary portion of one of the semicircular canals. Cupuloliths are implicated in *benign paroxysmal positional vertigo.

curare *n.* an extract from the bark of South American trees (*Strychnos* and *Chondodendron* species) that relaxes and paralyses voluntary muscle. Used for centuries as an arrow poison by South American Indians, curare was formerly employed to control the muscle spasms of tetanus and as a muscle relaxant in surgical operations.

curettage *n.* the scraping of the skin or the internal surface of an organ or body cavity by means of a spoon-shaped instrument (**curette**), usually to remove diseased tissue or to obtain a specimen for diagnostic purposes (*see also* DILATATION AND CURETTAGE). Curettage of the skin is combined with cauterization; it may be used for the removal of *basal cell carcinoma, seborrhoeic *keratoses, etc., and usually causes little scarring.

curette *n.* a spoon-shaped instrument for scraping tissue from a cavity (*see* CURETTAGE, DILATATION AND CURETTAGE).

curie *n.* a former unit for expressing the activity of a radioactive substance. It has been replaced by the *becquerel. Symbol: Ci.

Curling's ulcers *see* STRESS ULCERS. [T. B. Curling (1811–88), British surgeon]

Curschmann's spirals elongated *casts of the smaller bronchi, which are coughed up in bronchial asthma. They unroll to a length of 2 cm or more and have a central core ensheathed in mucus and cell debris. [H. Curschmann (1846–1910), German physician]

Cushing's syndrome the condition resulting from excess amounts of *corticosteroid hormones in the body. Symptoms include weight gain, reddening of the face and neck, excess growth of body and facial hair, raised blood pressure, loss of mineral from the bones (osteoporosis), raised blood glucose levels, and sometimes mental disturbances. The syndrome may be due to overstimulation of the adrenal glands by excessive amounts of the hormone ACTH, secreted either by a tumour of the pituitary gland (**Cushing's disease**) or by a malignant tumour in the lung or elsewhere. Other causes include a benign or malignant tumour of the adrenal gland(s), resulting in excess activity of the gland, and prolonged therapy with high doses of corticosteroid drugs. [H. W. Cushing (1869–1939), US surgeon]

Cushing's ulcers *see* STRESS ULCERS. [H. W. Cushing]

cusp *n.* **1.** any of the cone-shaped prominences on teeth, especially the molars and premolars. **2.** a pocket or fold of the membrane (endocardium) lining the heart or of the layer of the wall of a vein, several of which form a *valve. When the blood flows backwards the cusps fill up and become distended, so closing the valve.

cutaneous *adj.* relating to the skin.

cutaneous T-cell lymphoma a group of lymphomas in which abnormal T *lymphocytes are concentrated in the skin. The most common form is *mycosis fungoides.

cuticle *n.* 1. the *epidermis of the skin. 2. a layer of solid or semisolid material that is secreted by and covers an *epithelium. 3. a layer of cells, such as the outer layer of cells in a hair.

cutis *n. see* SKIN.

CVP *see* CENTRAL VENOUS PRESSURE.

CVS *see* CHORIONIC VILLUS SAMPLING.

cyan- (cyano-) *combining form denoting* blue.

cyanide *n.* any of the notoriously poisonous salts of hydrocyanic acid. Cyanides combine with and render inactive the enzymes of the tissues responsible for cellular respiration, and therefore they kill extremely quickly; unconsciousness is followed by convulsions and death. Hydrogen cyanide vapour is fatal in less than a minute when inhaled. Sodium or potassium cyanide taken by mouth may also kill within minutes. Prompt treatment with sodium nitrite and sodium thiosulphate or dicobalt *edetate may save life. Cyanides give off a smell of bitter almonds.

cyanocobalamin *n. see* VITAMIN B$_{12}$.

cyanopsia *n.* a condition in which everything looks bluish.

cyanosis *n.* a bluish discoloration of the skin and mucous membranes resulting from an inadequate amount of oxygen in the blood. Cyanosis is associated with heart failure, lung diseases, the breathing of oxygen-deficient atmospheres, and asphyxia. Cyanosis is also seen in *blue babies, because of congenital heart defects. —**cyanotic** *adj.*

cyberknife *n.* a frameless stereotactic radiotherapy system produced from a small *linear accelerator, which has a robotic arm that allows the beam to be directed from any direction, and which monitors movement of implanted markers to deliver real-time *image-guided radiotherapy.

cybernetics *n.* the science of communication processes and automatic control systems in both machines and living things: a study linking the working of the brain and nervous system with the functioning of computers and automated feedback devices. *See also* BIONICS.

cycl- (cyclo-) *combining form denoting* 1. cycle or cyclic. 2. the ciliary body. Example: **cyclectomy** (excision of).

cyclamate *n.* either of two compounds, sodium or calcium cyclamate, that are thirty times as sweet as sugar and, unlike saccharin, stable to heat. Cyclamates were used as sweetening agents in the food industry until 1969, when their use was banned because they were suspected of causing cancer.

cyclitis *n.* inflammation of the *ciliary body of the eye (*see* UVEITIS). *See also* FUCHS' HETEROCHROMIC CYCLITIS.

cyclizine *n.* a drug with *antihistamine properties, used to prevent and relieve nausea and vomiting in motion sickness, vertigo, and disorders of the inner ear. It is administered by mouth or injection; common side-effects are drowsiness and dizziness. Trade name: **Valoid**.

cycloablation *n.* the destruction of part of the *ciliary body of the eye to reduce the production of aqueous humour and hence reduce intraocular pressure. This technique is used in the treatment of advanced glaucoma resistant to other forms of treatment.

cyclocryotherapy *n.* the destruction of part of the *ciliary body (*see* CYCLOABLATION) by freezing. It is used to reduce intraocular pressure in the control of glaucoma.

cyclodialysis *n.* separation of the *ciliary body from its attachment to the sclera, producing a cleft between the two (**cyclodialysis cleft**). This may be the result of trauma or it may be performed as part of an operation in the treatment of glaucoma.

cyclopenthiazide *n.* a *diuretic used to treat fluid retention (oedema), high blood pressure (hypertension), and heart failure. It is administered by mouth and may cause a fall in blood pressure on standing up and reduced blood potassium levels. Trade name: **Navidrex**.

cyclopentolate *n.* a drug, similar to *atropine, that is used in eye drops to paralyse the ciliary muscles and dilate the pupil for eye examinations. Trade names: **Minims Cyclopentolate Hydrochloride, Mydrilate**.

cyclophoria *n.* a type of squint (*see* STRABISMUS) in which the eye, when tested, tends to rotate slightly clockwise or anticlockwise.

cyclophosphamide *n.* an *alkylating agent used to treat a variety of cancers, including chronic lymphocytic leukaemia, lymphomas, and solid tumours, often in combination with other *cytotoxic drugs. It also has *immunosuppressant properties and is used in treating conditions, notably rheumatoid arthritis, requiring a reduced immune response. Cyclophosphamide is administered by mouth or intravenously; common side-effects are nausea, vomiting, and – particularly at high doses – hair loss. *See also* MESNA.

cyclophotoablation *n.* the use of light or lasers to destroy the *ciliary body of the eye in order to reduce production of aqueous humour and hence reduce intraocular pressure. It is used in the treatment of glaucoma.

cycloplegia *n.* paralysis of the ciliary muscle of the eye (*see* CILIARY BODY). This causes inability to alter the focus of the eye and is usually accompanied by paralysis of the muscles of the iris, resulting in fixed dilation of the pupil (**mydriasis**). It is induced by the use of atropine or similar drugs in order to inactivate the muscle in cases of inflammation of the iris and ciliary body and to objectively assess the refractive status of the eye, particularly in children. It may also occur after injuries to the eye.

cycloserine *n.* an *antibiotic, active against a wide range of bacteria, that may be used as supporting treatment in tuberculosis. It is administered by mouth; side-effects, which can be severe, include headache, dizziness, drowsiness, convulsions, and mental confusion.

cyclosporin *n. see* CICLOSPORIN.

cyclothymia (cyclothymic disorder) *n.* the occurrence of mood swings from cheerfulness to misery. These fluctuations are not as great as those of *bipolar affective disorder. They may represent a personality trait for which *psychotherapy is sometimes helpful.

cyclotron *n.* a machine in which charged particles following a spiral path within a magnetic field are accelerated by an alternating electric field. It produces very high-energy charged particles for radiotherapy (*proton therapy), which has been used in the treatment of certain cancers, particularly of the eye. Cyclotrons are used in the preparation of radioisotopes for imaging, particularly those for PET scanning (*see* POSITRON EMISSION TOMOGRAPHY).

cyesis *n. see* PREGNANCY.

cyproheptadine *n.* a potent *antihistamine used to treat allergies, such as hay fever and urticaria; it also inhibits the effects of *serotonin and is used to prevent migraine attacks. Cyproheptadine is administered by mouth; drowsiness is a common side-effect. Trade name: **Periactin**.

cyproterone (cyproterone acetate) *n.* a steroid drug that inhibits the effects of male sex hormones (*see* ANTI-ANDROGEN). It is used to treat hypersexuality disorders and advanced prostate cancer in men; combined with ethinylestradiol as **co-cyprindiol** (Dianette), it is used to treat acne and hirsuitism in women. Cyproterone is administered by mouth and common side-effects include tiredness, loss of strength, inhibition of sperm formation, infertility, and breast enlargement (gynaecomastia). Because of a risk of liver damage, liver function tests should be carried out before and during treatment. Trade names: **Androcur, Cyprostat**.

cyrtometer *n.* a device for measuring the shape of the chest and its movements during breathing.

cyst *n.* 1. an abnormal sac or closed cavity lined with *epithelium and filled with liquid or semisolid matter. There are many varieties of cysts occurring in different parts of the body. **Retention cysts** arise when the outlet of a glandular duct is blocked, as in *sebaceous cysts. Some cysts are congenital, due to abnormal embryonic development; for example, *dermoid cysts. Others are tumours containing cells that secrete mucus or other substances, and another type of cyst is formed by parasites in the body (*see* HYDATID). Cysts may occur in the jaws: a **dental cyst** occurs at the apex of a tooth, a **dentigerous cyst** occurs around the crown of an unerupted tooth, and an **eruption cyst** forms over an erupting tooth. *See also* FIMBRIAL CYST, OVARIAN CYST, PSEUDOCYST. 2. a dormant stage produced during the life cycle of certain protozoan parasites of the alimentary canal, including *Giardia* and *Entamoeba*. Cysts, passed out in the faeces, have tough outer coats that protect the parasites from unfavourable conditions. The parasites emerge from their cysts when they are eaten by a new host. **3.** a structure formed by and surrounding the larvae of certain parasitic worms.

cyst- (cysto-) *combining form denoting* **1.** a bladder, especially the urinary bladder. Example: **cystoplasty** (plastic surgery of). **2.** a cyst.

cystadenoma *n.* an *adenoma showing a cystic structure.

cystalgia *n.* pain in the urinary bladder. This is common in *cystitis and when there are stones in the bladder and is occasionally present in bladder cancer. Treatment is directed to the underlying cause.

cystectomy *n.* surgical removal of the urinary bladder. This is necessary in the treatment of certain bladder conditions, notably cancer, and necessitates subsequent *urinary diversion. The ureters draining the urine from the kidneys are reimplanted into an isolated segment of intestine (usually the ileum), which is brought to the skin surface as a spout (*see* ILEAL CONDUIT). Alternatively, in **bladder replacement**, a segment of ileum or colon is reconstructed to form a pouch (the **Studer pouch** is created from approximately 50 cm of ileum), which is anastomosed to the urethra and acts as a reservoir for the urine. Emptying may be achieved by abdominal straining or *intermittent self-catheterization.

cysteine *n.* a sulphur-containing *amino acid that is an important constituent of many enzymes. The disulphide (S–S) links between adjacent cysteine molecules in polypeptide chains contribute to the three-dimensional molecular structure of proteins.

cystic *adj.* **1.** of, relating to, or characterized by cysts. **2.** of or relating to the gall bladder or urinary bladder.

cystic duct *see* BILE DUCT.

cysticercosis *n.* a disease caused by the presence of tapeworm larvae (*see* CYSTICERCUS) of the species *Taenia solium* in any of the body tissues. Humans become infected on ingesting tapeworm eggs in contaminated food or drink. The presence of cysticerci in the muscles causes pain and weakness; in the brain the symptoms are more serious, including mental deterioration, paralysis, giddiness, epileptic attacks,

and convulsions, which may be fatal. There is no specific treatment for this cosmopolitan disease although surgical removal of cysticerci may be necessary to relieve pressure on the brain.

cysticercus (bladderworm) *n.* a larval stage of some *tapeworms in which the scolex and neck are invaginated into a large fluid-filled cyst. The cysts develop in the muscles or brain of the host following ingestion of tapeworm eggs. *See* CYSTICERCOSIS.

cystic fibrosis (fibrocystic disease of the pancreas, mucoviscidosis) a hereditary disease affecting cells of the exocrine glands (including mucus-secreting glands, sweat glands, and others). The faulty gene responsible for the most common form of the disease has been identified as lying on chromosome no. 7 and is recessive, i.e. both parents of the patient can be *carriers without being affected by the disease. Affected individuals have abnormalities in a protein, **cystic fibrosis transmembrane conductance regulator** (**CFTR**), that enables the transport of chloride ions across cell membranes: this results in the production of thick mucus, which obstructs the intestinal glands (causing meconium *ileus in newborn babies), pancreas (causing deficiency of pancreatic enzymes resulting in *malabsorption and *failure to thrive), and bronchi (causing *bronchiectasis). Respiratory infections, which may be severe, are a common complication. Common agents include *Haemophilus, *Pseudomonas, *Staphylococcus, and *Burkholderia cepacia.* The sweat contains excessive amounts of sodium and chloride, which is an aid to diagnosis.

Treatment consists of minimizing the effects of the disease by administration of pancreatic enzymes and physiotherapy for the lungs and by preventing and combating secondary infection. Sputum viscosity can be reduced by nebulized recombinant human *DNAse. *Genetic counselling is essential, as each subsequent child of carrier parents has a one in four chance of being affected (*see also* MOUTHWASH TEST, PREIMPLANTATION GENETIC DIAGNOSIS). Some patients are benefiting from revolutionary new treatments, including transplantation of heart and lungs and treatment aimed at altering the genetic content of the faulty cells (*see* GENE THERAPY).

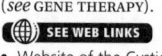 **SEE WEB LINKS**

• Website of the Cystic Fibrosis Trust

cystic hygroma a collection of fluid behind the neck of a fetus, occasionally extending laterally to involve the sides of the neck (*see* HYDROPS FETALIS). In its mildest form it is evidenced by an increased nuchal translucency (*see* NUCHAL TRANSLUCENCY SCANNING). Cystic hygroma may be a diagnostic feature of chromosomal abnormality (e.g. Down's syndrome, Turner's syndrome).

cystine *n. see* AMINO ACID.

cystinosis *n.* an inborn defect in the metabolism of amino acids, leading to abnormal accumulation of the amino acid cystine in the blood, kidneys, and lymphatic system. *See also* FANCONI SYNDROME.

cystinuria *n.* an *inborn error of metabolism resulting in excessive excretion of the amino acid cystine in the urine due to a defect of reabsorption by the kidney tubules. It may lead to the formation of cystine stones in the kidney.

cystitis *n.* inflammation of the urinary bladder, often caused by infection (most commonly by the bacterium *Escherichia coli*). It is usually accompanied by the desire to pass urine frequently, with a degree of burning. More severe attacks are often associated with the painful passage of blood in the urine, which is accompanied by a cramplike pain in the lower abdomen persisting after the bladder has been emptied. An acute attack is treated by antibiotic administration and a copious fluid intake. *See also* INTERSTITIAL CYSTITIS.

cystitome *n.* a small knife with a tiny curved or hooked blade, used to cut the lens capsule in the type of operation for cataract in which the capsule is left behind (extracapsular *cataract extraction).

cystocele *n.* prolapse of the base of the bladder in women. It is usually due to weakness of the pelvic floor after childbirth and causes bulging of the anterior wall of the vagina on straining. When accompanied by stress incontinence of urine, surgical repair (anterior *colporrhaphy) is indicated.

cystography *n.* X-ray examination of the urinary bladder after the injection of a contrast medium. The X-ray images thus obtained are known as **cystograms**. Cystography is most commonly performed to detect reflux of urine from the bladder to the ureters, usually in children (*see* VESICOURETERIC REFLUX). If films are taken during voiding then the urethra can also be observed (*see* URETHROGRAPHY). The examination can also be performed in conjunction with manometry (*see* BLADDER PRESSURE STUDY).

cystoid macular oedema swelling of the central area of the retina (macula), usually occurring as a result of trauma, posterior *uveitis, or ocular surgery.

cystolithiasis *n.* the presence of stones (calculi) in the urinary bladder. The stones are either formed in the bladder, due to obstruction, urinary retention, and infection (**primary calculi**), or pass to the bladder after being formed in the kidneys (**secondary calculi**). They cause pain, the passage of bloody urine, and interruption of the urinary stream and should be removed surgically. *See* CALCULUS.

cystometer *n.* an apparatus for measuring the pressure within the bladder. Modern investigations also include measurement of urine flow, and the resultant bladder pressure/flow study (**urodynamic investigation**) provides useful information regarding bladder function.

cystopexy (vesicofixation) *n.* a surgical operation to fix the urinary bladder (or a portion of it) in a different position. It may be performed as part of the repair or correction of a prolapsed bladder.

cystoplasty *n.* the operation of enlarging the capacity of the bladder by incorporating a segment of bowel. In a **clam cystoplasty**, the bladder is cut across longitudinally from one side of the neck to the other side through the dome (fundus) of the bladder and a length of the ileum or colon is inserted as a patch. In the operation of **ileocaecocystoplasty**, the dome is removed by cutting across the bladder transversely or sagittally above the openings of the ureters; it is replaced by an isolated segment of caecum and terminal ileum. In **ileocystoplasty** the bladder is enlarged by an opened-out portion of small intestine. The bladder may be totally replaced by a reservoir constructed from either small or large intestine (*see* CYSTECTOMY).

cystosarcoma phylloides a malignant tumour of the connective tissue of the breast: it accounts for approximately 1% of all breast cancers. Such tumours may show a wide variation in cell structure and they often present as a large mass but without distant spread. The best treatment for a localized tumour is simple *mastectomy.

cystoscopy *n.* examination of the bladder by means of an instrument (**cystoscope**) inserted via the urethra. The cystoscope consists of either a metal sheath surrounding a telescope and light-conducting bundles or a flexible tube with built-in optical fibres for viewing and illumination. Irrigating fluid is conducted through a channel into the bladder. When using the rigid instrument, additional channels are available for the catheters to be inserted into the ureters, diathermy electrodes for removing polyps, etc., or biopsy forceps for taking specimens of tumours or other growths. When using the flexible cystoscope, only small instruments can be passed through the additional channel, such as biopsy forceps, diathermy electrodes, or laser fibres for the destruction of tumours or stones.

cystostomy *n.* the operation of creating an artificial opening between the bladder and the anterior abdominal wall. This provides a temporary or permanent drainage route for urine.

cystotomy *n.* surgical incision into the urinary bladder, usually by cutting through the abdominal wall above the pubic symphysis (**suprapubic cystotomy**). This is necessary for such operations as removing stones or tumours from the bladder and for gaining access to the prostate gland in the operation of transvesical *prostatectomy.

cyt- (cyto-) *combining form denoting* 1. cell(s). 2. cytoplasm.

cytarabine *n.* an *antimetabolite that interferes with pyrimidine synthesis and is used to suppress the symptoms of acute myeloblastic leukaemia. It is administered by subcutaneous, intravenous, or *intrathecal injection and can damage the normal bone marrow, leading to various blood cell disorders. Other side-effects are nausea, vomiting, mouth ulcers, and diarrhoea. Trade name: **DepoCyte**.

-cyte *combining form denoting* a cell. Examples: **chondrocyte** (cartilage cell); **osteocyte** (bone cell).

cytidine *n.* a compound containing cytosine and the sugar ribose. *See also* NUCLEOSIDE.

cytochemistry *n.* the study of chemical compounds and their activities in living cells.

cytochrome *n.* a compound consisting of a protein linked to *haem. Cytochromes act as electron transfer agents in biological oxidation-reduction reactions, particularly those associated with the mitochondria in cellular respiration. *See* ELECTRON TRANSPORT CHAIN.

cytogenetics *n.* a science that links the study of inheritance (genetics) with that of cells (cytology); it is concerned mainly with the study of the *chromosomes, especially their origin, structure, and functions.

cytokine inhibitor any one of a group of agents that inhibit the activity of cytokines, especially *tumour necrosis factor alpha (TNF-α). They include *infliximab, *etanercept, and **adalimumab** (Humira), known as **anti-TNF drugs**, which are used as *disease-modifying antirheumatic drugs.

cytokines *pl. n.* protein molecules, released by cells when activated by antigen, that are involved in cell-to-cell communications, acting as enhancing mediators for immune responses through interaction with specific cell-surface receptors on leucocytes. Kinds of cytokines include *interleukins (produced by leucocytes), *lymphokines (produced by lymphocytes), *interferons, and *tumour necrosis factor.

cytokinesis *n.* division of the cytoplasm of a cell, which occurs at the end of cell division, after division of the nucleus, to form two daughter cells. *Compare* KARYOKINESIS.

cytology *n.* the study of the structure and function of cells. The examination of cells under a microscope is used in the diagnosis of various diseases. These cells are obtained by scraping an organ, as in **cervical cytology** (*see* CERVICAL SMEAR, LIQUID-BASED CYTOLOGY), by aspiration (*see* ASPIRATION CYTOLOGY), or they are collected from cells already shed (**exfoliative cytology**). *See also* BIOPSY. —**cytological** *adj.*

cytolysis *n.* the breakdown of cells, particularly by destruction of their outer membranes.

cytomegalovirus (CMV) *n.* a member of the herpes group of viruses (*see* HERPESVIRUS). It commonly occurs in humans and normally produces symptoms milder than the common cold. However, in individuals whose immune systems are compromised (e.g. by cancer or AIDS) it can cause more severe effects (such as *retinitis), and it has been found to be the cause of congenital handicap in infants born to women who have contracted the virus during pregnancy.

cytometer *n.* an instrument for determining the number of cells in a given quantity of fluid, such as blood, cerebrospinal fluid, or urine. *See* HAEMOCYTOMETER.

cytomorphosis *n.* the changes undergone by a cell in the course of its life cycle.

cytopenia *n.* a deficiency of one or more of the various types of blood cells. *See* EOSINOPENIA, ERYTHROPENIA, LYMPHOPENIA, NEUTROPENIA, PANCYTOPENIA, THROMBOCYTOPENIA.

cytophotometry *n.* the study of chemical compounds in living cells by means of a **cytophotometer**, an instrument that measures light intensity through stained areas of cytoplasm.

cytoplasm *n.* the jelly-like substance that surrounds the nucleus of a cell. *See also* ECTOPLASM, ENDOPLASM, PROTOPLASM. —**cytoplasmic** *adj.*

cytoplasmic inheritance the inheritance of characters controlled by genes present in the cell cytoplasm rather than by genes on the chromosomes in the cell nucleus. An example of cytoplasmic inheritance is that controlled by mitochondrial genes (*see* MITOCHONDRION).

cytosine *n.* one of the nitrogen-containing bases (*see* PYRIMIDINE) that occurs in the nucleic acids DNA and RNA.

cytosome *n.* the part of a cell that is outside the nucleus.

cytotoxic drug any drug that damages or destroys cells: usually refers to those drugs used to treat various types of cancer. There are various classes of cytotoxic drugs, including *alkylating agents (e.g. *chlorambucil, *cyclophosphamide, *melphalan), *antimetabolites (e.g. *fluorouracil, *methotrexate, *mercaptopurine), *anthracycline antibiotics (e.g. *doxorubicin, *daunorubicin, *dactinomycin), *vinca alkaloids, and platinum compounds (e.g. *carboplatin, *cisplatin). Other cytotoxic drugs include *taxanes and *topoisomerase inhibitors, and some *monoclonal antibodies (e.g. *bevacizumab, *trastuzumab) have cytotoxic activity. All these drugs offer successful treatment in some conditions and help reduce symptoms and prolong life in others. Cytotoxic drugs destroy cancer cells by interfering with cell division, but they also affect normal cells, particularly in bone marrow (causing *myelosuppression), hair follicles (causing hair loss), the stomach lining (resulting in severe nausea and vomiting), mouth (causing soreness), and fetal tissue (they should not be taken during the later stages of pregnancy). Dosage must therefore be carefully controlled. *See also* CHEMOTHERAPY.

cytotoxic T cell a type of T *lymphocyte that destroys cancerous cells, virus-infected cells, and *allografts. Cytotoxic T cells recognize peptide antigens attached to proteins that are encoded by the *HLA system.

cytotrophoblast *n. see* TROPHOBLAST.

dabigatran etexilate a drug used for the prevention of venous thromboembolism following hip or knee replacement surgery: it directly inhibits the action of *thrombin. It is administered by mouth; the most common side-effect is haemorrhage. Trade name: **Padaxa**.

dacarbazine *n.* a drug administered by injection in the treatment of melanoma and (in combination with other *cytotoxic drugs) soft tissue sarcomas and Hodgkin's disease. Side-effects include severe nausea and vomiting and *myelosuppression.

dacry- (**dacryo-**) *combining form denoting* 1. tears. 2. the lacrimal apparatus.

dacryoadenitis *n.* inflammation of the tear-producing (lacrimal) gland (*see* LACRIMAL APPARATUS).

dacryocystitis *n.* inflammation of the lacrimal sac (in which tears collect), usually occurring when the duct draining the tears into the nose is blocked (*see* LACRIMAL APPARATUS).

dacryocystorhinostomy (**DCR**) *n.* an operation to relieve blockage of the nasolacrimal duct (which drains tears into the nose), in which a communication is made between the lacrimal sac and the nose by removing the intervening bone. *See* DACRYOCYSTITIS, LACRIMAL APPARATUS.

dactinomycin (**actinomycin D**) *n.* a *cytotoxic drug (an antibiotic) used mainly to treat cancers in children. It is administered intravenously; side-effects include nausea, vomiting, diarrhoea, blood disorders, and bone-marrow damage. Trade name: **Comegen Lyovac**.

dactyl- *combining form denoting* the digits (fingers or toes). Examples: **dactylomegaly** (abnormally large size of); **dactylospasm** (painful contraction of).

dactylitis *n.* inflammation of a finger or toe caused by bone infection (as in tuberculous *osteomyelitis) or rheumatic disease or seen in infants with sickle-cell disease.

dactylology *n.* the representation of speech by finger movements: sign language.

dalteparin sodium *see* LOW-MOLECULAR-WEIGHT HEPARIN.

Daltonism (**protanopia**) *n.* red-blindness: a defect in colour vision in which a person cannot distinguish between reds and greens. The term has been used to refer to *colour blindness in general. [J. Dalton (1766–1844), British chemist]

damp *n.* (in mining) any gas encountered underground other than air. *See* BLACKDAMP, FIREDAMP.

danazol *n.* a synthetic *progestogen that inhibits the secretion by the pituitary gland of gonadotrophins. It may be used to treat endometriosis and severe urticaria and is administered by mouth. Possible side-effects include nausea, rashes, swelling of the feet and ankles, weight gain, oiliness of the skin, and, in women, menstrual disturbances, excessive growth of facial and body hair, and irreversible voice changes. Because of the severity of these effects, danazol is now rarely used in gynaecology. Trade name: **Danol**.

Dance's sign *see* SIGN OF DANCE.

D and C *see* DILATATION AND CURETTAGE.

dandruff *n.* visible scaling from the surface of the scalp. It is extremely common, occurring in about 50% of the population, and is associated with the presence of the yeast *Malassezia furfur*. It is the precursor of seborrhoeic *eczema of the scalp, in which there is a degree of inflammation in addition to the greasy scaling. Dandruff can be controlled by shampoos containing tar, selenium sulphide, pyrithione zinc, or imidazole antifungals. Medical name: **pityriasis capitis**.

Dandy-Walker syndrome a form of *cerebral palsy in which the *cerebellum is usually the part of the brain affected. It leads to unsteadiness of balance and an abnormal gait and may be associated with *hydrocephalus. [W. E. Dandy (1886–1946) and A. E. Walker (1907–95), US surgeons]

dangerous drugs *see* MISUSE OF DRUGS ACT 1971.

dantrolene *n.* a *muscle relaxant drug used to relieve spasticity in such conditions as cerebral palsy, multiple sclerosis, and spinal cord injury. It is administered by mouth; possible side-effects include weakness, dizziness, drowsiness, and diarrhoea; liver damage sometimes occurs. Dantrolene, given intravenously, is also used to treat malignant hyperthermia, a serious complication of anaesthesia. Trade names: **Dantrium, Dantrium Intravenous**.

dantron (danthron) *n.* a stimulant *laxative administered by mouth for treating constipation in terminally ill patients; it sometimes colours the urine pink or red. It is usually combined with a faecal softener (e.g. in **co-danthramer, co-danthrusate**).

dapsone *n.* a drug (*see* SULPHONE) used to treat *leprosy and dermatitis herpetiformis. It is administered by mouth; the most common side-effects are allergic skin reactions.

dark adaptation the changes that take place in the retina and pupil of the eye enabling vision in very dim light. Dark adaptation involves activation of the *rods – the cells of the retina that function best in dim light – and the reflex enlargement of the pupil (*see* PUPILLARY REFLEX). *Compare* LIGHT ADAPTATION.

dasatinib *n. see* TYROSINE KINASE INHIBITOR.

data protection safeguards relating to the use of personal information about a living person. The relevant statute is the Data Protection Act 1998, which sets out eight principles of lawful data protection. Under the Act individuals have a basic right to control information stored about them, i.e. if they are the 'subject' of data. Data may be factual or express opinions and in paper or electronic form. Information concerning health is considered 'sensitive personal data' under the legislation. Information must be accurate and cannot be used or passed on to others without the knowledge of the subject, who can then object. Holders of information are required to be registered with a local data controller, who in turn must inform the *Information Commissioner, who oversees the implementation of legislation and enforces

the rules. Individuals about whom information is held can request to view a copy of the information relevant to them (a 'subject access request') and a response is required within 40 days of the request. If inaccurate or misleading information is being held, the subject can ask that the data be amended. Specific exceptions include information held by the police or relating to state security and medical research, but not medical information that may affect employment or promotion.

daunorubicin *n.* an *anthracycline antibiotic that interferes with DNA synthesis and is used in the treatment of acute leukaemias and AIDS-related Kaposi's sarcoma. It is administered by intravenous infusion. Possible side-effects include loss of hair and damage to bone marrow and heart muscle. Trade name: **DaunoXome**.

da Vinci robot *see* PROSTATECTOMY.

dawn phenomenon (Somogyi effect) the phenomenon of high fasting blood-sugar levels in the morning due to an unrecognized hypoglycaemic episode during the night in a person with diabetes. The low blood sugar has resulted in an outpouring of regulatory hormones, such as adrenaline and glucagon, which have raised the blood sugar to supranormal levels by the time of waking. It is important to recognize the cause, since increasing the evening insulin dose, thinking this will bring the morning sugars down, could actually cause a more severe nocturnal hypoglycaemic attack, which the body may not be able to counteract: coma might ensue. The condition can be tested for by measuring blood sugars at the time of the assumed low level.

day blindness (hemeralopia) comparatively good vision in poor light but poor vision in good illumination. The condition is usually congenital and associated with poor *visual acuity and defective colour vision. Acquired cases occur when the *cones (light-sensitive cells) are selectively destroyed by disease. *Compare* NIGHT BLINDNESS.

day-case surgery surgical procedures that can be performed in a single day, without the need to admit the patient for an overnight stay in hospital. Modern techniques of surgery and anaesthesia now enable many surgical cases of minor and intermediate degrees of severity to be treated in this way: examples include many breast lesions, dilatation and curettage, and operations for hernia and varicose veins. Special units are established in many hospitals.

day hospital a hospital in which patients spend a substantial part of the day under clinical supervision but do not stay overnight. Day hospitals are mainly used for the assessment, treatment, and rehabilitation of elderly patients and those with mental disorders. Patients may attend on one or more days during the week.

D cells *see* ISLETS OF LANGERHANS.

DCIS *see* DUCTAL CARCINOMA IN SITU.

DCR *see* DACRYOCYSTORHINOSTOMY.

D-dimer *n.* a protein measured in a blood test to diagnose thrombosis. Although a negative result practically rules out thrombosis, a positive result can indicate thrombosis but also has other potential causes. Its main use, therefore, is to exclude thromboembolic disease where the probability is low. This test is now widely used in protocols for the diagnosis of *pulmonary embolism.

DDT (chlorophenothane, dicophane) *n.* a powerful insecticide that was formerly widely used against lice, fleas, flies, bed bugs, cockroaches, and other disease-carrying and destructive insects. It is a relatively stable compound that is stored in animal fats, and the quantities now present in the environment – in the form of stores accumulated in animal tissues – have led to its use being restricted. Acute poisoning, from swallowing more than 20 g, produces nervous irritability, muscle twitching, convulsions, and coma, but only a few fatalities have been reported.

de- *prefix denoting* **1.** removal or loss. Examples: **demineralization** (of minerals from bones or teeth); **devascularization** (of blood supply). **2.** reversal.

deafness *n.* partial or total loss of hearing in one or both ears. **Conductive deafness** is due to a defect in the conduction of sound from the external ear to the inner ear. This may be due to perforations of the eardrum, fluid or infection in the middle ear (*see* GLUE EAR, OTITIS (MEDIA)), or disorders of the small bones in the middle ear (*ossicles). **Sensorineural** (or **perceptive**) **deafness** may be due to a lesion of the *cochlea in the inner ear, the cochlear nerve, or the auditory centres in the brain. It may be present from

birth (for example if the mother was affected with German measles during pregnancy). In adults it may be brought on by injury, disease (e.g. *Ménière's disease), or prolonged exposure to loud noise; progressive sensorineural deafness (**presbyacusis**) is common with advancing age.

The type of deafness can be diagnosed by various hearing tests (*see* RINNE'S TEST, WEBER'S TEST, AUDIOGRAM), and the treatment depends on the cause. *See also* COCHLEAR IMPLANT, HEARING AID, HEARING THERAPY.

(⊕) SEE WEB LINKS
- Website of the British Deaf Association: includes information on British Sign Language
- Website of the Royal National Institute for Deaf People

deamination *n.* a process, occurring in the liver, that occurs during the metabolism of amino acids. The amino group ($-NH_2$) is removed from an amino acid and converted to ammonia, which is ultimately converted to *urea and excreted.

death *n.* absence of vital functions. Death is diagnosed by permanent cessation of the heartbeat. **Brain death** is defined as permanent functional death of the centres in the brainstem that control breathing, heart rate, and other vital reflexes (including pupillary responses). Many decisions in medicine depend on death being clearly defined and objectively observed. Particular problems arise when a potential organ donor is being kept artificially alive. Legally, two independent medical opinions are required before brain death is agreed and organs can be removed for transplantation. In medical ethics, death is relevant because it elucidates debates about *personhood and prompts consideration of the duties owed to the living and the deceased. Religious perspectives on death may inform the ways in which people perceive the withdrawal of medical treatment and organ donation.

death certificate a legal document, signed by a doctor, stating (in Part 1) the immediate cause of a person's death followed by diseases underlying the condition. For example, if the immediate cause of death was a myocardial infarction, the underlying disease might have been ischaemic heart disease or hypertension. Other diseases, which were not directly linked with the immediate cause of death but may have contributed to the patient's overall condition, are mentioned in Part 2 of the certificate. The document usually states the decedent's gender and date and place of death; other details, such as occupation, may also be included. The death certificate forms a vital record in most countries throughout the world; without a death certificate, there can be no funeral. In the United Kingdom, this information is registered at St. Catherine's House, London. Following the case of Dr Harold Shipman and the subsequent public inquiry, legislative change has introduced greater checks on, and scrutiny of, death certification by doctors.

debridement *n.* the process of cleaning an open wound by removal of foreign material and dead tissue, so that healing may occur without hindrance.

dec- (deca-) *prefix denoting* ten.

decalcification *n.* loss or removal of calcium salts from a bone or tooth.

decapitation *n.* removal of the head, usually the head of a dead fetus to enable delivery to take place. This procedure is very rare nowadays, being undertaken only in dire circumstances when the fetal head is too large to pass through the birth canal, the mother's life is endangered, and Caesarean section impossible.

decapsulation *n. see* DECORTICATION.

decay *n.* (in bacteriology) the decomposition of organic matter due to microbial action.

deception *n.* the act of deliberately misleading, misrepresenting, or withholding information. Respect for patient *autonomy and the importance of trust in therapeutic relationships require that doctors should always strive to be honest with patients. *See also* THERAPEUTIC PRIVILEGE.

decerebrate *adj.* denoting a neurological state in which the functions of the higher centres of the brain are eliminated. This is brought about in experimental animals by cutting across the brain below the cerebrum, but certain injuries to the brain in humans may cause the same severe neurological signs as occur in a decerebrate animal.

deci- *prefix denoting* a tenth.

decibel (dB) *n.* one tenth of a bel: a unit for comparing levels of power (especially sound) on a logarithmic scale. A power source of intensity P has a power level of $10 \log_{10} P/P_0$

decibels, where P_0 is the intensity of a reference source. The decibel is much more widely used than the bel. Silence is 0 dB; a whisper has an intensity of 30 dB, normal speech 60 dB, a shout 90 dB, and a jet aircraft 120 dB.

decidua *n.* the modified mucous membrane that lines the wall of the uterus during pregnancy and is shed with the afterbirth at parturition (*see* ENDOMETRIUM). There are three regions: the **decidua capsularis**, a thin layer that covers the embryo; the **decidua basalis**, where the embryo is attached; and the **decidua parietalis**, which is not in contact with the embryo. —**decidual** *adj.*

deciduous teeth *see* PRIMARY TEETH.

de Clérambault syndrome *see* EROTOMANIA. [G. G. de Clérambault (1872–1934), French physician]

declive *n.* an area of the upper surface of the *cerebellum, posterior to the culmen and anterior to the folium of the middle lobe.

decomposition *n.* the temperature-dependent gradual disintegration of dead organic matter, usually foodstuffs or tissues, by the chemical action of bacteria and/or fungi.

decompression *n.* **1.** the reduction of pressure on an organ or part of the body by surgical intervention. Surgical decompression can be effected at many sites: the pressure of tissues on a nerve may be relieved by incision; raised pressure in the fluid of the brain can be lowered by cutting into the *dura mater; and cardiac compression – the abnormal presence of blood or fluid round the heart – can be cured by cutting the sac (pericardium) enclosing the heart. **2.** the gradual reduction of atmospheric pressure for deep-sea divers, who work at artificially high pressures. *See* COMPRESSED AIR ILLNESS.

decompression sickness *see* COMPRESSED AIR ILLNESS.

decongestant *n.* an agent that reduces or relieves nasal congestion. Nasal decongestants are *sympathomimetic or *antimuscarinic drugs applied locally, in the form of nasal sprays or drops.

decontamination *n.* the process of cleaning surgical instruments to remove adherent protein prior to sterilization in an autoclave.

decortication *n.* **1.** the removal of the outside layer (cortex) from an organ or structure, such as the kidney. **2.** an operation for removing the blood clot and scar tissue that forms after bleeding into the chest cavity (haemothorax). **3. (decapsulation)** the surgical removal of a *capsule from an organ; for example, the stripping of the membrane that envelops the kidney or of the inflammatory capsule that encloses a chronic abscess, as in the treatment of *empyema.

decubitus 1. *n.* the recumbent position. **2.** *adj.* describing a radiograph taken with the patient lying on his side and the X-ray beam travelling horizontally. Such films reveal *free gas in the peritoneal cavity following perforation of a hollow organ and *fluid levels in the bowel when it is obstructed. *Compare* AN-TEROPOSTERIOR, POSTEROANTERIOR.

decubitus ulcer *see* PRESSURE SORE.

decussation *n.* a point at which two or more structures of the body cross to the opposite side. The term is used particularly for the point at which nerve fibres cross over in the central nervous system.

deep transverse arrest mechanical obstruction of labour in which the fetal head is unable to rotate from occipitotransverse to occipitoanterior position (*see* OCCIPUT).

deep vein thrombosis (DVT) *see* PHLE-BOTHROMBOSIS.

deer fly *see* CHRYSOPS.

defecation *n.* a bowel movement in which faeces are evacuated through the rectum and anus. The amount and composition of the food eaten determine to a large degree the bulk of the faeces, and the transit time through the intestinal tract determines the water content. *See* CONSTIPATION, DIARRHOEA.

defence mechanism the means whereby an undesirable impulse or emotion can be avoided or controlled. Defence mechanisms are regarded as normal forms of self-protection; however, used excessively, they can become pathological. Many defence mechanisms have been described, including *repression, *projection, *reaction formation, *sublimation, and *splitting.

defensive medicine health care that becomes distorted by fear of legal action so that medical decisions are taken with a view to protecting the professional against legal liability. *See also* NEGLIGENCE.

deferent *adj.* **1.** carrying away from or down from. **2.** relating to the vas deferens.

defervescence *n.* the disappearance of a fever, a process that may occur rapidly or take several days, depending upon the cause and treatment given.

defibrillation *n.* administration of a controlled electric shock to restore normal heart rhythm in cases of cardiac arrest due to ventricular *fibrillation. The apparatus used is a *defibrillator.

defibrillation gel pads *see* COUPLING AGENTS.

defibrillator *n.* the apparatus used for *defibrillation, which may be internal (*see* IMPLANTABLE CARDIOVERTOR DEFIBRILLATOR) or external. External defibrillators may be fully automated (*see* AUTOMATED EXTERNAL DEFIBRILLATOR), semiautomated, or manual and usually deliver the electric current via two defibrillation paddles. They are now all manufactured to deliver a biphasic current waveform (until recently they were all monophasic). The efficacy of the first shock during *cardiac arrest is higher with biphasic systems, which also use less battery power per shock.

defibrination *n.* the removal of *fibrin, one of the plasma proteins that causes coagulation, from a sample of blood. It is normally done by whisking the blood with a bundle of fine wires, to which the strands of fibrin that form in the blood adhere.

deficiency *n.* (in genetics) *see* DELETION.

deficiency disease any disease caused by the lack of an essential nutrient in the diet. Such nutrients include *vitamins, *essential amino acids, and *essential fatty acids.

degarelix *n.* a *gonadotrophin-releasing-hormone antagonist used in the treatment of prostate cancer. It is administered by subcutaneous injection; side-effects include hot flushes and pain at the injection site. Trade name: **Firmagon**.

degeneration *n.* the deterioration and loss of specialized function of the cells of a tissue or organ. The changes may be caused by a defective blood supply or by disease. Degeneration may involve the deposition of calcium salts, fat (*see* FATTY DEGENERATION), or fibrous tissue in the affected organ or tissue. *See also* INFILTRATION.

deglutition *n.* *see* SWALLOWING.

dehiscence *n.* a splitting open, as of a surgical wound.

dehydration *n.* **1.** loss or deficiency of water in body tissues. The condition may result from inadequate water intake and/or from excessive removal of water from the body; for example, by sweating, vomiting, or diarrhoea. Symptoms include great thirst, nausea, and exhaustion. The condition is treated by drinking plenty of water; severe cases require *oral rehydration therapy or intravenous administration of water and salts (which have been lost with the water). **2.** the removal of water from tissue during its preparation for microscopical study, by placing it successively in stronger solutions of ethyl alcohol. Dehydration follows *fixation and precedes *clearing.

dehydroepiandrosterone (DHEA) *n.* a weak androgen produced and secreted by the adrenal glands after the stage of adrenal maturation known as *adrenarche. It is produced from 17-hydroxypregnenolone and itself is largely converted to **dehydroepiandrosterone sulphate** and **androstenedione**. All three of these molecules can cause a degree of mild *androgenization but can also be converted in the circulation to the more potent androgens *testosterone and *dihydrotestosterone.

dehydrogenase *n. see* OXIDOREDUCTASE.

déjà vu a vivid psychic experience in which immediately contemporary events seem to be a repetition of previous happenings. It is a symptom of some forms of *epilepsy. *See also* JAMAIS VU.

delayed suture (delayed primary closure) a technique used in the closure of contaminated wounds and wounds associated with tissue necrosis, such as are produced by missile injuries. The superficial layers of the wound are left open, to be closed later when the tissues have been cleaned.

deletion (deficiency) *n.* (in genetics) a type of mutation involving the loss of DNA. The deletion may be small, affecting only a portion of a single gene, or large, resulting in loss of a part of a chromosome and affecting many genes.

Delhi boil *see* ORIENTAL SORE.

deliberate self-harm any attempt at self-injury or self-poisoning, which often occurs in the context of acute stress, personality disorder, depression, and alcoholism. It is also occasionally known as **parasuicide**: the patient is considered to have performed a suicidal act but without the intention to kill him- or herself. Treatment consists of various forms of *psychotherapy, a *psychosocial assessment, and occasionally *antipsychotic medication, *lithium, or *SSRIs. If the attempt is serious, immediate treatment may be necessary in a medical ward or (more rarely), if suicidal intent persists, in a psychiatric ward. Patients who do not have a mental disorder should be assessed using the criteria set out in the Mental Capacity Act 2005 and, if found to have *capacity, are entitled to consent to or refuse treatment like any other capacitous adult. *See also* SUICIDE.

delirium *n.* an acute disorder of the mental processes accompanying organic brain disease. It may be manifested by delusions, disorientation, hallucinations, or extreme excitement and occurs in metabolic disorders, intoxication, deficiency diseases, and infections.

delirium tremens an acute confusional state often seen as a withdrawal syndrome in chronic alcoholics (*see* ALCOHOLISM) and caused by sudden cessation of drinking alcohol. It can be precipitated by a head injury or an acute infection causing abstinence from alcohol. Features include anxiety, tremor, sweating, and vivid and terrifying visual and sensory hallucinations, often of animals and insects. Without medical treatment severe cases may end fatally.

delivery *n. see* LABOUR.

dellen *pl. n.* localized areas of reduced corneal thickness, usually at the limbus (the junction of the cornea with the sclera), due to local dehydration. They may occur after surgery to correct a squint, due to elevated conjunctiva at the limbus causing poor wetting of the adjacent cornea.

deltoid *n.* a thick triangular muscle that covers the shoulder joint (see illustration). It is responsible for raising the arm away from the side of the body.

delusion *n.* a belief that is held with unshakable conviction, cannot be altered by rational argument, and is outside the person's normal cultural or subcultural belief system. The belief is usually wrong, but can occasionally be true. The abnormal pathology lies in the irrational way in which the person comes to the belief. In mental illness it may be a false belief that the individual is persecuted by others, is very powerful, is guilty of something they have not actually done, is poor, or is a victim of physical disease (*see* PARANOIA). Delusions may be a symptom of *schizophrenia, *mania, or an organic psychosis.

delusional infestation (delusional parasitosis, Ekbom's syndrome) a *monodelusional disorder in which patients believe they or their environment are infested by parasites. These can range from rats in the patient's house to microspores in the air. Classically patients believe they have insects underneath their skin. Many present the alleged parasite as a specimen for examination. If compliance can be established, most patients respond well to *antipsychotic medication.

delusional perception a *Schneiderian first-rank symptom in which a person believes that a normal percept (product of perception) has a special meaning for him or her. For example, a cloud in the sky may be misinterpreted as meaning that someone has sent that person a message to save the world. While the symptom is particularly indicative of *schizophrenia, it also occurs in other psychoses, including *mania (in which it often has grandiose undertones).

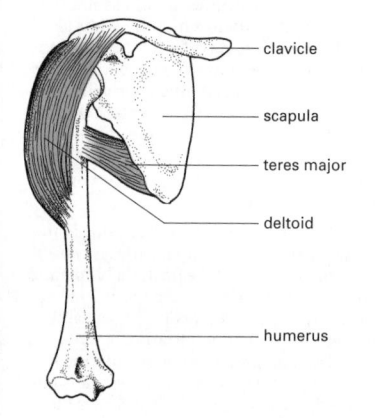

The deltoid muscle.

delusion of reference a *delusion in which the patient believes that unsuspicious occurrences refer to him or her in person. Patients may, for example, believe that certain news bulletins have a direct reference to them, that music played on the radio is played for them, or that car licence plates have a meaning relevant to them. **Ideas of reference** differ from delusions of reference in that insight is retained.

demeclocycline *n.* a *tetracycline antibiotic that is used to treat infections caused by *Chlamydia*, rickettsiae, and mycoplasmas. It is also used to treat *syndrome of inappropriate secretion of antidiuretic hormone. Demeclocycline is administered by mouth; common side-effects are nausea, diarrhoea, and symptoms resulting from the growth of organisms not sensitive to the drug. Trade name: **Ledermycin.**

dementia *n.* a chronic and progressive deterioration of behaviour and higher intellectual function due to organic brain disease. It is marked by memory disorders, changes in personality, deterioration in personal care, impaired reasoning ability, and disorientation. Dementia is usually a condition of old age, but it can occur in young or middle-aged people. The most common causes are *Alzheimer's disease, frontotemporal dementia (e.g. *Pick's disease), and dementia due to diffuse *cortical Lewy body disease. Another common form, **multi-infarct dementia**, results from the destruction of brain tissue by a series of small strokes. It is important to distinguish these organic conditions from psychological disorders that can cause similar symptoms such as *depression (*see* PSEUDODEMENTIA).

demi- *prefix denoting* half.

Demodex *n.* a genus of harmless parasitic mites, the follicle mites, found in the hair follicles and associated sebaceous glands of the face. They resemble tiny worms, about 0.4 mm in length, and their presence may give rise to dermatitis.

demography *n.* the study of populations on a national, regional, or local basis in terms of age, sex, and other *variables, including patterns of migration and survival. It is used in *public health medicine to help identify health needs and *risk factors. *See also* BIOSTATISTICS.

demulcent *n.* a soothing agent that protects the mucous membranes and relieves irritation. Demulcents form a protective film and are used in mouth washes, gargles, etc., to soothe irritation or inflammation in the mouth.

demyelination *n.* damage to the *myelin sheaths surrounding the nerve fibres in the central or peripheral nervous system. This in turn affects the function of the nerve fibres, which the myelin normally supports. Demyelination may be a primary disorder, as in *multiple sclerosis. There may be associated nerve-fibre damage.

denaturation *n.* the changes in the physical and physiological properties of a protein that are brought about by heat, X-rays, or chemicals. These changes include loss of activity (in the case of enzymes) and loss (or alteration) of antigenicity (in the case of *antigens).

dendrite *n.* one of the shorter branching processes of the cell body of a *neuron, which makes contact with other neurons at synapses and carries nerve impulses from them into the cell body.

dendritic cell a type of haemopoietic cell with specialized antigen-presenting functions. *See* ANTIGEN-PRESENTING CELL.

dendritic ulcer a branching ulcer of the surface of the cornea caused by *herpes simplex virus. A similar appearance may be produced by a healing corneal abrasion. Dendritic ulcers tend to recur because the virus lies dormant in the corneal sensory nerves; years may elapse between recurrences.

denervation *n.* interruption of the nerve supply to the muscles and skin. The muscle is paralysed and its normal tone (elasticity) is lost. The muscle fibres atrophy (shrink) and are replaced by fat. A denervated area of skin loses all forms of sensation and its subsequent ability to heal and renew its tissues may be impaired.

dengue (breakbone fever) *n.* a disease caused by arboviruses and transmitted to humans principally by the mosquito *Aëdes aegypti*. Symptoms, which last for a few days, include severe pains in the joints and muscles, headache, sore throat, fever, running of the eyes, and an irritating rash. These symptoms recur in a usually milder form after an interval of two or three days. Death rarely occurs, but the patient is left debilitated and requires considerable convalescence. A more severe form, **dengue haemorrhagic fever**, characterized by a breakdown of the blood-clotting mechanism with internal bleeding, can affect children. Dengue occurs throughout the tropics and subtropics. Patients are given aspirin and codeine to relieve the pain and calamine lotion is helpful in easing the irritating rash.

denominator *n.* the part of the fetus that is used to describe positions for *presentation. For vertex (back of the head) presentation, it is the *occiput; for breech presentation, the sacrum; for face presentation, the mentum (chin).

dens *n.* a tooth or tooth-shaped structure.

dense deposit disease *see* MESANGIO-CAPILLARY GLOMERULONEPHRITIS.

dens invaginatus literally, an infolded tooth: a specific type of tooth malformation that mainly affects upper lateral incisors to varying degrees.

dent- (denti-, dento-) *combining form denoting* the teeth. Example: **dentoalveolar** (relating to the teeth and associated jaw).

dental care professional any of several professionals supporting a dentist, formerly referred to as **dental auxiliaries** and **professionals complementary to dentistry**. A **dental hygienist** performs scaling and instruction in oral hygiene under the prescription of the dentist. A **dental nurse** helps the dentist at the chairside by preparing materials, passing instruments, and aspirating fluids from the patient's mouth. A **dental technician** constructs dentures, crowns, and orthodontic appliances in the laboratory for the dentist. A **clinical dental technician** provides dentures directly to patients. A **dental therapist** performs non-complex treatment under the prescription of a dentist. Dental care professionals are required to be statutorily registered in the UK.

dental caries decay and crumbling of the substance of a tooth. Dental caries is caused by the metabolism of the bacteria in *plaque attached to the surface of the tooth. Acid formed by bacterial breakdown of sugar in the diet causes demineralization of the enamel of the tooth. If no preventive measure or treatment is carried out it spreads into the dentine and progressively destroys the tooth. It is the most common cause of toothache, and once infection has spread to the pulp it may extend through the root canal into the periapical tissues to cause an *apical abscess.

Frequent intake of sugar is a major cause, and the disease is more common in young people and has a predilection for specific sites. Dental caries can be most effectively prevented by restricting the frequency of sugar intake and avoiding sweet food and drinks at bedtime. The resistance of enamel to dental caries can be increased by the application of *fluoride salts to the tooth surface from toothpastes or mouth rinses. *Fluoridation of water also makes teeth resistant to caries during the period of tooth development. Once caries has spread into the dentine, treatment usually consists of removing the decayed part of the tooth using a *drill and replacing it with a *filling.

dental chair the chair on which a patient lies for dental treatment. Electric switches change the position of the patient, and the chair is frequently attached to the *dental unit.

dental floss fine thread, usually of nylon, used to clean some surfaces of teeth. A thicker version is known as **dental tape**.

dental handpiece a piece of dental equipment (high-speed or low-speed) for holding a dental *bur or *file. It is made of corrosion-resistant materials to allow sterilization. *See* DRILL.

dental implant *see* IMPLANT.

dental nerve either of two nerves that supply the teeth; they are branches of the trigeminal nerve. The **inferior dental nerve** supplies the lower teeth and for most of its length exists as a single large bundle; thus anaesthesia of it has a widespread effect (*see* INFERIOR DENTAL BLOCK). The **superior dental nerve**, which supplies the upper teeth, breaks into separate branches at some distance from the teeth and it is possible to anaesthetize these individually with less widespread effect for the patient.

dental nurse *see* DENTAL CARE PROFESSIONAL.

dental pantomogram (DPT) a special form of tomogram (*see* TOMOGRAPHY) that provides a picture of all the teeth of both jaws on one film. Newer equipment can produce three-dimensional images of part of the jaw.

dental unit a major fixed piece of dental equipment to which are attached the dental drills, aspirator, compressed air syringe, and ultrasonic scaler. It is frequently integral with the *dental chair.

dentate *adj.* **1.** having teeth. **2.** serrated; having toothlike projections.

dentifrice *n.* a paste or powder for cleaning the teeth. *See* TOOTHPASTE.

dentine *n.* a hard tissue that forms the bulk of a tooth. The dentine of the crown is covered by enamel and that of the root by cementum. The dentine is permeated by fine tubules, which near the centre of the tooth contain cellular processes from the pulp. Exposed dentine is sensitive to touch, heat, and cold.

dentinogenesis *n.* the formation of *dentine by *odontoblasts. Although dentinogenesis continues throughout life, very little dentine is formed later than a few years after tooth eruption unless it is stimulated by caries, abrasion, or trauma. **Dentinogenesis imperfecta** is a hereditary condition in which dentine formation is disturbed; this may result in loss of overlying enamel and excessive wear of the dentine.

dentist *n.* a member of the dental profession, who in the UK must be registered with the General Dental Council.

dentistry *n.* the study, management, and treatment of diseases and conditions affecting the mouth, jaws, teeth, and their supporting tissues. Subdisciplines are: dental public health, *endodontics, oral medicine, oral surgery, *orthodontics, *paediatric dentistry, *periodontology, preventive dentistry, *prosthodontics, and restorative dentistry.

dentition *n.* the arrangement of teeth in the mouth. The **primary dentition** comprises the teeth of young children. It consists of 20 teeth, made up of incisors, canines, and molars only. The lower incisor erupts first at about 6 months of age, and all the primary teeth have usually erupted by the age of 2½ years. The lower incisors are shed first at about 7 years of age, and from this time until about 13 years old both primary and permanent teeth are present; i.e. there is a **mixed dentition**. The **permanent dentition** consists of up to 32 teeth, made up of incisors, canines, premolars, and molars. The first tooth to erupt is the first molar (at the age of 6 years) and most permanent teeth have appeared by the age of 14 years, although the third molars may not erupt until the age of 18–21 years. See illustrations overleaf.

Dent's disease a rare X-linked (*see* SEX-LINKED) recessive inherited condition usually

d

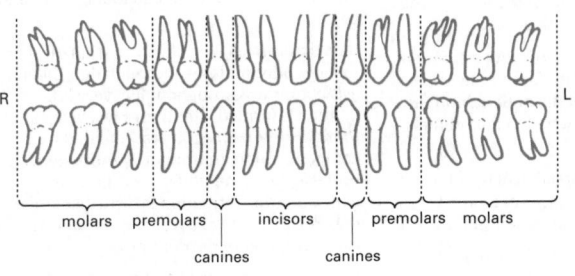

molars | incisors | molars
canines | canines

Primary dentition.

R | molars | premolars | incisors | premolars | molars | L
canines | canines

Permanent dentition.

presenting in childhood or early adult life with polyuria, microscopic haematuria, renal stone disease, or rickets. The majority of patients have a mutation of the gene encoding chloride channel 5 (*CLCN5*); others have a defect of the *OCRL1* gene, normally associated with **Lowe's syndrome**, but do not present with the cataracts, mental retardation, and tubular acidosis associated with this condition. In still others the genetic defect has yet to be defined but is not associated with either *CLCN5* or *OCRL1*. Patients with Dent's disease have evidence of proximal tubular dysfunction. [C. E. Dent (1911–76), British physician]

denture *n.* a removable replacement for one or more teeth carried on some type of plate or frame. A **complete denture** replaces all the teeth in one jaw. It is usually made entirely of acrylic resin. A **partial denture** replaces some teeth because others still remain. It is designed to restore function with the least potential damage to the remaining teeth. The framework of the denture base is often made of metal (*cobalt-chromium) because of its strength. (*See also* PROSTHESIS.) **Denture sore mouth** is inflammation of the gum under the denture, caused by a mixed infection of *Candida* and bacteria under a poorly cleaned denture or

removable orthodontic appliance. **Denture hyperplasia** is an overgrowth of fibrous tissue covered by mucous membrane, resulting from chronic irritation by a denture.

Denys-Drash syndrome a rare disorder consisting of the triad of *nephroblastoma (Wilms' tumour), congenital nephropathy, and intersex disorders, resulting from mutations in the Wilm's tumour suppressor gene (*WT1*). Incomplete forms exist; congenital nephropathy, with diffuse mesangial sclerosis, is the constant feature with either Wilms' tumour or intersex disorders, usually in the form of male *pseudohermaphroditism. [P. Denys (20th century), French physician; A. Drash (20th century), British physician]

deodorant *n.* an agent that reduces or removes unpleasant body odours by destroying bacteria that live on the skin and break down sweat. Deodorant preparations often contain an antiseptic.

deontology 1. a theoretical approach to ethical questions in which moral obligation is seen as arising from certain unvarying rules and principles, which are universal, i.e. they should be followed irrespective of consequences (*compare* CONSEQUENTIALISM). Such an approach is central to *Kantian ethics, although deontological approaches may require that moral deliberation should always include consideration of likely consequences. **2.** the branch of *ethics concerned with the nature of *duty and obligation. —**deontological** *adj.*

deoxycholic acid *see* BILE ACIDS.

deoxycorticosterone *n.* a hormone, synthesized and released by the adrenal cortex, that regulates salt and water balance. *See also* CORTICOSTEROID.

deoxyribonuclease *n.* an enzyme, located in the *lysosomes of cells, that splits DNA at specific places in the molecule.

deoxyribonucleic acid *see* DNA.

Department of Health (DH) a department of central government that supports the Secretary of State for Health in meeting his or her obligations, which include the *National Health Service, the promotion and protection of the health of the nation, and social care, including the oversight of personal social services provided by local authorities. The department is staffed by civil servants, including health professionals, based in two main offices and in public health groups in the government offices of the regions. Although mainly concerned with the NHS, the department also oversees private and voluntary provision of health services. Equivalent departments support the ministers responsible for health services in Scotland, Wales, and Northern Ireland.

(((🌐))) **SEE WEB LINKS**

• DH website: provides information on a wide range of public health issues

dependence (drug dependence) *n.* the physical and/or psychological effects produced by the habitual taking of certain drugs, characterized by a compulsion to continue taking the drug; in ICD-10 (*see* INTERNATIONAL CLASSIFICATION OF DISEASES) it is known as **drug dependency syndrome**. In **physical dependence** withdrawal of the drug causes specific symptoms (**withdrawal symptoms**), such as sweating, vomiting, or tremors, that are reversed by further doses. Substances that may induce physical dependence include alcohol and the 'hard' drugs morphine, heroin, and cocaine. Dependence on 'hard' drugs carries a high mortality, partly because overdosage may be fatal and partly because their casual injection intravenously may lead to infections such as *hepatitis and *AIDS. Treatment is

difficult and requires specialist skills. Much more common is **psychological dependence**, in which repeated use of a drug induces reliance on it for a state of wellbeing and contentment, but there are no physical withdrawal symptoms if use of the drug is stopped. Substances that may induce psychological dependence include nicotine in tobacco, cannabis, and many 'soft' drugs, such as barbiturates and amphetamines.

depersonalization *n.* a state in which a person feels himself becoming unreal or strangely altered, or feels that his mind is becoming separated from his body. Minor degrees of this feeling are common in normal people under stress. Severe feelings of depersonalization occur in anxiety neurosis, in states of *dissociation, in depression and schizophrenia, and in epilepsy (particularly temporal-lobe epilepsy). *See also* DEREALIZATION, OUT-OF-BODY EXPERIENCE.

depilatory *n.* an agent applied to the skin to remove hair.

depolarization *n.* the sudden surge of charged particles across the membrane of a nerve cell or a muscle cell that accompanies a physicochemical change in the membrane and cancels out, or reverses, its resting potential to produce an *action potential. The passage of a *nerve impulse is a rapid wave of depolarization along the membrane of a nerve fibre.

depot injection the administration of a sustained-action drug formulation that allows slow release and gradual absorption, so that the active agent can act for much longer periods than is possible with standard injections. Depot injections are usually given deep into a muscle; some contraceptive hormones are available in a depot formulation.

depressant *n.* an agent that reduces the normal activity of any body system or function. Drugs such as general *anaesthetics, *barbiturates, and opioids are depressants of the central nervous system and respiration. *Cytotoxic drugs, such as azathioprine, are depressants of the levels of white blood cells.

depression *n.* **1.** a mental state characterized by excessive sadness. **2.** a mood disorder characterized by the pervasive and persistent presence of core and somatic symptoms on most days for at least 2 weeks. Core symptoms include low mood and loss or impairment of motivation, energy, interest, and enjoyment. Somatic symptoms include impaired memory and concentration, loss of appetite and libido, insomnia, early morning wakening (more than 2 hours earlier than normal), physical and mental activity that is either agitated and restless or slow and retarded, and a diurnal variation of mood (usually patients feel particularly depressed in the mornings). Additional symptoms include automatic negative thoughts, pessimistic views of oneself, the future, and the present (**Beck's triad of depression**), suicidal *ideation, tearfulness, *alexithymia, and a poor frustration tolerance. A single period of experiencing these symptoms is called a **major depressive episode**; experiencing one or more of such episodes (without mania) is known as **major depression**, **major depressive disorder**, or **clinical depression**. Depression may or may not be triggered by stressful events or trauma. Risk factors include genetic and social elements (e.g. poverty, lack of confidants, substance abuse) and psychological elements (e.g. the presence of personality disorder, a history of abuse or *dysthymia). Treatment is with *antidepressant drugs, *cognitive behavioural therapy, and/or *psychotherapy. Severe cases may need *electroconvulsive therapy. The course of the illness can be a single episode or recurrent episodes, or it may become chronic. **~depressive** *adj.*

depressor *n.* 1. a muscle that causes lowering of part of the body. The **depressor labii inferioris** is a muscle that draws down and everts the lower lip. 2. a nerve that lowers blood pressure.

derealization *n.* a feeling of unreality in which the environment is experienced as unreal and as flat, dull, or strange. The experience is unwelcome and often frightening. It occurs in association with *depersonalization or with the conditions that cause depersonalization, for example schizophrenia, anxiety, depression, or *dissociative disorder.

derm- (**derma-, dermo-, dermat(o)-**) *combining form denoting* the skin.

-derm *combining form denoting* 1. the skin. 2. a germ layer.

Dermacentor *n.* a genus of hard *ticks, worldwide in distribution, the adults of which are parasites of humans and other mammals. The wood tick, *D. andersoni*, transmits Rocky Mountain spotted fever to humans in the western USA and the dog tick,

D. variabilis, is the vector of this disease in the east.

dermal *adj.* relating to or affecting the skin, especially the *dermis.

Dermanyssus *n.* a genus of widespread parasitic mites. The red poultry mite, *D. gallinae*, is a common parasite of wild birds in temperate regions but can also infest poultry. It occasionally attacks and takes a blood meal from humans, causing itching and mild dermatitis.

dermatitis *n.* an inflammatory condition of the skin caused by outside agents (*compare* ECZEMA, an endogenous disease in which such agents do not play a primary role). **Irritant contact dermatitis** may occur in anyone who has sufficient contact with such irritants as acids, alkalis, solvents, and (especially) detergents. It is the commonest cause of **occupational dermatitis** in hairdressers, nurses, cooks, etc. (*See also* NAPKIN RASH.) In **allergic contact dermatitis** skin changes resembling those of eczema develop as a delayed (type IV) reaction to a particular allergen, which may be present at low concentrations. Common examples include nickel dermatitis (from costume jewellery, clothing fasteners, zips, etc.) and fragrance allergy (from toiletries, deodorants, perfumes, etc.). Treatment of dermatitis depends on removing the cause, which is not always possible.
  Dermatitis herpetiformis is an uncommon very itchy rash with symmetrical blistering, especially on the knees, elbows, buttocks, and shoulders. It is associated with *gluten sensitivity and responds well to treatment with dapsone or a gluten-free diet.

Dermatobia *n.* a genus of nonbloodsucking flies inhabiting lowland woods and forests of South and Central America. The parasitic maggots of *D. hominis* can cause a serious disease of the skin in humans (*see* MYIASIS). The maggots burrow into the skin, after emerging from eggs transported by bloodsucking insects (e.g. mosquitoes), and produce painful boil-like swellings. Treatment involves surgical removal of the maggots.

dermatochalasis *n.* redundant eyelid skin, which may cause drooping of the upper lid. It usually occurs as a result of ageing. *Compare* BLEPHAROCHALASIS.

dermatofibrosarcoma protuberans a tumour probably derived from *histiocytes that may occur in any part of the body. It is locally invasive but tends not to metastasize. It often recurs locally despite excision.

dermatoglyphics *n.* **1.** the patterns of finger, palm, toe, and sole prints. These patterns are formed by skin ridges, the distribution of which is unique to each individual. Abnormalities are found in those with chromosomal variants, such as *Down's syndrome. **2.** the study of these patterns. In addition to its use in medicine, dermatoglyphics is also of value in criminology and is of interest to anthropologists. *See also* FINGERPRINT.

dermatology *n.* the medical specialty concerned with the diagnosis and treatment of skin disorders. —**dermatological** *adj.* —**dermatologist** *n.*

dermatome *n.* **1.** a surgical instrument used for cutting thin slices of skin in some skin grafting operations. **2.** that part of the segmented mesoderm in the early embryo that forms the deeper layers of the skin (dermis) and associated tissues. *See* SOMITE.

dermatomyositis *n.* an inflammatory disorder of the skin and underlying tissues, including the muscles (in the absence of a rash it is known as *polymyositis). The condition is one of the *connective-tissue diseases. A pink/purple skin eruption occurs on the face, scalp, neck, shoulders, and knuckles (known as **Gottron's papules**) and is later accompanied by severe swelling. Dermatomyositis is often associated with internal cancer in adults, though not in children.

Dermatophagoides *n.* a genus of *mites that have been detected in samples of dust taken from houses in various parts of Europe. House-dust mites feed on human skin and scales and cause dermatitis of the scalp. Waste products from the mites produce an allergic response in susceptible people that is an important trigger for some forms of *rhinitis and *asthma.

dermatophyte *n.* a fungus belonging to any one of the three genera (*Microsporum*, *Trichophyton*, and *Epidermophyton*) that can feed on *keratin and cause various forms of *ringworm (tinea); these infections may be referred to as **dermatophytoses**.

dermatosis *n.* any disease of skin, particularly one without inflammation. In **juvenile plantar dermatosis**, which affects children up to the age of 14, the skin on the front of

the sole becomes red, glazed, and symmetrically cracked. This condition, which settles spontaneously after a number of years, is believed to be related to the wearing of trainers.

dermis (corium) *n.* the true *skin: the thick layer of living tissue that lies beneath the epidermis. It consists mainly of loose connective tissue within which are blood capillaries, lymph vessels, sensory nerve endings, sweat glands and their ducts, hair follicles, sebaceous glands, and smooth muscle fibres. —**dermal** *adj.*

dermographism *n.* a common local reaction caused by stroking the skin, which develops itchy *weals. People with such highly sensitive skin can 'write' on it with a finger or blunt instrument. A rare delayed form exists. Dermographism can be confirmed with a calibrated instrument called a **dermographometer**. Antihistamines are first-line treatment.

dermoid cyst (dermoid) a benign tumour – a type of *teratoma – containing developmentally mature skin complete with hair follicles and sebaceous glands, and often pockets of sebum, blood, fat, bone, nails, teeth, eyes, cartilage, and thyroid tissue, which may give rise to symptoms of thyrotoxicosis. It is usually found at sites marking the fusion of developing sections of the body in the embryo and is the most common benign ovarian tumour in girls and young women. Sometimes a dermoid cyst may develop after an injury. Treatment is complete surgical removal, preferably in one piece and without any spillage of cyst contents. Tumours in the skin are best removed by a plastic surgeon. Because of the risks of surgery and anaesthesia to pregnant women, it is usually considered more feasible to remove bilateral dermoid cysts of the ovaries discovered during pregnancy only if they grow beyond 6 cm in diameter. The procedure is usually performed through laparotomy or very carefully through laparoscopy and should preferably be done in the second trimester.

descemetocele *n.* thinning of the *stroma of the cornea to such an extent that *Descemet's membrane is all that is maintaining the integrity of the eyeball. It occurs in severe ulceration of the cornea.

Descemet's membrane the membrane that forms the deepest layer of the *stroma of the cornea of the eye. The endothelium lies between it and the aqueous humour. [J. Descemet (1732–1810), French anatomist]

desensitization *n.* **1.** (**hyposensitization**) a method for reducing the effects of a known allergen by injecting, over a period, gradually increasing doses of the allergen, until resistance is built up. *See* ALLERGY. **2.** a technique used in the *behaviour therapy of phobic states. The thing that is feared is very gradually introduced to the patient, first in imagination and then in reality. At the same time the patient is taught relaxation to inhibit the development of anxiety (*see* RELAXATION THERAPY). In this way he is able to cope with progressively closer approximations to the feared object or situation.

desert *n.* the state of deserving something. In medical ethics it is controversial to argue that some patients may be more deserving of treatment than others on the basis of their past or present conduct. *See also* NEED.

desferrioxamine *n.* a drug that combines with iron in body tissues and fluids and is used to treat iron poisoning, iron overload (including that resulting from prolonged or constant blood transfusion, as for thalassaemia), diseases involving iron storage in parts of the body (*see* HAEMOCHROMATOSIS), and for the diagnosis of such diseases. It is administered by subcutaneous infusion; reactions and pain sometimes occur. Trade name: **Desferal**.

designer drug a psychoactive drug produced by minor chemical modification of existing illegal substances so as to circumvent prohibitive legislation. These drugs are manufactured in secret laboratories for profit, without regard to any probable medical and social dangers to the consumers.

desmoid tumour a dense connective-tissue tumour with a dangerous propensity for repeated local recurrence after treatment. Intra-abdominal desmoids have an association with familial adenomatous *polyposis (FAP).

desmoplasia *n.* **1.** the proliferation of *fibroblasts to produce a fibrous *stroma in response to a malignant tumour. It is a feature of the more aggressive tumours. **2.** the formation of fibrous *adhesions. —**desmoplastic** *adj.*

desmopressin *n.* a synthetic derivative of *vasopressin that causes a decrease in urine output and is used to treat diabetes insipidus and nocturnal *enuresis. It is also effective in mild haemophilia and von Willebrand's disease. Side-effects include stomach cramps, headache, and flushing of the skin. It is taken orally, sublingually, intranasally, or by injection. Trade names: **DDAVP**, **DesmoMelt**, **Desmotabs**, **Desmospray**, **Octim**.

desmosome *n.* an area of contact between two adjacent cells, occurring particularly in epithelia. The cell membranes at a desmosome are thickened and fine fibres (**tonofibrils**) extend from the desmosome into the cytoplasm.

desogestrel *n.* a *progestogen used in various *oral contraceptives, either alone (**Cerazette**) or in combination with ethinylestradiol (**Marvelon**, **Mercilon**).

desquamation *n.* the process in which the outer layer of the *epidermis of the skin is removed by scaling.

detached retina *see* RETINAL DETACHMENT.

detergent *n.* a synthetic cleansing agent that removes all impurities from a surface by reacting with grease and suspended particles, including bacteria and other microorganisms. Detergents are used for cleansing or as *antiseptics and *disinfectants.

detoxication (**detoxification**) *n.* **1.** the process whereby toxic substances are removed or toxic effects neutralized. It is one of the functions of the liver. **2.** the period of withdrawal when a person stops long-term consumption of alcohol or some other drug. Withdrawal symptoms (e.g. *delirium tremens) may occur during detoxication.

detrition *n.* the process of wearing away solid bodies (e.g. bones) by friction or use.

detrusor *n.* the muscle of the urinary bladder wall. The functioning of the detrusor and urethral sphincter is assessed by a urodynamic investigation (*see* URODYNAMICS). This is used to diagnose dysfunction, absent and exaggerated reflexes, and overactivity of the muscle. Neurogenic detrusor overactivity is due to neurological damage, as occurs in multiple sclerosis.

detumescence *n.* **1.** the reverse of erection, whereby the erect penis or clitoris becomes flaccid after orgasm. **2.** subsidence of a swelling.

deut- (deuto-, deuter(o-)) *combining form denoting* two, second, or secondary.

deuteranopia *n.* a defect in colour vision in which reds, yellows, and greens are confused. It is thought that the mechanisms for perceiving red light and green light are in some way combined in people with this defect. *Compare* PROTANOPIA, TRITANOPIA. *See also* COLOUR BLINDNESS.

deutoplasm *n. see* YOLK.

developmental delay considerable delay in the physical or mental development of children when compared with their peers. There are many causes. **Global delay** describes the state of a child whose overall development is slow in all areas.

developmental disorder any one of a group of conditions in infancy or childhood, that are characterized by delays in biologically determined psychological functions, such as language. They are more common in males than females and tend to follow a course of handicap with gradual improvement. They are classified into **pervasive** conditions, in which many types of development are involved (e.g. *autism), and **specific** disorders, in which the handicap is an isolated problem (such as *dyslexia).

developmental milestones skills gained by a developing child, which should be achieved by a given age. Examples of such milestones include smiling by six weeks and sitting unsupported by six months. Failure to achieve a particular milestone by a given age is indicative of *developmental delay. See table overleaf.

deviance *n.* variation from normal behaviour beyond the limits acceptable to the majority of the conforming peer group; particularly (though not exclusively) applied to sexual habits (*see also* SEXUAL DEVIATION).

deviation *n.* **1.** (in ophthalmology) any abnormal position of one or both eyes. For example, if the eyes are both looking to one side when the head is facing forwards, they are said to be **deviated** to that side. Such deviations of both eyes may occur in brain disease. Deviations of one eye, such as *dissociated vertical deviation, come into the category of squint (*see* STRABISMUS). **2.** *see* SEXUAL DEVIATION.

Devic's disease *see* NEUROMYELITIS OPTICA. [E. Devic (1869–1930), French physician]

devitalization *n.* (in dentistry) removal of a diseased pulp from a tooth. In primary teeth the coronal pulp alone may be removed, while the pulp in the root is kept alive or root canal treatment undertaken. For permanent teeth, *see* ROOT CANAL TREATMENT.

dew-point hygrometer *see* HYGROMETER.

DEXA (dual-energy X-ray absorptiometry) a method of measuring bone density based on the proportion of a beam of photons that passes through the bone. The results of a DEXA scan are expressed as a *T score. *See also* OSTEOPOROSIS.

dexamethasone *n.* a *corticosteroid drug used principally to treat severe allergies, eye inflammation, rheumatic and other inflammatory conditions, and congenital adrenal hyperplasia. It is administered by mouth, by injection into a joint, or as eye drops; side-effects include sodium and fluid retention, muscle weakness, convulsions, vertigo, headache, and hormonal disturbances (including menstrual irregularities). Dexamethasone is also used in a series of tests for Cushing's syndrome (*see* DEXAMETHASONE SUPPRESSION TESTS). Trade names: **Maxidex**, **Minims Dexamethasone**.

dexamethasone suppression tests (DSTs) tests based on the principle that appropriate doses of *dexamethasone can suppress the output of cortisol from the adrenal glands in the normal state and that this ability is reduced or lost in *Cushing's syndrome. In the **overnight DST** 1 mg of dexamethasone is administered at midnight and the serum cortisol level is measured at 9.00 am the next morning. Failure to suppress cortisol output may indicate Cushing's syndrome but also occurs in patients with obesity and depressive illness. In the **low-dose DST** (0.5 mg dexamethasone every 6 hours for 48 hours), cortisol suppression occurs in patients with obesity and depression but not in those with Cushing's syndrome. In the **high-dose DST** (2 mg dexamethasone every 6 hours for 48 hours), cortisol is suppressed in patients with Cushing's disease (in which excess amounts of ACTH are secreted by the pituitary gland) but not in those with Cushing's syndrome due to other causes. Although the low- and high-dose tests are unreliable, all three tests should be performed to aid the diagnosis of Cushing's syndrome.

Developmental milestones.

	6 weeks Supine infant	6–9 months Sitting infant	1 year Standing/walking infant	18–24 months Mobile toddler	3–4 years Communicating child
Gross motor	Symmetrical movements of all limbs When prone raises head	Supports head Sits unaided (6 m) Stands holding on (7 m) Pulls to standing (9 m)	Walks holding onto furniture (9 m) Walks if led A few steps unsupported (12 m)	Walks with normal gait Climbs steps Kicks ball (20 m)	Hops on one foot
Fine motor/vision	Fixes and follows gaze	Reaches for objects Palmar grasp Transfers objects hand to hand Bangs toys together	Pincer grip (10 m)	Scribbles (14 m) Builds tower of six blocks (24 m)	Copies circle (3 y) Copies square (4 y) Builds bridge or steps with blocks when shown
Language/hearing	Normal cry Responds to sounds	Turns to a voice (7 m) Nonspecific babble (10 m) Turns to own name	Understands simple commands: 'No' Says a few words appropriately: 'Mama' 'Dada' (13 m) Turns to own name	Combines two different words (20 m) Points to one named body part	Gives first and last name Recognizes colours (3 y) Speech fully comprehensible (4 y)
Social	Regards face Smiles responsively	Puts solid food in mouth (6 m) Waves goodbye (8 m)	Drinks from cup (12 m) Wary of strangers	Feeds self with spoon Removes clothing Asserts own wishes Symbolic play with miniature toys	Washes hands with help Eats with knife and fork Make-believe play Shows sympathy appropriately Likes hearing and telling stories

(Median ages of achievement of each skill in brackets)

dexamfetamine (dexamphetamine) *n.* *see* AMPHETAMINES.

dextr- (dextro-) *combining form denoting* 1. the right side. Example: **dextroposition** (displacement to the right). 2. (in chemistry) dextrorotation.

dextran *n.* a carbohydrate, consisting of branched chains of glucose units, that is a storage product of bacteria and yeasts. Preparations of dextran solution are used in transfusions, to increase the volume of plasma.

dextrin *n.* a carbohydrate formed as an intermediate product in the digestion of starch by the enzyme amylase. Dextrin is used in the preparation of pharmaceutical products (as an *excipient) and surgical dressings.

dextrocardia *n.* a congenital defect in which the position of the heart is a mirror image of its normal position, with the apex of the ventricles pointing to the right. It may be associated with other congenital defects and is often combined with **situs invertus**, in which the appendix and liver lie on the left side of the abdomen and the stomach lies on the right side. Isolated dextrocardia produces no adverse effects.

dextrose *n.* *see* GLUCOSE.

DHEA *see* DEHYDROEPIANDROSTERONE.

DI *see* ARTIFICIAL INSEMINATION.

di- *prefix denoting* two or double.

dia- *prefix denoting* 1. through. 2. completely or throughout. 3. apart.

diabetes *n.* any disorder of metabolism causing excessive thirst and the production of large volumes of urine. Used alone, the term most commonly refers to *diabetes mellitus. *See also* DIABETES INSIPIDUS, HAEMOCHROMATOSIS (BRONZE DIABETES). —**diabetic** *adj., n.*

diabetes insipidus a rare metabolic disorder in which the patient produces large quantities of dilute urine and is constantly thirsty. It is due to deficiency of the pituitary hormone *vasopressin (antidiuretic hormone), which regulates reabsorption of water in the kidneys, and is treated by administration of the hormone. *See also* WATER-DEPRIVATION TEST.

diabetes mellitus a disorder of carbohydrate metabolism in which sugars in the body are not oxidized to produce energy due to lack of the pancreatic hormone *insulin. The accumulation of sugar leads to its appearance in the blood (**hyperglycaemia**), then in the urine; symptoms include thirst, loss of weight, and the excessive production of urine. The use of fats as an alternative source of energy leads to disturbances of the *acid-base balance, the accumulation of ketones in the bloodstream (*ketosis), and eventually to **diabetic coma**. There appears to be an inherited tendency to diabetes; the disorder may be triggered by various factors, including physical stress.

Diabetes that starts in childhood or adolescence is usually more severe than that beginning in middle or old age. It is known as **type 1** (or **insulin-dependent) diabetes mellitus** as patients have little or no ability to produce the hormone and are entirely dependent on insulin injections for survival. In **type 2** (**noninsulin-dependent** or **maturity-onset) diabetes mellitus**, which usually occurs after the age of 40 but can develop in young people (*see* MATURITY-ONSET DIABETES OF THE YOUNG), the pancreas retains some ability to produce insulin but this is inadequate for the body's needs; alternatively, the body becomes resistant to the effects of insulin. Patients may require treatment with *oral hypoglycaemic drugs or insulin. *Gestational diabetes develops during pregnancy. In all types of diabetes the diet must be carefully controlled, with adequate carbohydrate for the body's needs. Lack of balance in the diet or in the amount of insulin taken leads to *hypoglycaemia. Long-term complications of diabetes include damage to blood vessels, which can affect the eyes (diabetic *retinopathy), kidneys (*diabetic nephropathy), and nerves (*diabetic neuropathy).

Diabetes UK the main British support charity for patients with diabetes and workers in the diabetes field.

(((🌐))) SEE WEB LINKS

- Website of Diabetes UK: provides information on living with type 1 and type 2 diabetes (including recipes)

diabetic amyotrophy an acute mononeuropathy of the femoral nerve, usually of microvascular origin, associated with chronic poor diabetic control. Symptoms are thigh pain and progressive weakness of knee extension. Examination reveals wasting of the quadriceps muscle group and loss of the knee jerk. It may affect both legs and recovery is usually slow. Treatment is with physiotherapy and improved control of the diabetes; the condition never seems to recur in the same leg. The main *differential diagnosis is of compression of the nerve roots in the spinal canal.

diabetic glomerulosclerosis the characteristic microscopic changes seen in a diabetic kidney after many years of progressive damage.

diabetic hand syndrome the combination of features, often found in the hands of long-standing diabetic subjects, consisting of *Dupuytren's contractures, knuckle pads, *carpal tunnel syndrome, *cheiroarthropathy, and sclerosing *tenosynovitis.

diabetic holiday foot syndrome a condition in which patients with diabetic sensory polyneuropathy (see DIABETIC NEUROPATHY) suffer significant trauma to their insensate feet through holiday activities. These may include walking on hot flagstones or sand and wearing ill-fitting shoes. The condition may be prevented with prior education and advice and by maintaining safe footcare practices.

diabetic honeymoon period a well-recognized period just after the diagnosis of type 1 *diabetes mellitus when only very low insulin doses are required to control the condition. It lasts from months to a few years but inevitably ends, when dose requirements will increase quite quickly.

diabetic ketoacidosis (DKA) a metabolic state resulting from a profound lack of insulin, usually found only in type 1 *diabetes mellitus. Inability to inhibit glucose production from the liver results in *hyperglycaemia, which can be extreme and lead to severe dehydration. The concurrent failure to suppress fatty-acid production from adipose tissue results in the excess conversion of fatty acids to ketones in the liver (*ketosis) and the development of a metabolic *acidosis, which can be severe. Patients often present with vomiting (from the ketosis), which contributes to the dehydration. The condition is treated as a medical emergency with intravenous fluid and insulin; patients should be monitored in high-dependency units.

diabetic nephropathy progressive damage to the kidneys seen in some people with long-standing diabetes. Excessive leakage of protein into the urine is followed by gradual decline of the kidney function and even kidney failure. *See also* DIABETIC GLOMERULOSCLEROSIS.

diabetic neuropathy progressive damage to the nerves seen in some people with long-standing diabetes. It most commonly affects the legs, causing pain or numbness working up from the feet. There is no cure but drugs can sometimes be used to control the discomfort experienced, and good diabetic control may prevent worsening. *See also* DIABETIC HOLIDAY FOOT SYNDROME.

diabetic retinopathy *see* RETINOPATHY.

diabetologist *n.* a doctor who specializes in the diagnosis and treatment of *diabetes mellitus and the prevention of its long-term complications. In the UK most diabetologists are also endocrinologists.

diaclast *n.* a surgical instrument used for the destruction of the skull of a fetus. This rare procedure enables a dead fetus to be delivered through the birth canal (see DECAPITATION).

diagnosis *n.* the process of determining the nature of a disorder by considering the patient's *signs and *symptoms, medical background, and – when necessary – results of laboratory tests and X-ray examinations. Unlike therapeutic procedures, diagnostic processes usually do not directly benefit the patient in terms of treatment. *See also* DIFFERENTIAL DIAGNOSIS, PRENATAL DIAGNOSIS. *Compare* PROGNOSIS. —**diagnostic** *adj.*

Diagnostic and Statistical Manual of Mental Disorders *see* DSM.

diagnostic peritoneal lavage the instillation of saline directly into the abdominal cavity and its subsequent aspiration a few minutes later. If the fluid is bloodstained on recovery an intra-abdominal haemorrhage is indicated. This is a useful diagnostic tool in trauma patients.

diakinesis *n.* the final stage in the first prophase of *meiosis, in which homologous chromosomes, between which crossing over has occurred, are ready to separate.

dialysate *n.* fluid used in the dialysis process. In *haemodialysis the dialysate is purified tap water to which has been added a precise amount of electrolyte solution. In *peritoneal dialysis the dialysate is a commercially produced fluid containing electrolytes with glucose, glucose polymers, or amino acids.

dialyser (dialyzer) *n.* a medical device designed to allow controllable transfer of solutes and water across a semipermeable membrane separating blood and *dialysate solutions flowing countercurrent to each other. Most modern dialysers are based on hollow-fibre technology and are tube-shaped. Blood enters the top of the tube and travels, by capillary action, down a large number of hollow microfibres, which are embedded in polyurethane at each end of the dialyser tube for support. Dialysate enters the tube from the side, near the bottom of the tube. It runs in the opposite direction to the blood, around the hollow fibres and separated from the blood by the semipermeable membrane that constitutes the microfibre wall. A number of different dialyser membranes are in use, displaying a wide variety of permeabilities (related to pore size), biocompatibilities (not activating *cytokine or alternate pathway *complement responses in the blood), and costs.

dialysis *n.* a method of separating particles of different dimensions in a liquid mixture, using a thin semipermeable membrane whose pores are too small to allow the passage of large particles, such as proteins, but large enough to permit the passage of dissolved crystalline material. A solution of the mixture is separated from distilled water by the membrane; the solutes pass through the membrane into the water while the proteins, etc., are retained. The principle of dialysis is used in the *dialyser (*see also* HAEMODIALYSIS). The peritoneum is used as an autogenous semipermeable membrane in the technique of *peritoneal dialysis.

diamorphine *n.* the chemical name for heroin: a powerful opioid analgesic (*see* OPIATE) that is administered orally or by injection for the relief of acute and chronic pain, especially in terminal illness, and pulmonary oedema.

Dianette *n. see* CYPROTERONE.

diapedesis *n.* migration of cells through the walls of blood capillaries into the tissue spaces. Diapedesis is an important part of the reaction of tissues to injury (*see* INFLAMMATION).

diaphoresis *n.* the process of sweating, especially excessive sweating. *See* SWEAT.

diaphoretic (sudorific) *n.* a drug that causes an increase in sweating. *Antipyretic

drugs have diaphoretic activity, which helps reduce the body temperature in fevers.

diaphragm *n.* **1.** (in anatomy) a thin musculomembranous dome-shaped muscle that separates the thoracic and abdominal cavities. The diaphragm is attached to the lower ribs at each side and to the breastbone and the backbone at the front and back. It bulges upwards against the heart and the lungs, arching over the stomach, liver, and spleen. There are openings in the diaphragm through which the oesophagus, blood vessels, and nerves pass. The diaphragm plays an important role in *breathing. It contracts with each inspiration, becoming flattened downwards and increasing the volume of the thoracic cavity. With each expiration it relaxes and is restored to its dome shape. **2.** a hemispherical rubber cap fitted inside the vagina over the neck (cervix) of the uterus as a contraceptive. When combined with the use of a chemical spermicide the diaphragm provides reliable contraception with a failure rate as low as 2–10 pregnancies per 100 woman-years.

diaphyseal aclasia *see* EXOSTOSIS.

diaphysis *n.* the body, or shaft, of a long bone, which ossifies from a primary centre. It comprises a thick cylinder of compact bone surrounding a large medullary cavity. *Compare* EPIPHYSIS, PHYSIS. —**diaphyseal** *adj.*

diaphysitis *n.* inflammation of the diaphysis (shaft) of a bone, through infection or rheumatic disease. It may result in impaired growth of the bone and consequent deformity.

diarrhoea *n.* frequent bowel evacuation or the passage of abnormally soft or liquid faeces. It may be caused by intestinal infections, other forms of intestinal inflammation (such as *colitis or *Crohn's disease), *malabsorption, anxiety, and the *irritable bowel syndrome. Severe or prolonged diarrhoea may lead to excess losses of fluid, salts, and nutrients in the faeces.

diarthrosis (synovial joint) *n.* a freely movable joint. The ends of the adjoining bones are covered with a thin cartilaginous sheet, and the bones are linked by a ligament (**capsule**) lined with *synovial membrane, which secretes synovial fluid (see illustration overleaf). Such joints are classified according to the type of connection between the bones and the type of movement allowed. *See*

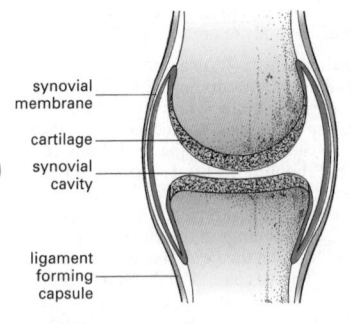

synovial
membrane

cartilage

synovial
cavity

ligament
forming
capsule

A diarthrosis.

ARTHRODIC JOINT, CONDYLARTHROSIS,
ENARTHROSIS, GINGLYMUS, SADDLE JOINT, TRO-
CHOID JOINT.

diaschisis *n.* a temporary loss of reflex activity in the brainstem or spinal cord following destruction of the cerebral cortex. As
time passes this state of suppressed reflex
activity is replaced by one of unduly exaggerated reflexes and spasticity of the limbs.

diastase *n.* an enzyme that hydrolyses
starch in barley grain to produce maltose
during the malting process. It has been used
to aid the digestion of starch in some digestive disorders.

diastema *n.* a space between two teeth.

diastole *n.* the period between two contractions of the heart, when the muscle of
the heart relaxes and allows the chambers to
fill with blood. The term usually refers to
ventricular diastole, which lasts about 0.5
seconds in a normal heart rate of about
70/minute. During exertion this period
shortens, so allowing the heart rate to increase. *See also* BLOOD PRESSURE, SYSTOLE.
—**diastolic** *adj.*

diastolic dysfunction impairment of
heart function due to increased stiffness of
the left *ventricle, which results in reduced
capacity of the heart to fill with blood during
diastole. *Compare* SYSTOLIC DYSFUNCTION.

diastolic pressure *see* BLOOD PRESSURE.

diathermy *n.* the production of heat
in a part of the body by means of a high-
frequency electric current passed between
two electrodes placed on the patient's skin.
The principle of diathermy is also utilized in
various surgical instruments to coagulate

tissues and seal off blood vessels, thus effecting *haemostasis. Examples include
diathermy knives, **forceps**, and **scissors**.
Diathermy snares and **needles** can be used
to destroy unwanted tissue and to remove
small superficial neoplasms. In **bipolar
diathermy** electric current passes between
the two electrodes of the instrument. In
monopolar diathermy the instrument is one
electrode, the other being a large pad applied to another part of the patient's body.
See also ELECTROSURGERY.

diathesis *n.* a higher than average tendency to acquire certain diseases, such as allergies, rheumatic diseases, or gout. Such
diseases may run in families, but they are
not inherited.

diazepam *n.* a long-acting *benzodiazepine used for the short-term relief of
acute anxiety and insomnia and in the treatment of delirium tremens, status epilepticus,
and febrile convulsions; it is also used as a
*premedication. Diazepam is administered
by mouth, injection, or rectally and can
cause dependence; side-effects include
drowsiness and lethargy, confusion, and
muscle weakness.

diazoxide *n.* a *vasodilator used to lower
blood pressure in the emergency treatment
of patients with hypertension (as in kidney
disease); it is administered by intravenous
injection, usually in combination with other
antihypertensive drugs. Diazoxide is also
given by mouth to treat conditions in which
the levels of blood sugar are chronically low
(including *insulinoma). Trade name: **Eu-
demine**.

DIC *see* DISSEMINATED INTRAVASCULAR COAGU-
LATION.

dicephalus *n. see* CRANIOPAGUS.

dichorionicity *n. see* CHORIONICITY, TWINS.
—**dichorionic** *adj.*

dichromatic *adj.* describing the state of
colour vision of those who can appreciate
only two of the three primary colours. People
with such vision match any given colour by a
mixture of the two they can distinguish.
Compare TRICHROMATIC.

Dick test an obsolete immunological test
for susceptibility to *scarlet fever. [G. F. Dick
(1881–1967) and G. R. H. Dick (1881–1963),
US physicians]

diclofenac *n.* an anti-inflammatory drug

(*see* NSAID) used to relieve joint pain in osteoarthritis, rheumatoid arthritis, ankylosing spondylitis, and acute gout and also for pain relief after surgery. It is administered by mouth, injection, or in suppositories; possible side-effects include abdominal pain, nausea, and diarrhoea; gastric ulceration can be prevented by administering diclofenac in combination with *misoprostol (as **Arthrotec**). Trade names: **Dyloject**, **Motifene**, **Voltarol**, etc.

dicophane *n. see* DDT.

dicrotism *n.* a condition in which the pulse is felt as a double beat for each contraction of the heart. It may be seen in typhoid fever. —**dicrotic** *adj.*

dicycloverine (dicyclomine) *n.* an *antimuscarinic drug that reduces spasms of smooth muscle and is used as an *antispasmodic to relieve irritable bowel syndrome and related conditions. It is administered by mouth; side-effects include dry mouth, thirst, and dizziness. Trade name: **Merbentyl**.

didanosine (ddI) *n.* an antiretroviral drug that interferes with the action of the enzyme *reverse transcriptase, by means of which HIV, the cause of AIDS, is able to incorporate itself into the human host cell. The drug is administered by mouth, in combination with other antiretroviral drugs, to treat HIV infection and AIDS. Possible side-effects include damage to nerves, severe pancreatitis, nausea, vomiting, and headache. Trade name: **Videx**.

DIDMOAD syndrome *see* WOLFRAM SYNDROME.

didym- (didymo-) *combining form denoting* the testis.

dieldrin *n.* an insecticide that attacks the central nervous system of insects and has proved useful in the control of various beetles, flies, and larvae that attack crops. Because of its persistence in and contamination of the environment, its use in the UK is now severely restricted.

diencephalon *n.* an anatomical division of the forebrain, consisting of the epithalamus, thalamus (dorsal thalamus), hypothalamus, and ventral thalamus (subthalamus). *See* BRAIN.

diet *n.* the mixture of foods that a person eats. A **balanced diet** contains the correct proportions of all the nutrients, i.e. vitamins, minerals (calcium, phosphorus, potassium, sodium, chlorine, sulphur, magnesium, and the *trace elements), and *dietary fibre, as well as water, carbohydrates and fats (which provide energy), and proteins (required for growth and maintenance).

dietary fibre (roughage) the part of food that cannot be digested and absorbed to produce energy. Dietary fibre falls into four groups: **cellulose**, **hemicelluloses**, **lignins**, and **pectins**. Highly refined foods, such as sucrose, contain no dietary fibre. Foods with a high fibre content include wholemeal cereals and flour, root vegetables, nuts, and fruit. Dietary fibre is considered by some to be helpful in the prevention of many of the diseases of Western civilization, such as *diverticulosis, constipation, appendicitis, obesity, and diabetes mellitus.

dietetics *n.* the application of the principles of *nutrition to the selection of food and the feeding of individuals and groups.

diethylcarbamazine *n.* an anthelmintic drug that destroys filariae and is therefore used in the treatment of filariasis and loiasis. It is administered as tablets. Side-effects may include headache, malaise, joint pains, nausea, and vomiting.

diethylstilbestrol (DES) *n.* a synthetic female sex hormone (*see* OESTROGEN) that was prescribed in the 1950s and 1960s to prevent miscarriage. It was subsequently found to increase the risk of cancers of the uterus, ovary, and breast, particularly the risk of *clear-cell carcinoma of the genital tract in the daughters of patients who were treated with it. Although licensed to treat breast cancer in postmenopausal women and prostate cancer, DES is rarely used because of its toxicity.

Dietl's crisis acute obstruction of a kidney causing severe pain in the loins. The obstruction usually occurs at the junction of the renal pelvis and the ureter, causing the kidney to become distended with accumulated urine (*see* HYDRONEPHROSIS). Sometimes the pelvis drains spontaneously, with relief of pain, but acute decompression of the kidney may be required with surgical relief of the obstruction (*pyeloplasty). [J. Dietl (1804–78), Polish physician]

Dieulafoy's lesion an abnormality of small blood vessels (microscopically, an arteriovenous malformation), identified most often in the mucosal lining of the upper stomach, that may cause severe spontaneous haemorrhage. It can rarely be found in the duodenum, colon, jejunum, or oesophagus. If detected endoscopically, curative therapy is often possible, although the abnormality is often difficult to see at gastroscopy. Surgical exploration may also be required if the bleeding is unresponsive to endoscopic treatment. [G. Dieulafoy (1839–1911), French physician]

differential diagnosis *diagnosis of a condition whose signs and/or symptoms are shared by various other conditions. For example, abdominal pain may be due to any of a large number of different disorders, most of which must be ruled out in arriving at a correct diagnosis.

differential leucocyte count (differential blood count) a determination of the proportions of the different kinds of white cells (leucocytes) present in a sample of blood. Usually 100 white cells are counted and classified under the microscope or by electronic apparatus, so that the results can readily be expressed as percentages of the total number of leucocytes and the absolute numbers per litre of blood. The information often aids diagnosis of disease.

differentiation *n.* 1. (in embryology) the process in embryonic development during which unspecialized cells or tissues become specialized for particular functions. 2. (in oncology) the degree of similarity of tumour cells to the structure of the organ from which the tumour arose. Tumours are classified as well, moderately, or poorly differentiated: well-differentiated tumours appear similar to the cells of the organ in which they arose; poorly differentiated tumours do not. Such classification is often of prognostic significance and determines the *grade of the tumour. Well-differentiated tumours are low-grade; poorly differentiated tumours are high-grade.

diffusion tensor imaging a variant of *diffusion weighted imaging in which both the direction and the amount of diffusion of water molecules in a tissue are coded in the image. This can be valuable in linear structures, such as nerves and muscle fibres. In the brain the major tracts and their communications can be studied with this technique (*see* TRACTOGRAPHY).

diffusion weighted imaging a method

of creating images by *magnetic resonance imaging that relies on the amount of available space that individual water molecules have to move in, which depends on the local microstructure. Pathological tissues generally are less organized, with more space for diffusion and a higher signal.

di George syndrome a hereditary condition resulting in an inability to fight infections (immunodeficiency) associated with absence of the parathyroid gland and the thymus, abnormalities of the heart, and low calcium levels. Affected children are prone to *Candida infections and often present with *failure to thrive. The condition has also been named **CATCH-22**: *C*ardiac abnormalities, *A*bnormal facies, *T*-cell deficiency (from absent thymus), *C*left palate, *H*ypocalcaemia, chromosome *22* (in which the defect lies). [A. M. di George (1921–), US paediatrician]

digestion *n.* the process in which ingested food is broken down in the alimentary canal into a form that can be absorbed and assimilated by the tissues of the body. Digestion includes mechanical processes, such as chewing, churning, and grinding food, as well as the chemical action of digestive enzymes and other substances (bile, acid, etc.). Chemical digestion begins in the mouth with the action of *saliva on food, but most of it takes place in the stomach and small intestine, where the food is subjected to *gastric juice, *pancreatic juice, and *succus entericus.

digit *n.* any one of the terminal divisions of a limb: a finger or toe.

digital *adj.* 1. (in anatomy) relating to a digit. 2. (in radiology) relating to or utilizing *digitization.

digital hearing aid *see* HEARING AID.

digital image an image made up of *pixels. Each pixel has numbers (digits) to describe its position and shade on the *grey scale. The more shades available, described by the number of computer bits required to store the shade of grey, the more accurately the image represents the original tissue contrast. An 8-bit computer image shows 2^8 (256) possible shades of grey, close to the maximum the human eye can differentiate. 12-bit (4096 levels of grey) images are of much higher quality and take up more memory. They can be manipulated more easily by computer using image enhancement techniques. *Compare* ANALOGUE IMAGE.

digitalis *n.* an extract from the dried leaves of foxgloves (*Digitalis* species), which contains various substances, including the *glycosides digitoxin and *digoxin (known as **cardiac glycosides**), which stimulate heart muscle and are used medicinally.

digitalization *n.* the administration of a derivative of *digitalis to a patient with heart failure until the optimum level has been reached in the heart tissues. At this stage the control of heart failure should be adequate and there should be few side-effects. The process of digitalization may take several days.

digital radiography (DR) an alternative to film radiography, by acquiring X-ray images from a large number of individual X-ray detectors on a matrix in a digital format directly. This contrasts with *computerized radiography, in which an *analogue image is taken and then put into a reader to be converted into a *digital image. The technique allows the storage of images and their subsequent retrieval, manipulation, and interpretation using computers (*see* PACS).

digital spot imaging (DSI) the production of static images using an *image intensifier and a digital camera, usually during a fluoroscopic examination. The images produced can be stored digitally (*see* DIGITIZATION) and either transferred to photographic film or viewed on a TV monitor.

digital subtraction a radiological technique that enhances X-ray images, most commonly of blood vessels (*see* ANGIOGRAPHY). A digitized image is taken before the contrast medium (a 'mask') is added, and this is subtracted by computer from the images taken after contrast injection. Only the outline of the blood vessel or other structure containing contrast medium remains on the image. The technique enables blood-vessel anatomy and blood supply to an organ to be demonstrated more clearly. The quality of the image is very dependent on the patient remaining still, since movement causes severe loss of image (movement *artifact). The technique can also be used in nuclear medicine using two different tracers to look for parathyroid gland tumours.

digitization *n.* (in radiology) the conversion of an *analogue image to a *digital image. The image is broken down to pixels and numerical values assigned to each pixel for its position and to describe its shade on the *grey scale. This allows storage, electronic manipulation, and transfer via computer links of any images, including radiographs or CT, MRI, or ultrasound scans.

digitoxin *n. see* DIGOXIN.

digoxin *n.* a cardiac glycoside – a drug extracted from *digitalis – that increases the force of heart muscle contraction and decreases heart rate. It is used mainly in the treatment of *supraventricular tachycardia (especially to control atrial fibrillation). Digoxin is administered by mouth or injection; possible side-effects include nausea, vomiting, loss of appetite, diarrhoea, abdominal pain, and abnormal heart activity. **Digitoxin** is a related drug with similar effects. Trade name: **Lanoxin**.

dihydrocodeine *n.* an opioid *analgesic used to relieve moderate to severe pain (*see* OPIATE). It is administered by mouth or injection and sometimes causes nausea, dizziness, and constipation. Dependence of the *morphine type can also occur, but this is rare. Dihydrocodeine may also be administered orally in combination with *paracetamol (as **co-dydramol** or **Remedeine**). Trade names: **DF 118 Forte**, **DHC Continus**.

dihydrofolate reductase inhibitor any of various drugs that interfere with the conversion of folate to its active form in the body. They include *pyrimethamine, *trimethoprim, and *methotrexate. When such drugs are necessary, folate deficiency is treated with *folinic acid rather than folic acid.

dihydrotestosterone (DHT) *n.* a product formed from the action of the enzyme 5α-reductase on *testosterone. Mostly derived from the peripheral conversion of testosterone, some DHT is also secreted directly by the testes. DHT is an estimated 2.5 times more potent than testosterone but is present in much smaller amounts in the circulation.

diiodotyrosine *n.* an iodine-containing substance produced in the thyroid gland from which the *thyroid hormones are derived.

dilaceration *n.* a condition affecting some teeth after traumatic injury, in which the incomplete root continues to form at an abnormal angle to the part already formed. In severe cases it may be necessary to remove the tooth.

dilatation *n.* the enlargement or expansion of a hollow organ (such as a blood vessel) or cavity.

dilatation and curettage (D and C) an operation in which the cervix (neck) of the uterus is dilated, using an instrument called a *dilator, and the lining (endometrium) of the uterus is lightly scraped off with a manual curette (*see* CURETTAGE) or removed by suction using an aspirator. It is performed for a variety of reasons, including the removal of any material remaining after miscarriage and obtaining an endometrial biopsy for histological examination.

dilator *n.* **1.** an instrument used to enlarge a body opening or cavity. For example, the male urethra may become narrowed by disease and it can sometimes be restored to its original size by inserting a dilator. Dilators (such as Hegar's dilator) are also used to enlarge the canal in the cervix of the uterus in the procedure of *dilatation and curettage. **2.** a drug, applied either locally or systemically, that causes expansion of a structure, such as the pupil of the eye or a blood vessel. *See also* VASODILATOR. **3.** a muscle that, by its action, opens an aperture or orifice in the body.

diltiazem *n.* a *calcium-channel blocker used in the prevention and treatment of angina and high blood pressure (hypertension). It acts as a vasodilator and is administered by mouth; side-effects include oedema, headache, nausea, dizziness, and skin rash. Trade names: **Adizem SR**, **Dilzem SR**, **Tildiem**, etc.

dimercaprol (BAL) *n.* a drug that combines with metals in the body and is used to treat poisoning by antimony, arsenic, bismuth, gold, and mercury. It is administered by intramuscular injection and commonly causes nausea, vomiting, and watering of the eyes.

dimethyl sulfoxide (DMSO) a drug that is instilled (in solution) into the bladder for the relief of symptoms of *interstitial cystitis. It may cause bladder spasms and hypersensitivity. DMSO is also combined with topically applied drugs to improve their absorption; it may cause skin irritation. Trade name: **Rimso-50**.

dimeticone (dimethicone) *n.* a silicone

preparation used to treat head lice; it forms a coating around the parasites that prevents their excretion of water. It is administered as a lotion and may cause skin irritation. Dimeticone is also included in various *barrier creams (with antiseptics and astringents) to prevent undue drying of the skin and protect it against irritating external agents. Trade name: **Hedrin**. *See also* SIMETICONE.

dinoprostone *n.* a *prostaglandin drug used mainly to induce labour. It is usually administered in a pessary or as a vaginal tablet or gel. Trade names: **Propess**, **Prostin E2**.

dioctyl sodium sulphosuccinate *see* DOCUSATE SODIUM.

diode laser a type of laser whose medical uses include treating diseases of the retina, by producing small burns in the retina (*see* PHOTOCOAGULATION), and selected cases of glaucoma (cyclophotocoagulation). It is also used for treating varicose veins (*see* ENDOVENOUS LASER TREATMENT).

dioptre *n.* the unit of measurement of the power of *refraction of a lens. One dioptre is the power of a lens that brings parallel light rays to a focus at a point one metre from the lens, after passing through it. A stronger lens brings light rays to a focus at a point closer to it than a weaker lens and has a higher dioptric power.

Dioralyte *n. see* ORAL REHYDRATION THERAPY.

dipeptidase *n.* an enzyme, found in digestive juices, that splits certain products of protein digestion (dipeptides) into their constituent amino acids. The latter are then absorbed by the body.

dipeptide *n.* a compound consisting of two amino acids joined together by a peptide bond (e.g. glycylalanine, a combination of the amino acids glycine and alanine). *See* DIPEPTIDASE.

diphenoxylate *n. see* CO-PHENOTROPE.

diphtheria *n.* an acute highly contagious infection, caused by the bacterium *Corynebacterium diphtheriae*, generally affecting the throat but occasionally other mucous membranes and the skin. The disease is spread by direct contact with a patient or carrier or by contaminated milk. After an incubation period of 2–6 days a sore throat, weakness, and mild fever develop. Later, a soft grey membrane forms across the throat, constricting the air passages and causing difficulty in breathing and swallowing; a *tracheostomy may be necessary. Bacteria multiply at the site of infection and release a toxin into the bloodstream, which damages heart and nerves. Death from heart failure or general collapse can follow within four days but prompt administration of antitoxin and penicillin arrests the disease. An effective immunization programme has now made diphtheria rare in most Western countries (*see also* SCHICK TEST).

diphtheroid *adj.* resembling diphtheria (especially the membrane formed in diphtheria) or the bacteria that cause it.

diphyllobothriasis *n.* an infestation of the intestine with the broad tapeworm, **Diphyllobothrium latum*, which sometimes causes nausea, malnutrition, diarrhoea, and anaemia resulting from impaired absorption of vitamin B_{12} through the gut. The infestation, common in Baltic countries, is contracted following ingestion of uncooked fish infected with the larval stage of the tapeworm. The tapeworm can be expelled from the gut with the anthelmintic *mepacrine.

Diphyllobothrium *n.* a genus of large tapeworms that can grow to a length of 3–10 m. The adult of *D. latum*, the broad (or fish) tapeworm, infects fish-eating mammals including humans, in whom it may cause serious anaemia (*see* DIPHYLLOBOTHRIASIS). The parasite has two intermediate hosts: a freshwater crustacean and a fish (*see also* PLEROCERCOID).

dipipanone *n.* a potent opioid *analgesic drug used in combination with *cyclizine (as **Diconal**) to relieve moderate or severe pain. It is administered by mouth and may cause drowsiness.

dipl- (**diplo-**) *combining form denoting* double.

diplacusis *n.* perception of a single sound as double owing to a defect of the *cochlea in the inner ear.

diplegia *n.* paralysis involving both sides of the body and affecting the legs more severely than the arms. **Cerebral diplegia** is a form of *cerebral palsy in which there is widespread damage, in both cerebral hemispheres, of the brain cells that control the movements of the limbs. —**diplegic** *adj.*

diplococcus *n.* any of a group of nonmotile parasitic spherical bacteria that occur in pairs. The group includes the *pneumococcus.

diploë *n.* the lattice-like tissue that lies between the inner and outer layers of the *skull.

diploid *adj.* describing cells, nuclei, or organisms in which each chromosome except the Y sex chromosome is represented twice. *Compare* HAPLOID, TRIPLOID. —**diploid** *n.*

diplopia *n.* double vision: the simultaneous awareness of two images of one object. It is usually due to limitation of movement of one eye so that the two eyes cannot simultaneously look at the same object. This may be caused by a defect of the nerves or muscles controlling eye movement or a mechanical restriction of eyeball movement in the orbit. Double vision that does not disappear on covering one eye can be caused by early cataract (*see also* POLYOPIA).

diplotene *n.* the fourth stage in the first prophase of *meiosis, in which *crossing over occurs between the paired chromatids of homologous chromosomes, which then begin to separate.

diprosopus *n.* a fetal monster with a single trunk and normal limbs but with some degree of duplication of the face.

dipsomania *n.* morbid and insatiable craving for alcohol, occurring in paroxysms. A small proportion of alcoholics show this symptom (*see* ALCOHOLISM). The term (meaning 'compulsive thirst') has occasionally been used in relation to individuals with schizophrenia, who drink water or juices excessively.

Diptera *n.* a large group of insects, including *mosquitoes, gnats, midges, house flies and *tsetse flies, that possess a single pair of wings. The mouthparts of many species, e.g. mosquitoes and tsetse flies, are specialized for sucking blood; these forms are important in the transmission of disease (*see* VECTOR). *See also* FLY.

Dipylidium *n.* a genus of tapeworms. *D. caninum*, a common parasite of the small intestine of dogs and cats, occasionally infects humans but usually produces no obvious symptoms. Fleas are the intermediate hosts, and children in close contact with pets become infected on ingesting fleas harbouring the parasite.

dipyridamole *n.* a drug that dilates the blood vessels of the heart and reduces platelet aggregation. It is given by mouth to prevent thrombosis around prosthetic heart valves. It may cause headache, stomach upsets, and dizziness. A combination of modified-release dipyridamole and aspirin (**Asasantin Retard**) is given to prevent recurrent stroke in patients who have had a transient ischaemic attack or an ischaemic stroke. Trade name: **Persantin**.

directly observed therapy (DOT) *see* TUBERCULOSIS.

director *n.* an instrument used to guide the extent and direction of a surgical incision.

Director of Public Health (DPH) a senior public health consultant or specialist in a primary care trust, health board, health authority, or a government office public health group. Responsibilities include advising on the health needs of the local population. *See also* PUBLIC HEALTH CONSULTANT, PUBLIC HEALTH SPECIALIST.

dis- *prefix denoting* separation.

disability *n.* a loss or restriction of functional ability or activity as a result of impairment of the body or mind. Social approaches to disability emphasize the effects that society collectively has in disabling people and denying opportunities, thereby extending beyond the medical condition or diagnostic label. *See also* HANDICAP.

disability living allowance a state benefit payable to those under 65 who have had a mental or physical disability requiring help for at least three months and are likely to need such help for at least a further six months. It has two components: a care component, payable at three rates to those needing help with personal care; and a mobility component, payable at two rates to those aged 3 years or over who need help with walking. The rates depend on the level of help required. People aged over 65 years with a disability and requiring help may be eligible for the **attendance allowance**.

Disability Rights Commission *see* EQUALITY AND HUMAN RIGHTS COMMISSION.

disabled persons' tax credit *see* WORKING TAX CREDIT.

disablement *n. see* HANDICAP.

disaccharide *n.* a carbohydrate consisting of two linked *monosaccharide units. The most common disaccharides are *maltose, *lactose, and *sucrose.

disarticulation *n.* separation of two bones at a joint. This may be the result of an injury or it may be done by the surgeon at operation in the course of amputation; for example of a limb, finger, or toe.

disc *n.* (in anatomy) a rounded flattened structure, such as an *intervertebral disc or the *optic disc.

disc cupping an abnormal enlargement of the central depression of the *optic disc due to loss of nerve fibres, as occurs in glaucoma.

discectomy *n.* surgical removal of part (**partial discectomy**) or all (**total discectomy**) of a diseased or damaged intervertebral disc. It is performed for the relief of neurological symptoms arising from a displaced intervertebral disc (*see* PROLAPSED INTERVERTEBRAL DISC) or as part of a more extensive procedure. *See also* MICRODISCECTOMY.

disc herniation displacement of an intervertebral disc through a tear in the fibrous outer coat of the disc. *See* PROLAPSED INTERVERTEBRAL DISC.

discoid lupus erythematosus (DLE) *see* LUPUS ERYTHEMATOSUS.

discontinuation syndrome symptoms that arise from the sudden cessation of certain centrally acting drugs, such as antidepressants, beta blockers, and antihypertensives. Experiences include a rebound effect in which the original symptoms return but are temporarily worse than before, flu-like symptoms and headaches, nausea, and giddiness that is usually short-lived and stops within 36 hours. This syndrome is not a sign of addiction and it does not indicate dependency.

discrimination *n.* treating individuals differently on the basis of morally insignificant characteristics, such as race, sex, or religion. In medicine, any discrimination of this kind (e.g. when deciding on treatments or allocating resources) offends against the ethical principle of *justice. Legally, discrimination can be direct (i.e. overtly differentiating between people and groups) or indirect (i.e. behaviour that will disproportionately affect particular people or some groups more than others). *See also* EQUALITY.

disease *n.* a disorder with a specific cause

(which may or may not be known) and recognizable signs and symptoms; any bodily abnormality or failure to function properly, except that resulting directly from physical injury (the latter, however, may open the way for disease).

disease-modifying antirheumatic drug (DMARD) any of various drugs used in the treatment of rheumatic disease: they affect the progression of the disease by suppressing the disease process. DMARDs include drugs affecting the immune response (immunomodulators), such as *immunosuppressants (e.g. methotrexate) and *cytokine inhibitors; *gold salts; *penicillamine; *sulfasalazine; and *hydroxychloroquine.

disimpaction *n.* the process of separating the broken ends of a bone when they have been forcibly driven together during a fracture.

disinfectant *n.* an agent that destroys or removes bacteria and other microorganisms. In medicine disinfectants are used to cleanse unbroken skin. An example is *cetrimide.

disinfection *n.* the process of eliminating infective microorganisms from contaminated instruments, clothing, or surroundings by using physical means or chemicals (*disinfectants).

disinfestation *n.* the destruction of insect pests and other animal parasites. This generally involves the use of insecticides applied either topically, as in delousing, or as a spray for eliminating an infestation of fleas or bed bugs in the home.

disjunction *n.* the separation of pairs of homologous chromosomes during meiosis or of the chromatids of a chromosome during *anaphase of mitosis or meiosis. *Compare* NONDISJUNCTION.

dislocation (luxation) *n.* displacement from their normal position of bones meeting at a joint such that there is complete loss of contact of the joint surfaces. It usually results from trauma (dislocation of the shoulder is common in sports injuries) but may be congenital, in which case it usually affects the hip (*see* CONGENITAL DISLOCATION OF THE HIP). In a traumatic dislocation the bones are restored to their normal positions by manipulation under local or general anaesthesia (*see* REDUCTION). *Compare* SUBLUXATION.

dismemberment *n.* the separating of body parts or the amputation of a leg, arm, or part of a limb.

disodium pamidronate *see* PAMIDRONATE.

disoma *n.* a double-bodied fetus with a single head.

disopyramide *n.* an *anti-arrhythmic drug used to treat supraventricular and ventricular arrhythmias. It is administered by mouth or injection; side-effects such as dry mouth, blurred vision, difficulty in urination, and digestive upsets may occur. Trade name: **Rythmodan**.

disorientation *n.* the state produced by loss of awareness of space, time, or personality. It can be the result of drugs, mental illness, or organic disease and is one of the symptoms tested for in the *mental state examination.

dispensary *n.* a place where medicines are made up by a pharmacist according to the doctor's prescription and dispensed to patients. A dispensary is often part of an outpatient department in a hospital.

dispensing practice (in Britain) a general practice with a dispensary on site to issue prescribed medications to patients. *See also* GENERAL PRACTITIONER.

displacement *n.* (in psychology) the substitution of one type of behaviour for another, usually the substitution of a relatively harmless activity for a harmful one; for example, kicking the cat instead of one's boss.

dissection *n.* the cutting apart and separation of the body tissues along the natural divisions of the organs and different tissues in the course of an operation. Dissection of corpses is carried out for the study of anatomy.

disseminated *adj.* widely distributed in an organ (or organs) or in the whole body. The term may refer to disease organisms or to pathological changes.

disseminated intravascular coagulation (DIC) a condition resulting from overstimulation of the blood-clotting mechanisms in response to disease or injury, such as severe infection, malignancy, acute leukaemia, burns, severe trauma, or severe haemorrhage during childbirth (*see also* ABRUPTIO PLACENTAE). The overstimulation results in generalized blood coagulation and excessive consumption of coagulation factors. The resulting deficiency of these may lead to spontaneous bleeding. Transfusions of plasma are given to replace the depleted clotting factors, and treatment of the underlying cause is essential.

disseminated sclerosis *see* MULTIPLE SCLEROSIS.

dissociated vertical deviation (DVD) a condition in which one eye looks upwards when the amount of light entering it is reduced, e.g. when it is covered. The eye returns to its original position when the cover is removed. DVD is an acquired condition chiefly associated with infantile esotropia (convergent *strabismus). The deviation is dissociated since there is no movement of the focusing (i.e. uncovered) eye during the deviation or return phase.

dissociation *n.* (in psychiatry) the process whereby thoughts and ideas can be split off from consciousness and may function independently, thus (for example) allowing conflicting opinions to be held at the same time about the same object. Dissociation may be the main factor in cases of dissociative *fugue and multiple personalities.

dissociative disorder any one of a group of mental disorders explained psychoanalytically as extreme *defence mechanisms. Symptoms include loss of memory for important personal details (*see* AMNESIA), wandering away from home (*see* FUGUE), the assumption of a new identity, and trancelike states with severely reduced response to external stimuli. *Conversion disorder is classified with dissociative disorders (as dissociative (conversion) disorders) in ICD-10 (*see* INTERNATIONAL CLASSIFICATION OF DISEASES).

distal *adj.* **1.** (in anatomy) situated away from the origin or point of attachment or from the median line of the body. For example, the term is applied to a part of a limb that is furthest from the body; to a blood vessel that is far from the heart; and to a nerve fibre that is far from the central nervous system. *Compare* PROXIMAL. **2.** (in dentistry) describing the surface of a tooth away from the midline of the jaw.

distichiasis *n.* a very rare condition in which there is an extra row of eyelashes behind the normal row. They may rub on the cornea.

distigmine *n.* a *parasympathomimetic drug used mainly to treat urinary retention after surgery. It is administered by mouth. Possible side-effects include nausea, vomiting, diarrhoea, and excessive salivation. Trade name: **Ubretid**.

distraction *n.* (in orthopaedics) increasing the distance between two points. In *limb lengthening procedures callus can be stretched longitudinally by increasing the distance between pins attached to the bone (*see* CALLOTASIS).

distraction test a hearing test used for screening infants between the ages of six and ten months. The infant is placed on its carer's knee, one examiner sits in front of the infant and gains its attention, and a second examiner is situated just behind the infant. At a given moment the first examiner becomes very still and the second examiner makes a sound at the level of the infant's ear to one side or the other. If the infant can hear it turns in the direction of the sound. The sounds made should be of different pitches and a given loudness.

district nurse a trained nurse with special training in *domiciliary services, usually employed by a primary care trust or health board. District nurses may also be allocated to a designated general practice, an arrangement known as *attachment.

disulfiram *n.* a drug used in the treatment of chronic alcoholism. It acts as a deterrent by producing unpleasant effects when taken with alcohol, including flushing, breathing difficulties, headache, palpitations, nausea, and vomiting. It is administered by mouth; common side-effects are fatigue, nausea, and constipation. Trade name: **Antabuse**.

dithranol *n.* a drug applied to the skin as an ointment, paste, cream, or scalp gel to treat *psoriasis. It may irritate the skin on application. Trade names: **Dithrocream**, **Micanol**, **Psorin**.

diuresis *n.* increased secretion of urine by the kidneys. This normally follows the drinking of more fluid than the body requires, but it can be stimulated by the administration of a *diuretic.

diuretic *n.* a drug that increases the volume of urine produced by promoting the excretion of salts and water from the kidney. The main classes of diuretics act by inhibiting the reabsorption of salts and water from the kidney tubules into the bloodstream.

Thiazide diuretics (e.g. *bendroflumethiazide, *chlortalidone) act at the distal convoluted tubules (*see* NEPHRON), preventing the reabsorption of sodium and potassium. **Potassium-sparing diuretics** (e.g. *amiloride, *spironolactone, *triamterene) prevent excessive loss of potassium at the distal convoluted tubules, and **loop diuretics** (e.g. *furosemide) prevent reabsorption of sodium and potassium in *Henle's loop. Diuretics are used to reduce the oedema due to salt and water retention in disorders of the heart, kidneys, liver, or lungs. Thiazides and potassium-sparing diuretics are also used – in conjunction with other drugs – in the treatment of high blood pressure. Treatment with thiazide and loop diuretics often results in potassium deficiency; this is corrected by simultaneous administration of potassium salts or a potassium-sparing diuretic.

diurnal *adj.* relating to the daylight hours; daily. *See* CIRCADIAN.

divarication *n.* the separation or stretching of bodily structures. **Rectus divarication** is stretching of the *rectus abdominis muscle, a common condition associated with pregnancy or obesity.

divaricator *n.* **1.** a scissor-like surgical instrument used to divide portions of tissue into two separate parts during an operation. **2.** a form of retractor used to open out the sides of an abdominal incision and facilitate access.

divergence *n.* (in ophthalmology) simultaneous abduction of the eyes. **Divergence excess** is a divergent squint (*see* STRABISMUS) in which the eyes are deviated outwards more when looking in the distance than when looking at near objects. **Divergence insufficiency** is a convergent squint (*see* STRABISMUS) in which the eyes are deviated slightly inwards only when looking in the distance.

diverticular disease a condition in which there are diverticula (*see* DIVERTICULUM) in the colon associated with symptoms. A minority of patients may develop *diverticulitis or its complications: abscess, haemorrhage, fistulae, *stricture, and *intestinal obstruction. Symptoms in uncomplicated disease may include lower abdominal pain and altered stool frequency or consistency. The pain is often due to spasm of the muscle of the intestine, but many other factors are usually involved. The cause of the disease is unknown but may be linked to diets lacking roughage or fibre in childhood.

diverticulitis *n.* inflammation of a *diverticulum, most commonly of one or more colonic diverticula. This type of diverticulitis is caused by infection and causes lower abdominal pain often associated with diarrhoea ; it may lead to complications, including abscess formation and perforation, which usually require surgical management. A Meckel's diverticulum sometimes becomes inflamed due to infection, causing symptoms similar to *appendicitis. Diverticula elsewhere in the alimentary tract are usually not subject to diverticulitis. *Compare* DIVERTICULAR DISEASE.

diverticulosis *n.* a condition in which diverticula exist in a segment of the intestine without evidence of inflammation (*compare* DIVERTICULITIS).

diverticulum *n.* (*pl.* **diverticula**) a sac or pouch formed at weak points in the walls of the alimentary tract. They may be caused by increased pressure from within (**pulsion diverticula**) or by pulling from without (**traction diverticula**). A **pharyngeal diverticulum** occurs in the pharynx and may cause difficulty in swallowing. **Oesophageal diverticula** occur in the middle or lower oesophagus (gullet); they may be associated with muscular disorders of the oesophagus but rarely cause symptoms. **Gastric diverticula**, which are rare, affect the stomach (usually the upper part) and cause no symptoms. **Duodenal diverticula** occur on the concave surface of the duodenal loop; they are usually asymptomatic but a small minority may be associated with *dyspepsia, choledocholithiasis, and an increased risk of pancreatitis. **Jejunal diverticula** affect the small intestine, are often multiple, and may give rise to abdominal discomfort, diarrhoea, and *malabsorption due to overgrowth of bacteria within them. **Meckel's diverticulum** occurs in the ileum, about 35 cm from its termination, as a congenital abnormality. It may become inflamed, mimicking *appendicitis; if it contains embryonic remnants of stomach mucosa it may form a *peptic ulcer, causing pain, bleeding, or perforation. **Colonic diverticula**, affecting the colon (particularly the left side), become commoner with increasing age and often cause no symptoms. However they are sometimes associated with abdominal pain or altered bowel habit (*see* DIVERTICULAR DISEASE) or

they may become inflamed (*see* DIVERTICULI-
TIS).

division *n.* **1.** the separation of an organ
or tissue into parts by surgery. **2.** *see* CELL DI-
VISION.

Dix-Hallpike test (Hallpike test) a test
for *benign paroxysmal positional vertigo
(BPPV), performed with the patient first sitting upright on an examination couch and
then lying supine with the head and neck extended beyond the edge of the couch. The
patient's head is rotated to the left (or right)
and supported by the examiner while the patient assumes the supine position and keeps
his or her eyes focused on the examiner's
eyes. The test is then repeated with the other
ear facing down. In patients with BPPV, after
a short delay rotatory *nystagmus is seen, in
association with severe vertigo and nausea,
which gradually abates. The effect diminishes with repeated manoeuvres. In conditions affecting the cerebellum or brainstem,
the nystagmus occurs immediately, in any
direction, and does not diminish, and patients do not feel especially nauseated. [M. R.
Dix and C. S. Hallpike (20th century), British
otologists]

dizygotic twins *see* TWINS.

DLE discoid lupus erythematosus. *See*
LUPUS ERYTHEMATOSUS.

DMARD *see* DISEASE-MODIFYING ANTI-
RHEUMATIC DRUG.

DMD (Duchenne muscular dystrophy) *see*
MUSCULAR DYSTROPHY.

DMSA *d*imercapto*s*uccinic *a*cid, which
when labelled with *technetium-99m is used
as a tracer to obtain *scintigrams of the kidney, by means of a *gamma camera. DMSA
binds to the proximal tubules of the kidney.
It is used particularly to show scarring, resulting from infection, and to assess the relative quantity of functioning tissue in each
kidney.

DNA (deoxyribonucleic acid) the genetic
material of nearly all living organisms, which
controls heredity and is located in the cell
nucleus (*see* CHROMOSOME, GENE). DNA is a
*nucleic acid composed of two strands made
up of units called *nucleotides (see illustration). The two strands are wound around
each other into a double helix and linked together by hydrogen bonds between the
bases of the nucleotides (*see* BASE PAIRING).
The genetic information of the DNA is con-

tained in the sequence of bases along the
molecule (*see* GENETIC CODE); changes in the
DNA cause *mutations. The DNA molecule
can make exact copies of itself by the process
of *replication, thereby passing on the genetic information to the daughter cells when
the cell divides.

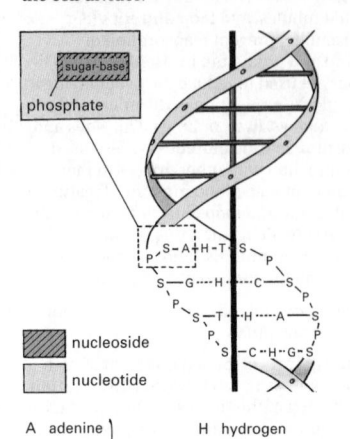

A	adenine		H	hydrogen
G	guanine	bases	S	deoxyribose sugar
T	thymine		P	phosphate
C	cytosine		----	hydrogen bond

nucleoside

nucleotide

DNA. Structure of part of a DNA molecule.

DNA polymerase inhibitor any one of a
class of antiviral drugs that inhibit the action
of DNA polymerase enzymes, which are used
by viruses to form their own DNA. These
drugs prevent, to a varying degree, the reproduction of viruses. They include *aciclovir,
*foscarnet, *ganciclovir, and *valaciclovir.

DNA repair a variety of mechanisms that
help to ensure that the genetic sequence, as
expressed in the DNA, is maintained and
that errors that occur during DNA replication, by mutation, are not allowed to accumulate. An error in the genetic sequence
could cause cell death by interfering with the
replication process. DNA repair involves the
action of enzymes, which detect damage to
DNA and effect the repair. Some genetic diseases, including *ataxia telangiectasia and
*xeroderma pigmentosum, are due to defi-
ciencies in these enzymes.

DNAR order Do Not Attempt Resuscitation order: an instruction, usually made by a
patient while he or she has capacity and

recorded in their notes, requesting that doctors desist from performing resuscitation in the event of physiological failure. By respecting a patient's choice with regard to resuscitation, a doctor is respecting that patient's *autonomy. If resuscitation is considered *futile, a decision not to attempt it may be taken; ideally, this should be communicated to the patient and the reasons explained sensitively.

DNAse *n.* an enzyme that catalyses the cleavage of DNA. A genetically engineered form, recombinant human DNAse (**dornase alfa**), is used in the treatment of *cystic fibrosis to reduce the viscosity of the sticky secretions in the lungs. Administered by inhalation via a jet nebulizer, it appears to hydrolyse extracellular DNA that accumulates with other neutrophil debris in the airways. Trade name: **Pulmozyme**.

dobutamine *n.* an *inotropic *sympathomimetic drug (a β_1 agonist) used to increase the force of contraction of the ventricles and improve the heart output, for example in patients who have had a *myocardial infarction or in cases of shock. It is given by intravenous infusion.

docetaxel *n.* a *taxane used in the treatment of breast cancer, advanced or metastatic *non-small-cell lung cancer, and metastatic prostate cancer that is resistant to hormonal treatment. It is administered by intravenous infusion; side-effects are as for all *cytotoxic drugs, but also typically include hypersensitivity reactions, neuropathy, and leg oedema. Trade name: **Taxotere**.

Doctor *n.* **1.** the title given to a recipient of a higher university degree than a Master's degree (this is usually a Doctor of Philosophy (PhD or DPhil) degree). The degree *Medicinae Doctor* (MD) is awarded by some British universities as a research degree to those with a first degree in medicine. In the US, the degree is awarded on qualification. **2.** a courtesy title given to a qualified medical practitioner, i.e. one who has been registered by the *General Medical Council (GMC). Most doctors in the UK obtain bachelors' degrees in medicine and surgery (MB, BS) or the diplomas of the conjoint boards of the Royal Colleges of Physicians and Surgeons of England and Scotland or the Society of Apothecaries (e.g. LRCP, MRCS, LMSSA): these degrees or diplomas and one year's hospital experience are required by the GMC before they will register a person as a doctor.

Normally it is compulsory to have undertaken year 1 of the medical *Foundation Programme (or two full-time **preregistration appointments**) in at least two specialties at hospitals recognized for this purpose. The doctor has the title **F1 doctor**, **house officer** (or **physician** or **surgeon**), **resident**, or **intern** and is debarred from independent practice. Surgeons in the UK do not use the title Doctor and are referred to, as a mark of distinction, as Mr, Mrs, or Ms. Qualified dentists also use the courtesy title Doctor. *See also* CONSULTANT.

doctrine of double effect where it is foreseen that a single action will have both a good and a bad outcome, a person may perform such an action provided that (a) he or she intends only the positive outcome, (b) the bad outcome is not disproportionate to the good, and (c) the good outcome is not a direct consequence of the bad. The classic example occurs where a terminally ill patient requires high doses of opiates for pain relief that may also depress respiratory function and hasten his or her death. In such a case the law holds that the doctor may supply the necessary dosage without this being considered tantamount to *euthanasia, even though the outcome will be the same, i.e. the morality of the action does not lie in its consequences (*see* CONSEQUENTIALISM).

docusate sodium (dioctyl sodium sulphosuccinate) a stimulant *laxative and softening agent that is used to relieve constipation and prepare the bowel for radiological examination. It is administered by mouth or enema and may cause abdominal cramps. It is also used in ear drops to soften earwax. Trade names: **Dioctyl**, **Docusol**, **Norgalax Micro-enema**.

dolasetron *n. see* ONDANSETRON.

dolich- (dolicho-) *combining form denoting* long. Example: **dolichocolon** (abnormally long colon).

dolichocephaly *n.* the condition of having a relatively long narrow skull, with a *cephalic index of 75 or less. The head of a fetus in a breech presentation is often dolichocephalic. —**dolichocephalic** *adj.*

dolor *n.* pain: one of the classical signs of inflammation in a tissue, the other three being *calor (heat), *rubor (redness), and *tumor (swelling). The pain in inflammation is thought to be due to the release of chemicals from damaged cells.

dolorimetry *n.* the measurement of pain. *See* ALGESIMETER.

domiciliary consultation 1. a house call by a *general practitioner made at the request of a patient or the patient's carer. It is commonly referred to as a **home visit**. 2. (in Britain) an arrangement in the *National Health Service whereby a hospital specialist, at the request of a general practitioner, visits to advise on the diagnosis or treatment of a patient who, on medical grounds, is unable to attend hospital. The specialist receives special remuneration for this service.

domiciliary midwife *see* COMMUNITY MIDWIFE.

domiciliary services (in Britain) health and social services that are available in the home and are distinguished from hospital-based services. They include the services of such personnel as community nurses employed by care trusts (*see* DISTRICT NURSE, COMMUNITY MIDWIFE, HEALTH VISITOR) and social workers and care assistants employed by social service departments of local authorities. The term **community services** is applied to these services.

dominant *adj.* (in genetics) describing a gene (or its corresponding characteristic) whose effect is shown in the individual whether its *allele is the same or different. If the allele is different it is described as *recessive and its effect is masked. In genetic diseases showing **autosomal dominant** inheritance, the defective gene is dominant and will therefore be inherited by 50% of the offspring (of either sex) of a person with the disease. It will always be expressed in these offspring (since the normal allele inherited from the unaffected parent is recessive). —**dominant** *n.*

domperidone *n.* an antiemetic drug used especially to reduce the nausea and vomiting caused by other drugs (e.g. anticancer drugs). It inhibits the effects of *dopamine, acting to close the sphincter muscle at the upper opening of the stomach (the cardia) and to relax the sphincter at the lower opening (the pylorus). It is administered by mouth or suppository; possible side-effects include breast enlargement and pain. Trade name: **Motilium**.

donepezil *n. see* ACETYLCHOLINESTERASE INHIBITOR.

donor *n.* a person who makes his own tissues or organs available for use by someone else. For example, a donor may provide blood for transfusion (*see* BLOOD DONOR), a kidney for transplantation, or sex cells for *artificial insemination or *oocyte donation.

donor insemination *see* ARTIFICIAL INSEMINATION.

Do Not Attempt Resuscitation order (DNAR order) *see* DNAR ORDER.

dopa *n.* dihydroxyphenylalanine: a physiologically important compound that forms an intermediate stage in the synthesis of catecholamines (dopamine, adrenaline, and noradrenaline) from the essential amino acid tyrosine. It also plays a role itself in the functioning of certain parts of the brain. The laevorotatory form, *levodopa, is administered for the treatment of *parkinsonism, in which there is a deficiency of the neurotransmitter *dopamine in the brain.

dopamine *n.* a *catecholamine derived from dopa that functions as a *neurotransmitter, acting on specific dopamine receptors and also on adrenoceptors throughout the body, especially in the *limbic system and *extrapyramidal system of the brain as well as the arteries and the heart. It also stimulates the release of noradrenaline from nerve endings. The effects vary with location and concentration. Dopamine is used to increase the strength of contraction of the heart in heart failure, shock, severe trauma, and septicaemia. It is administered by injection in carefully controlled dosage. Possible side-effects include unduly rapid or irregular heartbeat, nausea, vomiting, breathlessness, angina pectoris, and kidney damage.

Certain drugs (**dopamine receptor agonists**) have an effect on the body similar to that of dopamine. They include *apomorphine, *bromocriptine, *pergolide, *ropinirole, *cabergoline, and **pramipexole** (Mirapexin) and are used to treat *parkinsonism. Drugs that compete with dopamine to occupy and block the dopamine receptor sites in the body are known as **dopamine receptor antagonists**. They include some *antipsychotic drugs (e.g. the phenothiazines and *butyrophenones) and certain drugs (e.g. *domperidone and *metoclopramide) used to treat nausea and vomiting.

dopamine hypothesis the theory that schizophrenia is caused in part by abnormalities in the metabolism of *dopamine and can be treated in part by drugs that antagonize its action as a neurotransmitter.

Doppler ultrasound a diagnostic technique that utilizes the fact that the frequency of sound or light waves changes when they are reflected from a moving surface (the **Doppler effect**). It is used to study the flow in blood vessels and the movement of blood in the heart. The frequency detector may be part of an ultrasound imaging probe, which displays an image of the anatomy on a monitor. Simultaneously the Doppler signal from a particular point on the ultrasound image can be displayed next to the anatomical position using a split screen (**duplex imaging**). Using electronic techniques, direction and velocity of blood flow can each be allocated different colours and displayed on a colour monitor over the anatomical image (**colour flow ultrasound imaging**). **Power Doppler**, a modification of this technique, is more sensitive at detecting flow but does not give information on direction of flow. Doppler ultrasound is a valuable technique to detect vessel thrombosis, such as deep vein thrombosis, and can be safely used in pregnancy without the risk of ionizing radiation. Doppler measurement of the fetal middle cerebral vessels (**MCA Doppler**) can predict fetal anaemia as the resistance in these vessels is increased. This noninvasive technique has supplanted serial amniocentesis/fetal cord blood sampling in cases of *haemolytic disease of the newborn. Doppler of other fetal vessels (e.g. the ductus venosus) is used as a screening method for fetal chromosomal and cardiac defects and, later, fetal growth restriction. [C. J. Doppler (1803–53), Austrian physicist]

dornase alfa *n. see* DNAse.

dors- (dorsi-, dorso-) *combining form denoting* 1. the back. Example: **dorsalgia** (pain in). 2. dorsal.

dorsal *adj.* relating to or situated at or close to the back of the body or to the posterior part of an organ.

dorsiflexion *n.* backward flexion of the foot or hand or their digits; i.e. bending towards the upper surface.

dorsoventral *adj.* (in anatomy) extending from the back (dorsal) surface to the front (ventral) surface.

dorsum *n.* 1. the back. 2. the upper or posterior surface of a part of the body; for example, of the hand. *See also* DORSAL.

dorzolamide *n.* a *carbonic anhydrase inhibitor used to reduce intraocular pressure in the treatment of *glaucoma: it decreases the production of aqueous humour. Administered as eye drops (sometimes in combination with timolol) it may cause local burning or stinging, blurred vision, increased production of tears, dizziness, and pins and needles. Trade names: **Cosopt**, **Trusopt**.

dose *n.* a carefully measured quantity of a drug that is prescribed by a doctor to be given to a patient at any one time. The **median effective dose** (ED_{50}) is the dose of a drug that produces desired effects in 50% of individuals tested. *See also* LD_{50}.

dosimeter *n.* 1. a device used to measure the intensity of a radiation source. 2. a device to record the amount of radiation received by workers exposed to X-rays or other radiation. *See* THERMOLUMINESCENT DOSIMETER.

dosimetry *n.* 1. the calculation of appropriate radiation doses for treating given conditions, usually cancer in different parts of the body. *See* RADIOTHERAPY. 2. the measurement of the dose received by a patient having a diagnostic technique involving ionizing radiation or by a radiation worker in his or her employment.

dosulepin *n. see* ANTIDEPRESSANT.

DOT directly observed therapy: *see* TUBERCULOSIS.

double-blind trial *see* INTERVENTION STUDY.

double contrast a technique usually used in X-ray examinations of the bowel. Barium sulphate *contrast medium is used to coat the bowel wall. The bowel is then distended with gas. The X-ray images obtained give exquisite detail of the lining of the gut. *See also* BARIUM ENEMA, BARIUM SWALLOW AND MEAL.

double J stents *see* STENT.

double-outlet right ventricle (DORV) a congenital defect of the heart in which both the aorta and the pulmonary artery arise predominantly from the right ventricle anterior to the ventricular septum with an associated *ventricular septal defect (VSD). The relationship between the site of the VSD and the great arteries is important for surgical repair. DORV can be associated with chromosomal defects.

double uterus *see* UTERUS DIDELPHYS.

double vision *see* DIPLOPIA.

douche *n.* a stream of water used for cleaning any part of the body, most commonly the vagina. However, vaginal douching makes a woman more susceptible to infection; moreover, it is extremely unreliable as a method of contraception.

dowager's hump curvature of the spine in the cervical (neck) and upper thoracic region caused by osteoporosis. *Compare* BUFFALO HUMP.

Down's syndrome (Down syndrome) a condition resulting from a chromosomal abnormality most commonly due to the presence of three copies of chromosome 21 (**trisomy 21**), which is most likely to occur with advanced maternal age. Down's syndrome can also occur as a result of chromosomal rearrangement (*translocation) and as part of a *mosaicism, which are not related to maternal age. Affected individuals share certain clinical features, including a characteristic flat facial appearance with slanting eyes (as in Mongolian races, which gave the former name, **mongolism**, to the condition), broad hands with short fingers and a single crease across the palm, malformed ears, eyes with a speckled iris (**Brushfield spots**), short stature, and *hypotonia. Many individuals also have a degree of mental retardation, although the range of ability is wide and some individuals are of normal intelligence. The incidence of congenital heart defects is 40–50%, and other structural malformations (e.g. *duodenal atresia) and associated abnormalities (e.g. deafness, squints, obesity, type 2 diabetes) may also be present. *Prenatal diagnosis of Down's syndrome can be obtained by *amniocentesis and *chorionic villus sampling, which are invasive procedures, and about 33% of structural abnormalities in fetuses with Down's can be detected prenatally by *ultrasonography. *Prenatal screening tests (e.g. the *triple test) and soft *ultrasound markers (e.g. *nuchal translucency scanning) can estimate the risk of Down's syndrome being present. [J. L. H. Down (1828–96), British physician]

(()) SEE WEB LINKS

• Website of the Down's Syndrome Association

doxapram *n.* an *analeptic drug used to raise the level of consciousness in patients recovering from surgery and to treat respiratory failure. It is administered intravenously; possible side-effects include nausea, rapid heartbeat, dizziness, restlessness, and tremor. Trade name: **Dopram**.

doxazosin *n.* an *alpha blocker used to treat high blood pressure and to relieve urinary retention due to benign enlargement of the *prostate gland. It is administered by mouth. Possible side-effects include faintness on standing up, weakness, dizziness, and headache. Trade name: **Cardura**.

doxepin *n.* a tricyclic *antidepressant administered by mouth to relieve depression, especially when associated with anxiety; side-effects can include drowsiness, dry mouth, blurred vision, and digestive upsets. It is also applied topically as a cream to relieve itching associated with eczema. Trade names: **Sinequan**, **Xepin**.

doxorubicin *n.* an *anthracycline antibiotic isolated from *Streptomyces peucetius caesius* and used mainly in the treatment of acute leukaemias, Hodgkin's disease, non-Hodgkin's lymphoma, and various other forms of cancer. Doxorubicin acts by interfering with the production of DNA and RNA (*see also* CYTOTOXIC DRUG, TOPOISOMERASE INHIBITOR). It is administered by injection or infusion and can be given as a lipid formulation (**Caelyx**, **Myocet**; *see* LIPOSOME). Side-effects are those of other cytotoxic drugs; in addition, cardiotoxicity increases with cumulative dose of the drug. Use of alterative anthracyclines (e.g. epirubicin) or a liposomal preparation can reduce toxicity.

doxycycline *n.* a *tetracycline antibiotic used to treat infections caused by *Chlamydia*, rickettsiae, mycoplasmas, and *Brucella* as well as Lyme disease. It may also be used in the prevention and treatment of malaria and the treatment of mouth ulcers and oral herpes. It is administered by mouth and side-effects are those of the other tetracyclines. Trade names: **Periostat**, **Vibramycin-D**.

DPT *see* DENTAL PANTOMOGRAM.

DPT vaccine a combined vaccine against *d*iphtheria, whooping cough (*p*ertussis), and *t*etanus now replaced by the *DTaP/IPV/Hib and *DTaP/IPV vaccines. *See* IMMUNIZATION.

DR *see* DIGITAL RADIOGRAPHY.

drachm *n.* **1.** a unit of weight used in

pharmacy. 1 drachm = 3.883 g (60 grains). **2.** a unit of volume used in pharmacy. 1 fluid drachm = 3.696 ml (1/8 fluid ounce).

dracontiasis *n.* a tropical disease caused by the parasitic nematode *Dracunculus medinensis* (*see* GUINEA WORM) in the tissues beneath the skin. The disease is transmitted to humans via contaminated drinking water. The initial symptoms, which appear a year after infection, result from the migration of the worm to the skin surface and include itching, giddiness, difficulty in breathing, vomiting, and diarrhoea. Later a large blister forms on the skin, usually on the legs or arms, which eventually bursts and may ulcerate and become infected. Dracontiasis is common in India and West Africa but also occurs in Arabia, Iran, East Africa, and Afghanistan. Treatment involves extracting the worm or administering anthelmintics.

Dracunculus *n. see* GUINEA WORM.

dragee *n.* a *pill that has been coated with sugar.

drain **1.** *n.* a device, usually a tube or wick, used to draw fluid from an internal body cavity to the surface. A drain is sometimes inserted during an operation to ensure that any fluid formed immediately passes to the surface, so preventing an accumulation that may become infected or cause pressure in the operation site. Negative pressure (suction) can be applied through a tube drain to increase its effectiveness. **2.** *vb. see* DRAINAGE.

drainage *n.* the drawing off of fluid from a cavity in the body, usually fluid that has accumulated abnormally. For example, serous fluid may be drained from a swollen joint, pus removed from an internal abscess, or urine from an overdistended bladder. *See also* DRAIN.

drastic *n.* any agent causing a major change in a body system or function, e.g. strong laxatives.

draw-sheet *n.* a sheet placed beneath a patient in bed that, when one portion has been soiled or becomes uncomfortably wrinkled, may be pulled under the patient so that another portion may be used. The bed does not have to be remade, and the patient does not have to leave bed.

drepanocyte (sickle cell) *n. see* SICKLE-CELL DISEASE.

drepanocytosis *n. see* SICKLE-CELL DISEASE.

DRESS *d*rug *r*eaction with *e*osinophilia and *s*ystemic *s*ymptoms: a potentially fatal reaction to medications, also called **anticonvulsant** and **drug-induced hypersensitivity syndrome**. It is characterized by a nonspecific skin rash and variable other symptoms, such as fever, lymphadenopathy, full blood count abnormalities, organ (e.g. liver) dysfunction, and malaise. Common drug culprits include anticonvulsants and antibiotics, although many others have been reported to cause it. Prompt withdrawal of the suspected drug is critical for recovery, but sometimes the reaction can be prolonged, even after drug withdrawal.

dressing *n.* material applied to a wound or diseased part of the body, with or without medication, to give protection and assist healing.

drill *n.* (in dentistry) a rotary instrument used to remove tooth substance, particularly in the treatment of caries. It consists of a *dental handpiece that takes variously shaped *burs. Most drilling is done with an air-driven turbine handpiece, but some is performed with a much slower mechanically driven handpiece. Handpieces usually have a waterspray coolant and may have a fibre-optic light.

drip (intravenous drip) *n.* apparatus for the continuous injection (*transfusion) of blood, plasma, saline, glucose solution, or other fluid into a vein. The fluid flows under gravity from a suspended bottle through a tube ending in a hollow needle inserted into the patient's vein. The rate of flow can be adjusted according to the rate of drips seen in a transparent section of the tube, but many *infusions are now controlled by electronically regulated infusion pumps.

drom- (dromo-) *combining form denoting* movement or speed.

dropsy *n. see* OEDEMA.

Drosophila *n.* a genus of very small flies, commonly called fruit flies, that breed in decaying fruit and vegetables. *D. melanogaster* has been extensively used in genetic research as it has only four pairs of chromosomes and those in its salivary glands are easily recognizable. Adult *D. repleta* sometimes feed on faecal matter and may transmit disease organisms.

drug *n.* any substance that affects the structure or functioning of a living organism. Drugs are widely used for the prevention, diagnosis, and treatment of disease and for the relief of symptoms. The term 'medicine' is sometimes preferred for therapeutic drugs in order to distinguish them from drugs of abuse.

drug dependence *see* DEPENDENCE.

drug-eluting stent *see* STENT.

drusen *pl. n.* 1. (macular drusen) white or yellow deposits of *hyalin in *Bruch's membrane of the choroid. They may be associated with *macular degeneration. 2. (disc drusen) glistening nodules seen on an irregularly raised *optic disc. Consisting of excess *glia (produced congenitally) that has undergone degeneration and calcification, they can be confused with *papilloedema.

dry mouth a condition that occurs as a result of reduced salivary flow from a variety of causes, including therapeutic agents, *Sjögren's syndrome, connective tissue diseases, diabetes, excision or absence of a major salivary gland, or radiotherapy to the head that destroys the salivary glands. It causes swallowing and speech difficulties, inflamed gums, an increased incidence of dental caries, and loss of denture stability in people who have lost their teeth. Patients with their own teeth should be given strict dietary advice, chlorhexidine mouthwashes, and sugar-free nonacidic saliva substitutes; they require special monitoring by their dentist. Medical name: **xerostomia**.

dry socket a painful condition in which the normal healing of a tooth socket has been disturbed. Instead of being filled with a blood clot the socket is empty as a result of a nonspecific infection; treatment consists of chlorhexidine mouthwashes and the condition resolves in 10–14 days.

DSEK Descemet's stripping endothelial *keratoplasty.

DSI *see* DIGITAL SPOT IMAGING.

DSM Diagnostic and Statistical Manual of Mental Disorders: an influential publication of the American Psychiatric Association in which psychiatric disorders are classified and defined. The current (2000) version is the text revision (TR) of the DSM-IV, known as **DSM-IV-TR**.

DSTs *see* DEXAMETHASONE SUPPRESSION TESTS.

DTaP/IPV (dTaP/IPV) a booster vaccine given to children between 3 years 4 months and 5 years of age. It tops up protection against diphtheria, tetanus, pertussis (whooping cough), and polio.

DTaP/IPV/Hib a primary *immunization given to infants typically at 2, 3, and 4 months of age. It protects against five diseases: diphtheria, tetanus, pertussis (whooping cough), polio (inactivated polio vaccine), and *Haemophilus influenzae* type b infection (*see* HIB VACCINE).

DTPA *d*iethylene*t*riamine*p*enta*a*cetic *a*cid, which when labelled with *technetium-99m is used as a tracer to obtain *scintigrams of the kidney over a period of time, by means of a *gamma camera. DTPA is filtered out of the blood by the kidneys and passes into the urine; it is used to show function and reflux. It is particularly useful in assessing obstruction to urinary drainage from the kidneys.

Duane's syndrome an abnormality of the eye muscles leading most commonly to restricted abduction (outward movement of the eye away from the midline) of one eye. On attempted adduction (inward movement of the eye towards the midline) of that same eye there is retraction of the eye into the orbit and narrowing of the opening between the eyelids. [A. Duane (1858–1926), US ophthalmologist]

Duchenne muscular dystrophy *see* MUSCULAR DYSTROPHY. [G. B. A. Duchenne (1806–75), French neurologist]

duct *n.* a tubelike structure or channel, especially one for carrying glandular secretions.

ductal carcinoma in situ (DCIS) the earliest stage of breast cancer, detectable by mammography, which is confined to the lactiferous (milk) ducts of the breast. *See* CARCINOMA IN SITU.

ductions *pl. n.* movements of one eye, i.e. adduction (rotation towards the nose), abduction (rotation towards the temple), elevation, depression, intorsion, and extorsion.

ductless gland *see* ENDOCRINE GLAND.

ductule *n.* a small duct or channel.

ductus *n.* a duct. The **ductus deferens** is the *vas deferens.

ductus arteriosus a blood vessel in the fetus connecting the pulmonary artery directly to the ascending aorta, so bypassing the pulmonary circulation. It normally closes after birth. Failure of the ductus to close (**patent ductus arteriosus**) produces a continuous *murmur, and the consequences are similar to those of a *septal defect. It may close spontaneously in childhood but often requires surgical closure.

ductus venosus a blood vessel in the fetus that conveys oxygenated blood from the umbilical vein to the inferior vena cava and right atrium, where it passes through the *foramen ovale to the left atrium and left ventricle.

Dukes' staging a widely accepted histological classification of the extent of tumours of the colon and rectum, which is useful for prognosis. There have been modifications to the original classification. [Sir C. Dukes (1890–1977), British pathologist]

duloxetine *n. see* SNRI.

dumbness *n. see* MUTISM.

Dumdum fever *see* KALA-AZAR.

dumping syndrome a group of symptoms that sometimes occur after operations on the stomach, particularly *gastrectomy (**postgastrectomy syndrome**). In early dumping syndrome debilitating symptoms of abdominal cramps, flushing, sweating, diarrhoea, and palpitations begin about 30 minutes after a meal due to jejunal distension by hypertonic gastric contents. Late dumping syndrome is due to hypoglycaemia occurring 1–2 hours after a meal, especially one rich in carbohydrate. The patient feels faint, weak, and nauseous, has a rapid pulse, and may sweat and become pale. Avoidance of large carbohydrate meals and having small but frequent meals (six a day) may relieve the symptoms but further surgery is sometimes required.

Duncan disease *see* X-LINKED LYMPHO-PROLIFERATIVE SYNDROME. [Duncan family, in whom the disease was first studied]

duo- *combining form denoting* two.

duoden- (**duodeno-**) *combining form denoting* the duodenum. Example: **duodenectomy** (excision of).

duodenal atresia a condition in which the duodenum is narrowed, causing complete obstruction. It presents at birth with

vomiting, which is usually bile-stained, and is associated with other congenital abnormalities, particularly *Down's syndrome. Treatment is correction of any fluid imbalance followed by surgical repair.

duodenal ulcer an ulcer in the duodenum, caused by the action of acid and pepsin on the duodenal lining (mucosa) of a susceptible individual. It is usually associated with an increased output of stomach acid. Infection of the *antrum of the stomach with *Helicobacter pylori* is almost always present. Other causes include ingestion of aspirin or other *NSAIDs. Symptoms include pain in the upper abdomen, especially when the stomach is empty, which often disappears completely for weeks or months; vomiting may occur. Complications include bleeding (*see* HAEMATEMESIS), *perforation, and obstruction due to scarring (*see* PYLORIC STENOSIS). Symptoms are relieved by antacid medicines; most ulcers heal if treated by an *antisecretory drug, or if *H. pylori* is eradicated by a combination of a *proton-pump inhibitor (or an H_2-receptor antagonist) and antibiotics. Surgery (*see* GASTRECTOMY, VAGOTOMY) is now rarely required.

duodenoscope *n.* a fibreoptic or video instrument for examining the interior of the duodenum and for performing *ERCP.

duodenostomy *n.* an operation, now rarely performed, in which the duodenum is brought through the abdominal wall and opened, usually in order to introduce food. *See also* GASTRODUODENOSTOMY.

duodenum *n.* the first of the three parts of the small *intestine. It extends from the pylorus of the stomach to the jejunum. The duodenum receives bile from the gall bladder (via the common bile duct) and pancreatic juice from the pancreas. Its wall contains various glands (including *Brunner's glands) that secrete an alkaline juice, rich in mucus, that protects the duodenum from the effects of the acidic *chyme passing from the stomach. —**duodenal** *adj.*

duplex imaging *see* DOPPLER ULTRA-SOUND.

Dupuytren's contracture a flexion deformity of the fingers (usually the ring and little fingers) caused by a nodular *hypertrophy and *contracture of the *fascia in the palm. The characteristic sign is a nodule at the distal palmar crease or over the proximal phalanx of the finger. The condition is treated by surgical excision of the contracted and thickened tissue. [Baron G. Dupuytren (1777–1835), French surgeon]

dura (dura mater, pachymeninx) *n.* the thickest and outermost of the three *meninges surrounding the brain and spinal cord. It consists of two closely adherent layers, the outer of which is identical with the periosteum of the skull. The inner dura extends downwards between the cerebral hemispheres to form the **falx cerebri** and forwards between the cerebrum and cerebellum to form the **tentorium**. A thin film of fluid (not cerebrospinal fluid) separates the inner dura from the arachnoid.

dural *adj.* of, relating to, or affecting the *dura.

dutasteride *n.* a drug used in the treatment of benign prostatic hyperplasia (*see* PROSTATE GLAND). It is a 5α-reductase inhibitor, which blocks the conversion of testosterone to dihydrotestosterone. It has the same mode of action and side-effects as *finasteride. Trade name: **Avodart**.

duty *n.* what is owed to another person, creating an obligation or moral requirement to behave in one way rather than another. Duty may arise from rules or principles, such as the *four principles of medical ethics, or from particular relationships (e.g. doctor and patient or parent and child). Dilemmas may arise where these duties appear to conflict or are unclearly delineated. The idea of duty as an absolute *imperative that does not vary with circumstances is central to the tradition of *Kantian ethics (*see* DEONTOLOGY). Doctors also have legal duties towards their patients because of their *fiduciary relationship and assume a **duty of care** as soon as they start a consultation. If they fall short of their legal duty of care, doctors may be subject to a claim of negligence.

DVD *see* DISSOCIATED VERTICAL DEVIATION.

DVT (deep vein thrombosis) *see* PHLEBO-THROMBOSIS.

dwarfism *n.* abnormally short stature from any cause. The most common type is **achondroplastic dwarfism** (*see* ACHON-DROPLASIA). **Pituitary dwarfism** results from a deficiency of *growth hormone due to a defect in the pituitary gland; people with this type of dwarfism are well proportioned. **Primordial dwarfism** is due to a genetic defect in the response to growth hormone.

Dwarfism may also be associated with thyroid deficiency (*see* CRETINISM), in which both physical and mental development are arrested; chronic diseases such as rickets; renal failure; and intestinal malabsorption.

dydrogesterone *n.* a synthetic female sex hormone (*see* PROGESTOGEN) used (in conjunction with an oestrogen) in hormone replacement therapy. Dydrogesterone is administered by mouth and may cause mild nausea and breakthrough bleeding.

dynamic splintage a technique that retains the essentials of splinting but allows some controlled movement of the restrained body part.

dynamometer *n.* a device for recording the force of a muscular contraction. A small hand-held dynamometer may be used to record the strength of a patient's grip. A special optical dynamometer measures the action of the muscles controlling the shape of the lens of the eye.

dyne *n.* a unit of force equal to the force required to impart to a mass of 1 gram an acceleration of 1 centimetre per second per second. 1 dyne = 10^{-5} newton.

-dynia *combining form denoting* pain. Example: **proctodynia** (in the rectum).

dys- *prefix denoting* difficult, abnormal, or impaired. Examples: **dysbasia** (difficulty in walking); **dysgeusia** (impairment of taste).

dysaesthesia *n.* the abnormal and sometimes unpleasant sensation felt by a patient with partial damage to sensory nerve fibres when the skin is stimulated. *Compare* PARAESTHESIA.

dysarthria *n.* a speech disorder in which the pronunciation is unclear although the language content and meaning are normal.

dysbarism *n.* any clinical syndrome due to a difference between the atmospheric pressure outside the body and the pressure of air or gas within a body cavity (such as the paranasal sinuses or the middle ear). *See* COMPRESSED AIR ILLNESS.

dyschezia *n.* a form of constipation resulting from a long period of voluntary suppression of the urge to defecate. The rectum becomes distended with faeces and bowel movements are difficult or painful.

dyschondroplasia (Ollier's disease) *n.* a condition due to faulty ossification of cartilage, resulting in development of many benign cartilaginous tumours (*see* CHONDROMA). The bones involved may become stunted and deformed. There is an increased risk of developing malignant tumours (*see* CHONDROSARCOMA).

dyschromatopsia *n.* any defect of colour vision.

dyscoria *n.* any abnormality in the shape of the pupil.

dyscrasia *n.* an abnormal state of the body or part of the body, especially one due to abnormal development or metabolism. In classical medicine the term was used for the imbalance of the four humours (blood, phlegm, yellow bile, black bile), which was believed to be the basic cause of all diseases.

dysdiadochokinesis (adiadochokinesis) *n.* clumsiness in performing rapidly alternating movements. It is often recognized by asking the patient to tap alternately between the front and back of one hand and the back of the other hand. Impairment of this task is indicative of disease of the cerebellum or its intracerebral connections.

dysentery *n.* an infection of the intestinal tract causing severe diarrhoea with blood and mucus. **Amoebic dysentery** (**amoebiasis**) is caused by the protozoan *Entamoeba histolytica* and results in ulceration of the intestines and occasionally in the formation of abscesses in the liver (**amoebic** or **tropical abscesses**), lungs, testes, or brain. The parasite is spread by food or water contaminated by infected faeces. Symptoms appear days or even years after infection and include diarrhoea, indigestion, loss of weight, and anaemia. Prolonged treatment with drugs, including metronidazole, is usually effective in treating the condition. Amoebic dysentery is mainly confined to tropical and subtropical countries.

Bacillary dysentery is caused by bacteria of the genus *Shigella* and is spread by contact with a patient or carrier or through food or water contaminated by their faeces. Epidemics are common in overcrowded insanitary conditions. Symptoms, which develop 1–6 days after infection, include diarrhoea, nausea, cramp, and fever and they persist for about a week. An attack may vary from mild diarrhoea to an acute infection causing serious dehydration and bleeding from the gut. In most cases, provided fluid losses are replaced, recovery occurs within 7–10 days;

antibiotics may be given to eliminate the bacteria. *Compare* CHOLERA.

dysfunctional uterine bleeding *see* MENORRHAGIA.

dysgenesis *n.* faulty development. **Gonadal dysgenesis** is failure of the ovaries or testes to develop (*see* TURNER'S SYNDROME).

dysgerminoma (germinoma, gonocytoma) *n.* a malignant tumour of the ovary, thought to arise from primitive germ cells; it is homologous to the *seminoma of the testis. About 15% of such tumours affect both ovaries; outside the ovary they have been recorded in the anterior mediastinum and in the pineal gland. Dysgerminomas may occur from infancy to old age, but the average age of patients is about 20 years. Treatment is by oophorectomy, with chemotherapy for residual disease.

dysgraphia *n. see* AGRAPHIA.

dyshormonogenesis *n.* a collection of inherited disorders of thyroid hormone synthesis resulting in low levels of *thyroxine and *triiodothyronine and high levels of *thyroid-stimulating hormone, with consequent *goitre formation. The result may be *cretinism with a goitre or milder forms of *hypothyroidism with a goitre. Several different stages of the production pathway for thyroid hormones can be affected.

dyskaryosis *n.* the abnormal condition of a cell that has a nucleus showing the features characteristic of the earliest stage of malignancy, while retaining relatively normal cytoplasm. It may be seen, for example, in the squamous and columnar epithelial cells of a cervical smear (*see* CERVICAL SCREENING).

dyskinesia *n.* a group of involuntary movements that appear to be a fragmentation of the normal smoothly controlled limb and facial movements. They include *chorea, *dystonia, *athetosis, and those involuntary movements occurring as side-effects to the use of levodopa and the phenothiazines (*see* TARDIVE DYSKINESIA).

dyslexia *n.* a developmental disorder selectively affecting a child's ability to learn to read and write. The condition affects boys more often than girls and can create serious educational problems. It is sometimes called **specific dyslexia**, **developmental reading disorder**, or **developmental word blindness** to distinguish it from acquired difficulties with reading and writing. *Compare* ALEXIA. —**dyslexic** *adj.*

dysmenorrhoea *n.* menstruation that is associated with cramping low abdominal pain radiating into the lower back and thighs; the pain sometimes precedes menstrual flow. In **primary dysmenorrhoea** the painful periods begin soon after *menarche and are associated with increased production of *prostaglandin F$_{2\alpha}$ by the endometrium. **Secondary dysmenorrhoea** is caused by organic pelvic disease, such as fibroids or endometriosis.

dysmetabolic syndrome *see* METABOLIC SYNDROME.

dysmetria *n.* impaired coordination due to disorders of the cerebellum or its connections within the brainstem. In the *finger–nose test, the patient's finger over- or undershoots or passes the target because of failure to control the movement accurately.

dysmnesic syndrome a disorder of memory in which new information is not learned but old material is well remembered. *See* KORSAKOFF'S SYNDROME.

dysmorphic *adj.* describing a body characteristic that is abnormally formed. A dysmorphic feature can be a minor isolated feature, such a *clinodactyly, or it may be found in association with other features in more serious syndromes, such as *Down's syndrome.

dysmorphology *n.* the study of *malformations during embryogenesis.

dysmorphophobia (body dysmorphic disorder) *n.* a fixed distressing belief that one's body or part of one's body is deformed and repulsive, or an excessive fear that it might become so.

dysostosis *n.* the abnormal formation of bone or the formation of bone in abnormal places, such as a replacement of cartilage by bone.

dyspareunia *n.* painful sexual intercourse experienced by a woman. It may be related to *vaginismus or caused by underlying disease, such as endometriosis or pelvic inflammatory disease. *See* APAREUNIA.

dyspepsia (indigestion) *n.* disordered digestion: usually applied to pain or discomfort in the lower chest or upper abdomen after eating and sometimes accompanied by

nausea, vomiting, or a feeling of unease or fullness after eating. —**dyspeptic** *adj.*

dysphagia *n.* a condition in which the action of swallowing is either difficult to perform or in which swallowed material seems to be held up in its passage to the stomach, often described by the patient as a sticking sensation (*compare* ODYNOPHAGIA). It can be caused by painful conditions of the mouth and throat, obstruction of the pharynx or oesophagus by diseases of the wall (most seriously oesophageal carcinoma) or pressure from outside, or by abnormalities in the neurological coordination of the muscular activity of the pharynx or oesophagus, as a result of such disorders as motor neuron disease or multiple sclerosis.

dysphasia *n. see* APHASIA.

dysphonia *n.* difficulty in voice production. This may be due to a disorder of the larynx, pharynx, tongue, or mouth, or it may be *psychogenic. *Compare* DYSARTHRIA, APHASIA.

dysplasia (alloplasia, heteroplasia) *n.* a premalignant condition characterized by abnormal development of epithelium, bone, or other tissues. *See also* BRONCHOPULMONARY DYSPLASIA, FIBROUS DYSPLASIA. —**dysplastic** *adj.*

dysplastic kidneys any developmental abnormalities of the kidneys resulting from anomalous metanephric differentiation (*see* METANEPHROS). Most dysplastic kidneys are associated either with an abnormally located ureteral orifice or with urinary tract anomalies that are expected to produce unilateral, bilateral, or segmental urinary obstruction.

dyspnoea *n.* laboured or difficult breathing. (The term is often used for a sign of laboured breathing apparent to the doctor, **breathlessness** being used for the subjective feeling of laboured breathing.) Dyspnoea can be due to obstruction to the flow of air into and out of the lungs (as in bronchitis and asthma), various diseases affecting the tissue of the lung (including pneumoconiosis, emphysema, tuberculosis, and cancer), and heart disease.

dyspraxia *n. see* APRAXIA.

dyssocial *adj. see* ANTISOCIAL PERSONALITY DISORDER.

dysthymia *n.* a permanent state of mildly lowered mood. This never reaches the severity of clinical *depression but it can impair the person's quality of life. It is often associated with *emotionally unstable personality disorder. Treatment options include *psychotherapy and *SSRIs in high doses. —**dysthymic** *adj.*

dystocia *n.* difficult birth, caused by abnormalities in the fetus or the mother (*see* OBSTRUCTED LABOUR). Dystocia may arise due to uterine *inertia, which is more common in a first labour; abnormal fetal lie or presentation; absolute or relative *cephalopelvic disproportion; or (rarely) a massive fetal tumor, such as a sacrococcygeal teratoma. Oxytocin is commonly used to treat uterine inertia. However, pregnancies complicated by dystocia often end with assisted deliveries, including forceps, ventouse, or (commonly) Caesarean section. *See also* SHOULDER DYSTOCIA.

dystonia *n.* muscle dysfunction characterized by spasms or abnormal muscle contraction. One form is a postural disorder often associated with disease of the *basal ganglia in the brain. There may be spasm in the muscles of the face (*see* HEMIFACIAL SPASM), shoulders, neck, trunk, and limbs; the arm is often held in a rotated position and the head may be drawn back and to one side. Other forms of dystonia include *torticollis, *blepharospasm, and writer's *cramp. Dystonic conditions, including blepharospasm, may be helped by the injection of *botulinum toxin. —**dystonic** *adj.*

dystrophia myotonica (myotonic dystrophy) a type of *muscular dystrophy in which the muscle weakness and wasting is accompanied by an unnatural prolongation of the muscular contraction after any voluntary effort (*see* MYOTONIA). The muscles of the face, temples, and neck are especially wasted. Baldness, endocrine malfunction, and cataracts also occur. The disease can affect both sexes (it is inherited as an autosomal *dominant disorder). Genetic testing for mutations in the dystrophia myotonica protein kinase gene is now possible.

dystrophic calcification the calcification of injured or necrotic tissue in the absence of systemic *hypercalcaemia. Dystrophic calcification is a characteristic feature in some cancers of the breast, ovary, and thyroid gland. *Compare* METASTATIC CALCIFICATION.

dystrophy (dystrophia) *n.* a disorder of an organ or tissue, usually muscle, due to impaired nourishment of the affected part. The term is applied to several unrelated conditions; for example, *muscular dystrophy, *Fuchs' endothelial dystrophy, and **dystrophia adiposogenitalis** (*see* FRÖHLICH'S SYNDROME).

dysuria *n.* difficult or painful urination. This is usually associated with urgency and frequency of urination if due to *cystitis or *urethritis. The pain is burning in nature and is relieved by curing the underlying cause. A high fluid intake usually helps.

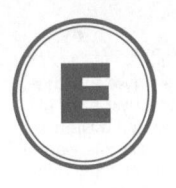

Eagle-Barrett syndrome *see* PRUNE BELLY SYNDROME.

Eales' disease inflammation of the blood vessels of the retina occurring in young adults. It is characterized by leakage from abnormal growths of new vessels as well as recurrent haemorrhages into the vitreous humour. [H. Eales (1852–1913), British physician]

ear *n.* the sense organ concerned with hearing and balance (see illustration). Sound waves, transmitted from the outside into the external auditory meatus, cause the eardrum (tympanic membrane) to vibrate. The small bones (ossicles) of the middle ear – the malleus, incus, and stapes – transmit the sound vibrations to the fenestra ovalis, which leads to the inner ear (*see* LABYRINTH). Inside the *cochlea the sound vibrations are converted into nerve impulses. Vibrations emerging from the cochlea could cause pressure to build up inside the ear, but this is released through the *Eustachian tube. The

*semicircular canals, *saccule, and *utricle – also in the inner ear – are all concerned with balance.

earache *n. see* OTITIS, OTALGIA.

eardrum *n. see* TYMPANIC MEMBRANE.

ear-lobe creases diagonal creases across the ear lobes, which have a statistically significant correlation with coronary atheroma. The reason is unknown.

early neonatal death *see* PERINATAL MORTALITY RATE.

early warning system (EWS) a system to detect deteriorating patients on the ward. Certain physical parameters are accorded scores: the higher the scores for individual patients, the greater the deterioration in their condition. Parameters scored include blood pressure, respiratory rate, pulse rate, blood oxygen saturation, and level of consciousness. Adjustments can be made for increased age.

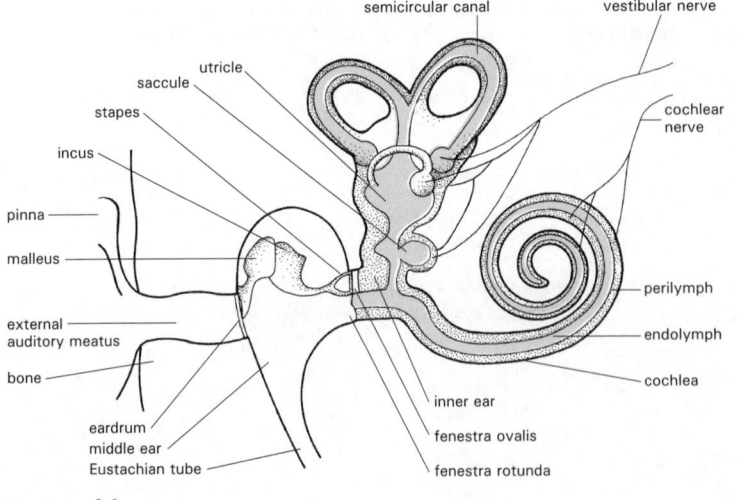

Structure of the ear.

earwax *n. see* CERUMEN.

Ebola virus a virus responsible for an acute infection in humans with features similar to those of *Marburg disease. Transmission is by contact with infected blood and other body fluids and the incubation period is 2–21 days (7 days on average). The mortality rate is 53–88%, but intensive treatment (including rehydration) in the early stages of the disease can halt its rapid and usually irreversible progression to haemorrhaging of internal organs. Sporadic but short-lived outbreaks have occurred in Africa since 1976, when the virus was first identified during an outbreak in the region of the Ebola river, in Zaïre (now Democratic Republic of Congo). An unknown species of animal – possibly a fruit bat – is assumed to act as a reservoir for the virus between outbreaks of the disease in humans.

Ebstein's anomaly a form of congenital heart disease affecting the right side of the heart: the tricuspid valve is displaced towards the apex to a varying extent, resulting in impaired right ventricular function. It can cause breathlessness, *failure to thrive, cyanosis, and abnormalities of heart rhythm, although if mild it may be asymptomatic. If mild, life expectancy is normal. If severe, corrective surgery may be necessary. [W. Ebstein (1836–1912), German physician]

eburnation *n.* the wearing down of the cartilage at the articulating surface of a bone, exposing the underlying bone and leading to bone sclerosis, in which the bone's surface becomes dense and smooth like ivory. This is an end result of *osteoarthritis.

EBV (EB virus) *see* EPSTEIN-BARR VIRUS.

ec- *prefix denoting* out of or outside.

ecbolic *n.* an agent, such as *oxytocin, that induces childbirth by stimulating contractions of the uterus.

ecchondroma *n.* (*pl.* **ecchondromata**) a benign cartilaginous tumour (*see* CHONDROMA) that protrudes beyond the margins of a bone. *Compare* ENCHONDROMA.

ecchymosis *n.* a *bruise: an initially bluish-black mark on the skin, resulting from the release of blood into the tissues either through injury or through the spontaneous leaking of blood from the vessels (as in some blood diseases).

eccrine *adj.* **1.** describing sweat glands that are distributed all over the body. Their ducts open directly onto the surface of the skin and they are densest on the soles of the feet and the palms of the hands. *Compare* APOCRINE. **2.** *see* MEROCRINE.

ecdemic *adj.* not occurring normally in the population of a country: applied sometimes to unusual diseases brought in from abroad by immigrants or travellers. *Compare* ENDEMIC.

ecdysis *n.* the act of shedding skin; *desquamation.

ECG *n. see* ELECTROCARDIOGRAM.

echinocacciasis (echinococcosis) *n. see* HYDATID DISEASE.

Echinococcus *n.* a genus of small parasitic tapeworms that reach a maximum length of only 8 mm. Adults are found in the intestines of dogs, wolves, or jackals. If the eggs are swallowed by a human, who can act as a secondary host, the resulting larvae penetrate the intestine and settle in the lungs, liver, or brain to form large cysts, usually 5–10 cm in diameter (*see* HYDATID DISEASE). Two species causing this condition are *E. granulosus* and *E. multilocularis.*

echoacousia *n.* a false sensation of echoing after normally heard sound owing to a defect of the cochlea in the inner ear.

echocardiography *n.* the use of *ultrasound waves to investigate and display the action of the heart as it beats. Used in the diagnosis and assessment of congenital and acquired heart diseases, it is safe, painless, and reliable and reduces the need for cardiac *catheterization. **M-mode echocardiography** uses a single beam of ultrasound. The image produced is not anatomical but permits precise measurement of cardiac dimensions and the diagnosis of valvular, myocardial, and pericardial disease. **2-D echocardiography** uses a pulsed array of ultrasound beams to build up a moving image on a TV monitor of the chambers and valves of the heart. In **Doppler echocardiography** ultrasound reflected from moving red blood cells is subject to the Doppler effect (change of frequency with velocity relative to the observer), which can be used to calculate blood flow and pressure within the heart and great vessels. It is useful in the diagnosis and assessment of valve disease and intracardiac shunts. In **transoesophageal echocardiography** (**TOE**) the ultrasound probe is mounted on an oesophageal endoscope. The examination from within the oesophagus allows the probe to be placed directly against the back of the heart, which enables improved visualization of the posterior structures.

echo de la pensée *see* THOUGHT ECHO.

echokinesis *n. see* ECHOPRAXIA.

echolalia *n.* pathological repetition of the words spoken by another person. It may be a symptom of language disorders, *autism, severe mental illness (e.g. catatonic schizophrenia), dementia, or *Tourette's syndrome.

echopraxia (echokinesis) *n.* pathological imitation of the actions of another person. It may be a symptom of *catatonia or of *latah.

echovirus *n.* one of a group of about 30 RNA-containing viruses, originally isolated from the human intestinal tract, that were found to produce pathological changes in cells grown in culture, although they were not clearly associated with any specific disease. These viruses – which were accordingly termed *e*nteric *c*ytopathic *h*uman *o*rphan viruses – are now more commonly known as *Coxsackie viruses. *Compare* REOVIRUS.

eclabium *n.* the turning outward of a lip.

eclampsia *n.* the occurrence of one or more convulsions not caused by other conditions, such as epilepsy or cerebral haemorrhage, in a woman with *pre-eclampsia. The onset of convulsions may be preceded by a sudden rise in blood pressure and/or a sudden increase in *oedema and development of *oliguria. The convulsions are usually followed by coma. Eclampsia is a threat to both mother and baby and must be treated immediately.

ECMO *see* EXTRACORPOREAL MEMBRANE OXYGENATION.

ECoG *see* ELECTROCOCHLEOGRAPHY.

ecology (bionomics) *n.* the study of the relationships between humans, plants and animals, and the environment, including the way in which human activities may affect other animal populations and alter natural surroundings. —**ecological** *adj.* —**ecologist** *n.*

econazole *n.* an antifungal drug used to treat ringworm and candidiasis. It is administered as a cream or vaginal pessary. Possible side-effects may include local irritation and burning. Trade names: **Ecostatin, Gyno-Pevaryl, Pevaryl**.

ecraseur *n.* a surgical device, resembling a *snare, that is used to sever the base of a tumour during its surgical removal.

ecstasy *n.* a sense of extreme wellbeing and bliss. The word applies particularly to *trance states dominated by religious thinking. While not necessarily pathological, it can be caused by epilepsy (especially of the temporal lobe) or by *schizophrenia or *mania.

Ecstasy *n.* the street name for methylene-dioxymethamphetamine (MDMA), a mildly hallucinogenic drug that generates feelings of euphoria in those who take it. Its most common side-effect is hyperthermia; drinking large quantities of water to combat the intense thirst produced by taking the drug may result in fatal damage to the body's fluid balance. Its manufacture, sale, use, and possession are illegal.

ECT *see* ELECTROCONVULSIVE THERAPY.

ect- (ecto-) *combining form denoting* outer or external.

ectasia (ectasis) *n.* the dilatation of a tube, duct, or hollow organ.

ecthyma *n.* an infection of the skin caused by *Streptococcus pyogenes, Staphylococcus aureus*, and other bacteria. The full thickness of the epidermis is involved (*compare* IMPETIGO, which is a superficial infection). Ecthyma heals slowly and causes scarring. It may be associated with poor hygiene or depressed immunity.

ectoderm *n.* the outer of the three *germ layers of the early embryo. It gives rise to the nervous system and sense organs, the teeth and lining of the mouth, and to the *epidermis and its associated structures (hair, nails, etc.). —**ectodermal** *adj.*

ectomorphic *adj.* describing a *body type that is relatively thin, with a large skin surface in comparison to weight. —**ectomorph** *n.* —**ectomorphy** *n.*

-ectomy *combining form denoting* surgical removal of a segment or all of an organ or part. Examples: **appendicectomy** (of the appendix); **prostatectomy** (of the prostate gland).

ectoparasite *n.* a parasite that lives on the outer surface of its host. Some ectoparasites, such as bed bugs, maintain only periodic contact with their hosts, whereas others, such as the crab louse, have a permanent association. *Compare* ENDOPARASITE.

ectopia *n*. 1. the misplacement, due either to a congenital defect or injury, of a bodily part. 2. the occurrence of something in an unnatural location (*see also* ECTOPIC BEAT, ECTOPIC PREGNANCY). —**ectopic** *adj*.

ectopic beat (extrasystole) a heartbeat due to an impulse generated somewhere in the heart outside the sinoatrial node. Ectopic beats are generally premature in timing; they are classified as **supraventricular** if they originate in the atria and **ventricular** if they arise from a focus in the ventricles. They may be produced by any heart disease, by nicotine from smoking, or by caffeine from excessive tea or coffee consumption; they are common in normal individuals. The patient may be unaware of their presence or may feel that his heart has 'missed a beat'. Ectopic beats may be suppressed by drugs such as quinidine, propranolol, and lidocaine; avoidance of smoking and reduction in excessive tea or coffee intake may help. *See* ARRHYTHMIA.

ectopic hormone a hormone produced by cells that do not usually produce it. Some tumour cells secrete hormones; for example, small-cell lung cancer cells secrete antidiuretic hormone and cause *hyponatraemia.

ectopic pregnancy (extrauterine pregnancy) the implantation of a fertilized egg cell at a site outside the uterus. This may happen if the fertilized egg cell remains in the ovary or in the Fallopian tube or if it lodges in the free abdominal cavity. The most common type of ectopic pregnancy is a **tubal pregnancy**, which occurs in Fallopian tubes that become blocked or inflamed. The growth of the fetus may cause the tube to rupture and bleed, causing severe haemorrhage. Early detection of the condition (e.g. by monitoring serum *human chorionic gonadotrophin and *transvaginal ultrasonography) allows conservative treatment in many cases; medical treatment, which preserves fertility, may also be possible. Laparoscopic surgery is the preferred surgical treatment.

ectoplasm *n*. the outer layer of cytoplasm in cells, which is denser than the inner cytoplasm (*endoplasm) and concerned with activities such as cell movement. —**ectoplasmic** *adj*.

ectro- *combining form denoting* congenital absence.

ectrodactyly *n*. congenital absence of all or part of one or more fingers.

ectromelia *n*. congenital absence or gross shortening (aplasia) of the long bones of one or more limbs. *See also* AMELIA, HEMIMELIA, PHOCOMELIA.

ectropion *n*. 1. turning out of the eyelid, away from the eyeball. The commonest type is **senile ectropion**, in which the lower eyelid droops because of laxity of the eyelid in old age. If the muscle that closes the eye (orbicularis oculi) is paralysed the lower lid also droops. Ectropion may also occur if scarring causes contraction of the surrounding facial skin. 2. (cervical ectopy) the replacement of the stratified squamous epithelium that normally lines the vaginal part of the cervix (ectocervix) by columnar epithelium, which has migrated from the *endocervix. As a result, the junction of squamous and columnar epithelia does not coincide with the opening of the cervix into the uterus. Cervical ectropion is caused by exposure to higher levels of oestrogen, which occurs normally at certain times (e.g. at puberty or in pregnancy) or with *anovulation. It usually causes no symptoms but in a few cases may be associated with postcoital bleeding and a mucoid vaginal discharge.

eczema *n*. a common itchy skin disease characterized by reddening (*erythema) and vesicle formation, which may lead to weeping and crusting. It is endogenous, or constitutional, i.e. outside agents do not play a primary role (*compare* DERMATITIS), but in some contexts the terms 'dermatitis' and 'eczema' are used interchangeably. There are five main types: (1) **atopic eczema**, which affects up to 20% of the population and is associated with asthma and hay fever; (2) **seborrhoeic eczema** (or **seborrhoeic dermatitis**), which involves the scalp, eyelids, nose, and lips, is associated with the presence of *Malassezia* yeasts and may also be seen in HIV infection; (3) **discoid** (or **nummular**) **eczema**, which is characterized by coin-shaped lesions and occurs in adults, especially on the limbs; (4) *pompholyx, affecting the palms and soles; (5) **gravitational** (or **stasis**) **eczema**, associated with poor venous circulation and incorrectly known as **varicose eczema**.

Treatment of eczema is with regular emollients and topical corticosteroids. Other treatments include topical *calcineurin inhibitors, phototherapy, and systemic immunosuppressants. There is emerging evidence that effective treatment of eczema helps to reduce the risk of subsequently developing asthma and hay fever. —**eczematous** adj.

eczema herpeticum (Kaposi's varicelliform eruption) a skin eruption, typically in children or young adults, of widespread *vesicles and ulcers caused by *herpes simplex. This is due to impaired barrier function in skin with eczema. Clinical features include fever, malaise, and lymphadenopathy. Rarely, the infection may become systemic and be life-threatening. Eczema herpeticum is commonly misdiagnosed as a bacterial infection. Treatment is with systemic antivirals and hospitalization may be required.

ED emergency department, also known as **A and E** (accident and emergency department): a hospital department that assesses and deals with the immediate problems of acutely ill and injured patients. *See also* A AND E MEDICINE.

edentulous adj. lacking teeth: usually applied to people who have lost some or all of their teeth.

edetate n. a salt of **ethylenediaminetetraacetic acid** (**EDTA**), which is used as a *chelating agent in the treatment of poisoning. **Dicobalt edetate** is an antidote to cyanide, administered by intravenous injection as soon as possible after poisoning. **Sodium calcium edetate** (Ledclair) is used to treat poisoning by heavy metals, especially lead; it is administered by intravenous infusion.

edrophonium n. an *anticholinesterase drug that is used after surgery to reverse the effects of nondepolarizing *muscle relaxants and in a test for diagnosis of *myasthenia gravis. It is administered by injection; side-effects can include nausea and vomiting, increased saliva flow, diarrhoea, and stomach pains.

EDTA (ethylenediaminetetraacetic acid) *see* EDETATE.

Edwards' syndrome a condition resulting from a genetic abnormality in which an extra chromosome is present – there are three no. 18 chromosomes instead of the usual two. Affected babies, who rarely survive, have a characteristic abnormally shaped head, low birth weight, prominent heels ('rocker-bottom feet'), heart abnormalities, and severe mental retardation. Prenatal screening (by *nuchal translucency scanning) and diagnosis (by *amniocentesis or *chorionic villus sampling) are possible. [J. H. Edwards (1928–), British geneticist]

EECP *see* ENHANCED EXTERNAL COUNTERPULSATION.

EEG (electroencephalogram) *see* ELECTROENCEPHALOGRAPHY.

EF *see* EJECTION FRACTION.

efalizumab n. a *monoclonal antibody used in the treatment of severe psoriasis that has not responded to orally administered drugs or to *PUVA; it inhibits activation of T *lymphocytes. Efalizumab is administered by subcutaneous injection; side-effects include flulike symptoms. Trade name: **Raptiva**.

effector n. any structure or agent that brings about activity in a muscle or gland, such as a motor nerve that causes muscular contraction or glandular secretion. The term is also used for the muscle or gland itself.

efferent adj. 1. designating nerves or neurons that convey impulses from the brain or spinal cord to muscles, glands, and other effectors; i.e. any motor nerve or neuron. 2. designating vessels or ducts that drain fluid (such as lymph) from an organ or part. *Compare* AFFERENT.

effleurage n. a form of *massage in which the hands are passed continuously and rhythmically over a patient's skin in one direction only, with the aim of increasing blood flow in that direction and aiding the dispersal of any swelling due to *oedema.

effusion n. 1. the escape of pus, serum, blood, lymph, or other fluid into a body cavity as a result of inflammation or the presence of excess blood or tissue fluid in an organ or tissue. 2. fluid that has escaped into a body cavity. Such effusions may be exudates (rich in protein) or transudates (low in protein).

eformoterol n. *see* FORMOTEROL.

eGFR estimated *glomerular filtration rate. Most estimates in clinical practice are based on the serum creatinine, age, gender, and race, with or without body weight. Examples are the *Cockcroft-Gault formula and **MDRD eGFR** (modification of diet in renal disease study method of estimating glomerular filtration rate).

EGFR *see* EPIDERMAL GROWTH FACTOR RECEPTOR.

egg cell *see* OVUM.

egg donation *see* OOCYTE DONATION.

ego *n.* (in psychoanalysis) the part of the mind that develops from a person's experience of the outside world and is most in touch with external realities. In Freudian terms the ego is said to reconcile the demands of the *id (the instinctive unconscious mind), the *superego (moral conscience), and reality.

Ehlers-Danlos syndrome any one of a rare group of inherited (autosomal *dominant or autosomal *recessive) disorders of the connective tissue involving abnormal or deficient *collagen, the protein that gives the body tissues strength. There are several types of differing severity. The skin of affected individuals is very elastic but also very fragile: it bruises easily and scars poorly, the scars often being paper-thin. The joints of those affected tend to be very mobile (double-jointed) and dislocate easily. In some types the uterus or bowel can rupture or the valves in the heart can be weaker than normal. [E. L. Ehlers (1863–1937), Danish dermatologist; H. A. Danlos (1844–1912), French dermatologist]

eidetic *adj. see* IMAGERY.

eikonometer *n.* an instrument for measuring the size of images on the retina of the eye.

Eisenmenger reaction (Eisenmenger syndrome) a condition in which *pulmonary hypertension is associated with a *septal defect, so that blood flows from the right to the left side of the heart or from the pulmonary artery to the aorta. This allows blue blood, poor in oxygen, to bypass the lungs and enter the general circulation. This reduces the oxygen content of the arterial blood in the aorta and its branches, resulting in a patient with a dusky blue appearance (*cyanosis) and an increased number of red blood cells (*polycythaemia). There is no curative treatment at this stage, but the patient may be helped by the control of heart failure

and polycythaemia. The condition may be prevented by appropriate treatment of the septal defect in early childhood before irreversible pulmonary hypertension develops. [V. Eisenmenger (1864–1932), German physician]

ejaculation *n.* the discharge of semen from the erect penis at the moment of sexual climax (orgasm) in the male. The constituents of semen are not released simultaneously, but in the following sequence: the secretion of *Cowper's glands followed by that of the *prostate gland and the spermatozoa and finally the secretion of the *seminal vesicles. *See also* PREMATURE EJACULATION.

ejection fraction (EF) the proportion or percentage of blood in the left *ventricle that is ejected with each heartbeat. It is commonly used to quantify left ventricular function, the normal value being 50% or greater.

Ekbom's syndrome 1. *see* RESTLESS LEGS SYNDROME. 2. *see* DELUSIONAL INFESTATION. [K. A. Ekbom (1907–77), Swedish neurologist]

elastic cartilage a type of *cartilage in which elastic fibres are distributed in the matrix. It is yellowish in colour and is found in the external ear.

elastic tissue strong extensible flexible *connective tissue rich in yellow **elastic fibres**. These fibres are long, thin, and branching and are composed primarily of an albumin-like protein, **elastin**. Elastic tissue is found in the dermis of the skin, in arterial walls, and in the walls of the alveoli of the lungs.

elastin *n.* protein forming the major constituent of *elastic tissue fibres.

elastography *n.* an ultrasonic imaging technique that displays the elasticity of soft tissues, most commonly using *ultrasound although *magnetic resonance imaging can be used to gather similar information. It has been found useful in demonstrating abnormalities of muscle, liver, and breast tissue.

elastosis *n.* degeneration of the yellow fibres in connective tissues and skin (*see* ELASTIC TISSUE).

elation (exaltation) *n.* a state of cheerful excitement and enthusiasm. Marked elation of mood is a characteristic of *mania or *hypomania.

elbow *n.* the hinge joint (*see* GINGLYMUS) between the bones of the upper arm (humerus) and the forearm (radius and ulna). It is a common site of fractures and dislocation.

electrocardiogram (ECG) *n.* a tracing of the electrical activity of the heart recorded by *electrocardiography (see illustration). It aids in the diagnosis of heart disease, which may produce characteristic changes in the ECG. *See* QRS COMPLEX, Q–T INTERVAL, S–T SEGMENT.

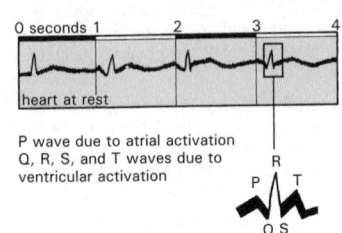

P wave due to atrial activation
Q, R, S, and T waves due to ventricular activation

A typical electrocardiogram.

electrocardiography *n.* a technique for recording the electrical activity of the heart. Electrodes connected to the recording apparatus (**electrocardiograph**) are placed on the skin of the four limbs and chest wall; the record itself is called an *electrocardiogram (ECG). In conventional **scalar electrocardiography** 12 leads (*see* LEAD²) are recorded, but more may be employed in special circumstances (for example, an oesophageal lead, from an electrode within the gullet, may be used in the analysis of arrhythmias).

electrocardiophonography *n.* a technique for recording heart sounds and murmurs simultaneously with the ECG, which is used as a reference tracing. The sound is picked up by a microphone placed over the heart. The tracing is a **phonocardiogram**. It provides a permanent record of heart sounds and murmurs and is useful in their analysis.

electrocautery *n.* the destruction of diseased or unwanted tissue by means of a needle or snare that is electrically heated. Warts, polyps, and other growths can be burned away by this method.

electrocoagulation *n.* the coagulation of body tissues by means of a high-frequency electric current concentrated at one point as

it passes through them. Electrocoagulation, using a *diathermy knife, permits bloodless incisions to be made during operation.

electrocochleography (ECoG) *n.* a test to measure electrical activity produced within the *cochlea in response to a sound stimulus. It is used in the diagnosis of Ménière's disease and other forms of sensorineural *deafness.

electroconvulsive therapy (ECT) a treatment for severe depression and occasionally for *puerperal psychosis and *mania. A convulsion is produced by passing an electric current through the brain. The convulsion is modified by giving a *muscle relaxant drug and an *anaesthetic, so that in fact only a few muscle twitches are produced. The procedure can temporarily cause confusion, loss of memory, and headache, which almost always pass off within a few hours. These side-effects are reduced by unilateral treatment, in which the current is passed only through the nondominant hemisphere of the brain. A course of ECT usually entails between 6 and 10 treatments; sometimes up to 16 treatments are given to achieve remission of depression. ECT is effective in about 50% of patients in whom no other treatment was successful, but the beneficial effect on mood does not always last. Occasionally **maintenance ECT** (usually involving one treatment every 2–4 weeks) is given to avoid relapse after a completed course of ECT. Under the Mental Health Acts 1983 and 2007, special legal provision applies to ECT.

electrodesiccation *n.* *see* FULGURATION.

electroencephalogram (EEG) *n.* *see* ELECTROENCEPHALOGRAPHY.

electroencephalography *n.* the technique for recording the electrical activity from different parts of the brain and converting it into a tracing called an **electroencephalogram (EEG)**. The machine that records this activity is known as an **encephalograph**. The pattern of the EEG reflects the state of the patient's brain and his level of consciousness in a characteristic manner. Electroencephalography is mostly used in the diagnosis and management of epilepsy and sleep disorders.

electroglottography *n.* a method of assessing laryngeal function using external recording electrodes.

electrokymography *n.* the technique of recording the movements of an organ, especially the heart, by means of a *fluoroscope and a photoelectric recording system.

electrolarynx *n.* a battery-powered electrical vibrator that helps people to speak after *laryngectomy.

electrolyte *n.* a solution that produces ions (an ion is an atom or group of atoms that conduct electricity); for example, sodium chloride solution consists of free sodium and free chloride ions. In medical usage electrolyte usually means the ion itself; thus the term **serum electrolyte level** means the concentration of separate ions (sodium, potassium, chloride, bicarbonate, etc.) in the circulating blood. Concentrations of various electrolyte levels can be altered by many diseases, in which electrolytes are lost from the body (as in vomiting or diarrhoea) or are not excreted and accumulate (as in renal failure). When electrolyte concentrations are severely diminished they can be corrected by administering the appropriate substance by mouth or by intravenous drip. When excess of an electrolyte exists it may be removed by *dialysis or by special resins in the intestine, taken by mouth or by enema. *See also* ANION.

electromyography *n.* continuous recording of the electrical activity of a muscle by means of electrodes inserted into the muscle fibres. The tracing is displayed on an oscilloscope. The technique is used for diagnosing various nerve and muscle disorders and assessing progress in recovery from some forms of paralysis.

electron microscope a microscope that uses a beam of electrons as a radiation source for viewing the specimen. The resolving power (ability to register fine detail) is a thousand times greater than that of an ordinary light microscope. The specimen must be examined in a vacuum, which necessitates special techniques for preparing it, and the electrons are usually focused onto a fluorescent screen (for direct viewing) or onto a photographic plate (for a photograph, or **electron micrograph**). A **transmission electron microscope** is used to examine thin sections at high magnification. A **scanning electron microscope** reveals the surfaces of objects at various magnifications; its great depth of focus is advantageous.

electron transport chain a series of en-zymes and proteins in living cells through which electrons are transferred, via a series of oxidation-reduction reactions. This ultimately leads to the conversion of chemical energy into a readily usable and storable form. The most important electron transport chain is the **respiratory chain**, present in mitochondria and functioning in cellular respiration.

electronvolt *n.* a unit of energy (symbol: eV) equal to the increase in the energy of an electron when it passes through a rise in potential of one volt. In clinical imaging, the energy of gamma rays is usually expressed in **kiloelectronvolts** (symbol: kV; 1 kV = 1000 eV).

electrooculography *n.* a method of recording eye movements and to assess the resting potential of the retina. Tiny electrodes are attached to the skin at the inner and outer corners of the eye, and as the eye moves an alteration in the potential between these electrodes is recorded. The recording itself is called an **electrooculogram** (**EOG**).

electrophoresis *n.* the technique of separating electrically charged particles, particularly proteins, in a solution by passing an electric current through the solution. The rate of movement of the different components depends upon their charge, so that they gradually separate into bands. Electrophoresis is widely used in the investigation of body chemicals, such as the analysis of the different proteins in blood serum.

electrophysiological study (**EPS**) an assessment of the electrical system of the heart by means of thin preshaped wires passed into the heart via the femoral vein. An *electrocardiogram is recorded from various points within the heart, and the reaction of the heart to timed electrical stimuli is observed. The information obtained guides treatment of arrhythmia, particularly *radiofrequency ablation.

electroretinography *n.* a method of recording changes in the electrical potential of the retina when it is stimulated by light; the recording itself is called an **electroretinogram** (**ERG**). One electrode is placed on the eye in a contact lens and the other is usually attached to the back of the head. In retinal disease the pattern of electrical change is altered. The technique is useful in diagnosing retinal diseases when opacities, such as cataract, make it difficult to view the retina or when the disease produces little visible change in the retina.

electrosurgery *n.* the use of a high-frequency electric current from a fine wire electrode (a *diathermy knife) to cut tissue. The ground electrode is a large metal plate. When used correctly, little heat spreads to the surrounding tissues, in contrast to *electrocautery.

electrotherapy *n.* the passage of electric currents through the body's tissues to stimulate the functioning of nerves and the muscles that they supply. The technique is used to treat the muscles of patients with various forms of paralysis due to nerve disease or muscle disorder. *See also* FARADISM, GALVANISM.

electuary *n.* a pharmaceutical preparation in which the drug is made up into a paste with syrup or honey.

elephantiasis *n.* gross enlargement of the skin and underlying connective tissues caused by obstruction of the lymph vessels, which prevents drainage of lymph from the surrounding tissues. Inflammation and thickening of the walls of the vessels and their eventual blocking is commonly caused by the parasitic filarial worms *Wuchereria bancrofti* and *Brugia malayi*. The parts most commonly affected are the legs but the scrotum, breasts, and vulva may also be involved. Elastic bandaging is applied to the affected parts and the limbs are elevated and rested. Larval forms in the blood are killed with diethylcarbamazine. *See also* FILARIASIS.

elevator *n.* **1.** an instrument that is used to raise a depressed broken bone, for example in the skull or cheek. A specialized **periosteal elevator** is used in orthopaedics to strip the fibrous tissue (periosteum) covering bone. **2.** a lever-like instrument used to ease a tooth or root out of its socket during extraction.

elimination *n.* (in physiology) the entire process of excretion of metabolic waste products from the blood by the kidneys and urinary tract.

ELISA *see* ENZYME-LINKED IMMUNOSORBENT ASSAY.

ELISPOT *e*nzyme-*l*inked *i*mmunosorbent *spot* assay, used in monitoring the immune response. It specifically enumerates *cytokine-producing cells. Each spot that develops in the assay represents a single reactive cell.

elixir *n.* a preparation containing alcohol (ethanol) or glycerine, which is used as the vehicle for bitter or nauseous drugs.

elliptocytosis *n.* the presence of significant numbers of abnormal elliptical red cells (**elliptocytes**) in the blood. Elliptocytosis may occur as a hereditary disorder or be a feature of certain blood diseases, such as *myelofibrosis or iron-deficiency *anaemia.

Elschnig pearls round or oval transparent cystic structures on the posterior capsule due to proliferation of lens epithelial cells following extracapsular *cataract extraction. They can grow to occlude the pupil and cause reduction in vision. [A. Elschnig (1863–1939), German ophthalmologist]

elutriation *n.* the separation of a fine powder from a coarser powder by mixing them with water and decanting the upper layer while it still contains the finer particles. The heavier coarse particles sink to the bottom more rapidly.

em- *prefix. see* EN-.

emaciation *n.* wasting of the body, caused by such conditions as malnutrition, tuberculosis, cancer, or parasitic worms.

emasculation *n.* strictly, surgical removal of the penis. The term is often used to mean loss of male physical and emotional characteristics, either as a result of removal of the testes (castration) or of emotional stress.

embalming *n.* the preservation of a dead body by the introduction of chemical compounds that delay putrefaction. Embalming is employed mainly so that a body can be transported long distances and funeral rites can be conducted without undue haste. In the USA it is a routine hygienic measure.

embedding *n.* (in microscopy) the fixing of a specimen within a mass of firm material in order to facilitate the cutting of thin sections for microscopical study. The embedding medium, e.g. paraffin wax for light microscopy or Araldite for electron microscopy, helps to keep the specimen intact.

embolectomy *n.* surgical removal of an *embolus in order to relieve arterial obstruction. The embolus may be removed by cutting directly into the affected artery (**arteriotomy**). In some instances it is removed by a balloon *catheter, which is manipulated beyond the embolus from a small arteriotomy in an accessible artery. The catheter is then withdrawn carrying the embolus with it. In some cases of pulmonary embolism, embolectomy may be life saving. It may also prevent gangrene in cases of a limb artery embolus.

embolism *n.* the condition in which an embolus becomes lodged in an artery and obstructs its blood flow. The most common form of embolism is *pulmonary embolism, in which a blood clot is carried in the circulation to lodge in the pulmonary artery. An embolus in any other artery constitutes a **systemic embolism**. In this case a common source of the embolus is a blood clot within the heart in mitral valve disease or following *myocardial infarction. The clinical features depend upon the site at which an embolus lodges (for example, a stroke may result from a cerebral embolism and gangrene caused by a limb embolism). Treatment is by *anticoagulant therapy with heparin and warfarin. Major embolism is treated by *embolectomy or *thrombolysis to remove or dissolve the embolus. *See also* AIR EMBOLISM.

embolization (therapeutic embolization) *n.* the introduction of embolic material to reduce or completely obstruct blood flow in such conditions as congenital arteriovenous malformations (*see* ANGIOMA), angiodysplasia, malignant tumours, or arterial rupture. Under X-ray screening control, a catheter is guided to the artery supplying the affected area and occluding material, such as microspheres, metallic coils, or PVA (polyvinyl alcohol) foam, is injected. The procedure may treat the underlying problem or simplify subsequent surgery. *See also* UTERINE ARTERY EMBOLIZATION.

embolus *n.* (*pl.* **emboli**) material, such as a blood clot, fat, air, amniotic fluid, or a foreign body, that is carried by the blood from one point in the circulation to lodge at another point (*see* EMBOLISM).

embrasure *n.* the space formed between adjacent teeth.

embrocation *n.* a lotion rubbed onto the body to treat sprains and strains.

embryo *n.* an animal at an early stage of development, before birth. In humans the term refers to the products of conception within the uterus up to the eighth week of development, during which time all the main organs are formed (see illustration). *Compare* FETUS. —**embryonic** *adj.*

embryology *n.* the study of growth and development of the embryo and fetus from fertilization of the ovum until birth. —**embryological** *adj.*

embryonic disc the early embryo before the formation of *somites. It is a flat disc of tissue bounded dorsally by the amniotic cav-

An embryo.

ity and ventrally by the yolk sac. The formation of the *primitive streak and *archenteron in the embryonic disc determines the orientation of the embryo, which then becomes progressively elongated.

embryo transfer the transfer of an embryo from an in vitro culture into the uterus. *See also* IN VITRO FERTILIZATION.

EMDR *see* EYE MOVEMENT DESENSITIZATION AND REPROCESSING THERAPY.

emergency contraception *see* POST-COITAL CONTRACEPTION.

emesis *n. see* VOMITING.

emetic *n.* an agent that causes vomiting. Substances such as common salt, which irritate the stomach nerves if taken in sufficient quantities, cause vomiting. Some emetics, e.g. *ipecacuanha, are used as *expectorants at low doses.

eminence *n.* a projection, often rounded, on an organ or tissue, particularly on a bone. An example is the **iliopubic eminence** on the hip bone.

emissary veins a group of veins within the skull that drain blood from the venous sinuses of the dura mater to veins outside the skull.

emission *n.* the flow of semen from the erect penis, usually occurring while the subject is asleep (**nocturnal emission**).

EMLA cream a cream containing a *e*utectic *m*ixture of *l*ocal *a*naesthetics (*lidocaine and *prilocaine; hence the name). Applied to the skin as a thick coating and left on for 90 minutes, it gives a helpful degree of local anaesthesia, allowing blood samples to be taken and facilitating biopsy procedures in young children.

emmetropia *n.* the state of refraction of the normal eye, in which parallel light rays are brought to a focus on the retina with the accommodation relaxed. Distant objects are seen clearly without any effort to focus. *Compare* AMETROPIA, HYPERMETROPIA, MYOPIA.

emollient *n.* an agent that soothes and softens the skin. Emollients are fats and oils, such as lanolin and liquid paraffin; they are used alone as moisturizers to lessen the need for active drug therapy (such as corticosteroids for eczema) and in skin preparations as a base for a more active drug, such as an antibiotic.

emotion *n.* a state of arousal that can be experienced as pleasant or unpleasant. Emotions can have three components: **subjective**, **physiological**, and **behavioural**. For example, fear can involve an unpleasant subjective experience, an increase in physiological measures such as heart rate, sweating, etc., and a tendency to flee from the fear-provoking situation.

emotionally unstable personality disorder a *personality disorder characterized by a tendency to act impulsively without consideration of the consequences, unpredictable and capricious mood, a tendency towards outbursts of emotion, inability to control behavioural explosions, quarrelsome behaviour, and conflict with others. There is an **impulsive type**, with particular emphasis on impulsivity and quarrelsome behaviour, especially when criticized; and a **borderline type**, with an emphasis on disturbance and uncertainty about self-image (including sexual preference), liability to become involved in intense and unstable relationships, excessive efforts to avoid abandonment, recurrent threats or acts of self-harm, and chronic feelings of emptiness. Treatments include cognitive analytical therapy (*see* COGNITIVE THERAPY), *antipsychotic medication, and occasionally *SSRIs and *lithium.

empathy *n.* the ability to imagine and understand the thoughts, perspective, and emotions of another person. In counselling and psychotherapy empathy is often considered to be one of the necessary qualities enabling a successful therapeutic relationship. *See also* ALEXITHYMIA.

emphysema *n.* air in the tissues. In **pulmonary emphysema** the air sacs (*alveoli) of the lungs are enlarged and damaged, which reduces the surface area for the exchange of oxygen and carbon dioxide. Severe emphysema causes breathlessness, which is made worse by infections. There is no specific treatment, and the patient may become dependent on oxygen. The mechanism by which emphysema develops is not understood, although it is known to be particularly common in men in Britain and is associated with chronic bronchitis, smoking, and advancing age. *See also* CHRONIC OBSTRUCTIVE PULMONARY DISEASE.

In **surgical emphysema** air may escape into the tissues of the chest and neck from leaks in the lungs or oesophagus; occasionally air escapes into other tissues during surgery, and bacteria may form gas in soft tissues. The presence of air or gas gives the affected tissues a characteristic crackling feeling to the touch, and it may be visible on X-rays. When air moves to the mediastinum the condition is known as *pneumomediastinum. It is easily absorbed once the leak or production is stopped.

empirical *adj.* describing a system of treatment based on experience or observation, rather than of logic or reason.

employment and support allowance the allowance payable to people under state retirement age who are unable to work because of illness or disability; it replaced *incapacity benefit in 2008. Entitlement depends on either an adequate record of National Insurance contributions or satisfying income-related criteria. An assessment-phase allowance is paid during the first 13 weeks of a claim, and eligible claimants are paid the main-phase rate following a work capability assessment.

empty sella syndrome a congenital malformation of the bony structure (the *sella turcica) that houses the pituitary gland such that the space is largely filled with cerebrospinal fluid, which squashes the usually spherical gland into a flattened shape against the floor of the sella. It is usually associated with enlargement of the sella, which can be seen on lateral X-ray. Only 10% of cases of this condition have defective pituitary function.

empyema (pyothorax) *n.* pus in the *pleural cavity, usually secondary to infection in the lung or in the space below the diaphragm. Empyema is a life-threatening condition, which can be relieved by aspiration or drainage of the pus or by decapsulation (*see* DECORTICATION).

emulsion *n.* a preparation in which fine droplets of one liquid (such as oil) are dispersed in another liquid (such as water). In pharmacy medicines are prepared in the form of emulsions to disguise the taste of an oil, which is dispersed in a flavoured liquid.

en- (em-) *prefix denoting* in; inside.

enalapril *n.* a drug used in the treatment of high blood pressure (hypertension) and heart failure. It inhibits the action of angiotensin (*see* ACE INHIBITOR), which results in decreased vasopressor (blood-vessel constricting) activity and decreased aldosterone secretion. It is administered by mouth; side-effects can include a persistent dry cough, a drastic fall in blood pressure, headache, dizziness, fatigue, and diarrhoea. Trade name: **Innovace**.

enamel *n.* the extremely hard outer covering of the crown of a *tooth. It is formed before tooth eruption by *ameloblasts and consists of crystalline *hydroxyapatite.

enarthrosis *n.* a ball-and-socket joint: a type of *diarthrosis (freely movable joint), e.g. the shoulder joint and the hip joint. Such a joint always involves a long bone, which is thus allowed to move in all planes.

encapsulated *adj.* (of an organ, tumour, bacterium, etc.) enclosed in a *capsule.

encephal- (encephalo-) *combining form denoting* the brain.

encephalin (enkephalin) *n.* a peptide occurring naturally in the brain and having effects resembling those of morphine or other opiates. *See also* ENDORPHIN.

encephalitis *n.* inflammation of the brain. It may be caused by a viral or bacterial infection or it may be part of an allergic response to a systemic viral illness or vaccination (*see* ENCEPHALOMYELITIS). **Viral encephalitis** is endemic in some parts of the world; it may also occur epidemically or sporadically. One form – **encephalitis lethargica** – reached epidemic proportions shortly after World War I and was marked by headache and drowsiness, progressing to coma (hence its popular name – **sleepy sickness**). Encephalitis can cause postencephalitic *parkinsonism. Another type of encephalitis that occurs sporadically is due to the herpes simplex virus.

encephalocele *n. see* NEURAL TUBE DEFECTS.

encephalography *n.* any of various techniques for recording the structure of the brain or the activity of the brain cells. Examples are *electroencephalography and *pneumoencephalography.

encephalomyelitis *n.* an acute inflammatory disease affecting the brain and spinal cord. It is sometimes part of an overwhelming virus infection but **acute disseminated encephalomyelitis** (ADEM) is a form of delayed tissue hypersensitivity provoked by a mild infection or vaccination 7–10 days earlier. Survival through the acute phase of the illness is often followed by a remarkably complete recovery.

encephalomyelopathy *n.* any condition in which there is widespread disease of the brain and spinal cord. **Necrotizing encephalomyelopathy of childhood** is a progressive illness with extensive destruction of nerve cells throughout the central nervous system. It is thought to be caused by a disorder of metabolism.

encephalon *n. see* BRAIN.

encephalopathy *n.* any of various diseases that affect the functioning of the brain. *See* HEPATIC ENCEPHALOPATHY, SPONGIFORM ENCEPHALOPATHY, WERNICKE'S ENCEPHALOPATHY.

enchondroma *n.* (*pl.* **enchondromata**) a benign cartilaginous tumour (*see* CHONDROMA) occurring within cortical bone, usually in the short tubular bones of the hands and feet. Such tumours are usually solitary and asymptomatic, but an enlarging lesion may fracture (the usual reason for presentation). When multiple tumours occur the condition is known as **enchondromatosis**. *Compare* ECCHONDROMA.

encopresis *n.* incontinence of faeces. The term is used for faecal soiling in a child who has gained bowel control but passes formed stools in unacceptable places. The underlying problem is behavioural and treatment is difficult, often requiring the input of a child psychiatrist. Encopresis must be distinguished from chronic constipation with overflow.

encysted *adj.* enclosed in a cyst.

end- (endo-) *combining form denoting* within or inner. Example: **endonasal** (within the nose).

endarterectomy *n.* a surgical 're-bore' of an artery that has become obstructed by *atheroma with or without a blood clot (thrombus); the former operation is known as **thromboendarterectomy**. The inner part of the wall is removed together with any clot that is present. This restores patency and arterial blood flow to the tissues beyond the obstruction. The technique is most often applied to obstruction of the carotid arteries (**carotid endarterectomy**) or of the arteries that supply the legs.

endarteritis *n.* chronic inflammation of the inner (intimal) portion of the wall of an artery, which most often results from late syphilis. Thickening of the wall produces progressive arterial obstruction and symptoms from inadequate blood supply to the affected part (*ischaemia). The arteries to the brain are often involved, giving rise to meningovascular syphilis. Endarteritis of the aorta may obstruct the mouths of the coronary arteries, supplying the heart. Endarteritis of the arteries to the wall of the aorta (the vasa vasorum) contributes to *aneurysm formation. The syphilitic infection may be eradicated with penicillin.

end artery the terminal branch of an artery, which does not communicate with other branches. The tissue it supplies is therefore probably completely dependent on it for its blood supply.

endemic *adj.* occurring frequently in a particular region or population: applied to diseases that are generally or constantly found among people in a particular area. *Compare* ECDEMIC, EPIDEMIC, PANDEMIC.

endemic syphilis *see* BEJEL.

endocarditis *n.* inflammation of the lining of the heart cavity (endocardium) and valves. It is most often due to rheumatic fever or results from bacterial infection (**bacterial endocarditis**). Temporary or permanent damage to the heart valves may result. The main features are fever, changing heart murmurs, heart failure, and *embolism. Treatment consists of rest and antibiotics; surgery may be required to repair damaged heart valves.

endocardium *n.* a delicate membrane, formed of flat endothelial cells, that lines the heart and is continuous with the lining of arteries and veins. At the openings of the heart cavities it is folded back on itself to form the cusps of the valves. It presents a smooth slippery surface, which does not impede blood flow. —**endocardial** *adj.*

endocervicitis *n.* inflammation of the mucous membrane that lines the cervix (neck) of the uterus, usually caused by infection. Surface cells (columnar epithelium) may die, resulting in a new growth of healthy epithelium over the affected area. The condition is accompanied by a thick mucoid discharge.

endocervix *n.* the mucous membrane lining the cervix (neck) of the uterus, which (like the *endometrium) is covered with stratified columnar *epithelium.

endochondral *adj.* within the material of a cartilage.

endocrine gland (ductless gland) a gland that manufactures one or more *hormones and secretes them directly into the bloodstream (and not through a duct to the exterior). Endocrine glands include the pituitary, thyroid, parathyroid, and adrenal glands, the ovary and testis, the placenta, and part of the pancreas.

endocrinology *n.* the study of the *endocrine glands and the substances they secrete (*hormones). —**endocrinologist** *n.*

endoderm *n.* the inner of the three *germ layers of the early embryo, which gives rise to the lining of most of the alimentary canal and its associated glands, the liver, gall bladder, and pancreas. It also forms the lining of the bronchi and alveoli of the lung and most of the urinary tract. —**endodermal** *adj.*

endodermal sinus tumour a rare tumour of fetal remnants of the ovaries or testes. In women it is an aggressive malignant ovarian tumour that develops in adolescence and may secrete alpha-fetoprotein and human chorionic gonadotrophin, which can be used as *tumour markers. It is treated by oophorectomy with adjuvant chemotherapy.

endodontics *n.* the study, treatment, and prevention of diseases of the pulp of teeth and their sequelae. A major part of treatment is *root canal treatment.

endogenous *adj.* **1.** arising within or derived from the body. *Compare* EXOGENOUS. **2.** formerly (until the 1980s), denoting a type of *depression (also known as **melancholia**) that was thought to arise totally biologically and therefore without any particular triggers. It stood in contrast to **reactive depression**, which was supposed to have been primarily triggered by stress or trauma. Today this differentiation is not usually made as the validity of separating these two types of depression could not be proven.

endolymph *n.* the fluid that fills the membranous *labyrinth of the ear.

endolymphatic duct a blind-ended duct that leads from the sacculus and joins a duct

from the utriculus of the membranous *labyrinth of the ear.

endolymphatic sac a dilatation at the end of the *endolymphatic duct that removes waste products from the inner ear.

endometrial ablation the removal of the entire endometrium by means of an ablative technique under hysteroscopic control, usually performed as a day case or in a specialized out-patient clinic. It is an alternative to the more traditional hysterectomies that were undertaken for the relief of *menorrhagia. Methods for hysteroscopic endometrial ablation introduced in the 1980s included Nd:YAG (neodymium:yttrium–aluminium–garnet) laser ablation, *transcervical resection of the endometrium (TCRE), and rollerball *electrocoagulation (RBE). These first-generation procedures remain the gold standard for the hysteroscopic treatment of menorrhagia. Since the 1990s, the second generation of hysteroscopic ablation techniques have been developed. These include balloon thermal coagulation, in which a heated balloon is inserted into the uterus and destroys the endometrium; **microwave endometrial ablation** (**MEA**), which vaporizes the endometrial tissue; and **Novasure**, which destroys the endometrium by *radiofrequency ablation. About 75% of women obtain satisfactory improvement in their symptoms after these procedures.

endometrial cancer a malignant tumour of the lining (*endometrium) of the uterus. Risk factors are nulliparity (never having given birth), obesity, and tamoxifen use as chemotherapy for breast cancer. The presenting symptom is usually *postmenopausal bleeding, but this cancer may present with postmenopausal discharge or *pyometra. The tumour invades the *myometrium and spreads down to the cervix and through the Fallopian tubes to the ovaries and peritoneal cavity and through the lymphatics to pelvic and aortic nodes. Prognosis depends on tumour differentiation, depth of myometrial invasion, extent of tumour spread, and involvement of retroperitoneal nodes. Treatment is total abdominal *hysterectomy and bilateral *salpingo-oophorectomy, with *lymphadenectomy and radiotherapy if indicated.

endometrial hyperplasia an increase in the thickness of the cells of the *endometrium, usually due to prolonged exposure to unopposed oestrogen, which can be endogenous, as in anovular menstrual cycles; or exogenous, deriving, for example, from *hormone replacement therapy or an oestrogen-secreting tumour. It is classified as simple, complex, or atypical. Endometrial hyperplasia most commonly presents with abnormal uterine bleeding and accounts for 15% cases of postmenopausal bleeding. It may also be asymptomatic, and in some cases regresses spontaneously without ever being detected. The presence of atypical cells may lead to *endometrial cancer. Treatment can include progestogen therapy or surgery (*see* ENDOMETRIAL ABLATION); hysterectomy is advised when atypical changes are present.

endometrioma *n.* a complex *ovarian cyst, usually with 'chocolate' material (altered blood) inside and associated with *endometriosis. A history of cyclical enlargement of the nodule and painful periods is highly suggestive. There is a characteristic ground-glass appearance on transvaginal ultrasound and these cysts may be associated with a raised *CA125 level. Endometriomas are not amenable to medical therapy and should be surgically excised.

endometriosis *n.* the presence of fragments of endometrial tissue at sites in the pelvis outside the uterus or, rarely, throughout the body (e.g. in the lung, rectum, or umbilicus). It is thought to be caused by retrograde *menstruation. When the tissue has infiltrated the wall of the uterus (myometrium) the condition is known as **adenomyosis**. Symptoms vary, but typically include pelvic pain, severe *dysmenorrhoea, *dyspareunia, infertility, and a pelvic mass (or any combination of these). Medical treatment is aimed at suppressing ovulation using *gonadorelin analogues, combined oral contraceptives, or the intrauterine system (*see* IUS). High-dose progestogens suppress *gonadotrophins (FSH and LH), shrink implanted endometrial tissue, and reduce retrograde menstruation. They have a similar efficacy to other medical treatments, are cheaper, and have fewer side-effects than gonadorelin analogues. Surgical treatment may also be necessary, usually by laser or ablative therapy via the laparoscope. More radical surgical treatment in the form of a total hysterectomy and bilateral salpingo-oophorectomy is sometimes required.

endometritis *n.* inflammation of the *endometrium due to acute or chronic infection. It may be caused by foreign bodies, bacteria, viruses, or parasites. In the acute phase it may occur in the period immediately after childbirth (puerperium) but the chronic phase may not be associated with pregnancy (as in tuberculous endometritis). Chronic endometritis in women with IUDs may be responsible for the contraceptive action.

endometrium *n.* the mucous membrane lining the uterus, which is covered with columnar *epithelium. It becomes progressively thicker and more glandular and has an increased blood supply in the latter part of the menstrual cycle. This prepares the endometrium for implantation of the embryo, but if this does not occur much of the endometrium breaks down and is lost in menstruation. If pregnancy is established the endometrium becomes the *decidua, which is shed after birth. —**endometrial** *adj.*

endomorphic *adj.* describing a *body type that is relatively fat, with highly developed viscera and weak muscular and skeletal development. —**endomorph** *n.* —**endomorphy** *n.*

endomorphin *n.* *see* ENDORPHIN.

endomyocarditis *n.* an acute or chronic inflammatory disorder of the muscle and lining membrane of the heart. When the membrane surrounding the heart (pericardium) is also involved the condition is termed **pancarditis**. The principal causes are rheumatic fever and virus infections. There is enlargement of the heart, murmurs, embolism, and frequently arrhythmias. The treatment is that of the cause and complications. *See also* ENDOCARDITIS.

A chronic condition, **endomyocardial fibrosis**, is seen in Black Africans: the cause is unknown.

endomysium *n.* the fine connective tissue sheath that surrounds a single *muscle fibre.

endoneurium *n.* the layer of fibrous tissue that separates individual fibres within a *nerve.

endoparasite *n.* a parasite that lives inside its host, for example in the liver, lungs, gut, or other tissues of the body. *Compare* ECTOPARASITE.

endopeptidase *n.* a digestive enzyme (e.g. *pepsin) that splits a whole protein into small peptide fractions by splitting the linkages between peptides in the interior of the molecule. *Compare* EXOPEPTIDASE. *See also* PEPTIDASE.

endophthalmitis *n.* inflammation, usually due to infection, within the eye.

endophytic *adj.* describing growth inwards from an epithelial surface due to invasion of the surrounding tissues. Endophytic growth is characteristic of carcinomas. *Compare* EXOPHYTIC.

endoplasm *n.* the inner cytoplasm of cells, which is less dense than the *ectoplasm and contains most of the cell's structures. —**endoplasmic** *adj.*

endoplasmic reticulum (ER) a system of membranes present in the cytoplasm of cells. ER is described as **rough** when it has *ribosomes attached to its surface and **smooth** when ribosomes are absent. It is the site of manufacture of proteins and lipids and is concerned with the transport of these products within the cell (*see also* GOLGI APPARATUS).

endopyelotomy *n.* a procedure for relieving obstruction of the junction between the kidney pelvis and ureter. An incision is made, via an endoscope, through the skin and proximal ureter into the obstructed region, using electrocautery, laser, or an endoscopic scalpel. Following this, *balloon dilation is usually performed and a *stent inserted.

end organ a specialized structure at the end of a peripheral nerve, acting as a receptor for a particular sensation. Taste buds, in the tongue, are end organs subserving the sense of taste.

endorphin (endomorphin) *n.* one of a group of chemical compounds, similar to the *encephalins, that occur naturally in the brain and have pain-relieving properties similar to those of the opiates. They are also responsible for sensations of pleasure. The endorphins are derived from a substance found in the pituitary gland known as **beta-lipotrophin**; they are thought to be concerned with controlling the activity of the endocrine glands.

endoscope *n.* any instrument used to obtain a view of the interior of the body. Examples of endoscopes include the *auriscope and the *gastroscope. Essentially, most endoscopes consist of a tube with a light at the end and an optical system or a miniature video camera for transmitting an image to the examiner's eye. *See also* FIBRESCOPE. —**endoscopic** *adj.* —**endoscopy** *n.*

endoscopic retrograde cholangiopan-creatography *see* ERCP.

endoscopic sinus surgery (ESS) surgery of the *paranasal sinuses using endoscopes. **Functional endoscopic sinus surgery** (**FESS**) clears inflamed tissue from routes of sinus drainage and aeration to allow the other sinuses to return to normal.

endospore *n.* the resting stage of certain bacteria, particularly species of the genera *Bacillus* and *Clostridium*. In adverse conditions the bacterium can become enclosed within a tough protective coat, allowing the cell to survive. On return of favourable conditions the spore changes back to the vegetative form.

endostapler *n.* a stapling instrument (*see* STAPLE) used endoscopically for fixing tissues or joining them together.

endosteum *n.* the membrane that lines the marrow cavity of a bone.

endothelin *n.* any one of a class of peptide hormones, consisting of chains of 21 amino acids, that are synthesized by endothelial cells, often of large blood vessels. They are the most powerful known stimulants of smooth muscle (such as that in the walls of arteries) and are believed to be important causes of hypertension. The drug **bosentan** (Tracleer), which blocks receptors for endothelin-1, is administered by mouth for the treatment of pulmonary hypertension. A similar drug is **ambrisentan** (Volibris).

endothelioma *n.* any tumour arising from or resembling endothelium. It may arise from the linings of blood or lymph vessels (**haemangioendothelioma** and **lymphangioendothelioma** respectively); from the linings of the pleural cavity or the peritoneal cavity (*see* MESOTHELIOMA); or from the meninges (*see* MENINGIOMA).

endothelium *n.* the single layer of cells that lines the heart, blood vessels, and lymphatic vessels. It is derived from embryonic mesoderm. The **corneal endothelium** is the innermost layer of the *cornea. *Compare* EPITHELIUM. —**endothelial** *adj.*

endothermic *adj.* describing a chemical reaction associated with the absorption of heat. *Compare* EXOTHERMIC.

endotoxin *n.* a poison generally harmful to all body tissues, contained within certain Gram-negative bacteria and released only when the bacterial cell is broken down or dies and disintegrates. *Compare* EXOTOXIN.

endotracheal *adj.* within or through the trachea (windpipe). *See* INTUBATION.

endovascular *adj.* within a blood vessel: describing procedures for imaging the circulation or for treating vascular disorders from within the circulation, including *angioplasty, the placement of *stents in aneurysms (*see* ENDOVASCULAR ANEURYSM REPAIR), and *embolization. Endovascular procedures are usually performed by an interventional radiologist or a vascular surgeon.

endovascular aneurysm repair (EVAR) a recently developed technique that involves the insertion into an *aneurysm of a number of covered metal *stents, which line the aneurysm and thereby exclude it from the circulation, preventing further expansion and rupture. The delivery system containing the stents is introduced through the common femoral artery. *Fluoroscopy provides real-time imaging to guide placement of the stents and ensure they are in the correct anatomical position.

endovenous laser treatment (EVLT) a minimally invasive procedure to treat *varicose veins. A laser fibre (usually an 810-nm *diode laser) contained within a sheath is fed into the vein by ultrasound guidance and slowly withdrawn as it is fired, thereby delivering laser energy that causes irreversible destruction and eventual ablation of the vein.

end-plate *n.* the area of muscle cell membrane immediately beneath the motor nerve ending at a *neuromuscular junction. Special receptors in this area trigger muscular contraction when the nerve ending releases its *neurotransmitter.

end-stage renal failure (ESRF, CKD 5) the most advanced stage of kidney failure, which is reached when the *glomerular filtration rate (GFR) falls to 15 ml/min (normal GFR = 100 ml/min).

enema *n.* (*pl.* **enemata** or **enemas**) a quantity of fluid infused into the rectum through a tube passed into the anus. An **evacuant enema** (soap or olive oil) is used to remove faeces. A **therapeutic enema** is used to insert drugs into the rectum, commonly

corticosteroids or aminosalicylates in the treatment of *proctocolitis. *See also* BARIUM ENEMA, SMALL-BOWEL ENEMA.

enervation *n.* 1. weakness; loss of strength. 2. the surgical removal of a nerve.

engagement *n.* (in obstetrics) the stage of pregnancy that occurs when the presenting part of the fetus has descended into the mother's pelvis. Engagement of the fetal head occurs when the widest part has passed through the pelvic inlet.

enhanced external counterpulsation (EECP) a novel treatment for patients with intractable angina. Specially designed inflatable trousers are inflated rhythmically in time with ventricular *diastole. Theoretically this imparts additional energy to the circulating blood volume when the heart is relaxed, and this may improve blood flow down severely narrowed coronary arteries. It is also claimed to have beneficial effects on blood flow to other organs. Despite promising clinical trials, this technique has not been widely adopted.

enkephalin *n. see* ENCEPHALIN.

enophthalmos *n.* a condition in which the eye is abnormally sunken into the socket. It may follow fractures of the floor of the orbit that allow the eye to sink downwards and backwards.

enoxaparin sodium *see* LOW-MOLECULAR-WEIGHT HEPARIN.

enoximone *n.* an *inotropic drug used in the treatment of congestive heart failure to increase the force and output of the heart. It is administered by intravenous injection or infusion. Trade name: **Perfan**.

ensiform cartilage *see* XIPHOID PROCESS.

ENT *see* OTORHINOLARYNGOLOGY.

Entamoeba *n.* a genus of widely distributed amoebae, of which some species are parasites of the digestive tract of humans. *E. histolytica* invades and destroys the tissues of the intestinal wall, causing amoebic *dysentery and ulceration of the gut wall (*see also* AMOEBOMA); infection of the liver with this species (amoebic hepatitis) is common in tropical countries. *E. coli* is a harmless intestinal parasite; *E. gingivalis*, found within the spaces between the teeth, is associated with periodontal disease and gingivitis.

enter- (**entero-**) *combining form denoting*

the intestine. Example: **enterolith** (calculus in).

enteral *adj.* of or relating to the intestinal tract.

enteral feeding *see* NUTRITION.

enteralgia *n. see* COLIC.

enterectomy *n.* surgical removal of part of the small intestine.

enteric *adj.* relating to or affecting the intestine.

enteric-coated *adj.* describing tablets that are coated with a substance that enables them to pass through the stomach and into the intestine unchanged. Enteric-coated tablets contain drugs that are destroyed by the acid contents of the stomach.

enteric fever *see* PARATYPHOID FEVER, TYPHOID FEVER.

enteritis *n.* inflammation of the small intestine, usually causing diarrhoea. **Infective enteritis** is caused by viruses or bacteria; **radiation enteritis** is caused by X-rays used for radiation therapy of pelvic and other malignancies. It can cause fistula or stricture formation and malabsorption. *See also* CROHN'S DISEASE (REGIONAL ENTERITIS), GASTROENTERITIS.

enterobiasis (oxyuriasis) *n.* a disease, common in children throughout the world, caused by the parasitic nematode *Enterobius vermicularis* (*see* THREADWORM) in the large intestine. The worms do not cause any serious lesions of the gut wall although, rarely, they may provoke appendicitis. The emergence of the female from the anus at night irritates and inflames the surrounding skin, causing the patient to scratch and thereby contaminate fingers and nails with infective eggs. The eggs may reinfect the same child or be spread to other children. Worms may occasionally enter the vulva and cause a discharge from the vagina. Enterobiasis responds well to treatment with *piperazine compounds.

Enterobius (Oxyuris) *n. see* THREADWORM.

enterocele *n.* a hernia of the *pouch of Douglas (between the rectum and uterus) into the upper part of the posterior vaginal wall. It may contain loops of small bowel.

enterocentesis *n.* a former name for a surgical procedure in which a hollow needle is pushed through the wall of the stomach or

intestines to release an abnormal accumulation of gas or fluid or to introduce a catheter for feeding (*see* GASTROSTOMY, ENTEROSTOMY).

enteroclysis *n. see* SMALL-BOWEL ENEMA.

Enterococcus *n.* a genus of spherical Gram-positive bacteria formerly classified as species of *Streptococcus. They are normal inhabitants of the human and animal intestine but a few species, notably *E. faecalis* and *E. faecium*, can cause infections in humans. They are responsible for some hospital-acquired infections and have been found in teeth with persisting disease after root canal treatment. Enterococci have the ability to survive under adverse (starvation) conditions and are therefore difficult to eradicate; there is concern at the development of strains resistant to glycopeptide antibiotics, such as *vancomycin (**glycopeptide-resistant enterococci**, **GRE**).

enterocolitis *n.* inflammation of the colon and small intestine. *See also* COLITIS, ENTERITIS, NECROTIZING ENTEROCOLITIS.

enterogastrone *n.* a hormone from the small intestine (duodenum) that inhibits the secretion of gastric juice by the stomach. It is released when the stomach contents pass into the small intestine.

enterogenous *adj.* borne by or carried in the intestine.

enterokinase *n.* the former name for *enteropeptidase.

enterolith *n.* a stone within the intestine. It usually builds up around a gallstone or a swallowed fruit stone.

enteropathy *n.* disease of the small intestine. *See also* COELIAC DISEASE (GLUTEN-SENSITIVE ENTEROPATHY).

enteropeptidase *n.* an enzyme secreted by the glands of the small intestine that acts on trypsinogen to produce *trypsin.

enterorrhaphy *n.* the surgical procedure of stitching an intestine that has either perforated or been divided during an operation.

enteroscope *n.* an illuminated optical instrument (*see* ENDOSCOPE) used to inspect the interior of the small intestine. The image is transmitted through digital video technology. The examination can be performed using the oral and/or anal approach. The double balloon (**push and pull**) type, about 280 cm long with a distal balloon combined with an *overtube with a proximal balloon, is introduced under direct vision. Double balloon inflation and deflation helps in progression of the endoscope through the small intestine and is the predominant type in current use. The **sonde** (or **push**) type, about 280 cm long, has a single inflatable balloon that helps pull the instrument through the length of the intestine using peristalsis. It is now rarely used in clinical practice. The enteroscope is useful in diagnosing the cause of obscure gastrointestinal haemorrhage of the small intestine or of *strictures. It may also be used to treat bleeding lesions, remove small intestinal polyps, and to obtain tissue samples in suspected cases of malabsorption, inflammation, or intestinal tumours. —**enteroscopy** *n.*

enterostomy *n.* an operation in which the small intestine is brought through the abdominal wall and opened (*see* DUODENOSTOMY, JEJUNOSTOMY, ILEOSTOMY) or is joined to the stomach (**gastroenterostomy**) or to another loop of small intestine (**enteroenterostomy**).

enterotomy *n.* surgical incision into the intestine.

enterotoxin *n.* a poisonous substance that has a particularly marked effect upon the gastrointestinal tract, causing vomiting, diarrhoea, and abdominal pain.

enterovirus *n.* any virus that enters the body through the gastrointestinal tract, multiplies there, and then (generally) invades the central nervous system. Enteroviruses include *Coxsackie viruses and *polioviruses.

enterozoon *n.* any animal species inhabiting or infecting the gut of another. *See also* ENDOPARASITE.

enthesis *n.* (*pl.* **entheses**) **1.** the site of insertion of tendons or ligaments into bones. **2.** the insertion of synthetic inorganic material to replace lost tissue.

enthesopathy *n.* any rheumatic disease resulting in inflammation of *entheses. Ankylosing *spondylitis, *psoriatic arthritis, and *Reiter's syndrome are examples.

entoptic phenomena visual sensations caused by changes within the eye itself, rather than by the normal light stimulation process. The commonest are tiny floating spots (**floaters**) that most people can see occasionally, especially when gazing at a brightly illuminated background (such as a blue sky).

entrapment neuropathy pain, muscle wasting, and paralysis resulting from pressure on a nerve in conditions in which it is subjected to compression by surrounding structures. *See* CARPAL TUNNEL SYNDROME.

entropion *n.* inturning of the eyelid towards the eyeball. The lashes may rub against the eye and cause irritation (*see* TRICHIASIS). The commonest type is **spastic entropion** of the lower eyelid, due to spasm of the muscle that closes the eye (orbicularis oculi). Entropion may also be caused by scarring of the lining membrane (conjunctiva) of the lid.

enucleation *n.* the complete removal of an organ, tumour, or cyst leaving surrounding structures intact. In ophthalmology it is an operation in which the eyeball is removed but the other structures in the socket (e.g. eye muscles) are left in place. Commonly a plastic ball is temporarily buried in the socket to give a better cosmetic result prior to fitting an artificial eye.

enuresis *n.* the involuntary passing of urine. The most common form is bedwetting (**nocturnal enuresis**) by children (the majority of children are dry during the day by the age of three years and at night by four). Nocturnal enuresis is occasionally caused by underlying disorders of the urinary tract, particularly infection, but in the majority of children the problem is behavioural; there is often a family history. The condition usually settles spontaneously as the child grows older, but it may persist into teenage – and rarely adult – life. It can be treated by behavioural techniques, such as the use of a nocturnal alarm (*see* BELL AND PAD) or *reinforcement of periods of continence with a reward system, or by drug treatment. Enuresis that starts in adulthood is usually associated with a disorder of the bladder, a side-effect of medication, or a neurological disease, such as multiple sclerosis. *See also* INCONTINENCE. —**enuretic** *adj.*

environment *n.* any or all aspects of the surroundings of an organism, both internal and external, which influence its growth, development, and behaviour.

Environmental Health Officer (EHO) a person, employed by a local authority, with special training in such aspects of environmental health as housing, pollution, and food safety (formerly known as a **Public Health Inspector**). EHOs work closely with other professionals within the local authority and with other agencies, including the *Health Protection Agency.

environmental hearing aid any of various devices for helping people with hearing difficulties. Environmental aids include *assistive listening devices and **alerting devices**, such as door bells with visible as well as audible alarms, infrared links to televisions, and vibrating alarm clocks.

enzyme *n.* a protein that, in small amounts, speeds up the rate of a biological reaction without itself being used up in the reaction (i.e. it acts as a catalyst). An enzyme acts by binding with the substance involved in the reaction (the **substrate**) and converting it into another substance (the **product** of the reaction). An enzyme is relatively specific in the type of reaction it catalyses; hence there are many different enzymes for the various biochemical reactions. Each enzyme requires certain conditions for optimum activity, particularly correct temperature and pH, the presence of *coenzymes, and the absence of specific inhibitors. Enzymes are unstable and are easily inactivated by heat or certain chemicals. They are produced within living cells and may act either within the cell (as in cellular respiration) or outside it (as in digestion). The names of enzymes usually end in '-ase'; enzymes are named according to the substrate upon which they act (as in lactase), or the type of reaction they catalyse (as in hydrolase).
Enzymes are essential for the normal functioning and development of the body. Failure in the production or activity of a single enzyme may result in metabolic disorders; such disorders are often inherited and some have serious effects. —**enzymatic** *adj.*

enzyme-linked immunosorbent assay (ELISA) a sensitive technique for measuring the amount of a substance. An antibody that will bind to the substance is produced; the amount of an easily measured enzyme that then binds to the antibody complex enables accurate measurement.

EOG *see* ELECTROOCULOGRAPHY.

eosin *n.* a red acidic dye, produced by the reaction of bromine and fluorescein, used to stain biological specimens for microscopical examination. Eosin may be used in conjunction with a contrasting blue alkaline dye

taken up by different parts of the same specimen.

eosinopenia *n.* a decrease in the number of eosinophils in the blood.

eosinophil *n.* a variety of white blood cell distinguished by a lobed nucleus and the presence in its cytoplasm of coarse granules that stain orange-red with *Romanowsky stains. Eosinophils are capable of ingesting foreign particles, is present in large numbers in lining or covering surfaces within the body, is involved in allergic responses, and may be involved in host defence against parasites. There are normally $40–400 \times 10^6$ eosinophils per litre of blood. *See also* POLYMORPH.

eosinophilia *n.* an increase in the number of eosinophils in the blood. Eosinophilia occurs in response to certain drugs and in a variety of diseases, including allergies, parasitic infestations, and certain forms of leukaemia.

eparterial *adj.* situated on or above an artery.

ependyma *n.* the extremely thin membrane, composed of cells of the *glia (**ependymal cells**), that lines the ventricles of the brain and the choroid plexuses. It is responsible for helping to form cerebrospinal fluid. —**ependymal** *adj.*

ependymoma *n.* a cerebral tumour derived from the glial (non-nervous) cells lining the cavities of the ventricles of the brain (*see* EPENDYMA). It may obstruct the flow of cerebrospinal fluid, causing a *hydrocephalus.

ephebiatrics (hebiatrics) *n.* the branch of medicine concerned with the common disorders of adolescents. *Compare* PAEDIATRICS.

ephedrine *n.* a drug that causes constriction of blood vessels and widening of the bronchial passages (*see* SYMPATHOMIMETIC). It is used mainly as a nasal *decongestant, being administered as nasal drops, but is also injected intravenously to reverse hypotension following epidural or spinal anaesthesia. It may cause nausea, insomnia, headache, and dizziness.

epi- *prefix denoting* above or upon.

epiblepharon *n.* a fold of skin, present from birth, stretching across the eye just above the lashes of the upper eyelid or in front of them in the lower lid. It may cause the lower lashes to turn upwards or inwards against the eye. It usually disappears within the first year of life.

epicanthus (epicanthic fold) *n.* (*pl.* **epicanthi**) a vertical fold of skin from the upper eyelid that covers the inner corner of the eye. Epicanthi are normal in many Asian peoples and occur abnormally in certain congenital conditions, e.g. *Down's syndrome. —**epicanthal**, **epicanthic** *adj.*

epicardia *n.* the part of the *oesophagus, about 2 cm long, that extends from the level of the diaphragm to the stomach.

epicardium *n.* the outermost layer of the heart wall, enveloping the myocardium. It is a serous membrane that forms the inner layer of the serous *pericardium. —**epicardial** *adj.*

epicondyle *n.* the protuberance above a *condyle at the end of an articulating bone.

epicranium *n.* the structures that cover the cranium, i.e. all layers of the scalp.

epicranius *n.* the muscle of the scalp. The **frontal** portion, at the forehead, is responsible for raising the eyebrows and wrinkling the forehead; the **occipital** portion, at the base of the skull, draws the scalp backwards.

epicritic *adj.* describing or relating to sensory nerve fibres responsible for the fine degrees of sensation, as of temperature and touch. *Compare* PROTOPATHIC.

epidemic *n.* a sudden outbreak of infectious disease that spreads rapidly through the population, affecting a large proportion of people. The commonest epidemics today are of influenza. *Compare* ENDEMIC, PANDEMIC. —**epidemic** *adj.*

epidemiology *n.* the study of the distribution of diseases and determinants of disease in populations. Originally restricted to the study of epidemic infectious diseases, such as smallpox and cholera, it now covers all forms of disease that relate to the environment and ways of life. It thus includes the study of the links between smoking and cancer, and diet and coronary disease, as well as *communicable diseases.

epidermal growth factor receptor (**EGFR**) a protein on the surface of cells (*see* RECEPTOR) that binds with epidermal *growth factor and is therefore involved in cell division. EGFR is expressed at increased levels in numerous tumours, particularly of the head and neck, and in colorectal cancer, in which it can be a target for antibody therapy with *cetuximab. *Tyrosine kinase inhibitors acting specifically on the EGFR include **gefitinib** (Iressa) and **erlotinib** (Tarceva) in lung and pancreatic cancer.

epidermis *n.* the outer layer of the *skin, which is divided into four layers (see illustration). The innermost **Malpighian** or **germinative layer** (**stratum germinativum**) consists of continuously dividing cells. The other three layers are continually renewed as cells from the germinative layer are gradually pushed outwards and become progressively impregnated with keratin (*see* KERATINIZATION). The outermost layer (**stratum corneum**) consists of dead cells whose cytoplasm has been entirely replaced by keratin. It is thickest on the soles of the feet and palms of the hands. —**epidermal** *adj.*

epidermoid *adj.* having the appearance of epidermis (the outer layer of the skin): used

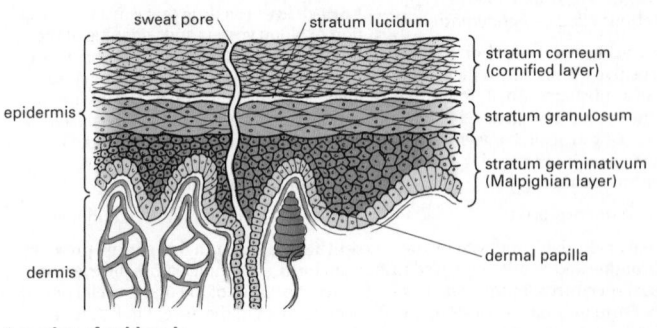

A section of epidermis.

to describe certain tumours of tissues other than the skin.

epidermoid cyst *see* SEBACEOUS CYST.

epidermolysis bullosa any one of a group of genetically determined disorders characterized by blistering of skin and mucous membranes that occurs secondarily to minor mechanical trauma. Many different types exist: milder cases are restricted to skin and mucosal fragility; other types may be complicated by the development of skin squamous cell carcinomas (dystrophic) or death in early childhood due to overwhelming sepsis or airway involvement.

Epidermophyton *n.* a genus of fungi that grow on the skin, causing *ringworm. *See also* DERMATOPHYTE.

epidiascope *n.* an apparatus for projecting a greatly magnified image of an object, such as a specimen on a microscope slide, on to a screen.

epididymectomy *n.* the surgical removal or excision of the epididymis.

epididymis *n.* (*pl.* **epididymides**) a highly convoluted tube, about seven metres long, that connects the *testis to the vas deferens. The spermatozoa are moved passively along the tube over a period of several days, during which time they mature and become capable of fertilization. They are concentrated and stored in the lower part of the epididymis until ejaculation. —**epididymal** *adj.*

epididymitis *n.* inflammation of the epididymis. The usual cause is infection spreading down the vas deferens from the bladder or urethra, resulting in pain, swelling, and redness of the affected half of the scrotum. The inflammation may spread to the testicle (**epididymo-orchitis**). Treatment is by administration of antibiotics and analgesics.

epididymovasostomy *n.* the operation of connecting the vas deferens to the epididymis to bypass obstruction of the latter. It is performed in an attempt to cure *azoospermia caused by this blockage.

epidural (extradural) *adj.* on or over the dura mater (the outermost of the three membranes covering the brain and spinal cord). The **epidural space** is the space between the dura mater of the spinal cord and the vertebral canal. The spinal epidural space is used for anaesthetizing spinal nerve roots (*see* EPIDURAL ANAESTHESIA).

epidural anaesthesia suppression of sensation in the lower part of the body by the injection of a local anaesthetic into the *epidural space. The injection site is often the sacral or caudal regions of the vertebral column, and a special blunt needle with a side-hole is used to reduce the chance of penetrating the dura. A fine catheter is passed through the needle to enable repeated or continuous injections of anaesthetic solution. Epidural anaesthesia is particularly useful for providing pain relief during childbirth or to reduce the need for deep general anaesthesia.

epigastrium *n.* the upper central region of the *abdomen. —**epigastric** *adj.*

epigastrocele *n.* a *hernia through the upper central abdominal wall.

epiglottis *n.* a thin leaf-shaped flap of cartilage, covered with mucous membrane, situated immediately behind the root of the tongue. It covers the entrance to the *larynx during swallowing.

epiglottitis *n.* an infection of the epiglottis, which swells and causes obstruction of the upper airways. Epiglottitis usually occurs in children between one and seven years old, who complain of drooling and breathing difficulties and are acutely unwell. The main bacterium that causes epiglottitis is *Haemophilus influenzae*, and the infection has become much less common since the *Hib vaccine was introduced. Treatment consists of antibiotics and, if necessary, intubation. Children should be nursed in intensive care until the infection is under control.

epikeratophakia *n.* eye surgery to correct errors of *refraction in which the curvature of the cornea is altered using donor corneal tissue, which has been frozen and shaped using a lathe to produce a tissue lens that is then sutured onto the cornea.

epilation *n.* the removal of a hair by its roots. This can be done mechanically (by plucking, waxing, or threading) or by use of topical creams, electrolysis, and lasers.

epilepsy *n.* a disorder of brain function characterized by recurrent seizures that have a sudden onset. The term **idiopathic** is used to describe epilepsy that is not associated with structural damage to the brain. Seizures may be generalized or partial. **Generalized epilepsy** may take the form of tonic-clonic or absence seizures. In **tonic-clonic** (or **major**)

seizures (formerly called **grand mal**), the patient falls to the ground unconscious with the muscles in a state of spasm. The lack of any respiratory movement may result in a bluish discoloration of the skin and lips (cyanosis). This – the tonic phase – is replaced by convulsive movements (the clonic phase) when the tongue may be bitten and urinary incontinence may occur. Movements gradually cease and the patient may rouse in a state of confusion, complaining of headache, or may fall asleep. **Absence seizures** (formerly called **petit mal** in children) consist of brief spells of unconsciousness lasting for a few seconds, during which posture and balance are maintained. The eyes stare blankly and there may be fluttering movements of the lids and momentary twitching of the fingers and mouth. The electroencephalogram characteristically shows bisynchronous spike and wave discharges (3 per second) during the seizures and at other times. Attacks are sometimes provoked by overbreathing or intermittent photic stimulation. As the stream of thought is completely interrupted, children with frequent seizures may have learning difficulties. This form of epilepsy seldom appears before the age of three or after adolescence. It often subsides spontaneously in adult life, but it may be followed by the onset of major or partial epilepsy.

In **partial** (or **focal**) **seizures**, the nature of the seizure depends upon the location of the damage in the brain. For example, a simple partial motor seizure consists of convulsive movements that might spread from the thumb to the hand, arm, and face (this spread of symptoms is called the **Jacksonian march**); there is no loss of awareness. **Complex partial seizures** are commonly caused by damage to the cortex of the temporal lobe or the adjacent parietal lobe of the brain: this form of epilepsy is often called **temporal lobe** (or **psychomotor**) **epilepsy**. Symptoms may include *hallucinations of smell, taste, sight, and hearing, paroxysmal disorders of memory, and *automatism. Throughout an attack the patient is in a state of clouded awareness and afterwards may have no recollection of the event (*see also* DÉJÀ VU, JAMAIS VU). A number of these symptoms are due to scarring and atrophy (mesial temporal sclerosis) affecting the temporal lobe.

The different forms of epilepsy can be controlled by the use of antiepileptic drugs (*see* ANTICONVULSANT). Surgical resection of focal epileptogenic lesions in the brain is appropriate in a strictly limited number of cases. —**epileptic** *adj., n.*

(⊕) SEE WEB LINKS

• Website of Epilepsy Action: includes practical advice for people living with epilepsy

epileptogenic *adj.* having the capacity to provoke epileptic seizures.

epiloia *n. see* TUBEROUS SCLEROSIS.

epimysium *n.* the fibrous elastic tissue that surrounds a *muscle.

epinephrine *n. see* ADRENALINE.

epineural *adj.* derived from or situated on the neural arch of a vertebra.

epineurium *n.* the outer sheath of connective tissue that encloses the bundles (fascicles) of fibres that make up a *nerve.

epinucleus *n.* tissue surrounding the relatively hard lens nucleus, between the nucleus and the softer cortex of the lens.

epiphenomenon *n.* an unusual symptom or event that may occur simultaneously with a disease but is not necessarily directly related to it. *Compare* COMPLICATION.

epiphora *n.* watering of the eye, in which tears flow onto the cheek. It is due to some abnormality of the tear drainage system (*see* LACRIMAL APPARATUS).

epiphysis *n.* (*pl.* **epiphyses**) **1.** the end of a long bone, which is initially separated by cartilage from the shaft (diaphysis) of the bone and develops separately. It eventually fuses with the diaphysis to form a complete bone. *See also* PHYSIS. **2.** *see* PINEAL GLAND. —**epiphyseal** *adj.*

epiphysitis *n.* inflammation of the end (epiphysis) of a long bone. It may result in retardation of growth and deformity of the affected bone.

epiplo- *combining form denoting* the omentum. Example: **epiplocele** (hernia containing omentum).

epiploon *n. see* OMENTUM.

epiretinal membrane (**cellophane maculopathy**) a transparent membrane that forms on the retina, over the *macula. Contraction of this causes wrinkling of the retina (**macular pucker**) and hence distorted vision.

epirubicin *n. see* ANTHRACYCLINE.

episclera *n.* the outermost covering of the *sclera of the eye, which provides nutritional support to the sclera.

episcleritis *n.* inflammation of the *episclera, resulting in a red painful eye that is sensitive to light. It is usually a benign condition, which will settle without treatment.

episio- *combining form denoting* the vulva. Example: **episioplasty** (plastic surgery of).

episiotomy *n.* an incision into the tissues surrounding the opening of the vagina (perineum) during a difficult birth, at the stage when the infant's head has partly emerged through the opening of the birth passage. The aim is to enlarge the opening in a controlled manner so as to make delivery easier and to avoid extensive tearing of adjacent tissues.

epispadias *n.* a congenital abnormality in which the opening of the *urethra is on the dorsal (upper) surface of the penis. Surgical correction is carried out in infancy.

epistasis *n.* **1.** the stopping of a flow or discharge, as of blood. **2.** a type of gene action in which one gene can suppress the action of another (nonallelic) gene. The term is sometimes used for any interaction between nonallelic genes. —**epistatic** *adj.*

epistaxis *n.* bleeding from the nose, which is a very common condition. Although there is usually no obvious underlying cause, epistaxis can be caused by low-grade bacterial infection of the front of the nose, hypertension, clotting disorders, or tumours of the nose or sinuses. Treatments include pinching the bottom part of the nostrils together, cauterizing the bleeding vessel, or packing the nose with preformed packs, antiseptic gauze, or specially designed inflatable balloons. Occasionally surgery is required to interrupt the flow of blood to the nose. *See* LITTLE'S AREA, KIESSELBACH'S PLEXUS.

epithalamus *n.* part of the forebrain, consisting of a narrow band of nerve tissue in the roof of the third ventricle (including the region where the choroid plexus is attached) and the *pineal gland. *See also* BRAIN.

epithalaxia *n.* loss of layers of epithelial cells from the lining of the intestine.

epithelial ingrowth abnormal healing of a corneal wound or incision in which the conjunctival/corneal epithelium invades the internal surface of the healing wound. The

consequences of this can be devastating to the eye and difficult to treat.

epithelioma *n.* a tumour of *epithelium, the covering of internal and external surfaces of the body: a former name for *carcinoma.

epithelium *n.* the tissue that covers the external surface of the body and lines hollow structures (except blood and lymphatic vessels). It is derived from embryonic ectoderm and endoderm. Epithelial cells may be flat and scalelike (**squamous**), **cuboidal**, or **columnar**. The latter may bear cilia or brush borders or secrete mucus or other substances (*see* GOBLET CELL). The cells rest on a common **basement membrane**, which separates epithelium from underlying *connective tissue. Epithelium may be either **simple**, consisting of a single layer of cells; **stratified**, consisting of several layers; or **pseudostrati-**

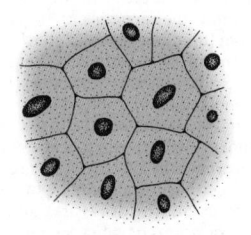

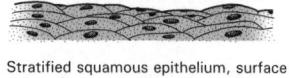

Stratified squamous epithelium, surface view above and sectional view below

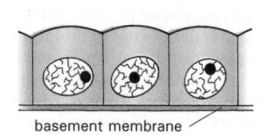

basement membrane

Simple cuboidal epithelium

goblet cell

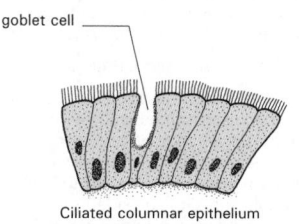

Ciliated columnar epithelium

Types of epithelium.

fied, in which the cells appear to be arranged in layers but in fact share a common basement membrane (see illustration). *See also* ENDOTHELIUM, MESOTHELIUM. —**epithelial** *adj.*

epitrichium (periderm) *n.* the most superficial layer of the skin, one cell in thickness, that is only present early in embryonic development. It protects the underlying *epidermis until it is fully formed.

Epley particle repositioning manoeuvre a series of head and body movements used to move microscopic debris from the posterior *semicircular canal in the inner ear. It is used in the treatment of *benign paroxysmal positional vertigo.

EPO *see* ERYTHROPOIETIN.

epoetin (recombinant human erythropoietin) *n.* any of three forms of *erythropoietin produced by genetic engineering – **epoetin alfa** (Binocrit, Eprex), **epoetin beta** (NeoRecormon), or **epoetin zeta** (Retacrit) – used for treating anaemia associated with chronic renal failure or induced by chemotherapy. **Darbepoetin alfa** (Aranesp) and **methoxy polyethylene glycol-epoetin beta** (**pegzerepoetin alfa**; Mircera) are derivatives of epoetin with similar uses but longer duration of action. The drugs are administered by intravenous or subcutaneous injection and side-effects include diarrhoea, raised blood pressure, headache, and flulike symptoms.

eponychium *n. see* NAIL.

eponym *n.* a disease, structure, or species named after a particular person, usually the person who first discovered or described it. Eponyms are widespread in medicine, but they are being replaced as more descriptive terms become necessary. Thus the eponyms islets of Langerhans, aqueduct of Sylvius, and Hashimoto's disease are more likely to be designated in text books as pancreatic islands, cerebral aqueduct, and autoimmune thyroiditis, respectively. —**eponymous** *adj.*

epoophoron *n. see* PAROOPHORON.

epoprostenol *n.* a prostaglandin drug (*see* PROSTACYCLIN) used immediately before and during renal dialysis to prevent clotting of blood in the shunt and also to treat primary *pulmonary hypertension. It is administered by intravenous infusion and side-effects include flushing, headache, and hypotension. Trade name: **Flolan**.

EPS *see* ELECTROPHYSIOLOGICAL STUDY.

Epstein-Barr virus (EB virus, EBV, human herpesvirus 4, HHV-4) the virus, belonging to the *herpesvirus group, that is the causative agent of *glandular fever. It attacks B *lymphocytes. EB virus is also implicated in hepatitis and in certain cancers (e.g. *Burkitt's lymphoma and *Hodgkin's disease). [Sir M. A. Epstein (1921–) and Y. M. Barr (1932–), British pathologists]

epulis *n.* a swelling on the gum. Most such swellings are due to fibrous hyperplasia, but an epulis may be the opening of a *sinus tract.

Epworth Sleepiness Scale a questionnaire to assess the likelihood of falling asleep. It is used to help distinguish snoring from *obstructive sleep apnoea.

equality *n.* in medical ethics, the principle that cases with an equal moral status should be treated equally. This means, most obviously, that patients with the same clinical needs should not be treated differently on morally irrelevant grounds, such as race (*see* DISCRIMINATION), and are afforded identical rights, respect, and value. However, there is much debate over what characteristics are morally important when medical resources need to be rationed; for example, whether a patient's age or *quality of life is morally important. *See* JUSTICE.

Equality and Human Rights Commission a nondepartmental public body set up in 2007 to reduce discrimination and promote equality in regard to race, disability, sex, sexual orientation, religion and belief, and human rights. It replaced the **Commission for Racial Equality**, the **Disability Rights Commission**, and the **Equal Opportunities Commission**.

equi- *combining form denoting* equality.

equinia *n. see* GLANDERS.

equipoise *n.* a state of genuine and substantial uncertainty as to which of two or more courses of action will be best for a patient. Equipoise is an important ethical principle in research, specifically in the design of clinical trials. It is generally held that the random allocation of patients to one or other arm of a trial is ethically acceptable only where there is a genuine uncertainty (equipoise) as to which treatment will most benefit trial participants. Knowingly to assign an individual to inferior or ineffective treatment (such as a placebo) would offend against the principle that his or her *best interests are paramount. A distinction is sometimes made between **clinical equipoise**, which refers to uncertainty across the medical profession as a whole, and **theoretical equipoise**, which refers to the uncertainty of an individual doctor. In addition, patients may not share the state of equipoise; for example, if a patient has his or her own preferences and there are significant side-effects influencing the choice of treatment, it would be *paternalistic and counter to *beneficence not to respect that patient's wishes.

Erb's palsy weakness or paralysis of the shoulder and arm usually caused by injury to the upper roots of the *brachial plexus during traumatic childbirth. This may happen if, during a difficult delivery, excess traction applied to the head damages the fifth and sixth cervical roots of the spinal cord. The muscles of the shoulder and the flexors of the elbow are paralysed and the arm hangs at the side internally rotated at the shoulder with the forearm pronated (**waiter's-tip deformity**). Recovery may be spontaneous, but in some cases nerve grafts or muscle transfers are required. [W. H. Erb (1840–1921), German neurologist]

ERCP (endoscopic retrograde cholangiopancreatography) the technique in which a catheter is passed through a *duodenoscope into the *ampulla of Vater of the common bile duct and injected with a radio-opaque medium to outline the pancreatic duct and bile ducts radiologically. Magnetic resonance cholangiopancreatography (MRCP; *see* CHOLANGIOGRAPHY) is often used first in the diagnosis of obstructive jaundice and pancreatic disease, followed by ERCP for confirmation and therapeutic intervention by removal of stones from the bile duct, biopsy from suspected lesions, or insertion of a *stent. *See also* PAPILLOTOMY.

erectile *adj.* capable of causing erection or becoming erect. The penis is composed largely of erectile tissue.

erectile dysfunction inability in a male to obtain and/or maintain a penile erection to enable vaginal penetration for sexual intercourse. There are many causes and contributing factors; often a combination of physical causes and psychological factors is responsible for the condition. The physical causes include peripheral vascular disease, diabetes mellitus, certain medications, hy-

pogonadism or other endocrine disorders, and anatomical abnormalities of the penis. Treatments that work by increasing blood flow to the cavernous sinuses of the penis include oral *sildenafil and injectable *alprostadil. Penile *prostheses are surgically inserted into the penis.

erection *n.* the sexually active state of the penis, which becomes enlarged and rigid (due to the erectile tissue being swollen with blood) and capable of penetrating the vagina. The term is also applied to the clitoris in a state of sexual arousal.

erepsin *n.* a mixture of protein-digesting enzymes (*see* PEPTIDASE) secreted by the intestinal glands. It is part of the *succus entericus.

erethism *n.* **1.** a state of abnormal mental excitement or irritability. **2.** rapid response to a stimulus.

erg *n.* a unit of work or energy equal to the work done when the point of application of a force of 1 dyne is displaced through a distance of 1 centimetre in the direction of the force. 1 erg = 10^{-7} joule.

ERG *see* ELECTRORETINOGRAPHY.

erg- (ergo-) *combining form denoting* work or activity.

ergocalciferol *n. see* VITAMIN D.

ergograph *n.* an apparatus for recording the work performed by the muscles of the body when undergoing activity. Ergographs are useful for assessment of the capabilities of athletes undergoing training.

ergometrine *n.* a drug that stimulates contractions of the uterus. Combined with *oxytocin (in **Syntometrine**), it is administered by intramuscular injection to assist the final stage of labour and to control bleeding following incomplete miscarriage.

ergonomics *n.* the study of humans in relation to their work and working surroundings. This broad science involves the application of psychological as well as physiological principles to the design of buildings, machinery, vehicles, packaging, implements, and anything else with which people come into contact.

ergosterol *n.* a plant sterol that, when irradiated with ultraviolet light, is converted to ergocalciferol (vitamin D_2). *See* VITAMIN D.

ergot *n.* a fungus (*Claviceps purpurea*) that

grows on rye. It produces several important alkaloids, chemically related to LSD, including *ergotamine and *ergometrine, which are used in medicine in the treatment of migraine and in childbirth. Eating bread made with rye infected with the fungus has led to sporadic outbreaks of *ergotism over the centuries.

ergotamine *n.* a drug that causes constriction of blood vessels and is used to relieve migraine. It is administered in combination with caffeine (in **Cafergot**) or cyclizine and caffeine (in **Migril**) by mouth or in suppositories. Common side-effects are nausea and vomiting, and ergotism may develop as a result of high doses; because of this it has largely been superseded by *5HT$_1$ agonists.

ergotism *n.* poisoning caused by eating rye infected with the fungus *ergot. The chief symptom is gangrene of the fingers and toes, with diarrhoea and vomiting, nausea, and headache. In the Middle Ages the disease was known as **St Anthony's fire**, because of the inflamed appearance of the tissues afflicted with gangrene and the belief that a pilgrimage to St Anthony's tomb would result in cure.

erlotinib *n. see* EPIDERMAL GROWTH FACTOR RECEPTOR, TYROSINE KINASE INHIBITOR.

erogenous *adj.* describing certain parts of the body, the physical stimulation of which leads to sexual arousal.

erosion *n.* 1. an eating away of surface tissue by physical or chemical processes, including those associated with inflammation. In the skin an erosion represents a superficial type of ulceration and therefore heals quite readily. 2. (in dentistry) loss of surface tooth substance, usually caused by repeated application of acid, which softens the enamel. It may result from excessive intake of fruit juice, carbonated drinks, or acidic fruits or by regurgitation of acid from the stomach, as in bulimia nervosa, hiatus hernia, alcoholism, or stress (*see* GASTRO-OESOPHAGEAL REFLUX DISEASE). The teeth become very sensitive. The cause should be corrected; severe cases may require extensive dental restorations.

erot- (**eroto-**) *combining form denoting* sexual desire or love. Example: **erotophobia** (morbid dread of).

eroticism *n.* 1. those elements in thought,

imagination, pictorial imagery, literature, or the arts that tend to arouse sexual excitement or desire. 2. sexual interest or excitement prompted by contemplation or stimulation of areas of the body not normally associated with sexuality. The terms **anal eroticism** and **oral eroticism** are used both in a theoretical Freudian sense and in reference to adult physical sexual activity.

erotomania (**de Clérambault syndrome**) *n.* a delusion that the individual is loved by some person, often a person of importance. It can be a symptom of a *monodelusional disorder or part of a mental illness, such as dementia or schizophrenia.

eructation *n.* belching: the sudden raising of gas from the stomach.

eruption *n.* 1. the outbreak of a rash. A **bullous eruption** is an outbreak of blisters. 2. (in dentistry) the emergence of a growing tooth from the gum into the mouth.

erysipelas *n.* a streptococcal infection of the skin, especially the face, characterized by redness and swelling; it usually has a sharply defined margin, which can differentiate erysipelas from the otherwise similar *cellulitis. The patient is ill, with a high temperature. Phenoxymethylpenicillin (*penicillin V) is the treatment of choice.

erysipeloid *n.* an infection of the skin and underlying tissues with *Erysipelothrix insidiosa*, developing usually in people handling fish, poultry, or meat. Infection enters through scratches or cuts on the hands, and is normally confined to a finger or hand, which becomes reddened; sometimes systemic illness develops. Treatment is with penicillin.

Erysipelothrix *n.* a genus of Gram-positive nonmotile rod-shaped bacteria with a tendency to form filaments. They are parasites of mammals, birds, and fish. *E. insidiosa* (formerly *E. rhusiopathiae*) is a widely distributed species causing the disease *erysipeloid.

erythema *n.* flushing of the skin due to dilatation of the blood capillaries in the dermis. It may be physiological or a sign of inflammation or infection. **Erythema nodosum** is characterized by tender bruiselike swellings on the shins and is often associated with streptococcal infection. In **erythema multiforme** the eruption, which can take various forms, is characterized by so-called 'target lesions' that may be recurrent and follow herpes simplex infection (especially in children) or medications (especially in adults). **Erythema ab igne** is a reticular pigmented rash on the lower legs or elsewhere caused by persistent exposure to radiant heat. **Erythema infectiosum (fifth disease, slapped cheek syndrome)** is a common benign infectious disease of children caused by human *parvovirus B19. It is characterized by fever and a rash, first on the cheeks and later on the trunk and extremities, that disappears after several days.

erythr- (erythro-) *combining form denoting* 1. redness. Example: **erythuria** (excretion of red urine). 2. erythrocytes.

erythrasma *n.* a chronic skin infection due to the bacterium *Corynebacterium minutissimum*, occurring in such areas as the armpits, groin, and toes, where skin surfaces are in contact. It fluoresces coral-pink under *Wood's light and can be treated with topical or systemic antibiotics.

erythroblast *n.* any of a series of nucleated cells (*see* NORMOBLAST, PROERYTHROBLAST) that pass through a succession of stages of maturation to form red blood cells (*erythrocytes). Erythroblasts are normally present in the blood-forming tissue of the bone marrow, but they may appear in the circulation in a variety of diseases (*see* ERYTHROBLASTOSIS). *See also* ERYTHROPOIESIS.

erythroblastosis *n.* the presence in the blood of the nucleated precursors of the red blood cells (*erythroblasts). This may occur when there is an increase in the rate of red cell production, as in haemorrhagic or haemolytic *anaemia, or in infiltrations of the bone marrow by tumours, etc.

erythroblastosis foetalis a severe but rare haemolytic *anaemia affecting newborn infants due to destruction of the infant's red blood cells by factors present in the mother's serum. It is usually caused by incompatibility of the rhesus blood groups between mother and infant (*see* RHESUS FACTOR).

erythrocyanosis *n.* mottled purplish discoloration on the legs and thighs, usually of adolescent girls or obese boys before puberty. The disorder sometimes occurs in older women and is worse in cold weather. Weight loss is the best treatment because it reduces the insulating effect of a thick layer of fat.

erythrocyte (red blood cell) *n.* a *blood cell containing the red pigment *haemoglobin, the principal function of which is the transport of oxygen. A mature erythrocyte has no nucleus and its shape is that of a biconcave disc, approximately 7 μm in diameter. There are normally about 5×10^{12} erythrocytes per litre of blood. *See also* ERYTHROPOIESIS.

erythrocyte sedimentation rate *see* ESR.

erythrocytic *adj.* describing those stages in the life cycle of the malarial parasite (*see* PLASMODIUM) that develop inside the red blood cells (*see* TROPHOZOITE). *Compare* EXOERYTHROCYTIC.

erythroderma (exfoliative dermatitis) *n.* abnormal reddening, flaking, and thickening of the skin affecting a wide area of the body. Commoner after the age of 50, erythroderma affects men three times as often as women; it may result from pre-existing skin disease, such as eczema or psoriasis, or be caused by drugs or lymphoma. This clinical picture is a form of acute skin failure.

erythroedema *n.* *see* PINK DISEASE.

erythrogenesis *n.* a former name for *erythropoiesis.

erythromelalgia *n.* painful paroxysmal dilation of the blood vessels of the skin, usually affecting the extremities; the skin feels hot. Some patients may respond to aspirin.

erythromycin *n.* an antibiotic used to treat respiratory and other infections caused by a wide range of bacteria. It is administered by mouth or intravenous infusion or (for treating acne) topically. Side-effects are rare and mild, though nausea, vomiting, and diarrhoea occur occasionally. Trade names: **Erymax, Erythrocin, Erythroped, Stiemycin**.

erythron *n.* circulating mature red blood cells and that part of the blood-forming system of the body that is directed towards the production of red blood cells. The erythron is not a single organ but is dispersed throughout the blood-forming tissue of the *bone marrow. *See also* ERYTHROPOIESIS.

erythropenia *n.* a reduction in the number of red blood cells (*erythrocytes) in the blood. This usually, but not invariably, occurs in *anaemia.

erythroplasia *n.* an abnormal red patch of skin that occurs particularly in the mouth or on the genitalia and is precancerous. *Compare* LEUKOPLAKIA.

erythropoiesis *n.* the process of red blood cell (*erythrocyte) production, which normally occurs in the blood-forming tissue of the *bone marrow. The ultimate precursor of the red cell is the *haemopoietic stem cell, but the earliest precursor that can be identified microscopically is the *proeryth-roblast. This divides and passes through a series of stages of maturation termed respectively early, intermediate, and late *normo-blasts, the latter finally losing its nucleus to become a mature red cell. *See also* HAEMOPOIESIS.

erythropoietin (EPO) *n.* a hormone se-creted by certain cells in the kidney in re-sponse to a reduction in the amount of oxygen reaching the tissues. Erythropoietin increases the rate of red cell production (*erythropoiesis) and is the mechanism by which the rate of erythropoiesis is con-trolled. Genetically engineered forms of the hormone are used for treating certain anaemias (*see* EPOETIN, ESA).

erythropsia *n.* red vision: a symptom sometimes experienced after removal of a cataract and also in snow blindness.

ESA erythropoiesis-stimulating agent: a substance similar to the hormone *erythro-poietin, which stimulates red blood cell pro-duction (erythropoiesis). Examples include the commercial *epoetin products.

eschar *n.* a scab or slough, as produced by the action of heat or a corrosive substance on living tissue.

Escherichia *n.* a genus of Gram-negative, generally motile, rodlike bacteria that have the ability to ferment carbohydrates, usually with production of gas, and are found in the intestines of humans and many animals. *E. coli* – a lactose-fermenting species – is usu-ally not harmful but some strains cause gas-trointestinal infections. Ingestion of the pathogenic serotype *E. coli O157*, derived from infected meat, causes colitis with bloody diarrhoea, which may give rise to the complications of *haemolytic uraemic syn-drome or thrombocytopenic *purpura (*see also* FOOD POISONING). *E. coli* is widely used in laboratory experiments for bacteriological and genetic studies.

escitalopram *n. see* SSRI.

esophoria *n.* a tendency to squint in

which the eye, when covered, tends to turn inwards towards the nose. The eye always straightens on removal of the cover. *See also* HETEROPHORIA.

esotropia *n.* convergent squint (*see* STRA-BISMUS).

espundia (mucocutaneous leishmaniasis) *n.* a disease of the skin and mucous mem-branes caused by the parasitic protozoan *Leishmania braziliensis* (*see* LEISHMANIASIS). Occurring in South and Central America, es-pundia takes the form of ulcerating lesions on the arms and legs; the infection may also spread to the mucous membranes of the nose and mouth, causing serious destruction of the tissues.

ESR (erythrocyte sedimentation rate) the rate at which red blood cells (erythrocytes) settle out of suspension in blood plasma, measured under standardized conditions. The ESR increases if the level of certain pro-teins in the plasma rises, as in rheumatic dis-eases, chronic infections, and malignant disease, and thus provides a simple but valu-able screening test for these conditions.

essence *n.* a solution consisting of an es-sential oil dissolved in alcohol.

essential *adj.* describing a disorder that is not apparently attributable to an outside cause; for example, essential *hypertension.

essential amino acid an *amino acid that is essential for normal growth and de-velopment but cannot be synthesized by the body. Essential amino acids are normally ob-tained from protein-rich foods in the diet, such as liver, eggs, and dairy products. There are nine essential amino acids: tryptophan, lysine, phenylalanine, histidine (essential only for children), threonine, valine, methio-nine, leucine, and isoleucine.

essential fatty acid (omega fatty acid) one of a group of *unsaturated fatty acids that are essential for growth but cannot be synthesized by the body. They belong to the n-3 (or omega-3) and n-6 (or omega-6) classes of polyunsaturated fatty acids and in-clude **linoleic** (omega-6), **linolenic** (omega-3), and **arachidonic** (omega-6) **acids**. Linoleic acid occurs in corn oil, soyabean oil, and many other plant fats and oils; arachi-donic acid can be synthesized from it in the body. Linolenic acid occurs in certain plant oils and in fish. Both omega-3 and omega-6 acids should be consumed in the diet.

essential oil a volatile oil derived from an aromatic plant. Essential oils are used in various pharmaceutical preparations.

esterase *n.* an enzyme that catalyses the hydrolysis of esters into their constituent acids and alcohols. For example, fatty-acid esters are broken down to form fatty acids plus alcohol.

ESWL extracorporeal shock-wave lithotripsy. *See* LITHOTRIPSY.

etanercept *n.* a *cytokine inhibitor that is used in the treatment of severe rheumatoid and psoriatic arthritis and severe psoriasis that have not responded to other treatments. It is administered by subcutaneous injection; side-effects include nausea and vomiting, headache, and fever. Trade name: **Enbrel**.

ethambutol *n.* a drug used in the treatment of tuberculosis, in conjunction with other drugs. It is administered by mouth and occasionally causes visual disturbances, which cease when the drug is withdrawn. Allergic rashes and digestive upsets may also occur.

ethanol (ethyl alcohol) *n. see* ALCOHOL.

ether *n.* a volatile liquid formerly used as an anaesthetic administered by inhalation, but now replaced by safer and more efficient drugs. Ether irritates the respiratory tract and affects the circulation.

ethical erosion an empirically observed phenomenon whereby medical students and doctors become less morally sensitive and ethically aware due to increasing cynicism, the negative effects of health-care training and practice, and the desire to 'fit in' with others in the profession.

ethics *n.* **1.** the branch of philosophy concerned with the content of moral judgments (**normative ethics**) and their nature and meaning (**metaethics**). *See also* CONSEQUENTIALISM, KANTIAN ETHICS, NARRATIVE ETHICS. **2.** the principles, values, virtues, or rules of conduct accepted within a particular profession or field of activity. *See* BIOETHICS, MEDICAL ETHICS.

ethics committee a group usually including lay people, medical and health-care professionals, and other experts set up to review health-care practice. There are two types of ethics committee. A **research ethics committee** reviews research that involves the use of human subjects. It is responsible for safeguarding the rights and welfare of patients by ensuring that they are adequately informed of the procedures involved in a research project (including the use of dummy or placebo treatments as controls), that the tests and/or therapies are relatively safe, and that no-one is pressurized into participating in research. There are legal as well as professional requirements to seek ethics committee approval, e.g. when carrying out clinical trials of drugs. The National Research Ethics Service (*see* NATIONAL PATIENT SAFETY AGENCY) coordinates the ethical review and governance of research, referring submissions to research ethics committees (RECs) throughout the UK. The second type of ethics committee is a **clinical ethics committee**, which provides a resource to healthcare professionals about ethical issues in clinical practice. There is neither an obligation for trusts to have a clinical ethics committee nor for clinicians to refer cases to such committees where they exist, although clinical ethics committees are an increasing presence in the NHS.

ethinylestradiol *n.* a synthetic female sex hormone (*see* OESTROGEN) used mainly, in combination with a progestogen, in *oral contraceptives (e.g. **Femodene**, **Marvelon**). Alone, it is used for treating menopausal symptoms, hypogonadism, and menstrual disorders in women and advanced prostate cancer in men. *See also* CYPROTERONE.

ethmoid bone a bone in the floor of the cranium that contributes to the nasal cavity and orbits. The part of the ethmoid forming the roof of the nasal cavity – the **cribriform plate** – is pierced with many small holes through which the olfactory nerves pass. *See also* NASAL CONCHA, SKULL.

ethnology *n.* the study of the different human racial, cultural, and religious groups and their variations: a branch of anthropology that deals mainly with differences between groups and how these are reflected in people's behavior and attitudes.

ethosuximide *n.* an *anticonvulsant drug used mainly to control absence seizures. It is administered by mouth; side-effects such as drowsiness, depression, and digestive disturbances may occur but are usually temporary. Trade names: **Emeside**, **Zarontin**.

etidronate (disodium etidronate) *n. see* BISPHOSPHONATES.

etiology *n. see* AETIOLOGY.

etoposide *n.* a *cytotoxic drug derived from an extract of the mandrake plant that interferes with DNA replication (*see* TOPO-ISOMERASE INHIBITOR). It is administered intravenously or by mouth, primarily in the treatment of bronchial carcinoma, lymphomas, and testicular tumours. Side-effects include alopecia, nausea, and marrow suppression. Trade names: **Etopophos**, **Vepesid**.

etoricoxib *n. see* COX-2 INHIBITOR.

etynodiol (**ethynodiol**) *n.* a synthetic female sex hormone (*see* PROGESTOGEN) that is used in progestogen-only *oral contraceptives. Side-effects can include breast swelling, weight gain, fluid retention, and breakthrough bleeding. Trade name: **Femulen**.

eu- *prefix denoting* 1. good, well, or easy. 2. normal.

eubacteria *pl. n.* a very large group of bacteria with rigid cell walls and – typically – flagella for movement. The group comprises the so-called 'true' bacteria, excluding those, such as spirochaetes and mycoplasmas, with flexible cell walls.

eucalyptol *n.* a volatile oil that has a mild irritant effect on the mucous membranes of the mouth and digestive system. It is taken as pastilles or inhaled as vapour to relieve catarrh. Large doses may cause nausea, vomiting, and diarrhoea.

euchromatin *n.* chromosome material (*see* CHROMATIN) that stains most deeply during mitosis and represents the major genes. *Compare* HETEROCHROMATIN.

eugenics *n.* the 'science' that is concerned with the improvement of the human race by means of the principles of genetics. It is strongly associated with ideas of selective breeding, discrimination, and immoral regimes, such as the Nazi government in Germany. Discomfort remains about any system of eugenics. Interventions used in reproductive medicine, such as *preimplantation genetic diagnosis, antenatal screening, diagnostic testing, and abortion, are regarded by some with suspicion as the potential first step towards a eugenic society. —**eugenic** *adj.*

euglycaemia *n. see* NORMOGLYCAEMIA.

euphoria *n.* a state of optimism, cheerfulness, and wellbeing. A morbid degree of euphoria is characteristic of *mania and *hypomania. *See also* ECSTASY, ELATION.

euplastic *adj.* describing a tissue that heals quickly after injury.

euploidy *n.* the condition of cells, tissues, or organisms in which there is one complete set of chromosomes or a whole multiple of this set in each cell. *Compare* ANEUPLOIDY. —**euploid** *adj., n.*

European Resuscitation Council the supervisory body of *advanced life-support courses in Europe, responsible for updating the content of the courses based on best evidence from all countries represented.

Eustachian tube the tube that connects the middle *ear to the pharynx. It allows the pressure on the inner side of the eardrum to remain equal to the external pressure. [B. Eustachio (1520–74), Italian anatomist]

euthanasia *n.* the act of taking life to relieve suffering. In **voluntary euthanasia** a person asks for, or consents to, measures to be taken to end his or her life. This may be accomplished by active steps, usually the administration of a drug, or passively, for example by deliberately withholding treatment. Voluntary euthanasia is lawful in a number of European jurisdictions, e.g. the Netherlands, Belgium, and Switzerland. **Involuntary** (or **compulsory**) **euthanasia** is where society or those acting on authority give instructions to end the lives of individuals, such as infants, who cannot express their wishes or have not given consent. *See also* ARTIFICIAL NUTRITION AND HYDRATION; ASSISTED SUICIDE; DOCTRINE OF DOUBLE EFFECT; EXTRAORDINARY MEANS.

euthymia *n.* a normal (i.e. nondepressed) mood state, often referred to in *mental state examinations. The term also refers to a neutral mood state in a person with bipolar affective disorder. —**euthymic** *adj.*

euthyroid *adj.* having a thyroid gland that functions normally. *Compare* HYPERTHYROIDISM, HYPOTHYROIDISM. —**euthyroidism** *n.*

euthyroid sick syndrome (**sick euthyroid syndrome**) a syndrome characterized by alteration in the thyroid function tests in which the level of triiodothyronine is markedly reduced, thyroxine is slightly reduced, and thyroid-stimulating hormone is reduced or normal. This syndrome is commonly seen in nonthyroidal illness, due to altered metabolism and transport of the thyroid hormones, but is sometimes mistaken for primary hypothyroidism.

evacuator *n.* a device for sucking fluid out of a cavity. In its simplest form it consists of a hollow rubber bulb that is attached, via a valve system, to a tube inserted into the cavity. Another valve leads to a discharge tube. Evacuators may be used to empty the bladder of unwanted material during such operations as the removal of a calculus or transurethral *prostatectomy.

evagination *n.* the protrusion of a part or organ from a sheathlike covering or by eversion of its inner surface.

EVAR *see* ENDOVASCULAR ANEURYSM REPAIR.

evening primrose oil oil pressed from the seeds of the evening primrose plant (*Oenothera biennis*), which has been used medicinally for centuries. The oil is rich in the polyunsaturated fatty acid linoleic acid (*see* ESSENTIAL FATTY ACID) and also contains gamma-linolenic acid. The latter component is claimed by some to be the active ingredient of the oil but this is not proven. Symptom relief has been reported for rheumatoid arthritis, breast pain, premenstrual syndrome, eczema, diabetic neuropathy, cancer, hypercholesterolaemia, and heart disease, although study results have been negative or mixed.

eventration *n.* **1.** protrusion of the intestines through the abdominal wall. **2.** abnormal elevation of part of the diaphragm due to a congenital weakness (but without true herniation), as observed by X-ray.

event sampling (in psychology) a way of recording behaviour in which the presence of a particular kind of behaviour is noted whenever it occurs. It is used for precise descriptions of behaviour and for following the course of *behaviour modification. *See also* TIME SAMPLING.

eversion *n.* a turning outward; in **eversion of the cervix** the edges of the cervix (neck) of the uterus turn outward.

evisceration *n.* **1.** (in surgery) the removal of the viscera. **2.** (in ophthalmology) an operation in which the contents of the eyeball are removed, the empty outer envelope (sclera) being left behind. *Compare* ENUCLEATION.

EVLT *see* ENDOVENOUS LASER TREATMENT.

Ewing's sarcoma a malignant tumour of bone occurring in children and young adults. Distinguished from *osteosarcoma by J. Ewing in 1921, it commonly arises in the femur but is liable to spread to other bones and to the lung. It usually presents with pain, often associated with fever and *leucocytosis. The tumour is sensitive to radiotherapy, and systemic therapy with *cytotoxic drugs has greatly improved its prognosis. [J. Ewing (1866–1943), US pathologist]

EWS *see* EARLY WARNING SYSTEM.

ex- (exo-) *prefix denoting* outside or outer.

exaltation *n. see* ELATION.

exanthem *n.* a rash or eruption (usually maculopapular), such as that occurring in measles. **Exanthem subitum** is another name for *roseola (infantum). —**exanthematous** *adj.*

excavator *n.* **1.** a spoon-shaped surgical instrument that is used to scrape out diseased tissue, usually for laboratory examination. **2.** a type of hand instrument with spoon ends used for removing decayed dentine from teeth. It may also be used as a *curette.

exchange transfusion a technique for treating *haemolytic disease in newborn infants. Using a syringe with a three-way tap, blood is withdrawn from the baby (via the umbilical vein), ejected, and replaced by an equal amount of donor blood compatible with the mother's blood, without detaching the syringe. By many repetitions of this exchange, red blood cells liable to be destroyed and bilirubin released from those already destroyed are removed, while keeping the baby's blood volume and number of red cells constant. Exchange transfusion can also be used in *sickle-cell disease, as a temporary treatment during a crisis, or in neonatal jaundice.

excimer laser a form of ultraviolet laser that can remove very thin sheets of tissue. This can be used to alter the curvature of the corneal surface, for example to treat long- or short-sightedness (*see* LASEK, LASIK), or to remove diseased (e.g. calcified) tissue from the corneal surface. *See* KERATECTOMY.

excipient *n.* a substance that is combined with a drug in order to render it suitable for administration; for example in the form of pills. Excipients should have no pharmacological action themselves.

excise *vb.* to cut out tissue, an organ, or a tumour from the body. —**excision** *n.*

excitation *n.* (in neurophysiology) the triggering of a conducted impulse in the membrane of a muscle cell or nerve fibre. During excitation a polarized membrane becomes momentarily depolarized and an *action potential is set up.

excoriation *n.* the destruction and removal of the surface of the skin or the covering of an organ by scraping, the application of a chemical, or other means.

excrescence *n.* an abnormal outgrowth on the surface of the body, such as a wart.

excreta *n.* any waste material discharged from the body, especially faeces.

excretion *n.* the removal of the waste products of metabolism from the body, mainly through the action of the *kidneys. Excretion also includes the loss of water, salts, and some urea through the sweat glands and carbon dioxide and water vapour from the lungs, and the term is also used to include the egestion of faeces.

exemestane *n. see* AROMATASE INHIBITOR.

exenteration *n.* (in ophthalmology) an operation in which all the contents of the eye socket (orbit) are removed, leaving only the bony walls intact. The bone is covered by a skin graft. This operation is sometimes necessary when there is a malignant tumour in the orbit.

exercise *n.* any activity resulting in physical exertion that is intended to maintain physical fitness, to condition the body, or to correct a physical deformity. Exercises may be done actively by the person or passively by a therapist. **Aerobic exercises** are intended to increase oxygen consumption (as in running) and to benefit the lungs and cardiovascular system, in contrast to *isometric exercises. In **isotonic exercises**, the muscles contract and there is movement, but the force remains the same; this improves joint mobility and muscle strength.

exflagellation *n.* the formation and release of mature flagellated male sex cells (*see* MICROGAMETE) by the *microgametocytes of the malarial parasite (*see* PLASMODIUM). The process, which is completed in 10–15 minutes, occurs after the microgametocytes have been transferred from a human to the stomach of a mosquito.

exfoliation *n.* **1.** flaking off of the upper layers of the skin. **2.** separation of a surface epithelium from the underlying tissue. **3.** the natural shedding of primary teeth. —**exfoliative** *adj.*

exhalation (**expiration**) *n.* the act of breathing air from the lungs out through the mouth and nose. *See* BREATHING.

exhibitionism *n.* exposure of the genitals to another person, as a sexually deviant act. The word is often broadened to mean public flaunting of any quality of the individual.

exo- *prefix. see* EX-.

exocoelom *n. see* EXTRAEMBRYONIC COELOM.

exocrine gland a gland that discharges its secretion by means of a duct, which opens onto an epithelial surface. An exocrine gland may be **simple**, with a single unbranched duct, or **compound**, with branched ducts and multiple secretory sacs. The illustration shows some different types of these glands. Examples of exocrine glands are the sebaceous and sweat glands. *See also* SECRETION.

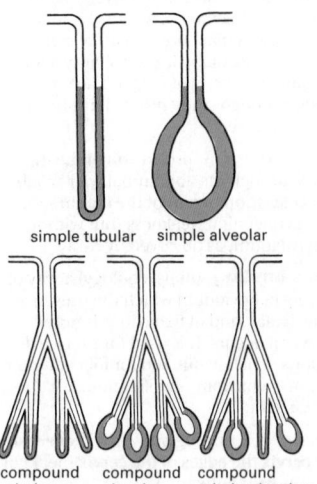

simple tubular   simple alveolar

compound tubular   compound alveolar   compound tubulo-alveolar

Types of exocrine glands.

exoenzyme *n.* an *enzyme that acts outside the cell that produced it. Examples of exoenzymes are the digestive enzymes.

exoerythrocytic *adj.* describing those

stages in the life cycle of the malarial parasite (*see* PLASMODIUM) that develop in the cells of the liver. Each parasite (*sporozoite) divides repeatedly to produce a schizont containing many merozoites.

exogenous *adj.* originating outside the body or part of the body: applied particularly to substances in the body that are derived from the diet rather than built up by the body's own processes of metabolism. *Compare* ENDOGENOUS.

exomphalos (umbilical hernia) *n.* a congenital defect in which the abdominal wall fails to close during fetal development and bowel, covered by peritoneum, herniates through the umbilical cord. Unlike *gastroschisis, it is associated with other structural fetal abnormalities. It can be corrected by surgery.

exopeptidase *n.* an enzyme (e.g. *trypsin) that takes part in the digestion of proteins by splitting off the terminal amino acids of a polypeptide chain. *Compare* ENDOPEPTIDASE. *See also* PEPTIDASE.

exophoria *n.* a tendency to squint in which the eye, when covered, tends to turn outwards. The eye always straightens on removal of the cover. *See also* HETEROPHORIA.

exophthalmic goitre (Graves' disease) *see* THYROTOXICOSIS.

exophthalmometer (proptometer) *n.* an instrument for measuring the distance from the edges of the bony orbits to the corneas to ascertain the degree of *exophthalmos in Graves' disease (*see* THYROTOXICOSIS).

exophthalmos *n.* protrusion of the eyeballs in their sockets. This can result from injury or disease of the eyeball or socket but is most commonly associated with overactivity of the thyroid gland (*see* THYROTOXICOSIS).

exophytic *adj.* describing growth outwards from an epithelial surface. Exophytic growth is characteristic of benign epithelial tumours but carcinomas may also have an exophytic growth component. *Compare* ENDOPHYTIC.

exosmosis *n.* outward osmotic flow. *See also* OSMOSIS.

exostosis *n.* a benign outgrowth of bone with a cap of cartilage, arising from a bony surface. It is a stalklike *osteochondroma. **Hereditary multiple exostoses** (**diaphyseal aclasia**, **familial osteochondroma**) is a hereditary (autosomal *dominant) abnormality of cartilage and bone growth that results in the formation of multiple exostoses, most commonly at the ends of the long bones.

exothermic *adj.* describing a chemical reaction in which energy is released in the form of heat. *Compare* ENDOTHERMIC.

exotic *adj.* describing a disease occurring in a region of the world far from where it might be expected. Thus malaria and leishmaniasis are regarded as exotic when they are diagnosed in patients in Britain.

exotoxin *n.* a highly potent poison, often harmful to only a limited range of tissues, that is produced by a bacterial cell and secreted into its surrounding medium. It is generally unstable, being rendered inactive by heat, light, and chemicals. Exotoxins are produced by such bacteria as those causing *botulism, *diphtheria, and *tetanus. *Compare* ENDOTOXIN.

exotropia *n.* divergent squint (*see* STRABISMUS).

expectorant *n.* a drug that enhances the expulsion of sputum from the air passages. *Mucolytic expectorants act by decreasing the viscosity of the bronchial secretions so that they are easier to cough up. Drugs such as *ipecacuanha and ammonium chloride are claimed to be **stimulant expectorants** in small quantities: they irritate the lining of the stomach, which is said to provide a stimulus for the reflex production of sputum by the glands in the bronchial mucous membrane. At higher doses they produce vomiting.

expectoration *n.* the act of spitting out material brought into the mouth by coughing.

expiration *n.* **1.** the act of breathing out air from the lungs: exhalation. **2.** dying.

explant 1. *n.* live tissue transferred from the body (or any organism) to a suitable artificial medium for culture. The tissue grows in the artificial medium and can be studied for diagnostic or experimental purposes. Tumour growths are sometimes examined in this way. **2.** *n.* silicone rubber material sutured to the outside of the eyeball over a retinal tear or hole (*see* PLOMBAGE). The resulting indent allows the retina to reattach. **3.** *vb.* to transfer live tissue for culture outside the body. —**explantation** *n.*

exploitation *n.* taking unfair advantage of another's misfortune, weakness, or *vulnerability. In medical ethics, the principle of *nonmaleficence means that doctors have an active duty to avoid any exploitation of their patients. This is usually held to require that professional boundaries are maintained and to prohibit personal or sexual relationships between professionals and their patients. Another example of potential exploitation is the practice of holding clinical trials and conducting research in developing countries when the treatments being tested are designed for sale and use in the West and will not be made available to those who acted as research participants or subjects.

exploration *n.* (in surgery) an investigative operation on a wound, tissue, or cavity. It may be undertaken to determine the cause of symptoms. —**exploratory** *adj.*

exposure *n.* (in behaviour therapy) a method of treating fears and phobias that involves confronting the individual with the situation he has been avoiding, so allowing the fears to wane by *habituation. It can be achieved gradually by *desensitization or *graded self-exposure or suddenly by *flooding.

expressed emotion a measure of the degree of warmth or hostility in a relationship between two people, assessed when one person is talking about the other. High levels of criticism and hostility from family members can worsen the prognosis of mentally ill patients, especially in schizophrenia; increased expressed emotion may be addressed with specialized *family therapy.

expulsive haemorrhage sudden bleeding from the choroid, usually during a surgical procedure or trauma. This may force the ocular tissue out of the wound and is potentially one of the most devastating intraoperative complications of ocular surgery.

exsanguination *n.* **1.** depriving the body of blood; for example, as a result of an accident causing severe bleeding or – very rarely – through uncontrollable bleeding during a surgical operation. **2.** a technique for providing a bloodless field to facilitate delicate or haemorrhagic operative procedures. **3.** the removal of blood from a part (usually a limb) prior to stopping the inflow of blood (by tourniquet). —**exsanguinate** *vb.*

exsiccation *n.* drying up, as may occur in tissues deprived of an adequate supply of water during dehydration or starvation.

exstrophy *n.* a severe congenital abnormality in which the bladder fails to close during development: the baby is born with an absent lower abdominal wall and the internal surface of the posterior bladder wall is exposed. It is associated with *epispadias, total urinary incontinence, and undescended testes.

exsufflation *n.* the forcible removal of secretions from the air passages by some form of suction apparatus.

extension *n.* **1.** the act of extending or stretching, especially the muscular movement by which a limb is straightened. **2.** the application of *traction to a fractured or dislocated limb in order to restore it to its normal position.

extensor *n.* any muscle that causes the straightening of a limb or other part.

exteriorization *n.* a surgical procedure in which an organ is brought from its normal site to the surface of the body. This may be done as a temporary or permanent measure; for example, the intestine may be brought to the surface of the abdomen (*see* COLOSTOMY). The process is also sometimes used in physiological experiments on animals.

external fixator an apparatus consisting of a rigid frame that connects pins passed through the skin into the bone above and below a fracture. This immobilizes the fracture, and is used particularly to treat some compound fractures. An external fixator is also used for *limb lengthening.

exteroceptor *n.* a sensory nerve, ending in the skin or a mucous membrane, that is responsive to stimuli from outside the body. *See also* CHEMORECEPTOR, RECEPTOR.

extinction *n.* (in psychology) the weakening of a conditioned reflex that takes place if it is not maintained by *reinforcement. This is used as a method of treatment when undesirable behaviour (e.g. destructiveness) is reduced simply by withdrawing whatever rewards it (e.g. the fuss made by other people).

extirpation *n.* the complete surgical removal of tissue, an organ, or a growth.

extra- *prefix denoting* outside or beyond.

extra-articular *adj.* not involving a joint.

The term is commonly used to specify a fracture pattern or the position of a bone tumour. *See also* INTRA-ARTICULAR, PERI-ARTICULAR.

extracellular *adj.* situated or occurring outside cells; for example, **extracellular fluid** is the fluid surrounding cells.

extracorporeal *adj.* situated or occurring outside the body. **Extracorporeal circulation** is the circulation of the blood outside the body, as through a *heart-lung machine or in *haemodialysis.

extracorporeal membrane oxygenation (ECMO) a technique that is accepted as a rescue treatment for otherwise fatal respiratory failure in newborn babies or infants due to prematurity or overwhelming septicaemia (e.g. meningitis). It involves modified prolonged *cardiopulmonary bypass to support gas exchange, which allows the lungs to rest and recover. ECMO is only available in selected high-technology centres.

extract *n.* a preparation containing the pharmacologically active principles of a drug, made by evaporating a solution of the drug in water, alcohol, or ether.

extraction *n.* **1.** the surgical removal of a part of the body. Extraction of teeth is usually achieved by applying *elevators and extraction *forceps to the crown or root of the tooth to dislocate it from its socket. When this is not possible, for example because the tooth or root is deeply buried within the bone, extraction is performed surgically by removing bone and, where necessary, dividing the tooth. **2.** the act of pulling out a baby from the body of its mother during childbirth.

extractor *n.* an instrument used to pull out a natural part of the body, to remove a foreign object, or to assist delivery of a baby (*see* VENTOUSE (VACUUM EXTRACTOR)).

extradural *adj. see* EPIDURAL.

extraembryonic coelom (exocoelom) the cavity, lined with mesoderm, that surrounds the embryo from the earliest stages of development. It communicates temporarily with the coelomic cavity within the embryo (peritoneal cavity). Late in pregnancy it becomes almost entirely obliterated by the growth of the *amnion, which fuses with the *chorion.

extraembryonic membranes the membranous structures that surround the embryo and contribute to the placenta and umbilical cord. They include the *amnion, *chorion, *allantois, and *yolk sac. In humans the allantois is always very small and by the end of pregnancy the amnion and chorion have fused into a single membrane and the yolk sac has disappeared.

extraordinary means life-prolonging treatments that are not regarded as beneficial (i.e. they do nothing to promote recovery or relieve suffering) and that may even be burdensome to the patient. It has been argued that there is no moral obligation to prolong life and/or to impose greater suffering by extraordinary means. 'Extraordinary' does not mean unusual: treatments that are considered routine may be classed as extraordinary when they are no longer clinically effective or are considered *futile. Another way to describe the appropriateness of such interventions is to talk of 'proportionate' and 'disproportionate' means. *See* ARTIFICIAL NUTRITION AND HYDRATION.

extrapleural *adj.* relating to the tissues of the chest wall outside the parietal *pleura.

extrapyramidal effects symptoms caused by a reduction of dopamine activity in the extrapyramidal system due to the adverse effects of *dopamine receptor antagonists, notably phenothiazine *antipsychotic drugs. These effects include *parkinsonism, *akathisia, and *dyskinesia.

extrapyramidal system the system of nerve tracts and pathways connecting the cerebral cortex, basal ganglia, thalamus, cerebellum, reticular formation, and spinal neurons in complex circuits not included in the *pyramidal system. The extrapyramidal system is mainly concerned with the regulation of stereotyped reflex muscular movements.

extrasystole *n. see* ECTOPIC BEAT.

extrauterine *adj.* outside the uterus.

extravasation *n.* the leakage and spread of blood or fluid from vessels into the surrounding tissues, which follows injury, burns, inflammation, and allergy.

extraversion *n. see* EXTROVERSION.

extrinsic muscle a muscle, such as any of those controlling movements of the eyeball, that has its origin some distance from the part it acts on. *See also* EYE.

extroversion *n.* **1. (extraversion)** an enduring personality trait characterized by interest in the outside world rather than the self. People high in extroversion (**extroverts**), as measured by questionnaires and tests, are gregarious and outgoing, prefer to change activities frequently, and are not susceptible to permanent *conditioning. Extroversion was first described by Carl Jung as a tendency to action rather than thought, to scientific rather than philosophical interests, and to emotional rather than intellectual reactions. Eysenck used it as one of the main personality traits in his widely used personality questionnaire. *Compare* INTROVERSION. **2.** a turning inside out of a hollow organ, such as the uterus (which sometimes occurs after childbirth).

extrovert *n. see* EXTROVERSION.

extrusion *n.* (in dentistry) **1.** the forced eruption of a tooth either by means of an orthodontic appliance or surgically; for example, to realign a tooth that has failed to erupt or has been accidentally forced into the jaw. **2.** the partial displacement of a tooth from its socket as a result of traumatic injury.

exudation *n.* the slow escape of liquid (called the **exudate**) that is rich in proteins and contains white cells through the walls of intact blood vessels, usually as a result of inflammation. Exudation is a normal part of the body's defence mechanisms.

eye *n.* the organ of sight: a three-layered roughly spherical structure specialized for receiving and responding to light. The outer

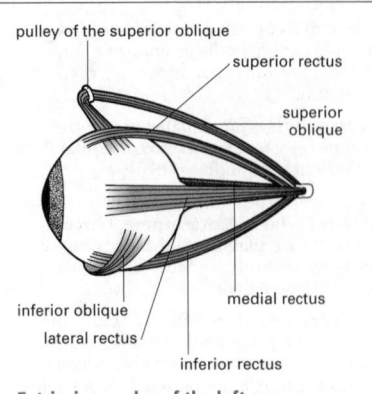

Extrinsic muscles of the left eye.

fibrous coat consists of the sclera and the transparent cornea; the middle vascular layer comprises the choroid, ciliary body, and iris; and the inner sensory layer is the retina (see illustration below).

Light enters the eye through the cornea, which refracts the light through the aqueous humour onto the lens. By adjustment of the shape of the lens (*see* ACCOMMODATION) light is focused through the vitreous humour onto the retina. In the retina light-sensitive cells (*see* CONE, ROD) send nerve impulses to the brain via the optic nerve. The arrangement of the two eyes at the front of the head provides *binocular vision. Each eye is contained in an *orbit, and movement of the eye within the orbit is controlled by extrinsic eye muscles (see illustration above).

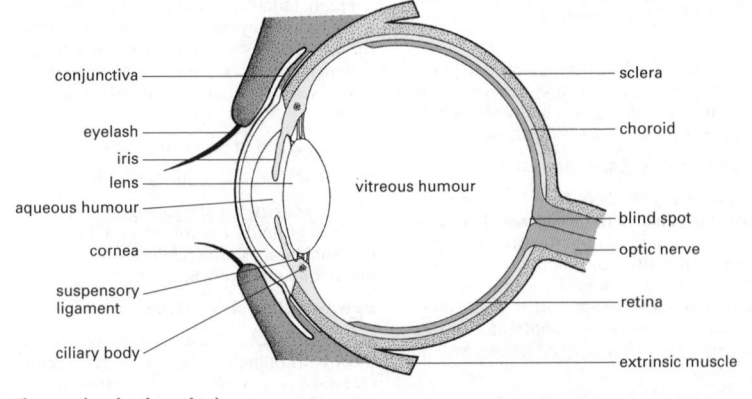

The eye (sagittal section).

eyeball *n.* the body of the *eye, which is roughly spherical, is bounded by the *sclera, and lies in the *orbit. It is closely associated with accessory structures – the eyelids, conjunctiva, and lacrimal (tear-producing) apparatus – and its movements are controlled by three pairs of extrinsic eye muscles (see illustration).

eyebrow *n.* the small fringe of hair on the bony ridge just above the eye. It helps to prevent moisture from running into the eye. Anatomical name: **supercilium**.

eyelash *n.* one of the long stiff hairs that form a row projecting outwards from the front edge of the upper and lower eyelids. The eyelashes help keep dust away from the eye. Anatomical name: **cilium**.

eyelid *n.* the protective covering of the eye. Each eye has two eyelids consisting of skin, muscle, connective tissue (**tarsus**), and sebaceous glands (**meibomian** or **tarsal glands**). Each eyelid is lined with membrane (*conjunctiva) and fringed with eyelashes. Stimulation of the pain receptors in the cornea causes the eyelids to close in a reflex action. Inflammation of a meibomian gland can result in a *chalazion. Anatomical names: **blepharon, palpebra**.

eye movement desensitization and reprocessing therapy (EMDR) a type of psychotherapy used for the treatment of significant anxiety or distress caused by traumatic events or post-traumatic stress disorder. The aim is to separate the emotional from the actual memory of the event in order to reduce the anxiety related to the memory.

eyepiece *n.* the lens or system of lenses of an optical instrument, such as a microscope, that is nearest to the eye of the examiner. It usually produces a magnified image of the previous image formed by the instrument. *Compare* OBJECTIVE.

eyespot *n.* a small light-sensitive area of pigment found in some protozoans and other lower organisms.

eyestrain *n.* a sense of fatigue brought on by use of the eyes for prolonged close work or in persons who have an uncorrected error of *refraction or an imbalance of the muscles that move the eyes. Symptoms are usually aching or burning of the eyes, accompanied by headache and even general fatigue if the eyes are not rested. Medical name: **asthenopia**.

e

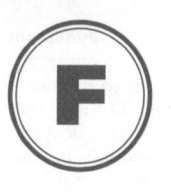

Fabry disease (Anderson-Fabry disease) an inherited disorder – an X-linked recessive condition (*see* SEX-LINKED) – characterized by deficiency of the enzyme α-galactosidase. It causes accumulation of glycosphingolipid (*see* CEREBROSIDE) in the body, leading to prominent and progressive involvement of the skin (with the formation of *angiokeratomas), heart, kidneys, and nervous system. The disease is treated with genetically engineered enzyme replacement therapy. [J. Fabry (1860–1930), German dermatologist]

face-bow *n.* (in dentistry) an instrument for transferring the jaw relationship of a patient to an *articulator to allow reproduction of the lateral and protrusive movements of the lower jaw.

face-lift *n.* plastic surgery designed to correct sagging facial tissues. Eyelid drooping can be corrected at the same procedure.

facet *n.* a small flat surface on a bone or tooth, especially a surface of articulation.

facial nerve the seventh *cranial nerve (VII): a mixed sensory and motor nerve that supplies the muscles of facial expression, the taste buds of the front part of the tongue, the sublingual salivary glands, and the lacrimal glands. A small branch to the middle ear regulates the tension on the ear ossicles.

facial paralysis paralysis of the facial nerve, causing weakness and loss of function of the muscles it serves. It occurs in *Bell's palsy. The commonest cause is infection with the herpes simplex virus.

-facient *suffix denoting* causing or making. Example: **abortifacient** (causing abortion).

facies *n.* **1.** facial expression, often a guide to a patient's state of health as well as emotions. The typical facies seen in a patient with enlarged adenoids is a vacant look, with the mouth drooping open. A **Hippocratic facies** is the sallow face, sagging and with listless staring eyes, that indicates approaching death. **2.** (in anatomy) a specified surface of a bone or other body part.

facilitation *n.* (in neurology) the phenom-

enon that occurs when a neuron receives, through a number of different synapses, impulses that are not powerful enough individually to start an *action potential but whose combined activity brings about some *depolarization of the membrane. In this facilitated state any small additional depolarization will suffice to trigger off an impulse in the cell.

facio- *combining form denoting* the face. Examples: **faciobrachial** (relating to the face and arm); **faciolingual** (relating to the face and tongue); **facioplegia** (paralysis of).

factitious *adj.* produced artificially, either deliberately or by accident, and therefore not to be taken into account when the results of an experiment are considered or a diagnosis is being made. A **factitious disorder** is one in which a person makes up physical or psychological symptoms to gain sympathy and attention.

factor *n.* (in biochemistry) a substance that is essential to a physiological process, often a substance the nature of which is unknown. *See also* COAGULATION FACTORS, GROWTH FACTOR.

Factor V Leiden an inherited mutation in the gene coding for coagulation Factor V, which results in an increased susceptibility to develop venous *thrombosis.

Factor VIII (antihaemophilic factor) a *coagulation factor normally present in blood. Deficiency of the factor, which is inherited by males from their mothers, results in *haemophilia A. *See also* VON WILLEBRAND'S DISEASE.

Factor IX (Christmas factor) a *coagulation factor normally present in blood. Deficiency of the factor results in *haemophilia B.

Factor XI a *coagulation factor normally present in blood. Deficiency of the factor is inherited, but rarely causes spontaneous bleeding. However, bleeding does occur after surgery or trauma to the blood vessels.

facultative *adj.* describing an organism

that is not restricted to one way of life. A **facultative parasite** can live either as a parasite or, in different conditions, as a nonparasite able to survive without a host. *Compare* OBLIGATE.

FAD (flavin adenine dinucleotide) a *coenzyme, derived from riboflavin, that takes part in many important oxidation-reduction reactions. It consists of two phosphate groups, adenine, and ribose.

fading *n*. (in behaviour modification) *see* PROMPTING.

faecal impaction *see* CONSTIPATION, IMPACTED.

faecal incontinence *see* INCONTINENCE.

faecalith (faecolith, coprolith) *n*. a hard mass of faeces within the colon, vermiform appendix, or rectum, due to chronic constipation: a cause of inflammation.

faecal occult blood test (FOBT) a non-invasive test used to identify microscopic blood (*see* OCCULT) in faeces. It is widely used as a screening test for colorectal cancer.

faeces *n*. the waste material that is eliminated through the anus. It is formed in the *colon and consists of a solid or semisolid mass of undigested food remains (chiefly cellulose) mixed with *bile pigments (which are responsible for the colour), bacteria, various secretions (e.g. mucus), and some water. —**faecal** *adj*.

Fahrenheit temperature temperature expressed on a scale in which the melting point of ice is assigned a temperature of 32° and the boiling point of water a temperature of 212°. For most medical purposes the Celsius (centigrade) scale has replaced the Fahrenheit scale. The formula for converting from Fahrenheit (F) to Celsius (C) is: C = $5/9(F − 32)$. *See also* CELSIUS TEMPERATURE. [G. D. Fahrenheit (1686–1736), German physicist]

failure to thrive (FTT) failure of an infant to grow satisfactorily compared with the average for that community. It is detected by regular measurements and plotting on *centile charts. It can be the first indication of a serious underlying condition, such as kidney or heart disease or malabsorption, or it may result from problems at home, particularly *nonaccidental injury.

fainting *n*. *see* SYNCOPE.

fairness *n*. *see* EQUALITY, JUSTICE.

falciform ligament a fold of peritoneum separating the right and left lobes of the liver and attaching it to the diaphragm and the anterior abdominal wall as far as the umbilicus.

Fallopian tube (oviduct, uterine tube) either of a pair of tubes that conduct ova (egg cells) from the ovary to the uterus (*see* REPRODUCTIVE SYSTEM). The ovarian opens into the abdominal cavity via a funnel-shaped structure with finger-like projections (**fimbriae**) surrounding the opening. Movements of the fimbriae at ovulation assist in directing the ovum to the Fallopian tube. The ovum is fertilized near the ovarian end of the tube. [G. Fallopius (1523–63), Italian anatomist]

falloposcope *n*. a narrow flexible fibreoptic *endoscope used to view the inner lining of the Fallopian tubes (*see* FALLOPOSCOPY).

falloposcopy *n*. observation of the interior of a Fallopian tube using a *falloposcope introduced via a hysteroscope (*see* HYSTEROSCOPY).

Fallot's tetralogy *see* TETRALOGY OF FALLOT.

false negative a result of a diagnostic test or procedure that wrongly indicates the absence of a disease or other condition. *See* SENSITIVITY.

false positive a result of a diagnostic test or procedure that wrongly indicates the presence of a disease or other condition. *See* SENSITIVITY.

false pregnancy *see* PSEUDOCYESIS.

false rib *see* RIB.

falx (falx cerebri) *n*. (*pl*. **falces**) a sickle-shaped fold of the *dura mater that dips inwards from the skull in the midline, between the cerebral hemispheres.

familial *adj*. describing a condition or character that is found in some families but not in others. It is often inherited.

familial adenomatous polyposis (FAP) *see* POLYPOSIS.

familial hypercholesterolaemia *see* HYPERCHOLESTEROLAEMIA.

familial mixed hyperlipidaemia *see* HYPERLIPIDAEMIA.

family doctor *see* GENERAL PRACTITIONER.

family planning 1. the use of *contraception to limit or space out the numbers of children born to a couple. 2. provision of contraceptive methods within a community or nation. *See also* GENETIC COUNSELLING.

family practitioner *see* GENERAL PRACTITIONER.

family therapy a form of *psychotherapy based on the belief that psychological problems are the products of abnormalities in communication between family members. All family members are therefore seen together, when possible, in order to clarify and modify the ways they relate together (*see* GENOGRAM, PARADOX).

famotidine *n.* an H_2-receptor antagonist (*see* ANTIHISTAMINE) used for the treatment of duodenal ulcers and conditions of excessive gastric acid secretion, such as the Zollinger-Ellison syndrome. It is administered by mouth; side-effects are headache, diarrhoea, and dizziness. Trade name: **Pepcid**.

Fanconi's anaemia an autosomal *recessive disorder characterized by severe aplastic *anaemia (failure of the bone marrow to produce blood cells, either red or white) and an increased predisposition to malignancy. It also causes mental retardation, poor growth, skeletal abnormalities, and kidneys of an unusual shape or in an unusual position. The condition is due to a defect in one of a group of genes known as Fanconi's anaemia (*FA*) genes. Children are usually diagnosed between five and ten years of age. The only treatment available is *haemopoietic stem cell transplantation; without this, most affected individuals die by the age of 30 from bone marrow failure or leukaemia. [G. Fanconi (1892–1979), Swiss paediatrician]

Fanconi syndrome a disorder of the proximal kidney tubules, which may be inherited or acquired and is most common in children. It is characterized by the urinary excretion of large amounts of amino acids, glucose, and phosphates (though blood levels of these substances are normal). Symptoms may include osteomalacia, rickets, muscle weakness, and *cystinosis. Treatment is directed to the cause. [G. Fanconi]

Fansidar *n. see* PYRIMETHAMINE.

fantasy *n.* a complex sequence of imagination in which several imaginary elements are woven together into a story. An excessive preoccupation with one's fantasies may be symptomatic of a difficulty in coping with reality or part of a narcissistic personality disorder (*see* NARCISSISM). In psychoanalytic psychology, **unconscious fantasies** are believed to control behaviour, and psychological symptoms may be symbols of or defences against such fantasies (*see* SYMBOLISM).

FARA (cryptogenic) *f*ibrosing *a*lveolitis associated with *r*heumatoid *a*rthritis. *See* ALVEOLITIS.

farad *n.* the *SI unit of capacitance, equal to the capacitance of a capacitor between the plates of which a potential difference of 1 volt appears when it is charged with 1 coulomb of electricity. Symbol: F.

faradism *n.* the use of induced rapidly alternating electric currents to stimulate nerve and muscle activity. *See also* ELECTROTHERAPY.

farcy *n. see* GLANDERS.

farmer's lung an occupational lung disease caused by allergy to fungal spores that grow in inadequately dried stored hay, straw, or grain, which then becomes mouldy. It is an allergic *alveolitis, such as also results from sensitivity to many other allergens. An acute reversible form can develop a few hours after exposure; a chronic form, with the gradual development of irreversible breathlessness, occurs with or without preceding acute attacks. Avoidance of the allergen is the main principle of treatment, but most farmers are able to continue to farm by taking appropriate precautions.

fascia *n.* (*pl.* **fasciae**) connective tissue forming layers of variable thickness in all regions of the body. It is divided into **superficial fascia**, found immediately beneath the skin, and **deep fascia**, which envelops organs and tissues. Deep fascia includes the sheets of fibrous tissue that enclose muscles and muscle groups and separate them into layers.

fasciculation *n.* brief spontaneous contraction of a few muscle fibres, which is seen as a flicker of movement under the skin. It is most often associated with disease of the lower motor neurons (e.g. *motor neuron disease). Fasciculation may be seen in the calf muscles of normal individuals, especially after exercise.

fasciculus (fascicle) *n.* a bundle, e.g. of nerve or muscle fibres.

fasciitis *n.* inflammation of *fascia. It may result from bacterial infection or from a rheumatic disease, such as *Reiter's syndrome or ankylosing spondylitis. *See also* NECROTIZING FASCIITIS, PLANTAR FASCIITIS.

Fasciola *n.* a genus of *flukes. *F. hepatica*, the liver fluke, normally lives as a parasite of sheep and other herbivorous animals but sometimes infects humans (*see* FASCIOLIASIS).

fascioliasis *n.* an infestation of the bile ducts and liver with the liver fluke, *Fasciola hepatica*. Humans acquire the infection through eating wild watercress on which the larval stages of the parasite are present. The symptoms include fever, dyspepsia, vomiting, loss of appetite, abdominal pain, and coughing; the liver may also be extensively damaged (causing **liver rot**). Anthelmintics are used in the treatment of fascioliasis.

fasciolopsiasis *n.* a disease, common in the Far East, caused by the fluke *Fasciolopsis buski* in the small intestine. At the site of attachment of the adult flukes in the intestine there may be inflammation with some ulceration and bleeding. Symptoms include diarrhoea, and in heavy infections the patient may experience loss of appetite, vomiting, and (later) swelling of the face, abdomen, and legs. Death may follow in cases of severe ill health and malnutrition. The flukes can be removed with an anthelmintic (such as praziquantel).

Fasciolopsis *n.* a genus of large parasitic flukes widely distributed throughout eastern Asia and especially common in China. The adults of *F. buski*, the giant intestinal fluke, live in the human small intestine. Humans become infected with the fluke on eating uncooked water chestnuts contaminated with fluke larvae and the resulting symptoms can be serious (*see* FASCIOLOPSIASIS).

fasciotomy *n.* a procedure used to relieve or prevent *compartment syndrome by incising the fascial compartment containing the muscle(s) involved and the overlying skin. The wound is then allowed to close by secondary intention (*see also* DELAYED SUTURE), direct primary closure, or placement of a skin graft over the defect once the muscle swelling has resolved.

FASS (cryptogenic) *f*ibrosing *a*lveolitis associated with *s*ystemic *s*clerosis. *See* ALVEOLITIS.

fastigium *n.* **1.** the period during which a disease or fever is fully developed. **2.** the highest point in the roof of the fourth ventricle of the brain.

fat *n.* a substance that contains one or more fatty acids (in the form of *triglycerides) and is the principal form in which energy is stored by the body (in *adipose tissue). It also serves as an insulating material beneath the skin (in the subcutaneous tissue) and around certain organs (including the kidneys). Fat is one of the three main constituents of food (*see also* CARBOHYDRATE, PROTEIN); it is necessary in the diet to provide an adequate supply of *essential fatty acids and for the efficient absorption of fat-soluble vitamins from the intestine. Excessive deposition of fat in the body leads to *obesity. *See also* BROWN FAT, LIPID.

fatal familial insomnia an autosomal *dominant disorder due to a mutation in the gene for the *prion protein (PrP): it is an example of a *spongiform encephalopathy. Patients present with intractable progressive insomnia, disturbances of the autonomic nervous system, and eventually dementia.

fatigue *n.* **1.** mental or physical tiredness, following prolonged or intense activity. Muscle fatigue may be due to the waste products of metabolism accumulating in the muscles faster than they can be removed by the venous blood. Incorrect or inadequate food intake or disease may predispose a person to fatigue. **2.** the inability of an organism, an organ, or a tissue to give a normal response to a stimulus until a certain recovery period has elapsed.

fatigue fracture *see* STRESS FRACTURE.

fatty acid an organic acid with a long straight hydrocarbon chain and an even number of carbon atoms. Fatty acids are the fundamental constituents of many important lipids, including *triglycerides. Some fatty acids can be synthesized by the body; others, the *essential fatty acids, must be obtained from the diet. Examples of fatty acids are **palmitic acid**, **oleic acid**, and **stearic acid**. *See also* FAT, SATURATED FATTY ACID, UNSATURATED FATTY ACID.

fatty degeneration deterioration in the health of a tissue due to the deposition of abnormally large amounts of fat in its cells. The accumulation of fat in the liver and heart may seriously impair their functioning. The deposition of fat may be linked with incorrect diet, excessive alcohol consumption, or a shortage of oxygen in the tissues caused by poor circulation or a deficiency of haemoglobin.

fatty liver *see* NONALCOHOLIC FATTY LIVER DISEASE, ACUTE FATTY LIVER OF PREGNANCY.

fauces *n.* the opening leading from the mouth into the pharynx. It is surrounded by the **glossopalatine arch** (which forms the anterior pillars of the fauces) and the **pharyngopalatine arch** (the posterior pillars).

favism *n.* an inherited defect in the enzyme glucose-6-phosphate dehydrogenase causing the red blood cells to become sensitive to a chemical in fava beans (broad beans). Eating these beans results in destruction of red blood cells (haemolysis), which may lead to severe anaemia, requiring blood transfusion. Favism occurs most commonly in the Mediterranean and Middle East. *See also* GLUCOSE-6-PHOSPHATE DEHYDROGENASE DEFICIENCY.

FCE *see* FINISHED CONSULTANT EPISODE.

FDG *see* FLUORODEOXYGLUCOSE.

fear *n.* an emotional state evoked by the threat of danger and usually characterized by unpleasant subjective experiences as well as physiological and behavioural changes. Fear is often distinguished from *anxiety in having a specific object. Associated physiological changes can include increases in heart rate, blood pressure, sweating, etc. Behavioural changes can include an avoidance of fear-producing objects or situations and may be extremely disabling. Specific disabling fears are known as *phobias. *Beta blockers relieve the physiological manifestations of fear and are useful in the treatment of short-term fears, such as the fear of hearing the results of an examination. *Behaviour therapy or *cognitive behavioural therapy are treatments for disabling and persistent fears.

febricula *n.* a fever of low intensity or short duration.

febrifuge *n.* a treatment or drug that reduces or prevents fever. *See* ANTIPYRETIC.

febrile *adj.* relating to or affected with fever.

febrile convulsion (febrile seizure) an epileptic-type seizure associated with a fever. Such seizures affect up to 4% of children, usually aged between six months and

six years, and generally last less than 10 minutes. Seizures do not lead to mental retardation or cerebral palsy, although the risk of developing *epilepsy is around 2%, especially when other risk factors, such as family history, are present. Seizures may be recurrent, but the risk of this can be minimized by attempts to reduce the fever. The underlying infection is usually viral, but more serious conditions, such as meningitis, should be excluded.

feedback *n.* the coupling of the output of a process to the input. Feedback mechanisms are important in regulating many physiological processes; for example, the production of hormones and neurotransmitters. In **negative feedback**, a rise in the output of a substance will inhibit a further increase in its production, either directly or indirectly (*see* NEGATIVE FEEDBACK LOOP). In **positive feedback**, a rise in the output of a substance is associated with an increase in the output of another substance, either directly or indirectly.

Fehling's test a test for detecting the presence of sugar in urine, which has now been replaced by better and easier methods. [H. von Fehling (1812–85), German chemist]

Felty's syndrome a disorder characterized by enlargement of the spleen (*splenomegaly), rheumatoid arthritis, and a decrease in the number of neutrophils in the blood (*see* NEUTROPENIA). [A. R. Felty (1895–1964), US physician]

Femara *n. see* AROMATASE INHIBITOR.

feminist ethics an approach that is critical of the prevailing focus and methods of *medical ethics. In particular, it is argued that contemporary bioethics has replicated oppressive social structures, privilege, and power relationships at the expense of the marginalized. Moral problems are seen as determined from the social context in which they arise and narrative, care, and empowerment are usually integral to feminist analyses of ethical dilemmas.

feminization *n.* the development of female secondary sexual characteristics (enlargement of the breasts, loss of facial hair, and fat beneath the skin) in the male, either as a result of an endocrine disorder or of hormone therapy.

femoral *adj.* of or relating to the thigh or to the femur.

femoral artery an artery arising from the external iliac artery at the inguinal ligament. It is situated superficially, running down the front medial aspect of the thigh. Two-thirds of the way down it passes into the back of the thigh, continuing downward behind the knee as the **popliteal artery**.

femoral epiphysis *see* FEMUR.

femoral nerve the nerve that supplies the quadriceps muscle at the front of the thigh and receives sensation from the front and inner sides of the thigh. It arises from the second, third, and fourth lumbar nerves.

femoral triangle (**Scarpa's triangle**) a triangular depression on the inner side of the thigh bounded by the sartorius and adductor longus muscles and the inguinal ligament. The pulse can be felt here as the femoral artery lies over the depression.

femur (**thigh bone**) *n.* a long bone between the hip and the knee (see illustration). The head of the femur articulates with the acetabulum of the *hip bone. The **greater**

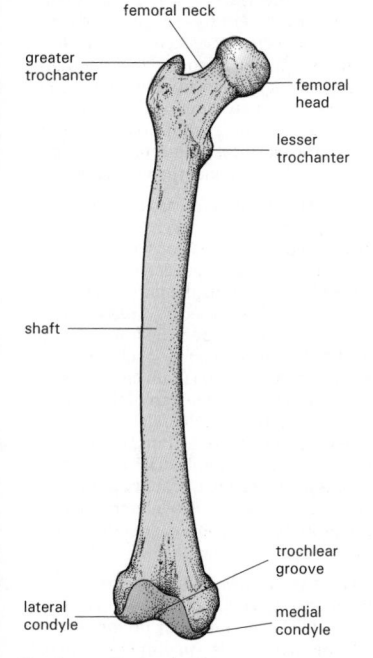

The femur (front view).

Labels: femoral neck; greater trochanter; femoral head; lesser trochanter; shaft; trochlear groove; lateral condyle; medial condyle

and **lesser trochanters** are protuberances on which the gluteus and psoas major muscles, respectively, are inserted. The **lateral** and **medial condyles** articulate with the *tibia, and the **trochlear groove** accommodates the kneecap (patella).

The narrowed end of the femur (**femoral neck**), which carries the head, is the commonest site of fracture of the leg in elderly women. Partial dislocation of the **femoral epiphysis**, the growth area of the upper end of the bone, leads to deformity of the head of the femur and premature degeneration of the hip joint.

fenbufen *n.* an anti-inflammatory drug (*see* NSAID) used to relieve inflammation and the resulting pain and stiffness. It is administered by mouth. Possible side-effects include rashes, nausea, and vomiting. Trade name: **Lederfen**.

fenestra *n.* (in anatomy) an opening resembling a window. The **fenestra ovalis** (**fenestra vestibuli**) – the oval window – is the opening between the middle *ear and the vestibule of the inner ear. It is closed by a membrane to which the stapes is attached. The **fenestra rotunda** (**fenestra cochleae**) – the round window – is the opening between the scala tympani of the cochlea and the middle ear. Sound vibrations leave the cochlea through the fenestra rotunda which, like the fenestra ovalis, is closed by a membrane.

fenestration *n.* a surgical operation in which a new opening is formed in the bony *labyrinth of the inner ear as part of the treatment of deafness due to *otosclerosis. It is rarely performed today, having been superseded by *stapedectomy.

fenofibrate *n. see* FIBRATES.

fenoprofen *n.* an *analgesic drug that also reduces inflammation (*see* NSAID) and is used to treat arthritic conditions. It is administered by mouth and may cause digestive upsets, drowsiness, dizziness, sweating, and headache. Trade name: **Fenopron**.

fentanyl *n.* a potent opioid analgesic (*see* OPIATE) used for the relief of severe pain (for example in cancer patients already receiving other opioids) and for pain relief during surgery. It is administered by mouth, intravenously, or skin patches. Trade names: **Abstral**, **Actiq**, **Durogesic DTrans**, **Effentora**, **Sublimaze**.

fermentation *n.* the biochemical process by which organic substances, particularly carbohydrate compounds, are decomposed by the action of enzymes to provide chemical energy. An example is **alcoholic fermentation**, in which enzymes in yeast decompose sugar to form ethyl alcohol and carbon dioxide.

ferning *n.* a test to determine if the amniotic membrane surrounding the fetus has ruptured in late pregnancy. A typical pattern of amniotic fluid crystallization occurs when the amniotic fluid dries.

ferri- (ferro-) *combining form denoting* iron.

ferric sulphate an iron salt used in solution to stop bleeding, for example in pulpotomy of primary teeth.

ferritin *n.* an iron-protein complex that is one of the forms in which iron is stored in the tissues.

ferrous sulphate an *iron salt administered by mouth to treat or prevent iron-deficiency anaemia. There are few serious side-effects; stomach upsets and diarrhoea may be prevented by taking the drug with meals. Similar preparations used to treat anaemia include **ferrous fumarate** (Fersaday, Fersamal, Galfer) and **ferrous gluconate**. Trade names: **Ironorm Drops, Feospan**.

fertility rate the number of live births occurring in a year per 1000 women of child-bearing age (usually 15 to 44 years). A less reliable measure of fertility can be obtained from the **live birth rate** (the number of live births per 1000 of the population) or the **natural increase** (the excess of live births over deaths). More rarely quoted are the **gross reproduction rate** (the rate at which the child-bearing female population is reproducing itself) and the **net reproduction rate**, which takes into account female mortality before the age of reproduction.

fertilization *n.* the fusion of a spermatozoon and an ovum. Rapid changes in the membrane of the ovum prevent other spermatozoa from penetrating. Penetration stimulates the completion of meiosis and the formation of the second polar body. Once the male and female pronuclei have fused the zygote starts to divide by cleavage.

FESS functional *endoscopic sinus surgery.

festination *n.* short tottering steps that become more rapid, due to a loss of postural reflexes and stooped posture. Festination is found in patients with *parkinsonism.

fetal alcohol syndrome a condition of newborn babies that results from the toxic effects on the fetus of maternal alcohol abuse. Babies have a low birth weight and growth is retarded; there may be head and facial abnormalities and possibly mental retardation. The greater the alcohol abuse, the more severe the fetal manifestations.

fetal blood sampling withdrawal of a sample of fetal blood, either from the umbilical vein during the antenatal period (*see* CORDOCENTESIS) or from a vein in the presenting part (usually the fetal scalp) during labour. The latter procedure is used to detect *hypoxia, by measuring the fetal pH and degree of *acidosis. The normal pH of fetal blood is 7.35 (range 7.45–7.25). The lower the pH, the more likely is the fetus to be suffering from hypoxia and acidosis, indicating an urgent need to deliver the baby.

fetal implant (fetal graft) the introduction of an ovum, fertilized in vitro and developed to the *blastocyst stage, into the uterus of a postmenopausal woman in order that she may become pregnant. Before this procedure, the woman's uterus must be prepared, by hormone therapy, to receive and nurture the blastocyst. Hormone treatment is continued throughout the pregnancy.

fetal transplant a research method in which specific cells are taken from a normal fetus, with the informed consent of the mother following her request for termination of pregnancy, for transplantation into a person suffering from a specific disease. These fetal cells would take over the function of the specific diseased or damaged cells of the host. Examples are fetal brain cells transplanted into the affected part of the brain in a patient suffering from Parkinson's disease, and fetal pancreatic cells transplanted into the pancreas of a juvenile diabetic. Other diseases are being investigated experimentally with a view to using fetal transplants. Such procedures involve major ethical considerations.

feticide *n.* the destruction of a fetus in the uterus, as by injection of potassium chloride into the fetal heart following premedication to the mother. This is usually performed to achieve a late-stage termination of pregnancy (after 21 weeks), for example because of major abnormalities in the fetus.

fetishism *n.* sexual attraction to an inappropriate object (known as a **fetish**). This may be a part of the body (e.g. the foot or the hair), clothing (e.g. underwear or shoes), or other objects (e.g. leather handbags or rubber sheets). In all these cases the fetish has replaced the normal object of sexual love, in some cases to the point at which sexual relationships with another person are impossible or are possible only if the fetish is either present or fantasized. Treatment can involve *psychotherapy or behaviour therapy using *aversion therapy and masturbatory conditioning of desirable sexual behaviour. *See also* SEXUAL DEVIATION.

feto- *combining form denoting* a fetus.

fetor (foetor) *n.* an unpleasant smell. **Fetor oris** is bad breath (*halitosis), which is most commonly caused by poor oral hygiene but can also occur in patients with acute appendicitis or uraemia. **Fetor hepaticus** is bad breath with a sweet faecal odour, occurring in patients with severe liver disease.

fetoscopy *n.* direct visualization of a fetus by passing a special fibreoptic endoscope (a **fetoscope**) through the abdomen of a pregnant woman into the amniotic cavity. Its original use as a technique for visualizing fetal malformations and sampling fetal blood for diagnosis of blood disorders has been abandoned with advances in high-resolution fetal imaging. It is now used to facilitate minimally invasive surgery on the fetus and placenta, either under local anaesthetic or by laparotomy on the mother; the fetoscope can be directed into place using *real-time imaging. Fetoscopic laser ablation of placental vessels is now commonly used in cases of twin-to-twin transfusion.

fetus (foetus) *n.* a mammalian *embryo during the later stages of development within the uterus. In human reproduction it refers to an unborn child from its eighth week of development. —**fetal** *adj.*

fetus papyraceous a twin fetus that has died in the uterus and become flattened and mummified.

Feulgen reaction a method of demonstrating the presence of DNA in cell nuclei. The tissue section under investigation is first hydrolysed with dilute hydrochloric acid and then treated with *Schiff's reagent. A purple coloration develops in the presence of DNA. [R. Feulgen (1884–1955), German chemist]

FEV *see* FORCED EXPIRATORY VOLUME.

fever (pyrexia) *n.* a rise in body temperature above the normal, i.e. above an oral temperature of 98.6°F (37°C) or a rectal temperature of 99°F (37.2°C). Fever is generally accompanied by shivering, headache, nausea, constipation, or diarrhoea. A rise in temperature above 105°F (40.5°C) may cause delirium and, in young children, *convulsions too. Fevers are usually caused by bacterial or viral infections and can accompany any infectious illness, from the common cold to *malaria. An **intermittent fever** is a periodic rise and fall in body temperature, often returning to normal during the day and reaching its peak at night, as in malaria. A **remittent fever** is one in which body temperature fluctuates but does not return to normal. *See also* RELAPSING FEVER.

FGF23 fibroblast growth factor 23: a hormone that is central to phosphate homeostasis. It is synthesized by osteoblasts and osteoclasts in response to high phosphate intake, hyperphosphataemia, or an increase in serum *calcitriol concentration. It inhibits phosphate reabsorption by the proximal tubule of the kidney and stimulates 24-hydroxylase, the enzyme that converts calcitriol and its precursor, 25-hydroxy vitamin D, into inactive metabolites. It may also have a negative effect on parathyroid hormone synthesis.

fibr- (fibro-) *combining form denoting* fibres or fibrous tissue.

fibrates *pl. n.* a class of drugs, chemically related to fibric acid, that are capable of reducing concentrations of triglycerides in the blood (*see* HYPERTRIGLYCERIDAEMIA); they may also reduce plasma *low-density lipoproteins and they tend to raise the levels of the beneficial *high-density lipoproteins. Fibrates are used for treating hyperlipidaemia; they include *bezafibrate, **ciprofibrate** (Modalim), **fenofibrate** (Lipantil, Supralip), and *gemfibrozil. Fibrates can have adverse effects on muscle (*see* MYOSITIS).

fibre *n.* **1.** (in anatomy) a threadlike structure, such as a muscle cell, a nerve fibre, or a collagen fibre. **2.** (in dietetics) *see* DIETARY FIBRE. —**fibrous** *adj.*

fibre optics the use of fibres for the transmission of light images. Synthetic fibres with special optical properties can be used in instruments to relay pictures of the inside of the body for direct observation or photography. *See* FIBRESCOPE. —**fibreoptic** *adj.*

fibrescope *n.* an *endoscope that uses *fibre optics for the transmission of images from the interior of the body. Fibrescopes have a great advantage over the older endoscopes as they are flexible and can be introduced into relatively inaccessible cavities of the body.

fibril *n.* a very small fibre or a constituent thread of a fibre (for example, a *myofibril of a muscle fibre). —**fibrillar, fibrillary** *adj.*

fibrillation *n.* chaotic electrical and mechanical activity of a heart chamber, which results in loss of synchronous contraction. The affected part of the heart then ceases to pump blood.

Fibrillation may affect the atria or ventricles independently. In **atrial fibrillation** (a common type of *arrhythmia), the chaotic electrical activity of the atria is conducted to the ventricles in a random manner resulting in a rapid and irregular pulse rate. The main causes are atherosclerosis, chronic rheumatic heart disease, and hypertensive heart disease. It may also complicate various other conditions, including chest infections and thyroid overactivity. The heart rate is controlled by the administration of *digoxin; in some cases the heart rhythm can be restored to normal by *cardioversion. Anticoagulant therapy with *warfarin reduces the risk of blood-clot formation, which could cause a stroke.

When **ventricular fibrillation** occurs the ventricles stop beating (*see* CARDIAC ARREST). It is most commonly the result of *myocardial infarction.

fibrin *n.* the final product of the process of *blood coagulation, produced by the action of the enzyme thrombin on a soluble precursor fibrinogen. The product thus formed (**fibrin monomer**) links up (polymerizes) with similar molecules to give a fibrous meshwork that forms the basis of a blood clot, which seals off the damaged blood vessel.

fibrinogen *n.* a substance (*coagulation factor), present in blood plasma, that is acted upon by the enzyme thrombin to produce the insoluble protein fibrin in the final stage of *blood coagulation. The normal

level of fibrinogen in plasma is 2–4 g/1 (4–6 g/l during pregnancy).

fibrinogenopenia *n.* a former name for *hypofibrinogenaemia.

fibrinoid *adj.* resembling the protein fibrin.

fibrinolysin *n. see* PLASMIN.

fibrinolysis *n.* the process by which blood clots are removed from the circulation, involving digestion of the insoluble protein *fibrin by the enzyme *plasmin. The latter exists in the plasma as an inactive precursor (plasminogen), which is activated in parallel with the *blood coagulation process. Normally a balance is maintained between the processes of coagulation and fibrinolysis in the body; an abnormal increase in fibrinolysis leads to excessive bleeding.

fibrinolytic *adj.* describing a group of drugs that are capable of breaking down the protein fibrin (*see* FIBRINOLYSIS), which is the main constituent of blood clots, and are therefore used to disperse blood clots (thrombi) that have formed within the circulation, most notably after myocardial infarction. They include *streptokinase, *urokinase, *alteplase, **reteplase** (Rapilysin), and **tenecteplase** (Metalyse). Possible side-effects include bleeding at needle puncture sites, headache, backache, blood spots in the skin, and allergic reactions.

fibroadenoma *n. see* ADENOMA.

fibroblast *n.* a widely distributed cell in *connective tissue that is responsible for the production of both the ground substance and of the precursors of collagen, elastic fibres, and reticular fibres.

fibrocartilage *n.* a tough kind of *cartilage in which there are dense bundles of fibres in the matrix. It is found in the intervertebral discs and pubic symphysis.

fibrocyst *n.* a benign tumour of fibrous connective tissue containing cystic spaces. —**fibrocystic** *adj.*

fibrocystic disease of the pancreas *see* CYSTIC FIBROSIS.

fibrocyte *n.* an inactive cell present in fully differentiated *connective tissue. It is derived from a *fibroblast.

fibrodysplasia *n.* abnormal development affecting connective tissue.

fibroelastosis *n.* overgrowth or disturbed growth of the yellow (elastic) fibres in *connective tissue, especially **endocardial fibroelastosis**, overgrowth and thickening of the inner layer of the heart's left ventricle.

fibroepithelial polyp a fibrous overgrowth covered by epithelium, often occurring inside the mouth in response to chronic irritation. It is sometimes called an *epulis.

fibroid 1. *n.* (leiomyoma, uterine fibroid) a benign tumour of fibrous and muscular tissue, one or more of which may develop within or attached to the outside of the uterus (see illustration). Fibroids that are large or distort the uterine cavity often cause pain and excessive menstrual bleeding. There may be difficulties with fertility and childbirth. Fibroids are more common in women over 30 years of age and they shrink after the menopause unless the woman is taking HRT. Medical treatment of fibroids includes administration of *gonadorelin analogues. Small fibroids can be destroyed by diathermy using a hysteroscope. Larger ones may be coagulated by laparoscopic use of the Nd:YAG *laser (**laparoscopic myolysis**) or removed by *myomectomy or *uterine artery embolization. Otherwise hysterectomy may be necessary. If discomfort and other symptoms are absent, surgery is not required.
2. *adj.* resembling or containing fibres.

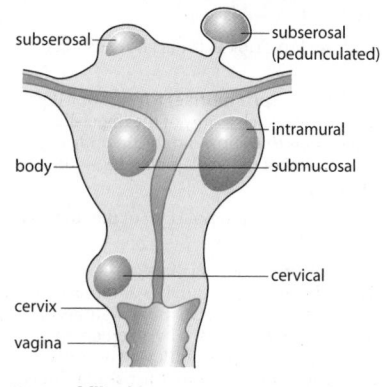

Types of fibroid.

fibroma *n.* (*pl.* **fibromas** or **fibromata**) a nonmalignant tumour of connective tissue.

fibromyalgia *n.* a disorder characterized by pain in the fibrous tissue components of muscles without any inflammation (*compare* FIBROMYOSITIS). Widespread aching and stiffness are accompanied by extreme fatigue and often associated with headache, numbness and tingling, and various other symptoms. Fibromyalgia is frequently triggered by anxiety, stress, sleep deprivation, and straining or overuse of muscles; it appears to be closely related to *CFS/ME/PVF.

fibromyositis *n.* general inflammation of fibromuscular tissue.

fibronectin *n.* a large glycoprotein that acts as a host defence mechanism. In the plasma it induces phagocytosis and on the cell surface it induces protein linkage which is important in the formation of new epithelium in wound healing. It is also involved in platelet aggregation. It is concentrated in connective tissue and the endothelium of the capillaries and is a component of the extracellular matrix.

fibroplasia *n.* the production of fibrous tissue, which is a part of the normal healing process. *See also* RETINOPATHY (OF PREMATURITY; RETROLENTAL FIBROPLASIA).

fibrosarcoma *n.* a malignant tumour of connective tissue, derived from *fibroblasts. Fibrosarcomas may arise in soft tissue or bone; they can affect any organ but are most common in the limbs, particularly the leg. They occur in people of all ages and may be congenital. The cells of these tumours show varying degrees of differentiation; the less well differentiated tumours containing elements of histiocytes have been recently reclassified as **malignant fibrous histiocytomas**.

fibrosis *n.* thickening and scarring of connective tissue, most often a consequence of inflammation or injury. **Pulmonary interstitial fibrosis** is thickening and stiffening of the lining of the air sacs (alveoli) of the lungs, causing progressive breathlessness. *See also* CYSTIC FIBROSIS, RETROPERITONEAL FIBROSIS. —**fibrotic** *adj.*

fibrositis *n.* inflammation of fibrous connective tissue, especially an acute inflammation of back muscles and their sheaths, causing pain and stiffness. *See also* MUSCULAR RHEUMATISM.

fibrous dysplasia a developmental abnormality in which changes occur in bony tissue. Trabecular bone is replaced by fibrous tissue, resulting in aching and a tendency to pathological fracture. In **monostotic fibrous dysplasia** one bone is affected; **polyostotic fibrous dysplasia** involves many bones. There is a small risk (5–10%) of malignant transformation (*fibrosarcoma).

fibula *n.* the long thin outer bone of the lower leg. The head of the fibula articulates with the *tibia just below the knee; the lower end projects laterally as the **lateral malleolus**, which articulates with one side of the *talus. —**fibular** *adj.*

fiduciary relationship a relationship in which one person holds a position of trust with respect to the other and is expected to act solely in the *best interests of that person and to treat information shared as confidential. In medicine, the doctor–patient relationship is a fiduciary relationship.

field of vision *see* VISUAL FIELD.

fifth disease *see* ERYTHEMA (INFECTIOSUM).

figlu test a test for folate or vitamin B$_{12}$ deficiency. A dose of the amino acid histidine, which requires the presence of folate or vitamin B$_{12}$ for its complete breakdown, is given by mouth. In the absence of these vitamins, *form*imino*glut*amic acid (figlu) – an intermediate product in histidine metabolism – accumulates and can be detected in the urine.

FIGO staging a classification drawn up by the International Federation of Gynaecology and Obstetrics to define the extent of the spread of cancers of the ovary, uterus, and cervix.

filament *n.* a very fine threadlike structure, such as a chain of bacterial cells. —**filamentous** *adj.*

filaria *n.* (*pl.* **filariae**) any of the long threadlike nematode worms that, as adults, are parasites of human connective and lymphatic tissues capable of causing disease. They include the genera *Brugia*, *Loa*, *Onchocerca*, and *Wuchereria*. Filariae differ from the intestinal nematodes (*see* HOOKWORM) in that they undergo part of their development in the body of a bloodsucking insect, e.g. a mosquito, on which they subsequently depend for their transmission to another human host. *See also* MICROFILARIA. —**filarial** *adj.*

filariasis *n.* a disease, common in the tropics and subtropics, caused by the presence in the lymph vessels of the parasitic nematode worms *Wuchereria bancrofti* and *Brugia malayi* (*see* FILARIA). The worms, which are transmitted to humans by various mosquitoes (including *Aëdes*, *Culex*, *Anopheles*, and *Mansonia*), bring about inflammation and eventual blocking of lymph vessels, which causes the surrounding tissues to swell (*see* ELEPHANTIASIS). The rupture of urinary lymphatics may lead to the presence of *chyle in the urine. Filariasis is treated with the drug *diethylcarbamazine.

file *n.* **1.** an instrument used to remove a sharp edge of bone. **2.** an instrument used in *endodontics to prepare the walls of a root canal for *root canal treatment. Files may be used by hand or in a *dental handpiece (rotary files); they are made from stainless steel or nickel-titanium alloy.

filiform *adj.* shaped like a thread; for example, the threadlike **filiform papillae** of the *tongue.

filling *n.* (in dentistry) the operation of inserting a specially prepared substance into a cavity drilled in a tooth, often in the treatment of dental caries. The filling may be **temporary** or **permanent**, and various materials may be used (*see* AMALGAM, CEMENT, COMPOSITE RESIN, GOLD).

filum *n.* a threadlike structure. The **filum terminale** is the slender tapering terminal section of the spinal cord.

FIM *see* FUNCTIONAL INDEPENDENCE MEASURE.

fimbria *n.* (*pl.* **fimbriae**) a fringe or fringe-like process, such as any of the finger-like projections that surround the opening of the ovarian end of the *Fallopian tube. —**fimbrial** *adj.*

fimbrial cyst a simple cyst of the *fimbria of the Fallopian tube.

finasteride *n.* a drug that causes shrinkage of the prostate gland. It is administered by mouth to relieve the symptoms of urinary retention caused by an enlarged gland obstructing the outflow of urine from the bladder and to reduce the risk of urinary retention. An *anti-androgen, the drug acts by reducing androgenic stimulation of the prostate, inhibiting the enzyme 5α-reductase, responsible for converting testosterone to its more active metabolite, *dihydrotestosterone, within the gland. It is sometimes also prescribed in men who have recurrent bleeding from the prostate. Side-effects include impotence and breast pain and enlargement. A low-dose formulation of finasteride is used to treat baldness in men. Trade names: **Propecia**, **Proscar**.

fine-needle aspiration cytology (FNA cytology) a technique in which a thin hollow needle is inserted into a mass to extract a tissue sample for microscopic examination. It is useful for detecting the presence of malignant cells, particularly in lumps of the breast and thyroid. *See also* ASPIRATION CYTOLOGY.

finger-flexion reflex *see* HOFFMANN'S SIGN.

finger–nose test a test for *ataxia or cerebral lesions. Using the index finger, the patient alternately touches his or her nose and then the examiner's finger, which is shifted to a new position for each of the patient's movements. The test is positive if the patient misses a target or develops a tremor as the target is approached (intention tremor).

fingerprint *n.* the distinctive pattern of minute ridges in the outer horny layer of the skin. Every individual has a unique pattern of loops (70%), whorls (25%), or arches (5%) (see illustration). Fingerprint patterns can show the presence of inherited disorders. *See also* DERMATOGLYPHICS.

finished consultant episode (FCE) the time a patient spends in the care of one consultant in one health-care provider. If a patient is transferred to a different hospital provider or a different consultant within the same hospital, a new episode begins.

firedamp *n.* (in mining) an explosive mixture of gases, usually containing a high proportion of methane, occasionally encountered in pockets underground. It can be distinguished from *blackdamp (choke-damp), which does not ignite.

first aid procedures used in an emergency to help a wounded or ill patient before the arrival of a doctor or admission to hospital.

first do no harm *see* PRIMUM NON NOCERE. *See also* NONMALEFICENCE.

first intention *see* INTENTION.

first-line treatment therapy that is the first choice for treating a particular condition; other (second-line) treatments are used only if first-line therapy has failed.

first-pass metabolism a process in which a drug administered by mouth is absorbed from the gastrointestinal tract and transported via the portal vein to the liver, where it is metabolized. As a result, in some cases only a small proportion of the active drug reaches the systemic circulation and its intended target tissue. First-pass metabolism can be bypassed by giving the drug via sublingual or buccal routes.

first-rank symptom *see* SCHNEIDERIAN FIRST- AND SECOND-RANK SYMPTOMS.

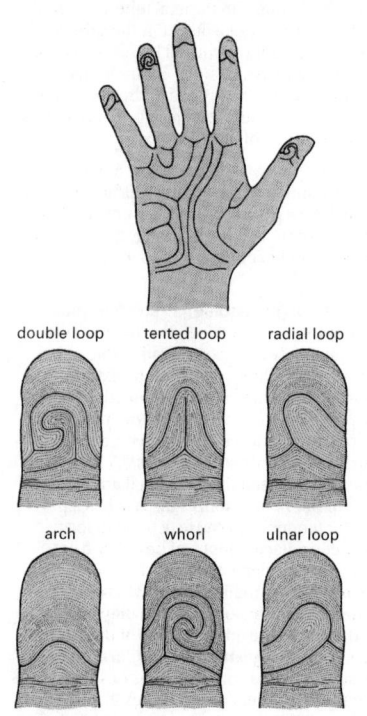

Fingerprint. Ridges on the hand, with details of the most common fingerprints.

FISH (fluorescence in situ hybridization) a technique that allows the nuclear DNA of *interphase cells or the DNA of *metaphase chromosomes, which are fixed to a glass microscope slide, to anneal with a fluorescent gene *probe. It is used for detecting and locating gene mutations and chromosome abnormalities.

fission *n.* a method of asexual reproduction in which the body of a protozoan or bacterium splits into two equal parts (**binary fission**), as in the *amoebae, or more than two equal parts (**multiple fission**), for example sporozoite formation in the malarial parasite (*see* PLASMODIUM). The resulting products of fission eventually grow into complete organisms.

fissure *n.* **1.** (in anatomy) a groove or cleft; e.g. the **fissure of Sylvius** is the groove that separates the temporal lobe of the brain from the frontal and parietal lobes. **2.** (in pathology) a cleftlike defect in the skin or mucous membrane caused by some disease process. *See* ANAL FISSURE. **3.** (in dentistry) a naturally occurring groove in the enamel on the surface of a tooth, especially a molar. It is a common site of dental caries.

fissure sealant (in dentistry) a material that is bonded to the enamel surface of teeth to seal the fissures, in order to prevent dental caries. Composite resins, unfilled resins, and glass ionomer cements have been used as fissure sealants.

fistula *n.* (*pl.* **fistulae**) **1.** an abnormal communication between two hollow organs, connecting two mucosa-lined surfaces, or between a hollow organ and the exterior. Many fistulae are caused by infection or injury. For example, an **anal fistula** may develop after an abscess in the rectum has burst (*see* ISCHIORECTAL ABSCESS), creating an opening between the anal canal and the surface of the skin. *Crohn's disease has a particular tendency to cause fistulae to form between adjacent loops of bowel or from bowel to bladder, vagina, or skin. Some fistulae result from malignant growths or ulceration: a carcinoma of the colon may invade and ulcerate the adjacent wall of the stomach, causing a **gastrocolic fistula**. Other fistulae develop as complications of surgery: after gall-bladder surgery, for example, bile may continually escape to the surface through the wound producing a **biliary fistula**. Fistulae may also be a form of congenital abnormality; examples include a **tracheo-oesophageal fistula** (between the windpipe and gullet) and a **rectovaginal fistula** (between the rectum and vagina). **2.** (arteriovenous fistula) a surgically created connection between an artery and a vein, usually in a limb, to create arterial and venous access for *haemodialysis. It can be a direct *anastomosis between the artery and

vein or a loop connecting the two, which may be autogenous or prosthetic.

fistulography *n.* imaging of a *fistula. X-rays can be used after injection of a radiopaque *contrast medium, usually through an opening in the skin after inserting a catheter, to see the extent of a fistula and the structures with which it communicates. In *haemodialysis patients, contrast is injected through a needle into the vessels around the surgical fistula to look for blockages or narrowings that are compromising flow. *Magnetic resonance imaging is the procedure of choice for examining fistulae around the rectum and anus.

fit *n.* a sudden attack. The term is commonly used specifically for the seizures of *epilepsy but it is also used more generally, e.g. a fit of coughing.

fixation *n.* **1.** (in psychoanalysis) a failure of psychological development, in which traumatic events prevent a child from progressing to the next developmental stage. This was formerly hypothesized to be a cause of mental illness and of personality disorder. *See also* PSYCHOSEXUAL DEVELOPMENT. **2.** a procedure for the hardening and preservation of tissues or microorganisms to be examined under a microscope. Fixation kills the tissues and ensures that their original shape and structure are retained as closely as possible. It also prepares them for sectioning and staining. The specimens can be immersed in a chemical *fixative or subjected to *freeze drying.

fixative (fixing agent) *n.* a chemical agent, e.g. alcohol or osmium tetroxide, used for the preservation and hardening of tissues for microscopical study. *See* FIXATION.

flaccid *adj.* **1.** flabby and lacking in firmness. **2.** characterized by a decrease in or absence of muscle tone. In **flaccid paralysis** there is absence of muscle tone in one or both limbs, and tendon reflexes are absent. It is a sign of damage to lower *motor neurons. *Compare* SPASTIC PARALYSIS. —**flaccidity** *n.*

flagellate *n.* a type of *protozoan with one or more fine whiplike threads (*see* FLAGELLUM) projecting from its body surface, by means of which it is able to swim. Some flagellates are parasites of humans and are therefore of medical importance. *See* TRYPANOSOMA, LEISHMANIA, GIARDIA, TRICHOMONAS.

flagellum *n.* (*pl.* **flagella**) a fine long whiplike thread attached to certain types of cell (e.g. spermatozoa and some unicellular organisms). Flagella are responsible for the movement of the organisms to which they are attached.

flail chest fracture of two or more ribs in two or more places, resulting from trauma. It produces an unstable 'flail' segment and is often associated with underlying lung trauma or pneumothorax. It leads to asphyxia unless corrected promptly.

flap *n.* **1.** (in surgery) a strip of tissue dissected away from the underlying structures but left attached at one end so that it retains its blood and nerve supply in a *pedicle. The flap is then used to repair a defect in another part of the body. The free end of the flap is sewn into the area to be repaired and after about three weeks, when the flap has 'healed into' its new site, the other end is detached and the remainder of the flap is sewn in. Flaps are commonly used by plastic surgeons in treating patients who have suffered severe skin and tissue loss after mutilating operations (e.g. mastectomy; *see* TRAM FLAP) or after burns or injuries not amenable to repair by split skin grafting (*see* SKIN GRAFT). Skin flaps may also be used to cover the end of a bone in an amputated limb. In neurosurgery combined skin and bone (**osteoplastic**) flaps are commonly raised to provide access to the cranium. **2.** (in dentistry) a piece of mucous membrane and periosteum attached by a broad base. It is lifted back to expose the underlying bone and enable a procedure such as surgical *extraction to be performed. It is subsequently replaced.

flare *n.* **1.** reddening of the skin that spreads outwards from a focus of infection or irritation in the skin. **2.** the red area surrounding an urticarial weal. **3.** (**aqueous flare**) the visible passage of a beam of light through the aqueous humour, which is a sign of inflammation of the anterior segment of the eye. The light is scattered by proteins in the aqueous humour that have exuded from blood vessels (*see* EXUDATION).

flashback *n.* **1.** vivid involuntary reliving of the perceptual abnormalities experienced during a previous episode of drug intoxication, including *hallucinations and *derealization, most commonly experienced with LSD. **2.** a symptom of *post-traumatic stress disorder characterized by the reliving of a traumatic experience.

flat-foot *n.* absence of the arch along the instep of the foot, so that the sole lies flat upon the ground. It is common in children until the age of 6 years, by which time the arch will usually have developed. Flat-foot that persists into adulthood may be due to an underlying bony disorder (**rigid flat-foot**) and may require surgery. Medical name: **pes planus**.

flat-panel detector a piece of equipment used instead of a conventional X-ray film to acquire the image in *digital radiography.

flatulence *n.* **1.** the expulsion of gas or air from the stomach through the mouth; belching. **2.** a sensation of abdominal distension. —**flatulent** *adj.*

flatus *n.* intestinal gas, passed through the rectum, composed partly of swallowed air and partly of gas produced by bacterial fermentation of intestinal contents. It consists mainly of hydrogen, carbon dioxide, and methane in varying proportions. Indigestible nonabsorbable carbohydrates in some foods (e.g. beans) cause increased volumes of flatus.

flatworm (**platyhelminth**) *n.* any of the flat-bodied worms, including the *flukes and *tapeworms. Both these groups contain many parasites of medical importance.

flav- (**flavo-**) *combining form denoting* yellow.

flavin adenine dinucleotide *see* FAD.

flavin mononucleotide *see* FMN.

flavivirus *n.* any member of a genus (and family) of *arboviruses that cause a wide range of diseases in vertebrates (including humans). Transmitted by ticks or mosquitoes, these include *yellow fever, *dengue, *Kyasanur Forest disease, *Russian spring-summer encephalitis, and *West Nile fever.

flavoprotein *n.* a compound consisting of a protein bound to either *FAD or *FMN (called **flavins**). Flavoproteins are constituents of several enzyme systems involved in intermediary metabolism.

flea *n.* a small wingless bloodsucking insect with a laterally compressed body and long legs adapted for jumping. Adult fleas are temporary parasites on birds and mammals and those species that attack humans (*Pulex*, *Xenopsylla*, and *Nosopsyllus*) may be important in the transmission of various diseases. Their bites are not only a nuisance but may become a focus of infection. Appropriate insecticide powders are used to destroy fleas in the home.

flecainide *n.* a drug used to control irregular heart rhythms (*see* ARRHYTHMIA). It is administered by mouth or intravenous injection. Possible side-effects include oedema, dizziness, vertigo, breathlessness, fever, and visual disturbances. Trade name: **Tambocor**.

Fleischer ring a deposit of iron in the form of a ring in the epithelium of the cornea, which is seen, for example, around the base of the 'cone' of the cornea in *keratoconus. It is best visualized using cobalt blue light. [B. Fleischer (1848–1904), German physician]

flexibilitas cerea *see* CATATONIA.

flexion *n.* the bending of a joint so that the bones forming it are brought towards each other. **Plantar flexion** is the bending of the toes (or fingers) downwards, towards the sole (or palm). *See also* DORSIFLEXION.

flexor *n.* any muscle that causes bending of a limb or other part.

flexure *n.* a bend in an organ or part, such as the **hepatic** and **splenic flexures** of the *colon. —**flexural** *adj.*

flight of ideas accelerated thinking that occurs in manic and hypomanic illness and attention-deficit/hyperactivity disorder. Speech is rapid, moving from one topic to another and reflecting casual associations between ideas (which may be linked, for example, by puns or rhymes).

floaters *pl. n.* opacities in the vitreous humour of the eye, which cast a shadow on the retina and are therefore seen as shapes or spots (**muscae volitantes**) against a bright background in good illumination. They are a form of *entoptic phenomenon.

floccillation (carphology) *n.* plucking at the bedclothes by a delirious patient.

flocculation *n.* a reaction in which normally invisible material leaves solution to form a coarse suspension or precipitate as a result of a change in physical or chemical conditions. *See also* AGGLUTINATION.

flocculent *adj.* describing a fluid containing woolly, fluffy, or flaky white particles, usually due to bacterial contamination.

flocculus *n.* a small ovoid lobe of the *cerebellum, overhung by the posterior lobe and connected centrally with the nodulus in the midline.

flooding *n.* **1.** excessive bleeding from the uterus, as in *menorrhagia or miscarriage. **2.** (in psychology) a method of treating *phobias in which the patient is exposed intensively and at length to the feared object, either in reality or fantasy. Although it is distressing and needs good motivation if treatment is to be completed, it is an effective and rapid form of therapy.

floppy baby syndrome *see* AMYOTONIA CONGENITA.

flow cytometry a technique in which cells are tagged with a fluorescent dye and then directed single file through a laser beam. The intensity of *fluorescence induced by the laser beam is proportional to the amount of DNA in the cells.

flowmeter *n.* an instrument for measuring the flow of a liquid or gas. Anaesthetic equipment has to be fitted with flowmeters so that the administration of anaesthetic gases in different proportions can be controlled. Flowmeters are widely used by asthma sufferers to measure their ability to expire air.

flucloxacillin *n.* a semisynthetic *penicillin that is effective against bacteria producing *penicillinase and is used to treat infections caused by penicillinase-producing staphylococci. It can be administered by mouth, injection, or intravenous infusion; possible side-effects are allergic reactions to penicillin, gastrointestinal disturbances, and (rarely) liver damage. Trade name: **Floxapen**.

fluconazole *n.* an antifungal drug used to treat candidiasis and other fungal infections. It is administered by mouth or intravenous infusion. Possible side-effects include nausea and vomiting. Trade name: **Diflucan**.

fluctuation *n.* the characteristic feeling of a wave motion produced in a fluid-filled part of the body by an examiner's fingers. If fluctuation is present when a swelling is examined, this is an indication that there is fluid within it and that the swelling is not due to a solid growth.

flucytosine *n.* an antifungal drug that is effective against systemic infections, including cryptococcosis and candidiasis. It is administered by intravenous infusion; side-effects may include nausea and vomiting, diarrhoea, rashes, and blood disorders. Trade name: **Ancotil**.

fludrocortisone *n.* a synthetic mineralocorticoid (*see* CORTICOSTEROID) used to treat disorders of the adrenal glands marked by deficient production of aldosterone. It is administered by mouth and side-effects include muscle weakness, bone disorders, digestive and skin disorders, and fluid retention. Trade name: **Florinef**.

fluid level the radiographic finding of a straight edge between fluid and gas within a hollow organ or cavity when a horizontal X-ray beam strikes the fluid surface tangentially. Multiple long fluid levels are seen in loops of small bowel that are obstructed. A fluid level in the lung suggests a cavity that is partially filled with fluid (e.g. an abscess).

fluke *n.* any of the parasitic flatworms belonging to the group Trematoda. Adult flukes, which have suckers for attachment to their host, are parasites of humans, occurring in the liver (**liver flukes**; *see* FASCIOLA), lungs (*see* PARAGONIMUS), gut (*see* HETEROPHYES), and blood vessels (**blood flukes**; *see* SCHISTOSOMA) and often cause serious disease. Eggs, passed out with the host's stools, hatch into larvae called *miracidia, which penetrate an intermediate snail host. Miracidia give rise asexually to *redia larvae and finally *cercariae in the snail's tissues. The released cercariae may enter a second intermediate host (such as a fish or crustacean); form a cyst (*metacercaria) on vegetation; or directly penetrate the human skin.

flumazenil *n.* a *benzodiazepine antagonist drug, used to reverse the sedative effects of benzodiazepines given during anaesthesia. It is administered by intravenous injection or infusion. Trade name: **Anexate**.

flunisolide *n.* an anti-inflammatory corticosteroid drug used in the prevention and treatment of hay fever. It is administered as a nasal spray; the most common side-effect is local irritation. Trade name: **Syntaris**.

fluocinolone *n.* a synthetic corticosteroid used topically to reduce inflammation in such skin conditions as eczema; it may also be used in the short-term treatment of psoriasis. It is applied to the skin as a cream, gel, or ointment. Side-effects include burning, itching, and local eruptions. Trade name: **Synalar**.

fluorescein sodium a water-soluble orange dye that glows with a brilliant green colour when blue light is shone on it. A dilute solution is used to detect defects in the surface of the cornea, since it stains areas where the *epithelium is not intact. In retinal *angiography it is injected into a vein and its circulation through the blood vessels of the retina is viewed and photographed by a special camera.

fluorescence *n.* the emission of light by a material as it absorbs radiation from outside. The radiation absorbed may be visible or invisible (e.g. ultraviolet rays or X-rays). *See* FLUOROSCOPE. —**fluorescent** *adj.*

fluorescence in situ hybridization *see* FISH.

fluoridation *n.* the addition of *fluoride to drinking water in order to reduce *dental caries. Drinking water with a fluoride ion content of one part per million is effective in reducing caries throughout life when given during the years of tooth development. *See also* FLUOROSIS.

fluoride *n.* a compound of fluorine. The incorporation of fluoride ions in the enamel of teeth makes them more resistant to *dental caries. The ions enter enamel during its formation, and after tooth eruption by surface absorption. The addition of fluoride to public water supplies is called *fluoridation. Fluoride may also be applied topically in toothpaste or by a dentist. If the water supply contains too little fluoride, fluoride salts may be given to children in the form of mouthwashes, drops, or tablets.

fluorodeoxyglucose (FDG) *n.* a variant of normal glucose in the body that is not metabolized and therefore accumulates in areas of high metabolism, such as tumours and areas of infection. It can be labelled with radioactive fluorine-18 and is in common use in PET scanning (*see* POSITRON EMISSION TOMOGRAPHY).

fluoropyrimidine *n.* any one of a class of *antimetabolite drugs used in the treatment of gastrointestinal malignancies and breast cancer. They include *fluorouracil and the orally administered drugs *capecitabine and **tegafur/uracil** (Uftoral).

fluoroscope *n.* historically, an instrument by which X-rays were projected through a patient onto a fluorescent screen enabling the resultant image to be viewed directly by the radiologist. However, this resulted in high radiation doses for the radiologist. For diagnostic purposes the screen has been replaced by the *image intensifier and TV monitor.

fluoroscopy *n.* the use of a *fluoroscope to visualize X-ray images. *Videofluoroscopy is synonymous with X-ray screening. It is valuable for observing moving structures (e.g. swallowed barium sulphate) or for guiding *interventional radiology procedures.

fluorosis *n.* the effects of high *fluoride intake. Dental fluorosis is characterized by mottled enamel, which is opaque and may be stained. Its incidence increases when the level of fluoride in the water supply is above 2 parts per million. The mottled enamel is resistant to dental caries. When the level is over 8 parts per million, systemic fluorosis may occur, with calcification of ligaments.

fluorouracil (5FU) *n.* a drug that prevents cell growth (*see* ANTIMETABOLITE) and is used in the treatment of solid tumours, such as cancers of the digestive system and breast (*see also* FOLINIC ACID). It is usually administered by intravenous infusion or injection; it is not well absorbed when taken by mouth, but oral *fluoropyrimidines (e.g. capecitabine and tegafur/uracil) are converted to 5FU in the liver. Side-effects may include digestive and skin disorders, mouth ulcers, hair loss, nail changes, and blood disorders (*see* MYELOSUPPRESSION). Fluorouracil is also applied as a cream (**Efudix**) to treat certain skin conditions, including skin cancer.

fluoxetine *n.* an *antidepressant drug that acts by prolonging the action of the neurotransmitter serotonin (5-hydroxytryptamine) in the brain (*see* SSRI). It is administered by mouth to treat depression, bulimia nervosa, and obsessive–compulsive disorder. Possible side-effects include nausea, vomiting, diarrhoea, allergic reactions (e.g. rash), insomnia, and anxiety. Trade name: **Prozac**.

flupentixol (flupenthixol) *n.* a thioxanthene *antipsychotic drug used to treat schizophrenia and other psychoses and depression. It is administered by mouth or intramuscular injection. Possible side-effects include abnormal involuntary movements (*see* EXTRAPYRAMIDAL EFFECTS). Trade names: **Depixol, Fluanxol**.

fluphenazine *n.* a phenothiazine *antipsychotic drug used for the treatment of schizophrenia and other psychotic disorders. It is administered by depot injection.

Side-effects include abnormal muscular movements (*see* EXTRAPYRAMIDAL EFFECTS). Trade name: **Modecate**.

flurazepam *n.* a benzodiazepine drug used for the short-term relief of insomnia and sleep disturbances (*see* HYPNOTIC). It is administered by mouth and sometimes causes morning drowsiness, dizziness, and muscle incoordination. Trade name: **Dalmane**.

flurbiprofen *n.* an analgesic that relieves inflammation (*see* NSAID), used in the treatment of rheumatoid arthritis, osteoarthritis, dysmenorrhoea, and other painful conditions and to prevent contraction of the pupil during eye surgery. Side-effects may include gastrointestinal upset, diarrhoea, and nausea. Trade names: **Froben, Ocufen**.

flush *n.* reddening of the face and/or neck. **Hectic flush** occurs in such wasting diseases as pulmonary tuberculosis. A **hot flush**, accompanied by a feeling of heat, occurs in some emotional disorders and during the menopause (*see* VASOMOTOR SYMPTOMS).

flutamide *n.* an *anti-androgen commonly used in the treatment of advanced prostate cancer, either alone or in combination with *gonadorelin analogues. It is taken by mouth; side-effects include gynaecomastia (breast enlargement) and diarrhoea.

fluticasone proprionate a corticosteroid used for the prophylaxis of asthma, the prophylaxis and treatment of hay fever and perennial rhinitis, and the treatment of dermatitis and eczema. It is administered by inhalation, nasal spray, or as a cream or ointment. Trade names: **Cutivate, Flixonase, Flixotide**.

flutter *n.* a disturbance of normal heart rhythm that – like *fibrillation – may affect the atria or ventricles. However, the arrhythmia is less rapid and less chaotic. The causes and treatment are similar to those of fibrillation. *See also* CARDIAC ARREST, DEFIBRILLATION.

fluvastatin *n. see* STATIN.

fluvoxamine *n.* an *antidepressant drug that acts by prolonging the action of the neurotransmitter serotonin (5-hydroxytryptamine) in the brain (*see* SSRI). It is taken by mouth to treat depression and obsessive–compulsive disorder; side-effects may include sleepiness, agitation, tremor, vomiting, and diarrhoea. Trade name: **Faverin**.

flux *n.* an abnormally copious flow from an organ or cavity. **Alvine flux** is *diarrhoea.

fly *n.* a two-winged insect belonging to a large group called the Diptera. The mouthparts of flies are adapted for sucking and sometimes also for piercing and biting. Fly larvae (maggots) may infest human tissues and cause disease (*see* MYIASIS).

FMN (flavin mononucleotide) a derivative of riboflavin (vitamin B$_2$) that is the immediate precursor of *FAD and functions as a *coenzyme in various oxidation-reduction reactions.

FNA *see* FINE-NEEDLE ASPIRATION CYTOLOGY.

FOBT *see* FAECAL OCCULT BLOOD TEST.

focal distance (of the eye) the distance between the lens and the point behind the lens at which light from a distant object is focused. In a normally sighted person the point of focus is on the retina, but in *myopia (short-sightedness) the focus is in front of the retina and in *hypermetropia (long-sightedness) the point of focus is beyond the retina.

focal segmental glomerulosclerosis (FSGS) a condition in which there is scarring in some (focal) glomeruli that affects only part (segmental) of the glomerular capillary tuft. Primary FSGS overlaps with *minimal change nephropathy and typically presents with the *nephrotic syndrome. Secondary FSGS has a wide range of causes, from viral infections, including HIV, to haemodynamic changes associated with reduced renal mass, hypertension, and obesity, and is usually associated with less severe proteinuria.

focus 1. *n.* the point at which rays of light converge after passing through a lens. 2. *n.* the principal site of an infection or other disease. 3. *n.* (in radiography) the point of origin of an X-ray beam. 4. *vb.* (in ophthalmology) to accommodate (*see also* ACCOMMODATION).

foetus *n. see* FETUS.

folate (pteroylglutamic acid) a B vitamin that is important in the synthesis of nucleic acids. The metabolic role of folate is interdependent with that of *vitamin B$_{12}$ (both are required by rapidly dividing cells) and a deficiency of one may lead to deficiency of the other. A deficiency of folate results in the condition of megaloblastic anaemia. Good sources of folate are liver, yeast extract, and green leafy vegetables. The actual daily requirement of folate is not known but the suggested daily intake is 200 µg/day for an adult, which should be doubled shortly before conception and during the first three months of pregnancy to prevent neural tube defects (e.g. spina bifida) and other congenital malformations (e.g. cleft lip and cleft palate) in the fetus.

fold *n.* (in anatomy and embryology) the infolding of two surfaces or membranes.

folic acid a synthetic form of *folate, which can be added to foods or used as a supplement for treating folate-deficient states.

folie à deux a condition in which two people who are closely involved with each other share one or more *delusions. Sometimes one member of the pair has developed a *psychosis and has imposed it on the other by a process of suggestion; sometimes both members are schizophrenic and elaborate their delusions or hallucinations together. More than two people may be involved (**folie à trois**, **folie à quatre**, etc.). Treatment usually involves separation of the affected people and management according to their individual requirements.

folinic acid a derivative of folic acid involved in purine synthesis. Administered by mouth or by injection or infusion in the form of its calcium or disodium salts, it is used to reverse the biological effects of methotrexate and other *dihydrofolate reductase inhibitors and so to prevent excessive toxicity. This action is termed **folinic acid rescue**. Folinic acid has a potentiating effect with *fluorouracil, with which it is often used. Trade names: **Isovorin**, **Refolinon**, **Sodiofolin**.

folium *n.* (*pl.* **folia**) a thin leaflike structure, such as any of the folds on the surface of the cerebellum.

follicle *n.* 1. (in anatomy) a small secretory cavity, sac, or gland, such as any of the cavities in the *ovary in which the ova are formed. *See also* GRAAFIAN FOLLICLE, HAIR FOLLICLE. 2. (in ophthalmology) any of the smooth translucent elevations of the conjunctiva produced by an immune response. They are usually associated with viral inflammation. —**follicular** *adj.*

follicle-stimulating hormone (FSH) a hormone (*see* GONADOTROPHIN) synthesized and released by the anterior pituitary gland. FSH stimulates ripening of the follicles in the ovary and formation of sperm in the testes. It is administered by injection to treat sterility due to lack of ovulation, amenorrhoea, and decreased sperm production. Stimulation of ovulation by FSH may, in some cases, lead to multiple pregnancy.

follicular cyst *see* OVARIAN CYST.

follicular occlusion tetrad the combination of major acne, *pilonidal sinus, chronic scalp *folliculitis, and *hidradenitis suppurativa.

folliculitis *n.* inflammation of hair follicles in the skin, commonly caused by bacterial infection. Folliculitis caused by *Malassezia* yeasts may be related to HIV infection.

fomentation *n. see* POULTICE.

fomes *n.* (*pl.* **fomites**) any object that is used or handled by a person with a *communicable disease and may therefore become contaminated with the infective organisms and transmit the disease to a subsequent user. Common fomites are towels, bedclothes, cups, and money.

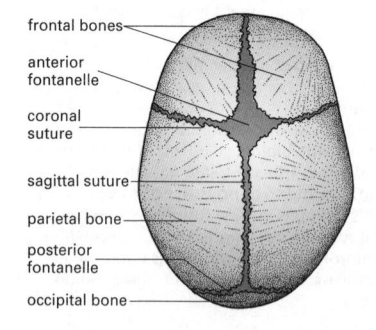

frontal bones
anterior fontanelle
coronal suture
sagittal suture
parietal bone
posterior fontanelle
occipital bone

Fontanelles (from above).

fontanelle *n.* an opening in the skull of a fetus or young infant due to incomplete *ossification of the cranial bones and the resulting incomplete closure of the *sutures. The **anterior fontanelle** occurs where the coronal, frontal, and sagittal sutures meet; the **posterior fontanelle** occurs where the sagittal and lambdoidal sutures meet (see illustration).

food poisoning an illness affecting the digestive system that results from eating food that is contaminated by bacteria or bacterial toxins, viruses, or (less commonly) by residues of insecticides (on fruit and vegetables) or poisonous chemicals such as lead or mercury. It can also be caused by eating poisonous fungi, berries, etc. Symptoms commence 1–24 hours after ingestion and include nausea, vomiting, diarrhoea, and abdominal pain. Food-borne infections are caused by bacteria of the genera *Salmonella*, *Campylobacter*, and *Listeria* in foods of animal origin. The disease is transmitted by human carriers who handle the food, by shellfish growing in sewage-polluted waters, or by vegetables fertilized by manure. Toxin-producing bacteria causing food poisoning include those of the genus *Staphylococcus*, which rapidly multiply in warm foods; pathogenic *Escherichia coli*; and the species *Clostridium perfringens*, which multiplies in reheated cooked meals. A rare form of food poisoning – *botulism – is caused by toxins produced by the bacterium *Clostridium botulinum*, which may contaminate badly preserved canned foods. *See also* GASTROENTERITIS.

foot *n.* the terminal organ of the lower limb. From a surgical point of view, the human foot comprises the seven bones of the *tarsus, the five metatarsal bones, and the phalangeal bones plus the surrounding tissues; anatomically, the bones and tissues of the ankle are excluded.

foramen *n.* (*pl.* **foramina**) an opening or hole, particularly in a bone. The **apical foramen** is the small opening at the apex of a tooth. The **foramen magnum** is a large hole in the occipital bone through which the spinal cord passes. The **foramen ovale** is the opening between the two atria of the fetal heart, which allows blood to flow from the right to the left side of the heart by displacing a membranous valve.

forced expiratory volume (FEV) the volume of air exhaled in a given period (usually limited to 1 second in tests of vital capacity). FEV is reduced in patients with obstructive airways disease and diminished lung volume.

forced preferential looking test (FPL test) a test used to evaluate the *visual acuity of infants and young children by observing whether the child looks at a blank screen or one with stripes, the spatial frequency of which can be changed.

forceps *n.* a pincer-like instrument designed to grasp an object so that it can be held firm or pulled. Specially designed forceps – of which there are many varieties – are used by surgeons and dentists in operations (see illustration). The forceps used in childbirth are so designed as to fit firmly round the baby's head without damaging it. Dental **extraction forceps** are specially designed to fit the various shapes of teeth. By having long handles and short beaks they provide considerable leverage.

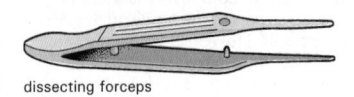

dissecting forceps

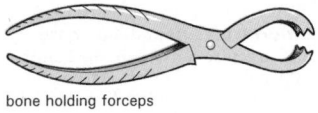

bone holding forceps

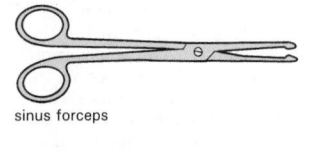

sinus forceps

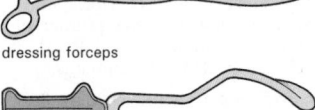

dressing forceps

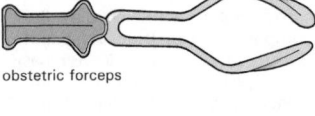

obstetric forceps

dental extraction forceps

Types of forceps.

forebrain *n.* the furthest forward division of the *brain, consisting of the *diencephalon and the two cerebral hemispheres.

foregut *n.* the front part of the embryonic gut, which gives rise to the oesophagus (gullet), stomach, and part of the small intestine (from which the liver and pancreas develop).

forensic medicine the branch of medicine concerned with the scientific investigation of the causes of injury and death in unexplained circumstances, particularly when criminal activity is suspected. Such investigations are carried out chiefly by pathologists at the request of a *coroner, in conjunction with other experts and police investigators.

forequarter amputation an operation involving removal of an entire arm, including the scapula and clavicle. It is usually performed for soft tissue or bone sarcomas arising from the upper arm or shoulder. *Compare* HINDQUARTER AMPUTATION.

foreskin *n. see* PREPUCE.

forewaters *n.* the *amniotic fluid that escapes from the uterus through the vagina when that part of the amnion lying in front of the presenting part of the fetus ruptures, either spontaneously or by *amniotomy. Spontaneous rupture is usual in labour but rupture may occur before labour starts (premature rupture of membranes).

formaldehyde *n.* the aldehyde derivative of formic acid, formerly used as a vapour to sterilize and disinfect rooms and such items as mattresses and blankets. The toxic vapour is produced by boiling *formalin in an open container or using it in a sealed autoclave.

formalin *n.* a solution containing 40% formaldehyde in water, used as a sterilizing agent and, in pathology, as a fixative. It is lethal to bacteria, viruses, fungi, and spores and is used to treat wools and hides to kill anthrax spores. Heating the solution produces the irritating vapour of *formaldehyde, which is also used for disinfection.

formal thought disorder thought disturbance characterized by disconnected thinking, manifested by rambling speech in which the patient's train of thought cannot be followed. Formal thought disorder was first described by the German psychiatrist Kurt Schneider and later elaborated on by various authors. Looking for evidence of formal thought disorder is part of every *mental state examination. It includes loosening of associations (*see* ASSOCIATION OF IDEAS), omissions, and *knight's-move thinking.

forme fruste an atypical form of a disease

in which the usual symptoms fail to appear and its progress is stopped at an earlier stage than would ordinarily be expected.

formication *n.* a prickling sensation said to resemble the feeling of ants crawling over the skin. It is sometimes a symptom of drug intoxication and has also been reported by patients with Parkinson's disease and multiple sclerosis.

formoterol (eformoterol) *n.* a *sympathomimetic drug (a β₂ agonist) used, with inhaled corticosteroids (*see also* BUDESONIDE), as a long-acting *bronchodilator to control chronic asthma and chronic obstructive pulmonary disease. Formoterol is formulated in powder or aerosol form for administration by inhaler. Side-effects include tremor, palpitations, and headache. Trade names: **Atimos Modulite, Foradil, Oxis Turbohaler**.

formulary *n.* a compendium of formulae used in the preparation of medicinal drugs.

fornix *n.* (*pl.* **fornices**) an arched or vault-like structure, especially the fornix cerebri, a triangular structure of white matter in the brain, situated between the hippocampus and hypothalamus. The **fornix of the vagina** is any of three vaulted spaces at the top of the vagina, around the cervix of the uterus. The superior (upper) and inferior (lower) **fornices of the conjunctiva** are the loose folds of conjunctiva reflected between the posterior aspect of the eyelid and the eyeball.

Forrest screening the UK national breast screening programme, introduced in 1988, in which regular *mammography is available for all women between the ages of 50 and 64. It enables the early diagnosis of breast cancer in order to improve treatment and reduce mortality. [Sir P. Forrest (1923–), Scottish surgeon]

forward parachute reflex a reflex action of the body that develops by five to six months and never disappears. If the body is held by the waist face down and lowered, the arms and legs extend automatically.

foscarnet *n.* an antiviral drug used in the treatment of herpes simplex and *cytomegalovirus retinitis that are resistant to *aciclovir, especially in patients with AIDS. It is administered by intravenous infusion. Possible side-effects include thirst and increased urine output, nausea and vomiting,

fatigue, headache, and kidney damage. Trade name: **Foscavir**.

fossa *n.* (*pl.* **fossae**) a depression or hollow. The **cubital fossa** is the triangular hollow at the front of the elbow joint; the **iliac fossa** is the depression in the inner surface of the ilium; the **pituitary fossa** is the hollow in the sphenoid bone in which the pituitary gland is situated; a **tooth fossa** is a pit in the enamel on the surface of a tooth.

foundation hospitals *see* FOUNDATION TRUSTS.

Foundation Programme a two-year programme of postgraduate medical training, introduced as part of the **Modernizing Medical Careers** initiative in 2005. Foundation year 1 replaced the old preregistration house officer year, and foundation year 2 replaced the first year of senior house officer training. *See also* DOCTOR.

foundation trusts (foundation hospitals) NHS organizations established under the Health and Social Care Act 2003. Foundation trusts have greater freedom than NHS acute and mental health trusts; they are accountable to their local communities, commissioners, parliament, and *Monitor. They are not under central government control and are not subject to performance management by *strategic health authorities. They are subject to inspection by the *Care Quality Commission, in the same way as other health-care providers. Foundation trusts have greater financial flexibility than NHS trusts, including greater access to capital funding and freedom to reinvest surpluses locally. In 2009 about half of eligible NHS trusts had achieved foundation status.

four principles an approach to medical ethics, proposed by Tom Beauchamp and James F. Childress, that identifies four basic tenets of ethical practice, namely: *autonomy, *beneficence, *nonmaleficence, and *justice. Although the four principles are often used as a framework for decision-making in Western medical ethics, there may be problems when principles conflict or their application is contested in practice.

fovea *n.* (in anatomy) a small depression, especially the shallow pit in the retina at the back of the eye. It contains a large number of *cones and is therefore the area of greatest acuity of vision: when the eye is directed at an object, the part of the image that is focused on the fovea is the part that is most accurately registered by the brain. *See also* MACULA (LUTEA).

foveola *n.* (in anatomy) a small depression.

FPL test *see* FORCED PREFERENTIAL LOOKING TEST.

fracture *n.* breakage of a bone, either complete or incomplete. A **simple fracture** involves a **clean** break with little damage to surrounding tissues and no break in the overlying skin. If the overlying skin is perforated and there is a wound extending to the fracture site, the fracture is **open**, and there is a risk of infection (*see* OSTEOMYELITIS). Treatment of a simple fracture includes realignment of the bone ends where there is displacement, immobilization by external splints or internal fixation, followed by *rehabilitation. *See also* COLLES' FRACTURE, COMMINUTED FRACTURE, GREENSTICK FRACTURE, PATHOLOGICAL FRACTURE, SCAPHOID FRACTURE, SMITH'S FRACTURE, STRESS FRACTURE.

fraenectomy *n.* an operation to remove the fraenum, including the underlying fibrous tissue.

fraenum (frenum, frenulum) *n.* **1.** any of the folds of mucous membrane under the tongue or between the gums and the upper or lower lips. **2.** any of several other structures of similar appearance.

fragile-X syndrome a major genetic disorder caused by a constriction near the end of the long arm of an *X chromosome. The fragile-X syndrome is second only to *Down's syndrome as a cause of mental retardation. Affected males have unusually high foreheads, unbalanced faces, large jaws, long protruding ears, and large testicles. They have an IQ below 50 and are prone to violent outbursts. Folic acid helps to control their behaviour. About one-third of the females with this mutation on one of their two X chromosomes also show developmental delay. Screening for the characteristic chromosome can be done by *amniocentesis or *chorionic villus sampling.

fragilitas *n.* abnormal brittleness or fragility, for example of the hair (**fragilitas crinium**) or the bones (**fragilitas ossium**; *see* OSTEOGENESIS IMPERFECTA).

framboesia *n. see* YAWS.

framycetin *n.* an antibiotic used mainly in the form of eye or ear drops (sometimes in combination with dexamethazone as **Sofradex**) to treat eye and ear infections. Local sensitivity sometimes occurs. Trade name: **Soframycin**.

Fraser guidelines *see* GILLICK COMPETENCE.

fraternal twins *see* TWINS.

freckle *n.* a small brown spot on the skin commonly found on exposed areas of red-haired or blond people. Freckles, which are harmless, appear where there is excessive production of the pigment melanin without any increase in numbers of melanocytes after exposure to sunlight. *Compare* LENTIGO.

free association (in *psychoanalysis) a technique in which the patient is encouraged to pursue a particular train of ideas as they enter consciousness. *See also* ASSOCIATION OF IDEAS.

free field audiogram *see* AUDIOGRAM.

free-floating anxiety an all-pervasive unfocused fear that is not produced by any appropriate cause or attached to any particular idea. Such anxiety is a feature of the *generalized anxiety disorder.

free gas the radiographic finding of gas outside the normal areas in the body where it would be expected, particularly in the peritoneal cavity. It is typically associated with perforation of a hollow organ containing gas, usually the bowel.

freeze drying a method for the *fixation of histological specimens, involving a minimum of chemical and physical change. Specimens are immersed in isopentane cooled to −190°C in liquid air. This fixes the tissue instantly, without the formation of large ice crystals (which would cause structural changes). The tissue is then dehydrated in a vacuum for about 72 hours at −32.5°C.

freeze etching a technique for preparing specimens for electron microscopy. The unfixed tissue is frozen and then split with a knife and a layer of ice is sublimed from the exposed surface. The resultant image is thus not distorted by chemical fixatives.

Frei test a rarely used diagnostic test for the sexually transmitted disease *lymphogranuloma venereum. A small quantity of the virus, inactivated by heat, is injected into the patient's skin. If the disease is present a small red swelling appears at the site of in-

290

jection within 48 hours. [W. S. Frei (1885–1943), German dermatologist]

fremitus *n.* vibrations or tremors in a part of the body, detected by feeling with the fingers or hand (*palpation) or by listening (*auscultation). The term is most commonly applied to vibrations perceived through the chest when a patient breathes, speaks (**vocal fremitus**), or coughs. The nature of the fremitus gives an indication as to whether the chest is affected by disease. For example, loss of vocal fremitus suggests the presence of fluid in the pleural cavity; its increase suggests consolidation of the underlying lung.

frenulum *n. see* FRAENUM.

frenum *n. see* FRAENUM.

frequency *n.* (of urine) the passage of urine more than seven times a day: a *lower urinary tract symptom that usually indicates genitourinary disorders and diseases but also accompanies *polyuria.

frequency distribution (in statistics) presentation of the characteristics (*variables) of a series of individuals (e.g. their heights, weights, or blood pressures) in tabular form or as a histogram (bar chart) so as to indicate the proportion of the series that have different measurements. A **normal** or **Gaussian distribution** is a continuous distribution that is symmetrical around the *mean value and is defined by its mean and *standard deviation; in a **skewed** or **asymmetrical distribution**, the measurements are clustered on one side of the mean and spread out over a wider range on the other.

Fresnel prism a flexible plastic prism that can be stuck to spectacle lenses to add a prism effect to spectacles. It may be used to correct double vision. [A. J. Fresnel (1788–1827), French physicist]

Freudian *adj.* relating to or describing the work and ideas of Austrian psychiatrist Sigmund Freud (1856–1939), inventor of psychoanalytic theory: applied particularly to the school of psychiatry based on his teachings (*see* PSYCHOANALYSIS).

friction murmur (friction rub) a scratching sound, heard over the heart with the aid of the stethoscope, in patients who have *pericarditis. It results from the two inflamed layers of the pericardium rubbing together during activity of the heart.

Friedreich's ataxia *see* ATAXIA. [N. Friedreich (1825–82), German neurologist]

frigidity *n.* an outdated term for lack of sexual desire or inability to achieve orgasm (almost always in women), now usually referred to as loss of libido or anorgasma, respectively.

fringe medicine *see* COMPLEMENTARY MEDICINE.

Fröhlich's syndrome a disorder of the *hypothalamus (part of the brain) affecting males: the boy is overweight with sexual development absent and disturbances of sleep and appetite. Medical name: **dystrophia adiposogenitalis**. [A. Fröhlich (1871–1953), Austrian neurologist]

Froin's syndrome a condition in which the cerebrospinal fluid (CSF) displays a combination of yellow colour and high protein content. It is characteristic of a block to the spinal circulation of CSF caused by a tumour. [G. Froin (1874–1932), French physician]

frontal *adj.* **1.** of or relating to the forehead (*see* FRONTAL BONE). **2.** denoting the *anterior part of a body or organ.

frontal bone the bone forming the forehead and the upper parts of the orbits; it contains several air spaces (**frontal sinuses**: *see* PARANASAL SINUSES). At birth the frontal bone consists of right and left halves, joined by a suture that usually closes during infancy. *See* SKULL.

frontal lobe the anterior part of each cerebral hemisphere (*see* CEREBRUM), extending as far back as the deep central sulcus (cleft) of its upper and outer surface. Immediately anterior to the central sulcus lies the motor cortex, responsible for the control of voluntary movement; the area further forward – the *prefrontal lobe – is concerned with behaviour, learning, judgment, and personality.

frontal sinus *see* PARANASAL SINUSES.

frostbite *n.* damage to the tissues caused by freezing. The affected parts, usually the nose, fingers, or toes, become pale and numb. Ice crystals form in the tissues, which may thus be destroyed, and amputation may become necessary. Frostbitten parts should not be rubbed, since there is no blood circulation in the tissues, but they may be gently warmed in tepid water. Precautions must be taken against bacterial infection, to which frostbitten skin is highly susceptible.

frozen shoulder (adhesive capsulitis) a well-defined disorder characterized by progressive pain and then stiffness of the shoulder that has no clear single cause and usually resolves spontaneously over about 18 months. Initial treatment during the painful inflammatory phase is with analgesics and anti-inflammatory drugs. During the stiff phase, when the pain and inflammation has settled, gentle physiotherapy and possible manipulation under anaesthesia is performed to help regain range of motion.

frozen watchfulness the state of a child who is unresponsive to its surroundings but is clearly aware of them. The child is usually expressionless and difficult to engage but of normal intelligence. Frozen watchfulness is usually a marker of *child abuse.

fructose *n.* a simple sugar found in honey and in such fruit as figs. Fructose is one of the two sugars in *sucrose. Fructose from the diet can be used to produce energy by the process known as *glycolysis, which takes place in the liver. Fructose is important in the diet of diabetics since, unlike glucose, fructose metabolism is not dependent on insulin.

fructosuria (levulosuria) *n.* the presence of fructose (levulose) in the urine.

frusemide *n. see* FUROSEMIDE.

FSGS *see* FOCAL SEGMENTAL GLOMERULO-SCLEROSIS.

FSH *see* FOLLICLE-STIMULATING HORMONE.

FTT *see* FAILURE TO THRIVE.

5FU *n. see* FLUOROURACIL.

Fuchs' endothelial dystrophy a hereditary condition in which the corneal endothelium looses its functional ability, usually with age. It may result in thickening and swelling of the cornea (*bullous keratopathy) and thus affect vision. **Cornea guttata**, small whitish deposits of hyalin, are seen on the inner surface of the cornea and signify a reduced number of endothelial cells. A corneal transplantation (*see* KERATOPLASTY) may become necessary in certain cases. [E. Fuchs (1851–1913), German ophthalmologist]

Fuchs' heterochromic cyclitis a condition characterized by chronic low-grade inflammation of the ciliary body and iris (anterior *uveitis) with depigmentation of the affected iris (*heterochromia). Glaucoma and cataract can develop in the affected eye.

fuchsin (magenta) *n.* any one of a group of reddish to purplish dyes used in staining bacteria for microscopic observation and capable of killing various disease-causing microorganisms. **Acid fuchsin (acid magenta)** is a mixture of sulphonated fuchsins; **basic fuchsin (basic magenta)** and **new (trimethyl) fuchsin** are basic histological dyes (basic fuchsin is also an antifungal agent).

Fuchs' spots pigmented lesions in the macular area of the retina that are seen in severely myopic (short-sighted) individuals. They are breaks in *Bruch's membrane allowing choroidal *neovascularization and can result in reduced vision. [E. Fuchs]

-fuge *combining form denoting* an agent that drives away, repels, or eliminates. Example: **febrifuge** (a drug that reduces fever).

fugue *n.* a period of memory loss during which the patient leaves his or her usual surroundings and wanders aimlessly. It is often preceded by psychological conflict and depression (*see* DISSOCIATIVE DISORDER) or it may be associated with organic mental disease or alcoholism.

fulguration (electrodesiccation) *n.* the destruction with a *diathermy instrument of warts, growths, or unwanted areas of tissue, particularly inside the bladder. This latter operation is performed via the urethra and viewed through a cystoscope.

fulminating (fulminant, fulgurant) *adj.* describing a condition or symptom that is of very sudden onset, severe, and of short duration.

fumigation *n.* the use of gases or vapours to bring about *disinfestation of clothing, buildings, etc. Sulphur dioxide, formaldehyde, and chlorine are common fumigating agents.

functional disorder a condition in which a patient complains of symptoms for which no physical cause can be found. Such a condition is frequently an indication of a psychiatric disorder. *Compare* ORGANIC DISORDER.

functional endoscopic sinus surgery (FESS) *see* ENDOSCOPIC SINUS SURGERY.

Functional Independence Measure (FIM) a table recommended by the WHO for assessing the degree of whole-person disability, being particularly useful for judging the extent of recovery from serious injury. It has five grades, ranging from 0 (fully independent) to 4 (completely dependent).

functional magnetic resonance imaging (fMRI) a type of *magnetic resonance imaging that measures the increased haemodynamic response seen with neural activity in the brain or spinal cord. fMRI has allowed major advances in **brain mapping** (i.e. matching sections of the brain with particular behaviours, thoughts, or emotions).

Functional Recovery Index an international index, published by the World Health Organization, that grades the degree of recovery after serious injury.

fundoplication n. a surgical operation for *gastro-oesophageal reflux disease in which the upper part of the stomach is wrapped around the lower oesophagus. **Nissen fundoplication** (named after Swiss surgeon Rudolf Nissen, 1896–1981) consists of a complete (360-degree) wrap; **toupe fundoplication** is a partial (270-degree) wrap. Fundoplication is now more often performed laparoscopically than via open surgery.

fundoscopy (ophthalmoscopy) n. examination of the interior of the eye by means of an *ophthalmoscope.

fundus n. 1. the base of a hollow organ: the part farthest from the opening; e.g. the fundus of the stomach, bladder, or uterus. 2. the interior concavity forming the back of the eyeball, opposite the pupil. **Fundus flavimaculatus** is a hereditary disease of the retina in which white material is deposited in the fundus at the level of the retinal pigment epithelium (see RETINA). It usually causes loss of central vision, but good vision may persist into adulthood. **Fundus albipunctatus** is a hereditary disease in which the fundus shows widespread distribution of uniform-sized white dots, resulting in poor *dark adaptation.

fungating adj. describing or relating to a mass of malignant tissue that has infiltrated the epithelium and broken through the skin surface. It may be infected, smell strongly, and cause pain and is most likely to occur in the advanced stages of cancer, particularly of the breast, head, or neck.

fungicide n. an agent that kills fungi. See also ANTIFUNGAL.

fungoid 1. adj. resembling a fungus. 2. n. a fungus-like growth.

fungus n. (pl. **fungi**) a simple organism (formerly regarded as a plant) that lacks the green pigment chlorophyll. Fungi include the *yeasts, rusts, moulds, and mushrooms. They live either as *saprophytes or as *parasites of plants and animals; some species infect and cause disease in humans. Some yeasts are a good source of vitamin B and many antibiotics are obtained from the moulds (see PENICILLIN). —**fungal** adj.

funiculitis n. inflammation of the spermatic cord. This usually arises in association with *epididymitis and causes pain and swelling of the involved cord. Treatment is by administration of antibiotics and analgesics.

funiculus n. 1. any of the three main columns of white matter found in each lateral half of the spinal cord. 2. a bundle of nerve fibres enclosed in a sheath; a fasciculus. 3. (formerly) the spermatic cord or umbilical cord.

funis n. (in anatomy) any cordlike structure, especially the umbilical cord.

funnel chest depression of the breastbone and inward curving of the costal cartilages articulating with it, resulting in deformity of the chest. It may displace the heart to the left and can cause slight breathlessness. Medical name: **pectus excavatum**.

furcation n. the place where the roots fork on a multirooted tooth.

furosemide (frusemide) n. a loop *diuretic used to treat fluid retention (oedema) associated with heart failure or kidney disease and also sometimes to treat high blood pressure. It is administered by mouth or injection; common side-effects are nausea and vomiting. Trade name: **Lasix**.

furuncle n. see BOIL.

furunculosis n. the occurrence of several *boils (furuncles) at the same time, usually caused by *Staphylococcus aureus* infection. Treatment includes thorough daily disinfection of the skin and incision (lancing), which may be more effective than antibiotic therapy. Diabetes mellitus should be excluded.

fusidic acid a steroid antibiotic used to treat skin and eye infections caused by staphylococci. It is administered topically and may cause hypersensitivity reactions.

Trade names: **Fucidin**, **Fucithalmic**. *See also* SODIUM FUSIDATE.

fusiform *adj.* spindle-shaped; tapering at both ends.

fusion *n.* the joining together of two structures. For example, the surgical fusion of two or more vertebrae is performed to stabilize an unstable spine. Fusion of the *epiphyses during growth is the cause of arrested growth of stature.

Fusobacterium *n.* a genus of Gram-negative rodlike bacteria with tapering ends. Most species are normal inhabitants of the mouth of animals and humans and produce no harmful effects, but anaerobic *Fusobac-terium* species are associated with *ulcerative gingivitis.

futile *adj.* describing an intervention that has little or no prospect of achieving its aim or intended purpose. In medical practice, claims of futility are often used to justify withholding or withdrawing medical treatment at the end of life. Claims that treatment is futile may be controversial because of the inherent uncertainty of prognoses, value judgments about quality of life, and contested therapeutic aims. Intensive care, for example, cannot be said to be futile simply on the grounds that the patient is unlikely to regain full health, since restoration of full health was never the intended purpose. —**futility** *n.*

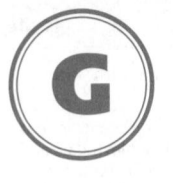

G

GABA *see* GAMMA-AMINOBUTYRIC ACID.

gabapentin *n.* an *anticonvulsant drug used to treat partial *epilepsy and neuropathic pain, including *peripheral neuropathy and postherpetic *neuralgia. It is administered by mouth; side-effects include gastrointestinal disturbances, dizziness, drowsiness, and shaky movements. **Pregabalin** (Lyrica) has similar uses and effects; it is also licensed to treat generalized anxiety disorder. Trade name: **Neurontin**.

GAD *see* GLUTAMIC ACID DECARBOXYLASE.

Gaffkya *n.* a genus of bacteria now classified as *Micrococcus*.

gag *n.* (in medicine) an instrument that is placed between a patient's teeth to keep his mouth open.

gag reflex (pharyngeal reflex) a normal reflex action caused by contraction of pharynx muscles when the soft palate or posterior pharynx is touched. The reflex is used to test the integrity of the *glossopharyngeal and *vagus nerves.

galact- (galacto-) *combining form denoting* 1. milk. Example: **galactosis** (formation of). 2. galactose.

galactagogue *n.* an agent that stimulates the secretion of milk or increases milk flow.

galactocele *n.* 1. a breast cyst containing milk, caused by closure of a milk duct. 2. an accumulation of milky liquid in the sac surrounding the testis (*see* HYDROCELE).

galactorrhoea *n.* pathological secretion of breast milk by women or men, usually as a result of a benign pituitary tumour (*see* PRO-LACTINOMA).

galactosaemia *n.* an inborn inability to utilize the sugar galactose, which in consequence accumulates in the blood. Untreated, affected infants fail to thrive and show developmental delay, but if galactose is eliminated from the diet growth and development may be normal.

galactose *n.* a simple sugar and a constituent of the milk sugar *lactose. Galactose

is converted to glucose in the liver. The enzyme necessary for this conversion is missing in infants with a rare inherited metabolic disease called *galactosaemia.

galantamine *n. see* ACETYLCHOLINESTER-ASE INHIBITOR.

galea *n.* 1. a helmet-shaped part, especially the **galea aponeurotica**, a flat sheet of fibrous tissue (*see* APONEUROSIS) that caps the skull and links the two parts of the *epicranius muscle. 2. a type of head bandage.

galenical *n.* a pharmaceutical preparation of a drug of animal or plant origin.

gall bladder a pear-shaped sac (7–10 cm long), lying underneath the right lobe of the liver, in which *bile is stored (see illustration). Bile passes (via the common hepatic duct) to the gall bladder from the liver, where it is formed, and is released into the duodenum (through the common bile duct) under the influence of the hormone *cholecystokinin, which is secreted when food is present in the duodenum. The gall bladder is a common site of stone formation (*see* GALL-STONE).

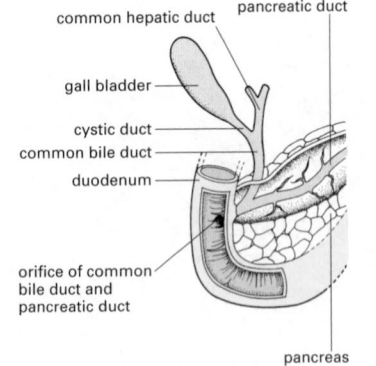

The gall bladder. Showing details of associated ducts.

gallium *n.* a silvery metallic element. A radioisotope of gallium can be used for the detection of lymphomas and areas of infection (such as an abscess) following intravenous injection. This technique is being replaced by other methods of imaging with lower radiation doses and better anatomical resolution.

gallop rhythm (triple rhythm) a third heart sound, which in association with a fast heart rate resembles the sound of a galloping horse. It is a sign of left ventricular failure (*see* HEART FAILURE).

gallstone *n.* a hard mass composed of bile pigments, cholesterol, and calcium salts, in varying proportions, that can form in the gall bladder. The formation of gallstones (**cholelithiasis**) occurs when the physical characteristics of bile alter so that cholesterol is less soluble or there is an excess of bile pigments. Diminished contractility of the gall bladder may also be a contributory factor, leading to biliary stasis. Gallstones may exist for many years without causing symptoms. However, they may cause severe pain (*see* BILIARY COLIC) or they may pass into the common bile duct and cause obstructive *jaundice or *cholangitis. Gallstones are usually diagnosed by ultrasonography, but those containing calcium may be seen on a plain X-ray (opaque stones). Symptomatic cholelithiasis is usually treated by surgical removal of the gall bladder (*see* CHOLECYSTECTOMY), usually laparoscopically. Nonsurgical treatments, such as stone-dissolving bile salts given by mouth or shattering by external ultrasound waves, have proved less successful and are not in widespread use.

galvanism *n.* (formerly) any form of medical treatment using electricity. **Interrupted galvanism** is a form of *electrotherapy in which direct current, in impulses lasting for 30 to 100 milliseconds, is used to stimulate the activity of nerves or the muscles they supply. *See also* FARADISM.

gamekeeper's thumb *see* SKIER'S THUMB.

gamete *n.* a mature sex cell: the *ovum of the female or the *spermatozoon of the male. Gametes are haploid, containing half the normal number of chromosomes.

gamete intrafallopian transfer (GIFT) a procedure for assisting conception, suitable only for women with healthy Fallopian tubes. In over 50% of women in whom infertility is diagnosed, the tubes are normal but some other factor, such as endometriosis, prevents conception. Using needle *aspira-

tion, under laparoscopic or ultrasonic guidance, ova are removed from the ovary. After being mixed with the partner's spermatozoa, they are introduced into a Fallopian tube, where fertilization takes place. The fertilized ovum can subsequently become implanted in the uterus.

gametocide *n.* a drug that kills *gametocytes. Drugs such as *primaquine destroy gametocytes of the malaria parasite (*see* PLASMODIUM), so interrupting the life cycle and preventing infection of the mosquito.

gametocyte *n.* any of the cells that are in the process of developing into gametes by undergoing *gametogenesis. *See also* OOCYTE, SPERMATOCYTE.

gametogenesis *n.* the process by which spermatozoa and ova are formed. In both sexes the precursor cells undergo *meiosis, which halves the number of chromosomes. However, the timing of events and the size and number of gametes produced are very different in the male and female. *See* OOGENESIS, SPERMATOGENESIS.

gamma-aminobutyric acid (GABA) an amino acid found in the central nervous system, predominantly in the brain, where it acts as an inhibitory *neurotransmitter.

gamma camera a piece of apparatus that detects radioactivity in the form of gamma rays emitted by radioactive isotopes that have been introduced into the body as *tracers. It contains an activated sodium iodide crystal (*see* SCINTILLATOR) and a large array of photomultiplier tubes. Using lead *collimators, the position of the source of the radioactivity can be plotted and displayed on a TV monitor or photographic film (*see* SCINTIGRAM).

gammaglobulin *n.* any of a class of proteins, present in the blood *plasma, identified by their characteristic rate of movement in an electric field (*see* ELECTROPHORESIS). Almost all gammaglobulins are *immunoglobulins. Injection of gammaglobulin provides temporary protection against *hepatitis A and reduces the incidence of coronary artery involvement in *Kawasaki disease. Infusions of gammaglobulin are used to treat immunodeficiencies or immune-mediated disorders, such as autoimmune haemolytic *anaemia or *idiopathic thrombocytopenic purpura. *See also* GLOBULIN.

gamma knife a device that allows high doses of radiation in the form of gamma rays to be accurately focused on pathological tissue, with less risk of damaging adjacent normal tissue compared with conventional radiotherapy. Multiple cobalt-60 sources deliver the gamma irradiation. The device is used in the treatment of vestibular schwannomas, certain brain tumours, vascular lesions of the brain, trigeminal neuralgia, and some forms of epilepsy.

gamma rays ionizing electromagnetic radiation of short wavelength given off by certain radioactive substances with equivalent properties to artificially produced X-rays. Gamma rays used in *nuclear medicine tend to have higher energy than diagnostic X-rays, with greater penetration; they are harmful to living tissues and can be used to sterilize certain materials and to kill bacteria as a means of food preservation. Higher energies are used in *radiotherapy with sufficient energy to kill tumour cells by causing breaks in DNA strands.

gamo- *combining form denoting* marriage.

ganciclovir *n.* an antiviral drug used to treat severe *cytomegalovirus (CMV) infections, including CMV retinitis, in immunocompromised patients. It is administered by intravenous infusion or as an eye gel. Possible side-effects include nausea, vomiting, diarrhoea, infertility, confusion, seizures, and disturbance of bone marrow blood-cell production. Trade names: **Cymevene**, **Virgan**.

gangli- (ganglio-) *combining form denoting* a ganglion.

ganglion *n.* (*pl.* **ganglia**) **1.** (in neurology) any structure containing a collection of nerve cell bodies and often also numbers of synapses. In the *sympathetic nervous system chains of ganglia are found on each side of the spinal cord, while in the *parasympathetic system ganglia are situated in or nearer to the organs innervated. Swellings in the posterior sensory *roots of the spinal nerves are termed ganglia; these contain cell bodies but no synapses. Within the central nervous system certain well-defined masses of nerve cells are called ganglia (or **nuclei**); for example, the *basal ganglia. **2.** an abnormal but harmless swelling (cyst) that sometimes forms in tendon sheaths, especially at the wrist.

ganglioside *n.* one of a group of *glycolipids found in the brain, liver, spleen, and red blood cells (they are particularly abundant in nerve cell membranes). Gangliosides are chemically similar to *cerebrosides but contain additional carbohydrate groups.

gangosa *n.* a lesion that occasionally appears in the final stage of *yaws, involving considerable destruction of the tissues of both the hard palate and the nose.

gangrene *n.* death and decay of part of the body due to deficiency or cessation of blood supply. The causes include disease, injury, or *atheroma in major blood vessels, frostbite or severe burns, and diseases such as *diabetes mellitus and *Raynaud's disease. **Dry gangrene** is death and withering of tissues caused simply by a cessation of local blood circulation. **Moist gangrene** (also known as **wet gangrene**) is death and putrefactive decay of tissue caused by bacterial infection. *See also* GAS GANGRENE.

Ganser syndrome a syndrome characterized by approximate answers, i.e. the patient gives grossly and absurdly false replies to questions, but the reply shows that the question has been understood. For example, the question "What colour is snow?" may elicit the reply "Green". This can be accompanied by odd behaviour or episodes of *stupor. The condition may be due to *conversion disorder or to conscious malingering, especially (historically) in prisoners. [S. J. M. Ganser (1853–1931), German psychiatrist]

Gardnerella *n.* a genus of anaerobic bacteria. *G. vaginalis* is a cause of *bacterial vaginosis and vaginitis and, in pregnant women, of late miscarriage and premature labour.

Gardner's syndrome a variant form of familial adenomatous *polyposis in which polyps in the colon are associated with fibromas and *osteomas (benign tumours), especially of the skull and jaw, and multiple *sebaceous cysts. [E. J. Gardner (1909–89), US physician]

gargoylism *n. see* HUNTER'S SYNDROME, HURLER'S SYNDROME.

Gartner's duct cysts vaginal cysts, usually small, that arise from **Gartner's duct** – remnants of the Wolffian duct (*see* MESONEPHROS) in females. No treatment is necessary if the cysts are small and not symptomatic, but surgical *marsupialization or excision may be required if they are large and cause obstruction. [H. T. Gartner (1785–1827), Danish surgeon and anatomist]

gas gangrene death and decay of wound tissue infected by the soil bacterium *Clostridium perfringens*. Toxins produced by the bacterium cause putrefactive decay of connective tissue with the generation of gas. Treatment is usually by surgery.

Gasterophilus *n.* a genus of widely distributed non-bloodsucking beelike flies. The parasitic maggots normally live in the alimentary canal of horses but, rarely, can also infect humans and cause an inflamed itching eruption of the skin (*see* CREEPING ERUPTION).

gastr- (gastro-) *combining form denoting* the stomach. Examples: **gastrocolic** (relating to the stomach and colon); **gastrointestinal** (relating to the stomach and intestines).

gastrectasia *n.* dilatation of the stomach. This may be caused by *pyloric stenosis or it may occur as a complication of some abdominal operations or trauma.

gastrectomy *n.* a surgical operation in which the whole or a part of the stomach is removed. **Total gastrectomy**, in which the oesophagus is joined to the jejunum, is usually performed for stomach cancer but occasionally for the *Zollinger-Ellison syndrome. In **partial** (or **subtotal**) **gastrectomy** the upper third or half of the stomach is joined to the duodenum or small intestine (**gastroenterostomy**); this operation was used in severe cases of *peptic ulcers before the advent of effective drug treatment and is still used to treat distal antral gastric cancers. After gastrectomy capacity for food is reduced, sometimes leading to weight loss. Other complications of gastrectomy include *dumping syndrome, ulceration at the anastomosis, anaemia, and *malabsorption.

gastric *adj.* relating to or affecting the stomach.

gastric banding a form of *bariatric surgery in which a band is placed around the stomach to effectively reduce its size and therefore restrict the amount of food it can accommodate. Weight loss should result. The procedure can be performed either in open operation or laparoscopically. The bands can be of a fixed size or adjustable (to vary calorie intake) by means of a small reservoir situated under the skin into which fluid can be injected or removed by the patient.

gastric bypass surgery any of several procedures of *bariatric surgery that allow food to bypass parts of the gut in order to reduce absorption of nutrients and calories. Such operations often lead to greater weight loss than restrictive procedures, such as *gastric banding and *stomach stapling, but complications of chronic malabsorption may occur and must be watched for.

gastric glands tubular glands that lie in the mucous membrane of the stomach wall. There are three varieties: the **cardiac, parietal (oxyntic)**, and **pyloric glands**, and they secrete *gastric juice.

gastric juice the liquid secreted by the *gastric glands of the stomach. Its main digestive constituents are hydrochloric acid, mucin, *rennin, and pepsinogen. The acid acts on pepsinogen to produce *pepsin, which functions best in an acid medium. The acidity of the stomach contents also kills unwanted bacteria and other organisms that have been ingested with the food. Gastric juice also contains *intrinsic factor, which is necessary for the absorption of vitamin B_{12}.

gastric stapling *see* STOMACH STAPLING.

gastric ulcer an ulcer in the stomach, caused by the action of gastic acid and, pepsin, on the stomach lining (mucosa). The output of stomach acid is not usually increased. Taking *NSAIDs (nonsteroidal anti-inflammatory drugs) and the presence of *Helicobacter pylori are important predisposing factors. Symptoms include vomiting and pain in the upper abdomen soon after eating, and such complications as bleeding (*see also* HAEMATEMESIS), *perforation, and obstruction due to scarring may occur. Symptoms are relieved by antacid medicines, but most ulcers heal if treated by an *antisecretory drug. Surgery may be required if the ulcer fails to heal. Since stomach cancer may mimic a gastric ulcer, all gastric ulcers should be examined by a *gastroscope and biopsies taken to aid in their differentiation.

gastrin *n.* a hormone produced in the mucous membrane of the pyloric region of the stomach (*see* G-CELL). Its secretion is stimulated by the presence of food. It is circulated in the blood to the rest of the stomach, where it stimulates the production of *gastric juice.

gastrinoma *n.* a rare tumour that secretes excess amounts of the hormone gastrin, causing the *Zollinger-Ellison syndrome. Such tumours most frequently occur in the pancreas; about half of them are malignant. Patients have very high levels of gastric acid and often present with complex and intractable gastroduodenal ulceration.

gastritis *n.* inflammation of the lining (mucosa) of the stomach. **Acute erosive (reactive) gastritis** is caused by ingesting excess alcohol or other irritating or corrosive substances, resulting in vomiting. **Chronic gastritis** is associated with smoking and chronic alcoholism and may be caused by bile entering the stomach from the duodenum, but most cases are caused by the bacterium *Helicobacter pylori*. It has no definite symptoms, but the patient may be liable to develop gastric ulcers or gastric cancer. **Atrophic gastritis**, in which the stomach lining is atrophied, may succeed chronic gastritis but may occur spontaneously as an *autoimmune disease, often in association with pernicious anaemia, and is strongly associated with the development of gastric cancer.

gastro- *combining form. see* GASTR-.

gastrocnemius *n.* a muscle that forms the greater part of the calf of the leg (see illustration). It flexes the knee and foot (so that the toes point downwards).

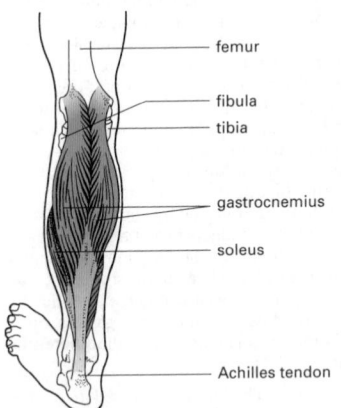

femur

fibula

tibia

gastrocnemius

soleus

Achilles tendon

Gastrocnemius and soleus muscles.

gastrocolic reflex a wave of peristalsis produced in the colon by introducing food into a fasting stomach.

gastroduodenoscope *n. see* GASTRO-SCOPE.

gastroduodenoscopy *n. see* OESOPHAGO-GASTRODUODENOSCOPY.

gastroduodenostomy *n.* a surgical operation in which the *duodenum (usually the third or fourth part) is joined to an opening made in the stomach in order to bypass an obstruction (such as *pyloric stenosis) or to facilitate the exit of food from the stomach after vagotomy. Much more commonly a *gastrojejunostomy or *gastroenterostomy is performed. *See also* DUODENOSTOMY.

gastroenteritis *n.* inflammation of the stomach and intestine. It is usually due to acute infection by viruses or bacteria or to food-poisoning toxins and causes nausea, vomiting, and diarrhoea. The illness usually lasts 3–5 days. Fluid loss is sometimes severe, especially in infants, and intravenous fluid replacement may be necessary. Viral or viral-type organisms (e.g. the *norovirus) are common causes of highly infectious gastroenteritis and, unlike bacterial pathogens, can be spread by aerosol or minimal contact and not necessarily by the faeco-oral route.

gastroenterology *n.* the study of gastrointestinal disease, which includes disease of any part of the digestive tract and also of the liver, biliary tract, and pancreas.

gastroenterostomy *n.* a surgical operation in which the small intestine is joined to an opening made in the stomach. The usual technique is *gastrojejunostomy to bypass obstruction (such as *pyloric stenosis).

Gastrografin *n.* trade name for meglumine diatrizoate, a water-soluble *contrast medium used in diagnostic radiology, usually in the gastrointestinal tract. It is used in some conditions as a laxative.

gastroileac reflex the relaxation of the *ileocaecal valve caused by the presence of food in the stomach.

gastrointestinal stromal tumour (GIST) a rare type of sarcoma arising from the gastrointestinal tract (usually the stomach), characterized by the presence of the receptor c-kit/CD117 on the surface of the tumour cells, which stimulates division of these cells. It displays a wide range of malignant behaviour. Specific treatment is available with *tyrosine kinase inhibitors.

gastrojejunostomy *n.* a surgical operation in which the *jejunum is joined to an opening made in the stomach. This is usually done in preference to *gastroduodenostomy. *See also* JEJUNOSTOMY.

gastrolith *n.* a stone in the stomach, which usually builds up around a *bezoar.

gastro-oesophageal reflux a condition in which the stomach contents reflux into the oesophagus because of permanent or intermittent impairment of the usual mechanisms preventing this. It may give rise to *oesophagitis. Patients may present not just with *heartburn but also with asthma or nocturnal cough and chronic throat symptoms. In severe cases there may be tooth *erosion.

gastro-oesophageal reflux disease (GORD) the syndrome caused by abnormal *gastro-oesophageal reflux, which includes symptoms of *heartburn, regurgitation, and *odynophagia, in which *oesophagitis may be present. It can lead to the development of *Barrett's oesophagus, a premalignant condition.

gastro-oesophagostomy *n.* a surgical operation in which the oesophagus (gullet) is joined to the stomach, bypassing the natural junction when this is obstructed by *achalasia, *stricture (narrowing), or cancer. This operation is rarely performed.

gastroparesis *n.* a condition in which the stomach fails to empty at an appropriate rate into the small intestine. Symptoms of bloating, nausea, early satiety, and vomiting are often intermittent in the early stages but can worsen to be a constant feature. It is most commonly seen in long-standing diabetes after the development of neuropathy affecting the parasympathetic nerves to the stomach.

gastropexy *n.* surgical attachment of the stomach to the abdominal wall.

gastroplasty *n.* surgical alteration of the shape of the stomach without removal of any part. The term was originally used for correction of an acquired deformity, e.g. narrowing due to a peptic ulcer, but has more recently been applied to techniques for reducing the size of the stomach in the treatment of morbid obesity, e.g. **vertical banded gastroplasty** (*see* STOMACH STAPLING) and *gastric banding.

gastroschisis *n.* a congenital defect in the abdominal wall, which during fetal development fails to close to the right of a normal umbilical cord. Bowel herniates through the defect and has no covering; free loops of bowel can be seen floating in the amniotic cavity on ultrasound. Treatment is surgical. *Compare* EXOMPHALOS.

gastroscope *n.* an illuminated optical telescope used to inspect the interior of the gullet (oesophagus), stomach, and duodenum. For many years these were rigid or semirigid instruments affording only limited views, but modern fully flexible instruments, which transmit the image using miniaturized video cameras, allow all areas of the oesophagus, stomach, and the first and second parts of the duodenum to be seen and photographed and specimens taken for microscopic examination. Therapeutic procedures (e.g. to arrest haemorrhage, remove a polyp, produce a *gastrostomy, dilate a stricture, or insert self-expandable metal stent) may be performed. As the same instruments can usually be introduced into the duodenum they are also known as **gastroduodenoscopes** or **oesophagogastroduodenoscopes**. —**gastroscopy** *n.*

gastrostomy *n.* a procedure in which an opening is made into the stomach from the outside. It is usually performed to allow food and fluid to be introduced into the stomach through a tube. It is indicated when swallowing is considered unsafe due to a neurological condition, such as stroke, multiple sclerosis, or motor neuron disease. It is often used temporarily after operations on the oesophagus or head and neck area until healing has occurred. Formerly a gastrostomy was always performed surgically, but it can now be done using an *endoscope (**percutaneous endoscopic gastrostomy, PEG**) or by direct puncture under radiological guidance (**radiologically inserted gastrostomy, RIG**).

gastrotomy *n.* a procedure during abdominal surgery in which the stomach is opened, usually to allow inspection of the interior (e.g. to find a point of bleeding), to remove a foreign body, or to allow the oesophagus to be approached from below (e.g. to pull down a tube through a constricting growth).

gastrula *n.* an early stage in the development of many animal embryos. It consists of a double-layered ball of cells formed by invagination and movement of cells in the preceding single-layered stage (blastula) in the process of **gastrulation**. It contains a central cavity, the *archenteron, which opens through the **blastopore** to the outside. True gastrulation only occurs in the embryos of amphibians and certain fish, but a similar process occurs in the embryonic disc in other vertebrates, including humans.

gating *n.* a method for acquiring images during specific parts of a fast-moving cycle, in particular the phases of contraction and relaxation of the heart, so that the appearance of the organ in each phase can be studied in isolation. The imaging is usually correlated with a physiological measure, such as an ECG trace. Gating is used in CT, MRI, and nuclear medicine.

Gaucher's disease a genetically determined (autosomal *recessive) disease resulting from the deposition of glucocerebrosides (*see* CEREBROSIDE) in the brain and other tissues (especially bone). It results in mental retardation, abnormal limb posture and spasticity, and difficulty with swallowing. Carrier detection and *preimplantation genetic diagnosis are possible; enzyme replacement therapy may be used in treatment. [P. C. E. Gaucher (1854–1918), French physician]

gauss *n.* a unit of magnetic flux density equal to 1 maxwell per square centimetre. 1 gauss = 10^{-4} tesla.

Gaussian distribution *see* FREQUENCY DISTRIBUTION, SIGNIFICANCE. [K. F. Gauss (1777–1855), German mathematician]

gauze *n.* thin open-woven material used in several layers for the preparation of dressings and swabs.

gavage *n.* forced feeding: any means used to get an unwilling or incapacitated patient to take in food by mouth, especially via a stomach tube.

GAVE (gastric antral vascular ectasia) a condition characterized by the presence of tortuous blood vessels (usually capillaries) in the lining of the stomach, which may involve a part or the whole of the stomach. It can be present diffusely in the lining of stomach or form a linear pattern (**watermelon stomach**). Various chronic medical conditions (e.g. *cirrhosis, *systemic sclerosis, and chronic renal failure) are often coexistent with this condition. It is often asymptomatic but can lead to anaemia requiring regular blood transfusions. Treatment can be difficult and involves optimal management of the underlying condition and direct endoscopic treatment of the lesions (*argon

plasma coagulation or laser thermocoagulation).

G-cell *n.* any of the cells of the mucous membrane of the stomach that are responsible for the production of *gastrin. They occur mainly in the gastric *antrum. Increased production of G-cells is associated with duodenal ulcer and the *Zollinger-Ellison syndrome: gastrin acts to increase the production of acid by the oxyntic cells of the gastric glands.

GCS *see* GLASGOW COMA SCALE.

gefitinib *n. see* EPIDERMAL GROWTH FACTOR RECEPTOR, TYROSINE KINASE INHIBITOR.

gel *n.* a colloidal suspension that has set to form a jelly. Some insoluble drugs are administered in the form of gels.

gelatin *n.* a jelly-like substance formed when tendons, ligaments, etc. containing *collagen (a protein) are boiled in water. Gelatin has been used in medicine as a source of protein in the treatment of malnutrition, in pharmacy for the manufacture of capsules and suppositories, and in bacteriology for preparing culture media.

gemcitabine *n.* a *cytotoxic drug that has an established role in the treatment of lung, pancreatic, bladder, and breast cancers. It is administered intravenously; side-effects are less severe than those of other *antimetabolites. Trade name: **Gemzar**.

gemeprost *n.* a *prostaglandin drug, administered as a vaginal pessary to terminate pregnancy. It causes powerful contractions of the uterus at any stage of pregnancy.

gemfibrozil *n.* a drug used to lower levels of *very low-density lipoproteins in patients with *hypertriglyceridaemia who have not responded to diet, weight reduction, or exercise (*see* FIBRATES). It is administered by mouth; side-effects include diarrhoea, abdominal pain, and nausea and vomiting. Trade name: **Lopid**.

gemmule *n.* one of the minute spines or surface extensions of a *dendrite, through which contact is made with another neuron at a *synapse.

gender identity disorder (GID) a condition in which an individual belongs to one gender on the basis of physical appearance and genetics but identifies psychologically with the other gender. The condition is diagnosed only if there is evidence of strong and persistent cross-gender identification and discomfort about one's sex, that these cause significant distress and social impairment, and that there is no concurrent endocrine disorder. *See also* TRANSSEXUALISM.

gene *n.* the basic unit of genetic material, which is carried at a particular place on a *chromosome. Originally it was regarded as the unit of inheritance and mutation but is now usually defined as a sequence of *DNA or *RNA that acts as the unit controlling the formation of a single polypeptide chain (*see* CISTRON). In diploid organisms, including humans, genes occur as pairs of *alleles. Various kinds of gene have been discovered: **structural genes** determine the biochemical makeup of the proteins; **regulator genes** control the rate of protein production (*see* OPERON). **Architectural genes** are responsible for the integration of the protein into the structure of the cell, and **temporal genes** control the time and place of action of the other genes and largely control the *differentiation of the cells and tissues of the body.

gene clone *see* CLONE.

General Dental Council a statutory body that controls the practice of dentistry in the UK.

general dental services a part of the NHS dental service. Dentists are included on the dental list of the appropriate primary care trust and are *independent contractors. Dental care is commissioned on the basis of units of dental activity, according to the complexity of the treatment.

generalized anxiety disorder a state of inappropriate and sometimes severe anxiety, without adequate cause, that lasts for at least six months. It affects about 2% of the population, women twice as often as men, and often develops in early adult life. It can, however, start at any age. There is a hereditary tendency to develop the disorder and about 25% of immediate relatives of sufferers are also affected. The disorder is thought to be caused by a disturbance of the functions of neurotransmitters, such as adrenaline or GABA, in the frontal lobes or the *limbic system of the brain. Symptoms affect all parts of the body. Palpitations, sweating, tremor, and dry mouth are core symptoms; additional symptoms include giddiness, *bruxism, restlessness, fatigability, breathlessness, lightheadedness, headaches, pins and needles, chest pain, fear of imminent death or loosing

control, diarrhoea, flushing, dysphagia, cramps, and muscle ache. Treatment includes *cognitive behavioural therapy and medication (*SSRIs or *SNRIs).

General Medical Council (GMC) the regulatory body of the medical profession in the UK, which was established in 1858 by the Medical Act and has statutory powers. It licenses doctors to practise medicine and has the power to revoke licences or place restrictions on practice. The governing body of the GMC, its Council, comprises 24 members, 12 of which are medically qualified and 12 of which are not. Its purpose is to protect, promote, and maintain the health and safety of the public by ensuring proper standards in the practice of medicine and medical education and training. Following various high-profile cases involving malpractice, there has been a shift in the role of the GMC from one of simple registration to that of *revalidation of doctors.

(((●))) **SEE WEB LINKS**
• GMC website: includes the Council's guide to Good Medical Practice

general paralysis of the insane (GPI, general paresis) a stage of tertiary *syphilis characterized by *dementia and spastic weakness of the limbs (paresis). Deafness, epilepsy, and *dysarthria may occur. The infecting organism can be detected in the brain cells and tests for syphilis in blood and cerebrospinal fluid are usually positive. When the symptoms are combined with those of *tabes dorsalis, the resulting condition is called **tabo-paresis**. The condition is now rare due to widespread treatment of earlier stages with penicillin and other antibiotics.

general practitioner (GP) a doctor working in the community who provides family health services to a local area. General practitioners (also known as **family doctors** or **family practitioners**) may work on their own or in a **group practice** in which they share premises and other resources with one or more other doctors. GPs are usually the first port of call for most patients with concerns about their health. They look after patients with wide-ranging medical conditions and can refer patients with more complex problems to specialists, such as hospital consultants. Some GPs with additional training and experience in a specific clinical area take referrals for assessment and treatment that may otherwise have been referred directly to hospital consultants; these are known as **GPs with a special interest** (**GPwSI** or **GPSI**). Most GPs work solely within the *National Health Service but a few work completely privately. There have been several models of providing general practice, including the now obsolete fundholding system. The current situation allows for GPs to provide general medical services (GMS), the terms and conditions of which are governed by a national contract (which was renegotiated in 2003), or personal medical services (PMS), the terms and conditions of which are governed by locally negotiated contracts within a broad framework. The new primary care contract (nGMS contract) came into force in April 2004, allowing GPs to opt out of weekend and night (*out-of-hours) service provision for patients registered with their practice. In this period, patient care is usually provided by an out-of-hours cooperative or deputizing service. At the same time the government also introduced the *Quality and Outcomes Framework (QOF) as a means to improve the quality of care provided. Most GPs are *independent contractors although more recently there has been an increase in the number of salaried GPs (employed by a *primary care trust). GPs may employ a variety of staff, including *practice nurses, *nurse practitioners, and counsellors.

general practitioner with special interest (GPwSI, GPSI) *see* GENERAL PRACTITIONER.

generic 1. *adj.* denoting a nonproprietary drug name, which is not protected by a trademark (*see* PROPRIETARY NAME). 2. *adj.* of or relating to a *genus. 3. *n.* a drug sold under its nonproprietary name.

-genesis *combining form denoting* origin or development. Example: **spermatogenesis** (development of spermatozoa).

gene therapy treatment directed to curing genetic disease by introducing normal genes into patients to overcome the effects of defective genes, using techniques of *genetic engineering. The most radical approach would be to do this at a very early stage in the embryo, so that the new gene would be incorporated into the germ cells (ova and sperm) and would therefore be inheritable. However, this approach is not considered to be either safe or ethical, because the consequences would affect all descendants of the patient, and it is not being pursued. In **somatic cell gene therapy** the healthy gene is inserted into *somatic cells (such as the *haemopoietic stem cells of the bone marrow) that give rise to other cells. All the surviving descendants of these modified cells will then be normal and, if present in sufficient numbers, the condition will be cured (the defective gene will, however, still be present in the germ cells).

At present, gene therapy is most feasible for treating disorders caused by a defect in a single recessive gene, so that the deficiency can be overcome by the introduction of a normal allele (therapy for disorders caused by dominant genes (e.g. Huntington's disease) would require the modification or replacement of the defective allele as its effect is expressed in the presence of a normal allele). Examples of such recessive disorders include *adenosine deaminase (ADA) deficiency and *cystic fibrosis. Gene therapy trials for the former condition have already begun: lymphocyte stem cells are isolated from the patient, using *monoclonal antibodies, and incubated with *retroviruses that have been genetically engineered to contain the normal ADA gene (*see* VECTOR). This gene thus becomes integrated into the stem cells, which – when returned to the patient's bone marrow – can then produce normal lymphocytes. A similar technique has been used in treating patients with *severe combined immune deficiency and is feasible for other blood disorders, such as sickle-cell anaemia and thalassaemia.

Clinical trials for the gene therapy of cystic fibrosis involve using *liposomes to introduce the normal gene into the lungs of sufferers via an inhaler.

Gene therapy for certain types of cancer is also undergoing clinical trials. Here the approach is aimed at introducing into the cancer cells tumour-suppressing genes, such as *$p53$ (which prevents uncontrolled cell division), or genes that direct the production of substances (such as *interleukin 2) that stimulate the immune system to destroy the tumour cells.

genethics *n.* the study of the social, moral, and political implications of knowledge and practice in genetics and genomics.

genetic code the code in which genetic information is carried by *DNA and *messenger RNA. This information determines the sequence of amino acids in every protein and thereby controls the nature of all proteins made by the cell. The genetic code is expressed by the sequence of *nucleotide bases in the nucleic acid molecule, a unit of three consecutive bases (a **codon**) coding for each amino acid. The code is translated into protein at the ribosomes (*see* TRANSCRIPTION, TRANSLATION). Any changes in the genetic code result in the insertion of incorrect amino acids in a protein chain, giving a *mutation.

genetic counselling the procedure by which patients and their families are given advice about the nature and consequences of inherited disorders, the possibility of becoming affected or having affected children, and the various options that are available to them for the prevention, diagnosis, and management of such conditions. Genetic counselling should be available at prenatal and postnatal clinics, and also through family planning clinics.

genetic drift the tendency for variations to occur in the genetic composition of small isolated inbreeding populations by chance. Such populations become genetically rather different from the original population from which they were derived.

genetic engineering (recombinant DNA technology) the techniques involved in altering the characteristics of an organism by inserting genes from another organism into its DNA. This altered DNA (known as **recombinant DNA**) is usually produced by isolating foreign genes, often by the use of *restriction enzymes, and inserting them into bacterial DNA, often using viruses as *vectors. Once inserted, the foreign gene may use the cell machinery of its host to synthesize the protein that it originally coded for in the organism it was derived from. For example, the human genes for *insulin, *interferon, and *growth hormone production have been incorporated into bacterial DNA and such genetically engineered bacteria are used in the commercial production of these substances. Some other applications of genetic engineering include DNA analysis, the production of *monoclonal antibodies, and – more recently – *gene therapy.

genetics *n.* the science of inheritance. It attempts to explain the differences and similarities between related organisms and the ways in which characters are passed from parents to their offspring. **Human** and **medical genetics** are concerned with the study of inherited diseases. *See also* CYTOGENETICS, MENDEL'S LAWS.

genetic screening *screening tests to discover individuals whose *genotypes are associated with specific diseases. Such individuals may later develop the disease itself or pass it on to their children (*see* CARRIER). The recent use of genetic screening to diagnose the sex of the fetus so that the parents may 'choose' the sex of their children has caused considerable controversy. *See also* MOUTHWASH TEST, PREIMPLANTATION GENETIC DIAGNOSIS.

geni- (**genio-**) *combining form denoting* the chin.

-genic *combining form denoting* **1.** producing. **2.** produced by.

genicular *adj.* relating to the knee joint: applied to arteries that supply the knee.

geniculum *n.* a sharp bend in an anatomical structure, such as the bend in the facial nerve in the medial wall of the middle ear.

genion *n.* (in *craniometry) the tip of the protuberance of the chin.

genioplasty *n.* an operation performed in plastic surgery to alter the size and shape of the chin. This can be built up with grafted bone, cartilage, or artificial material.

genital *adj.* relating to the reproductive organs or to reproduction.

genital herpes *see* HERPES.

genitalia *pl. n.* the reproductive organs of either the male or the female. However, the term is usually used in reference to the external parts of the reproductive system. *See also* VULVA.

genito- *combining form denoting* the reproductive organs. Examples: **genitoplasty** (plastic surgery of); **genitourinary** (relating to the reproductive and excretory systems).

genitourinary medicine the medical specialty concerned with the study and treatment of *sexually transmitted diseases.

genodermatosis *n.* any genetically determined skin disorder, such as *ichthyosis, *neurofibromatosis, or *xeroderma pigmentosum.

genogram *n.* in family *psychotherapy, a family tree and a family history of a particular psychological disorder, which are constructed in view of the whole family to help them understand each other better.

genome *n.* the total genetic material of an

organism, comprising the genes contained in its chromosomes; sometimes the term is used for the basic *haploid set of chromosomes of an organism. The human genome comprises 23 pairs of chromosomes (*see* HUMAN GENOME PROJECT).

genomics *n.* the branch of genetics concerned with the study of genomes. It includes both the mapping of genomes – and ultimately producing a DNA sequence for any particular organism or individual – and understanding how gene expression is controlled and gene products change under different conditions, including disease states.

genotype *n.* **1.** the genetic constitution of an individual or group, as determined by the particular set of genes it possesses. **2.** the genetic information carried by a pair of alleles, which determines a particular characteristic. **3.** a gene or pattern of genes the precise details of which are defined. *Compare* PHENOTYPE.

gentamicin *n.* an *aminoglycoside antibiotic used to treat serious infections caused by a wide range of bacteria. It can be administered by injection or infusion or applied as drops to the ears and eyes. Kidney and ear damage may occur at high doses. Trade names: **Cidomycin, Genticin**.

gentian violet 1. a dye used for staining tissues and microorganisms for microscopical study. **2.** *see* METHYL VIOLET.

genu *n.* **1.** the knee. **2.** any bent anatomical structure resembling the knee. —**genual** *adj.*

genuine stress incontinence *see* INCONTINENCE.

genus *n.* (*pl.* **genera**) a category used in the classification of animals and plants. A genus consists of several closely related and similar species; for example the genus *Canis* includes the dog, wolf, and jackal.

genu valgum abnormal in-curving of the legs at the knees, resulting in excessive separation of the feet when the knees are in contact. *See* KNOCK-KNEE.

genu varum abnormal outward curving of the legs at the knees, resulting in separation of the knees. *See* BOW-LEGS.

geo- *combining form denoting* the earth or soil.

geographical tongue a benign loss of papillae on the surface of the tongue taking the form of areas of *erythema that change from day to day. Medical names: **benign migratory glossitis, erythema migrans**.

geophagia *n.* the eating of dirt. *See* PICA.

ger- (**gero-, geront(o-)**) *combining form denoting* old age.

geriatrics *n.* the branch of medicine concerned with the diagnosis and treatment of disorders that occur in old age and with the care of the aged. *See also* GERONTOLOGY.

germ *n.* any microorganism, especially one that causes disease. *See also* INFECTION.

German measles a mild highly contagious virus infection, mainly of childhood, causing enlargement of lymph nodes in the neck and a widespread pink rash. The disease is spread by close contact with a patient. After an incubation period of 2–3 weeks a headache, sore throat, and slight fever develop, followed by swelling and soreness of the neck and the eruption of a rash of minute pink spots, spreading from the face and neck to the rest of the body. The spots disappear within seven days but the patient remains infectious for a further 3–4 days. An infection usually confers immunity. As German measles can cause fetal malformations during early pregnancy, girls should be immunized against the disease before puberty. Most children now receive immunization via the *MMR vaccine in their second year. Medical name: **rubella**. *Compare* SCARLET FEVER.

germ cell (**gonocyte**) any of the embryonic cells that have the potential to develop into spermatozoa or ova. The term is also applied to any of the cells undergoing gametogenesis and to the gametes themselves.

germicide *n.* an agent that destroys microorganisms, particularly those causing disease. *See* ANTIBIOTIC, ANTIFUNGAL, ANTISEPTIC, DISINFECTANT.

germinal *adj.* **1.** relating to the early developmental stages of an embryo or tissue. **2.** relating to a germ.

germinal epithelium the epithelial covering of the ovary, which was formerly thought to be the site of formation of *oogonia. It is now thought that the oogonia persist in a dormant state from the prenatal period until required in reproductive life.

germinal vesicle the nucleus of a mature

*oocyte, prior to fertilization. It is considerably larger than the nucleus of other cells.

germ layer any of the three distinct types of tissue found in the very early stages of embryonic development (*see* ECTODERM, ENDODERM, MESODERM). The germ layers can be traced throughout embryonic development as they differentiate to form the entire range of body tissues.

germ plasm the substance postulated by 19th century biologists (notably Weismann) to be transmitted via the gametes from one generation to the next and to give rise to the body cells.

gerontology *n.* the study of the changes in the mind and body that accompany ageing and the problems associated with them.

Gerstmann's syndrome a group of symptoms that represent a partial disintegration of the patient's recognition of his *body image. It consists of an inability to name the individual fingers, misidentification of the right and left sides of the body, and inability to write or make mathematical calculations (*see* ACALCULIA, AGRAPHIA). It is caused by disease in the association area of the dominant (usually left) parietal lobe of the brain. [J. G. Gerstmann (1887–1969), Austrian neurologist]

Gerstmann-Straussler-Scheinker syndrome an autosomal *dominant condition that is caused by a mutation in the *prion protein gene and resembles *Creutzfeldt-Jakob disease (CJD). Patients present with cerebellar dysfunction (*ataxia and *dysarthria) and later develop dementia. They continue to deteriorate over several years, in contrast with patients with CJD, who deteriorate rapidly over periods of less than 12 months. [J. G. Gerstmann]

gestaltism *n.* a school of psychology, originating in Germany, that regards mental processes as wholes (**gestalt**, from the German meaning 'form' or 'body') that cannot be broken down into constituent parts. From this was developed **gestalt therapy**, which aims at achieving a suitable gestalt within the patient that includes all facets of functioning.

gestation *n.* the period during which a fertilized egg cell develops into a baby that is ready to be delivered. Gestation averages 266 days in humans (or 280 days from the first day of the last menstrual period). *See also* PREGNANCY.

gestational diabetes mellitus diabetes or impaired glucose tolerance that is diagnosed during pregnancy (*see* GLUCOSE TOLERANCE TEST). Women at increased risk of gestational diabetes include those with a personal history of the condition or a family history of diabetes and those who have had a previously unexplained stillbirth. In most cases gestational diabetes resolves at the end of the pregnancy, but such women are at increased risk of developing type 2 diabetes thereafter. It is treated by dietary control with or without insulin or oral hypoglycaemic drugs. *See also* PREGESTATIONAL DIABETES MELLITUS.

gestational trophoblastic disease (GTD) a group of disorders spanning the conditions of complete and partial molar pregnancies (*see* HYDATIDIFORM MOLE) through to the malignant conditions of invasive mole, *choriocarcinoma, and the very rare placental site trophoblastic tumour (PSTT). If there is any evidence of persistence of GTD, most commonly defined as a persistent elevation of *human chorionic gonadotrophin, the condition is described as *gestational trophoblastic neoplasia.

gestational trophoblastic neoplasia (GTN) a group of disorders characterized by persistence of *gestational trophoblastic disease, with abnormal placental development and very high levels of *human chorionic gonadotrophin (hCG). The chorionic villi are fluid-filled with vacuolation of the placenta and destruction of the normal stroma. GTN is rare in the UK, with a calculated incidence of $1/714$ live births. It may develop after a molar pregnancy (*see* HYDATIDIFORM MOLE), a nonmolar pregnancy, or a live birth. The incidence after a live birth is estimated at $1/50,000$. A malignant condition may develop (*see* CHORIOCARCINOMA) if the abnormal tissue is not completely removed and the risk of this is monitored by the fall in hCG levels. Choriocarcinoma complicates approximately 3% of complete moles, although in 50% of cases of choriocarcinoma there is no history of immediately preceding trophoblastic disease. It may also occur following a normal pregnancy. In the UK, there is an effective registration and treatment programme. The programme has achieved impressive results, with high cure (98–100%) and low chemotherapy (5–8%) rates.

gestodene *n.* a *progestogen used in oral contraceptives in combination with *ethinylestradiol (an oestrogen). Trade names: **Femodene**, **Femodette**, **Katya 30/75**, **Sunya 20/75**, **Triadene**.

GFR *see* GLOMERULAR FILTRATION RATE.

Ghon's focus the lesion produced in the lung of a previously uninfected person by tubercle bacilli. It is a small focus of granulomatous inflammation, which may become visible on a chest X-ray if it grows large enough or if it calcifies. A Ghon focus usually heals without further trouble, but in some patients tuberculosis spreads from it via the lymphatics, the air spaces, or the bloodstream. [A. Ghon (1866–1936), Czech pathologist]

ghost vessels empty transparent blood vessels that persist in the cornea after regression of the inflammatory process that stimulated their development.

ghrelin *n.* a hormone produced by stomach cells that increases appetite and stimulates secretion of growth hormone (levels increase before meals and decrease thereafter). Its receptors and site of action are in the hypothalamus. Ghrelin levels are lower in obese individuals (suggesting that the hormone does not stimulate eating) and higher in patients with anorexia nervosa.

giant cell any large cell, such as a *megakaryocyte. Giant cells may have one or many nuclei.

giant-cell arteritis *see* ARTERITIS.

Giardia *n.* a genus of parasitic pear-shaped protozoa inhabiting the human small intestine. They have four pairs of *flagella, two nuclei, and two sucking discs used for attachment to the intestinal wall. *Giardia* is usually harmless but may occasionally cause diarrhoea (*see* GIARDIASIS).

giardiasis (lambliasis) *n.* a disease caused by the parasitic protozoan *Giardia lamblia* in the small intestine. Individuals become infected by eating food contaminated with cysts containing the parasite. Symptoms include diarrhoea, nausea, bellyache, and flatulence, as well as the passage of pale fatty stools (steatorrhoea). Large numbers of the parasite may interfere with the absorption of food through the gut wall. The disease occurs throughout the world and is particularly common in children; it responds well to oral doses of *metronidazole.

gibbus (gibbosity) *n.* a sharply angled curvature of the backbone, resulting from collapse of a vertebra. Infection with tuberculosis was a common cause.

Giemsa's stain a mixture of *methylene blue and *eosin, used for distinguishing different types of white blood cell and for detecting parasitic microorganisms in blood smears. It is one of the *Romanowsky stains. [G. Giemsa (1867–1948), German chemist]

GIFT *see* GAMETE INTRAFALLOPIAN TRANSFER.

gigantism *n.* abnormal growth causing excessive height, most commonly due to oversecretion during childhood of *growth hormone (somatotrophin) by the pituitary gland. In **eunuchoid gigantism** the tall stature is due to delayed puberty, which results in continued growth of the long bones before their growing ends (epiphyses) fuse. *See also* SOTOS SYNDROME.

GIK regime *see* ALBERTI REGIME.

Gilbert's syndrome familial unconjugated hyperbilirubinaemia: a condition due to an inherited congenital deficiency of the enzyme UDP glucuronyl transferase in the liver cells. Patients become mildly jaundiced, especially if they fast or have some minor infection. Occasionally they have mild abdominal discomfort. The jaundice can be diminished by small doses of phenobarbital, which stimulates enzyme activity. The condition is lifelong but harmless. [N. A. Gilbert (1858–1927), French physician]

Gilles de la Tourette syndrome *see* TOURETTE'S SYNDROME.

Gillick competence the means by which to assess legal *capacity in children under the age of 16 years, established in the case *Gillick v West Norfolk and Wisbech Area Health Authority* (1985) 2 A11 ER 402. Such children are deemed to be capable of giving valid *consent to advice or treatment without parental knowledge or agreement provided they have sufficient understanding to appreciate the nature, purpose, and hazards of the proposed treatment. In the Gillick case the criteria for deciding competence, set out by Lord Fraser, related specifically to contraceptive treatment. In addition to the elements of Gillick competence, the **Fraser guidelines** specified that a health professional must be convinced that the child was likely to begin, or to continue having, sexual intercourse with or without contraceptive treatment, that his or her physical and/or mental health would probably suffer in the absence of treatment, and it was in his or her best interests to provide treatment. The principle of Gillick competence applies to all treatment for those under the age of 16, not just contraceptive services. — **Gillick-competent** *adj.*

Gimbernat's ligament a portion of the medial end of the *inguinal ligament that is reflected along the upper part of the pubic bone. It is used to hold stitches during repairs of a femoral *hernia. [A. de Gimbernat (1734–1816), Spanish surgeon and anatomist]

gingiv- (gingivo-) *combining form denoting* the gums. Example: **gingivoplasty** (plastic surgery of).

gingiva *n.* (*pl.* **gingivae**) the gum: the layer of dense connective tissue and overlying mucous membrane that covers the alveolar bone and necks of the teeth. —**gingival** *adj.*

gingivectomy *n.* the surgical removal of excess gum tissue. It is a specific procedure of periodontal surgery.

gingivitis *n.* inflammation of the gums (*see* GINGIVA) caused by *plaque on the surfaces of the teeth at their necks. The gums are swollen and bleed easily. **Chronic gingivitis** is an early stage of *periodontal disease but is reversible with good oral hygiene. *Ulcerative gingivitis is painful and destructive. Gingival overgrowth may be caused by drug therapy, e.g. phenytoin.

ginglymus (hinge joint) *n.* a form of *diarthrosis (freely movable joint) that allows angular movement in one plane only, increasing or decreasing the angle between the bones. Examples are the knee joint and the elbow joint.

girdle *n.* (in anatomy) an encircling or arching arrangement of bones. *See also* PELVIC GIRDLE, SHOULDER GIRDLE.

GIST *see* GASTROINTESTINAL STROMAL TUMOUR.

glabella *n.* the smooth rounded surface of the *frontal bone in the middle of the forehead, between the two eyebrows.

gladiolus *n.* the middle and largest segment of the *sternum.

gland *n.* an organ or group of cells that is specialized for synthesizing and secreting certain fluids, either for use in the body or for excretion. There are two main groups of glands: the *exocrine glands, which discharge their secretions by means of ducts, and the *endocrine glands, which secrete their products – hormones – directly into the bloodstream. *See also* SECRETION.

glanders (equinia) *n.* an infectious disease of horses, donkeys, and mules that is caused by the bacterium *Pseudomonas mallei* and can be transmitted to humans. Symptoms include fever and inflammation (with possible ulceration) of the lymph nodes (a form of the disease known as **farcy**), skin, and nasal mucous membranes. In the untreated acute form death may follow in 2–20 days. In the more common chronic form, many patients survive without treatment. Administration of antibiotics is usually effective.

glandular fever an infectious disease, caused by the Epstein-Barr virus, that affects the lymph nodes in the neck, armpits, and groin; it mainly affects adolescents and young adults. After an incubation period of 5–7 days, symptoms commence with swelling and tenderness of the lymph nodes, fever, headache, a sore throat, lethargy, and loss of appetite. In some cases the liver is affected, causing *hepatitis, or the spleen is enlarged. Glandular fever is diagnosed by the presence of large numbers of *monocytes in the blood. Complications are rare but symptoms may persist for weeks before recovery. Medical name: **infectious mononucleosis**.

glans (glans penis) *n.* the acorn-shaped end part of the *penis, formed by the expanded end of the corpus spongiosum (erectile tissue). It is covered by the prepuce (foreskin), unless this has been removed by circumcision. The term glans is also applied to the end of the *clitoris.

glare *n.* the undesirable effects of scattered stray light on the retina, causing reduced contrast and visual performance as well as annoyance and discomfort. Glare is most commonly caused by cataract or corneal opacity

Glasgow Coma Scale (GCS, Glasgow scoring system) a numerical system used to estimate a patient's level of consciousness after head injury. Each of the following are numerically graded: eye opening (1–4), motor response (1–6), and verbal response

(1–5). The higher the score, the greater the level of consciousness: a score of 7 indicates a coma.

glass ionomer a dental filling material that is based on a *cement of a silicate glass and an organic acid.

glatiramer *n.* a drug that modifies the body's immune response and is used to reduce the frequency of relapses in people with relapsing/remitting multiple sclerosis. It is administered by subcutaneous injection; side-effects include flushing and palpitations. Trade name: **Copaxone**.

glaucoma *n.* a condition of the *optic disc in which a loss of retinal nerve fibres leads to loss of vision. The most significant and manageable risk factor is the pressure in the eye. There are two types of **primary glaucoma** (in which no other ocular disease is present): acute and chronic simple. In **acute** (or **angle-closure**) **glaucoma**, there is an abrupt rise in pressure due to sudden closure of the angle of the anterior chamber between the cornea and iris where aqueous humour usually drains from the eye. This is accompanied by sudden and severe pain with marked blurring of vision associated with inflammation of the anterior segment. In the more common **chronic simple** (or **open-angle**) **glaucoma**, the pressure increases gradually, usually without any symptoms, and the visual loss is insidious. The same type of visual loss may rarely occur in eyes with a normal pressure: this is called **normal** (or **low-tension**) **glaucoma**. Primary glaucoma occurs increasingly with age and is an important cause of blindness. **Secondary glaucoma** may occur when other ocular disease impairs the normal circulation of the aqueous humour and causes the intraocular pressure to rise.

In all types of glaucoma the aim of the treatment is to reduce the intraocular pressure. Drugs used for this purpose include beta blockers (e.g. timolol, levobunolol, carteolol), carbonic anhydrase inhibitors (e.g. brinzolamide, dorzolamide), alpha-receptor stimulants (e.g. apraclonidine, brimonidine), and prostaglandin analogues (e.g. latanoprost). They can be used in the form of eye drops. If the medical treatment is ineffective, surgery may be performed to make a new channel through which the aqueous humour may drain from the eye in sufficient quantities to allow the pressure to return to

normal. Such operations are known as **drainage** or **filtering operations**.

glaukomflecken *pl. n.* small anterior subcapsular lens opacities seen in acute (angle-closure) glaucoma.

Gleason grade the grade (from one to five) given to an area of prostate cancer, reflecting the level of differentiation of the tumour. Higher grades indicate poorer differentiation. [D. F. Gleason (1920–2008), US pathologist]

Gleason score a numerical score from two to ten, which is the sum of the two *Gleason grades given to the most common and second most common pattern of prostate cancer seen in the tumour.

gleet *n.* a discharge of purulent mucus from the penis or vagina resulting from chronic *gonorrhoea.

glenohumeral *adj.* relating to the glenoid cavity and the humerus: the region of the shoulder joint.

glenoid cavity (glenoid fossa) the socket of the shoulder joint: the pear-shaped cavity at the top of the *scapula into which the head of the humerus fits.

gli- (glio-) *combining form denoting* 1. glia. 2. a glutinous substance.

glia (neuroglia) *n.* the special connective tissue of the central nervous system, composed of different cells, including the *oligodendrocytes, *astrocytes, ependymal cells (*see* EPENDYMA), and *microglia, with various supportive and nutritive functions. Glial cells outnumber the neurons by between five and ten to one, and make up some 40% of the total volume of the brain and spinal cord. —**glial** *adj.*

gliadin *n.* a protein, soluble in alcohol, that is obtained from wheat. It is one of the constituents of *gluten.

glibenclamide *n.* a drug that reduces the level of sugar in the blood and is used to treat type 2 diabetes (*see* SULPHONYLUREA). It is administered by mouth. Side-effects include mild digestive upsets and skin reactions.

gliclazide *n.* a *sulphonylurea oral hypoglycaemic drug used in the treatment of type 2 diabetes. Trade name: **Diamicron**.

gliding joint *see* ARTHRODIC JOINT.

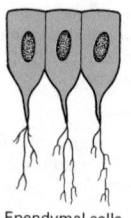

Ependymal cells

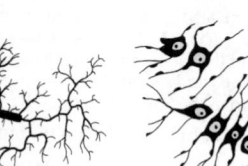

Protoplasmic astrocyte   Fibrous astrocyte

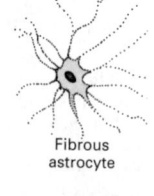

Microglia   Oligodendroglia

Types of glia.

glioblastoma (glioblastoma multiforme) *n.* the most aggressive type of brain tumour derived from non-nervous (glial) tissue (*see* ASTROCYTOMA). Its rapid enlargement destroys normal brain cells, with a progressive loss of function, and raises intracranial pressure, causing headache, vomiting, and drowsiness. Treatment is never curative and the prognosis is poor.

glioma *n.* any tumour of non-nervous cells (*glia) in the nervous system. The term is sometimes also used for all tumours that arise in the central nervous system, including *astrocytomas and *glioblastomas. Tumours of low-grade malignancy produce symptoms by pressure on surrounding structures; those of high-grade malignancy may be infiltrative.

gliosome *n.* a *lysosome in an *astrocyte.

glipizide *n.* a drug used to control high blood-glucose levels (hyperglycaemia) in patients with type 2 diabetes after diet control has failed (*see* SULPHONYLUREA). It is admin-

istered by mouth; side-effects are hypoglycaemia, nausea and vomiting, and skin rash. Trade names: **Glibenese**, **Minodiab**.

Glivec *n. see* IMATINIB.

global ethics an approach to moral problems acknowledging that ethical analysis is frequently culture-specific and geographically limited. The international and worldwide experience of health care is the subject of study and there is commonly close attention to inequities in health and health-care provision, with frequent emphasis on *human rights, *justice, and *equality.

globin *n.* a protein, found in the body, that can combine with iron-containing groups to form *haemoglobin (which is found in red blood cells) and *myoglobin (found in muscle).

globulin *n.* one of a group of simple proteins that are soluble in dilute salt solutions and can be coagulated by heat. A range of different globulins is present in the blood (the **serum globulins**, including alpha (α), beta (β), and *gamma (γ) globulins). Some globulins have important functions as antibodies (*see* IMMUNOGLOBULIN); others are responsible for the transport of lipids, iron, or copper in the blood. *See also* HORMONE-BINDING GLOBULINS.

globulinuria *n.* the presence in the urine of globulins.

globus *n.* a spherical or globe-shaped structure; for example the **globus pallidus**, part of the lenticular nucleus in the brain (*see* BASAL GANGLIA).

globus hystericus *see* GLOBUS PHARYNGEUS.

globus pharyngeus a common condition characterized by a sensation of a lump in the throat, in the midline just above the sternum; swallowing is not affected. The condition, formerly called **globus hystericus**, is sometimes related to *gastro-oesophageal reflux and tends to be worse during periods of stress.

glomangioma (glomus tumour) *n. see* GLOMUS.

glomerular filtration rate (GFR) the rate at which substances are filtered from the blood of the glomeruli into the Bowman's capsules of the *nephrons. It is calculated by measuring the *clearance of specific substances (e.g. creatinine) and is an index of renal function. *See* EGFR.

glomerulonephritis (glomerular nephritis, GN) *n.* inflammation of the glomeruli, although in practice the term is used for a number of glomerular conditions lacking microscopical signs of inflammation. For instance, *membranous nephropathy is often referred to as membranous glomerulonephritis. GN may be a primary disease, restricted in its clinical manifestations to the kidney, or part of a multisystem disorder, such as systemic *lupus erythematosus or *vasculitis. Its presentation may be acute, with a *nephritic or *nephrotic syndrome; subacute, with rapidly declining renal function over a period of days or weeks; or chronic, with signs of the disease picked up on routine medical examination. Abnormalities of urine analysis are to be expected, with blood, protein, and casts present in variable amounts. Arterial hypertension is a common associated finding. GN is classified according to the different patterns of histological injury seen on renal biopsy specimens; these are examined by light and electron microscopy and by immunofluorescent studies.

glomerulus *n.* (*pl.* **glomeruli**) **1.** the network of blood capillaries contained within the cuplike end (**Bowman's capsule**) of a *nephron. It is the site of primary filtration of waste products from the blood into the kidney tubule. **2.** any other small rounded mass.

glomus *n.* (*pl.* **glomera**) a small communication between a tiny artery and vein in the skin of the limbs. It is concerned with the regulation of temperature.

glomus jugulare a collection of *paraganglion cells in close relation to the internal jugular vein at its origin at the base of the skull. It is a site of origin for *glomus tumours (*see also* PARAGANGLIOMA).

glomus tumour 1. a benign tumour arising from *paraganglion cells associated with the vagus or glossopharyngeal nerves in the neck (*see* PARAGANGLIOMA). In the middle ear they are called **glomus tympanicum tumours**; around the jugular vein they are called **glomus jugulare tumours**. **2. (glomangioma)** a harmless but often painful tumour produced by malformation and overgrowth of a *glomus, usually in the skin at the ends of the fingers or toes. It may be cauterized or removed surgically.

gloss- (glosso-) *combining form denoting* the tongue. Examples: **glossopharyngeal** (relating to the tongue and pharynx); **glossoplasty** (plastic surgery of).

glossa *n. see* TONGUE.

glossectomy *n.* surgical removal of the tongue, an operation usually carried out for cancer in this structure.

Glossina *n. see* TSETSE.

glossitis *n.* inflammation of the tongue. Causes include anaemia, candidiasis, and vitamin deficiency. *See also* GEOGRAPHICAL TONGUE.

glossolalia *n.* nonsense speech that mimics normal speech in that it is appropriately formed into an imitation of syllables, words, and sentences. It can be uttered in *trance states and during sleep.

glossopharyngeal nerve the ninth *cranial nerve (IX), which supplies motor fibres to part of the pharynx and to the parotid salivary glands and sensory fibres to the posterior third of the tongue and the soft palate.

glossoplegia *n.* paralysis of the tongue.

glottis *n.* the space between the two *vocal folds. The term is often applied to the vocal folds themselves or to that part of the larynx associated with the production of sound.

gluc- (gluco-) *combining form denoting* glucose. Example: **glucosuria** (urinary excretion of).

glucagon *n.* a hormone, produced by the pancreas, that causes an increase in the blood sugar level and thus has an effect opposite to that of *insulin. Glucagon is administered by injection to counteract diabetic *hypoglycaemia.

glucagonoma *n.* a usually malignant pancreatic tumour of the alpha cells of the *islets of Langerhans that secretes excessive amounts of glucagon and causes impaired glucose tolerance or diabetes, a specific dermatitis, and weight loss.

glucagon stimulation test a test for *phaeochromocytomas not displaying typically high levels of plasma *catecholamines. An intravenous bolus of *glucagon is administered and the test is positive when there is a threefold increase in plasma catecholamine levels with a consequent rise in blood pressure. Protection from the blood-pressure rise can be given by pretreatment with alpha blockers. This test should not be performed in patients who suffer with angina.

glucocorticoid *n. see* CORTICOSTEROID.

glucokinase *n.* an enzyme (a *hexokinase), found in the liver, that catalyses the conversion of glucose to glucose-6-phosphate. This is the first stage of *glycolysis.

gluconeogenesis *n.* the biochemical process in which glucose, an important source of energy, is synthesized from non-carbohydrate sources, such as amino acids. Gluconeogenesis occurs mainly in the liver and kidney and meets the needs of the body for glucose when carbohydrate is not available in sufficient amounts in the diet.

glucosamine *n.* the amino sugar of glucose, i.e. glucose in which the hydroxyl group is replaced by an amino group. Glucosamine is a component of *mucopolysaccharides and *glycoproteins: for example, *hyaluronic acid, a mucopolysaccharide found in synovial fluid, and *heparin.

glucose (dextrose) *n.* a simple sugar containing six carbon atoms (a hexose). Glucose is an important source of energy in the body and the sole source of energy for the brain. Free glucose is not found in many foods (grapes are an exception); however, glucose is one of the constituents of both sucrose and starch, both of which yield glucose after digestion. Glucose is stored in the body in the form of *glycogen. The concentration of glucose in the blood is maintained at around 5 mmol/l by a variety of hormones, principally *insulin and *glucagon. If the blood-glucose concentration falls below this level neurological and other symptoms may result (*see* HYPOGLYCAEMIA). Conversely, if the blood-glucose level is raised above its normal level, to 10 mmol/l, the condition of *hyperglycaemia develops. This is a symptom of *diabetes mellitus.

glucose-6-phosphate dehydrogenase deficiency a hereditary disorder – an X-linked condition (*see* SEX-LINKED) – in which the absence of the enzyme glucose-6-phosphate dehydrogenase (G6PD), which functions in carbohydrate metabolism, results in the breakdown of the red blood cells (*haemolysis), usually after exposure to *oxidants, such as drugs, or infections. The breakdown causes acute attacks that are characterized by pallor, loin pain, and rigors. There are several varieties of G6PD defi-

ciency, which is most common in people of African, Middle Eastern, and Mediterranean descent. Treatment involves identifying and avoiding agents that trigger the haemolysis and treating acute attacks symptomatically. *See also* FAVISM.

glucose tolerance test (oral glucose tolerance test) the gold-standard diagnostic test for diabetes mellitus and the related condition, **impaired glucose tolerance** (IGT). After an overnight fast the blood-sugar level is measured (the fasting level). The patient is then given a drink containing 75 g glucose, and a further blood-sugar measurement is taken after two hours. Diabetes is diagnosed if the fasting level is above 7.0 mmol/l and/or the two-hour level is above 11.1 mmol/l. IGT is diagnosed when the fasting level is below 7.0 mmol/l and the two-hour level is between 7.0 mmol/l and 11.1 mmol/l. Many people with IGT progress to develop diabetes, but this can be prevented with adoption of a diabetic-type diet and weight loss (if overweight).

glucoside *n. see* GLYCOSIDE.

glucuronic acid a sugar acid derived from glucose. Glucuronic acid is an important constituent of *chondroitin sulphate (found in cartilage) and *hyaluronic acid (found in synovial fluid).

glue ear a common condition in which viscous fluid accumulates in the middle ear, causing *deafness. It is most frequently seen in children and is due to malfunction of the *Eustachian tube. Many cases resolve spontaneously; treatment, if required, consists of surgical incision of the eardrum (*myringotomy), drainage of the fluid, and the insertion of a *grommet. Medical names: **otitis media with effusion**, **secretory otitis media**.

glutamate dehydrogenase (glutamic acid dehydrogenase) an important enzyme involved in the *deamination of amino acids.

glutamic acid (glutamate) *see* AMINO ACID, NEUROTRANSMITTER.

glutamic acid decarboxylase (GAD) a common enzyme that, because of similarities to certain bacterial proteins, can provoke an autoimmune reaction against the beta cells of the pancreas progressing to type 1 *diabetes mellitus.

glutamic oxaloacetic transaminase (GOT) *see* ASPARTATE AMINOTRANSFERASE.

glutamic pyruvic transaminase (GPT) *see* ALANINE AMINOTRANSFERASE.

glutaminase *n.* an enzyme, found in the kidney, that catalyses the breakdown of the amino acid glutamine to ammonia and glutamic acid: a stage in the production of urea.

glutamine *n. see* AMINO ACID.

glutathione *n.* a peptide containing the amino acids glutamic acid, cysteine, and glycine. It functions as a *coenzyme in several oxidation-reduction reactions. Glutathione serves as an *antioxidant: it reacts with potentially harmful oxidizing agents and is itself oxidized (*see also* SELENIUM). This is important in ensuring the proper functioning of proteins, haemoglobin, membrane lipids, etc. High levels of glutathione in the blood are associated with longevity.

glutelin *n.* one of a group of simple proteins found in plants and soluble only in dilute acids and bases. An example is **glutenin**, found in wheat (*see* GLUTEN).

gluten *n.* a mixture of the two proteins **gliadin** and **glutenin**. Gluten is present in wheat and rye and is important for its baking properties: when mixed with water it becomes sticky and enables air to be trapped and dough to be formed. Sensitivity to gluten leads to *coeliac disease in children.

gluteus *n.* one of three paired muscles of the buttocks (**gluteus maximus**, **gluteus medius** and **gluteus minimus**). They are responsible for movements of the thigh. —**gluteal** *adj.*

glyc- (**glyco-**) *combining form denoting* sugar.

glycated haemoglobin (**glycosylated haemoglobin**) any derivative of haemoglobin in which a glucose molecule is attached to the haemoglobin molecule. The most abundant form of glycated haemoglobin is **haemoglobin A_{1c}** (**HbA_{1c}**), levels of which are significantly increased in diabetes. The percentage of the HbA molecules that become glycated is dependent on the general level of glucose in the plasma over the lifetime of the molecule (generally 3 months); this percentage is therefore used as the standard measure of the degree of control of *hyperglycaemia in a diabetic person over this period.

glycation *n.* the chemical linkage of glucose to a protein, to form a glycoprotein. Glycation of body proteins has been postulated as a cause of complications of diabetes mellitus. *See* ADVANCED GLYCATION END-PRODUCTS, GLYCATED HAEMOGLOBIN.

glyceride *n.* a *lipid consisting of glycerol (an alcohol) combined with one or more fatty acids. *See also* TRIGLYCERIDE.

glycerin (**glycerol**) *n.* a clear viscous liquid obtained by hydrolysis of fats and mixed oils and produced as a by-product in the manufacture of soap. It is used as an *emollient in many skin preparations, as a laxative (particularly in the form of *suppositories), and as a sweetening agent in the pharmaceutical industry.

glyceryl trinitrate (**nitroglycerin**) a drug that dilates blood vessels and is used mainly to prevent and treat angina (*see* VASO-DILATOR). It is administered by mouth (sublingual tablets or sprays), skin patches or ointment, intravenous infusion, or rectal ointment; large doses may cause flushing, headache, and fainting. Glyceryl trinitrate is also applied topically in the treatment of anal fissures. Trade names: **Glytrin Spray**, **Nitrolingual Pumpspray**, **Rectogesic**, **Suscard**, **Transiderm-Nitro**, etc.

glycine *n. see* AMINO ACID.

glycobiology *n.* the study of the chemistry, biochemistry, and other aspects of carbohydrates and carbohydrate complexes, especially *glycoproteins. Elucidation of the structure and role of the sugar molecules of glycoproteins has important medical implications and has led to the development of new drugs, such as *tissue-type plasminogen activators, drugs that affect the immune system, and antiviral drugs.

glycocholic acid *see* BILE ACIDS.

glycogen *n.* a carbohydrate consisting of branched chains of glucose units. Glycogen is the principal form in which carbohydrate is stored in the body: it is the counterpart of starch in plants. Glycogen is stored in the liver and muscles and may be readily broken down to glucose.

glycogenesis *n.* the biochemical process, occurring chiefly in the liver and in muscle, by which glucose is converted into glycogen.

glycogenolysis *n.* a biochemical process, occurring chiefly in the liver and in muscle, by which glycogen is broken down into glucose.

glycolipid *n.* a *lipid containing a sugar molecule (usually galactose or glucose). The *cerebrosides are examples of glycolipids.

glycolysis *n.* the conversion of glucose, by a series of ten enzyme-catalysed reactions, to lactic acid. Glycolysis takes place in the cytoplasm of cells and the first nine reactions (converting glucose to pyruvate) form the first stage of cellular *respiration. The process involves the production of a small amount of energy (in the form of ATP), which is used for biochemical reactions. The final reaction of glycolysis (converting pyruvate to lactic acid) provides energy for short periods of time when oxygen consumption exceeds demand; for example, during bursts of intense muscular activity. *See also* LACTIC ACID.

glycopeptide antibiotics *see* VANCO-MYCIN.

glycoprotein *n.* one of a group of compounds consisting of a protein combined with a carbohydrate (such as galactose or mannose). Examples of glycoproteins are certain enzymes, hormones, and antigens.

glycoside *n.* a compound formed by replacing the hydroxyl (–OH) group of a sugar by another group. (If the sugar is glucose the compound is known as a **glucoside**.) Glycosides found in plants include some pharmacologically important products, such as the **cardiac glycosides** *digoxin and digitoxin, derived from the foxglove (*Digitalis*). Other plant glycosides are natural food toxins, present in cassava, almonds, and other plant products, and may yield hydrogen cyanide if the plant is not prepared properly before eating.

glycosuria *n.* the presence of glucose in the urine in abnormally large amounts. Only very minute quantities of this sugar may be found normally in the urine. Higher levels may be associated with diabetes mellitus, kidney disease, and some other conditions.

glycosylated haemoglobin *see* GLY-CATED HAEMOGLOBIN.

GMC *see* GENERAL MEDICAL COUNCIL.

gnath- (**gnatho-**) *combining form denoting* the jaw. Example: **gnathoplasty** (plastic surgery of).

gnathion *n.* the lowest point of the midline of the lower jaw (mandible).

Gnathostoma *n.* a genus of parasitic nematodes. Adult worms are commonly found in the intestines of tigers, leopards, and dogs. The presence of the larval stage of *G. spinigerum* in humans, who are not the normal hosts, causes a skin condition called *creeping eruption.

gnotobiotic *adj.* describing germ-free conditions or a germ-free animal that has been inoculated with known microorganisms.

GnRH *see* GONADOTROPHIN-RELEASING HORMONE.

GnRH analogue *see* GONADORELIN ANALOGUE.

goblet cell a column-shaped secretory cell found in the *epithelium of the respiratory and intestinal tracts. Goblet cells secrete the principal constituents of mucus.

goitre *n.* a swelling of the neck due to enlargement of the thyroid gland. This may be due to lack of dietary iodine, which is necessary for the production of thyroid hormone: the gland enlarges in an attempt to increase the output of hormone. This was the cause of **endemic goitre**, formerly common in regions where the diet lacked iodine. **Sporadic goitre** may be due to simple overgrowth (hyperplasia) of the gland or to a tumour. In **exophthalmic goitre** (**Graves' disease**) the swelling is associated with overactivity of the gland and is accompanied by other symptoms (*see* THYROTOXICOSIS). Autoimmune thyroiditis can be associated with goitre (*see* HASHIMOTO'S DISEASE).

gold *n.* **1.** a bright yellow metal that is very malleable. In dentistry pure gold is now very rarely used as a filling. Gold alloys are used for *crowns, *inlays, and *bridges, either alone or veneered with a tooth-coloured material, but increasingly nonprecious alloys are being used. Gold alloys are now only rarely used as the metal framework for partial dentures, *cobalt-chromium alloys being used instead. **2.** (in pharmacology) any of several compounds of the metal gold, used in the treatment of rheumatoid arthritis. **Sodium aurothiomalate** (Myocrisin) is administered by intramuscular injection. Common side-effects include mouth ulcers, itching, blood disorders, skin reactions, and inflammation of the colon and kidneys. *Auranofin is a gold compound administered orally.

GOLD (Global Initiative for Chronic Obstructive Lung Disease) a body that works with health-care professionals and public health officials around the world to raise awareness of *chronic obstructive pulmonary disease (COPD) and to improve prevention and treatment of this disease. The publication of management guidelines has had a significant impact on a change in treatment for this condition worldwide.

Goldmann applanation tonometer *see* TONOMETER. [H. Goldmann (1899–1991), Swiss ophthalmologist]

golfer's elbow inflammation of the origin of the common flexor tendon on the medial epicondyle of the *humerus (medial epicondylitis), caused by overuse of the forearm muscles. Treatment is by rest, anti-inflammatory medication, or steroid injection. *Compare* TENNIS ELBOW.

Golgi apparatus a collection of vesicles and folded membranes in a cell, usually connected to the *endoplasmic reticulum. It stores and later transports the proteins manufactured in the endoplasmic reticulum. The Golgi apparatus is well developed in cells that produce secretions, e.g. pancreatic cells producing digestive enzymes. [C. Golgi (1844–1926), Italian histologist]

Golgi cells types of *neurons (nerve cells) within the central nervous system. **Golgi type I neurons** have very long axons that connect different parts of the system; **Golgi type II neurons**, also known as **microneurons**, have only short axons or sometimes none.

Golgi tendon organ *see* TENDON ORGAN.

Gomori's method a method of staining for the demonstration of enzymes, especially phosphatases and lipases, in histological specimens. [G. Gomori (1904–57), Hungarian histochemist]

gomphosis *n.* a form of *synarthrosis (immovable joint) in which a conical process fits into a socket. An example is the joint between the root of a tooth and the socket in the jawbone.

gonad *n.* a male or female reproductive organ that produces the gametes. *See* OVARY, TESTIS.

gonadal dysgenesis *see* TURNER'S SYNDROME.

gonadarche *n.* the period during which the gonads begin to secrete sex hormones, so triggering puberty. The timing for this event is controlled by the pituitary gland; gonadarche occurs usually between the ages of 10 and 11 in girls and 11 and 12 in boys.

gonadorelin analogue (GnRH analogue, LHRH analogue) any one of a group of analogues of *gonadotrophin-releasing hormone (gonadorelin), which stimulates the release of luteinizing hormone (LH) and follicle-stimulating hormone (gonadotrophins) from the pituitary gland. They are more powerful than the naturally occurring hormone, initially increasing the secretion of gonadotrophins by the pituitary: this acts to block the hormone receptors and to inhibit the release of further gonadotrophins, which suppresses production of oestrogens and androgens. Gonadorelin analogues include *buserelin, *goserelin, **leuprorelin** (Prostap), and **triptorelin** (Decapeptyl, Gonapeptyl Depot). Administered by subcutaneous or intramuscular injection or by nasal spray, they are used in the treatment of endometriosis, fibroids, and some types of infertility. GnRH analogues are also used in the treatment of advanced prostate cancer. After causing an initial rise in plasma testosterone for approximately ten days the level then falls to the same low level as that achieved by castration. Because the initial flare in testosterone may cause an acute enlargement of the cancer, *anti-androgens are given at the same time.

gonadotrophin (gonadotrophic hormone) *n.* any of several hormones synthesized and released by the pituitary gland that act on the testes or ovaries (gonads) to promote production of sex hormones and either sperm or ova. Their production is controlled by *gonadotrophin-releasing hormone. The main gonadotrophins are *follicle-stimulating hormone and *luteinizing hormone. They may be given by injection to treat infertility. *See also* HUMAN CHORIONIC GONADOTROPHIN.

gonadotrophin-releasing hormone (GnRH, gonadorelin) a peptide hormone produced in the hypothalamus and transported via the bloodstream to the pituitary gland, where it controls the synthesis and release of pituitary *gonadotrophins. It may be used to test the ability of the pituitary to produce gonadotrophins. *Gonadorelin analogues are used to treat endometriosis, fibroids, some types of infertility, and prostate cancer.

gonagra n. gout in the knee.

goni- (**gonio-**) *combining form denoting* an anatomical angle or corner.

goniometer n. an instrument for measuring angles, such as those made in joint movements.

gonion n. the point of the angle of the lower jawbone (mandible).

gonioscope n. a special kind of diagnostic contact lens used for viewing the structures at the angle of the anterior chamber of the eye (in front of the iris). These structures, at the periphery of the cornea, are not accessible to direct viewing.

goniotomy (trabeculotomy) n. a primary surgical procedure for treating congenital glaucoma (*see* BUPHTHALMOS). A fine knife is used to make an incision into the blocked *trabecular meshwork from within the eye, thus creating an opening through which the aqueous fluid can drain.

gonococcus n. (*pl.* **gonococci**) the causative agent of gonorrhoea: the bacterium *Neisseria gonorrhoeae.* —**gonococcal** *adj.*

gonocyte n. *see* GERM CELL.

gonorrhoea n. a sexually transmitted disease, caused by the bacterium *Neisseria gonorrhoeae,* that affects the genital mucous membranes of either sex. Symptoms develop about a week after infection and include pain on passing urine and discharge of pus (known as **gleet**) from the penis (in men) or vagina (in women); some infected women, however, experience no symptoms. If a pregnant woman has gonorrhoea, her baby's eyes may become infected during passage through the birth canal (*see* OPHTHALMIA NEONATORUM). In untreated cases, the infection may spread throughout the reproductive system, causing sterility; severe inflammation of the urethra in men can prevent passage of urine (a condition known as *stricture). Later complications include arthritis, inflammation of the heart valves (*endocarditis), and infection of the eyes, causing conjunctivitis. Treatment with ciprofloxacin, ofloxacin, or cefotaxime is usually effective.

good *adj.* positive, desirable, or morally admirable. The question of what is to be judged good is at the heart of medical ethics and ethics in general. Some theorists believe that one's intentions or will may or may not be good (*see* DEONTOLOGY), while others argue that only the consequences of actions may or may not be good (*consequentialism). Physicians have an explicit duty to do good for their patients (*see* BENEFICENCE). *See also* RIGHT.

Goodpasture's disease a rare autoimmune illness with production of antibodies directed against the glomerular basement membrane (anti-GBM antibodies). Classically patients present with lung haemorrhage and a rapidly progressive glomerulonephritis. Most cases will respond to aggressive treatment with plasma exchange and immunosuppression. [E. W. Goodpasture (1886–1960), US pathologist]

Goodpasture's syndrome any of various rare illnesses characterized by primary lung haemorrhage and rapidly progressive glomerulonephritis. They include *Goodpasture's disease and, more commonly, the systemic vasculitides (*see* VASCULITIS). [E. W. Goodpasture]

gooseflesh n. the reaction of the skin to cold or fear. The blood vessels contract and the small muscle attached to the base of each hair follicle also contracts, causing the hairs to stand up: this gives the skin an appearance of plucked goose skin.

GORD *see* GASTRO-OESOPHAGEAL REFLUX DISEASE.

Gordon's syndrome (pseudohypoaldosteronism type II, chloride shunt syndrome) an autosomal *dominant condition associated with increased chloride absorption in the distal tubule leading to a syndrome of mild volume expansion, hypertension, and metabolic acidosis with otherwise normal renal function. Plasma *renin and *aldosterone are suppressed as a result of the volume expansion. Other features can include short stature, intellectual impairment, muscle weakness, and renal stones.

gorget n. an instrument formerly used in the operation for removal of stones from the bladder. It is a *director or guide with a wide groove.

Gorlin's syndrome a genetic condition characterized by disorders of the skin, bones, and nervous system, with a markedly increased risk of developing multiple *basal cell carcinomas. [R. J. Gorlin (1923–), US pathologist]

goserelin *n.* a *gonadorelin analogue that is used in the treatment of endometriosis, prostate cancer, breast cancer, and fibroids, being administered by subcutaneous *depot injection at one- or three-monthly intervals. It is also used in the treatment of infertility by in vitro fertilization. Trade name: **Zoladex.**

Gottron's papules *see* DERMATOMYOSITIS.

Gott shunt a heparin-bonded shunt used to bypass sections of aorta that are being operated on. It is one of several shunts used in operations on the heart and arteries.

gouge *n.* a curved chisel used in orthopaedic operations to cut and remove bone.

goundou (anákhré) *n.* a condition following an infection with *yaws in which the nasal processes of the upper jaw bone thicken (*see* HYPEROSTOSIS) to form two large bony swellings, about 7 cm in diameter, on either side of the nose. The swellings not only obstruct the nostrils but also interfere with the field of vision. Initial symptoms include persistent headache and a bloody purulent discharge from the nose. Early cases can be treated with injections of penicillin; otherwise surgical removal of the growths is necessary. Goundou occurs in central Africa and South America.

gout *n.* a disease in which a defect in purine metabolism causes an excess of uric acid and its salts (urates) to accumulate in the bloodstream and the joints respectively. It results in attacks of acute gouty arthritis and chronic destruction of the joints and deposits of urates (**tophi**) in the skin and cartilage, especially of the ears. The excess of urates also damages the kidneys, in which stones may form. Treatment with drugs that increase the excretion of urates (*uricosuric drugs) or with *allopurinol, which slows their formation, can control the disease. Acute attacks of gout are treated with anti-inflammatory analgesics. *See also* PODAGRA.

governance *n.* the use of political power or authority to set, monitor, and enforce standards within systems or organizations. Within the UK National Health Service, there are two principal governance frameworks within which health-care professionals must

work: *clinical governance and **research governance**.

Graafian follicle a mature follicle in the ovary prior to ovulation, containing a large fluid-filled cavity that distends the surface of the ovary. The *oocyte develops inside the follicle, attached to one side. [R. de Graaf (1641–73), Dutch physician and anatomist]

grade *n.* **1.** the severity of a malignant tumour according to its degree of *differentiation. Low-grade tumours closely resemble normal tissues, are well differentiated, and have a good prognosis. High-grade tumours show a poor resemblance to normal tissues, are poorly differentiated, and have a poor prognosis. Benign tumours are not graded. **2.** the severity of a non-neoplastic disease.

graded self-exposure a technique used in the *behaviour therapy of phobias. A hierarchy of fears (increasingly fearful stimuli) is set up and the patients expose themselves to each level of the hierarchy in turn. Exposure continues until *habituation occurs; the patient then proceeds to the next highest level of the hierarchy. The patient is ultimately able to cope with the feared object or situation.

graft **1.** *n.* any organ, tissue, or object used for *transplantation to replace a faulty part of the body. A *skin graft is used to heal a damaged area of skin. A *bone graft can be performed using natural bone or a synthetic material. A kidney removed from a live or dead person and transplanted to another individual is described as a **kidney** (or **renal**) **graft**. Corneal grafts are taken from a recently dead individual to repair corneal opacity (*see* KERATOPLASTY). Diseased coronary arteries may be replaced by a *coronary artery bypass graft. Artificial grafts are used to replace diseased peripheral arteries and heart valves. **2.** *vb.* to transplant an organ or tissue. *See also* ALLOGRAFT, XENOGRAFT.

graft-versus-host disease (GVHD) a condition that occurs following bone marrow transplantation and sometimes blood transfusion, in which lymphocytes from the graft attack specific tissues in the host. The skin, gut, and liver are the most severely affected. Drugs that suppress the immune reaction, such as steroids and *ciclosporin, and antibodies directed against lymphocytes reduce the severity of the tissue damage.

Graham Steell murmur a soft high-pitched heart *murmur best heard over the second left intercostal space in early *diastole. It is a sign of *pulmonary regurgitation. [Graham Steell (1851–1942), British physician]

grain *n.* a unit of mass equal to 1/7000 of a pound (avoirdupois). 1 grain = 0.0648 gram.

gram *n.* a unit of mass equal to one thousandth of a kilogram. Symbol: g.

-gram *combining form denoting* a record; tracing. Example: **electrocardiogram** (record of an electrocardiograph).

gramicidin *n.* an antibiotic that acts against a wide range of bacteria. It is used in combination with other antibacterial drugs or steroids in topical preparations for the treatment of skin, ear, and eye infections.

Gram's stain a method of staining bacterial cells, used as a primary means of identification. A film of bacteria spread onto a glass slide is dried and heat-fixed, stained with a violet dye, treated with decolourizer (e.g. alcohol), and then counterstained with red dye. **Gram-negative** bacteria lose the initial stain but take up the counterstain, so that they appear red microscopically. **Gram-positive** bacteria retain the initial stain, appearing violet microscopically. These staining differences are based on variations in the structure of the cell wall in the two groups. [H. C. J. Gram (1853–1938), Danish physician]

grand mal (major epilepsy) *see* EPILEPSY.

grand multiparity the condition of a woman who has had five or more previous pregnancies. Such women are more prone to fetal malpresentations, postpartum haemorrhage, and rupture of the uterus.

granisetron *n. see* ONDANSETRON.

granular cast a cellular *cast derived from a kidney tubule. In certain kidney diseases, notably acute *glomerulonephritis, abnormal collections of renal tubular cells are shed from the kidney, often as a cast of the tubule. The casts can be observed on microscopic examination of the centrifuged deposit of a specimen of urine. Their presence in the urine indicates continued activity of the disease.

granulation *n.* the formation of a multicellular mass of tissue (**granulation tissue**) in response to an injury: this is an essential part of the healing process. Granulation tissue contains many new blood vessels and, in its later stages, large numbers of fibroblasts. The response is most frequently seen in healing open wounds and in the bases of ulcers.

granulocyte *n.* any of a group of white blood cells that, when stained with *Romanowsky stains, are seen to contain granules in their cytoplasm. They can be subclassified on the basis of the colour of the stained granules into *neutrophils, *eosinophils, and *basophils.

granulocytopenia *n.* a reduction in the number of *granulocytes (a type of white cell) in the blood. *See* NEUTROPENIA.

granuloma *n.* (*pl.* **granulomata** or **granulomas**) a localized collection of cells, usually produced in response to an infectious process, that is characterized by the presence of aggregates of epithelioid *histiocytes; giant cells, monocytes, or lymphocytes may also be present. The types of cells comprising a granuloma (of which there may be many or few) and their arrangement can assist in diagnosing the cause of the response; this is important in the diagnosis of tuberculosis, sarcoidosis, Crohn's disease, and the presence of certain foreign bodies (e.g. starch, talc). Other conditions giving rise to granulomata include syphilis, leprosy, and coccidioidomycosis, and a granuloma may also occur around the apex of a tooth root as a result of inflammation or infection of its pulp. —**granulomatous** *adj.*

granuloma annulare a chronic skin condition of unknown cause. In the common localized type there is a ring or rings of closely set papules, 1–5 cm in diameter, found principally on the hands and arms. The association with diabetes mellitus is controversial.

granuloma inguinale an infectious disease caused by *Calymmatobacterium granulomatis*, which is transmitted during sexual intercourse. A pimply rash on and around the genital organs develops into a granulomatous ulcer. The disease responds to treatment with tetracyclines and streptomycin.

granulomatosis *n.* any condition marked by multiple widespread *granulomata. *See also* WEGENER'S GRANULOMATOSIS.

granulopoiesis *n.* the process of production of *granulocytes, which normally occurs in the blood-forming tissue of the *bone marrow. Granulocytes are ultimately derived from a *haemopoietic stem cell, but the earliest precursor that can be identified microscopically is the *myeloblast. This divides and passes through a series of stages of maturation termed respectively *promyelocyte, *myelocyte, and *metamyelocyte, before becoming a mature granulocyte. *See also* HAEMOPOIESIS.

granzyme *n.* a *protease enzyme that is released by *cytotoxic T cells and *natural killer cells to induce death of virus-infected target cells.

graph- (grapho-) *combining form denoting* handwriting.

-graph *combining form denoting* an instrument that records. Example: **electrocardiograph** (instrument recording heart activity).

graphology *n.* the study of the characteristics of handwriting to obtain indications about a person's psychological make-up or state of health. It is possible to detect certain signs of physical disease, such as fine nervous tremors or irregularity of the pulse.

grasp reflex involuntary grasping in response to anything that touches the palm of the hand. This is a normal reflex in babies that is lost in early childhood. In adults it is a sign of damage to the *prefrontal lobes of the brain.

grattage *n.* the process of brushing or scraping the surface of a slowly healing ulcer or wound to remove *granulation tissue, which – though a stage in the healing process – sometimes overgrows or becomes infected and therefore delays healing. Grattage is used in the treatment of *trachoma.

gravel *n.* small stones formed in the urinary tract. The stones usually consist of calcareous debris or aggregations of other crystalline material. The passage of gravel from the kidneys is usually associated with severe pain (**ureteric colic**) and may cause blood in the urine. *See also* CALCULUS.

Graves' disease (exophthalmic goitre) *see* THYROTOXICOSIS. [R. J. Graves (1797–1853), Irish physician]

gravid *adj.* currently pregnant. The term **gravidity** is used to indicate the total number of pregnancies a woman has had, including the current pregnancy, previous live births, stillbirths, miscarriages, and abortions. *Compare* PARITY.

Grawitz tumour *see* RENAL CELL CARCI-NOMA. [P. A. Grawitz (1850–1932), German pathologist]

gray *n.* the *SI unit of absorbed dose of ionizing radiation, being the absorbed dose when the energy per unit mass imparted to matter by ionizing radiation is 1 joule per kilogram. It has replaced the rad. Symbol: Gy.

green monkey disease *see* MARBURG DISEASE.

greenstick fracture an incomplete break in a bone in which part of the outer shell (cortex) remains intact. It occurs in children, who have more flexible bones. *See also* FRACTURE.

grey matter the darker coloured tissues of the central nervous system, composed mainly of the cell bodies of neurons, branching dendrites, and glial cells (*compare* WHITE MATTER). In the brain grey matter forms the *cerebral cortex and the outer layer of the cerebellum; in the spinal cord the grey matter lies centrally and is surrounded by white matter.

grey scale (in radiology) a scale representing the possible gradient of densities from black to white for each *pixel in an image. In an *analogue image this gradient is smooth. A *digital image has many discrete steps. The more steps allowed, the closer to representing the true analogue image it comes, although more steps require more computer memory. Images can be manipulated by *windowing. This concept is particularly valuable in *computerized tomography. *See* HOUNSFIELD UNIT, DIGITIZATION.

Grey Turner sign a bluish bruiselike appearance around the flanks, which is seen in acute *pancreatitis. [G. Grey Turner (1877–1951), British surgeon]

gridiron incision an oblique incision made in the right lower quadrant of the abdomen, classically used for *appendicectomy.

gripe *n.* severe abdominal pain (*see* COLIC).

griseofulvin *n.* an antifungal drug administered by mouth or topically to treat fungal infections of the hair, skin, and nails, such as ringworm. Mild and temporary side-effects such as headache, skin rashes, and digestive upsets may occur. Trade name: **Grisol AF**.

groin *n.* the external depression on the front of the body that marks the junction of the abdomen with either of the thighs. *See also* INGUINAL.

grommet   *n.* a flanged metal or plastic tube that is inserted in the eardrum in cases of *glue ear. It allows air to enter the middle ear, bypassing the patient's own nonfunctioning *Eustachian tube.

ground substance   the matrix of *connective tissue, in which various cells and fibres are embedded.

group B streptococcus (GBS)   a Gram-positive bacterium that causes life-threatening infections in newborn infants following vaginal delivery (*see* STREPTOCOCCUS, LANCEFIELD CLASSIFICATION). 20% of pregnant women are carriers and have no symptoms; however, *vertical transmission of the bacterium from mother to fetus at the time of delivery may lead to neonatal sepsis, characterized by pneumonia, meningitis, and death in some cases. Antibiotic prophylaxis with penicillin is recommended for women with risk factors or who are known to be carriers.

group practice   *see* GENERAL PRACTITIONER.

group therapy   **1. (group psychotherapy)** *psychotherapy involving at least two patients and a therapist. The patients are encouraged to understand and to analyse their own and one another's problems. *See also* PSYCHODRAMA. **2.** therapy in which people with the same problem, such as *alcoholism or *phobias, meet and discuss together their difficulties and possible ways of overcoming them.

growth factor   any of various chemicals, particularly polypeptides, that have a variety of important roles in the stimulation of new cell growth and cell maintenance. They bind to the cell surface on receptors and are potential targets for anticancer therapy (*see* EPIDERMAL GROWTH FACTOR RECEPTOR). Specific growth factors can cause new cell proliferation (**epidermal growth factor, haemopoietic growth factor**) and the migration of cells (**fibroblast growth factor**) and play a role in wound healing (**platelet-derived growth factor; PDGF**). Some growth factors act in the embryonic stage of development; for example, *nerve growth factor. Some growth factors that induce cell proliferation are involved in the abnormal regulation of growth seen in cancer when produced in excessive amounts (e.g. **insulin-like growth factor, IGF-I**). Growth factors produced lo-

cally around a carcinoma (e.g. *vascular endothelial growth factor) are important in the encouragement of invasion by the tumour; other factors (e.g. autocrine motility factor, migration-stimulating factor) are also significant. *See also* BONE GROWTH FACTORS.

growth hormone (GH, somatotrophin**)** a hormone, synthesized and stored in the anterior pituitary gland, that promotes growth of the long bones in the limbs and increases protein synthesis (via *somatomedin). Its release is controlled by the opposing actions of **growth-hormone releasing hormone** and *somatostatin. Excessive production of growth hormone results in *gigantism before puberty and *acromegaly in adults. Lack of growth hormone in children causes *dwarfism. Synthetic human growth hormone (**somatotropin**) is used to treat a variety of conditions of growth-hormone deficiency. **Pegvisomant** is an analogue of human growth hormone that blocks GH receptors; it may be used to treat acromegaly.

growth plate   *see* PHYSIS.

grumous   *adj.* coarse; lumpy; clotted; often used to describe the appearance of the centre of wounds or diseased cells or the surface of a bacterial culture.

guanethidine   *n.* a drug that is occasionally used for the rapid reduction of high blood pressure resistant to other treatments (*see* SYMPATHOLYTIC). It is administered by intramuscular injection; common side-effects are diarrhoea, faintness, and headache. Trade name: **Ismelin**.

guanine   *n.* one of the nitrogen-containing bases (*see* PURINE) that occurs in the nucleic acids DNA and RNA.

guanosine   *n.* a compound containing guanine and the sugar ribose. *See also* NUCLEOTIDE.

gubernaculum   *n.* (*pl.* **gubernacula**) either of a pair of fibrous strands of tissue that connect the gonads to the inguinal region in the fetus. In the male they guide and possibly move the testes into the scrotum before birth. In the female the ovaries descend only slightly within the abdominal cavity and the gubernacula persist as the round ligaments connecting the ovaries and uterus to the abdominal wall.

guidewire   *n.* a piece of equipment used in interventional procedures, particularly in the *Seldinger technique. Guidewires often have multiple cores and a variety of coverings, depending on their functions, and they vary in stiffness. Their ends may be curved, to get past tight strictures, or J-shaped, to avoid accidentally puncturing a vessel wall or other structure while being pushed forward.

Guillain-Barré syndrome (postinfective polyneuropathy) a disease of the peripheral nerves in which there is numbness and weakness in the limbs. It usually develops 1–28 days after a respiratory or gastrointestinal infection (commonly with *Campylobacter*): antibodies directed against the pathogen's cell-surface antigens attack similar antigens on the myelin sheaths of the host's peripheral nerves. Involvement of the respiratory muscles may require mechanical ventilation. Recovery is variable and often prolonged (there is a 10% mortality rate). Treatment with immunoglobulins (intravenous) or with plasma exchange may speed recovery and reduce long-term disability. *See* POLYRADICULITIS. [G. Guillain (1876–1961) and A. Barré (1880–1967), French neurologists]

guillotine *n.* (in surgery) **1.** an instrument used for removing the tonsils. It is loop-shaped and contains a sliding knife blade. **2.** an encircling suture to control the escape of fluid or blood from an orifice or to close a gap.

guinea worm a nematode worm, *Dracunculus medinensis*, that is a parasite of humans. The white threadlike adult female, 60–120 cm long, lives in the connective tissues beneath the skin. It releases its larvae into a large blister on the legs or arms; when the limbs are immersed in water the larvae escape and are subsequently eaten by tiny water fleas (*Cyclops*), inside which their development continues. The disease *dracontiasis results from drinking water contaminated with *Cyclops*.

Gulf War syndrome a variety of symptoms, mainly neurological (including chronic fatigue, dizziness, amnesia, digestive upsets, and muscle wasting), that have been attributed to exposure of armed forces personnel to chemicals (e.g. insecticides) used during the Gulf War (1991) or possibly to the effects of vaccines and tablets given to protect personnel against the anticipated threat of chemical and biological warfare during the conflict. Medical research into the syndrome is continuing.

gullet *n. see* OESOPHAGUS.

gum *n.* (in anatomy) *see* GINGIVA.

gumboil *n.* the opening on the surface of the gum of a *sinus tract from a chronic abscess associated with the roots of a tooth. It may be accompanied by varying degrees of swelling, pain, and discharge.

gumma *n.* a small soft tumour, characteristic of the tertiary stage of *syphilis, that occurs in connective tissue, the liver, brain, testes, heart, or bone.

gumshield *n.* a soft flexible cover that fits over the teeth for protection in contact sports. The best type is specially made to fit the individual.

gunshot wound a common cause of both military and civil injuries. Gunshot wounds are usually produced by high-velocity missiles: deep-seated tissue destruction of thermal origin is a major complication.

gustation *n.* the sense of taste or the act of tasting.

gustatory *adj.* relating to the sense of taste or to the organs of taste.

gut *n.* **1.** *see* INTESTINE. **2.** *see* CATGUT.

Guthrie test (heel-prick blood test) a blood test performed on all newborn babies at the end of the first week of life. The blood is obtained by pricking the heel of the baby. The test can detect several *inborn errors of metabolism (including *phenylketonuria) and *hypothyroidism; it can also be used for detecting *cystic fibrosis, although this is not routinely offered. [R. Guthrie (1916–95), US paediatrician]

gutta *n.* (*pl.* **guttae**) (in pharmacy) a drop. Drops are the form in which medicines are applied to the eyes and ears.

gutta-percha *n.* the juice of an evergreen Malaysian tree, which is hard at room temperature but becomes soft and plastic when heated. On cooling, gutta-percha will retain any shape imparted to it when hot. It is used in dentistry in the form of gutta-percha points as the principal core of *root fillings.

guttate *adj.* describing lesions in the skin that are shaped like drops.

GVHD *see* GRAFT-VERSUS-HOST DISEASE.

gyn- (gyno-, gynaec(o)-) *combining form denoting* women or the female reproductive organs.

gynaecology *n.* the study of diseases of women and girls, particularly those affecting the female reproductive system. *Compare* OBSTETRICS. —**gynaecological** *adj.* —**gynaecologist** *n.*

gynaecomastia *n.* enlargement of the breasts in the male, due either to hormone imbalance or to drug (e.g. hormone) therapy.

gypsum *n. see* PLASTER OF PARIS.

gyr- (gyro-) *combining form denoting* 1. a gyrus. 2. a ring or circle.

gyrate atrophy a rare hereditary condition causing night blindness and constricted visual fields, usually developing in the first decade of life. Clinically it is characterized by a progressive atrophy of the choroid and retina.

gyrus *n.* (*pl.* **gyri**) a raised convolution of the *cerebral cortex, between two sulci (clefts).

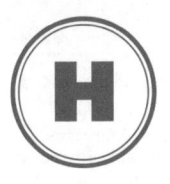

Haab's striae splits or tears in *Descemet's membrane occurring during infancy, commonly as a result of congenital glaucoma. [O. Haab (1850–1931), German ophthalmologist]

habit *n.* a sequence of learned behaviour occurring in a particular context or as a response to particular events. Habits are often the result of *conditioning, are performed automatically and unconsciously, and reduce decision-making. Habits, once established, often persist after the original causal factors no longer operate. Behavioural psychology is based on the premise that one form of conditioning can be replaced by another.

habituation *n.* 1. (in psychology) a simple type of learning consisting of a gradual waning response by the subject to a continuous or repeated stimulus that is not associated with *reinforcement. 2. (in pharmacology) the condition of being psychologically dependent on a drug, following repeated consumption, marked by reduced sensitivity to its effects and a craving for the drug if it is withdrawn. *See also* DEPENDENCE.

habitus *n.* an individual's general physical appearance, especially when this is associated with a constitutional tendency to a particular disease.

haem *n.* an iron-containing compound (a *porphyrin) that combines with the protein globin to form *haemoglobin, found in the red blood cells.

haem- (haema-, haemo-, haemat(o)-) *combining form denoting* blood. Examples: **haematogenesis** (formation of); **haemophobia** (fear of).

haemagglutination *n.* the clumping of red blood cells (*see* AGGLUTINATION). It is caused by an antibody–antigen reaction or some viruses and other substances.

haemagglutinin (HA, H) *n.* a glycoprotein projecting from the surface layer of the lipid bilayer envelope of *influenza virions. This protein is involved in virus binding and may influence virulence. It is a key target for

antibody attack and therefore is important in vaccination.

haemangioblastoma (Lindau's tumour) *n.* a tumour of the brain or spinal cord arising in the blood vessels of the meninges or brain. It is often associated with *phaeochromocytoma and *syringomyelia. *See also* VON HIPPEL-LINDAU DISEASE.

haemangioma *n.* a benign tumour of blood vessels. It often appears on the skin as a type of birthmark; the strawberry *naevus is an example. *See also* ANGIOMA.

Haemaphysalis *n.* a genus of hard *ticks. Certain species transmit tick *typhus in the Old World; *H. spinigera* transmits the virus causing *Kyasanur Forest disease in India.

haemarthrosis *n.* bleeding within a joint, which may follow injury or may occur spontaneously in bleeding disorders, such as *haemophilia. It is usually associated with swelling, warmth, and pain in the affected joint. Treatment includes immobilization, pressure bandaging, and correction of the blood disorder (if present). Aspiration of blood from a joint that is tensely swollen may relieve the pain.

haematemesis *n.* the act of vomiting blood. The blood may have been swallowed (e.g. following nosebleed or tonsillectomy) but more often arises from bleeding in the oesophagus, stomach, or duodenum. Common causes are gastric and duodenal ulcers, and varicose veins in the oesophagus. If much blood is lost, it may need to be replaced by blood transfusion. If bleeding does not stop spontaneously it may be arrested by coagulation of the bleeding point using a combination of mechanical methods (metallic clips), heat (*heater-probe, *argon plasma coagulation), the injection of *adrenaline (for bleeding peptic ulcers or vascular malformation) or a sclerosing material, the application of rubber bands (for oesophageal varices), or the injection of glue (for gastric varices). All of these techniques are applied through an *endoscope. *See also* MELAENA.

haemathidrosis (haematidrosis) *n. see* HAEMATOHIDROSIS.

haematin *n.* a chemical derivative of *haemoglobin formed by removal of the protein part of the molecule and oxidation of the iron atom from the ferrous to the ferric form.

haematinic *n.* a drug that increases the amount of *haemoglobin in the blood, e.g. *ferrous sulphate and other iron-containing compounds. Haematinics are used, often in combination with vitamins and folic acid, to prevent and treat anaemia due to iron deficiency. They are used particularly to prevent anaemia during pregnancy. Digestive disturbances sometimes occur with haematinics.

haematochesia *n.* the passage of fresh red blood through the rectum. Haematochesia occurs in patients with haemorrhoids, colorectal carcinoma, colitis, diverticulitis, angiodysplasia, and volvulus. Haematochesia also occurs as a result of severe haemorrhage in the upper gastrointestinal tract.

haematocoele *n.* a swelling caused by leakage of blood into a cavity, especially that of the tunica vaginalis, the membrane overlying the front and sides of the *testis. A **pelvic haematocoele** is a swelling near the uterus formed by the escape of blood, usually from a Fallopian tube in ectopic pregnancy.

haematocolpos *n.* distention of the vagina with blood due to an *imperforate hymen. *See* CRYPTOMENORRHOEA.

haematocrit *n. see* PACKED CELL VOLUME.

haematocyst *n.* a cyst that contains blood.

haematogenous (haematogenic) *adj.*
1. relating to the production of blood or its constituents; haematopoietic. **2.** produced by, originating in, or carried by the blood.

haematohidrosis (haemathidrosis, haematidrosis) *n.* the secretion of sweat containing blood.

haematology *n.* the study of blood and blood-forming tissues and the disorders associated with them. —**haematological** *adj.* —**haematologist** *n.*

haematoma *n.* an accumulation of blood within the tissues that clots to form a solid swelling. Injury, disease of the blood vessels,

or a clotting disorder of the blood are the usual causative factors. An **intracranial haematoma** causes symptoms by compressing the brain and by raising the pressure within the skull. A blunt injury to the head, especially the temple, may tear the middle meningeal artery, giving rise to a rapidly accumulating **extradural haematoma** requiring urgent surgical treatment. In elderly people a relatively slight head injury may tear the veins where they cross the space beneath the dura, giving rise to a **subdural haematoma**. Excellent results are obtained by surgical treatment. An **intracerebral haematoma** may be a consequence of severe head injury but is more often due to atheromatous disease of the cerebral arteries and high blood pressure resulting in bleeding into the brain. *See also* PERIANAL HAEMATOMA.

haematometra *n.* **1.** accumulation of menstrual blood in the uterus. **2.** any abnormally copious bleeding in the uterus.

haematomyelia *n.* bleeding into the tissue of the spinal cord. This may result in acutely developing symptoms that mimic *syringomyelia.

haematopoiesis *n. see* HAEMOPOIESIS.

haematoporphyrin *n.* a type of *porphyrin produced during the metabolism of haemoglobin.

haematosalpinx (haemosalpinx) *n.* the accumulation of menstrual blood in the *Fallopian tubes.

haematoxylin *n.* a colourless crystalline compound extracted from logwood (*Haematoxylon campechianum*) and used in various histological stains. When oxidized haematoxylin is converted to **haematein**, which imparts a blue colour to certain parts of cells, especially cell nuclei. **Heidenhain's iron haematoxylin** is used to stain sections that are to be photographed, since it gives great clarity at high magnification.

haematuria *n.* the passage of blood in the urine. This may be seen by the naked eye (**frank haematuria**) or urine microscopy (**microscopic haematuria**), or it may be detected by urinalysis sticks (**'dipstix' haematuria**). Haematuria is a very important symptom because it is associated with *transitional cell carcinoma, most commonly in the bladder, and kidney cancer. It may also be due to urinary-tract infections, stone disease, or some forms of *glomerulonephritis.

haemin *n.* a chemical derivative of haemoglobin formed by removal of the protein part of the molecule, oxidation of the iron atom, and combination with an acid to form a salt (*compare* HAEMATIN). **Chlorohaemin** forms characteristic crystals, the identification of which provides the basis of a chemical test for blood stains.

haemo- *combining form see* HAEM-.

Haemobartonella *n. see* BARTONELLA.

haemochromatosis (hereditary haemochromatosis, bronze diabetes, iron-storage disease) *n.* a hereditary disorder in which there is excessive absorption and storage of iron. This leads to damage and functional impairment of many organs, including the liver, pancreas, and endocrine glands. The main features are a bronze colour of the skin, diabetes, and liver failure. It is inherited as an autosomal *recessive trait in people of northern European descent and is due to mutations in the haemochromatosis gene (*HFE*) in the majority of cases. Iron may be removed from the body by blood letting or an iron *chelating agent may be administered. *Compare* HAEMOSIDEROSIS.

haemoconcentration *n.* an increase in the proportion of red blood cells relative to the plasma, brought about by a decrease in the volume of plasma or an increase in the concentration of red blood cells in the circulating blood (*see* POLYCYTHAEMIA). Haemoconcentration may occur in any condition in which there is a severe loss of water from the body. *Compare* HAEMODILUTION.

haemocytometer *n.* a special glass chamber of known volume into which diluted blood is introduced. The numbers of the various blood cells present are then counted visually, through a microscope. Haemocytometers have been largely replaced by electronic cell counters.

haemodiafiltration *n.* a form of renal replacement therapy that removes toxins by a combination of diffusion (as in conventional *haemodialysis), and convection (as in *haemofiltration), and is more efficient than either in the process.

haemodialysis *n.* a technique of removing waste materials or poisons from the blood using the principle of *dialysis. Haemodialysis is performed on patients whose kidneys have ceased to function; the process takes place in a *dialyser. The stream of blood taken from an artery is circulated through the dialyser on one side of a semipermeable membrane, while a solution of similar electrolytic composition to the patient's blood circulates on the other side. Water and waste products from the patient's blood filter through the membrane, whose pores are too small to allow passage of blood cells and proteins. The purified blood is then returned to the patient's body through a vein.

haemodilution *n.* a decrease in the proportion of red blood cells relative to the plasma, brought about by an increase in the total volume of plasma. This may occur in a variety of conditions, including pregnancy and enlargement of the spleen (*see* HYPERSPLENISM). *Compare* HAEMOCONCENTRATION.

haemofiltration *n.* the use of a transmembrane hydrostatic pressure to induce filtration of plasma water across the membrane of a **haemofilter**. Solutes dissolved in the plasma water accompany their solvent to a greater or lesser extent dependent on molecular weight and the characteristics of the filter membrane (pore size).

haemoglobin *n.* a substance contained within the red blood cells (*erythrocytes) and responsible for their colour, composed of the pigment **haem** (an iron-containing *porphyrin) linked to the protein **globin**. Haemoglobin has the unique property of combining reversibly with oxygen and is the medium by which oxygen is transported within the body. It takes up oxygen as blood passes through the lungs and releases it as blood passes through the tissues. Blood normally contains 12–18 g/dl of haemoglobin. *See also* MYOGLOBIN, OXYHAEMOGLOBIN.

haemoglobin A$_{1c}$ *see* GLYCATED HAEMOGLOBIN.

haemoglobinometer *n.* an instrument for determining the concentration of *haemoglobin in a sample of blood, which is a measure of its ability to carry oxygen.

haemoglobinopathy *n.* any of a group of inherited diseases, such as *thalassaemia and *sickle-cell disease, in which there is an abnormality in the production of haemoglobin.

haemoglobinuria *n.* the presence in the urine of free haemoglobin. The condition occurs if haemoglobin, released from disintegrating red blood cells, cannot be taken up rapidly enough by blood proteins. The condition sometimes follows strenuous exercise. It is also associated with certain infectious diseases (such as blackwater fever), ingestion of certain chemicals (such as arsenic), and injury.

haemogram *n.* the results of a routine blood test, including an estimate of the blood haemoglobin level, the *packed cell volume, and the numbers of red and white blood cells (*see* BLOOD COUNT). Any abnormalities seen in microscopic examination of the blood are also noted.

haemolysin *n.* a substance capable of bringing about destruction of red blood cells (*haemolysis). It may be an antibody or a bacterial toxin.

haemolysis *n.* the destruction of red blood cells (*erythrocytes). Within the body, haemolysis may result from defects within the red cells or from poisoning, infection, or the action of antibodies; it may occur in mismatched blood transfusions. It usually leads to anaemia. Haemolysis of blood specimens may result from unsatisfactory collection or storage or be brought about intentionally as part of an analytical procedure (*see* LAKING).

haemolytic *adj.* causing, associated with, or resulting from destruction of red blood cells (*erythrocytes). For example, a **haemolytic antibody** is one that causes destruction of red cells; a **haemolytic anaemia** is due to red-cell destruction (*see* ANAEMIA).

haemolytic disease of the newborn the condition resulting from destruction (haemolysis) of the red blood cells of the fetus by antibodies in the mother's blood passing through the placenta. When an exchange occurs between fetal and maternal blood (as at delivery, placental abruption, threatened miscarriage, or invasive procedures), the passage of red cells into the maternal circulation provokes an antibody response to the fetal red blood cell antigen in the mother. This most commonly happens when the red blood cells of the fetus are Rh positive (i.e. they have the *rhesus factor) but the mother's red cells are Rh negative. For the rhesus antigen, the primary IgM antibodies (*see* IMMUNOGLOBULIN) do not cross the placenta, but if the mother is exposed in another pregnancy, IgG antibodies do cross the placenta. This may result in very severe anaemia of the fetus, leading to heart failure with oedema (*hydrops fetalis) or

stillbirth. When the anaemia is less severe the fetus may reach term in good condition, but the accumulation of the bile pigment bilirubin from the destroyed cells causes severe jaundice after birth, which may require *exchange transfusion. If untreated, it may cause serious brain damage (*see* KERNICTERUS). Other red cell antigens that are clearly associated with fetal anaemia are D, Kell, and c.

A blood test early in pregnancy enables the detection of antibodies in the mother's blood and the adoption of various precautions for the infant's safety, including Doppler measurement of the fetal cerebral vessels (MCA Doppler; *see* DOPPLER ULTRASOUND) to detect fetal anaemia, which may require intrauterine transfusion. The incidence of the disease has been greatly reduced by preventing the formation of antibodies in a Rh-negative mother (*see* ANTI-D IMMUNOGLOBULIN).

haemolytic uraemic syndrome a condition in which sudden rapid destruction of red blood cells (*see* HAEMOLYSIS) causes acute renal failure due partly to obstruction of small arteries in the kidneys. The haemolysis also causes a reduction in the number of platelets, which can lead to severe haemorrhage. The syndrome may occur as a result of septicaemia following a respiratory or gastrointestinal infection (especially by pathogenic *Escherichia coli*), eclamptic fits in pregnancy (*see* ECLAMPSIA), or as a reaction to certain drugs. There may also be small sporadic outbreaks of the condition without any obvious cause.

haemoperfusion *n.* the passage of blood through a sorbent column with the aim of removing toxic substances. The commonest sorbent in use is charcoal, microencapsulated with cellulose nitrate. Haemoperfusion might be considered for the treatment of poisoning with carbamazepine, theophylline, barbiturates, and *Amanita* mushrooms.

haemopericardium *n.* the presence of blood within the membranous sac (pericardium) surrounding the heart, which may result from injury, tumours, rupture of the heart (e.g. following myocardial infarction), or a leaking aneurysm. The heart is compressed (*see* CARDIAC TAMPONADE) and the circulation impaired; a large fall in blood pressure and cardiac arrest may result. Surgical drainage of the blood may be life saving.

haemoperitoneum *n.* the presence of blood in the peritoneal cavity, between the lining of the abdomen or pelvis and the membrane covering the organs within.

haemophilia *n.* either of two hereditary disorders in which the blood clots very slowly, due to a deficiency of either of two *coagulation factors: **haemophilia A**, due to deficiency of Factor VIII (antihaemophilic factor); or **haemophilia B**, due to deficiency of Factor IX (Christmas factor). The patient may experience prolonged bleeding following any injury or wound, and in severe cases there is spontaneous bleeding into muscles and joints. Bleeding in haemophilia may be treated by recombinent-DNA-derived Factor VIII or plasma Factor VIII concentrate. Alternatively concentrated preparations of Factor VIII or Factor IX, obtained by freezing fresh plasma, may be administered (see CRYOPRECIPITATE). Haemophilia is controlled by a *sex-linked gene, which means that it is almost exclusively restricted to males: women can carry the gene – and pass it on to their sons – without being affected themselves. The genes encoding factors VIII and IX have been used in gene therapy trials for haemophilia. —**haemophiliac** *n.*

(🌐) SEE WEB LINKS
• Website of the Haemophilia Society

Haemophilus *n.* a genus of Gram-negative aerobic nonmotile parasitic rodlike bacteria frequently found in the respiratory tract. They can grow only in the presence of certain factors in the blood and/or certain coenzymes: they are cultured on fresh blood *agar. Most species are pathogenic: *H. aegyptius* causes conjunctivitis, and *H. ducreyi* soft sore (chancroid). *H. influenzae* is associated with acute and chronic respiratory infections (see also EPIGLOTTITIS) and is a common secondary cause of *influenza infections; *H. influenzae* type b is an important cause of bacterial *meningitis in young children (see HIB VACCINE).

haemophthalmia *n.* bleeding into the *vitreous humour of the eye: vitreous haemorrhage.

haemopneumothorax *n.* the presence of both blood and air in the pleural cavity, usually as a result of injury. Both must be drained out to allow the lung to expand normally. See also HAEMOTHORAX.

haemopoiesis (haematopoiesis) *n.* the process of production of blood cells and platelets which continues throughout life, replacing aged cells (which are removed from the circulation). In healthy adults, haemopoiesis is confined to the *bone marrow, but in embryonic life and in early infancy, as well as in certain diseases, it may occur in other sites (**extramedullary haemopoiesis**). See also ERYTHROPOIESIS, LEUCOPOIESIS, THROMBOPOIESIS. —**haemopoietic** *adj.*

haemopoietic stem cell the cell from which all classes of blood cells are derived. It cannot be identified microscopically, but can be defined by the presence of a combination of cell-surface proteins. It can be demonstrated by *tissue culture of the blood-forming tissue of the bone marrow, as well as by growth of human haemopoietic cells in immunodeficient mice strains, such as non-obese diabetic/severe combined immunodeficient (NOD/SCID). See also HAEMOPOIESIS.

haemoptysis *n.* the coughing up of blood. This symptom should always be taken seriously, however small the amount. In some patients the cause is not serious; in others it is never found. But it should always be reported to a doctor.

haemorrhage (bleeding) *n.* the escape of blood from a ruptured blood vessel, externally or internally. Arterial blood is bright red and emerges in spurts, venous blood is dark red and flows steadily, while damage to minor vessels may produce only an oozing. Rupture of a major blood vessel such as the femoral artery can lead to the loss of several litres of blood in a few minutes, resulting in *shock, collapse, and death, if untreated. See also HAEMATEMESIS, HAEMATURIA, HAEMOPTYSIS.

haemorrhagic *adj.* associated with or resulting from blood loss (see HAEMORRHAGE). For example, **haemorrhagic anaemia** is due to blood loss (see ANAEMIA).

haemorrhagic disease of the newborn a temporary disturbance in blood clotting caused by *vitamin K deficiency and affecting infants on the second to fourth day of life. It varies in severity from mild gastrointestinal bleeding to profuse bleeding into many organs, including the brain. It is more common in breast-fed and preterm infants. The condition can be prevented by giving all babies vitamin K, either by injection or orally, shortly after birth. Medical name: **melaena neonatorum**.

haemorrhoidectomy *n.* the surgical operation for removing *haemorrhoids, which are tied and then excised. Possible complications are bleeding or, later, anal stricture (narrowing). The operation is usually performed only for second- or third-degree haemorrhoids that have not responded to simple measures.

haemorrhoids (piles) *pl. n.* enlargement of the normal spongy blood-filled cushions in the wall of the anus (**internal haemorrhoids**), usually a consequence of prolonged constipation or, less often, diarrhoea. They most commonly occur at three main points equidistant around the circumference of the anus. Uncomplicated haemorrhoids are seldom painful; any pain is usually caused by an anal *fissure. The main symptom is bleeding, and in **first-degree haemorrhoids**, which never appear at the anus, bleeding at the end of defaecation is the only symptom. **Second-degree haemorrhoids** protrude beyond the anus as an uncomfortable swelling but return spontaneously; **third-degree haemorrhoids** remain outside the anus and need to be returned by manual pressure.

First- and second-degree haemorrhoids may respond to bowel regulation using a high-fibre diet with faecal softening agents. If bleeding persists, elastic bands may be applied or a sclerosing agent may be injected around the swollen cushions to make them shrivel up. Third-degree haemorrhoids often require surgery (*see* HAEMORRHOIDECTOMY), especially if they become *strangulated (producing severe pain and further enlargement).

External haemorrhoids are either prolapsed internal haemorrhoids or – more often – *perianal haematomas or the residual skin tags remaining after a perianal haematoma has healed.

haemosalpinx *n. see* HAEMATOSALPINX.

haemosiderin *n.* an iron-storage compound found mainly in the cells of the *macrophage-*monocyte system in the marrow, in the *Kupffer cells of the liver, and in the spleen. It contains around 30% iron by weight.

haemosiderosis *n.* the accumulation of *haemosiderin in various tissues.

haemostasis *n.* the arrest of bleeding, involving the physiological processes of *blood coagulation and the contraction of damaged blood vessels. The term is also applied to various surgical procedures (for example the application of *ligatures or *diathermy to cut vessels) used to stop bleeding.

haemostatic (styptic) *n.* an agent that stops or prevents haemorrhage; for example, *phytomenadione. Haemostatics are used to control bleeding due to various causes.

haemothorax *n.* blood in the pleural cavity, usually due to injury. If the blood is not drained dense fibrous *adhesions occur between the pleural surfaces, which can impair the normal movement of the lung. The blood may also become infected (*see* EMPYEMA).

haemozoin *n.* an iron-containing pigment present in the organisms that cause malaria (*Plasmodium* species).

hair *n.* a threadlike keratinized outgrowth of the epidermis of the *skin. It develops inside a tubular **hair follicle**. The part above the skin consists of three layers: an outer **cuticle**; a **cortex**, forming the bulk of the hair and containing the pigment that gives the hair its colour; and a central core (**medulla**), which may be hollow. The **root** of the hair, beneath the surface of the skin, is expanded at its base to form the **bulb**, which contains a matrix of dividing cells. As new cells are formed the older ones are pushed upwards and become keratinized to form the root and shaft. A hair may be raised by a small erector muscle in the dermis, attached to the hair follicle.

hairball *n. see* TRICHOBEZOAR.

hair follicle a sheath of epidermal cells and connective tissue that surrounds the root of a *hair.

hair papilla a projection of the dermis that is surrounded by the base of the hair bulb. It contains the capillaries that supply blood to the growing *hair.

hairy cell an abnormal white blood cell that has the appearance of an immature lymphocyte with fine hairlike cytoplasmic projections around the perimeter of the cell. It is found in a rare form of leukaemia (**hairy-cell leukaemia**) most commonly occurring in young men.

halfway house a residential home for a group of people where some professional supervision is available. It is used as a stage in the rehabilitation of recovering drug addicts and people who are mentally ill, usually when they have just been discharged from hospital or a rehabilitation facility and are able to work but are not yet ready for independent life.

halitosis *n.* bad breath. Causes of temporary halitosis include recently eaten strongly flavoured food, such as garlic or onions, and drugs such as paraldehyde. Other causes include mouth breathing, *periodontal disease, and infective conditions of the nose, throat, and lungs (especially *bronchiectasis). Constipation, indigestion, acute appendicitis, uraemia, and some liver diseases may also cause the condition. *See also* FETOR.

Hallpike test *see* DIX-HALLPIKE TEST.

hallucination *n.* a false perception of something that is not really there. Hallucinations may be visual, auditory, tactile, gustatory (of taste), or olfactory (of smell). They may be provoked by mental illness (such as *schizophrenia or severe anxiety disorders), *personality disorders, or physical disorders affecting the brain (such as temporal lobe *epilepsy sepsis, acute organic syndrome, or stroke) or they may be caused by drugs or sensory deprivation. Hallucinations should be distinguished from dreams and from *illusions (which are based upon real stimuli).

hallucinogen *n.* a drug that produces hallucinations, e.g. *cannabis and *lysergic acid diethylamide. Hallucinogens were formerly used to treat certain types of mental illness. —**hallucinogenic** *adj.*

hallux *n.* (*pl.* **halluces**) the big toe.

hallux rigidus painful stiffness and enlargement of the metatarsophalangeal joint, at the base of the big toe, resulting from osteoarthritis. Unlike *hallux valgus, men are more commonly affected than women. Conservative treatment is often successful, but in some cases surgery (e.g. *cheilectomy, *arthrodesis, or *arthroplasty) is required.

hallux valgus the most common foot deformity, usually affecting women, in which the big toe is displaced towards the others (i.e. away from the midline); it is associated with a *bunion. The second toe may become crowded by the big toe and a *hammer toe deformity often results. Treatment includes modified footwear and surgery.

hallux varus displacement of the big toe

away from the others (i.e. towards the middle).

haloperidol *n.* a *butyrophenone antipsychotic drug used to relieve anxiety and tension in the treatment of schizophrenia and other psychiatric disorders and also to treat tics and related movement disorders. It is administered by mouth or *depot injection; muscular incoordination and restlessness are common side-effects. Trade names: **Dozic**, **Haldol**, **Serenace**.

halophilic *adj.* requiring solutions of high salt concentration for healthy growth. Certain bacteria are halophilic. —**halophile** *n.*

halos *pl. n.* coloured rings seen around lights by people with acute congestive glaucoma and sometimes by people with cataract.

halothane *n.* a potent general *anaesthetic administered by inhalation, used for inducing and maintaining anaesthesia in all types of surgical operations. However, it may cause severe liver damage and is less widely used now than formerly.

hamartoma *n.* an overgrowth of mature tissue in which the elements show disordered arrangement and proportion in comparison to normal. The overgrowth is benign but malignancy may occur in any of the constituent tissue elements.

hamate bone (unciform bone) a hook-shaped bone of the wrist (*see* CARPUS). It articulates with the capitate and triquetral bones at the sides, with the lunate bone behind, and with the fourth and fifth metacarpal bones in front.

Hamman's sign a crunching sound synchronous with the heartbeat heard with a stethoscope in 45–50% of patients with *pneumomediastinum. [L. V. Hamman (1877–1946), US physician]

hammer *n.* (in anatomy) *see* MALLEUS.

hammer toe a deformity of a toe, most often the second, caused by fixed flexion of the proximal interphalangeal joint, which produces extension of distal interphalangeal and metatarsophalangeal joints. A corn often forms over the deformity, which may be painful. If severe pain does not respond to strapping or corrective footwear, it may be necessary to perform *arthrodesis at the affected joint.

hamstring *n.* any of the tendons at the

back of the knee. They attach the **hamstring muscles** (the biceps femoris, semitendinosus, and semimembranosus) to their insertions in the tibia and fibula.

hamulus *n.* (*pl.* **hamuli**) any hooklike process, such as occurs on the hamate, lacrimal, and sphenoid bones and on the cochlea.

HAN heroin-associated nephropathy: a syndrome of massive proteinuria, hypoalbuminuria, and hyperlipidaemia, with or without oedema, seen after prolonged intravenous addiction to heroin. Renal biopsies show the changes of *focal segmental glomerulosclerosis but the condition does not respond to immunosuppressant treatment and progresses to end-stage renal failure.

hand *n.* the terminal organ of the upper limb. From a surgical point of view, the human hand comprises the eight bones of the *carpus (wrist), the five metacarpal bones, and the phalangeal bones plus the surrounding tissues; anatomically, the bones and tissues of the wrist are excluded. The hand is a common site of infections and injuries, many of which are of industrial origin for which compensation may be claimed.

handedness *n.* the preferential use of one hand, rather than the other, in voluntary actions. Ambidexterity – the ability to use either hand with equal skill – is very rare. Over 95% of right-handed people and 50–70% of left-handed people have left-hemisphere dominance for language.

hand, foot, and mouth disease a self-limiting disease, mainly affecting young children, caused by *Coxsackie virus A16. A feeling of mild illness is accompanied by mouth ulcers and blisters on the hands and feet.

handicap *n.* partial or total inability to perform a social, occupational, or other activity that the affected person wants to do. It reflects the extent to which an individual is disadvantaged by some partial or total *disability when compared with those in a peer group who have no such disability. A handicap is usually related to an identifiable structural **impairment**. It may also reflect functional impairment, which may be unsuspected by the individual and discovered by clinical observation or testing. The alternative terms **abnormality**, **defect**, or **malformation** (for impairment) and **malfunction**

(for disability) are used by many authorities, which may sometimes cause confusion; in an attempt to resolve this, a working group of the *World Health Organization has suggested using the generic term **disablement**, but this has gained only limited acceptance. *See also* INTERNATIONAL CLASSIFICATION OF DISEASES.

Hand-Schüller-Christian disease *see* LANGERHANS CELL HISTIOCYTOSIS. [A. Hand (1868–1949), US paediatrician; A. Schüller (1874–1958), Austrian neurologist; H. A. Christian (1876–1951), US physician]

Hansen's bacillus *see* MYCOBACTERIUM. [G. H. A. Hansen (1841–1912), Norwegian physician]

Hansen's disease *see* LEPROSY.

hantavirus *n.* one of a genus of viruses that infect rats, mice, and voles and cause disease in humans when the secretions or excreta of these rodents are inhaled or ingested. The disease was first reported from the area of the Hantaan river, which separates North from South Korea, but hantavirus infections also occur in Japan, China, Russia, Europe, and the USA: in Britain it can affect farm, nature conservancy, and sewage workers and those engaged in water sports. The symptoms vary according to the strain of the infecting virus. Many patients have a mild influenza-like illness, but severe cases are characterized by high fever, headache, shock, nausea and vomiting, and *petechiae in the skin; there may be kidney pain and rapidly progressive kidney damage leading to kidney failure. A particularly virulent strain in the USA attacks the lungs, leading to rapid respiratory failure. The mortality rate in these severe cases is high.

haploid (monoploid) *adj.* describing cells, nuclei, or organisms that have a single set of unpaired chromosomes. In humans the gametes are haploid following *meiosis. *Compare* DIPLOID, TRIPLOID. —**haploid** *n.*

haplotype *n.* a complete set of *HLA antigens inherited from either parent.

happy puppet syndrome *see* ANGELMAN SYNDROME.

hapt- (hapto-) *combining form denoting* touch.

hapten *n. see* ANTIGEN.

haptoglobin *n.* a protein present in blood plasma that binds with free haemoglobin to form a complex that is rapidly removed from the circulation by the liver. Depletion of plasma haptoglobin is a feature of anaemias in which red blood cells are destroyed inside the circulation with the release of haemoglobin into the plasma and its loss in the urine.

harara *n.* a severe and itchy inflammation of the skin occurring in people continuously subjected to the bites of the *sandfly *Phlebotomus papatasii*. The incidence of this allergic skin reaction, prevalent in the Middle East, may be checked by controlling the numbers of sandflies.

harelip *n. see* CLEFT LIP.

Harrison's sulcus a depression on both sides of the chest wall of a child between the pectoral muscles and the lower margin of the ribcage. It is caused by exaggerated suction of the diaphragm when breathing in and develops in conditions in which the airways are partially obstructed (e.g. poorly treated asthma) or when the lungs are abnormally congested due to some congenital abnormality of the heart. [E. Harrison (1789–1838), British physician]

Hartmann's operation a method of reconstruction after surgical removal of distal colon and proximal rectum, in which the rectal stump is closed off and the divided end of the colon is brought out as a *colostomy. The technique allows for a second-stage joining up of the bowel ends with no colostomy. It is often used temporarily where primary anastomosis is unsafe (e.g. in cases of perforated *diverticular disease) or permanently as a palliative procedure (e.g. for unresectable colonic cancer). [H. Hartmann (1860–1952), French surgeon]

Hartmann's pouch a saclike dilatation of the gall-bladder wall near its outlet; it is a common site for finding *gallstones. [R. Hartmann (1831–93), German anatomist]

Hartmann's solution a *physiological solution used for infusion into the circulation. In addition to essential ions, it also contains glucose. [A. F. Hartmann (1898–1964), US paediatrician]

Hartnup disease a rare hereditary defect in the absorption of the amino acid tryptophan, leading to mental retardation, thickening and roughening of the skin on exposure to light, and lack of muscular coordination. The condition is similar to *pellagra. Treatment with nicotinamide is usually effective. [Hartnup, the family in whom it was first reported]

harvest mite *see* TROMBICULA.

Hashimoto's disease chronic inflammation of the thyroid gland (**thyroiditis**) due to the formation of antibodies against normal thyroid tissue (autoantibodies; *see* THYROID ANTIBODIES). Its features include a firm swelling of the thyroid and partial or total failure of secretion of thyroid hormones; often there are autoantibodies to other organs, such as the stomach. Women are more often affected than men and the condition often occurs in families. [H. Hashimoto (1881–1934), Japanese surgeon]

hashish *n. see* CANNABIS.

Hasson technique a technique used in laparoscopic surgery in which the skin, muscle, fascia, and peritoneum are incised under direct vision to allow the insertion of a blunt *trocar, through which the laparoscope is introduced. [H. M. Hasson (21st century), US gynaecologist]

haustrum *n.* one of the pouches on the external surface of the *colon.

Haversian canal one of the small canals (diameter about 50 μm) that ramify throughout compact *bone. *See also* HAVERSIAN SYSTEM. [C. Havers (1650–1702), English anatomist]

Haversian system one of the cylindrical units of which compact *bone is made. A **Haversian canal** forms a central tube, around which are alternate layers of bone matrix (**lamellae**) and **lacunae** containing bone cells. The lacunae are linked by minute channels (**canaliculi**).

hay fever a form of *allergy due to the pollen of grasses, trees, and other plants, characterized by inflammation of the membrane lining the nose and sometimes of the conjunctiva (*see* ALLERGIC CONJUNCTIVITIS). The symptoms of sneezing, running or blocked nose, and watering eyes are due to histamine release and often respond to treatment with *antihistamines. If the allergen is identified, it may be possible to undertake *desensitization. Medical name: **allergic rhinitis**.

hazardous substance (in occupational health) *see* COSHH.

HbA$_{1c}$ *see* GLYCATED HAEMOGLOBIN.

hCG *see* HUMAN CHORIONIC GONADO-TROPHIN.

HDL *see* HIGH-DENSITY LIPOPROTEIN.

HDU *see* HIGH-DEPENDENCY UNIT.

head *n.* **1.** the part of the body that contains the brain and the organs of sight, hearing, smell, and taste. **2.** the rounded portion of a bone, which fits into a groove of another to form a joint; for example, the head of the humerus or femur.

headache *n.* pain felt deep within the skull. Most headaches are caused by stress or fatigue but some are symptoms of serious intracranial disease. *See also* CLUSTER HEADACHE, MIGRAINE.

head injury an injury usually resulting from a blow to the head and often associated with brain injury. It may result in *contusion or – if the blood vessels in the head are torn – a *haematoma. The level of consciousness of a patient following a head injury can be monitored using the *Glasgow Coma Scale. Head injuries are an important cause of death due to accidents: legislation to impose protective headgear at industrial sites and on construction workers and motorcyclists has reduced their incidence.

head tilt, chin lift a manoeuvre for opening the airway of an unconscious patient. With the patient lying on his or her back, the neck is extended and the chin simultaneously pulled gently upwards to pull the tongue away from the back of the pharynx. This method is often used when mouth-to-mouth ventilation is to be given and is an alternative to the *jaw thrust manoeuvre.

Heaf test a skin test to determine whether or not an individual is immune to tuberculosis, carried out prior to vaccination. A spring-loaded gun mounted with very short needles produces a circle of six punctures in the forearm through which *tuberculin is introduced. If the test is positive a reaction causes the skin to become red and raised, indicating that the individual is immune. If the test is negative a vaccine (*BCG) should be given. [F. R. G. Heaf (20th century), British physician]

health *n.* according to the official definition of the World Health Organization, a state of complete physical, mental, and social wellbeing, not merely the absence of disease or infirmity.

Health and Safety Executive (HSE) (in Britain) a statutory body responsible for health and safety in the workplace (including factories, offices, and farms). *See also* COSHH.

(⊕) SEE WEB LINKS

- HSE website: provides guidance on a wide range of health and safety topics

health authority *see* NATIONAL HEALTH SERVICE, STRATEGIC HEALTH AUTHORITY.

health board a health authority in Wales (since 2003), Scotland, and Northern Ireland. *See* NATIONAL HEALTH SERVICE.

health care *see* PRIMARY CARE, SECONDARY CARE, TERTIARY CARE.

Healthcare Commission an independent organization established in 2004 that was responsible for promoting improvement in the quality of health care in England. The commission was abolished on 31 March 2009 and replaced by the *Care Quality Commission, which became operational on 1 April 2009.

health-care commissioning identifying services required to meet population health-care needs and obtaining such services from an appropriate service provider via allocation of resources and contracting arrangements. Commissioners monitor the quality of commissioned services, including adherence to any appropriate national standards. Most NHS commissioning is undertaken by *primary care trusts or *specialized commissioning groups.

health centre (in Britain) a building, owned or leased by a primary care trust or health authority, that houses personnel and/or services from one or more sections of the *National Health Service (e.g. *general practitioners, *district nurses, dentists, and *child health clinics. Services provided by local authorities, such as social services, may also operate from such a centre. A **GP-led health centre** (**polyclinic**) is one where a greater range of health services are available compared to conventional GP practices. They offer extended opening hours and other health services, such as ophthalmology and dentistry, as well as diagnostics, outpatient appointments, urgent care, and community services, such as community mental health care, community nursing, and management of long-term conditions. The main aim is to move more services into the community, thus making them easier to access for patients. Various models have been proposed for polyclinics, ranging from large premises housing many separate GP practices to more extensive facilities with additional services available. *See also* CHILDREN'S CENTRE.

health education methods used to inform people (either individually or collectively) and persuade and enable them to adopt lifestyles that the educators believe will improve health and to reject habits regarded as harmful to health. The term is also used in a broader sense to include instruction about bodily function, etc., so that the public is better informed about health issues. All children receive health education at school, often as part of a **personal, social, and health education** (**PSHE**) programme. *See also* HEALTH PROMOTION.

health inequalities differences in health-related *variables (e.g. life expectancy, all-age all-cause mortality, breast cancer incidence) between population groups (often defined by socio-economic group, sex, age, ethnic group, place of birth, place of residence, and income). Health inequalities between groups arise as a result of differences in constitutional factors (e.g. age, sex, ethnic group), educational attainment, health-related behaviour (e.g. smoking, diet) and access to services. Typically, socio-economic deprivation is associated with poorer health outcomes. Recent government policy has sought to reduce gaps in health outcomes between population groups, particularly those related to socio-economic group and income.

health promotion action to maintain the best possible health and quality of life of the members of the community and to stimulate their involvement in their personal health, both collectively and individually. Programmes may include interventions targeting individuals and their behavior, such as *health education, immunization, and *screening tests, and interventions targeting populations, such as environmental monitoring, housing, and water and food supplies.

health protection the branch of *public health medicine that is concerned with protecting the public from communicable diseases, chemicals and poisons, radiation, and other potential threats to health. *See* HEALTH PROTECTION AGENCY.

Health Protection Agency (HPA) a non-departmental public body set up as a special health authority in 2003 to protect the health of the UK population via advice and support to the NHS, local authorities, the *Department of Health, emergency services, and others. The HPA is involved in protecting people from communicable diseases and biological, chemical, poison, and radiation hazards. *See* CONSULTANT IN COMMUNICABLE DISEASE CONTROL.

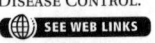 **SEE WEB LINKS**

• HPA website

health service manager an administrator with special training and skills in management who is concerned with the planning and provision of health services and with managing performance. Some managers enter the profession via the NHS Graduate Management Training Scheme; for others the basic training is in disciplines other than health; however, doctors, nurses, and others may fill such posts, sometimes combining them with professional appointments. *See also* NATIONAL HEALTH SERVICE.

Health Service Ombudsman an official responsible to Parliament and appointed to protect the interests of patients in relation to administration of and provision of health care by the *National Health Service. He or she can investigate complaints about the NHS when they cannot be resolved locally.

SEE WEB LINKS

• Website of the Health Service Ombudsman (England)
• Website of the Public Services Ombudsman for Scotland
• Website of the Public Services Ombudsman for Wales

health service planning balancing the health and health-care needs of a community, assessed by such indices as mortality, morbidity, and disability, with the resources available to meet these needs in terms of human resources (including ensuring the numbers in training grades meet future requirements) and technical resources, such as hospitals (capital planning), equipment, and medicines. *See also* CLINICAL AUDIT.

health visitor (public health nurse) a trained nurse with specialist qualifications in *health promotion and public health. The role of the health visitor takes place within the primary health-care team and focuses on families with children under five years old, but can be extended to other targeted groups in the population (e.g. the elderly) to meet health needs in the wider community. Health visitors seek to educate, in particular by drawing attention to unmet needs in terms of health and social care.

hearing aid a device to improve the hearing. Simple passive devices, such as ear trumpets, are now rarely used. An **analogue hearing aid** consists of a miniature microphone, an amplifier, and a tiny loudspeaker. The aid is powered by a battery and the whole unit is small enough to fit behind or within the ear inconspicuously. If necessary, aids can be built into the frames of spectacles. In a few cases of conductive hearing loss the loudspeaker is replaced by a vibrator that presses on the bone behind the ear and transmits the sound energy through the bones of the skull to the inner ear. **Digital hearing aids** are in some respects similar to analogue aids but in addition to the microphone, amplifier, and loudspeaker, they have digital-to-analogue converters and a tiny computer built into the casing of the aid. This enables the aid to be programmed to the patient's particular requirements and generally offers improved sound quality. *See also* BONE-ANCHORED HEARING AID, COCHLEAR IMPLANT, ENVIRONMENTAL HEARING AID, IMPLANTABLE HEARING AID.

hearing therapy the support and rehabilitation of people with hearing difficulties, tinnitus, or vertigo. It includes supplying help with acclimatizing to *hearing aids,

teaching lip-reading, advising on *environmental hearing aids, and offering general information and advice regarding the auditory system. Other functions are to explain such conditions as *Ménière's disease and *otosclerosis and to provide *tinnitus retraining therapy (TRT) and other forms of tinnitus management.

heart *n.* a hollow muscular cone-shaped organ, lying between the lungs, with the pointed end (**apex**) directed downwards, forwards, and to the left. The heart is about the size of a closed fist. Its wall consists largely of *cardiac muscle (myocardium), lined and surrounded by membranes (*see* ENDOCARDIUM, PERICARDIUM). It is divided by a **septum** into separate right and left halves, each of which is divided into an upper *atrium and a lower *ventricle (see illustration). Deoxygenated blood from the *venae cavae passes through the right atrium to the right ventricle. This contracts and pumps blood to the lungs via the *pulmonary artery. The newly oxygenated blood returns to the left atrium via the pulmonary veins and passes through to the left ventricle. This forcefully contracts, pumping blood out to the body via the *aorta. The direction of blood flow within the heart is controlled by *valves.

( ) SEE WEB LINKS

• Website of British Heart Foundation: provides information on the operation of the heart, keeping the heart healthy, and the main types of heart condition

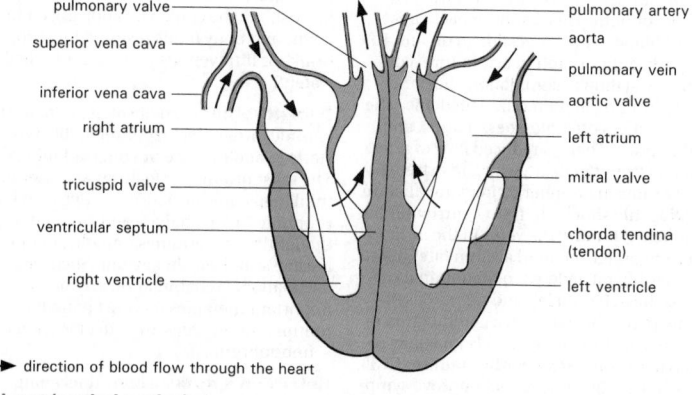

direction of blood flow through the heart

The heart (vertical section).

heart attack see MYOCARDIAL INFARCTION.

heart block a condition in which conduction of the electrical impulses generated by the natural pacemaker of the heart (the *sinoatrial node) is impaired. In **partial** or **incomplete heart block** conduction between atria and ventricles is delayed (**first degree heart block**) or not all the impulses are conducted from the atria to the ventricles (**second degree heart block**). In **third degree** or **complete heart block** no impulses are conducted and the ventricles beat at their own slow intrinsic rate (20–40 per minute).

Heart block may be congenital or it may be due to heart disease, including myocardial infarction, myocarditis, cardiomyopathy, and disease of the valves. It is most frequently seen in the elderly as the result of chronic degenerative scarring around the conducting tissue. There may be no symptoms, but when very slow heart and pulse rates occur the patient may develop heart failure or syncope (see STOKES-ADAMS SYNDROME). Symptoms may be abolished by the use of an artificial *pacemaker.

heartburn (pyrosis) n. discomfort or pain, usually burning in character, that is felt behind the breastbone and often appears to rise from the abdomen towards or into the throat. It may be accompanied by the appearance of acid or bitter fluid in the mouth (waterbrash) and is usually caused by regurgitation of stomach contents into the gullet.

heart failure a condition in which the pumping action of the heart is inadequate due to damaged heart valves, ventricular muscle, or both. This results in back pressure of blood, with congestion of organs. In **left ventricular** (or **left heart**) **failure**, congestion and fluid accumulation affect the lungs, resulting in pulmonary *oedema. The patient suffers breathlessness, cough, and *orthopnoea. There is reduced flow of arterial blood from the heart, which in extreme cases results in peripheral circulatory failure (**cardiogenic shock**). In **right ventricular** (or **right heart**) **failure**, the veins in the neck become engorged and fluid accumulates in the legs (peripheral oedema) or abdominal cavity (*ascites). If both left and right sides of the heart are affected then a combination of the above features is seen. This is usually referred to as **congestive cardiac failure** (**CCF**).

Diuretics (e.g. furosemide) improve symptoms. *ACE inhibitors, *beta blockers, and *spironolactone improve symptoms and life expectancy in patients with left ventricular failure. Heart surgery may be required for the correction of valve problems.

heart-lung machine an apparatus for taking over temporarily the functions of both the heart and the lungs during heart surgery. It incorporates a pump, to maintain the circulation, and equipment to oxygenate the blood. Blood is taken from the body by tubes inserted into the superior and inferior venae cavae, and the oxygenated blood is returned under pressure into a large artery, such as the femoral artery. The surgeon is therefore able to undertake the repair or replacement of heart valves or perform other surgical operations involving the heart and great blood vessels.

heart rate see PULSE.

heater-probe n. a device that can be passed through an endoscope to apply controlled heat in order to coagulate a bleeding peptic ulcer.

heat exhaustion fatigue and collapse due to the low blood pressure and blood volume that result from loss of body fluids and salts after prolonged or unaccustomed exposure to heat. It is most common in new arrivals in a hot climate and is treated by giving drinks or intravenous injections of salted water.

heatstroke (sunstroke) n. raised body temperature (pyrexia), absence of sweating, and eventual loss of consciousness due to failure or exhaustion of the temperature-regulating mechanism of the body. It is potentially fatal unless treated immediately: the body should be cooled by applying damp cloths and body fluids restored by giving drinks or intravenous injections of salted water.

hebephrenia n. an obsolescent name for a chronic form of *schizophrenia that typically starts in adolescence or young adulthood. The most prominent features are disordered thinking; inappropriate emotions with inappropriate *affect, naivity and vulnerability, thoughtless cheerfulness, apathy, or querulousness; and silly behaviour. Social and occupational rehabilitation are the most important therapies for most patients; *antipsychotic drugs are also efficacious. —**hebephrenic** adj.

Heberden's node a bony thickening arising at the terminal joint of a finger in *osteoarthritis. It is often inherited. [W. Heberden (1710–1801), British physician]

hectic *adj.* occurring regularly. A **hectic fever** is a fever that typically develops in the afternoons, in cases of pulmonary tuberculosis.

hecto- *prefix denoting* a hundred.

heel *n.* the part of the foot that extends behind the ankle joint, formed by the **heel bone** (*see* CALCANEUS).

heel-prick blood test *see* GUTHRIE TEST.

Hegar's sign an indication of pregnancy detectable between the 6th and 12th weeks: used before modern urine tests for pregnancy were available. If the fingers of one hand are inserted into the vagina and those of the other are placed over the pelvic cavity, the lower part of the uterus feels very soft compared with the body of the uterus above and the cervix below. [A. Hegar (1830–1914), German gynaecologist]

Heimlich manoeuvre *see* ABDOMINAL THRUSTS. [H. J. Heimlich (1920–), US physician]

helc- (**helco-**) *combining form denoting* an ulcer.

Helicobacter *n.* a genus of spiral flagellated Gram-negative bacteria. The species *H. pylori* (formerly classified as *Campylobacter pylori*) is found in the stomach within the mucous layer. It occurs in the majority of middle-aged people and causes progressive gastritis. It is almost invariably present in duodenal ulceration and usually in gastric ulceration. Eradication of the organism (using various combinations of antibiotics and *antisecretory drugs) leads to healing of the ulcer. *H. pylori* has also been implicated in some forms of stomach cancer and in heart disease. The role of other *Helicobacter* species in the causation of disease in humans is unclear.

helicopter-based emergency medical services *see* HEMS.

helicotrema *n.* the narrow opening between the scala vestibuli and the scala tympani at the tip of the *cochlea in the ear.

helio- *combining form denoting* the sun.

heliotherapy *n.* the use of sunlight to promote healing; sunbathing.

helix *n.* the outer curved fleshy ridge of the *pinna of the outer ear.

Heller's operation *see* ACHALASIA. [E. Heller (1877–1964), Austrian pathologist]

Heller's test a test for the presence of protein (albumin) in the urine. A quantity of urine is carefully poured onto the same quantity of pure nitric acid in a test tube. A white ring forms at the junction of the liquids if albumin is present. However, a similar result may be obtained if the urine contains certain drugs or is very concentrated. A dark brown ring indicates the presence of an abnormally high level of potassium indoxyl sulphate in the urine (*see* INDICANURIA). [J. F. Heller (1813–71), Austrian pathologist]

HELLP syndrome a form of severe *preeclampsia affecting many body systems and characterized by *h*aemolysis, *e*levated *l*iver enzymes, and a *l*ow *p*latelet count (hence the name). It constitutes an emergency requiring delivery as soon as the patient is stabilized.

Helly's fluid a mixture of potassium dichromate, sodium sulphate, mercuric chloride, formaldehyde, and distilled water, used in the preservation of bone marrow. [K. Helly (20th century), Swiss pathologist]

helminth *n.* any of the various parasitic worms, including the *flukes, *tapeworms, and *nematodes.

helminthiasis *n.* the diseased condition resulting from an infestation with parasitic worms (helminths).

helminthology *n.* the study of parasitic worms.

helper T cell a type of T *lymphocyte that plays a key role in cell-mediated immunity by recognizing foreign antigen on the surface of *antigen-presenting cells when this is associated with the individual's *MHC antigens, having been processed by antigen-presenting cells. Helper T cells stimulate the production of *cytotoxic T cells, which destroy the target cells.

hemeralopia *n. see* DAY BLINDNESS.

hemi- *prefix denoting* (in medicine) the right or left half of the body. Example: **hemianaesthesia** (anaesthesia of one side of the body).

hemiachromatopsia *n.* loss of colour appreciation in one half of the visual field.

hemianopia *n.* absence of half of the normal field of vision. The commonest type is **homonymous hemianopia**, in which the same half (right or left) is lost in both eyes. Sometimes the inner halves of the visual field are lost in both eyes, producing a **binasal hemianopia**, while in others the outer halves are lost, producing a **bitemporal hemianopia**. Very rarely both upper halves or both lower halves are lost, producing an **altitudinal hemianopia**.

hemiarthroplasty *n. see* ARTHROPLASTY.

hemiballismus *n.* a violent involuntary movement usually restricted to one arm and primarily involving the proximal muscles. It is a symptom of disease of the contralateral *basal ganglia; the commonest causes are stroke, haemorrhage, and trauma.

hemicolectomy *n.* surgical removal of about half the *colon (large intestine), usually the right section (**right hemicolectomy**) with subsequent joining of the *ileum to the transverse colon. This is performed for disease of the terminal part of the ileum (such as *Crohn's disease) or of the caecum or ascending colon (such as cancer or Crohn's disease).

hemicrania *n.* **1.** a headache affecting only one side of the head, usually *migraine. **2.** absence of half of the skull in a developing fetus.

hemifacial spasm a type of *dystonia that results in irregular spasms affecting the facial muscles on one side. It is usually due to irritation of the facial nerve by an overlying artery within the skull base. Treatment is with injections of *botulinum toxin.

hemihypertrophy *n.* a condition in which one side of the body is larger than the other. It is often benign but can be associated with *nephroblastoma.

hemimelia *n.* congenital absence or gross shortening (aplasia) of the distal portion of the arms or legs. Sometimes only one of the two bones of the distal arm (radius and ulna) or leg (tibia and fibula) may be affected. *See also* ECTROMELIA.

hemiparesis *n. see* HEMIPLEGIA.

hemiplegia (hemiparesis) *n.* paralysis of one side of the body. It is caused by disease affecting the opposite (contralateral) hemisphere of the brain.

hemisacralization *n.* fusion of the fifth lumbar vertebra to one side only of the sacrum. *See* SACRALIZATION.

hemisphere *n.* one of the two halves of the *cerebrum, not in fact hemispherical but more nearly quarter-spherical.

hemizygous *adj.* describing genes that are carried on an unpaired chromosome, for example the genes on the X chromosome in males. —**hemizygote** *n.*

hemlock *n.* the plant *Conium maculatum*, found in Britain and central Europe. It is a source of the poisonous alkaloid *coniine.

hemp *n. see* CANNABIS.

HEMS helicopter-based emergency medical services: a fast method for the provision of first aid and the rapid transport of the seriously injured (primary use) or the critically ill (secondary use) to a hospital.

Henle's loop the part of a kidney tubule that forms a loop extending towards the centre of the kidney. It is surrounded by blood capillaries, which absorb water and selected soluble substances back into the bloodstream. [F. G. J. Henle (1809–85), German anatomist]

Henoch-Schönlein purpura (Schönlein-Henoch purpura, anaphylactoid purpura) a common, and frequently recurrent, form of *purpura found especially (but not exclusively) in young children. It is characterized by red weals and a purple rash on the buttocks and lower legs due to bleeding into the skin from inflamed capillaries, together with arthritis, gastrointestinal symptoms, and (in some cases) nephritis. Glucocorticoids are often used for treatment. [E. H. Henoch (1820–1910), German paediatrician; J. L. Schönlein (1793–1864), German physician]

henry *n.* the *SI unit of inductance, equal to the inductance of a closed circuit with a magnetic flux of 1 weber per ampere of current. Symbol: H.

Hensen's node (primitive knot) the rounded front end of the embryonic *primitive streak. [V. Hensen (1835–1924), German pathologist]

heparin *n.* an *anticoagulant produced in liver cells, some white blood cells, and certain other sites, which acts by inhibiting the action of the enzyme *thrombin in the final stage of *blood coagulation. An extracted purified form of heparin is widely used for the prevention of blood coagulation both in patients with deep vein thrombosis and similar conditions and in blood collected for examination. The drug is administered by intravenous injection and the most important side-effect is bleeding. *See also* LOW-MOLECULAR-WEIGHT HEPARIN.

hepat- (hepato-) *combining form denoting* the liver. Examples: **hepatopexy** (surgical fixation of); **hepatorenal** (relating to the liver and kidney).

hepatalgia *n.* pain in or over the liver. It is usually caused by stretching of the outer covering (capsule) of the liver due to inflammation (especially liver abscess), the presence of enlarging primary or secondary liver malignancy, or swelling (as in cardiac failure or *steatosis).

hepatectomy *n.* the operation of removing the liver. **Partial hepatectomy** is the removal of one or more lobes of the liver; it may be carried out after severe injury or to remove a tumour localized in one part of the liver.

hepatic *adj.* relating to the liver.

hepatic duct *see* BILE DUCT.

hepatic encephalopathy (portosystemic encephalopathy) a condition in which brain function is impaired by the presence of toxic substances, absorbed from the colon, which are normally removed or detoxified by the liver. It occurs when the liver is severely damaged (as in cirrhosis) or bypassed. Symptoms include drowsiness, confusion, difficulty in performing tasks (e.g. writing), and coma. Treatment is mainly directed towards the underlying cause of liver failure or decompensation (e.g. arresting gastrointestinal haemorrhage, treating infection, etc). Supportive measures may include administering bowel cleansers (especially *lactulose, orally or by enema) and reducing protein and/or salt intake.

hepatic flexure the bend in the *colon, just underneath the liver, where the ascending colon joins the transverse colon.

hepaticostomy *n.* a surgical operation in which a temporary or permanent opening is made into the main duct carrying bile from the liver.

hepatic vein one of several short veins originating within the lobes of the liver as small branches, which unite to form the hepatic veins. These lead directly to the inferior vena cava, draining blood from the liver.

hepatitis *n.* inflammation of the liver caused by viruses, toxic substances (including alcohol), immunological abnormalities, or the excess deposition of fat (*see* NONALCOHOLIC FATTY LIVER DISEASE). **Infectious hepatitis** is caused by viruses, several types of which have been isolated as specific causes of the disease and can be detected by blood tests, including hepatitis A, hepatitis B, hepatitis C, hepatitis D, and hepatitis E. Other viral causes of hepatitis include the *Epstein-Barr virus. *See also* ENTAMOEBA.

Hepatitis A is transmitted by food or drink contaminated by a carrier or patient and commonly occurs where sanitation is poor. After an incubation period of 15–40 days, the patient develops fatigue, anorexia, nausea, vomiting, arthralgia, and fever. Yellow discoloration of the skin (*see* JAUNDICE) appears about a week later and persists for up to three weeks. The patient may be infectious throughout this period. Serious complications are unusual and an attack often confers immunity. Injection of *gammaglobulin provides temporary protection, but active immunization is preferable.

Hepatitis B (formerly known as **serum hepatitis**) is transmitted by infected blood or blood products contaminating hypodermic needles, blood transfusions, or tattooing needles, by unprotected sexual contact, or (rarely) by contact with any other body fluid. It often occurs in drug addicts. Symptoms, which develop suddenly after an incubation period of 1–6 months, include headache, fever, chills, general weakness, and jaundice. Treatment includes *interferon alfa and other oral antivirals (e.g. *lamivudine, *adefovir dipivoxil, entecavir). Most patients make a gradual recovery but the mortality rate is 5–20%. A vaccine is available.

Hepatitis C (formerly known as **non-A, non-B hepatitis**) has a mode of transmission similar to that of hepatitis B (predominantly intravenous drug abuse); symptoms include fatigue, sore bones, and dryness of the eyes. Treatment is with interferon alfa, peginterferon alfa, and ribavirin.

Hepatitis D is a defective virus and occurs only with or after infection with hepatitis B. Patients with D virus usually have severe chronic hepatitis.

Hepatitis E is transmitted by infected food or drink and can cause acute hepatitis; it is especially severe in a pregnant patient.

Chronic hepatitis continues for months or years, eventually leading to *cirrhosis (*see also* HEPATOMA). It is usually caused by persistent infection with a hepatitis virus (usually hepatitis B, C, or D), which may respond to treatment with interferon, or by autoimmune disease, treated by corticosteroids or immunosuppressant therapy.

hepatization *n.* the conversion of lung tissue, which normally holds air, into a solid liver-like mass during the course of acute lobar *pneumonia. In the early stages of lobar pneumonia, the lungs show red hepatization due to the presence of red and white blood cells in the alveolar spaces. As the disease progresses, the red cells are destroyed and phagocytosed, resulting in grey hepatization.

hepato- *combining form. see* HEPAT-.

hepatoblastoma *n.* a malignant tumour of the liver occurring in children, made up of embryonic liver cells. It is often confined to one lobe of the liver; such cases may be treated by a partial *hepatectomy.

hepatocellular *adj.* relating to or affecting the cells of the liver.

hepatocyte *n.* the principal cell type in the *liver: a large cell with many metabolic functions, including synthesis, storage, detoxification, and bile production.

hepatoma (hepatocellular carcinoma) *n.* a primary malignant tumour of the liver. Almost all patients have pre-existing *cirrhosis. It is the most common primary tumour of the liver, with the highest incidence in the Far East (Taiwan). In Western countries patients with cirrhosis due to chronic hepatitis B or C infection are at the highest risk. The higher incidence of hepatomas in non-Western societies is partly due to increased hepatitis B endemicity but other factors, including fungi (*see* AFLATOXIN) and other ingested toxins, do contribute towards some cases. Hepatomas often synthesize *alphafetoprotein, which circulates in the blood and is a useful marker for these tumours. The treatment options depend on the number and size of hepatomas and the synthetic function of the liver. They include liver transplantation, surgical resection, chemotherapy, and local ablative treatment. Hepatitis B vaccination has helped to reduce the incidence of hepatoma in parts of Asia and Africa.

hepatomegaly *n.* enlargement of the liver to such an extent that it can be felt below the rib margin. This may be due to congestion (as in heart failure), inflammation, infiltration (e.g. by fat), or tumour.

hepatorenal syndrome impairment of renal function, which can occur in acute or chronic liver disease. The condition is associated with intrarenal vasoconstriction and extrarenal vasodilation and hypotension, and the kidney disease is functional rather than structural in nature. There are two common clinical presentations. An acute form (type 1) is characterized by rapid spontaneous deterioration in renal function against a background of acute liver failure, acute alcoholic hepatitis, or acute decompensation of chronic cirrhotic liver disease. A chronic form (type 2) is characterized by insidious onset and slowly progressive deterioration in renal function. This is most often observed in patients with decompensated cirrhosis and portal hypertension. The prognosis of hepatorenal syndrome is extremely poor, and the best hope of survival is usually with liver transplantation.

hepatotoxic *adj.* damaging or destroying liver cells. Certain drugs, such as *paracetamol, can cause liver damage at high doses or with prolonged use.

hept- (hepta-) *prefix denoting* seven.

HER2 *h*uman *e*pidermal growth factor *r*eceptor *2*: a protein occurring in excessive amounts on the surface of tumour cells in highly malignant forms of breast cancer. It acts as an *epidermal growth factor receptor, which influences the growth and proliferation of the tumour. *See also* TRASTUZUMAB.

herbal medicine (herbalism) the use of plants or plant extracts for medicinal purposes in order to improve the body's natural functions and restore balance. Herbal medicines are given in many forms (liquids, infusions, tablets, topical preparations, etc.) and form part of an increasing number of complementary medical therapies. *See* PHYTOTHERAPY.

Herceptin *n. see* TRASTUZUMAB.

herd immunity the immunity of a group, community, or population to an infectious disease as a result of mass vaccination. The higher the percentage of the population vaccinated, the greater will be the resistance to the spread of infection within the population.

hereditary *adj.* transmitted from parents to their offspring; inherited.

hereditary multiple exostoses *see* EX-OSTOSIS.

hereditary nonpolyposis colorectal cancer (HNPCC, Lynch syndrome) an inherited disorder in which there is an increased incidence of colorectal *polyp formation, although to a lesser extent than in familial adenomatous *polyposis (FAP). HNPCC has also been associated with other types of tumour, particularly ovarian and endometrial tumours. This increased risk is due to inherited mutations that impair DNA mismatch repair.

heredity *n.* the process that causes the biological similarity between parents and their offspring. *Genetics is the study of heredity.

heredo- *combining form denoting* heredity.

Hering-Breuer reflex the normal physiological reflex to breathe out when the breath is held in inspiration and to breathe in when it is held in exhalation. [H. E. Hering (1866–1948), German physiologist; J. Breuer (1842–1925), German physician]

hermaphrodite *n.* an individual in which both male and female sex organs are present or in which the sex organs contain both ovarian and testicular cells. Human hermaphrodites are very rare. *See* INTERSEX. —**hermaphroditism** *n.*

hermeneutics *n.* the practice of interpreting and explaining, which derives from religious studies of important and historical texts. In *clinical ethics, it is the act of identifying values, weighing priorities, and making sense of diverse theories, principles, and guidance to reach a considered decision.

hernia *n.* the protrusion of an organ or tissue out of the body cavity in which it normally lies. An **inguinal hernia** (or **rupture**) occurs in the lower abdomen; a sac of peritoneum, containing fat or part of the bowel, bulges through a weak part (**inguinal canal**) of the abdominal wall. It may result from physical straining or coughing. A **scrotal hernia** is an inguinal hernia so large that it passes into the scrotum; a **femoral hernia** is

similar to an inguinal hernia but protrudes at the top of the thigh, through the point at which the femoral artery passes from the abdomen to the thigh. Other hernias of the abdominal wall include periumbilical, epigastric, and postsurgical hernias. A **diaphragmatic hernia** is the protrusion of an abdominal organ through the diaphragm into the chest cavity; the most common type is the **hiatus hernia**, in which the stomach passes partly or completely into the chest cavity through the hole (**hiatus**) for the oesophagus (gullet). This may be associated with *gastro-oesophageal reflux. *See also* EX-OMPHALOS.

Hernias may be complicated by becoming impossible to return to their normal site (**irreducible**); swollen and fixed within their sac (**incarcerated**); or cut off from their blood supply, becoming painful and eventually gangrenous (**strangulated**). The best treatment for hernias, especially if they are painful, is surgical repair (*see* HERNIOPLASTY).

hernia-en-glissade an inguinal *hernia that has an element of descent ('slide') of related structures alongside the sac.

hernio- *combining form denoting* a hernia.

hernioplasty *n.* the surgical operation to repair a hernia, in which the sac is excised (*herniotomy), the abnormal opening is sewn up, and the weakness strengthened, most commonly using a mesh of polypropylene.

herniorrhaphy *n.* surgical repair of a hernia. It can be performed through a *laparoscope. *See also* HERNIOPLASTY, HERNIOTOMY.

herniotomy *n.* excision of a hernial sac: the first stage of the surgical repair of a hernia. In infants and young muscular subjects it is all that is needed to cure the hernia.

heroin *n.* a white crystalline powder derived from *morphine that is a highly addictive drug of abuse. *See also* DIAMORPHINE.

heroin-associated nephropathy *see* HAN.

herpangina *n.* an acute viral infection, occurring predominantly in children, that causes a fever of sudden onset associated with malaise and acute ulceration of the soft palate and tonsillar area. It usually lasts 2–5 days.

herpes *n.* inflammation of the skin or mucous membranes that is caused by *herpesviruses and characterized by collections of small blisters. There are two types of **herpes simplex virus (HSV)**: type I causes the common **cold sore**, usually present on or around the lips; type II is mainly associated with **genital herpes** and is sexually transmitted. However, types I and II can both cause either genital herpes or cold sores, depending on the site of initial infection. HSV blisters are contagious through skin-to-skin contact and are recurrent in some people. HSV can also affect the conjunctiva (*see also* DENDRITIC ULCER).

Herpes zoster (shingles) is caused by the varicella-zoster virus, which also causes chickenpox. Following an attack of chickenpox, the virus lies dormant in the dorsal root ganglia of the spinal cord. Later, under one of a number of influences, the virus migrates down the sensory nerve to affect one or more *dermatomes on the skin in a band, causing the characteristic shingles rash. One side of the face or an eye (**ophthalmic zoster**) may be involved. Shingles may be chronically painful (**post-herpetic neuralgia**), especially in the elderly. *See also* RAMSAY HUNT SYNDROME.

Treatment of all forms of herpes is with an appropriate preparation of *aciclovir or related antiviral drugs; shingles may require potent analgesics and treatment of secondary bacterial infection.

herpesvirus *n.* one of a group of DNA-containing viruses causing latent infections in animals (including humans). The herpesviruses are the causative agents of *herpes and chickenpox. The group also includes the *cytomegalovirus and *Epstein-Barr virus. *Herpesvirus simiae* (**virus B**) causes an infection in monkeys similar to herpes simplex, but when transmitted to humans it can produce fatal encephalitis.

hertz *n.* the *SI unit of frequency, equal to one cycle per second. Symbol: Hz.

Herxheimer reaction *see* JARISCH-HERXHEIMER REACTION.

hesitation *n.* a *lower urinary tract symptom in which there is a delay between being ready to pass urine and the actual flow of urine.

heter- (**hetero-**) *combining form denoting* difference; dissimilarity.

heterochromatin *n.* chromosome material (*see* CHROMATIN) that stains most deeply when the cell is not dividing. It is

thought not to represent major genes but may be involved in controlling these genes, and also in controlling mitosis and development. *Compare* EUCHROMATIN.

heterochromia *n.* colour difference in the iris of the eye, which is usually congenital but is occasionally secondary to inflammation of the iris (as in *Fuchs' heterochromic cyclitis). In **heterochromia iridis** one iris differs in colour from the other; in **heterochromia iridum** one part of the iris differs in colour from the rest. —**heterochromic** *adj.*

heterogametic *adj.* describing the sex that produces two different kinds of gamete, which carry different *sex chromosomes, and that therefore determines the sex of the offspring. In humans men are the heterogametic sex: the sperm cells carry either an X or a Y chromosome. *Compare* HOMOGAMETIC.

heterogeneity *n.* (in oncology) variability or differences in the properties of cells within a tumour.

heterograft *n. see* XENOGRAFT.

heterophoria *n.* a tendency to squint. Normally both the eyes work together and look at the same point simultaneously, but if one eye is covered it will move out of alignment with the object the other eye is still viewing. When the cover is removed the eye immediately returns to its normal position. Most people have a small degree of heterophoria in which the covered eye turns outwards, away from the nose (**exophoria**; *compare* ESOPHORIA). Heterophoria may produce eyestrain because of the unconscious effort required to keep the two eyes aligned. *See also* STRABISMUS.

Heterophyes *n.* a genus of small parasitic *flukes occurring in Egypt and the Far East. Adult flukes of the species *H. heterophyes* live in the small intestine of humans and other fish-eating animals; in humans the flukes can produce serious symptoms (*see* HETEROPHYIASIS). The fluke has two intermediate hosts, a snail and a mullet fish.

heterophyiasis *n.* an infestation of the small intestine with the parasitic fluke *Heterophyes heterophyes*. Humans become infected on eating raw or salted fish that contains the larval stage of the fluke. The presence of adult flukes may provoke symptoms of abdominal pain and diarrhoea; if the eggs reach the brain, spinal cord, and heart (via the bloodstream) they produce serious lesions. Tetrachloroethylene may be used in treatment of the infection.

heteropsia *n.* different vision in each eye.

heterosis *n.* hybrid vigour: the increased sturdiness, resistance to disease, etc., of animals whose parents are genetically different compared both with their parents and with the offspring of genetically similar parents.

heterotopia (heterotopy) *n.* the displacement of an organ or part of the body from its normal position.

heterotrophic (organotrophic) *adj.* describing organisms (known as heterotrophs) that use complex organic compounds to synthesize their own organic materials. Most heterotrophs are **chemoheterotrophic**, i.e. they use the organic compounds as an energy source. This group includes the majority of bacteria and all animals and fungi. *Compare* AUTOTROPHIC.

heterotropia *n. see* STRABISMUS.

heterozygous *adj.* describing an individual in whom the members of a pair of genes determining a particular characteristic are dissimilar. *See* ALLELE. *Compare* HOMOZYGOUS. —**heterozygote** *n.*

hex- (hexa-) *combining form denoting* six.

hexacanth *n. see* ONCOSPHERE.

hexachromia *n.* the ability to distinguish only six of the seven colours of the spectrum, the exception being indigo. Most people cannot distinguish indigo from blue or violet.

hexamine *n. see* METHENAMINE.

hexokinase *n.* an enzyme that catalyses the conversion of glucose to glucose-6-phosphate. This is the first stage of *glycolysis.

hexosamine *n.* the amino derivative of a *hexose sugar. The two most important hexosamines are *glucosamine and galactosamine.

hexose *n.* a simple sugar with six carbon atoms. Hexose sugars are the sugars most frequently found in food. The most important hexose is *glucose.

5-HIAA *see* 5-HYDROXYINDOLEACETIC ACID.

hiatus *n.* an opening or aperture. For example, the diaphragm contains hiatuses for the oesophagus and aorta.

hiatus hernia *see* HERNIA.

Hib/MenC a combined vaccine that protects against *Haemophilus influenzae* type b infection (*see* HIB VACCINE) and meningococcal disease (*see* MENINGITIS C VACCINE). *See also* IMMUNIZATION.

Hib vaccine a vaccine that gives protection against the bacterium *Haemophilus influenzae* type b (Hib). Before the introduction of the vaccine in the UK in 1992, Hib was the commonest cause of meningitis in children under the age of 2 years. The vaccine, which has an excellent safety record, is currently given with the primary vaccines at two, three, and four months of age and as a booster at 12 months of age to extend protection against Hib meningitis. *See* IMMUNIZATION.

hiccup *n.* abrupt involuntary lowering of the diaphragm and closure of the sound-producing folds at the upper end of the trachea, producing a characteristic sound as the breath is drawn in. Hiccups, which usually occur repeatedly, may be caused by indigestion or more serious disorders, such as alcoholism. Medical name: **singultus**.

Hickman catheter a fine plastic cannula usually inserted into the subclavian vein in the neck to allow administration of drugs and repeated blood samples. The catheter is tunnelled for several centimetres beneath the skin to prevent infection entering the bloodstream. It is used most frequently in patients receiving long-term chemotherapy, particularly infusion regimes (e.g. fluorouracil).

hidr- (hidro-) *combining form denoting* sweat. Example: **hidropoiesis** (formation of).

hidradenitis suppurativa an unpleasant condition characterized by deep abscesses in the armpits, groin, and anogenital regions leading to sinuses and bridge scarring. It is regarded as part of the *follicular occlusion tetrad. It is three times more common in women and may be under androgen control. Treatment is with long-term antibiotics, anti-androgens, or occasionally surgery. The condition is difficult to treat but often resolves spontaneously after many years.

hidrosis *n.* 1. the excretion of sweat. 2. excessive sweating.

hidrotic *n.* an agent that causes sweating. *Parasympathomimetic drugs are hidrotics.

HIE *see* HYPOXIC-ISCHAEMIC ENCEPHALOPA-THY.

HIFU high-intensity focused *ultrasound: a minimally invasive technique that is undergoing clinical trials for the treatment of localized prostate cancer. An ultrasound probe is inserted into the rectum and precisely focuses a beam of high-intensity ultrasound on the cancerous tissue resulting in coagulative necrosis.

high-density lipoprotein (HDL) the smallest and densest of the *lipoproteins that carry cholesterol and triglycerides around the body, which is derived mainly from precursors produced in the liver. HDL has an important role in reverse cholesterol transfer, i.e. the removal of cholesterol from the circulation and the blood vessel walls and its transfer to the liver. Higher levels of HDL have been shown to be associated with lower levels of cardiovascular disease.

high-dependency unit (HDU) a hospital unit that provides specialist nursing care to seriously ill patients. The level of care given is greater than that available on general wards but less than in *intensive therapy units.

high-intensity focused ultrasound *see* HIFU, ULTRASOUND.

hilar cell tumour an androgen-producing tumour of the ovary found in older women and often resulting in *virilization. Such tumours are so called as they tend to occur around the area of the ovary where the blood vessels enter (the hilum). They are usually small and are treated by surgical removal, with resolution of most of the symptoms.

hilum *n.* (*pl.* **hila**) a hollow situated on the surface of an organ, such as the ovary, kidney, or spleen, at which structures such as blood vessels, nerve fibres, and ducts enter or leave it.

hindbrain (rhombencephalon) *n.* the part of the *brain comprising the cerebellum, pons, and medulla oblongata. The pons and medulla contain the nuclei of many of the cranial nerves, which issue from their surfaces, and the reticular formation. The fluid-filled cavity in the midline is the fourth *ventricle.

hindgut *n.* the back part of the embryonic gut, which gives rise to part of the large intestine, the rectum, bladder, and urinary ducts. *See also* CLOACA.

hindquarter amputation an operation involving removal of an entire leg and part or all of the pelvis associated with it. It is usually performed for soft tissue or bone sarcomas arising from the upper thigh, hip, or buttock. *Compare* FOREQUARTER AMPUTATION.

hinge joint *see* GINGLYMUS.

hip *n.* the region of the body where the thigh bone (femur) articulates with the *pelvis: the region on each side of the pelvis.

hip bone (innominate bone) a bone formed by the fusion of the ilium, ischium, and pubis. It articulates with the femur by the **acetabulum** of the ilium, a deep socket into which the head of the femur fits (*see* HIP JOINT). Between the pubis and ischium, below and slightly in front of the acetabulum, is a large opening – the **obturator foramen**. The right and left hip bones form part of the *pelvis.

hip girdle *see* PELVIC GIRDLE.

hip joint the ball-and-socket joint (*see* ENARTHROSIS) between the head of the femur and the acetabulum (socket) of the ilium (*see* HIP BONE). It is a common site of osteoarthritis and rheumatoid arthritis, which is often treated surgically (by *hip replacement). *See also* CONGENITAL DISLOCATION OF THE HIP.

Hippelates *n.* a genus of small flies. The adults of *H. pallipes* are suspected of transmitting *yaws in the West Indies. Other species of *Hippelates* may be involved in the transmission of conjunctivitis.

hippocampal formation a curved band of cortex lying within each cerebral hemisphere: in evolutionary terms one of the brain's most primitive parts. It forms a portion of the *limbic system and is involved in the complex physical aspects of behaviour governed by emotion and instinct.

hippocampus *n.* a swelling in the floor of the lateral *ventricle of the brain. It contains complex foldings of cortical tissue and is involved, with other connections of the *hippocampal formation, in the workings of the *limbic system. —**hippocampal** *adj.*

Hippocratic oath an oath that is often assumed to be taken but is actually rarely sworn by doctors. It is a code of behaviour and practice commonly attributed to the

Greek physician Hippocrates (460–370 BC), known as the 'Father of Medicine', and taken by the students of the medical school in Cos where he taught, but both the authorship and application of the oath to Hippocrates' students has been disputed. *See also* BENEFICENCE, MEDICAL ETHICS.

Hippuran *n.* trade name for sodium iodohippurate, used as a contrast medium in radiology of the urinary tract. Labelled with iodine-131, it can be used to measure renal function, although it has now largely been replaced by other agents.

hippus *n.* abnormal rhythmical variations in the size of the pupils, independent of the intensity of the light falling on the eyes. It is occasionally seen in various diseases of the nervous system.

hip replacement a surgical procedure developed for replacing a diseased hip joint with a prosthesis. A plastic or metal cup forms the socket, and the head of the femur is replaced by a metal ball on a stem placed inside the femur. There are many types of prosthesis, which can be fixed to the bone with or without cement. *See also* ARTHROPLASTY.

Hirschsprung's disease a congenital condition in which the rectum and sometimes part of the lower colon have failed to develop a normal nerve network. The affected portion does not expand or conduct the contents of the bowel, which accumulate in and distend the upper colon. Symptoms, which are usually apparent in the first weeks of life, are vomiting, constipation, abdominal distension, and intestinal obstruction. Diagnosis is by X-ray and by microscopic examination of samples of the bowel wall, which shows the absence of nerve cells. Treatment is by surgery to remove the affected segment and join the remaining (normal) colon to the anus. *See also* MEGACOLON. [H. Hirschsprung (1830–1916), Danish physician]

hirsutism *n.* the presence of coarse pigmented hair on the face, chest, upper back, or abdomen in a female as a result of *hyperandrogenism (excessive production of androgen). *See also* VIRILIZATION.

hirudin *n.* an *anticoagulant present in the salivary glands of *leeches and in certain snake venoms that prevents *blood coagulation by inhibiting the action of the enzyme *thrombin. The anticoagulants **lepirudin**

(Refludan) and **bivalirudin** (Angiox) are genetically engineered forms of hirudin from the medicinal leech.

hist- (histio-, histo-) *combining form denoting* tissue.

histaminase *n.* an enzyme, widely distributed in the body, that is responsible for the inactivation of histamine.

histamine *n.* a compound derived from the amino acid histidine. It is found in nearly all tissues of the body, associated mainly with the *mast cells. Histamine has pronounced pharmacological activity, causing dilation of blood vessels and contraction of smooth muscle (for example, in the lungs). It is an important mediator of inflammation and is released in large amounts after skin damage (such as that due to animal venoms and toxins), producing a characteristic skin reaction (consisting of flushing, a flare, and a weal). Histamine is also released in anaphylactic reactions and allergic conditions, including asthma, and gives rise to some of the symptoms of these conditions. *See also* ANAPHYLAXIS, ANTIHISTAMINE.

histamine acid phosphate a derivative of *histamine that was formerly used to test for acid secretion in the stomach in conditions involving abnormal gastric acid secretion, such as *Zollinger-Ellison syndrome.

histidine *n.* an *amino acid from which *histamine is derived.

histiocyte *n.* a fixed *macrophage, i.e. one that is stationary within connective tissue.

histiocytoma *n.* a tumour that contains *macrophages or *histiocytes, large cells with the ability to engulf foreign matter and bacteria. *See also* FIBROSARCOMA (MALIGNANT FIBROUS HISTIOCYTOMA).

histiocytosis *n.* any of a group of diseases in which there are abnormalities in certain large phagocytic cells (*histiocytes) due to (1) abnormal storage of fats, as in *Gaucher's disease; (2) inflammatory disorders, as in *Langerhans cell histiocytosis, which includes disorders previously called histiocytosis X; or (3) malignant proliferation of histiocytes.

histochemistry *n.* the study of the identification and distribution of chemical compounds within and between cells, by means of stains, indicators, and light and electron microscopy. —**histochemical** *adj.*

histocompatibility *n.* the form of *compatibility that depends upon tissue components, mainly specific glycoprotein antigens in cell membranes. A high degree of histocompatibility is necessary for a tissue graft or organ transplant to be successful. —**histocompatible** *adj.*

histogenesis *n.* the formation of tissues.

histogram *n.* a form of statistical graph in which values are plotted in the form of rectangles on a chart; a bar-chart.

histoid *adj.* **1.** resembling normal tissue. **2.** composed of one type of tissue.

histological grade the degree of *differentiation of a tumour. Typically, grade 1 resembles normal tissue (well-differentiated) and grade 3 is very abnormal (poorly differentiated) and has a poorer prognosis.

histology *n.* the study of the structure of tissues by means of special staining techniques combined with light and electron microscopy. —**histological** *adj.*

histone *n.* a simple protein that combines with a nucleic acid to form a *nucleoprotein.

Histoplasma *n.* a genus of parasitic yeast-like fungi. The species *H. capsulatum* causes the respiratory infection *histoplasmosis.

histoplasmin *n.* a preparation of antigenic material from a culture of the fungus *Histoplasma capsulatum*, used to test for the presence of the disease *histoplasmosis by subcutaneous injection.

histoplasmosis *n.* an infection caused by inhaling spores of the fungus *Histoplasma capsulatum*. The primary pulmonary form usually produces no symptoms or harmful effects and is recognized retrospectively by X-rays and positive *histoplasmin skin testing. Occasionally, progressive histoplasmosis, which resembles tuberculosis, develops. The fungus may spread via the bloodstream to attack other organs, such as the liver, spleen, lymph nodes, or intestine. Symptomatic disease is treated with intravenous amphotericin. The spores are found in soil contaminated with faeces, especially from chickens and bats. The disease is endemic in the northern and central USA, Argentina, Brazil, Venezuela, and parts of Africa.

histotoxic *adj.* poisonous to tissues: applied to certain substances and conditions.

HIV (human immunodeficiency virus) a

*retrovirus responsible for *AIDS. There are two varieties, HIV-1 and HIV-2; the latter is most common in Africa. *See also* HTLV.

HIVAN human immunodeficiency virus-associated nephropathy: a condition associated with HIV infection. The patient usually presents with nephrotic-range proteinuria (*see* NEPHROTIC SYNDROME) with microscopic haematuria, without oedema but with a rapid decline in renal function. Enlargement of the kidneys on ultrasound examination is a common finding, and HIVAN may precede other manifestations of HIV infection. Typical renal pathological findings are of a collapsing form of *focal segmental glomerulosclerosis. The clinical course is usually one of rapid decline in renal function.

hives *n. see* URTICARIA.

HLA system human leucocyte antigen system: a series of four gene families (termed A, B, C, and D) that code for polymorphic proteins expressed on the surface of most nucleated cells. Individuals inherit from each parent one gene (or set of genes) for each subdivision of the HLA system. If two individuals have identical HLA types, they are said to be histocompatible. Successful tissue transplantation requires a minimum number of HLA differences between donor and recipient tissues.

HMG CoA reductase *h*ydroxy*m*ethylglutaryl *co*enzyme *A* reductase: the key rate-limiting enzyme that is involved in the production of cholesterol in the liver. Inhibition of its action is the mechanism by which the *statin group of lipid-lowering agents work.

H1N1 *see* SWINE INFLUENZA.

H5N1 *see* AVIAN INFLUENZA.

HNPCC *see* HEREDITARY NONPOLYPOSIS COLORECTAL CANCER.

hobnail liver the liver of a patient with cirrhosis, which has a knobbly appearance caused by regenerating nodules separated by bands of fibrous tissue.

Hodgkin's disease a malignant disease of lymphatic tissue – a form of *lymphoma – usually characterized by painless enlargement of one or more groups of lymph nodes in the neck, axillae (armpits), groin, chest, or abdomen; the spleen, liver, bone marrow, and bones may also be involved. Apart from the enlarging nodes, there may also be weight loss, fever, profuse sweating at night, and itching (known as **B symptoms**). Hodgkin's disease is distinguished from other forms of lymphoma by the presence of large binucleate cells (**Reed-Sternberg cells**) in the affected lymph nodes. Treatment depends on the extent of disease and may include surgery, radiotherapy, drug therapy, or a combination of these. Drugs used in the treatment of the disease include vincristine, procarbazine, prednisolone, chlorambucil, and vinblastine. Many patients can be cured; in the early stages of the disease this may be in the order of 85% or more. [T. Hodgkin (1798–1866), British physician]

Hoffmann's sign (finger-flexion reflex) an abnormal reflex elicited by flicking the distal phalanx of the patient's middle finger sharply downwards. Hoffmann's sign is positive when there is a brisk flexion response in the index finger and thumb. It indicates an upper *motor neuron response due to a disorder at or above the cervical (neck) level of the spinal cord. [J. Hoffmann (1857–1919), German neurologist]

hole in the heart *see* SEPTAL DEFECT.

holistic *adj.* describing an approach to patient care in which the physical, mental, and social factors in the patient's condition are taken into account, rather than just the diagnosed disease. The term is applied to a range of orthodox and complementary methods of treatment. *See also* COMPLEMENTARY MEDICINE.

Hollister ring a watertight adherent ring placed around an intestinal *stoma and incorporating a flange to which a disposable plastic bag could be attached. It was the forerunner of modern disposable stoma bags.

Holmes-Adie syndrome *see* ADIE'S SYNDROME.

holmium:YAG laser a type of *YAG laser that uses a short-pulsed high-energy beam with a wavelength of 2100 nm to cut, perforate, and fragment tissue. It has a penetration of 0.4 mm. This laser is used in the fragmentation of urinary tract calculi (stones) and in *enucleation of the prostate gland.

holo- *combining form denoting* complete or entire.

holocrine *adj.* describing a gland or type

of secretion in which the entire cell disintegrates when the product is released.

Homans' sign a test for deep vein thrombosis of the calf. With the patient lying supine, the examiner squeezes the calf firmly and dorsiflexes the foot; the test is positive if deep-seated pain is felt in the calf. [J. Homans (1877–1954), US physician]

home delivery *see* COMMUNITY MIDWIFE.

home help *see* CARE ASSISTANT.

homeo- (homoeo-) *combining form denoting* similar; like.

homeopathy (homoeopathy) *n.* a complementary therapy based on the theory that 'like cures like'. It involves treating a condition with a tiny dose of a substance that in larger doses would normally cause or aggravate that condition. The dose (so diluted as to be indistinguishable from pure water) is activated by shaking in an exact way. Homeopathy was developed by a German doctor, Samuel Hahnemann (1755–1843), in 1796. —**homeopathic** *adj.* —**homeopathist** *n.*

homeostasis *n.* the physiological process by which the internal systems of the body (e.g. blood pressure, body temperature, *acid-base balance) are maintained at equilibrium, despite variations in the external conditions. —**homeostatic** *adj.*

home visit *see* DOMICILIARY CONSULTATION.

homo- *combining form denoting* the same or common.

homocysteine *n.* a sulphur-containing amino acid that is an intermediate in the synthesis of *cysteine. A deficiency in the enzyme cystathionine synthetase results in elevated levels in the blood of homocysteine and homocystine (an oxidized form of homocysteine), resulting in elevated urinary levels (*see* HOMOCYSTINURIA). It is becoming increasingly recognized that elevated levels of homocysteine in the blood are a risk factor for vascular disease independent of diabetes, hypertension, elevated levels of cholesterol in the blood, and smoking. Levels are also elevated in vitamin B_{12} deficiency.

homocystinuria *n.* an *inborn error of metabolism, inherited as an autosomal *recessive trait, caused by an enzyme deficiency resulting in an excess of *homocysteine in the blood and the presence of homocystine in the urine. Clinically affected individuals are mentally retarded, excessively tall with long fingers (due to overgrowth of bones), generally have loose ligaments (which may result in dislocation of the lens), and have a tendency to form blood clots in the veins and arteries, leading to strokes. Treatment is by diet, which may allow for normal development if the disease is recognized early enough, and high-dose vitamin B_6 therapy.

homoeopathy *n. see* HOMEOPATHY.

homogametic *adj.* describing the sex that produces only one kind of gamete, which carries the same *sex chromosome, and that therefore does not determine the sex of the offspring. In humans women are the homogametic sex: each egg cell carries an X chromosome. *Compare* HETEROGAMETIC.

homogenize *vb.* to reduce material to a uniform consistency, e.g. by crushing and mixing. Organs and tissues are homogenized to determine their overall content of a particular enzyme or other substance. **—homogenization** *n.*

homogentisic acid a product formed during the metabolism of the amino acids phenylalanine and tyrosine. In normal individuals homogentisic acid is oxidized by the enzyme **homogentisic acid oxidase**. In rare cases this enzyme is lacking and a condition known as *alcaptonuria, in which large amounts of homogentisic acid are excreted in the urine, results.

homograft *n. see* ALLOGRAFT.

homoiothermic *adj.* warm-blooded: able to maintain a constant body temperature independently of, and despite variations in, the temperature of the surroundings. Mammals (including humans) and birds are homoiothermic. *Compare* POIKILOTHERMIC. **—homoiothermy** *n.*

homolateral *adj. see* IPSILATERAL.

homologous *adj.* **1.** (in anatomy) describing organs or parts that have the same basic structure and evolutionary origin, but not necessarily the same function or superficial structure. *Compare* ANALOGOUS. **2.** (in genetics) describing a pair of chromosomes of similar shape and size and having identical gene loci. One member of the pair is derived from the mother; the other from the father.

homonymous *adj.* describing a visual defect in which the visual field to one side of

the body is restricted in both eyes (*see* HEMIANOPIA).

homozygous *adj.* describing an individual in whom the members of a pair of genes determining a particular characteristic are identical. *See* ALLELE. *Compare* HETEROZYGOUS. **—homozygote** *n.*

homunculus *n.* **1.** (manikin) a dwarf with no deformity or abnormality other than small size. **2.** (manikin) a small jointed anatomical model of a man. **3.** (in early biological theory) a miniature human being thought to be contained within each of the reproductive cells.

honeycomb lung the honeycomb pattern seen on X-ray at the later stages of chronic lung conditions, in which the lungs become less elastic and more fibrotic. Once the honeycomb appearance is visible on the X-ray, the lungs are likely to progress to respiratory failure.

HONK *see* HYPEROSMOLAR NON-KETOTIC STATE.

hook *n.* a surgical instrument with a bent or curved tip, used to hold, lift, or retract tissue at operation.

hookworm *n.* either of two nematode worms, *Necator americanus* or *Ancylostoma duodenale*, which live as parasites in the human intestine. Both species, also known as the New and Old World hookworms respectively, are of great medical importance (*see* HOOKWORM DISEASE).

hookworm disease a condition resulting from an infestation of the small intestine by hookworms. Hookworm larvae live in the soil and infect humans by penetrating the skin. The worms travel to the lungs in the bloodstream and from there pass via the windpipe and gullet to the small intestine. Heavy hookworm infections may cause considerable damage to the wall of the intestine, leading to a serious loss of blood; this, in conjunction with malnutrition, can provoke severe anaemia. Symptoms include itching and rash at the site of infection, followed by abdominal pain, diarrhoea, debility, and mental inertia. More serious effects can include difficulty in breathing, heart enlargement, and irregular heartbeat. The disease occurs mostly in the tropics and subtropics; mebendazole is used in treatment.

hordeolum *n. see* STYE.

horizontal transmission the spread of an infectious agent from one person or group to another, usually through contact with contaminated material, such as sputum or faeces. *Compare* VERTICAL TRANSMISSION.

hormone *n.* a substance that is produced in one part of the body (by an *endocrine gland, such as the thyroid, adrenal, or pituitary), passes into the bloodstream and is carried to other (distant) organs or tissues, where it acts to modify their structure or function. Examples of hormones are corticosteroids (from the adrenal cortex), adrenaline (from the adrenal medulla), androgens and oestrogens (from the testis and ovary, respectively), thyroid hormone (from the thyroid gland), and insulin (from the islets of Langerhans). The *pituitary gland secretes a variety of hormones, whose release is controlled by specific releasing hormones.

hormone-binding globulins a family of plasma proteins whose function is to bind free hormone molecules to varying degrees and thus reduce their function. Alterations in levels of the binding globulins, for example during pregnancy or ill health, can result in variations in assays of hormone levels in individuals. Examples include **thyroid-binding globulin**, **sex-hormone-binding globulin**, and **corticosteroid-binding globulin**.

hormone replacement therapy (HRT) the use of female hormones for the relief of symptoms resulting from cessation of ovarian function, either at the time of the natural *menopause or following surgical removal of the ovaries. Oestrogenic hormones may be prescribed orally, transdermally (as skin patches or gel), or by subcutaneous implant. The combination of progestogen with oestrogen is preferred if the woman has retained her uterus, since administration of oestrogen alone might cause overstimulation of the endometrium or even cancer. HRT is effective against *vasomotor symptoms (e.g. hot flushes) and genitourinary atrophy (causing vaginal dryness); for the best results it should be started as soon as the symptoms first appear. Because studies indicate that HRT may increase the risk of breast cancer, stroke, and other conditions associated with ageing, it should be used only in the short term (no more than five years) in women over 50 and is no longer recommended for the prevention of osteoporosis.

horn *n.* (in anatomy) a process, outgrowth, or extension of an organ or other structure. It is often paired. In the spinal cord crescent-shaped areas of grey matter (seen in cross section) are known as the dorsal and ventral horns.

Horner's syndrome a syndrome consisting of a constricted pupil (miosis), drooping of the upper eyelid (*ptosis), and an absence of sweating over the affected side of the face. The symptoms are due to a disorder of the sympathetic nerves in the brainstem or cervical (neck) region. [J. F. Horner (1831–86), Swiss ophthalmologist]

horseshoe kidney an anatomical variation in kidney development whereby the lower poles of both kidneys are joined together. This usually causes no trouble but it may be associated with impaired drainage of urine from the kidney by the ureters, which cross in front of the united lower segment.

hospice *n.* an institution that provides palliative or end-of-life care for people with terminal illnesses. Most modern hospices are modelled on St Christopher's Hospice, founded in London in 1967 by Dame Cicely Saunders. They specialize in symptom management and maintaining the psychological wellbeing of patients. Support for the families of the patients is also a feature of the services provided by most hospices. **Hospice at Home** services provide specialist palliative care for terminally ill patients in their own homes.

hospital *n.* an institution providing medical or psychiatric care and treatment of patients. Such care may be residential (in-patient), including the care of patients for a whole day and their return home at night (day care). Out-patient services include consultation with specialists by prior appointment, X-rays, laboratory tests, physiotherapy, and accident and emergency services for those requiring urgent care. Most health districts have a **district general hospital** (**DGH**), which provides sufficient basic services for the population of the district. Some larger hospitals have resources that are more highly specialized, to meet the needs of a wider population, providing so-called **regional** or **supraregional** (**national**) services. Such hospitals often provide training for medical students (**teaching** or **university hospitals**) and for postgraduate education. Some smaller hospitals – known as **community hospitals** – may be staffed by general practitioners and are intended for people for whom home care is not practicable on social grounds. Since 1991 hospitals have become self-governing NHS acute *trusts, their income deriving chiefly from contracts to provide services to *primary care trusts. *Foundation trusts are hospitals with greater freedoms and flexibilities than acute trusts.

Hospital Episode Statistics (HES) (in England) a database containing data on all admissions to NHS hospitals and admissions of NHS patients treated elsewhere. *See* RECORD LINKAGE.

hospital fatality rate *see* CASE FATALITY RATE.

hospital infection *see* NOSOCOMIAL INFECTION.

hospital social worker a social worker employed to assist hospital patients with social problems that may arise through illness. *See also* SOCIAL SERVICES.

host *n.* an animal or plant in or upon which a *parasite lives. An **intermediate host** is one in which the parasite passes its larval or asexual stages; a **definitive host** is one in which the parasite develops to its sexual stage.

Hounsfield unit the numerical unit assigned electronically to each *pixel in a computerized tomography (CT) image, according to its X-ray density. The fixed points on the scale are arbitrarily assigned as −1000 for air and 0 for water. The CT image is viewed in a 'window'. The range of Hounsfield units displayed (window width) and the centre point of the range of interest (window level) can be varied by the radiologist in order to observe specific tissues (*see* WINDOWING). The unit was named after Sir Godfrey Hounsfield (1919–2004), who developed CT scanning in the 1950s. Symbol: HU.

hourglass stomach a deformity of the stomach in which the 'waist' is constricted by fibrosis caused by a chronic peptic ulcer, producing an upper and a lower cavity separated by a narrow channel.

house-dust mite *see* DERMATOPHAGOIDES.

housemaid's knee (prepatellar bursitis) inflammation and resultant swelling of the bursa in front of the kneecap, usually due to repetitive friction and pressure over the kneecap, as from frequent episodes of prolonged kneeling. Treatment includes pressure bandaging, *NSAIDs, and avoidance of kneeling. *See* BURSITIS.

house officer/physician/surgeon *see* DOCTOR.

HPA *see* HEALTH PROTECTION AGENCY.

HPV *see* HUMAN PAPILLOMAVIRUS.

H₂-receptor antagonist *see* ANTIHISTAMINE.

HRT *see* HORMONE REPLACEMENT THERAPY.

HSE *see* HEALTH AND SAFETY EXECUTIVE.

5HT 5-hydroxytryptamine (*see* SEROTONIN).

5HT₁ agonist (triptan) any one of a class of drugs that stimulate *serotonin (5-hydroxytryptamine) receptors and are effective in the relief of *migraine headaches by causing constriction of cerebral blood vessels. The group includes **almotriptan** (Almogran), **naratriptan** (Naramig), *sumatriptan, and **zolmitriptan** (Zomig).

HTLV human T-cell leukaemia/lymphoma virus (or lymphocytotrophic virus) – a family of viruses that includes HTLV-I, which causes lymphoma. *HIV (the AIDS virus) was formerly called HTLV-III.

HU *see* HOUNSFIELD UNIT.

Hudson-Stähli line a linear horizontal yellowish line seen in the deep epithelium of ageing corneas. [A. C. Hudson (1875–1962), British ophthalmologist; J. Stähli (20th century), Swiss ophthalmologist]

Hughes syndrome *see* ANTIPHOSPHOLIPID ANTIBODY SYNDROME. [G. Hughes (21st century), British physician]

human chorionic gonadotrophin (hCG) a hormone, similar to the pituitary *gonadotrophins, that is produced by the placenta during pregnancy. hCG maintains the secretion of *progesterone by the corpus luteum of the ovary, the secretion of pituitary gonadotrophins being blocked during pregnancy. Large amounts are excreted in the urine, and this is used as the basis for most *pregnancy tests. Serum hCG monitoring is used for tracking early pregnancy and detecting *ectopic pregnancies (in which the level will not double over a 48-hour period, as it does with normal pregnancies). The level of hCG in the serum is also one of the indicators used in *prenatal screening tests: levels are higher in pregnancies affected by Down's syndrome in comparison with normal pregnancies (see also PAPP-A, TRIPLE TEST). Levels of hCG are very high in *gestational trophoblastic neoplasia. Some malignant tumours (e.g. malignant teratoma, endodermal sinus tumour) secrete hCG, which can be used as a *tumour marker. A preparation of hCG is given by injection to treat fertility problems due to ovulation disorders and to induce *superovulation in in vitro fertilization.

human chorionic somatomammotrophin see HUMAN PLACENTAL LACTOGEN.

Human Fertilization and Embryology Act 1990 an Act of Parliament that makes provisions for human embryos and children produced as a result of assisted conception. The 1990 Act was reviewed and significantly amended by the Human Fertilization and Embryology Act 2008. The increasing developments in reproductive medicine mean that it is no longer possible to define legal parentage solely on a genetic basis. Under the Act, a person must give written informed *consent before tissue is removed for use in assisted conception. The legal mother is defined as the woman who has given birth to the child, regardless of genetic parentage, unless the child is subsequently adopted or (in the case of children born to *surrogate mothers) a *section 30 order is made. The legal father is generally the genetic father except when the latter is a licensed sperm donor or when the donor's sperm is used after his death. When a woman conceives as a result of assisted conception, her spouse may be regarded as the child's legal father, even if he is not the genetic father, as long as he consented to her treatment.

The Act also established the **Human Fertilization and Embryology Authority**, which controls, regulates, and reviews practice and research involving the use of embryos and issues licences for research and for treatment in assisted conception. It also maintains a register of persons whose gametes are used for assisted conception and of children born as a result.

( ) SEE WEB LINKS

• Website of the Human Fertilization and Embryology Authority: provides information and guidance for patients, professionals, donors, and donor-conceived people

Human Genome Project a massive international research project to isolate all the genes in human DNA and determine the sequence of genes on human chromosomes.

The project began in 1988 and the full draft sequence was published in 2001; the high-quality sequence was completed in 2003. The human genome comprises some 3×10^9 nucleotide base pairs (see DNA) forming 22,000–25,000 genes, distributed among 23 pairs of chromosomes. Knowledge of the entire human genome has already resulted in the identification of the genes associated with many hereditary disorders and revealed the existence of a genetic basis or component for many other diseases not previously known to have one. Theoretically, this would enable the development of targeted drugs and the large-scale genetic screening of populations. See PHARMACOGENOMICS, TARGETED AGENT.

human immunodeficiency virus see HIV.

humanity n. 1. the state or quality of being human. In most ethical traditions, membership of the human species is seen as conferring a unique moral status, so that human life is considered inherently and particularly valuable and worthy of protection (see SANCTITY OF LIFE). Humanity may be defined in terms of a unique capacity to feel, reason, evoke emotional responses, or form relationships (see PERSONHOOD). 2. compassion or benevolence.

human leucocyte antigen system see HLA SYSTEM.

human menopausal gonadotrophins commercially available preparations of *follicle-stimulating hormone and *luteinizing hormone (**menotrophin**; Merional, Menopur) or follicle-stimulating hormone alone (**urofollitropin**; Fostimon). Administered by intramuscular or subcutaneous injection, they are used mainly to treat infertility in women with gonadotrophin deficiency due to hypopituitarism and to stimulate super-ovulation in women undergoing in vitro fertilization.

human papillomavirus (HPV) a virus – a member of the *papovavirus group – that causes warts, including genital warts. There are over 50 strains of HPV: certain strains are considered to be causative factors in the development of anal and genital cancers, especially cervical cancer, but additional factors are necessary before the cells become malignant. HPV is one of the most common sexually transmitted infections. In women the presence of HPV may be detected on colposcopic examination, although techniques using DNA amplification (*see* POLYMERASE CHAIN REACTION) give more accurate results and suggest that up to 40% of a normal, apparently healthy, female population may harbour these viruses. In women with an abnormal cervical smear, the DNA test is found to be positive in a much higher percentage and is therefore a useful indicator of a high risk of developing cancer of the cervix. The **HPV vaccine** provides protection against strains of HPV associated with cervical cancer and other precancerous conditions (Ceravix, Gardasil) and against genital warts (Gardasil).

human placental lactogen (human chorionic somatomammotrophin) a protein hormone of 190 amino acids produced by the placenta during most but not all pregnancies. Despite its name it does not appear to have a role in lactation and its exact function remains obscure. It does, however, seem to contribute to the development of diabetes in some pregnancies.

human rights a legal framework adopted by the United Nations following World War II that sought to define and promote fundamental entitlements, conditions, and freedoms to be afforded to all human beings. In the UK the Human Rights Act 1998 enacts the provisions of the 1950 European Convention on Human Rights, which sets out, via fourteen articles, an individual's rights, entitlements, and freedoms.

Human Tissue Authority the UK government agency, established by the Human Tissue Act 2004, that regulates the removal, use, and storage of human organs and tissue from both the living and the deceased for certain purposes as defined by the statute. These purposes include clinical research, clinical audit, and medical education. Anyone handling such material for those purposes should have a licence issued by the authority. Membership of the authority comprises clinical, scientific, academic, and lay representatives.

(⊕) SEE WEB LINKS
• Website of the Human Tissue Authority

humectant 1. *n.* a substance that is used for moistening. 2. *adj.* causing moistening.

humerus *n.* the bone of the upper arm (see illustration). The **head** of the humerus articulates with the *scapula at the shoulder joint. At the lower end of the shaft the

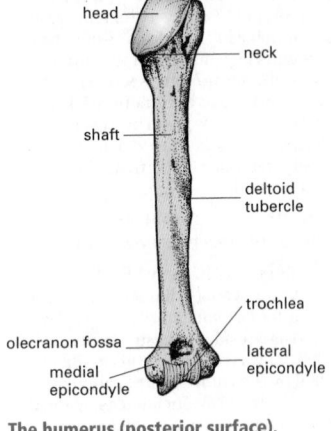

The humerus (posterior surface).

trochlea articulates with the *ulna and part of the radius. The radius also articulates with a rounded protuberance (the **capitulum**) close to the trochlea. Depressions (**fossae**) at the front and back of the humerus accommodate the ulna and radius, respectively, when the arm is flexed or straightened.

humoral *adj.* circulating in the bloodstream; humoral *immunity requires circulating antibodies.

humour *n.* a body fluid. *See* AQUEOUS HUMOUR, VITREOUS HUMOUR.

hunchback deformity *see* KYPHOS.

Hunner's ulcer *see* INTERSTITIAL CYSTITIS. [G. L. Hunner (1868–1957), US urologist]

Hunter's syndrome a hereditary disorder caused by deficiency of an enzyme that results in the accumulation of protein–carbohydrate complexes and fats in the cells of the body (*see* MUCOPOLYSACCHARIDOSIS). This leads to mental retardation, enlargement of the liver and spleen, and prominent coarse facial features (**gargoylism**). The disease is *sex-linked, being restricted to males, although females can be *carriers. Medical name: **mucopolysaccharidosis type II**. [C. H. Hunter (1872–1955), US physician]

Huntington's disease (Huntington's chorea) a hereditary disease caused by a defect in a single gene that is inherited as an autosomal *dominant characteristic, therefore tending to appear in half of the children of the parents with this condition. Symptoms, which begin to appear in early middle age, include unsteady gait and jerky involuntary movements (*see* CHOREA), accompanied later by behavioural changes, and progressive dementia. There is a defect in the Huntington gene on chromosome 4; *genetic screening is possible for those at risk. [G. Huntington (1850–1916), US physician]

Hurler's syndrome a hereditary disorder caused by deficiency of an enzyme that results in the accumulation of protein–carbohydrate complexes and fats in the cells of the body (*see* MUCOPOLYSACCHARIDOSIS). This leads to severe mental retardation, enlargement of the liver and spleen, heart defects, deformities of the bones, and coarsening and thickening of facial features (**gargoylism**). A bone marrow transplant offers the only hope of treatment. Medical name: **mucopolysaccharidosis type I**. [G. Hurler (1889–1965), Austrian paediatrician]

Hürthle cell tumour a malignant tumour of the thyroid gland that arises from **Hürthle** (or **Askanazy**) **cells**, altered follicular cells of the gland that have large nuclei and stain deeply with eosin (these cells are also found in benign nodules and Hashimoto's disease). Hürthle cell carcinoma is not as common as papillary, follicular, or anaplastic thyroid carcinomas (*see* THYROID CANCER). [K. W. Hürthle (1860–1945), German histologist]

Hutchinson's teeth narrowed and notched permanent incisor teeth: a sign of congenital *syphilis. [J. Hutchinson (1828–1913), British surgeon]

hyal- (hyalo-) *combining form denoting* 1. glassy; transparent. 2. hyalin. 3. the vitreous humour of the eye.

hyalin *n.* a clear glassy material produced as the result of degeneration in certain tissues, particularly connective tissue and epithelial cells.

hyaline cartilage the most common type of *cartilage: a bluish-white elastic material with a matrix of chondroitin sulphate in which fine collagen fibrils are embedded.

hyaline membrane disease *see* RESPIRATORY DISTRESS SYNDROME.

hyalitis *n.* inflammation of the *vitreous humour of the eye. *See also* ASTEROID HYALOSIS.

hyaloid artery a fetal artery lying in the

*hyaloid canal of the eye and supplying the lens.

hyaloid canal a channel within the vitreous humour of the *eye. It extends from the centre of the optic disc, where it communicates with the lymph spaces of the optic nerve, to the posterior wall of the lens.

hyaloid membrane the transparent membrane that surrounds the *vitreous humour of the eye, separating it from the retina.

hyaluronic acid an acid *mucopolysaccharide that acts as the binding and protective agent of the ground substance of connective tissue. It is also present in the synovial fluid around joints and in the vitreous and aqueous humours of the eye.

hyaluronidase *n.* an enzyme that depolymerizes *hyaluronic acid and therefore increases the permeability of connective tissue. Hyaluronidase is found in the testes, in semen, and in other tissues.

hybrid *n.* the offspring of a cross between two genetically unlike individuals. A hybrid, whose parents are usually of different species or varieties, is often sterile.

HYCOSY (hysterosalpingo-contrast sonography) an out-patient technique that tests for blocked Fallopian tubes. Using *transvaginal ultrasonography following the injection of an echo contrast medium through the cervix, flow along the tubes can be reliably visualized. *See also* DOPPLER ULTRASOUND.

hydatid *n.* a bladder-like cyst formed in various human tissues following the growth of the larval stage of an *Echinococcus* tapeworm. *E. granulosus* produces a single large fluid-filled cyst, called **unilocular hydatid**, which gives rise internally to smaller daughter cysts. The entire hydatid is bound by a fibrous capsule. *E. multilocularis* forms aggregates of many smaller cysts with a jelly-like matrix, called an **alveolar hydatid**, and enlarges by budding off external daughter cysts. Alveolar hydatids are not delimited by fibrous capsules and produce malignant tumours, which invade and destroy human tissues. *See also* HYDATID DISEASE.

hydatid disease (hydatidosis, echinococciasis, echinococcosis) a condition resulting from the presence in the liver, lungs, or brain of *hydatid cysts. The cysts of *Echinococcus multilocularis* form malignant tumours;

those of *E. granulosus* exert pressure as they grow and thereby damage surrounding tissues. The presence of hydatids in the brain may result in blindness and epilepsy, and the rupture of any cyst can cause severe allergic reactions including fever and *urticaria. Treatment may necessitate surgical removal of the cysts. Spread of hydatid disease, particularly common in sheep-raising countries, can be prevented by the deworming of dogs.

hydatidiform mole a collection of fluid-filled sacs that develop when the membrane (chorion) surrounding the embryo degenerates in early pregnancy with proliferation of the *trophoblast. These sacs give the placenta the appearance of a bunch of grapes and a characteristic snowstorm appearance on ultrasound. The levels of hCG are abnormally high. Hydatidiform mole can be subdivided into complete and partial mole based on genetic and histological features. Complete moles show no evidence of fetal tissue; there is usually evidence of a fetus or fetal red blood cells with a partial mole. The widespread use of ultrasound has led to earlier diagnosis and has changed the pattern of molar pregnancy. The majority of women present with symptoms of early pregnancy failure. *See* GESTATIONAL TROPHOBLASTIC DISEASE.

hydatidosis *n. see* HYDATID DISEASE.

hydr- (hydro-) *combining form denoting* water or a watery fluid.

hydraemia *n.* the presence in the blood of more than the normal proportion of water.

hydralazine *n.* a *vasodilator drug used, usually in conjunction with *diuretics, to treat hypertension. It is given by mouth or by intravenous injection or infusion; side-effects, including rapid heart rate, headache, faintness, and digestive upsets, can occur, especially at high doses. Trade name: **Apresoline**.

hydramnios *n. see* POLYHYDRAMNIOS.

hydrargyria *n. see* MERCURIALISM.

hydrarthrosis *n.* swelling at a joint caused by excessive synovial fluid. The condition usually involves the knees and may be recurrent. Often no cause is apparent; in some cases rheumatoid arthritis develops later.

hydrocalycosis *n. see* CALIECTASIS.

hydrocele *n.* the accumulation of watery liquid in a sac, usually the sac surrounding the testes. This condition is characterized by painless enlargement of the scrotum; it is treated surgically, by drainage of the fluid or removal of the sac.

hydrocephalus *n.* an abnormal increase in the amount of cerebrospinal fluid within the ventricles of the brain. In childhood, before the sutures of the skull have fused, hydrocephalus makes the head enlarge. In adults, because of the unyielding nature of the skull, hydrocephalus raises the intracranial pressure with consequent drowsiness and vomiting. Hydrocephalus may be caused by obstruction to the outflow of cerebrospinal fluid (CSF) from the ventricles (**obstructive hydrocephalus**), a failure of its reabsorption into the cerebral sinuses, or increased production of CSF (**communicating hydrocephalus**). *Spina bifida may be associated with hydrocephalus in childhood. Treatment involves treating the underlying cause and, if necessary, diverting the excess cerebrospinal fluid into the abdominal cavity, where it is absorbed. This is achieved by tunnelling a thin tube from the ventricles to the abdomen (**ventriculo-peritoneal shunt**) or to the atrium of the heart (**ventriculo-atrial shunt**).

hydrochloric acid a strong acid present, in a very dilute form, in gastric juice. The secretion of excess hydrochloric acid by the stomach results in the condition *hyperchlorhydria.

hydrochlorothiazide *n.* a thiazide *diuretic used in combination with other drugs (e.g. *amiloride) to treat fluid retention (oedema) and high blood pressure.

hydrocortisone *n.* a pharmaceutical preparation of the steroid hormone *cortisol. Hydrocortisone is used in the treatment of adrenal failure (*Addison's disease), shock, and inflammatory, allergic, and rheumatic conditions (including rheumatoid arthritis, colitis, and eczema). It may be given by mouth, by intramuscular, intravenous, or intra-articular injection, or in the form of a cream, ointment, or eye or ear drops. Possible side-effects of hydrocortisone therapy include peptic ulcers, bone and muscle damage, suppression of growth in children, and the signs of *Cushing's syndrome. Trade names: **Dioderm**, **Hydrocortistab**, **Locoid**, **Mildison**, **Solu-Cortel**.

hydrocyanic acid (prussic acid) an intensely poisonous volatile acid that can cause death within a minute if inhaled. It has a smell of bitter almonds. *See* CYANIDE.

hydrogenase *n.* an enzyme that catalyses the addition of hydrogen to a compound in reduction reactions.

hydrogen bond a weak electrostatic bond formed by linking a hydrogen atom between two electronegative atoms (e.g. nitrogen or oxygen). The large number of hydrogen bonds in proteins and nucleic acids are responsible for maintaining the stable molecular structure of these compounds.

hydrogen peroxide an oxidizing agent used (in the form of a solution or cream) as a skin disinfectant for cleansing wounds and treating superficial bacterial infections. Diluted hydrogen peroxide solution is used as a deodorant mouthwash for treating oral infections (e.g. ulcerative gingivitis). Strong solutions irritate the skin. Trade names: **Crystacide, Peroxyl**.

hydrolase *n.* an enzyme that catalyses the hydrolysis of compounds. Examples are the *peptidases.

hydroma *n. see* HYGROMA.

hydronephrosis *n.* distension and dilatation of the pelvis of the kidney. This is due to an obstruction to the free flow of urine from the kidney. An obstruction at or below the neck of the bladder will result in hydronephrosis of both kidneys. The term **primary pelvic hydronephrosis** is used when the obstruction, usually functional, is at the junction of the renal pelvis and ureter. Surgical relief by *pyeloplasty is advisable to avoid the back pressure atrophy of the kidney and the complications of infection and stone formation. —**hydronephrotic** *adj.*

hydropericarditis *n. see* HYDROPERICARDIUM.

hydropericardium *n.* accumulation of a clear serous fluid within the membranous sac surrounding the heart. It occurs in many cases of *pericarditis (**hydropericarditis**). If the heart is compressed the fluid is withdrawn (aspirated) via a needle inserted into the pericardial sac through the chest wall (**pericardiocentesis**). *See also* HYDROPNEU-MOPERICARDIUM.

hydroperitoneum *n. see* ASCITES.

hydrophobia *n. see* RABIES.

hydrophthalmos *n. see* BUPHTHALMOS.

hydropneumopericardium *n.* the presence of air and clear fluid within the pericardial sac around the heart, which is most commonly due to entry of air during pericardiocentesis (*see* HYDROPERICARDIUM). The presence of air does not affect the management of the patient.

hydropneumoperitoneum *n.* the presence of fluid and gas in the peritoneal cavity. This may be due to the introduction of air through an instrument being used to remove the fluid; because of a perforation in the digestive tract that has allowed the escape of fluid and gas; or rarely because gas-forming bacteria are growing in the peritoneal fluid.

hydropneumothorax *n.* the presence of air and fluid in the pleural cavity. If the patient is shaken the fluid makes a splashing sound (called a **succussion splash**). An *effusion of serous fluid commonly complicates a *pneumothorax, and must be drained.

hydrops *n.* an abnormal accumulation of fluid in body tissues or cavities. For example, **corneal hydrops** is the sudden painful accumulation of fluid in the cornea seen in *keratoconus. It results in a sudden reduction of vision. *See also* HYDROPS FETALIS, MÉNIÈRE'S DISEASE (ENDOLYMPHATIC HYDROPS).

hydrops fetalis the accumulation of fluid in fetal tissues or body cavities. This may take the form of a *cystic hygroma. In its most severe form, excessive fluid collects in the peritoneal cavity (*see* ASCITES), the pleural and pericardial cavities, and the soft tissues (*see* OEDEMA). Hydrops may occur at any stage of gestation but is not usually seen until 16–18 weeks; the earlier it presents, the worse the prognosis. There are several causes of hydrops, one of which is severe anaemia associated with rhesus factor incompatibility (*see* HAEMOLYTIC DISEASE OF THE NEWBORN). Other (nonimmune) causes include congenital heart defects, fetal arrhythmias, chromosomal abnormalities, and fetal infection with human *parvovirus B19. Treatment before birth with intrauterine blood transfusions to the fetus may be undertaken in specialized fetal medicine units; without treatment the mortality is high. Prenatal ultrasound scanning enables early recognition of hydrops fetalis and has been enhanced with the introduction of MCA Doppler (*see* DOPPLER ULTRASOUND).

hydrosalpinx *n.* the accumulation of fluid

in one of the *Fallopian tubes due to inflammation and subsequent obstruction, usually as a result of pelvic infection.

hydrotherapy *n.* the use of water in the treatment of disorders, as by exercising in remedial swimming pools as part of the *rehabilitation of arthritic or partially paralysed patients.

hydrothorax *n.* fluid in the pleural cavity. *See also* HYDROPNEUMOTHORAX.

hydrotubation *n.* the introduction of a fluid (usually a dye) through the cervix (neck) of the uterus under pressure to allow visualization, by *laparoscopy, of the passage of the dye through the Fallopian tubes. It is used to test whether or not the tubes are blocked in the investigation of infertility.

hydroureter *n.* an accumulation of urine in one of the tubes (ureters) leading from the kidneys to the bladder. The ureter becomes swollen and the condition usually results from obstruction of the ureter by a stone or a pelvic mass.

hydroxocobalamin *n.* a cobalt-containing drug administered by intramuscular injection to treat conditions involving vitamin B_{12} deficiency, such as pernicious anaemia. Trade names: **Cobalin-H**, **Neo-Cytamen**.

hydroxyapatite *n.* **1.** the crystalline component of bones and teeth, consisting of a complex form of calcium phosphate. **2.** a biocompatible ceramic material that is a synthetic form of natural hydroxyapatite. Some joint replacement prostheses are coated with synthetic hydroxyapatite, which encourages bone to grow on to the implant. The material is also used in some forms of middle-ear surgery.

hydroxycarbamide (hydroxyurea) *n.* a drug that prevents cell growth and is used mainly to treat chronic myeloid leukaemia and *myelodysplastic syndromes but also to reduce the frequency of sickle-cell crises (*see* SICKLE-CELL DISEASE). It is administered by mouth. Hydroxycarbamide may lower the white cell content of the blood due to its effects on the bone marrow. Trade names: **Hydrea**, **Siklos**.

hydroxychloroquine *n.* a drug similar to *chloroquine, used mainly to treat lupus erythematosus and rheumatoid arthritis (*see* DISEASE-MODIFYING ANTIRHEUMATIC DRUG). It is administered by mouth; side-effects such as skin reactions, headache, and digestive upsets may occur and prolonged use can lead to eye damage. Trade name: **Plaquenil**.

5-hydroxyindoleacetic acid (5-HIAA) a metabolite of *serotonin, the most common secretion product of *carcinoid tumours. Measured over 24 hours in the urine, this is the most reliable screening test for such tumours.

hydroxyproline *n.* a compound, similar in structure to the *amino acids, found only in *collagen.

5-hydroxytryptamine *n. see* SEROTONIN.

hydroxyurea *n. see* HYDROXYCARBAMIDE.

hydroxyzine *n.* an *antihistamine drug with sedative properties, used to relieve anxiety, tension, and agitation and to treat pruritus (itching). It is administered by mouth and may cause drowsiness, headache, dry mouth, and gastrointestinal upsets. Trade names: **Atarax**, **Ucerax**.

hygiene *n.* the science of health and the study of ways of preserving it, particularly by promoting cleanliness.

hygr- (hygro-) *combining form denoting* moisture.

hygroma (hydroma) *n.* a type of cyst. It may develop from the liquified remains of a subdural *haematoma (**subdural hygroma**). *See also* CYSTIC HYGROMA.

hygrometer *n.* an instrument for measuring the relative humidity of the atmosphere, i.e. the ratio of the moisture in the air to the moisture it would contain if it were saturated at the same temperature and pressure. In the **dew-point hygrometer** a polished surface is reduced in temperature until the water vapour from the atmosphere forms on it. The temperature of this dew point enables the relative humidity of the atmosphere to be calculated. In the **wet-and-dry bulb hygrometer**, there are two thermometers mounted side by side, the bulb of one being surrounded by moistened muslin. The thermometer with the wet bulb will register a lower temperature than that with the dry bulb owing to the cooling effect of the evaporating water. The temperature difference enables the relative humidity to be calculated.

hymen *n.* the membrane that covers the opening of the vagina at birth but usually perforates spontaneously before puberty. If the initial opening is small it may tear, with slight loss of blood, at the first occasion of sexual intercourse.

Hymenolepis *n.* a genus of small widely distributed parasitic tapeworms. The dwarf tapeworm, *H. nana,* only 40 mm in length, lives in the human intestine. Fleas can be important vectors of this species, and children in close contact with flea-infested dogs are particularly prone to infection. *H. diminuta* is a common parasite of rodents; humans occasionally become infected on swallowing stored cereals contaminated with insect pests – the intermediate hosts for this parasite. Symptoms of abdominal pain, diarrhoea, loss of appetite, and headache are obvious only in heavy infections of either species. Treatment involves a course of *anthelmintics.

hymenotomy *n.* incision of the hymen at the entrance to the vagina. This operation may be performed on a young girl if the membrane completely closes the vagina and thus impedes the flow of menstrual blood. It is also carried out to alleviate dyspareunia (painful intercourse).

hyo- *combining form denoting* the hyoid bone. Example: **hyoglossal** (relating to the hyoid bone and tongue).

hyoglossus *n.* a muscle that serves to depress the tongue. It has its origin in the hyoid bone.

hyoid bone a small isolated U-shaped bone in the neck, below and supporting the tongue. It is held in position by muscles and ligaments between it and the styloid process of the temporal bone.

hyoscine (scopolamine) *n.* an *antimuscarinic drug that prevents muscle spasm. **Hyoscine butylbromide** (Buscopan) is administered by mouth in the treatment of spasm in the digestive system and difficult or painful menstruation. **Hyoscine hydrobromide** (Joy Rides, Kwells, Scopoderm TTS) is used for preoperative medication and to treat motion sickness. It is administered by mouth, injection, or skin patches. Side-effects of both drugs are rare but can include dry mouth, blurred vision, difficulty in urination, and increased heart rate.

hyp- (hypo-) *prefix denoting* **1.** deficiency, lack, or small size. Example: **hypognathous** (having a small lower jaw). **2.** (in anatomy) below; beneath. Example: **hypoglossal** (under the tongue).

hypalgesia *n.* an abnormally low sensitivity to pain.

hyper- *prefix denoting* **1.** excessive; abnormally increased. **2.** (in anatomy) above.

hyperacusis *n.* abnormally acute hearing or painful sensitivity to sounds.

hyperadrenalism *n.* overactivity of the adrenal glands. *See* CUSHING'S SYNDROME.

hyperaemia *n.* the presence of excess blood in the vessels supplying a part of the body. In **active hyperaemia** (**arterial hyperaemia**) the arterioles are relaxed and there is an increased blood flow. In **passive hyperaemia** the blood flow from the affected part is obstructed.

hyperaesthesia *n.* excessive sensibility, especially of the skin.

hyperaldosteronism *n. see* ALDOSTERONISM.

hyperalgesia *n.* an abnormal state of increased sensitivity to painful stimuli.

hyperandrogenism *n.* excessive secretion of androgen in women. It is associated with *hirsutism, acne, sparse or infrequent menstruation (oligomenorrhoea), absent or infrequent ovulation, infertility, endometrial *hyperplasia, *hyperlipidaemia, *hyperglycaemia, and hypertension; all these conditions may be the result of mutations in specific genes. *See also* VIRILIZATION.

hyperbaric *adj.* at a pressure greater than atmospheric pressure.

hyperbaric oxygenation a technique for exposing a patient to oxygen at high pressure. It is used to treat carbon monoxide poisoning, gas gangrene, compressed air illness, and acute breathing difficulties. It is also used in some cases during heart surgery.

hyperbilirubinaemia *n.* an excess of the *bile pigment bilirubin in the blood. Normally there is under 0.8 mg bilirubin per 100 ml blood (17 μmol/l); when the concentration of bilirubin is above 1–1.5 mg per 100 ml (20–30 μmol/l), visible *jaundice occurs. Hyperbilirubinaemia can occur in isolation and in the absence of significant liver disease. *Gilbert's syndrome or red cell *haemolysis are usual causes. *See also* VAN DEN BERGH'S TEST.

hypercalcaemia *n.* the presence in the blood of an abnormally high concentration of calcium. There are many causes, including excessive ingestion of vitamin D, overactivity of the *parathyroid glands, and malignant disease. Malignant hypercalcaemia results from the secretion by the tumour of substances (most commonly *parathyroid hormone-related protein) that stimulate bone resorption or from bone metastases causing localized destruction and release of calcium into the bloodstream. Hypercalcaemia may also occur as an inherited congenital condition, for example **familial benign** (or **hypocalciuric**) **hypercalcaemia** or *Williams syndrome. *Compare* HYPOCALCAEMIA.

hypercalcaemic nephropathy defects of kidney function related to a high serum calcium, irrespective of cause. Impaired urine-concentrating ability and reduction in glomerular filtration rate are common features. Histologically, calcific deposits in the kidneys (*nephrocalcinosis) may be seen in cases of long-standing hypercalcaemia.

hypercalcinuria (hypercalcuria) *n.* the presence in the urine of an abnormally high concentration of calcium.

hypercapnia (hypercarbia) *n.* the presence in the blood of an abnormally high concentration of carbon dioxide.

hyperchloraemia *n.* the presence in the blood of an abnormally high concentration of chloride.

hyperchlorhydria *n.* a greater than normal secretion of hydrochloric acid by the stomach, usually associated with a *duodenal ulcer. Extremely high levels of acid secretion are found in the *Zollinger-Ellison syndrome.

hypercholesterolaemia *n.* the presence of elevated concentrations of *cholesterol in the blood (*see also* HYPERLIPIDAEMIA), which predisposes to atheromatous disease (*see* ATHEROMA). **Familial hypercholesterolaemia** is an autosomal *dominant condition in which raised levels of *low-density lipoprotein (LDL) result from a mutation in the LDL receptor gene, producing a deficiency of LDL receptors, which normally remove cholesterol from the circulation. The *heterozygous state, with LDL levels of 5–10 mmol/1, may not be detected until adulthood; usual signs are tendon *xanthomas on the backs of the hands and a *corneal arcus. The *homozygous state is much more serious as cardiovascular complications can occur in childhood, due to massively in-

creased total cholesterol levels (>12 mmol/1).

hyperchromatism *n.* the property of the nuclei of certain cells (for example, those of tumours) to stain more deeply than normal. —**hyperchromatic** *adj.*

hyperdactylism (polydactylism) *n.* the condition of having more than the normal number of fingers or toes. The extra digits are commonly undersized (rudimentary) and are usually removed surgically shortly after birth.

hyperdynamia *n.* excessive activity of muscles.

hyperemesis gravidarum persistent vomiting during pregnancy, which causes weight loss and ketosis. In severe cases, if inadequately or inappropriately treated, it may cause liver damage and Wernicke's encephalopathy; in such cases it may be necessary to terminate the pregnancy.

hyperextension *n.* extension of a joint or limb beyond its normal limit.

hyperglycaemia *n.* an excess of glucose in the bloodstream. It may occur in a variety of diseases, most notably in *diabetes mellitus, due to insufficient insulin in the blood and excessive intake of carbohydrates. Untreated it may progress to diabetic coma.

hyperhidrosis (hyperidrosis) *n.* excessive sweating, which may occur in certain diseases, such as thyrotoxicosis or fevers, or following the use of certain drugs. More commonly, however, there is no underlying cause for this condition. There are many successful treatments, including topical preparations, antimuscarinic drugs, and injections of *botulinum toxin.

hyperinsulinism *n.* **1.** excessive secretion of the hormone insulin by the islet cells of the pancreas. **2.** metabolic disturbance due to administration of too much insulin.

hyperkalaemia *n.* the presence in the blood of an abnormally high concentration of *potassium, usually due to failure of the kidneys to excrete it. *See also* ELECTROLYTE.

hyperkeratosis *n.* thickening of the outer horny layer of the skin. It may occur as an inherited disorder, affecting the palms and soles.

hyperkinesia *n.* a state of overactive restlessness in children. —**hyperkinetic** *adj.*

hyperkinetic disorder *see* ATTENTION-DEFICIT/HYPERACTIVITY DISORDER.

hyperlipidaemia (hyperlipaemia) *n.* the presence in the blood of an abnormally high concentration of cholesterol (*see* HYPERCHOLESTEROLAEMIA) and/or triglycerides (*see* HYPERTRIGLYCERIDAEMIA) in the form of lipoproteins, which predisposes to *atherosclerosis and coronary heart disease. **Familial mixed hyperlipidaemia** is an autosomal *dominant condition that occurs in 1 in 200 people and in up to 20% of those with early-onset cardiovascular disease. It is marked by elevation of triglycerides, *low-density lipoprotein, and/or *very low-density lipoprotein coupled with a reduction in *high-density lipoprotein.

hyperlipoproteinaemia *n.* the presence in the blood of abnormally high concentrations of *lipoproteins.

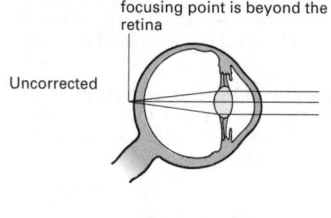

focusing point is beyond the retina

Uncorrected

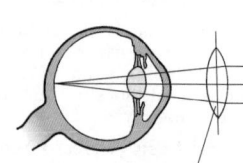

Corrected

convex lens converges light rays falling on the eye

Hypermetropia (long-sightedness).

hypermetropia (long-sightedness) *n.* the condition in which parallel light rays are brought to a focus behind the retina when the *accommodation is relaxed (see illustration). Moderate degrees of hypermetropia may not cause blurred vision in children and young adults because of their ability to accommodate, but for older people and those with greater degrees of hypermetropia near vision is more blurred than distance vision. Normal vision can be restored by wearing spectacles with convex lenses. *Compare* EMMETROPIA, MYOPIA.

hypermotility *n.* excessive movement or activity, especially of the stomach or intestine.

hypernatraemia *n.* the presence in the blood of an abnormally high concentration of *sodium. *See also* ELECTROLYTE.

hypernephroma *n. see* RENAL CELL CARCINOMA.

hyperopia *n.* the usual US term for *hypermetropia.

hyperosmia *n.* an abnormally acute sense of smell.

hyperosmolar non-ketotic state (hyperosmolar non-ketosis, HONK) a state of extreme hyperglycaemia seen in type 2 diabetes that is due to increased production of glucose in the liver, reduced muscle usage, and often an excessive intake of sugary drinks in an attempt to combat what is thought by the patient to be a viral illness. There is excessive urine output and steadily worsening dehydration, but no acidosis or ketosis (*compare* DIABETIC KETOACIDOSIS). Even with treatment (including intravenous fluids and insulin) mortality can be as high as 15%.

hyperostosis *n.* excessive enlargement of the outer layer of a bone. The condition is harmless and is usually recognized as an incidental finding on X-ray. It commonly affects the frontal bone of the skull (**hyperostosis frontalis**). **Infantile cortical hyperostosis** (or **Caffey's disease**) affects infants under six months. There is periodic swelling of the long bones, jaw, and shoulder blade, with pain and a fever. The condition settles spontaneously.

hyperparathyroidism *n.* excessive secretion of *parathyroid hormone, usually due to a small tumour in one of the parathyroid glands. It results in *hypercalcaemia. *See also* VON RECKLINGHAUSEN'S DISEASE.

hyperphagia *n.* pathological overeating due to a loss of the normal regulatory processes.

hyperpiesia *n. see* HYPERTENSION.

hyperplasia *n.* the increased production and growth of normal cells in a tissue or organ without an increase in the size of the cells. The affected part becomes larger but retains its normal form. Hyperplasia can be physiological, as in the breasts during pregnancy, or pathological, as in benign prostatic hyperplasia (*see* PROSTATE GLAND). *See also* ENDOMETRIAL HYPERPLASIA. *Compare* HYPER-TROPHY, NEOPLASIA.

hyperpnoea *n.* an increase in the rate of breathing that is proportional to an increase in metabolism; for example, on exercise. *Compare* HYPERVENTILATION.

hyperpraxia *n.* excessive motor activity, such as is seen in *mania and *attention-deficit/hyperactivity disorder.

hyperprolactinaemia *n. see* PROLACTIN.

hyperpyrexia *n.* a rise in body temperature above 106°F (41.1°C). *See* FEVER.

hypersensitive *adj.* prone to respond abnormally to the presence of a particular antigen, which may cause a variety of tissue reactions ranging from *serum sickness to an allergy (such as hay fever) or, at the severest, to anaphylactic shock (*see* ANAPHYLAXIS). It is thought that when the normal antigen-antibody defence reaction is followed by tissue damage this may be due to an abnormality in the working of the *complement system. *See also* ALLERGY, IMMUNITY. —**hypersensitivity** *n.*

hypersomnia *n.* sleep lasting for exceptionally long periods, as occurs in some cases of brain inflammation.

hypersplenism *n.* a decrease in the numbers of red cells, white cells, and platelets in the blood resulting from destruction or pooling of these cells by an enlarged spleen. Hypersplenism may occur in any condition in which there is enlargement of the spleen (*see* SPLENOMEGALY).

hypersthenia *n.* an abnormally high degree of strength or physical tension in all or part of the body.

hypertelorism *n.* an abnormally increased distance between two organs or parts, commonly referring to widely spaced eyes (**ocular hypertelorism**). *See* CROUZON SYNDROME, SOTOS SYNDROME.

hypertension *n.* high *blood pressure, i.e. elevation of the arterial blood pressure above the normal range expected in a particular age group. Hypertension may be of unknown cause (**essential hypertension** or **hyperpiesia**). It may also result from kidney disease, including narrowing (stenosis) of the renal artery (*renovascular hypertension), endocrine diseases (such as Cushing's disease or phaeochromocytoma) or disease

of the arteries (such as coarctation of the aorta), when it is known as **secondary** or **symptomatic hypertension.**

Complications that may arise from hypertension include atherosclerosis, heart failure, cerebral haemorrhage, and kidney failure, but treatment may prevent their development. Hypertension is symptomless until the symptoms of its complications develop. Some cases of hypertension may be cured by eradicating the cause. Most cases, however, depend upon long-term drug therapy to lower the blood pressure and maintain it within the normal range. The drugs used include thiazide *diuretics, *ACE inhibitors, *calcium-channel blockers, *beta blockers, and *alpha blockers. Combinations of drugs may be needed to obtain optimum control. *See also* MALIGNANT HYPERTENSION, PORTAL HYPERTENSION, PULMONARY HYPERTENSION.

hyperthermia (hyperthermy) *n.* **1.** exceptionally high body temperature (about 41°C or above). *See* FEVER. **2.** treatment of disease by inducing fever. *Compare* HYPO-THERMIA.

hyperthyroidism *n.* overactivity of the thyroid gland, either due to a tumour, overgrowth of the gland, or Graves' disease. *See* THYROTOXICOSIS.

hypertonia (hypertonicity) *n.* exceptionally high tension in muscles.

hypertonic *adj.* **1.** describing a solution that has a greater osmotic pressure than another solution. *See* OSMOSIS. **2.** describing muscles that demonstrate an abnormal increase in *tonicity.

hypertrichosis *n.* excessive growth of hair (*see* HIRSUTISM).

hypertriglyceridaemia *n.* an excess of *triglyceride lipids in the serum, which can be caused by a genetic predisposition with or without a high-fat diet (*see also* LIPOPROTEIN LIPASE), excessive alcohol intake, or poorly controlled diabetes mellitus. The condition can predispose to cardiovascular disease and, in its extreme form, to acute pancreatitis. Lipid-lowering drugs, including *fibrates and *nicotinic acid, are used in treatment.

hypertrophic cardiomyopathy a familial condition affecting the heart, characterized by unexplained thickening (hypertrophy) of the wall of the left ventricle. In many cases this is an incidental finding and patients have a good outcome. However, more severely affected patients may suffer chest pain, tachyarrhythmia (*see* AR-RHYTHMIA), heart failure, and sudden death. In some cases there is focal thickening of muscle around the left ventricular outflow tract (**asymmetric septal hypertrophy**, ASH), and this can result in restriction of blood flow to the body (**hypertrophic obstructive cardiomyopathy**, HOCM). The diagnosis is made by electrocardiography and echocardiography. Usually drug treatment is sufficient to control symptoms, but some patients require cardiac *catheterization or surgical treatment. Those deemed at highest risk of sudden death may require an *implantable cardiovertor defibrillator.

hypertrophy (hypertrophia) *n.* increase in the size of a tissue or organ brought about by the enlargement of its cells rather than by cell multiplication (as during normal growth and tumour formation). Hypertrophy can be a physiological response to normal stimuli, as in the enlargement of skeletal muscles in response to increased work. Pathological hypertrophy occurs in response to abnormal stimuli, as in cardiac muscle as a result of hypertension or aortic valve stenosis (*see also* HYPERTROPHIC CARDIOMYOPATHY). *Compare* HYPERPLASIA. —**hypertrophic** *adj.*

hypertropia *n. see* STRABISMUS.

hyperuricaemia (lithaemia) *n.* the presence in the blood of an abnormally high concentration of uric acid. *See* GOUT.

hyperuricuria (lithuria) *n.* the presence in the urine of an abnormally high concentration of uric acid.

hyperventilation *n.* breathing at an abnormally rapid rate at rest. This causes a reduction of the carbon dioxide concentration of arterial blood, leading to dizziness, tingling (paraesthesiae) in the lips and limbs, tetanic cramps in the hands, and tightness across the chest. If continued, hyperventilation may cause loss of consciousness. This sequence of events occurs in the **hyperventilation syndrome** (**HVS**), which has been estimated to contribute to 10% of out-patient referrals to hospital.

hypervitaminosis *n.* the condition resulting from excessive consumption of vitamins. This is not serious in the case of water-soluble vitamins, when any intake in excess of requirements is easily excreted in the urine. However, the fat-soluble vitamins

A and D are toxic if taken in excessive amounts.

hypervolaemia *n.* an increase in the volume of circulating blood.

hyphaema *n.* a collection of blood in the anterior chamber (in front of the iris) of the eye.

hyphedonia *n.* a lower than normal capacity for achieving enjoyment.

hypn- (hypno-) *combining form denoting* 1. sleep. 2. hypnosis.

hypnagogic *adj. see* IMAGERY.

hypnagogic hallucinations vivid and intense auditory or visual hallucinations occurring at the beginning or the end of sleep. They occur in 30–60% of patients with *narcolepsy.

hypnopompic *adj. see* IMAGERY.

hypnosis *n.* a sleeplike state, artificially induced in a person by a **hypnotist**, in which the mind is more than usually receptive to suggestion and memories of past events – apparently forgotten – may be elicited by questioning. Hypnotic suggestion may be used for a variety of therapeutic purposes; as a form of psychotherapy it is known as **hypnotherapy**.

hypnotherapy *n.* any form of psychotherapy that utilizes *hypnosis.

hypnotic (soporific) *n.* a drug that produces sleep by depressing brain function. Hypnotics include benzodiazepines (such as *loprazolam, *nitrazepam, and *temazepam) and drugs that act at benzodiazepine receptor sites, such as **zaleplon** (Sonata), **zolpidem** (Stilnoct), and **zopiclone** (Zimovane). Hypnotics are used for the short-term treatment of insomnia and sleep disturbances. Some of them (e.g. nitrazepam, *flurazepam) may cause hangover effects in the morning.

hypnotism *n.* the induction of *hypnosis.

hypo- *prefix. see* HYP-.

hypoaesthesia *n.* a condition in which the sense of touch is diminished; uncommonly this may be extended to include other forms of sensation.

hypobaric *adj.* at a pressure lower than that of the atmosphere.

hypocalcaemia *n.* the presence in the blood of an abnormally low concentration of calcium. *See* TETANY. *Compare* HYPERCAL-CAEMIA.

hypocapnia *n. see* ACAPNIA.

hypochloraemia *n.* the presence in the blood of an abnormally low concentration of chloride.

hypochlorhydria *n.* reduced secretion of hydrochloric acid by the stomach. *See* ACHLORHYDRIA.

hypochondria *n.* preoccupation with the physical functioning of the body and with imagined ill health. In the most severe form there are delusions of ill health, often associated with underlying illness, such as *depression. When symptoms reach the level sufficient to be classified as a disorder, it is called **hypochondriasis** (in *DSM-IV-TR) or **hypochondriacal disorder** (in ICD-10). Treatment with reassurance, *antidepressant drugs, and/or psychotherapy is usual, but the condition is often chronic. —**hypochondriac** *adj., n.*

hypochondrium *n.* the upper lateral portion of the *abdomen, situated beneath the lower ribs. —**hypochondriac** *adj.*

hypocretin *n.* a recently discovered neuropeptide that originates in the hypothalamus. Low levels of hypocretin in the cerebrospinal fluid are found in most patients with *narcolepsy and may also be found in patients who have suffered with stroke, brain tumours, head injuries, and infections of the nervous system.

Hypoderma *n.* a genus of non-bloodsucking beelike insects – the warble flies – widely distributed in Europe, North America, and Asia. Cattle are the usual hosts for the parasitic maggots, but rare and accidental infections of humans have occurred (*see* MYIASIS), especially in farm workers. The maggots migrate beneath the skin surface, producing an inflamed linear lesion similar to that of *creeping eruption.

hypodermic *adj.* beneath the skin: usually applied to subcutaneous *injections. The term is also applied to the syringe used for such injections, and sometimes – loosely – to any injection.

hypodipsia *n.* pathological failure to drink enough to maintain the body's normal plasma osmolality. Like its most extreme form, **adipsia**, it is most commonly due to lesions of the thirst centre in the anterior hypothalamus.

hypodontia *n.* congenital absence of some of the teeth.

hypofibrinogenaemia (fibrinogenopenia) *n.* a deficiency of the clotting factor *fibrinogen in the blood, which results in an increased tendency to bleed. It may occur as an inherited disorder in which either production of fibrinogen is impaired or the fibrinogen produced does not function in the normal way (**dysfibrinogenaemia**). Alternatively, it may be acquired. For example, it is the commonest cause of blood coagulation failure during pregnancy, when the blood fibrinogen level falls below the normal pregnancy level of 4–6 g/l as a result of *disseminated intravascular coagulation (DIC). This usually occurs as a complication of severe *abruptio placentae, prolonged retention of a dead fetus, or amniotic fluid embolism.

hypogammaglobulinaemia *n.* a deficiency of the protein *gammaglobulin in the blood. It may occur in a variety of inherited disorders or as an acquired defect, as in chronic lymphocytic *leukaemia (CLL). Since gammaglobulin consists mainly of antibodies (*immunoglobulins), hypogammaglobulinaemia results in an increased susceptibility to infections.

hypogastrium *n.* that part of the central *abdomen situated below the region of the stomach. —**hypogastric** *adj.*

hypogeusia *n.* a condition in which the sense of taste is abnormally weak. *See also* HYPOAESTHESIA.

hypoglossal nerve the twelfth *cranial nerve (XII), which supplies the muscles of the tongue and is therefore responsible for the movements of talking and swallowing.

hypoglycaemia *n.* a deficiency of glucose in the bloodstream, causing muscular weakness and incoordination, mental confusion, and sweating. If severe it may lead to **hypoglycaemic coma**. Hypoglycaemia most commonly occurs in *diabetes mellitus, as a result of insulin overdosage and insufficient intake of carbohydrates. It is treated by administration of glucose: by injection if the patient is in a coma, by mouth otherwise. *See also* REACTIVE HYPOGLYCAEMIA. —**hypoglycaemic** *adj.*

hypoglycaemic unawareness a serious

condition in which a diabetic patient loses the earliest warning signs of an approaching hypoglycaemic episode. Patients thus may suffer a severe attack, with confusion, seizures, or even coma and death, because they fail to take the necessary measures to abort the episode. The condition is more common in longstanding diabetes and in those who experience many hypoglycaemic episodes. It necessitates a temporary driving ban until awareness can be regained, usually by avoidance of further attacks for a period of time.

hypogonadism *n.* impaired function of the gonads (testes or ovaries), causing absence or inadequate development of the *secondary sexual characteristics. This may be due to a disorder of the gonads or to lack of secretion of the pituitary *gonadotrophins (**hypogonadotrophic hypogonadism**).

hypohidrosis *n. see* ANHIDROSIS.

hypoinsulinism *n.* a deficiency of insulin due either to inadequate secretion of the hormone by the pancreas or to inadequate treatment of diabetes mellitus.

hypokalaemia *n.* the presence of abnormally low levels of potassium in the blood: occurs in dehydration. *See* ELECTROLYTE.

hypokalaemic nephropathy abnormalities seen with chronic hypokalaemia (usually K^+ <3.0 mmol/l) and manifest by impaired urine-concentrating ability and reduced capacity to excrete sodium. Histological changes include cytoplasmic vacuolation of the renal tubules and medullary fibrosis.

hypomania *n.* a mild degree of *mania. Elated mood leads to faulty judgment; behaviour lacks the usual social restraints and the sexual drive is increased; there is a reduced need for sleep; speech is rapid and pressured; the individual is energetic but not persistent and tends to be irritable or possibly aggressive. The abnormality is not as great as in mania and the patient may appear normal and 'a bit of a character' to those who do not know him or her (*see* ELATION, EUPHORIA). Treatment follows the same principles as for mania, and it may be difficult to prevent an individual from damaging his or her own interests with extravagant behaviour; hospitalization would indicate that the severity of mania had been reached. —**hypomanic** *adj.*

hyponatraemia *n.* the presence in the blood of an abnormally low concentration of *sodium: occurs in dehydration. *See* ELECTROLYTE.

hypoparathyroidism *n.* subnormal activity of the parathyroid glands, causing a fall in the blood concentration of calcium and muscular spasms (*see* TETANY).

hypopharynx (laryngopharynx) *n.* the part of the pharynx that lies below the level of the hyoid bone.

hypophysectomy *n.* the surgical removal or destruction of the pituitary gland (hypophysis) in the brain. The operation may be conducted by opening the skull or by the insertion of special needles that produce a very low temperature (*see* CRYOSURGERY). Radiotherapy (e.g. by insertion of needles of *yttrium-90) can also be used to destroy parts of the pituitary.

hypophysis *n. see* PITUITARY GLAND.

hypophysitis *n.* a rare condition of inflammation of the *pituitary gland (hypophysis). The main cause is an infiltration by lymphocytes, most commonly during or just after pregnancy. This usually presents as a mass lesion of the pituitary with visual-field loss and headache or with anterior *hypopituitarism, which may be total or just involve particular hormone systems. Around 50% of cases are associated with other autoimmune endocrine diseases, and antipituitary antibodies have been identified.

hypopiesis *n.* abnormally reduced blood pressure in the absence of organic disease (*see* HYPOTENSION).

hypopituitarism *n.* subnormal activity of the pituitary gland, causing *dwarfism in childhood and a syndrome of impaired sexual function, pallor, and premature ageing in adult life (*see* SIMMONDS DISEASE).

hypoplasia *n.* underdevelopment of an organ or tissue. **Dental hypoplasia** is the defective formation of parts of a tooth, for example due to systemic upset while the tooth is being formed. **Pulmonary hypoplasia** is deficient lung development in a fetus or newborn infant for gestational age, with a decrease in lung size or volume. —**hypoplastic** *adj.*

hypoplastic left heart a congenital heart disorder in which the left side of the heart, particularly the left ventricle, is underdeveloped. The first part of the aorta may also be abnormal. Affected babies usually develop severe heart failure within the first few days of life. Diagnosis can be confirmed on *echocardiography. Prognosis is generally very poor – most babies die within the first few weeks – but milder cases may be amenable to surgery. It is the commonest cause of death in the neonatal period due to heart disease.

hypoplastic leukaemia a stage of *leukaemia in which there is a decrease in the number of white cells, red cells, and platelets in the blood and reduced *haemopoiesis in the bone marrow.

hypopnoea *n.* an episode during sleep in which there is a reduction in the nasal airflow to less than 50% of normal, but more than 30% (*see* APNOEA), for more than 10 seconds. *See also* OBSTRUCTIVE SLEEP APNOEA.

hypopraxia *n.* **1.** a condition of diminished and enfeebled activity. **2.** a lack of interest in, or a disinclination for, activity; listlessness.

hypoproteinaemia *n.* a decrease in the quantity of protein in the blood. It may result from malnutrition, impaired protein production (as in liver disease), or increased loss of protein from the body (as in the *nephrotic syndrome). It results in swelling (*oedema), because of the accumulation of fluid in the tissues, and increased susceptibility to infections. *See also* HYPOGAMMA-GLOBULINAEMIA.

hypoprothrombinaemia *n.* a deficiency of the clotting factor *prothrombin in the blood, which results in an increased tendency to bleed. It may occur as an inherited defect or as the result of liver disease, vitamin K deficiency, or anticoagulant treatment.

hypopyon *n.* pus in the anterior chamber (in front of the iris) of the eye. Seen in severe cases of *uveitis or other ocular infections, it can be a sign of endophthalmitis following intraocular surgery.

hyposensitive *adj.* less than normally responsive to the presence of antigenic material. *Compare* HYPERSENSITIVE. —**hyposensitivity** *n.*

hyposensitization *n. see* DESENSITIZATION.

hyposmia *n.* reduction in the sense of smell. *See* ANOSMIA.

hypospadias *n.* a congenital abnormality in which the opening of the *urethra is on the underside of the penis: either on the glans penis (**glandular hypospadias**), at the junction of the glans with the shaft (**coronal hypospadias**), or on the shaft itself (**penile hypospadias**). All varieties can be treated surgically, and neither micturition nor sexual function need be impaired. *See* MAGPI OPERATION.

hypostasis *n.* accumulation of fluid or blood in a dependent part of the body, under the influence of gravity, in cases of poor circulation. Hypostatic congestion of the lung bases may be seen in debilitated patients who are confined to bed. It predisposes to pneumonia (hypostatic pneumonia) but it may be prevented by careful nursing and physiotherapy. A similar condition (**lividity**) occurs after death when blood pools in the dependent parts of the body after the circulation has ceased. —**hypostatic** *adj.*

hyposthenia *n.* a state of physical weakness or abnormally low muscular tension.

hyposthenuria *n.* the secretion of urine of low specific gravity. The inability to concentrate the urine occurs in patients at the final stage of chronic renal failure.

hypotension *n.* a condition in which the arterial *blood pressure is abnormally low, which is most commonly experienced when rising from a sitting or lying position (**postural** or **orthostatic hypotension**). Severe cases may manifest as *shock.

hypothalamus *n.* the region of the forebrain in the floor of the third ventricle, linked with the thalamus above and the *pituitary gland below (*see* BRAIN). It contains several important centres controlling body temperature, thirst, hunger, and eating, water balance, and sexual function. It is also closely connected with emotional activity and sleep and functions as a centre for the integration of hormonal and autonomic nervous activity through its control of the pituitary secretions (*see* NEUROENDOCRINE SYSTEM, PITUITARY GLAND). —**hypothalamic** *adj.*

hypothenar *adj.* describing or relating to the fleshy prominent part of the palm of the hand below the little finger. *Compare* THENAR.

hypothermia *n.* **1.** accidental reduction of body temperature below the normal range in the absence of protective reflex actions, such as shivering. Often insidious in onset, it is particularly liable to occur in babies and the elderly if they are living in poorly heated homes and have inadequate clothing. **2.** deliberate lowering of body temperature for therapeutic purposes. This may be done during surgery, in order to reduce the patient's requirement for oxygen.

hypothetical imperative *see* IMPERATIVE.

hypothyroidism *n.* subnormal activity of the thyroid gland. If present at birth and untreated it leads to *cretinism. In adult life it causes mental and physical slowing, undue sensitivity to cold, slowing of the pulse, weight gain, and coarsening of the skin (**myxoedema**). The condition can be treated by administration of thyroxine.

hypotonia *n.* a state of reduced tension in muscle.

hypotonic *adj.* **1.** describing a solution that has a lower osmotic pressure than another solution. *See* OSMOSIS. **2.** describing muscles that demonstrate diminished *tonicity.

hypotony *n.* a very low intraocular pressure, usually as a result of trauma or surgery to the eye.

hypotrichosis *n.* a condition in which less hair develops than normal.

hypotropia *n. see* STRABISMUS.

hypoventilation *n.* breathing at an abnormally shallow and slow rate, which results in an increased concentration of carbon dioxide in the blood. **Alveolar hypoventilation** may be primary, which is very rare, or secondary, which can be due to destructive lesions of the brain or to an acquired blunting of respiratory drive arising from failure of the respiratory pump.

hypovitaminosis *n.* a deficiency of a vitamin caused either through lack of the vitamin in the diet or from an inability to absorb or utilize it.

hypovolaemia (oligaemia) *n.* a decrease in the volume of circulating blood. *See* SHOCK.

hypoxaemia *n.* reduction of the oxygen concentration in the arterial blood, recognized clinically by the presence of central and peripheral *cyanosis. When the partial

pressure of oxygen (pO_2) falls below 8.0 kPa (60 mmHg), the condition is defined as respiratory failure.

hypoxia *n.* a deficiency of oxygen in the tissues. *See also* ANOXIA, HYPOXAEMIA.

hypoxic-ischaemic encephalopathy (HIE, birth asphyxia, perinatal asphyxia) brain damage in a newborn infant as a result of the brain receiving inadequate oxygen. HIE may cause seizures and, if severe, death within minutes of oxygen deprivation. If the infant survives there can be significant long-term consequences, such as developmental delay, mental retardation, or cerebral palsy.

hypsarrhythmia *n.* a severe abnormality on an EEG (*see* ELECTROENCEPHALOGRAPHY) that demonstrates a chaotic pattern of brain activity. It is usually characteristic of *infantile spasms.

hyster- (hystero-) *combining form denoting* **1.** the uterus. **2.** hysteria.

hysterectomy *n.* the surgical removal of the uterus, either through an incision in the abdominal wall (**abdominal hysterectomy**) or through the vagina (**vaginal hysterectomy**). **Subtotal hysterectomy** (rarely performed now) involves removing the body of the uterus but leaving the neck (cervix); in **total hysterectomy** the entire uterus is removed. Hysterectomy is performed for cancerous conditions affecting the uterus and for nonmalignant conditions (e.g. fibroids) in which there is excessive menstrual bleeding. Abdominal hysterectomy carries a higher risk of morbidity than vaginal hysterectomy; the latter is therefore the preferred route unless contraindicated.

hysteria *n.* **1.** formerly, a neurosis characterized by emotional instability, repression, dissociation, some physical symptoms (*see* HYSTERICAL), and vulnerability to suggestion. Two types were recognized: **conversion hysteria**, now known as *conversion disorder; and **dissociative hysteria**, comprising a group of conditions now generally regarded as *dissociative disorders. *See also* NEUROSIS. **2.** a state of great emotional excitement.

hysterical *adj.* **1.** formerly, describing a symptom that is not due to organic disease, is produced unconsciously, and from which the individual derives some gain. What were known as hysterical symptoms are characteristic of *conversion disorder. **2.** describing a kind of *personality disorder characterized by instability and shallowness of feelings and by superficiality and a tendency to manipulate in personal relationships.

hysterosalpingography *n.* X-ray imaging of the uterus and Fallopian tubes following injection of water or a soluble *contrast medium.

hysterosalpingosonography *n. see* HYCOSY.

hysteroscopy *n.* visualization of the interior of the uterus using a **hysteroscope** (a type of *endoscope). It can also be used for therapeutic procedures, such as polypectomy. —**hysteroscopic** *adj.*

hysterotomy *n.* an operation for removal of the fetus by incision of the uterus through the abdomen before the 24th week of gestation; after this time the operation is called *Caesarean section. Hysterotomy is now rarely performed owing to improvements in the efficiency of drugs now available for inducing abortion, e.g. *mifepristone.

-iasis *combining form denoting* a diseased condition. Example: **leishmaniasis** (disease caused by *Leishmania* species).

iatro- *combining form denoting* **1.** medicine. **2.** doctors.

iatrogenic *adj.* describing a condition or disease that has resulted from treatment and/or the actions of health-care professionals, for example an unforeseen or inevitable side-effect, hospital-acquired infection, or post-operative complication.

IBD *see* INFLAMMATORY BOWEL DISEASE.

IBS *see* IRRITABLE BOWEL SYNDROME.

ibuprofen *n.* an anti-inflammatory drug (*see* NSAID), used in the treatment of arthritic conditions and for pain relief (as in dysmenorrhoea and migraine). It is administered by mouth and sometimes causes skin rashes and digestive upsets. Trade names: **Brufen**, **Fenbid**, **Nurofen**, etc.

ICD **1.** *see* INTERNATIONAL CLASSIFICATION OF DISEASES. The latest version is **ICD-10**. **2.** *see* IMPLANTABLE CARDIOVERTOR DEFIBRILLATOR.

ICF International Classification of Functioning, Disabilities and Health. *See* INTERNATIONAL CLASSIFICATION OF DISEASES.

ICG angiography indocyanine green *angiography.

ichor *n.* a watery material oozing from wounds or ulcers.

ichthyosis *n.* a genetically determined skin disorder (*see* GENODERMATOSIS) in which there is abnormal scaling of the skin (the scaly condition of the skin is reflected in the name of this disorder, which is derived from the Greek word for fish). Ichthyosis may be caused by a variety of genetic defects in skin shedding; the pattern of scaling varies according to the underlying defect. The commonest form, **ichthyosis vulgaris**, is inherited as an autosomal *dominant and occurs in 1 in 300 of the population. **Lamellar ichthyosis** is a very rare condition in which the skin, particularly on the palms and soles, is thickened and lizard-like. Treat-

ment of ichthyosis is mainly by the regular use of emollients. *See also* XERODERMA.

icodextrin *n.* a glucose polymer solution produced by the hydrolysis of cornstarch and containing a spectrum of polymer molecules with an average molecular weight of 16,200 Da. It is used in the dialysate treatment of renal failure by *peritoneal dialysis. It exerts a strong osmotic effect, allowing removal of fluid without exposing the peritoneum to high levels of glucose. It is of most use when the dialysate is required to remain within the body for a long period, for instance overnight during chronic ambulatory peritoneal dialysis or during the day with automated peritoneal dialysis.

ICSH (interstitial-cell-stimulating hormone) *see* LUTEINIZING HORMONE.

ICSI (intracytoplasmic sperm injection) a technique of assisted conception that has revolutionized the treatment of severe male infertility. Spermatozoa are aspirated or extracted from the testis or epididymis (*see* MESA, PESA) and a single sperm is injected into the cytoplasm of a secondary *oocyte in vitro. The fertilized ovum is then implanted into the uterus.

icterus *n. see* JAUNDICE.

ictus *n.* a stroke or any sudden attack, such as a subarachnoid haemorrhage. The term is often used for an epileptic seizure, stressing the suddenness of its onset.

id *n.* (in psychoanalysis) a part of the unconscious mind governed by the instinctive forces of *libido and the death instinct (governing aggression, etc.). These violent forces seek immediate release in action or in symbolic form. The id is therefore said to be governed by the pleasure principle and not by the demands of reality or of logic. In the course of individual development some of the functions of the id are taken over by the *ego.

-id *suffix denoting* relationship or resemblance to. Example: **spermatid** (a stage of sperm formation).

idea of reference *see* DELUSION OF REFERENCE.

ideation *n.* the process of thinking or of having *imagery or ideas. The presence or absence of **suicidal ideation** is tested as part of every *mental state examination and risk assessment.

identical twins *see* TWINS.

ideo- *combining form denoting* 1. the mind or mental activity. 2. ideas.

ideomotor *adj.* describing or relating to a motor action that is evoked by an idea. **Ideomotor apraxia** is the inability to translate the idea of a complex behaviour into action.

idio- *combining form denoting* peculiarity to the individual.

idiopathic *adj.* denoting a disease or condition the cause of which is not known or that arises spontaneously. —**idiopathy** *n.*

idiopathic intracranial hypertension *see* BENIGN INTRACRANIAL HYPERTENSION.

idiopathic pulmonary fibrosis (IPF) the same clinical entity as cryptogenic fibrosing *alveolitis. This term has been in use in North America for some years and is now commonly used in the UK.

idiopathic thrombocytopenic purpura (ITP) an *autoimmune disease in which platelets are destroyed, leading to spontaneous bruising (*see* PURPURA). Acute ITP is a relatively mild disease of children, who usually recover without treatment. A chronic form of the disease, typically affecting adults, is more serious, requiring treatment with corticosteroids or, if there is no response, with splenectomy. If both fail, immunosuppressant drugs may be effective. Platelet concentrates are used for life-threatening bleeding.

idiosyncrasy *n.* an unusual and unexpected sensitivity exhibited by an individual to a particular drug or food. Drug idiosyncrasy commonly takes the form of undue susceptibility or hypersensitivity, so that the standard dose causes an excessive effect; the normal effect is produced by a small fraction of the standard dose. —**idiosyncratic** *adj.*

idioventricular *adj.* affecting or peculiar to the ventricles of the heart. The term is most often used to describe the very slow beat of the heart's ventricles under the influence of their own natural subsidiary pacemaker (**idioventricular rhythm**). An accelerated idioventricular rhythm of 80–120 beats per minute is often seen in patients a few hours after being admitted with a heart attack (*see* MYOCARDIAL INFARCTION). Its presence is a good sign since it usually indicates restoration of blood flow down the occluded coronary artery.

idoxuridine *n.* an iodine-containing antiviral drug that inhibits the growth of viruses and is used to treat herpes simplex infections. It is administered topically and may cause irritation and stinging on application.

ifosfamide *n.* a *cytotoxic drug (an *alkylating agent) used in the treatment of malignant disease, particularly sarcomas, testicular tumours, and lymphomas. It is administered intravenously by injection or infusion. Side-effects include nausea, vomiting, alopecia, and haemorrhagic cystitis; concomitant administration of *mesna is recommended to prevent cystitis.

Ig *see* IMMUNOGLOBULIN.

IgA nephropathy *see* BERGER'S NEPHROPATHY.

IGF insulin-like growth factor, which includes IGF-I and IGF-II. *See* GROWTH FACTOR, SOMATOMEDIN.

IGRT *see* IMAGE-GUIDED RADIOTHERAPY.

IGT impaired glucose tolerance (*see* GLUCOSE TOLERANCE TEST).

IL-2 *n. see* INTERLEUKIN.

ile- (ileo-) *combining form denoting* the ileum. Examples: **ileocaecal** (relating to the ileum and caecum); **ileocolic** (relating to the ileum and colon).

ileal conduit a segment of small intestine (ileum) used to convey urine from the ureters to the exterior into an appliance (*see also* URINARY DIVERSION). The ureters are implanted into an isolated segment of bowel, usually ileum but sometimes sigmoid colon, one end of which is brought through the abdominal wall to the skin surface. This end forms a spout, or **stoma**, which projects into a suitable urinary appliance. The ureters themselves cannot be used for this purpose as they tend to narrow and retract if brought through the skin. The operation is performed if the bladder has to be removed or bypassed; for example, because of cancer.

ileal pouch (perineal pouch) a reservoir made from loops of ileum to replace a surgically removed rectum, avoiding the need for a permanent *ileostomy. This is commonly constructed in patients who have had their colon surgically removed for various disorders (e.g. ulcerative colitis, familial adenomatous polyposis).

ileectomy *n.* surgical removal of the ileum (small intestine) or part of the ileum.

ileitis *n.* inflammation of the ileum (small intestine). It may be caused by *Crohn's disease, tuberculosis, the bacterium *Yersinia enterocolitica*, or typhoid or it may occur in association with ulcerative *colitis (when it is known as **backwash ileitis**).

ileocaecal valve a valve at the junction of the small and large intestines consisting of two membranous folds that close to prevent the backflow of food from the colon and caecum to the ileum.

ileocolitis *n.* inflammation of the ileum and the colon (small and large intestines). The commonest causes are *Crohn's disease and tuberculosis.

ileocolostomy *n.* a surgical operation in which the ileum is joined to some part of the colon. It is usually performed when the right side of the colon has been removed or if it is desired to bypass either the terminal part of the ileum or right side of the colon.

ileocystoplasty *n. see* CYSTOPLASTY.

ileorectal anastomosis (ileoproctostomy) a surgical operation in which the ileum is joined to the rectum, usually after surgical removal of the colon (*see* COLECTOMY).

ileostomy *n.* a surgical operation in which the ileum is brought through the abdominal wall to create an artificial opening (**stoma**) through which the intestinal contents can discharge, thus bypassing the colon. Various types of bag may be worn to collect the effluent. The operation is usually performed in association with *colectomy; or to allow the colon to rest and heal in cases of colitis; or following injury or surgery to the colon.

ileum *n.* the lowest of the three portions of the small *intestine. It runs from the jejunum to the *ileocaecal valve. —**ileal**, **ileac** *adj.*

ileus *n.* intestinal obstruction, usually obstruction of the small intestine (ileum). **Par-**alytic or **adynamic ileus** is functional obstruction of the ileum due to loss of intestinal movement (peristalsis), which may be caused by abdominal surgery (*see* LAPAROTOMY); spinal injuries; electrolyte abnormalities, particularly of potassium (hypokalaemia); or peritonitis. Treatment consists of intravenous administration of fluid and nutrients and removal of excess stomach secretions by nasogastric tube until peristalsis returns (the 'drip and suck' approach). If possible, the underlying condition is treated. Mechanical obstruction of the ileum may be caused by a gallstone entering the bowel through a fistula or widened bile duct (**gallstone ileus**); thickened *meconium in newborn babies with *cystic fibrosis (**meconium ileus**); or intestinal worms, usually the threadworm *Enterobius vermicularis* (**verminous ileus**).

ili- (ilio-) *combining form denoting* the ilium.

iliac arteries the arteries that supply most of the blood to the lower limbs and pelvic region. The right and left **common iliac arteries** form the terminal branches of the abdominal aorta. Each branches into the **external iliac artery** and the smaller **internal iliac artery**.

iliacus *n.* a flat triangular muscle situated in the area of the groin. This muscle acts in conjunction with the *psoas muscle to flex the thigh.

iliac veins the veins draining most of the blood from the lower limbs and pelvic region. The right and left **common iliac veins** unite to form the inferior vena cava. They are each formed by the union of the **internal** and **external iliac veins**.

iliopsoas *n.* a composite muscle made up of the *iliacus and *psoas muscles, which have a common tendon.

ilium *n.* the haunch bone: a wide bone forming the upper part of each side of the *hip bone (*see also* PELVIS). There is a concave depression (**iliac fossa**) on the inside of the pelvis; the right iliac fossa provides space for the vermiform appendix. —**iliac** *adj.*

illusion *n.* a false perception due to misinterpretation of the stimuli arising from an object. For example, a patient may misinterpret a curtain cord as a snake. Illusions can occur in normal people, when they are usually spontaneously corrected. They may also occur in almost any psychiatric syndrome. *Compare* HALLUCINATION.

image-guided radiotherapy (IGRT) the process of imaging during a course of radiation treatment to verify the internal position of the target in comparison to the initial planning scan. This enables adjustment of *treatment fields to improve coverage and allows the use of smaller treatment volumes. The possible methods for IGRT include **cone beam CT**, *tomotherapy, *cyberknife, and ultrasound and kilovoltage X-rays of implanted fiducial markers.

image intensifier an electronic device that provides a TV image from an X-ray source. The X-rays strike a fluorescent screen, giving off electrons, which are accelerated using an electron lens before striking a second fluorescent screen, which is usually attached to a video camera. The acceleration of the electrons amplifies the signal from the original image, giving a brighter picture, so that the radiation dose can be reduced. Images can be taken from the camera to be observed in real time on a video monitor or, using a brief higher-dose exposure, to provide a more detailed static image (*see* DIGITAL SPOT IMAGING).

imagery *n.* the production of vivid mental representations by the normal processes of thought. **Hypnagogic imagery** occurs just before falling asleep, and the images are often very distinct. **Hypnopompic imagery** occurs in the state between sleep and full wakefulness. Like hypnagogic imagery, the experiences may be very vivid. **Eidetic imagery**, commoner in children than adults, is the production of images of exceptional clarity, which may be recalled long after being first experienced.

imaging *n.* (in radiology) the production of images of organs or tissues by a range of techniques. These images are used by physicians in diagnosis and in monitoring the effects of treatment. They can also be used to guide *interventional radiology techniques. *See also* COMPUTERIZED TOMOGRAPHY, MAGNETIC RESONANCE IMAGING, ULTRASONOGRAPHY.

imago *n.* (in psychoanalysis) the internal unconscious representation of an important person in the individual's life, particularly a parent.

imatinib *n.* a *cytotoxic drug that works by inhibiting tyrosine kinases, enzymes that are

active in some cancer cells (*see* TYROSINE KINASE INHIBITOR). Imatinib is used in the treatment of chronic myeloid leukaemia in which the *Philadelphia chromosome is present, *myeloproliferative disorders associated with abnormalities of the platelet-derived growth factor receptor gene, *gastrointestinal stromal tumours (GIST), and acute lymphoblastic leukaemia. The drug is administered by mouth; the commonest side-effects are intestinal upset, fluid retention, and muscle pain and cramps. Trade name: **Glivec**.

imidazole *n.* one of a group of chemically related antifungal drugs that are also effective against a wide range of bacteria; some (e.g. *tiabendazole and *mebendazole) are also used as anthelmintics. The group includes *econazole, *clotrimazole, *ketoconazole, and *miconazole. They are administered by mouth or externally as creams.

imipramine *n.* a drug administered by mouth to treat depression (*see* ANTIDEPRESSANT) and, in children, bedwetting. Its effects may be slow to develop; common side-effects include dry mouth, blurred vision, constipation, sweating, and rapid heartbeat.

imiquimod *n.* a drug used for treating anogenital warts, superficial basal cell carcinoma, and actinic *keratosis. It is administered as a cream. Trade name: **Aldara**.

imitation *n.* acting in the same way as another person, either temporarily or permanently. It can be used in therapy (*see* MODELLING).

immersion foot *see* TRENCH FOOT.

immobilization *n.* the procedure of making a normally movable part of the body, such as a joint, immovable. This helps infected, diseased, or injured tissue (bone, joint, or muscle) to heal. Immobilization may be temporary (for example, by means of a plaster of Paris cast on a limb) or it may be permanent. Permanent immobilization of a joint is achieved by means of *arthrodesis.

immune *adj.* protected against a particular infection by the presence of specific antibodies against the organisms concerned. *See* IMMUNITY.

immune response the response of the *immune system to antigens. There are two types of immune response produced by two populations of *lymphocytes. B lymphocytes (or B cells) are responsible for **humoral immunity**, producing free antibodies that circulate in the bloodstream; and T lymphocytes (or T cells) are responsible for **cell-mediated immunity** (*see* HELPER T CELL, CYTOTOXIC T CELL, SUPPRESSOR T CELL).

immune system the organs responsible for *immunity. The primary *lymphoid organs are the thymus and the bone marrow; the secondary lymphoid organs are the lymph nodes and lymphoid aggregates (spleen, tonsils, gastrointestinal lymph tissue, and Peyer's patches).

immunity *n.* the body's ability to resist infection, afforded by the presence of circulating *antibodies and white blood cells. Healthy individuals protect themselves by means of physical barriers, phagocytic cells, *natural killer cells, and various blood-borne molecules. All of these mechanisms are present prior to exposure to infectious agents and are part of **natural** (or **innate**) **immunity**. Antibodies are manufactured specifically to deal with the antigens associated with different diseases as they are encountered. **Active immunity** arises when the body's own cells produce, and remain able to produce, appropriate antibodies following an attack of a disease or deliberate stimulation (*see* IMMUNIZATION). **Passive immunity**, which is only short-lived, is provided by injecting ready-made antibodies in *antiserum taken from another person or an animal already immune. Babies have passive immunity, conferred by antibodies from the maternal blood and *colostrum, to common diseases for several weeks after birth. *See also* IMMUNE RESPONSE.

immunization *n.* the production of *immunity by artificial means. Passive immunity, which is temporary, may be conferred by the injection of an *antiserum, but the production of active immunity calls for the use of treated antigens, to stimulate the body to produce its own antibodies: this is the procedure of *vaccination (also called **inoculation**). The material used for immunization (the *vaccine) may consist of live bacteria or viruses so treated that they are harmless while remaining antigenic or completely dead organisms or their products (e.g. toxins) chemically or physically altered to produce the same effect.

immuno- *combining form denoting* immunity or immunological response.

immunoassay *n.* any of various techniques for determining the levels of antigen and antibody in a tissue. *See* IMMUNOELECTROPHORESIS, IMMUNOFLUORESCENCE, RADIOIMMUNOASSAY.

immunocompromised *adj.* describing patients in whom the immune response is reduced or defective due to *immunosuppression. Such patients are vulnerable to opportunistic infections.

immunodeficiency *n.* deficiency in the *immune response. This can be acquired, as

Age	Vaccine
2 months	DTaP/IPV/Hib pneumococcal vaccine
3 months	DTaP/IPV/Hib meningitis C vaccine (MenC)
4 months	DTaP/IPV/Hib MenC pneumococcal vaccine
12 months	Hib/MenC
13 months	MMR pneumococcal vaccine
3 years 4 months–5 years	DTaP/IPV MMR
Girls aged 12 to 13 years	HPV
13–18 years	Td/IPV

Childhood immunization schedule.

in *AIDS, but there are many varieties of primary immunodeficiency occurring as inherited disorders characterized by *hypo-gammaglobulinaemia or defects in T-cell function, or both.

immunoelectrophoresis *n.* a technique for identifying antigenic fractions in a serum. The components of the serum are separated by *electrophoresis and allowed to diffuse through agar gel towards a particular anti-serum. Where the antibody meets its anti-gen, a band of precipitation occurs. *See also* PRECIPITIN.

immunofluorescence *n.* a technique for observing the amount and/or distribution of antibody or antigen in a tissue section. The antibodies are labelled (directly or indirectly) with a fluorescent dye (e.g. fluorescein) and applied to the tissue, which is observed through an ultraviolet microscope. In **direct immunofluorescence** the antibody is la-belled before being applied to the tissue. In **indirect immunofluorescence** the antibody is labelled after it has bound to the antigen, by means of fluorescein-labelled anti-immunoglobulin serum. —**immunofluo-rescent** *adj.*

immunogenicity *n.* the property that en-ables a substance to provoke an immune re-sponse, including foreignness (*see* ANTIGEN), size, route of entry into the body, dose, num-ber and length of exposures to the antigen, and host genetic make-up.

immunoglobulin (Ig) *n.* one of a group of structurally related proteins (*gammaglobu-lins) that act as antibodies. Several classes of Ig with different functions are distinguished – IgA, IgD, IgE, IgG, and IgM. They can be separated by *immunoelectrophoresis. *See* ANTIBODY.

immunological tolerance a failure of the body to distinguish between materials that are 'self', and therefore to be tolerated, and those that are 'not self', against which it mounts an *immune response. Tolerance re-sults from the interaction of antigens with lymphocytes under conditions in which the lymphocytes are not activated but rendered unresponsive.

immunology *n.* the study of *immunity and all of the phenomena connected with the defence mechanisms of the body. —**im-munological** *adj.*

immunosuppressant *n.* a drug, such as

*azathioprine or *cyclophosphamide, that reduces the body's resistance to infection and other foreign bodies by suppressing the immune system. Immunosuppressants are used to maintain the survival of organ and tissue transplants and to treat various *auto-immune diseases, including rheumatoid arthritis (*see* DISEASE-MODIFYING ANTI-RHEUMATIC DRUG). *Ciclosporin is the im-munosuppressant usually used in organ transplant recipients. Because immunity is lowered during treatment with immunosup-pressants, there is an increased susceptibil-ity to infection and certain types of cancer.

immunosuppression *n.* suppression of the *immune response, usually by disease (e.g. AIDS) or by drugs (e.g. steroids, azathio-prine, ciclosporin).

immunotherapy *n.* the prevention or treatment of disease using agents that may modify the immune response. It is a largely experimental approach, studied most widely in the treatment of leukaemias (especially hairy-cell leukaemia), melanoma, and renal cell carcinoma. *See* BIOLOGICAL RESPONSE MODIFIER.

immunotoxin *n.* one of a class of com-pounds being studied for the treatment of certain cancers. Therapeutic immunotoxins combine *monoclonal antibodies, which can specifically target cancerous cells, with a highly toxic compound (such as *ricin) that inactivates the cells' *ribosomes and thus in-hibits protein synthesis. Because the toxin does not attack the whole cell only tiny amounts are required.

immunotransfusion *n.* the transfusion of an *antiserum to treat or give temporary protection against a disease.

impacted *adj.* firmly wedged. An **im-pacted tooth** (usually a wisdom tooth) is one that cannot erupt into a normal position be-cause it is obstructed by other tissues. **Im-pacted faeces** are so hard and dry that they cannot pass through the anus without spe-cial measures being taken (*see* CONSTIPA-TION). An **impacted fracture** is one in which the bone ends are driven into each other. —**impaction** *n.*

impaired glucose tolerance (IGT) *see* GLUCOSE TOLERANCE TEST.

impairment *n. see* HANDICAP.

impalpable *adj.* describing a structure within the body that cannot be detected (or that can be detected only with difficulty) by feeling with the hand.

imperative *n.* in ethics, a rule, principle, or law used to direct or guide one's actions. *Kantian ethics distinguishes between **categorical** and **hypothetical imperatives**. Whereas the latter are merely prudent or expedient and will vary with circumstances, the former are binding moral *duties and it is rational that they are applicable to all situations and people. *See also* DEONTOLOGY.

imperforate *adj.* lacking an opening. Occasionally girls at puberty are found to have an **imperforate hymen** (a fold of membrane close to the vaginal orifice), which impedes the flow of menstrual blood.

imperforate anus (proctatresia) partial or complete obstruction of the anus: a condition, discovered at birth, due to failure of the anus to develop normally in the embryo. There are several different types of imperforate anus; these include **developmental anal stenosis**, **persistent anal membrane**, and **covered anus** (due to fused genital folds). If the anal canal fails to develop, the rectum ends blindly above the muscles of the perineum. Most mild cases of imperforate anus can be treated by a simple operation. If the defect is extensive a temporary opening is made in the colon (*see* COLOSTOMY), with later surgical reconstruction of the rectum and anus.

impetigo *n.* a superficial bacterial infection of the skin. **Nonbullous impetigo** is caused by *Staphylococcus aureus*, *Streptococcus* species, or both organisms; it mainly affects young children and is highly contagious, with yellowish-brown crusting. **Bullous impetigo** is caused by *Staph. aureus*; it is characterized by blisters, is less contagious than the nonbullous form, and occurs at any age. Treatment of impetigo is with topical or systemic antibiotics.

implant *n.* **1.** a drug (such as a subcutaneous hormone implant), a prosthesis (such as an artificial hip, an **intraocular lens implant** (*see* CATARACT), a *breast implant, a *cochlear implant, or an *artificial heart implant), or a radioactive source (such as radium needles) that is put into the body. **2.** (in dentistry) a rigid structure that is embedded in bone or under its periosteum to provide support for replacement teeth on a *denture or a *bridge. Recent types (**osseointegrated implants**) consist of a number of

special titanium alloy inserts (fixtures), placed in the jawbone, onto which abutments are fitted after the bone has healed. Later an artificial-tooth superstructure is bolted onto the abutments. Osseointegrated implants are also used to retain facial *prostheses. *See also* OSSEOINTEGRATION.

implantable cardiovertor defibrillator (ICD) a self-contained device, similar to a *pacemaker, that monitors heart rhythm and delivers an electric shock to correct life-threatening arrhythmia. *See also* DEFIBRILLATOR.

implantable hearing aid a form of hearing aid in which a small electrical vibrator is surgically attached to the auditory *ossicles. An external device with a microphone and an electronic processing unit passes information to the implanted device using radiofrequency waves. The external part is located behind the pinna and is powered by batteries. Trade name: **Soundbridge (Vibrant Soundbridge)**.

implantation *n.* **1.** (nidation) the attachment of the early embryo to the lining of the uterus, which occurs at the *blastocyst stage of development, six to eight days after ovulation. The site of implantation determines the position of the placenta. **2.** the placing of a substance (e.g. a drug) or an object (e.g. an artificial pacemaker) within a tissue. **3.** the surgical replacement of damaged tissue with healthy tissue (*see* TRANSPLANTATION).

impotence *n.* inability of a man to have sexual intercourse (*coitus). *See* ERECTILE DYSFUNCTION.

impression *n.* (in dentistry) a mould made of the teeth and surrounding soft tissues or of a toothless jaw. A soft impression material (e.g. silicone or alginate) is placed over the teeth or jaw and sets within several minutes, producing an elastic mould. Impressions may also be taken with hard-setting materials (e.g. plaster or zinc oxide–eugenol cement). After removal from the mouth a plaster model is made; on this are constructed *restorations of teeth, *dentures, or *orthodontic appliances.

imprinting *n.* **1.** (in animal behaviour) a rapid and irreversible form of learning that takes place in some animals during the first hours of life. Animals attach themselves in this way to members of their own species, but if they are exposed to creatures of a different species during this short period, they

become attached to this species instead.
2. (in genetics) a phenomenon whereby gene expression depends on whether the chromosome is maternal or paternal in origin. For example, both *Prader-Willi syndrome and *Angelman syndrome are caused by a *deletion of the same part of chromosome 15. When the deletion involves the chromosome 15 that came from the father, the child has Prader-Willi syndrome; inheritance of the same deletion from the mother results in Angelman syndrome.

impulse *n.* (in neurology) *see* NERVE IMPULSE.

IMRT *see* INTENSITY-MODULATED RADIOTHERAPY.

in- (im-) *prefix denoting* **1.** not. **2.** in; within; into.

inanition *n.* a condition of exhaustion caused by lack of nutrients in the blood. This may arise through starvation, malnutrition, or intestinal disease.

inappetence *n.* lack of desire, usually for food.

in articulo mortis Latin: at the moment of death.

inborn error of metabolism any one of a group of inherited conditions in which there is a disturbance in either the structure, synthesis, function, or transport of protein molecules. There are over 1500 inborn errors of metabolism; examples are *phenylketonuria, *homocystinuria, and *hypogammaglobulinaemia.

inbreeding *n.* the production of offspring by parents who are closely related; for example, who are first cousins or siblings. The amount of inbreeding in a population is largely controlled by culture and tradition. *Compare* OUTBREEDING.

incapacity benefit a state benefit payable to those under the state retirement age who are incapable of work because of an illness or disability but who do not qualify for statutory sick pay. It was replaced by the *employment and support allowance, paid to new claimants since 2008.

incarcerated *adj.* confined or constricted so as to be immovable: applied particularly to a type of *hernia.

incidence rate a measure of morbidity based on the number of new episodes of ill-ness arising in a population over a period of time. It can be expressed in terms of affected persons or episodes per 1000 individuals at risk. *Compare* PREVALENCE.

incidentaloma *n.* a growth found incidentally on (usually) an adrenal gland (**adrenal incidentaloma**) during CT or MRI scanning of the abdomen or thorax for other clinical reasons. These growths are rarely significant, particularly if small, but they may be pathological if the patient has symptoms (e.g. hypertension, flushing) that could be attributable to an adrenal tumour.

incision *n.* **1.** the surgical cutting of soft tissues, such as skin or muscle, with a knife or scalpel. **2.** the cut so made.

incisor *n.* any of the four front teeth in each jaw, two on each side of the midline. *See also* DENTITION.

incisure *n.* (in anatomy) a notch, small hollow, or depression.

inclusion bodies particles occurring in the nucleus and cytoplasm of cells usually as a result of virus infection. Their presence can sometimes be used to diagnose such an infection.

inclusion conjunctivitis a sexually transmitted disease caused by *Chlamydia trachomatis*. It can be transmitted to infants at birth, with the disease clinically apparent 5–13 days after birth. Diagnosis is by cell culture. Treatment in the newborn is with topical erythromycin; adults require oral tetracycline or doxycycline for three weeks.

income support an income-related benefit payable to those whose income and savings do not exceed a specified maximum level and who do not work full-time.

incompatibility *n. see* COMPATIBILITY.

incompetence *n.* **1.** impaired function of the valves of the heart or veins, which allows backward leakage of blood. *See* AORTIC REGURGITATION, MITRAL REGURGITATION, VARICOSE VEINS. **2.** (incapacity) impairment of mental functioning such that a person is unable to understand, retain, and weigh up information so as to communicate a choice or preference. **3.** inability to fulfil the responsibilities and meet the standards of care expected of individuals working in a professional role in health care.

incontinence *n.* **1.** (urinary incontinence) the inappropriate involuntary passage of urine, resulting in wetting. **Stress incontinence** is the loss of urine on exertion (e.g. coughing and straining). It is common in women in whom the muscles of the pelvic floor are weakened after childbirth. **Urodynamic stress incontinence** (formerly called **genuine stress incontinence**) in women is due to a simultaneous rise in bladder and abdominal pressure that exceeds urethral pressure without a contraction of the detrusor muscle of the bladder. **Overflow incontinence** is leakage from a full bladder, which occurs most commonly in elderly men with bladder outlet obstruction or in patients with neurological conditions affecting bladder control. **Urge incontinence** is leakage of urine that accompanies an intense desire to pass water with failure of restraint. It is frequently caused by overactivity of the *detrusor muscle. *See also* ENURESIS. **2.** (faecal incontinence, anal incontinence) inability to control bowel movements, causing involuntary loss of faeces or flatus that is adversely affecting the patient's quality of life.

(((⊕))) SEE WEB LINKS

• Website of the Bladder and Bowel Foundation

incoordination *n.* (in neurology) an impairment in the performance of precise movements. These are dependent upon the normal function of the whole nervous system, and incoordination may result from a disorder in any part of it, especially the *cerebellum. *See* APRAXIA, ATAXIA, DYSMETRIA.

incubation *n.* **1.** the process of development of an egg or a culture of bacteria. **2.** the care of a premature baby in an *incubator.

incubation period (latent period) **1.** the interval between exposure to an infection and the appearance of the first symptoms. **2.** (in bacteriology) the period of development of a bacterial culture.

incubator *n.* a transparent container for keeping premature babies in controlled conditions and protecting them from infection. Other forms of incubator are used for cultivating bacteria in Petri dishes and for hatching eggs.

incus *n.* a small anvil-shaped bone in the middle *ear that articulates with the malleus and the stapes. *See* OSSICLE.

independent contractors (in Britain) *general practitioners, *dentists, and others who are not employees of the *National Health Service but who receive payment to provide an agreed level of service.

Independent Mental Capacity Advocate (IMCA) a person who must, by virtue of the *Mental Capacity Act 2005, be contacted to represent the *best interests of a patient who lacks *capacity and has no family or friends by acting as a proxy in medical decision-making. IMCAs are available via the local **Independent Mental Capacity Advocacy Service.**

Inderal *n. see* PROPRANOLOL.

indican *n.* a compound excreted in the urine as a detoxification product of *indoxyl. Indican is formed by the conjugation of indoxyl with sulphuric acid and potassium on the decomposition of tryptophan.

indicanuria *n.* the presence in the urine of an abnormally high concentration of *indican. This may be a sign that the intestine is obstructed.

indication *n.* (in medicine) **1.** a strong reason for believing that a particular course of action is desirable. In a wounded patient, the loss of blood, which would lead to circulatory collapse, is an indication for blood transfusion. **2.** any of the conditions for which a particular drug treatment may be prescribed, as defined by its *licence. *Compare* CONTRAINDICATION.

indigestion *n. see* DYSPEPSIA.

indinavir *n. see* PROTEASE INHIBITOR.

indocyanine green angiography *see* ANGIOGRAPHY.

indole *n.* a derivative of the amino acid tryptophan, excreted in the urine and faeces. Abnormal patterns of urinary indole excretion are found in some mentally retarded patients.

indolent *adj.* describing a disease process that is failing to heal or has persisted. The term is applied particularly to ulcers of skin or mucous membrane.

indometacin (indomethacin) *n.* an anti-inflammatory drug (*see* NSAID), used mainly for the relief of pain and severe inflammation in the treatment of rheumatic disease and similar disorders. It is administered either by mouth or in suppositories; common side-effects are headache, dizziness, and digestive upsets. It is also used in the treatment of patent *ductus arteriosus, being administered by intravenous injection. Trade name: **Indocid PDA**.

indoramin *n.* an *alpha blocker drug used to treat high blood pressure and to relieve urinary retention due to benign enlargement of the *prostate gland. It is administered by mouth. Possible side-effects can include drowsiness, nasal congestion, dry mouth, and failure of ejaculation. Trade names: **Baratol, Doralese**.

indoxyl *n.* an alcohol derived from *indole by bacterial action. It is excreted in the urine as *indican.

induced abortion *see* ABORTION.

induction *n.* **1.** (in obstetrics) the starting of labour by artificial means. **Medical induction** is carried out using such drugs as *prostaglandins or *oxytocin, which stimulate uterine contractions. **Surgical induction** is performed by *amniotomy (artificial rupture of membranes), usually supplemented by oxytocic drugs. Induction of labour is carried out if the wellbeing or life of mother or child is threatened by continuance of the pregnancy. **2.** (in anaesthesia) initiation of *anaesthesia. General anaesthesia is usually induced by the intravenous injection of short-acting *anaesthetics, e.g. thiopental.

induction loop system (loop system) a device for helping people with some types of *hearing aid or *cochlear implant to hear more effectively in certain situations. Electrical signals from a television, sound system, or microphone are passed through an amplifier to a wire that is positioned in a loop encompassing the desired listening area. This creates an electromagnetic field that can be picked up by a coil within the hearing aid or cochlear implant. Induction loops are installed in such places as public buildings, lecture theatres, classrooms, and churches. *See also* ASSISTIVE LISTENING DEVICE.

induration *n.* abnormal hardening of a tissue or organ. *See also* SCLEROSIS.

indusium *n.* a thin layer of grey matter covering the upper surface of the *corpus callosum between the two cerebral hemispheres.

industrial disease *see* OCCUPATIONAL DISEASE.

industrial injuries disablement benefit a state benefit payable to a person disabled by injury or a prescribed industrial disease sustained or contracted in the course of employment (*see* OCCUPATIONAL DISEASE, PRESCRIBED DISEASE). The benefit is payable as a weekly amount. The amount of the benefit depends on the degree of disablement as determined following assessment by a specialist. To be entitled to benefit, the disablement must be assessed as being at least 20% of total disability (1% in the case of pneumoconiosis, byssinosis, and diffuse mesothelioma). The benefit is payable if the claimant is still suffering disability two months or more after the date of the accident or onset of the disease. It is payable for a period assessed as the time for which the claimant is likely to suffer the disability. The assessment can be reviewed if the claimant's condition deteriorates or if he or she is still disabled at the end of the period of assessment.

inertia *n.* (in physiology) sluggishness or absence of activity in certain smooth muscles. In **uterine inertia** the muscular wall of the uterus fails to contract adequately during labour, making the process excessively long. This inertia may be present from the start of labour or it may develop because of exhaustion following strong contractions. *See also* SHOULDER DYSTOCIA.

in extremis Latin: at the point of death.

infant *n.* a child incapable of any form of independence from its mother: the term is usually used to refer to a child under one year of age, especially a premature or newborn child. In legal use the term denotes a child up to the age of seven years.

infanticide *n.* (in Britain) under the terms of the Infanticide Act 1938, the killing of an infant by the natural mother within 12 months of birth. The crime is distinguished from murder and treated more leniently at law because it is believed that the postnatal period may result in disturbance to a woman's balance of mind due to childbirth and/or lactation. Under such circumstances a woman would not be charged with murder but with infanticide. The law relating to infanticide is considered by many to be outdated and has been the subject of formal review following a report from the Law Commission.

infantile *adj.* **1.** denoting conditions occurring in adults that are recognizable in childhood, e.g. poliomyelitis (**infantile**

375

paralysis) and **infantile scurvy**. **2**. of, relating to, or affecting infants.

infantile spasms (salaam attacks) a rare but serious form of epilepsy that usually begins between three and eight months of age. The spasms are involuntary flexing movements of the arms, legs, neck, and trunk; each spasm lasts 1–3 seconds and is associated with flushing of the face, and runs of spasms occur over a period of several minutes. They may occur many times in one day. The baby fails to respond to human contact and development is usually profoundly slowed. An EEG pattern of *hypsarrhythmia is usual and diagnostic. Diagnosis may be delayed as spasms are sometimes confused with colic. Immediate recognition and treatment with antiepileptic medication, corticosteroids, or ACTH offers a chance of arresting the disease, but outcome depends primarily on the nature of the underlying brain abnormality.

infantilism *n.* persistence of childlike physical or psychological characteristics into adult life.

infant mortality rate (IMR) the number of deaths of children under one year of age per 1000 live births in a given year. Included in the IMR are the **neonatal mortality rate** (calculated from deaths occurring in the first four weeks of life) and **postneonatal mortality rate** (from deaths in the remainder of the first year). Neonatal deaths are further subdivided into **early** (first week) and **late** (second, third, and fourth weeks). In prosperous countries neonatal deaths account for about two-thirds of infant mortalities, the majority being in the first week (in the UK the major cause is prematurity and related problems). The IMR is usually regarded more as a measure of social affluence than a measure of the quality of antenatal and/or obstetric care; the latter is more truly reflected in the *perinatal mortality rate.

infarct *n. see* INFARCTION.

infarction *n.* the death of part or the whole of an organ that occurs when the artery carrying its blood supply is obstructed by a blood clot (thrombus) or an *embolus. For example, *myocardial infarction, affecting the muscle of the heart, follows coronary thrombosis. A small localized area of dead tissue produced as a result of an inadequate blood supply is known as an **infarct**. Infarcts also arise when venous outflow from an organ or tissue is obstructed, as occurs when the ovary or testis twist on their vascular pedicles (stalks), or when the sigmoid colon twists in *volvulus.

infection *n.* invasion of the body by harmful organisms (pathogens), such as bacteria, fungi, protozoa, rickettsiae, or viruses. The infective agent may be transmitted by a patient or *carrier in airborne droplets expelled during coughing and sneezing or by direct contact, such as kissing or sexual intercourse (*see* SEXUALLY TRANSMITTED DISEASE); by animal or insect *vectors; by ingestion of contaminated food or drink; or from an infected mother to the fetus during pregnancy or birth. Pathogenic organisms present in soil, organisms from animal intermediate hosts, or those living as *commensals on the body can also cause infections. Organisms may invade via a wound or bite or through mucous membranes. After an *incubation period symptoms appear, usually consisting of either localized inflammation and pain or more remote effects. Treatment with antibiotics is usually effective against most infections, but there are few specific treatments for many of the common viral infections, including the common cold (*see* ANTIVIRAL DRUG, INTERFERON).

infectious disease *see* COMMUNICABLE DISEASE.

infectious mononucleosis *see* GLANDULAR FEVER.

inferior *adj.* (in anatomy) lower in the body in relation to another structure or surface.

inferior dental block a type of injection to anaesthetize the inferior *dental nerve. Inferior dental block is routinely performed to allow dental procedures to be carried out on the lower teeth on one side of the mouth.

inferior dental canal a bony canal in the *mandible on each side. It carries the inferior *dental nerve and vessels and for part of its length its outline is visible on a radiograph.

inferiority complex **1**. an unconscious and extreme exaggeration of feelings of insignificance or inferiority, which may be shown by behaviour that is defensive or compensatory (such as aggression). **2**. (in psychoanalysis) a *complex said to result from the conflict between Oedipal wishes (*see* OEDIPUS COMPLEX) and the reality of the child's lack of power. This gives rise to repressed feelings of personal inferiority.

infertility *n.* inability in a woman to conceive or in a man to induce conception after regular unprotected sexual intercourse for two years. Female infertility may be due to failure to ovulate, to obstruction of the *Fallopian tubes, or to disease of the lining of the uterus (endometrium). Possible treatments (depending on the cause) include administration of drugs (such as *clomifene or *gonadorelin analogues), surgery (*see* SALPINGOGRAPHY, SALPINGOSTOMY, SALPINGOLYSIS) to restore patency of the Fallopian tubes, *gamete intrafallopian transfer (GIFT), and *in vitro fertilization. Causes of male infertility include decreased numbers or motility of spermatozoa (*see* OLIGOSPERMIA) and total absence of sperm (*see* AZOOSPERMIA). *See also* ANDROLOGY, STERILITY.

infestation *n.* the presence of animal parasites either on the skin (for example ticks) or inside the body (for example tapeworms).

infibulation *n. see* (FEMALE) CIRCUMCISION.

infiltration *n.* **1.** the abnormal entry of a substance (**infiltrate**) into a cell, tissue, or organ. Examples of infiltrates are blood cells, cancer cells, fat, starch, or calcium and magnesium salts. **2.** the injection of a local anaesthetic solution into the tissues to cause local *anaesthesia. Infiltration anaesthesia is routinely used to anaesthetize upper teeth to allow dental procedures to be carried out.

inflammation *n.* the body's response to injury, which may be acute or chronic. **Acute inflammation** is the immediate defensive reaction of tissue to any injury, which may be caused by infection, chemicals, or physical agents. It involves pain, heat, redness, swelling, and loss of function of the affected part. Blood vessels near the site of injury are dilated, so that blood flow is locally increased. White blood cells enter the tissue and begin to engulf bacteria and other foreign particles. Similar cells from the tissues (*see* MACROPHAGE) remove and consume the dead cells, sometimes with the production of pus, enabling the process of healing to commence. In certain circumstances healing does not occur and **chronic inflammation** ensues.

inflammatory bowel disease (IBD) a group of chronic intestinal diseases characterized by relapsing and remitting inflammation of the gastrointestinal tract. The most common types are ulcerative *colitis and *Crohn's disease.

infliximab *n.* a *monoclonal antibody that inhibits the activity of *tumour necrosis factor (TNF-α; *see* CYTOKINE INHIBITOR). It is used to treat severe Crohn's disease and ulcerative colitis, and rheumatoid arthritis, ankylosing spondylitis, and psoriatic arthritis that have failed to respond to treatment with corticosteroids or immunosuppressants and antirheumatic drugs, respectively. It is also used to treat *graft-versus-host disease in haemopoietic stem cell transplantation. Infliximab is administered by intravenous infusion; side-effects include intestinal upset, flushing, and allergic reactions. Trade name: **Remicade**.

influenza *n.* a highly contagious virus infection that affects the respiratory system. Types A and B are the forms that most commonly cause outbreaks in humans. The viruses are transmitted by coughing and sneezing. Symptoms commence after an incubation period of 1–4 days and include headache, fever, loss of appetite, weakness, and general aches and pains. They may continue for about a week. With bed rest and aspirin most patients recover, but a few may go on to develop pneumonia, either a primary influenzal viral pneumonia or a secondary bacterial pneumonia. Either of these may lead to death from haemorrhage within the lungs. The main bacterial organisms responsible for secondary infection are *Streptococcus pneumoniae*, *Haemophilus influenzae*, and *Staphylococcus aureus*, against which appropriate antibiotic therapy must be given.

An influenzal infection provides later protection only against the specific strain of virus concerned; the same holds true for immunization. Strains are classified according to the presence of different subtypes of two glycoproteins (antigens) on the viral surface: *haemagglutinin (H) and *neuraminidase (N). Small changes in the structure of these antigens, which occur frequently in influenza A and B viruses, require the continual development of new vaccines to protect against annual outbreaks of the disease. Major changes in antigenic structure occur much more rarely, when there is genetic recombination between strains that can infect more than one species (most strains of the virus are highly species-specific). However, when it does occur, it could result in the development of hybrid strains causing new forms of influenza that are difficult to contain; the pandemic of 1918–19 is thought to have arisen in this way (see also AVIAN INFLUENZA, SWINE INFLUENZA).

Information Commissioner the person in charge of the independent public agency set up to regulate the use and storage of personal data under the Data Protection Act 1998 (see DATA PROTECTION). The office of the Information Commissioner both regulates the use of data under the Act and judges any enforcement action required as a result of noncompliance with the principles of the statute. The Independent Commissioner's office also promotes public access to official information under the Freedom of Information Act 2000.

informed consent the principle that requires clinicians to provide sufficient information to patients or potential research participants in order to render their *consent lawful. Informed consent is sometimes said to be tautologous in that, under UK law, information is a *sine qua non* of consent.

infra- *prefix denoting* below.

infrared radiation the band of electromagnetic radiation that is longer in wavelength than the red of the visible spectrum. Infrared radiation is responsible for the transmission of radiant heat. It may be used in physiotherapy to warm tissues, reduce pain, and improve circulation, but is not as effective as *diathermy for deep structures. Special photographic film, which is sensitive to infrared radiation, is used in *thermography.

infundibulum *n.* any funnel-shaped channel or passage, particularly the hollow conical stalk that extends downwards from the hypothalamus and is continuous with the posterior lobe of the pituitary gland.

infusion *n.* 1. the slow injection of a substance, usually into a vein (**intravenous (IV) infusion**). This is a common method for replacing water, electrolytes, and blood products and is also used for the continuous administration of drugs (e.g. antibiotics, painkillers) or *nutrition. See also DRIP. 2. the process whereby the active principles are extracted from plant material by steeping it in water that has been heated to boiling point (as in the making of tea). 3. the solution produced by this process.

ingesta *pl. n.* food and drink that is introduced into the alimentary canal through the mouth.

ingestion *n.* 1. the process by which food is taken into the alimentary canal. It involves chewing and swallowing. 2. the process by which a phagocytic cell takes in solid material, such as bacteria.

ingravescent *adj.* gradually increasing in severity.

ingrowing toenail downward curving of the sides of a toenail, which causes chafing of the skin alongside the nail resulting in inflammation around the base of the nail.

inguinal *adj.* relating to or affecting the region of the groin (inguen).

inguinal canal either of a pair of openings that connect the abdominal cavity with the scrotum in the male fetus. The inguinal canals provide a route for the descent of the testes into the scrotum, after which they normally become obliterated.

inguinal hernia see HERNIA.

inguinal ligament (Poupart's ligament) a ligament in the groin that extends from the anterior superior iliac spine to the pubic tubercle. It is part of the *aponeurosis of the external oblique muscle of the abdomen.

INH see ISONIAZID.

inhalation *n.* 1. (**inspiration**) the act of breathing air into the lungs through the mouth and nose. See BREATHING. 2. a gas, vapour, or aerosol breathed in for the treatment of conditions of the respiratory tract. —**inhaler** *n.*

inherited thrombophilias see THROMBOPHILIA.

inhibition *n.* 1. (in physiology) the prevention or reduction of the functioning of an organ, muscle, etc., by the action of certain nerve impulses. 2. (in psychoanalysis) an inner command that prevents one from doing something forbidden. Some inhibitions are essential for social adjustment, but excessive inhibitions can severely restrict one's life.

inhibitor *n.* a substance that prevents the occurrence of a given process or reaction. See also MAO INHIBITOR.

inion *n.* the projection of the occipital bone that can be felt at the base of the skull.

initiation *n.* (in oncology) the first step in the development of cancer (*see* CARCINOGENESIS).

initiator (in oncogenesis) *n.* a substance that induces an irreversible change in a cell's DNA that can result in a cancer. An example is dimethylbenzanthracene. *Compare* PROMOTER.

injection *n.* introduction into the body of drugs or other fluids by means of a syringe, usually drugs that would be destroyed by the digestive processes if taken by mouth. Common routes for injection are into the skin (**intracutaneous** or **intradermal**); below the skin (**subcutaneous**), e.g. for insulin; into a muscle (**intramuscular**), for drugs that are slowly absorbed; and into a vein (**intravenous, IV**), for drugs to be rapidly absorbed. *Enemas are also regarded as injections.

injury scoring system (injury severity scale, ISS) a system used, particularly in *triage, for grading the severity of an injury. *See also* ABBREVIATED INJURY SCALE.

inlay *n.* **1.** a substance or piece of tissue placed within a tissue, generally to replace a defect. For example, a bone graft may be inlaid into an area of missing or damaged bone, or an aortic prosthesis placed using an inlay technique within an aneurysm. **2.** (in dentistry) a rigid restoration inserted into a tapered cavity in a tooth. It is held in place with a cement *lute. While cast gold has been the most widely used material, porcelain and composite resin are also used.

inlet *n.* an aperture providing the entrance to a cavity, such as that of the pelvis.

innate *adj.* describing a condition or characteristic that is present in an individual at birth and is inherited from his parents. *See also* CONGENITAL.

inner ear *see* LABYRINTH.

innervation *n.* the nerve supply to an area or organ of the body, which can carry either motor impulses to the structure or sensory impulses away from it towards the brain.

innominate artery (brachiocephalic artery) a short artery originating as the first large branch of the *aortic arch, passing upwards to the right, and ending at the lower neck near the right sternoclavicular joint. Here it divides into the right common carotid and the right subclavian arteries.

innominate bone *see* HIP BONE.

innominate vein (brachiocephalic vein) either of two veins, one on each side of the neck, formed by the junction of the external jugular and subclavian veins. The two veins join to form the superior vena cava.

INO internuclear ophthalmoplegia (*see* OPHTHALMOPLEGIA).

ino- *combining form denoting* **1.** fibrous tissue. **2.** muscle.

inoculation *n.* the introduction of a small quantity of material, such as a vaccine, in the process of *immunization: a more general name for *vaccination.

inoculum *n.* any material that is used for inoculation.

inosine pranobex a *antiviral drug that is administered by mouth to treat herpes simplex infections (cold sores and genital herpes) and genital warts. Trade name: **Imunovir.**

inositol *n.* a compound, similar to a hexose sugar, that is a constituent of some cell phospholipids. Inositol is present in many foods, in particular in the bran of cereal grain. It is sometimes classified as a vitamin but it can be synthesized by most animals and there is no evidence that it is an essential nutrient in humans.

inositol triphosphate (IP$_3$) a short-lived biochemical *second messenger formed from *phospholipid in the cell membrane when a chemical messenger (e.g. a hormone or serotonin) binds to receptors on the cell surface. Inositol triphosphate triggers the rapid release of calcium into the cell fluid, which initiates various cellular processes, such as smooth muscle contraction and the release of glucose, histamine, etc. Inositol triphosphate exists for only a few seconds before being converted to inositol by the action of a sequence of enzymes.

inotropic *adj.* affecting the contraction of heart muscle. Drugs such as *dobutamine, *dopamine, and *enoximone have positive inotropic action, stimulating heart muscle contractions and causing the heart rate to increase. *Beta-blocker drugs, such as *propranolol, have negative inotropic action, reducing heart muscle contractions and causing the heart rate to decrease.

Inoue balloon *see* MITRAL STENOSIS, VALVULOPLASTY.

in-patient *n.* a patient who is admitted to a bed in a hospital ward and remains there for a period of time for treatment, examination, or observation. *Compare* OUT-PATIENT.

inquest *n.* an official judicial enquiry into the cause of a person's death: carried out when the death is sudden or takes place under suspicious circumstances. The results of medical and legal investigations that have been carried out are considered by a *coroner, sitting with or without a jury, and made publicly known. *See also* AUTOPSY.

INR international normalized ratio: the ratio of a patient's *prothrombin time (PT) to a standardized 'normal' PT. For example, an INR of 2 indicates that a patient's blood takes twice the normal time to clot. It is used to monitor anticoagulant dosage.

insanity *n.* a degree of mental illness such that the affected individual is not responsible for his actions or is not capable of entering into a legal contract. The term is a legal rather than a medical one.

insect *n.* a member of a large group of mainly land-dwelling *arthropods. The body of the adult is divided into a head, thorax, and abdomen. The head bears a single pair of sensory antennae; the thorax bears three pairs of legs and, in most insects, wings (these are absent in some parasitic groups, such as lice and fleas). Some insects are of medical importance. Various bloodsucking insects transmit tropical diseases, for example the female *Anopheles* mosquito transmits malaria and the tsetse fly transmits sleeping sickness. The bites of lice can cause intense irritation and, secondarily, bacterial infection. The organisms causing diarrhoea and dysentery can be conveyed to food on the bodies of flies. *See also* MYIASIS.

insecticide *n.* a preparation used to kill insects. Ideally, an insecticide should have no toxic effects when ingested by human beings or animals, but modern powerful compounds have inherent dangers and have caused fatalities. Some insect powders contain organic phosphorus compounds and fluorides; when ingested accidentally they may cause damage to the nervous system. The use of such compounds is generally under strict control. *See also* DDT, DIELDRIN.

insemination *n.* introduction of semen into the vagina. *See also* ARTIFICIAL INSEMINATION, INTRAUTERINE INSEMINATION.

insertion *n.* (in anatomy) the point of attachment of a muscle (e.g. to a bone) that is relatively movable when the muscle contracts. *Compare* ORIGIN.

insight *n.* one's level of awareness of one's illness. Insight can be fully or partially intact or absent. Full insight requires an understanding that one has an illness, seeks help, and complies with treatment. Insight can be impaired temporarily through drug intoxication or through medical or mental illness or permanently after brain damage or in some cases of *dementia. The term is also applied in psychology to the patient's accuracy of understanding the development of his or her personality and problems; in this sense insight can be enhanced by psychotherapy.

insolation *n.* exposure to the sun's rays. *See also* HEATSTROKE.

insomnia *n.* inability to fall asleep or to remain asleep for an adequate length of time. Insomnia may be associated with physical disease, particularly if there are painful symptoms, or psychological conditions, such as depression, anxiety, or stress.

inspiration *n. see* INHALATION.

inspissated *adj.* (of secretions, etc.) thickened or dried by evaporation or dehydration.

instillation *n.* **1.** the application of liquid medication drop by drop, as into the eye. **2.** the medication, such as eye drops, applied in this way.

instinct *n.* **1.** a complex pattern of behaviour innately determined, which is characteristic of all individuals of the same species. The behaviour is released and modified by environmental stimuli, but its pattern is relatively uniform and predetermined. **2.** an innate drive that urges the individual towards a particular goal (for example, *libido in psychoanalytic psychology).

institutionalization *n.* a condition produced by long-term residence in an impersonal institution (such as some residential care homes and orphanages) where stimulation is lacking. The individual adapts to the behaviour characteristic of the institution to such an extent that he or she is handicapped in other environments. The features often include apathy, dependence, social withdrawal or awkwardness, and a lack of personal responsibility. The effects of institutionalization on mental health can be significant and informed the move towards more care in the community.

insufficiency *n.* inability of an organ or part, such as the heart or kidney, to carry out its normal function.

insufflation *n.* the act of blowing gas or a powder, such as a medication, into a body cavity.

insula *n.* an area of the *cerebral cortex that is overlapped by the sides of the deep lateral sulcus (cleft) in each hemisphere.

insulin *n.* a protein hormone, produced in the pancreas by the beta cells of the *islets of Langerhans, that is important for regulating the amount of sugar (glucose) in the blood. Insulin secretion is stimulated by a high concentration of blood sugar. Lack of this hormone gives rise to *diabetes mellitus, in which large amounts of sugar are present in the blood and urine. This condition may be treated successfully by insulin injections (*see* INSULIN ANALOGUES, INSULIN PEN, ISOPHANE INSULINS). *See also* CONTINUOUS SUBCUTANEOUS INSULIN INFUSION.

insulin analogues a group of synthetic human insulins with specific alterations in their amino-acid sequences designed to modify their rate of absorption from the injection site (subcutaneous tissue). Some are absorbed much more rapidly and have a shorter duration of action than the older insulins; others are absorbed more slowly but at a constant rate, to prevent peaks in the plasma insulin levels associated with hypoglycaemia. These analogues include the short-acting **insulin aspart**, **insulin glulisine**, and **insulin lispro** and the long-acting **insulin detemir** and **insulin glargine**.

insulinase *n.* an enzyme, found in such tissues as the liver and kidney, that is responsible for the normal breakdown of insulin in the body.

insulinoma *n.* an insulin-producing and usually benign tumour of the beta cells in the *islets of Langerhans of the pancreas. Symptoms can include sweating, faintness, episodic loss of consciousness, and other features of *hypoglycaemia (*see* WHIPPLE'S TRIAD). Single tumours can be removed surgically. Multiple very small tumours scattered throughout the pancreas cannot be treated by surgery but do respond to drugs that poison the beta cells, including *diazoxide.

insulin pen a penlike device designed to inject a measured dose of insulin. The dose can be 'dialled up' and then safely injected from a 3-ml cartridge contained within. The pen can be capped off and easily stored in a pocket or small bag; some types are disposable, while others can be refilled.

insulin resistance diminution in the response of the body's tissues to insulin, so that higher concentrations of serum insulin are required to maintain normal circulating glucose levels. Eventually the islet cells can no longer produce adequate amounts of insulin for effective glucose lowering, resulting in hyperglycaemia. Insulin resistance is one of the risk factors for cardiovascular disease. *See also* DIABETES MELLITUS, METABOLIC SYNDROME.

insulin shock a condition in which excess insulin in the body decreases the amount of glucose in the blood (*see* HYPOGLYCAEMIA). If not treated with glucose or glucagon, coma and death can occur.

insulin stress test an important but potentially dangerous test of anterior pituitary function involving the deliberate induction of a hypoglycaemic episode with injected insulin and the subsequent measurement of plasma cortisol and growth hormone at regular intervals over the next three hours. The stress of the hypoglycaemia should induce a rise in the levels of these hormones unless the anterior pituitary or the adrenal glands are diseased. The test can induce epileptic seizures or angina in those with a predisposition and should not be performed in susceptible individuals. It is often combined with the thyrotrophin-releasing hormone (TRH) test and the gonadotrophin-releasing hormone (GnRH) test in what is known as the **triple test**.

insult *n.* an injury or physical trauma.

Intal *n. see* CROMOGLICATE.

integrated care pathway a multidisciplinary plan for delivering health and social care to patients with a specific condition or set of symptoms. Such plans are often used for the management of common conditions and are intended to improve patient care by reducing unnecessary deviation from best practice. *See* CLINICAL GOVERNANCE.

integrated governance *see* CLINICAL GOVERNANCE.

integration *n.* the blending together of

the *nerve impulses that arrive through the thousands of synapses at a nerve cell body. Impulses from some synapses cause *excitation, and from others *inhibition; the overall pattern decides whether an individual nerve cell is activated to transmit a message or not.

integument *n.* **1.** the skin. **2.** a membrane or layer of tissue covering any organ of the body.

intelligence quotient (IQ) an index of intellectual development. In childhood and adult life it represents intellectual ability relative to the rest of the population; in children it can also represent rate of development (*mental age as a percentage of chronological age). Most *intelligence tests are constructed so that the resulting intelligence quotients in the general population have a *mean of about 100 and a *standard deviation of about 15. An IQ of below 80 is considered to be indicative of *learning disability.

intelligence test a standardized assessment procedure for the determination of intellectual ability. The score produced is usually expressed as an *intelligence quotient. Most tests present a series of different kinds of problems to be solved. The best known are the Wechsler Adult Intelligence Scale (WAIS), the Wechsler Intelligence Scale for Children (WISC), and the Stanford Binet Intelligence Scale. Scores on intelligence tests are used for such purposes as the diagnosis of *mental retardation and the assessment of intellectual deterioration.

intensity-modulated radiotherapy (IMRT) radiotherapy using multiple beams with variable intensity across each field, resulting in dose distributions that can fit to concave shapes and thus reduce dose to surrounding healthy tissues and organs. It can be used to treat a wide range of cancers and can enable safe delivery of higher doses to tumours.

intensive therapy unit (ITU, intensive care unit**)** a hospital unit designed to give intensive care, provided by specialist multidisciplinary staff, to a selected group of seriously ill patients or to those in need of special postoperative techniques (e.g. heart or chest patients).

intention *n.* **1.** a process of healing. Healing by **first intention** is the natural healing of a wound or surgical incision when the edges are brought together under aseptic condi-

tions and *granulation tissue forms. In healing by **second intention** the wound edges are separated and the cavity is filled with granulation tissue over which epithelial tissue grows from the wound edges. In healing by **third intention** the wound ulcerates, granulations are slow to form, and a scar forms at the wound site. **2.** evaluation of a person's aims or purpose in undergoing an action, which is important for the assessment and attribution of responsibility in ethicolegal questions and defined legally for the purposes of criminal law. *See also* DOCTRINE OF DOUBLE EFFECT.

intention tremor *see* TREMOR.

inter- *prefix denoting* between. Examples: **intercostal** (between the ribs); **intertrochanteric** (between the trochanters).

intercalated *adj.* describing structures, tissues, etc., that are inserted or situated between other structures.

intercellular *adj.* situated or occurring between cells.

intercostal muscles muscles that occupy the spaces between the ribs and are responsible for controlling some of the movements of the ribs. The superficial **external intercostals** lift the ribs during inspiration; the deep **internal intercostals** draw the ribs together during expiration.

intercurrent *adj.* going on at the same time: applied to an infection contracted by a patient who is already suffering from an infection or other disease.

interferon *n.* a substance that is produced by cells infected with a virus and has the ability to inhibit viral growth (*see* CYTOKINES). Interferon is active against many different viruses, but particular interferons are effective only in the species that produces them. There are three types of human interferon: **alpha** (from white blood cells), **beta** (from fibroblasts), and **gamma** (from lymphocytes).

Human interferon can be produced in bacterial host cells by *genetic engineering for clinical use. **Interferon alfa** (IntronA, Roferon-A) is used in treating hepatitis B and C and certain lymphomas and other cancers, **peginterferon alfa** (Pegasys, ViraferonPeg) is used for hepatitis B and C, and **interferon beta** (Avonex, Betaferon, Extavia, Rebif) for multiple sclerosis. They are administered by injection; side-effects, including flulike symptoms, lethargy, and depression, may be severe.

interkinesis *n.* **1.** the resting stage between the two divisions of *meiosis. **2.** *see* INTERPHASE.

interleukin *n.* any of a family of proteins that control some aspects of haemopoiesis and the immune response (*see* CYTOKINES). Many interleukins are currently characterized. **Interleukin 2** (**IL-2**) stimulates T lymphocytes to become *natural killer cells, active against cancer cells, and is being investigated for the treatment of cancer: recombinant interleukin 2 (**aldesleukin**, Proleukin), administered by subcutaneous injection, can be of benefit in the treatment of renal cell carcinoma.

intermediate care a health and social care service that aims to facilitate earlier discharge from hospital or prevent admission to hospital by providing support at a level between *primary care and *secondary care. Intermediate care is provided on a short-term basis, usually no longer than six weeks.

intermenstrual bleeding bleeding arising from the genital tract in a woman with a regular menstrual cycle, not occurring at menstruation or following sexual intercourse.

intermittency *n.* a *lower urinary tract symptom in which the flow of urine is not continuous but stops and starts.

intermittent auscultation a method of fetal monitoring in *labour, with *auscultation of the fetal heart for one minute through a uterine contraction every 15 minutes during the first stage, and after every other contraction, or every five minutes, in the second stage of labour.

intermittent claudication *see* CLAUDICATION.

intermittent fever a fever that rises, subsides, then returns again. *See* MALARIA.

intermittent pneumatic compression a technique to prevent thrombosis in bedridden patients. It uses an inflatable device that squeezes the calf when it inflates, preventing pools of blood forming behind the valves in the veins, thus mimicking the effects of walking.

intermittent self-catheterization (**clean intermittent self-catheterization**, **ISC**, **CISC**) a procedure in which the patient periodically passes a disposable catheter through the urethra into the bladder for the purpose of emptying it of urine. It is increasingly used in the management of patients of both sexes (including children) with chronic *retention and large residual urine volumes, often due to *neuropathic bladder. ISC may prevent back pressure and dilatation of the upper urinary tract with consequent infection and incontinence.

intern *n.* *see* DOCTOR.

International Classification of Diseases (**ICD**) a list of all known diseases and syndromes, including mental and behavioural disorders, published by the *World Health Organization every ten years (approximately). Over the years the classification has moved from being disease-orientated to include a wider framework of illness and other health problems. The latest version, **ICD-10**, was published in 1992 and employs alphanumeric coding. It is used in many countries as the principal means of classifying both mortality and morbidity experience and allows comparison of morbidity and mortality rates nationally and internationally. A parallel list, the **International Classification of Functioning, Disabilities and Health** (**ICF**), has also been compiled and is being used alongside the ICD. *See also* HANDICAP.

SEE WEB LINKS
• The standard international classification for statistical, administrative, and epidemiological purposes, as supplied by the World Health Organization

International Prostate Symptom Score (**IPSS**) a self-administered questionnaire completed by men with *lower urinary tract symptoms that gives a numerical score (on a scale of 0 to 35) to indicate the severity of their symptoms.

interneuron *n.* a neuron in the central nervous system that acts as a link between the different neurons in a *reflex arc. It usually possesses numerous branching processes (dendrites) that make possible extensive and complex circuits and pathways within the brain and spinal cord.

internode *n.* the length of *axon covered with a myelin sheath. Internodes are separated by nodes of Ranvier, where the sheath is absent.

internuclear ophthalmoplegia (INO) *see* OPHTHALMOPLEGIA.

interobserver error (in statistical surveys) *see* VALIDITY.

interoceptor *n.* any *receptor organ composed of sensory nerve cells that respond to and monitor changes within the body, such as the stretching of muscles or the acidity of the blood.

interparietal bone (inca bone, incarial bone) the bone lying between the *parietal bones, at the back of the skull.

interpeduncular *adj.* situated between the peduncles of the cerebrum or cerebellum.

interphase (interkinesis) *n.* the period when a cell is not undergoing division (mitosis), during which activities such as DNA synthesis occur.

intersex *n.* the condition of possessing the characteristics of both sexes, making it difficult to establish the sex of the individual at birth from the appearance of his or her genitals. *See* HERMAPHRODITE, PSEUDOHERMAPHRODITISM. —**intersexuality** *n.*

interstice *n.* a small space in a tissue or between parts of the body. —**interstitial** *adj.*

interstitial cells cells that form part of the connective tissue (**interstitium**) between other tissues, especially the cells interspersed between the seminiferous tubules of the *testis (also called **Leydig cells**). They secrete *androgens in response to stimulation by *luteinizing hormone from the anterior pituitary gland.

interstitial-cell-stimulating hormone *see* LUTEINIZING HORMONE.

interstitial cystitis a chronic nonbacterial inflammation of the bladder accompanied by an urgent desire to pass urine frequently and bladder pain; it is sometimes associated with an ulcer in the bladder wall (**Hunner's ulcer**). The cause is unknown and *contracture of the bladder eventually occurs. Treatment is by distension of the bladder under spinal or epidural anaesthetic, instillation of anti-inflammatory solutions into the bladder, and administration of steroids or *NSAIDs. Bladder enhancement or augmentation (*see* CYSTOPLASTY) may be required for a contracted bladder.

interstitial nephritis disease of the *tubulointerstitium of the kidney. Acute interstitial nephritis (AIN) represents in many cases an allergic reaction to drugs (especially ampicillin, cefalexin, NSAIDs, allopurinol, and furosemide). AIN can also be associated with acute infections and autoimmune disease. Thirst and polyuria may be prominent, and renal function severely affected. In allergic cases, the use of steroids hastens recovery after the allergen has been removed. Chronic interstitial nephritis (CIN) is associated with progressive scarring of the tubulointerstitium, often with lymphocyte infiltration. Primary causes of CIN include gout, radiation nephropathy, sarcoidosis, *analgesic nephropathy, reflux nephropathy, chronic hypokalaemia and hypercalcaemia, and *Aristolochia*-associated nephropathies. Management of CIN involves removal of the precipitating cause, where identified, and control of hypertension.

interstitial pneumonitis an alternative name for cryptogenic fibrosing *alveolitis (CFA, or idiopathic pulmonary fibrosis, IPF), used by lung pathologists to classify the different cellular types of the disease. The most common cellular pattern seen on CT scanning is **usual interstitial pneumonitis** (**UIP**). Use of the latter abbreviation is increasing in clinical contexts: the diagnosis CFA/UIP or just UIP now often appears in hospital notes and discharge letters. A differing cellular pattern with cellular infiltrate is seen in patients with **nonspecific interstitial pneumonitis** (**NSIP**).

intertrigo *n.* superficial inflammation of two skin surfaces that are in contact, such as between the thighs or under the breasts, particularly in obese people. It is caused by friction and sweat and is often aggravated by infection, especially with *Candida*.

interventional cardiology a subspecialty of cardiology concerned with the treatment of heart conditions using cardiac *catheterization techniques under local anaesthetic and X-ray control, including *percutaneous coronary intervention and percutaneous balloon mitral *valvuloplasty.

interventional radiology the performance of therapeutic or diagnostic procedures under the control of an appropriate imaging technique. Guidance is commonly by X-ray fluoroscopy, ultrasound, or computerized tomography, and recently also by magnetic resonance imaging. Procedures commonly performed include the placing of vascular catheters, drainage of fluid collections or abscesses, stenting of obstructions to the gastrointestinal tract or blood vessels, embolization, cryotherapy, and radiofrequency ablation. Imaging is also used in many forms of *minimally invasive surgery.

intervention study a comparison of the outcome between two or more groups of patients that are deliberately subjected to different regimes to test a hypothesis, usually of treatment (in a **clinical trial**). Wherever possible those entering the trial should be allocated to their respective groups by means of random numbers, and one such group (**controls**) should have no active treatment (**randomized controlled trial**). Ideally neither the patient nor the person assessing the outcome should be aware of which group each patient is allocated to. In a **blind trial**, the patients are not aware of their group; in a **double-blind trial**, neither the patients nor the doctor or observer are aware of the therapy group. The groups may exchange treatment after a prearranged period (**cross-over trial**). Randomized controlled trials are increasingly used to assess new treatments against current standards; for example, to compare new chemotherapeutic agents to established treatment (the control group). To be ethically sound, there must not be evidence at the time of the study to show conclusively which arm of the trial is the best (*see* EQUIPOISE).

intervertebral disc the flexible plate of fibrocartilage that connects any two adjacent vertebrae in the backbone. At birth the central part of the disc – the **nucleus pulposus** – consists of a gelatinous substance, which gradually becomes replaced by cartilage with age. The intervertebral discs account for one quarter of the total length of the backbone; they act as shock absorbers, protecting the brain and spinal cord from the impact produced by running and other movements. A tear in the outer fibrous portion of the disc results in displacement of the nucleus pulposus to varying degrees: protrusion, prolapse (*see* PROLAPSED INTERVERTEBRAL DISC), extrusion, or sequestration.

intestinal flora bacteria normally present in the intestinal tract. Some are responsible for the synthesis of *vitamin K. By producing a highly acidic environment in the intestine they may also prevent infection by pathogenic bacteria that cannot tolerate such conditions.

intestinal juice *see* SUCCUS ENTERICUS.

intestinal obstruction partial or complete blockage of the bowel producing symptoms of vomiting, distension, and abdominal pain due to failure to pass intestinal contents. The causes may be acute (e.g. incarcerated hernia) or chronic (e.g. tumours, Crohn's disease). Conservative management is by nasogastric suction ('suck') and replacement of water and electrolytes ('drip'), but most cases require surgical cure by removing the underlying cause.

intestine (bowel, gut) *n.* the part of the *alimentary canal that extends from the stomach to the anus. It is divided into two main parts – the small intestine and the large intestine. The **small intestine** is divided into the *duodenum, *jejunum, and *ileum. It is here that most of the processes of digestion and absorption of food take place. The surface area of the inside of the small intestine is increased by the presence of finger-like projections called **villi** (see illustration). Glands in the mucous layer of the intestine secrete digestive enzymes and mucus. The **large intestine** consists of the *caecum, vermiform *appendix, *colon, and *rectum. It is largely concerned with the absorption of water from the material passed from the small intestine. The contents of the in-

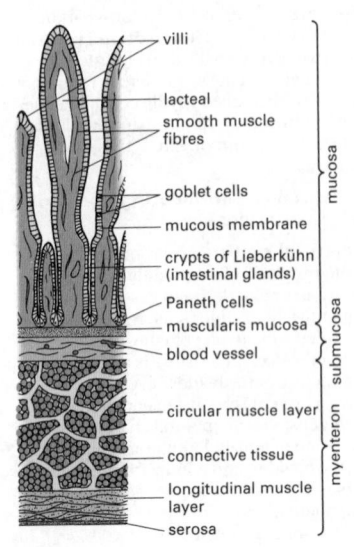

Intestine. Longitudinal section through the ileum.

testines are propelled forwards by means of rhythmic muscular contractions (*see* PERISTALSIS). —**intestinal** *adj*.

intima (tunica intima) *n*. **1.** the inner layer of the wall of an *artery or *vein. It is composed of a lining of endothelial cells and an elastic membrane. **2.** the inner layer of various other organs or parts.

intolerance *n*. the inability of a patient to tolerate a particular drug, manifested by various adverse reactions.

intoxication *n*. the symptoms of poisoning due to ingestion of any toxic material, including alcohol and heavy metals.

intra- *prefix denoting* inside; within. Examples: **intralobular** (within a lobule); **intraosseous** (within the bone marrow); **intrauterine** (within the uterus).

intra-articular *adj*. within a joint. The term is commonly used to specify a fracture pattern, the location of a soft-tissue injury, or the route of injection of a drug. *See also* EXTRA-ARTICULAR, PERIARTICULAR.

intracameral *adj*. within a chamber, such as the anterior or posterior chamber of the eye. In **intracameral anaesthesia** an anaesthetic agent is injected into the anterior chamber of the eye, usually during surgery.

intracellular *adj*. situated or occurring inside a cell or cells.

intracorneal *adj*. within the cornea.

intracranial *adj*. within the skull.

intracranial hypotension headache an increasingly recognized type of persistant headache in a patient with no history of headaches. Features include headache that is worse on standing and resolves on lying flat. It may be associated with other symptoms, such as dizziness, tinnitus, and (rarely) *diplopia. The commonest cause is a complication of lumbar puncture, but it may occur spontaneously (**spontaneous intracranial hypotension**) after a dural tear resulting in a leak of cerebrospinal fluid. Treatment is with bed rest and increased intake of fluids; caffeine orally or intravenously is also used. In cases that do not resolve, an epidural blood patch procedure is performed, in which a small quantity of the patient's blood is slowly injected into the *epidural space to seal the leak.

intracytoplasmic sperm injection *see* ICSI.

intradermal *adj*. within the skin. An **intradermal injection** is made into the skin.

intramuscular *adj*. within a muscle. An **intramuscular injection** is made into a muscle.

intraobserver error (in statistical surveys) *see* VALIDITY.

intraocular *adj*. of or relating to the area within the eyeball. An **intraocular lens implant** is a plastic lens placed inside the eye after *cataract extraction to replace the natural lens.

intraosseous needle a wide-bore needle for insertion directly into the bone marrow of (usually) the tibia in children, used only in emergencies when no other means of intravenous access can be gained. Intraosseous needles enable fluids and drugs to be given rapidly. They are only for use with unconscious patients and must be removed when alternative access is obtained.

intrapartum *adj*. occurring during labour or childbirth.

intrastromal *adj*. (in ophthalmology) within the *stroma of the cornea.

intrastromal keratomileusis an operation to correct severe degrees of myopia (short-sightedness). A disc of corneal tissue (from the *stroma of the cornea) is removed, frozen, and remodelled on a lathe, then replaced into the cornea to alter its curvature and thus reduce the myopia. *Excimer laser treatment, which is easier to perform, has now replaced this (*see* LASIK).

intrathecal *adj*. **1.** within the *meninges of the spinal cord. An **intrathecal injection** is made into the meninges. **2.** within a sheath, e.g. a nerve sheath.

intrauterine contraceptive device *see* IUCD.

intrauterine fetal death death of a fetus in the uterus after 24 weeks of gestation. *See* STILLBIRTH.

intrauterine growth restriction (IUGR) failure of a fetus to achieve its growth potential, resulting in the birth of a baby whose birth weight is abnormally low in relation to its gestational age (*see* SMALL FOR GESTATIONAL AGE). Causes include *uteroplacental insufficiency, maternal disease (e.g. infection, malnutrition, high blood pressure, smoking, and alcoholism), poor socioeconomic conditions, multiple pregnancy (e.g. twins), and fetal disease or chromosomal abnormalities. It may be associated with *preterm birth.

intrauterine insemination (IUI) a procedure for assisting conception in which carefully washed spermatozoa are injected into the uterus through the vagina at the time of ovulation, which is induced and monitored (using ultrasound) to determine the day of insemination. This procedure is used in cases of male infertility due to inability of the sperm to penetrate the cervical mucus or the barriers surrounding the ovum, in which case the sperm may be treated in vitro to improve their motility and *acrosome reaction. IUI is also used for donor insemination.

intravenous *adj.* into or within a vein. *See* INFUSION, INJECTION.

intravenous feeding *see* NUTRITION.

intravenous pyelography (IVP) *see* PYELOGRAPHY.

intravenous urography (IVU) a series of X-ray images of the urinary tract following the injection into a vein of a radiopaque *contrast medium. This material is concentrated and excreted by the kidneys, and the IVU reveals details of the kidneys, ureters, and the bladder. An IVU provides information about kidney function and may reveal the presence of stones, tumours, obstructions, or anatomical abnormalities in the urinary tract. *See also* PYELOGRAPHY.

intraventricular haemorrhage (IVH) *see* PERIVENTRICULAR HAEMORRHAGE.

intraversion *n. see* INTROVERSION.

intra vitam Latin: during life.

intravitreal *adj.* within the vitreous humour of the eye.

intrinsic factor a glycoprotein secreted in the stomach. The secretion of intrinsic factor is necessary for the absorption of *vitamin B_{12}; a failure of secretion of intrinsic factor leads to a deficiency of the vitamin and the condition of *pernicious anaemia.

intrinsic muscle a muscle that is contained entirely within the organ or part it acts on. For example, there are intrinsic

muscles of the tongue, whose contractions change the shape of the tongue.

intro- *prefix denoting* in; into.

introitus *n.* (in anatomy) an entrance into a hollow organ or cavity.

introjection *n.* (in psychoanalysis) the process of adopting, or of believing that one possesses, the qualities of another person. This can be a form of *defence mechanism.

intromission *n.* the introduction of one organ or part into another, e.g. the penis into the vagina.

introversion *n.* 1. (intraversion) an enduring personality trait characterized by interest in the self rather than the outside world. People high in introversion (**introverts**), as measured by questionnaires and psychological tests, tend to have a small circle of friends, like to persist in activities once they have started, and are highly susceptible to permanent *conditioning. Introversion was first described by Carl Jung as a tendency to distancing oneself from others, to philosophical interests, and to reserved defensive reactions. *Compare* EXTROVERSION. 2. a turning inwards of a hollow organ (such as the uterus) on itself.

introvert *n. see* INTROVERSION.

intubation *n.* the introduction of a tube into part of the body for the purpose of diagnosis or treatment. Thus **gastric intubation** may be performed to keep the stomach empty during and after abdominal surgery and to provide feeding and drugs when the patient is unable to swallow. In **endotracheal intubation** an endotracheal tube is inserted through the mouth into the trachea to maintain an airway in an unconscious or anaesthetized patient. It requires expert knowledge for insertion, using a laryngoscope, and has a small cuff at the far end for inflation inside the trachea. It affords the best level of protection of the airway from vomitus.

intumescence *n.* a swelling or an increase in the volume of an organ.

intussusception *n.* the telescoping (**invagination**) of one part of the bowel into another: most common in young children under the age of four. As the contents of the intestine are pushed onwards by muscular contraction more and more intestine is dragged into the invaginating portion, resulting in obstruction. Symptoms include intermittent screaming and pallor, vomiting, and the passing of bloody mucus ('redcurrent jelly') with the stools; if the condition does not receive prompt surgical treatment, shock from gangrene of the bowel may result. A barium or Gastrografin enema may confirm the diagnosis and in many cases may relieve the intussusception.

inulin *n.* a carbohydrate with a high molecular weight, used in a test of kidney function called **inulin clearance**. Inulin is filtered from the bloodstream by the kidneys. By injecting it into the blood and measuring the amount that appears in the urine over a given period, it is possible to calculate how much filtrate the kidneys are producing in a given time.

inunction *n.* the rubbing in with the fingers of an ointment or liniment.

invagination *n.* **1.** the infolding of the wall of a solid structure to form a cavity. This occurs in some stages of the development of embryos. **2.** *see* INTUSSUSCEPTION.

invasion *n.* the spread of *cancer into neighbouring normal structures; it is one of the cardinal features of malignancy.

inversion *n.* **1.** the turning inwards or inside-out of a part or organ: commonly applied to the state of the uterus after childbirth when its upper part is pulled through the cervical canal. **2.** a chromosome mutation in which a block of genes within a chromosome are in reverse order, due to that section of the chromosome becoming inverted. The centromere may be included in the inverted segment (**pericentric inversion**) or not (**paracentric inversion**).

invertebrate **1.** *n.* an animal without a backbone. The following are invertebrate groups of medical importance: *insects, *ticks, *nematodes, *flukes, and *tapeworms. **2.** *adj.* not possessing a backbone.

in vitro Latin: describing biological phenomena that are made to occur outside the living body (traditionally in a test-tube).

in vitro fertilization (IVF) fertilization of an ovum outside the body, the resultant *zygote being incubated to the *blastocyst stage and then implanted in the uterus. The technique, pioneered in Britain, resulted in 1978 in the birth of the first **test-tube baby**. IVF may be undertaken when a woman has blocked Fallopian tubes, unexplained infer-

tility, endometriosis, or ovulation disorders; it is also carried out for purposes of surrogacy and egg donation. The mother-to-be is given hormone therapy causing a number of ova to mature at the same time (*see* SUPEROVULATION). Several of them are then removed from the ovary through a laparoscope. The ova are mixed with spermatozoa and incubated in a culture medium until the blastocyst is formed. The blastocyst is then implanted in the mother's uterus and the pregnancy proceeds normally. IVF is regulated by the *Human Fertilization and Embryology Act 1990 via the Human Fertilization and Embryology Authority.

in vivo Latin: describing biological phenomena that occur or are observed occurring within the bodies of living organisms.

involucrum *n.* a growth of new bone, formed from the *periosteum, that sometimes surrounds a mass of infected and dead bone in osteomyelitis.

involuntary muscle muscle that is not under conscious control, such as the muscle of the gut, stomach, blood vessels, and heart. *See also* CARDIAC MUSCLE, SMOOTH MUSCLE.

involution *n.* **1.** the shrinking of the uterus to its normal size after childbirth. **2.** atrophy of the corpus luteum, which occurs after pregnancy or if implantation of the embryo does not occur. **3.** atrophy of an organ in old age.

iodine *n.* an element required in small amounts for healthy growth and development. An adult body contains about 30 mg of iodine, mostly concentrated in the thyroid gland: this gland requires iodine to synthesize *thyroid hormones. A deficiency of iodine leads to *goitre. The daily requirement of iodine in an adult is thought to be about 140 µg per day; dietary sources of iodine are sea food and vegetables grown in soil containing iodide and also iodized table salt. Iodine is used in the diagnosis and treatment of diseases of the thyroid gland (*see* LUGOL'S IODINE, RADIOACTIVE IODINE THERAPY) and also as an antiseptic and skin disinfectant (in the form of **povidone-iodine**). Water-soluble contrast media used in X-ray examinations are organic chemicals containing iodine, which is radiopaque due to its high atomic weight. Symbol: I.

iodism *n.* iodine poisoning. The main features are a characteristic staining of the mouth and odour on the breath. Vomited material may be yellowish or bluish. There is pain and burning in the throat, intense thirst, and diarrhoea, with dizziness, weakness, and convulsions. Emergency treatment includes administration of starch or flour in water and lavage with sodium thiosulphate solution.

IOL intraocular lens implant. *See* CATARACT.

ion *n.* an atom or group of atoms that has lost one or more electrons, making it electrically charged and therefore more chemically active. *See* ANION, CATION, ELECTROLYTE, IONIZATION.

ion channel a protein that spans a cell membrane to form a water-filled pore through which ions (e.g. calcium $[Ca^{2+}]$, sodium $[Na^+]$, potassium $[K^+]$) can pass into or out of the cell.

ionization *n.* the process of producing *ions. Some molecules ionize in solution (*see* ELECTROLYTE). Ions can also be produced when **ionizing radiation** dislodges one or more electrons from an atom or molecule. This can be harmful to DNA in cells, resulting in tumours or genetic defects.

iontophoresis *n.* the technique of introducing through the skin, by means of an electric current, charged particles of a drug, so that it reaches a deep site. The method has been used to transfer salicylate ions through the skin in the treatment of deep rheumatic pain. *See also* CATAPHORESIS.

IOUS *intra*operative *u*ltrasound examination (*see* ULTRASONOGRAPHY).

ipecacuanha *n.* a plant extract used in small doses, usually in the form of tinctures and syrups, as an *expectorant to relieve coughing and to induce vomiting. Ipecacuanha irritates the digestive system, and high doses may cause severe digestive upsets.

IPF *see* IDIOPATHIC PULMONARY FIBROSIS.

ipratropium *n.* an *antimuscarinic drug used as a bronchodilator in the treatment of chronic reversible airways obstruction (*see* BRONCHOSPASM) and to relieve rhinorrhoea resulting from *rhinitis. Ipratropium is administered by inhalation or nasal spray; side-effects include dry mouth and nasal dryness. Trade names: **Atrovent**, **Ipratropium Steri-Neb**, **Respontin**, **Rinatec**.

ipsilateral (ipselateral, homolateral) *adj.* on or affecting the same side of the body: ap-

plied particularly to paralysis (or other symptoms) occurring on the same side of the body as the brain lesion that caused them. *Compare* CONTRALATERAL.

IPSS *see* INTERNATIONAL PROSTATE SYMPTOM SCORE.

IQ *see* INTELLIGENCE QUOTIENT.

irbesartan *n. see* ANGIOTENSIN II ANTAGONIST.

irid- (irido-) *combining form denoting* the iris.

iridectomy *n.* an operation on the eye in which a part of the iris is removed.

iridencleisis *n.* an operation for *glaucoma, now rarely performed, in which a small incision is made beneath the *conjunctiva close to the cornea and part of the iris is drawn into it. The iris acts like a wick and keeps the incision open for the drainage of fluid from the anterior chamber of the eye to the tissue beneath the conjunctiva.

iridium-192 *n.* a radioactive isotope of the metallic element iridium. It is the most common source used for intracavitary *brachytherapy. Symbol: Ir-192.

iridocyclitis *n.* inflammation of the iris and ciliary body of the eye. *See* UVEITIS.

iridodialysis *n.* a tear, caused by injury to the eye, in the attachment of the iris to the ciliary body. Usually a dark crescentic gap is seen at the edge of the iris where the tear has occurred, and the pupil pulls away from the site of the tear.

iridodonesis *n.* tremulousness of the iris when the lens is moved. It is due to absence of support from the lens, against which the iris normally lies, and occurs when the lens is absent or dislocated from its normal position.

iridoplegia *n.* paralysis of the iris, which is usually associated with *cycloplegia and results from injury, inflammation, or the use of pupil-dilating eye drops. In the case of injury, the pupil is usually larger than normal and moves little, if at all, in response to light and drugs.

iridotomy *n.* an operation on the eye in which an incision is made in the iris using a knife or a *YAG laser.

irinotecan *n. see* TOPOISOMERASE INHIBITOR.

iris *n.* the part of the eye that regulates the amount of light that enters. It forms a coloured muscular diaphragm across the front of the lens; light enters through a central opening, the **pupil**. A ring of muscle round the margin contracts in bright light, causing the pupil to become smaller (*see* PUPILLARY REFLEX). In dim light a set of radiating muscles contract and the constricting muscles relax, increasing the size of the pupil. The outer margin of the iris is attached to the *ciliary body.

iris bombé an abnormal condition of the eye in which the iris bulges forward towards the cornea. It is due to pressure from the aqueous humour behind the iris when its passage through the pupil to the anterior chamber of the eye is blocked (**pupil-block glaucoma**).

Irish Sign Language (ISL) *see* SIGN LANGUAGE.

iritis *n.* inflammation of the iris. *See* UVEITIS.

IRMER Ionising Radiation (Medical Exposures) Regulations 2000. *See* RADIATION PROTECTION.

iron *n.* an element essential to life. The body of an adult contains on average 4 g of iron, over half of which is contained in *haemoglobin in the red blood cells, the rest being distributed between *myoglobin in muscles, *cytochromes, and iron stores in the form of *ferritin and *haemosiderin. Iron is an essential component in the transfer of oxygen in the body. The absorption and loss of iron is very finely controlled. A good dietary source is meat, particularly liver. The recommended daily intake of iron is 10 mg per day for men and 12 mg per day for women during their reproductive life. A deficiency of iron may lead to *anaemia. Symbol: Fe.

Many preparations of iron are used to treat iron-deficiency anaemia. These include preparations taken by mouth, such as *ferrous sulphate, and those administered by injection, such as *iron dextran.

iron dextran a drug containing *iron and *dextran, administered by intramuscular injection or intravenous infusion to treat iron-deficiency anaemia. Side-effects can include pain at the site of injection, rapid beating of the heart, and allergic reactions. Trade name: **CosmoFer**.

iron lung *see* VENTILATOR.

iron-storage disease *see* HAEMOCHROMATOSIS.

irradiation *n.* **1.** exposure of the body's tissues to ionizing radiation (*see* IONIZATION). The source may be background radiation, diagnostic X-rays, radiotherapy, or nuclear accidents. **2.** exposure of a substance or object to ionizing radiation. Irradiation of food with gamma rays, which kill bacteria, is a technique used in food preservation.

irreducible *adj.* unable to be replaced in a normal position: applied particularly to a type of *hernia.

irrigation *n.* the process of washing out a wound or hollow organ with a continuous flow of water or medicated solution. Techniques are available for washing out the entire intestinal tract (**whole-gut irrigation**) as a prelude to surgery on the lower intestine.

irritability *n.* (in physiology) the property of certain kinds of tissue that enables them to respond in a specific way to outside stimuli. Irritability is shown by nerve cells, which can generate and transmit electrical impulses when stimulated appropriately, and by muscle cells, which contract when stimulated by nerve impulses.

irritable bowel syndrome (IBS) a common condition in which abdominal pain, bloating, or discomfort is associated with an alteration in the bowel habit, in the absence of an organic cause. The symptoms are caused by abnormal muscular contractions in the intestine and heightened sensitivity to such stimuli as stretching or distension. The cause is unknown, but the condition is often associated with stress or anxiety and may follow severe infection of the intestine (**postinfectious irritable bowel syndrome**). Tests may be needed to rule out organic disease. Treatment is based on removing anxiety (psychotherapy), dietary adjustment and faecal softening agents, and drugs to reduce spasm or diminish pain sensitivity.

irritant *n.* any material that causes irritation of a tissue, ranging from nettles (causing pain and swelling) to tear gas (causing watering of the eyes). Chronic irritation by various chemicals can give rise to *dermatitis.

isch- (ischo-) *combining form denoting* suppression or deficiency.

ischaemia *n.* an inadequate flow of blood

to a part of the body, caused by constriction or blockage of the blood vessels supplying it. Ischaemia of heart muscle produces *angina pectoris. Ischaemia of the calf muscles of the legs on exercise (causing intermittent *claudication) or at rest (producing *rest pain) is common in elderly subjects with atherosclerosis of the vessels at or distal to the point where the aorta divides into the iliac arteries. —**ischaemic** adj.

ischi- (**ischio-**) combining form denoting the ischium.

ischiorectal abscess an abscess in the space between the sheet of muscle that assists in control of the rectum (levator ani) and the pelvic bone. It may occur spontaneously, but is often secondary to an anal fissure, thrombosed *haemorrhoids, or other disease of the anus (such as Crohn's disease). Symptoms are severe throbbing pain near the anus with swelling and fever; it may cause an anal *fistula. Pus is drained from the abscess by surgical incision.

ischium n. a bone forming the lower part of each side of the *hip bone (see also PELVIS). —**ischiac**, **ischial** adj.

island n. (in anatomy) an area of tissue or group of cells clearly differentiated from surrounding tissues.

islet n. (in anatomy) a small group of cells that is structurally distinct from the cells surrounding it.

islet cell transplantation a new technique still under evaluation for curing type 1 *diabetes mellitus, which involves the injection of donated cells from the pancreatic *islets of Langerhans into the liver, where it is hoped they will seed and survive. The transplanted cells then take over insulin production from the recipient's diseased pancreas.

islet cell tumour any tumour arising in a cell of the pancreatic *islets of Langerhans. These tumours, which include *insulinomas, *glucagonomas, and *somatostatinomas, form one of the two major subclasses of gastrointestinal neuroendocrine tumours, the other being the *carcinoid tumours.

islets of Langerhans small groups of endocrine cells scattered through the material of the *pancreas. There are three main histological types: alpha (α) cells, which secrete *glucagon; beta (β) cells, which produce *insulin; and D cells, which release *somato-

statin and *pancreatic polypeptide. [P. Langerhans (1847–88), German physician and anatomist]

iso- combining form denoting equality, uniformity, or similarity.

isoagglutinin (**isohaemagglutinin**) n. one of the antibodies occurring naturally in the plasma that cause *agglutination of red blood cells of a different group.

isoagglutinogen n. one of the *antigens naturally occurring on the surface of red blood cells that is attacked by an isoagglutinin in blood plasma of a different group, so causing *agglutination.

isoantibody n. an *antibody that occurs only in some individuals of a species against the components of foreign tissues from an individual of the same species.

isoantigen n. an antigenic substance that occurs only in some individuals of a species. Thus the antigens of the *HLA system are isoantigens, as are the agglutinogens of the different *blood groups.

isodactylism n. a congenital defect in which all the fingers are the same length.

isoenzyme (**isozyme**) n. a physically distinct form of a given enzyme. Isoenzymes catalyse the same type of reaction but have slight physical and immunological differences. Isoenzymes of dehydrogenases, oxidases, transaminases, phosphatases, and proteolytic enzymes are known to exist.

isohaemagglutinin n. see ISOAGGLUTININ.

isoimmunization n. the development of antibodies (**isoantibodies**) within an individual against antigens from another individual of the same species.

isolation n. **1.** the separation of a person with an infectious disease from noninfected people. See also QUARANTINE. **2.** (in surgery) the separation of a structure from surrounding structures by the use of instruments.

isoleucine n. an *essential amino acid. See also AMINO ACID.

isomerase n. any one of a group of enzymes that catalyse the conversion of one isomer of a compound into another.

isometheptene n. a *sympathomimetic drug used in the treatment of migraine attacks, in combination with paracetamol (as

Midrid). It is administered by mouth. Possible side-effects include dizziness.

isometric exercises (isometrics) a system of exercises based on the principle of **isometric contraction** of muscles. This occurs when the fibres are called upon to contract and do work, but despite an increase in tension do not shorten in length. It can be induced in muscles that are used when a limb is made to pull or push against something that does not move. The exercises increase fitness and build muscle.

isometropia *n.* an equal power of *refraction in both eyes.

isomorphism *n.* the condition of two or more objects being alike in shape or structure. It can exist at any structural level, from molecules to whole organisms. —**isomorphic, isomorphous** *adj.*

isoniazid (isonicotinic acid hydrazide, INH) *n.* a drug used in the treatment of *tuberculosis, usually taken by mouth. Because tuberculosis bacteria soon become resistant to isoniazid, it is given in conjunction with other antibiotics. Side-effects include peripheral neuropathy, especially in patients with diabetes or alcohol dependence, which can be countered by including pyridoxine (vitamin B_6) in the preparation.

isophane insulins a group of insulins in which the insulin molecules are combined with *protamine molecules to slow down their rate of absorption from the injection site. The insulin is released steadily from the skin into the bloodstream to stabilize blood sugar over a longer period. Mixtures of isophane and fast-acting insulins are also available (**biphasic insulin aspart, biphasic insulin lispro**).

isosorbide dinitrate a drug used for the prevention and treatment of angina; it acts by relaxing the smooth muscle of both arteries and veins, thus causing dilatation (*see* VASODILATOR). It is administered by mouth (as tablets or a spray) or by intravenous infusion; side-effects include headache, flushing, dizziness, and hypotension. Trade names: **Angitak, Isoket, Isoket Retard**.
   Isosorbide dinitrate is converted in the body to the active form of the drug, **isosorbide mononitrate**, which is available as a preventative oral treatment for angina. Trade names: **Elantan, Imdur, Ismo, Isodur, Isotard, Monomax**, etc.

isosthenuria *n.* inability of the kidneys to produce either a concentrated or a dilute urine. This occurs in the final stages of renal failure.

isotonic *adj.* **1.** describing solutions that have the same osmotic pressure. *See* OSMOSIS. **2.** describing muscles that have equal *tonicity.

isotonic exercises *see* EXERCISE.

isotope *n.* any one of the different forms of an element, possessing the same number of protons (positively charged particles) in the nucleus, and thus the same atomic number, but different numbers of neutrons. Isotopes therefore have different atomic weights. Radioactive isotopes decay into other isotopes or elements, emitting alpha, beta, or gamma radiation. Some radioactive isotopes may be produced artificially by bombarding elements with neutrons. These are known as **nuclides** and are used extensively in *radiotherapy for the treatment of cancer.

isotretinoin *n.* a drug related to vitamin A (*see* RETINOID) that is administered orally in the treatment of severe acne that has failed to respond to other treatment and topically for mild to moderate acne. Possible side-effects include dry skin, nose bleeds, eyelid and lip inflammation, muscle, joint, and abdominal pains, diarrhoea, and some disturbances of vision. Trade names: **Isotrex, Roaccutane**.

isotropic *adj.* (in computerized tomography or magnetic resonance imaging) denoting the acquisition of data when the slice thickness is similar in size to that of an individual *pixel, i.e. the *voxel is a cube. Computerized reconstruction in any plane will not suffer any loss of detail. The concept is particularly applicable for *multidetector computerized tomography, in which slice thickness of less than 1 mm is used.

isozyme *n. see* ISOENZYME.

ispaghula husk a bulking agent (*see* LAXATIVE) used to treat constipation, *diverticular disease, *irritable bowel syndrome, and other conditions of disturbed bowel habit. It is administered by mouth. Trade names: **Fibrelief, Fybogel, Isogel, Ispagel Orange, Regulan**.

ISS *see* INJURY SCORING SYSTEM.

isthmus *n.* a constricted or narrowed part of an organ or tissue, such as the band of thyroid tissue connecting the two lobes of the thyroid gland.

itch *n.* discomfort or irritation of the skin, prompting the sufferer to scratch or rub the affected area. It is an important symptom of skin disease. *See* PRURITUS.

-itis *combining form denoting* inflammation of an organ, tissue, etc. Examples: **arthritis** (of a joint); **peritonitis** (of the peritoneum).

itraconazole *n.* an antifungal drug that is administered by mouth or intravenous infusion to treat a wide variety of fungal infections, including candidiasis and ringworm. Side-effects include nausea and abdominal pain. Trade name: **Sporanox**.

ITU *see* INTENSIVE THERAPY UNIT.

IUCD (intrauterine contraceptive device) a plastic or metal coil, spiral, or other shape, about 25 mm long, that is inserted into the cavity of the uterus to prevent conception. Its exact mode of action is unknown but it is thought to interfere with implantation of the embryo. Early IUCDs (such as the Lippes loop) were made of plastic; later variants (such as the Gravigard) are covered with copper, which slowly dissolves and augments the contraceptive action. About one-third of women fitted with an IUCD find the side-effects (heavy menstrual bleeding or back pain) unacceptable, but most have no complaints. The unwanted pregnancy rate is about 2 per 100 woman-years. If pregnancy should occur there is normally no need to remove the device (it may, however, be shed spontaneously). *See also* IUS, POSTCOITAL CONTRACEPTION.

IUGR *see* INTRAUTERINE GROWTH RESTRICTION.

IUI *see* INTRAUTERINE INSEMINATION.

IUS (intrauterine system) a hormonal contraceptive device consisting of a plastic T-shaped frame that is inserted into the uterus. It carries a progestogen (*levonorgestrel) in a sleeve around its stem and has two fine threads attached to its base, by which it can be removed. It provides a long-term method of contraception that is also reversible. The IUS is also used in the treatment of menorrhagia. Trade name: **Mirena**.

IV intravenous. *See* INFUSION, INJECTION.

ivermectin *n.* a drug used in the treatment of *onchocerciasis. It acts by killing the immature forms (*microfilariae) of the parasite. Ivermectin is also used to treat creeping eruption, strongyloidiasis, and scabies. It is administered by mouth; side-effects, which are mild, include itching and swollen lymph nodes.

IVF *see* IN VITRO FERTILIZATION.

IVU *see* INTRAVENOUS UROGRAPHY.

Ixodes *n.* a genus of widely distributed parasitic ticks. Several species are responsible for transmitting *Lyme disease, *tularaemia, Queensland tick typhus, and *Russian spring-summer encephalitis. The bite of a few species can give rise to a serious paralysis, caused by a toxin in the tick's saliva.

ixodiasis *n.* any disease caused by the presence of *ticks.

Ixodidae *n.* a family of *ticks.

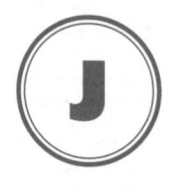

Jacksonian march *see* EPILEPSY. [J. H. Jackson (1835–1911), British neurologist]

Jacquemier's sign a bluish or purplish coloration of the vagina: a possible indication of pregnancy. [J. M. Jacquemier (1806–79), French obstetrician]

jactitation *n.* restless tossing and turning of a person suffering from a severe disease, frequently one with a high fever.

Jaeger test types a card with text printed in type of different sizes, used for testing acuity of near vision. [E. R. Jaeger von Jastthal (1818–84), Austrian ophthalmologist]

jamais vu one of the manifestations of temporal lobe *epilepsy, in which there is a sudden feeling of unfamiliarity with everyday surroundings.

Janeway lesions red spots on the palm of the hands caused by a bacterial infection of the heart (*see* ENDOCARDITIS). [E. G. Janeway (1841–1911), US physician]

Jarisch-Herxheimer reaction (**Herxheimer reaction**) exacerbation of the symptoms of syphilis that may occur on starting antibiotic therapy for the disease. The effect is transient and requires no treatment. [A. Jarisch (1850–1902), Austrian dermatologist; K. Herxheimer (1861–1944), German dermatologist]

jaundice *n.* a yellow discoloration of the skin or whites of the eyes, indicating excess bilirubin (a bile pigment) in the blood. Jaundice is classified into three types. **Obstructive jaundice** occurs when bile made in the liver fails to reach the intestine due to obstruction of the *bile ducts (e.g. by gallstones or a tumour) or to *cholestasis. The urine is dark, the faeces pale, and the patient may itch. **Hepatocellular jaundice** is due to disease of the liver cells, such as *hepatitis, when the liver is unable to utilize the bilirubin, which accumulates in the blood. The urine may be dark but the faeces retain their colour. **Haemolytic jaundice** occurs when there is excessive destruction of red cells in the blood (*see* HAEMOLYSIS). Urine and faeces retain their normal colour. Medical name: **icterus**.

jaw *n.* either the *maxilla (upper jaw) or the *mandible (lower jaw). The jaws form the framework of the mouth and provide attachment for the teeth.

jaw-jerk reflex an abnormal reflex elicited by lightly placing the index finger across the chin of the patient and tapping it with a tendon hammer while the jaw hangs loosely open. A brisk upward movement of the jaw indicates an upper *motor neuron disorder above the brainstem.

jaw thrust a manoeuvre for opening the airway of an unconscious patient. The flats of the hands are placed on the cheeks with the fingers hooked under the angles of the jaw so that the jaw can be pulled upwards to separate the tongue from the back of the pharynx. The tongue often falls onto the back of the pharynx in unconsciousness, causing obstruction to the airway. This method is particularly useful when spinal injury is suspected and movement of the neck is undesirable. This is an alternative to the *head tilt, chin lift manoeuvre.

jaw wiring a radical but reversible approach to obtain weight loss in which the jaws are wired together surgically to restrict food intake to simple fluids. Success can be dramatic but weight is often regained once the restriction is removed and normal eating habits are resumed. *See also* BARIATRIC SURGERY.

JCA *see* JUVENILE CHRONIC ARTHRITIS.

jejun- (**jejuno-**) *combining form denoting* the jejunum.

jejunal biopsy removal of a piece of the lining (mucosa) of the upper small intestine. This can be done by a surgical operation but is usually performed by an *enteroscope or less usually a special metal capsule (Crosby capsule), swallowed by the patient. When the capsule is in the *jejunum a small knife within it is triggered by suction on an attached tube, cutting off a small piece of mucosa. The specimen is then examined microscopically to assist in the diagnosis of *coeliac disease, *Crohn's disease, *Whipple's disease, or intestinal infections, or its enzyme content may be measured chemically to detect, for example, *lactase deficiency.

jejunal ulcer *see* PEPTIC ULCER, ZOLLINGER-ELLISON SYNDROME.

jejunectomy *n.* surgical removal of the jejunum or part of the jejunum.

jejunoileostomy *n.* an operation in which the jejunum is joined to the ileum (small intestine), when either the end of the jejunum or the beginning of the ileum has been removed or is to be bypassed. It is usually performed for intestinal disease (e.g. Crohn's disease). It was formerly used for the treatment of obesity but has been abandoned because of serious side-effects.

jejunostomy *n.* a surgical operation in which the jejunum is brought through the abdominal wall and opened. It can enable the insertion of a catheter into the jejunum for short-term infusion of nutrients or other substances. In **feeding jejunostomy** a tube is directly inserted into the jejunum (surgically or endoscopically) to enable the introduction of nutrients directly into the small bowel. This is useful in cases of operations on the stomach and duodenum and recurrent vomiting not responding to medical treatment. **Percutaneous endoscopic gastrojejunostomy** (**PEGJ**) usually involves placement of a jejunal tube extension after insertion of a PEG tube (*see* GASTROSTOMY).

jejunotomy *n.* a surgical incision into the jejunum in order to inspect the interior or remove something from within it.

jejunum *n.* part of the small *intestine. It comprises about two-fifths of the whole small intestine and connects the duodenum to the ileum. —**jejunal** *adj.*

jerk *n.* the sudden contraction of a muscle in response to a nerve impulse. Examples are the *ankle jerk and the **knee jerk** (*see* PATELLAR REFLEX). Eliciting these and other jerks is a means of testing the nerve pathways, via the spinal cord, which are involved in *reflexes.

JGA *see* JUXTAGLOMERULAR APPARATUS.

jigger *n. see* TUNGA.

Jod-Basedow phenomenon a collection of symptoms that includes skin rash, conjunctivitis, salivary gland inflammation, and hyperthyroidism due to the intake of high doses of iodine (German *Jod*, hence the name). [K. A. von Basedow (1799–1854), German physician]

joint *n.* the point at which two or more bones are connected. The opposing surfaces of the two bones are lined with cartilaginous, fibrous, or soft (synovial) tissue. The three main classes of joint are *diarthrosis (freely movable), *amphiarthrosis (slightly movable), and *synarthrosis (immovable).

joule *n.* the *SI unit of work or energy, equal to the work done when the point of application of a force of 1 newton is displaced through a distance of 1 metre in the direction of the force. In electrical terms the joule is the work done per second when a current of 1 ampere flows through a resistance of 1 ohm. Symbol: J. *See also* CALORIE.

jugular *adj.* relating to or supplying the neck or throat.

jugular vein any one of several veins in the neck. The **internal jugular** is a very large paired vein running vertically down the side of the neck and draining blood from the brain, face, and neck. It ends behind the sternoclavicular joint, where it joins the subclavian vein. The **external jugular** is a smaller paired vein running superficially down the neck to the subclavian vein and draining blood from the face, scalp, and neck. Its tributary, the **anterior jugular**, runs down the front of the neck.

jugular venous pressure (**JVP**) the pressure in the internal jugular vein, which is an indirect measurement of *central venous pressure (CVP) in the right atrium. In clinical practice the JVP is estimated by visual inspection at the bedside with the patient reclining at 45 degrees.

jugum *n.* (in anatomy) a ridge or furrow that connects two parts of a bone.

jumper's knee (patellar tendinitis) a form of *tendinitis that is common in athletes and dancers. Repeated sudden contracture of the quadriceps muscle at take-off causes inflammation of the attachment of the patellar tendon to the lower end of the patella. Treatment includes rest, physiotherapy, and anti-inflammatory medication.

junction *n.* (in anatomy) the point at which two different tissues or structures are in contact. *See also* NEUROMUSCULAR JUNCTION.

justice *n.* the moral requirement to treat people fairly and impartially and with a proper regard for their entitlements and deserts – although the ways in which ethicists and philosophers define fairness, entitlements, and deserts varies considerably. Justice is common to many theories of ethics and is one of the *four principles of medical ethics. Issues of justice are mainly, but not exclusively, concerned with the fair allocation of medical resources when these are limited and is encapsulated in theories of distributive justice (*see* DESERT, EQUALITY, NEED, RATIONING).

juvenile chronic arthritis (JCA, Still's disease) any one of a group of conditions characterized by inflammation of the joints lasting longer than six weeks and occurring before the age of 16. The causes are unknown but immunological and infective mechanisms are suspected. JCA can affect either four or fewer joints (**pauciarticular JCA**) or more than four (**polyarticular JCA**). There are two recognized types of pauciarticular JCA: type 1, which generally affects girls below the age of four; and type 2 (**juvenile-onset spondylarthropathy**), which generally affects boys over the age of nine. There are also two types of polyarticular JCA, depending on the presence or absence of a particular antibody in the blood. There is a great range of severity of these diseases. Treatment consists of pain management and

prevention of subsequent deformity or limitation of movement (e.g. contractures).

juvenile-onset spondylarthropathy
see JUVENILE CHRONIC ARTHRITIS.

juvenile polyp *see* POLYP.

juxta- *combining form denoting* proximity to. Example: **juxta-articular** (near a joint).

juxtaglomerular apparatus (JGA) a microscopic structure within the kidney that is important in regulating blood pressure, body fluid, and electrolytes. It is situated in each nephron, between the afferent arteriole of the glomerulus and the returning distal convoluted tubule of the same nephron. The JGA consists of specialized cells within the distal tubule (the **macula densa**), which detect the amount of sodium chloride passing through the tubule and can secrete locally acting vasoconstrictor substances that act on the associated afferent arteriole to induce a reduction in filtration pressure (tubuloglomerular feedback). Modified cells within the afferent arterioles secrete *renin in response to a fall in perfusion pressure or feedback from the macula densa and form a central role in the renin-*angiotensin-aldosterone axis. **Mesangial cells** support and connect the macula densa and the specialized cells in the afferent arteriole and have sympathetic innervation, facilitating the renin response to sympathetic nervous stimulation.

JVP *see* JUGULAR VENOUS PRESSURE.

Kahn reaction a test for syphilis, in which antibodies specific to the disease are detected in a sample of the patient's blood by means of a *precipitin reaction. This test is not as reliable as some. [R. L. Kahn (20th century), US bacteriologist]

kala-azar (visceral leishmaniasis, Dumdum fever) *n.* a tropical disease caused by the parasitic protozoan *Leishmania donovani*. The parasite, which is transmitted to humans by *sandflies, invades the cells of the lymphatic system, spleen, and bone marrow. Symptoms include enlargement and subsequent lesions of the liver and spleen; anaemia; a low *leucocyte count; weight loss; and irregular fevers. The disease occurs in Asia, South America, the Mediterranean area, and Africa. Drugs containing antimony, with supplementary pentamidine, are used in the treatment of this potentially fatal disease.

kallidin *n.* a naturally occurring polypeptide consisting of ten amino acids. Kallidin is a powerful vasodilator and causes contraction of smooth muscle; it is formed in the blood under certain conditions. *See* KININ.

kallikrein *n.* one of a group of enzymes found in the blood and body fluids that act on certain plasma globulins to produce bradykinin and kallidin. *See* KININ.

Kallmann's syndrome a familial condition that is the most common form of isolated *gonadotrophin deficiency; it is combined with underdevelopment of the olfactory lobes, causing *anosmia. The syndrome is caused by a gene *deletion on the short arm of the X chromosome. Patients often present with delayed puberty. There is an association with *ichthyosis, mental retardation, obesity, renal and skeletal abnormalities, and undescended testes, but these features are very variable. [F. J. Kallmann (1897–1965), US geneticist]

Kantian ethics an approach to moral questions deriving from the teachings and writing of the German philosopher Immanuel Kant (1724–1804). It is characterized by an emphasis on the rational endeavour of determining what is right. In particular, attention to the inner morality of the individual is integral to achieving freedom (*see* AUTONOMY). Moral determination depends on reason (rather than personal wants or feelings) and the absolute nature of *duty, which is always applicable (*see* IMPERATIVE). Kantian ethics deny *consequentialism; acts are to be judged by their accordance with universal principles rather than their good or bad consequences (*see* DEONTOLOGY). The Kantian tradition has been influential in medical ethics and finds translation in normative professional codes, and its insistence that every human life must be treated as an end in itself and not simply as a means continues to inform contemporary ethical practice.

kaolin *n.* a white clay that contains aluminium and silicon and is purified and powdered for use as an adsorbent. It may be used in the form of an oral suspension to treat chronic diarrhoea. Kaolin is also used in dusting powders and poultices.

Kaposi's sarcoma a malignant tumour arising from blood vessels in the skin and appearing as purple to dark brown plaques or nodules. It is common in Africa and is sometimes seen in those of Mediterranean extraction, but more commonly occurs in patients with *AIDS. The tumour evolves slowly; radiotherapy is the treatment of choice for localized lesions but chemotherapy may be of value in metastatic disease. Highly active antiretroviral therapy (*see* ANTIRETROVIRAL DRUG) should be started in those with HIV infection as a first-line treatment. [M. Kaposi (1837–1902), Hungarian dermatologist]

Kartagener's syndrome a hereditary condition in which the heart and other internal organs lie on the opposite side of the body to the norm (i.e. the heart lies on the right; *see* DEXTROCARDIA); it is associated with chronic sinusitis and bronchiectasis. [M. Kartagener (1897–1975), German physician]

kary- (karyo-) *combining form denoting* a cell nucleus.

karyokinesis *n.* division of the nucleus of

a cell, which occurs during cell division before division of the cytoplasm (**cytokinesis**). *See* MITOSIS.

karyolysis *n.* the breakdown of a cell nucleus, which occurs during cell *necrosis and is preceded by fragmentation of the nucleus (**karyorrhexis**).

karyoplasm *n. see* NUCLEOPLASM.

karyosome *n.* the dense mass of *chromatin found in the cell nucleus, which is composed mainly of chromosomes.

karyotype 1. *n.* the *chromosome set of an individual or species described in terms of both the number and structure of the chromosomes. 2. *n.* the representation of the chromosome set in a diagram. 3. *vb.* to determine the karyotype of a cell, as by microscopic examination.

katathermometer *n.* a thermometer used to measure the cooling power of the air surrounding it, having its bulb covered with water-moistened material. The instrument is brought to a steady temperature of 100°F and then exposed to the air. The time taken for the temperature recorded by the thermometer to fall to 95°F gives an index of the air's cooling power.

Kawasaki disease (Kawasaki syndrome, mucocutaneous lymph node syndrome) a condition of unknown cause affecting young children, usually less than five years old and most commonly of Japanese or Korean descent, and characterized by fever, conjunctivitis, a sore throat, and a generalized rash and reddening of the palms and soles. This is followed by peeling of the fingers and toes. The fever usually persists for 1–2 weeks. In approximately one-fifth of children there is involvement of the coronary arteries and heart muscle (myocardium), resulting in *myocarditis and *aneurysms of the coronary arteries. About 2% of cases are fatal. The aneurysms will usually resolve spontaneously but slowly. Treatment involves aspirin therapy, and *gammaglobulin reduces the risk of coronary artery disease. [T. Kawasaki (20th century), Japanese physician]

Kayser-Fleischer ring a brownish-yellow ring in the outer rim of the cornea of the eye. It is a deposit of copper granules and is diagnostic of *Wilson's disease. When well developed it can be seen by unaided observation, but faint Kayser-Fleischer rings may only be detected by specialized *slit-lamp ophthalmological examination. [B. Kayser (1869–1954), German ophthalmologist; B. Fleischer (1848–1904), German physician]

Kegel exercises (pelvic-floor exercises) active rehabilitation of the pelvic-floor muscles, which leads to a cure in 50–80% of patients with stress incontinence. [A. H. Kegel (20th century), US gynaecologist]

Kehr's sign pain in the left shoulder caused by irritation of the undersurface of the diaphragm by blood leaking from a ruptured spleen. The pain impulses are referred along the *phrenic nerve. [H. Kehr (1862–1913), German surgeon]

Kell antigens a group of antigens that may or may not be present on the surface of red blood cells, forming the basis of a *blood group. This group is important in blood transfusion reactions. [Mrs Kell (20th century), patient in whom they were first demonstrated]

Keller's operation an operation for *hallux valgus (*see also* BUNION) or *hallux rigidus that involves an excision *arthroplasty of the metatarsophalangeal joint, at the base of the big toe. The toe will be slightly shorter and floppy, but usually this improves alignment and range of movement. [W. L. Keller (1874–1959), US surgeon]

keloid *n.* an overgrowth of fibrous scar tissue following trauma to the skin. It does not resolve spontaneously but may be flattened by silicone gels, applied pressure, injections of potent corticosteroids, or intralesional excision (or combinations of these). Keloid formation is particularly common at certain sites, such as the breastbone or ear lobe; surgical excision of benign (nonmalignant) lesions from such sites is therefore best avoided. *See also* SCAR.

kelvin *n.* the *SI unit of temperature, formally defined as the fraction 1/273.16 of the temperature of the triple point of water. A temperature in kelvins is equal to a Celsius temperature plus 273.15°C. Symbol: K.

Kemp echoes *see* OTOACOUSTIC EMISSIONS.

kerat- (kerato-) *combining form denoting* 1. the cornea. Example: **keratopathy** (disease of). 2. horny tissue, especially of the skin.

keratalgia *n.* pain arising from the cornea.

keratectasia *n.* bulging of the cornea at

the site of scar tissue (which is thinner than normal corneal tissue).

keratectomy *n.* an operation in which a part of the cornea is removed, usually a superficial layer. This procedure is now frequently done by an *excimer laser, either to correct refractive errors (myopia, hypermetropia), by reshaping the surface of the cornea (**photorefractive keratectomy**; PRK), or to remove diseased corneal tissue (**phototherapeutic keratectomy**). *See also* AUTOMATED LAMELLAR KERATECTOMY.

keratin *n.* one of a family of proteins that are the major constituents of the nails, hair, and the outermost layers of the skin. The cytoplasm of epithelial cells, including *keratinocytes, contains a network of keratin filaments.

keratinization (cornification) *n.* the process by which cells become horny due to the deposition of *keratin within them. It occurs in the *epidermis of the skin and associated structures (hair, nails, etc.), where the cells become flattened, lose their nuclei, and are filled with keratin as they approach the surface.

keratinocyte *n.* a type of cell that makes up 95% of the cells of the epidermis. Keratinocytes migrate from the deeper layers of the epidermis and are finally shed from the surface of the skin.

keratitis *n.* inflammation of the *cornea of the eye. It may be due to physical or chemical agents (abrasions, exposure to dust, chemicals, ultraviolet light, etc.) or result from infection. The eye waters and is very painful, and vision is blurred. In **disciform keratitis** a disc-shaped patch of oedema and inflammation develops in the cornea, usually as an immune response to viral infection, commonly herpes simplex. **Filamentary keratitis** is associated with small mucoid deposits of epithelial filaments on the surface of the cornea, which come off to leave small corneal erosions that cause severe pain until they heal.

keratoacanthoma *n.* a firm nodule that appears singly on the skin, grows to 1–2 cm across in about six weeks, and disappears gradually during the next few months. Men are affected more often than women, commonly between the ages of 50 and 70. Keratoacanthomas occur mainly on the face; the cause is not known. Spontaneous healing may leave an unsightly scar; therefore

treatment by curettage and cautery, or excision, may be required. The precise relationship of keratoacanthoma to *squamous cell carcinoma is controversial.

keratocele (descemetocele) *n.* outward bulging of the base of a deep ulcer of the cornea. The deep layer of the cornea (Descemet's membrane) is elastic and relatively resistant to perforation; it therefore bulges when the overlying cornea has been destroyed.

keratoconjunctivitis *n.* combined inflammation of the cornea and conjunctiva of the eye. **Keratoconjunctivitis sicca** is dryness of the cornea and conjunctiva due to deficiency production of tears. It may be associated with systemic disorders, such as *Sjögren's syndrome, systemic lupus, systemic sclerosis, and sarcoidosis.

keratoconus *n.* conical cornea: a slowly progressive abnormality in the cornea, which changes from its normal gradual curve to a more conical shape, causing distortion of vision.

keratoglobus (megalocornea) *n.* a congenital disorder of the eye in which the whole cornea bulges forward in a regular curve. *Compare* KERATOCONUS.

keratomalacia *n.* a progressive nutritional disease of the eye due to vitamin A deficiency. The cornea softens and may even perforate. This condition is very serious and blindness is usually inevitable. *See also* XEROPHTHALMIA.

keratome *n.* any instrument designed for cutting the cornea. The simplest type has a flat triangular blade attached at its base to a handle, the other two sides being very sharp and tapering to a point. Power-driven keratomes have oscillating or rotating blades. An automated keratome is used in *automated lamellar keratectomy.

keratometer (ophthalmometer) *n.* an instrument for measuring the radius of curvature of the cornea. Usually the vertical and horizontal curvatures are measured. All keratometers work on the principle that the size of the image of an object reflected from a convex mirror (in this case, the cornea) depends on the curvature of the mirror. The steeper the curve, the smaller the image. The keratometer is used for assessing the degree of curvature of the cornea in different meridians. —**keratometry** *n.*

keratomileusis *n. see* INTRASTROMAL KERATOMILEUSIS, LASIK (LASER IN SITU KERATOMILEUSIS).

keratopathy *n.* any disorder relating to the cornea. *See* BAND KERATOPATHY, BULLOUS KERATOPATHY.

keratoplasty (**corneal graft**) *n.* an eye operation in which any diseased part of the cornea is replaced by clear corneal tissue from a donor. In **penetrating keratoplasty** all layers of the cornea are replaced, in **lamellar keratoplasty** only the superficial layers are replaced, and in **Descemet's stripping endothelial keratoplasty** (**DSEK**) the endothelium only is replaced.

keratoprosthesis *n.* an optically clear prosthesis that is implanted into the cornea to replace an area that has become opaque. Due to its poor success rate, it is used only as a last resort in an attempt to restore some sight to patients with severe disease where corneal transplantation (*see* KERATOPLASTY) is unlikely to succeed.

keratoscope (**Placido's disc**) *n.* an instrument for detecting abnormal curvature of the cornea. It consists of a black disc, about 20 cm in diameter, marked with concentric white rings. The examiner looks through a small lens in the centre at the reflection of the rings in the patient's cornea. A normal cornea will reflect regular concentric images of the rings; a cornea that is abnormally curved (for example in *keratoconus) or scarred reflects distorted rings. Modern keratoscopes can print out a contour map of the corneal surface.

keratosis *n.* a horny overgrowth of the skin. **Actinic** (or **solar**) **keratoses** are red spots with a scaly surface, found in older fair-skinned people who have been chronically overexposed to the sun. They may occasionally become a *squamous cell carcinoma. **Seborrhoeic keratoses** (also known as **seborrhoeic warts**) never become malignant. They are superficial yellowish or brown spots, crusty or greasy-looking, occurring especially on the trunk in middle age, that become warty over the years.

keratosis obturans an abnormal buildup of *keratin and dead skin cells within the ear canal that can block the canal, cause conductive hearing loss (*see* DEAFNESS), and erode the bone of the ear canal. It is associated with *bronchiectasis and chronic sinusitis.

keratotomy *n.* an incision into the cornea. *See* ARCUATE KERATOTOMY, RADIAL KERATOTOMY.

keratouveitis *n.* inflammation involving both the cornea (*see* KERATITIS) and the uvea (*see* UVEITIS).

kerion *n.* an uncommon and severe form of *ringworm of the scalp consisting of a painful inflamed mass. It is caused by a type of fungus (e.g. *Trichophyton tonsurans*).

Kerley B lines fine horizontal lines seen in the angle between the diaphragm and the chest wall on an AP (*anteroposterior) chest X-ray. It is a sign of pulmonary *oedema and therefore heart failure. [P. J. Kerley (20th century), British radiologist]

kernicterus *n.* staining and subsequent damage of the brain by bile pigment (bilirubin), which may occur in severe cases of *haemolytic disease of the newborn. Immature brain cells in the *basal ganglia are affected, and as brain development proceeds a pattern of *cerebral palsy emerges at about six months, with uncoordinated movements, deafness, disturbed vision, and feeding and speech difficulties.

Kernig's sign a symptom of *meningitis in which the hamstring muscles in the legs are so stiff that the patient is unable to extend his legs at the knee when the thighs are held at a right angle to the body. [V. Kernig (1840–1917), Russian physician]

Kernohan's phenomenon (**Kernohan's syndrome**) *hemiplegia that is *ipsilateral to the brain lesion that caused it, due to pressure of the lesion (which is often a haematoma) on surrounding structures in the brain. It is unusual because normally a lesion of the brain causes dysfunction in the *contralateral limbs. [J. W. K. Kernohan (20th century), US pathologist]

ketoacidosis *n.* a condition in which *acidosis is accompanied by *ketosis, such as occurs in diabetes mellitus (*see* DIABETIC KETOACIDOSIS). Symptoms include nausea and vomiting, abdominal tenderness, confusion or coma, extreme thirst, and weight loss.

ketoconazole *n.* an antifungal drug (*see* IMIDAZOLE) used in the treatment of such fungal diseases as *candidiasis, *histoplasmosis, and *blastomycosis that are resistant to other antifungals. It is taken by mouth; side-effects include abdominal pain, itching, nausea, and vomiting, and it may cause liver damage. Ketoconazole may also be applied topically for fungal skin infections. Trade name: **Nizoral**.

ketogenesis *n.* the production of *ketone bodies. These are normal products of lipid metabolism and can be used to provide energy. The condition of *ketosis can occur when excess ketone bodies are produced.

ketogenic diet a diet that promotes the formation of *ketone bodies in the tissues. A ketogenic diet is one in which the principal energy source is fat rather than carbohydrate.

ketonaemia *n.* the presence in the blood of *ketone bodies.

ketone *n.* any member of a group of organic compounds consisting of a carbonyl group (=CO) flanked by two alkyl groups. The ketones acetoacetic acid, acetone, and β-hydroxybutyrate (known as **ketone** (or **acetone**) **bodies**) are produced during the metabolism of fats. *See also* KETOSIS.

ketonuria (acetonuria) *n.* the presence in the urine of *ketone (acetone) bodies. This may occur in diabetes mellitus, starvation, or after persistent vomiting and results from the partial oxidation of fats. Ketone bodies may be detected by adding a few drops of 5% sodium nitroprusside solution and a solution of ammonia to the urine; the gradual development of a purplish-red colour indicates their presence.

ketoprofen *n.* an anti-inflammatory drug (*see* NSAID) administered by mouth, intramuscular injection, rectal suppository, or topically to treat various arthritic and rheumatic diseases and to relieve pain. Gas-

tric bleeding and ulceration may occur. Trade names: **Orudis**, **Oruvail**.

ketose *n.* a simple sugar that terminates with a keto group (–C=O); for example, *fructose.

ketosis *n.* raised levels of *ketone bodies in the body tissues. Ketone bodies are normal products of fat metabolism and can be oxidized to produce energy. Elevated levels arise when there is an imbalance in fat metabolism, such as occurs in diabetes mellitus or starvation. Ketosis may result in severe *acidosis. *See also* KETONURIA.

keV *symbol for* kiloelectronvolt. *See* ELECTRONVOLT.

keyhole surgery *see* MINIMALLY INVASIVE SURGERY.

khat (**qat**, **kat**) *n.* the leaves of the shrub *Catha edulis*, which contain a stimulant. In Yemen these leaves are wrapped around betel nuts and chewed: this habit is associated with the development of oral *leukoplakia.

kidney *n.* either of the pair of organs responsible for the excretion of nitrogenous wastes, principally urea, from the blood (see illustration). The kidneys are situated at the back of the abdomen, below the diaphragm, one on each side of the spine; they are supplied with blood by the renal arteries. Each kidney is enclosed in a fibrous capsule and is composed of an outer **cortex** and an inner **medulla**. The active units of the kidney are the *nephrons, within the cortex and medulla, which filter the blood under pressure and then reabsorb water and selected substances back into the blood. The *urine thus formed is conducted from the nephrons

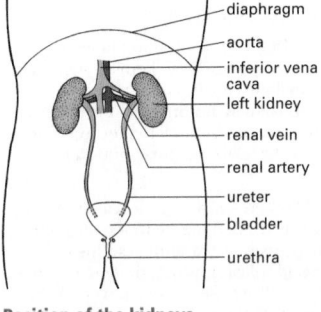

Position of the kidneys.

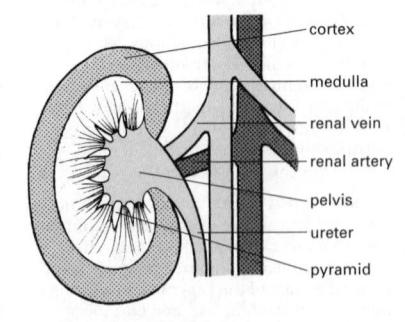

Section through a kidney.

via the renal tubules into the **renal pelvis** and from here to the ureter, which leads to the bladder. *See also* HAEMODIALYSIS, HORSE-SHOE KIDNEY, RENAL FUNCTION TESTS.

(⊕) SEE WEB LINKS
- Website of the National Kidney Federation: includes basic information on the kidneys and a guide to kidney diseases, their symptoms, and treatment

Kienböck's disease necrosis of the *lunate bone of the wrist caused by interruption of its blood supply (*see* OSTEOCHON-DRITIS, OSTEONECROSIS). It usually follows chronic stress or injury to the wrist and presents with pain and stiffness, with reduced grip strength. Initially, X-rays may show no abnormality; if the disease is suspected, a bone scan or MRI is indicated. Treatment is with rest, splintage, and *NSAIDs, but some cases require surgical shortening of the radius or *arthrodesis of the wrist. [R. Kienböck (1871–1953), Austrian radiologist]

Kiesselbach's plexus a collection of capillaries in the mucosa at the anterior part of the nasal septum. Nosebleeds frequently have their origin from this plexus. *See* EPISTAXIS; LITTLE'S AREA. [W. Kiesselbach (1839–1902), German laryngologist]

kilo- *prefix denoting* a thousand.

kilocalorie *n.* one thousand calories. *See* CALORIE.

kilogram *n.* the *SI unit of mass equal to 1000 grams and defined in terms of the international prototype (a cylinder of platinum-iridium alloy) kept at Sèvres, near Paris. Symbol: kg.

kilovolt *n.* one thousand *volts (symbol: kV). In radiography, the kilovoltage of the X-ray machine determines the maximum energy of the X-rays produced. The setting is important in controlling the exposure of the film and is generally higher when more penetration is required, depending on the thickness of the body part being imaged. *See also* MILLIAMP.

Kimmelstiel-Wilson lesion a nodular form of glomerulosclerosis associated with diabetic nephropathy. *See also* DIABETIC GLOMERULOSCLEROSIS. [P. Kimmelstiel and C. Wilson (20th century), US physicians]

kin- (kine-) *combining form denoting* movement.

kinaesthesia *n.* the sense that enables the brain to be constantly aware of the position and movement of muscles in different parts of the body. This is achieved by means of *proprioceptors, which send impulses from muscles, joints, and tendons. Without this sense, coordinated movement would be impossible with the eyes closed.

kinaesthesiometer *n.* an instrument for measuring a patient's awareness of the muscular and joint movements of his own body: used during the investigation of nervous and muscular disorders and certain forms of brain damage.

kinanaesthesia *n.* inability to sense the positions and movements of parts of the body, with consequent disordered physical activity.

kinase *n.* **1.** an agent that can convert the inactive form of an enzyme (*see* PROENZYME) to the active form. **2.** an enzyme that catalyses the transfer of phosphate groups. An example is *phosphofructokinase.

kinematics *n.* the study of motion and the forces required to produce it. This includes the different forces at work during the movement of a single part of the body, and more complex movements such as running and climbing.

kineplasty *n.* a method of amputation in which the muscles and tendons of the affected limb are arranged so that they can be integrated with a specially made artificial replacement. This enables direct movement of the artificial hand or limb by the muscles.

-kinesis *combining form denoting* movement.

kinetochore *n. see* CENTROMERE.

King-Kopetzky syndrome *see* OBSCURE AUDITORY DYSFUNCTION.

kinin *n.* one of a group of naturally occurring polypeptides that are powerful *vasodilators, which lower blood pressure, and cause contraction of smooth muscle. The kinins **bradykinin** and **kallidin** are formed in the blood by the action of proteolytic enzymes (**kallikreins**) on certain plasma globulins (**kininogens**). Kinins are not normally present in the blood, but are formed under certain conditions; for example when tissue is damaged or when there are changes in the pH and temperature of the blood. They are thought to play a role in inflammatory response.

KIRs killer cell immunoglobulin-like receptors, which are present on the surface of *natural killer cells.

kiss of life *see* MOUTH-TO-MOUTH RESUSCITATION.

Klatskin tumour *see* CHOLANGIOCARCINOMA. [G. Klatskin (20th century), US physician]

Klebsiella *n.* a genus of Gram-negative rodlike nonmotile bacteria, mostly lactose-fermenting, found in the respiratory, intestinal, and urinogenital tracts of animals and humans. The species *K. oxytoca* is associated with human urinary infections; *K. pneumoniae* is associated with pneumonia and other respiratory infections. The species *K. rhinoscleromatis* causes *rhinoscleroma, a chronic infection of the nose and pharynx.

Klebs-Loeffler bacillus *see* CORYNEBACTERIUM. [T. Klebs (1834–1913) and F. A. J. Loeffler (1852–1915), German bacteriologists]

Kleine-Levin syndrome a rare episodic disorder characterized by periods (usually of a few days or weeks) in which sufferers eat enormously, sleep for most of the day and night, and may become more dependent or aggressive than normal. Between episodes they are usually quite unaffected. The disorder almost always resolves spontaneously. [W. Kleine (20th century), German neuropsychiatrist; M. Levin (20th century), US neurologist]

klepto- *combining form denoting* stealing.

kleptomania *n.* a pathologically strong impulse to steal, often in the absence of any desire for the stolen object(s). It is sometimes associated with *depression.

Klinefelter's syndrome a genetic disorder in which there are three sex chromosomes, XXY, rather than the normal XX or XY. Affected individuals are apparently male, but are tall and thin, with small testes, failure of normal sperm production (azoospermia), enlargement of the breasts (gynaecomastia), and absence of facial and body hair. [H. F. Klinefelter (1912–90), US physician]

Klumpke's paralysis a partial paralysis of the arm caused by injury to a baby's *brachial plexus during birth. This may result from an obstetric manoeuvre in which the arm is raised at the shoulder to an extreme degree, which damages the lower cervical (neck) and upper thoracic (chest) nerve roots of the spinal cord. It results in weakness and wasting of the muscles of the hand. [A. Klumpke (1859–1927), French neurologist]

K-nail *n.* *see* KÜNTSCHER NAIL.

kneading *n.* *see* PETRISSAGE.

knee *n.* the hinge joint (*see* GINGLYMUS) between the end of the femur, the top of the tibia, and the back of the *patella (kneecap). It is commonly involved in *sports injuries (such as a torn meniscus or ligament) and is a common site of osteoarthritis and rheumatoid arthritis; it can be replaced by an artificial joint (*see also* ARTHROPLASTY).

knee-elbow position the buttocks-up position assumed by patients undergoing anorectal examinations, now commonly performed in the left lateral position. It is also useful for helping patients dispel excess flatus following colonoscopy.

knee jerk *see* PATELLAR REFLEX.

knight's-move thinking a form of *formal thought disorder, common in psychosis, in which connections between sentences or parts of sentences are without a coherent train of thought.

knock-knee *n.* abnormal in-curving of the legs, resulting in a gap between the ankles when the knees are in contact. In severe cases there is stress on the knee, ankle, and foot joints, resulting eventually in degenerative arthritis. The condition may be corrected by *osteotomy. Medical name: **genu valgum**.

Kobberling-Dunnigan syndrome *see* LIPODYSTROPHY.

Kocher manoeuvre a method for *reduction of an anteriorly dislocated shoulder by manipulation. Longitudinal traction is applied to the elbow, pulling down the shoulder, then the forearm, bent at the elbow, is externally rotated to 90°. [E. T. Kocher (1841–1917), Swiss surgeon]

Kocher's incision an oblique incision made in the right upper quadrant of the abdomen, classically used for open *cholecystectomy. [E. T. Kocher]

Koch's bacillus *see* MYCOBACTERIUM. [R. Koch (1843–1910), German bacteriologist]

Koebner phenomenon (isomorphic response) a phenomenon that occurs in skin diseases, especially psoriasis and lichen planus, in which the characteristic lesions of the disease appear in linear form in response to such trauma as cuts, burns, or scratches. [H. Koebner (1834–1904), German dermatologist]

Koeppe nodule a type of nodule occurring in the iris at the pupil margin in both granulomatous and nongranulomatous *uveitis . [L. Koeppe (20th century), German ophthalmologist]

Köhler's disease *osteonecrosis of the *navicular bone of the foot (*see* OSTEOCHONDRITIS). It occurs in children aged 3–7 years, causing pain and limping, and is treated by strapping the foot, rest, and anti-inflammatory drugs. [A. Köhler (1874–1947), German physician]

koilonychia *n.* the development of thin (brittle) concave (spoon-shaped) nails, a common disorder that can occur with anaemia due to iron deficiency, though the cause is not known. Any underlying disease should be treated.

Koplik's spots small red spots with bluish-white centres that often appear on the mucous membranes of the mouth in *measles. [H. Koplik (1858–1927), US physician]

koro *n.* a state of acute anxiety, seen especially in certain cultures (such as that of the Chinese of SE Asia), characterized by a sudden belief that the penis is shrinking into the abdomen and will disappear: the sufferer is convinced that disappearance of the penis means death. Occasionally women have a similar belief that their breasts are disappearing into their body. It is usually treated with tranquillizing drugs and reassurance.

Korsakoff's syndrome an organic disorder affecting the brain that results in a memory defect in which new information fails to be learnt although events from the past are still recalled; *disorientation in time and place; and a tendency to unintentionally invent material to fill memory blanks (*see* CONFABULATION). The commonest cause of the condition is *alcoholism, especially when this has led to deficiency of thiamine (vitamin B_1). Large doses of thiamine are given as treatment. The condition often becomes chronic. [S. S. Korsakoff (1854–1900), Russian neurologist]

Kostmann's syndrome (severe congeni-tal neutropenia) a hereditary (autosomal *recessive) disorder characterized by severe *neutropenia. This results in frequent bacterial infections, and death often occurs before the age of 6 months.

KRAS *n.* an important *oncogene for the causation of human lung and colorectal cancer.

kraurosis *n.* shrinking of a body part, usually the vulva in elderly women (**kraurosis vulvae**).

Krebs cycle (citric acid cycle) a complex cycle of enzyme-catalysed reactions, occurring within the cells of all living animals, in which acetate, in the presence of oxygen, is broken down to produce energy in the form of *ATP (via the *electron transport chain) and carbon dioxide. The cycle is the final step in the oxidation of carbohydrates, fats, and proteins; some of the intermediary products of the cycle are used in the synthesis of amino acids. [Sir H. A. Krebs (1900–81), British biochemist]

Krukenberg's spindle a vertical linear deposit of brown pigment on the inner surface of the cornea (corneal endothelium), appearing in cases of pigment dispersion syndrome. [F. E. Krukenberg (1871–1946), German pathologist]

Krukenberg tumour a rapidly developing malignant growth in one or (more often) both ovaries. It is caused by the *transcoelomic spread of a primary growth in the stomach or intestine, typically an adenocarcinoma. [F. E. Krukenberg]

krypton-81m *n.* a radioactive gas that is the shortest-lived isotope in medical use (half-life 13 seconds). It can be used to investigate the *ventilation of the lungs. The patient breathes a small quantity of the gas, the arrival of which in different parts of the lungs is recorded by means of a *gamma camera. This is often performed as part of *ventilation-perfusion scanning to look for pulmonary emboli. *See also* RUBIDIUM-81.

KUB X-ray an abdominal plain X-ray film that is longer than normal to enable it to include the *k*idneys, *u*reters, and the entire *b*ladder.

Kugelberg-Wellander disease (juvenile spinal muscular atrophy) *see* SPINAL MUSCULAR ATROPHY. [E. Kugelberg and L. Wellander (20th century), Swedish neurologists]

Küntscher nail (K-nail) a metal rod that is inserted down the middle of the femur (thigh bone) to stabilize a transverse fracture of the shaft. [G. Küntscher (1902–72), German orthopaedic surgeon]

Kupffer cells phagocytic cells that line the sinusoids of the *liver (*see* MACROPHAGE). They are particularly concerned with the formation of *bile and are often seen to contain fragments of red blood cells and pigment granules that are derived from the breakdown of haemoglobin. [K. W. von Kupffer (1829–1902), German anatomist]

kuru (trembling disease) *n.* a disease that involves a progressive degeneration of the nerve cells of the central nervous system, particularly in the region of the brain that controls movement. Muscular control becomes defective and shiver-like tremors occur in the trunk, limbs, and head. Death usually occurs within 9–12 months. Thought to be caused by a *prion and transmitted by cannibalism, kuru was largely limited to the Fore tribe of New Guinea and mainly affected women and children, reaching high levels in the mid-20th century. It has died out since cannibalism is no longer practised. *See also* SPONGIFORM ENCEPHALOPATHY.

Kussmaul breathing the slow deep respiration associated with acidosis. [A. Kussmaul (1822–1902), German physician]

kV *symbol for* *kilovolt.

Kveim test a test used for the diagnosis of *sarcoidosis. Tissue from a lymph node of a person suffering from the disease is injected intradermally; the development of a granuloma at the injection site indicates that the subject has sarcoidosis. [M. A. Kveim (20th century), Norwegian physician]

kwashiorkor *n.* a form of malnutrition due to a diet deficient in protein and energy-producing foods, common among certain African tribes. Kwashiorkor develops when, after prolonged breast feeding, the child is weaned onto an inadequate traditional family diet. The diet is such that it is physically impossible for the child to consume the required quantity in order to obtain sufficient protein and energy. Kwashiorkor is most common in children between the ages of one and three years. The symptoms are *oedema, loss of appetite, diarrhoea, general discomfort, and apathy; the child fails to thrive and

there is usually associated gastrointestinal infection.

Kyasanur Forest disease a tropical disease, common in southern India, caused by a virus transmitted to humans through the bite of the forest-dwelling tick *Haemaphysalis spinigera*. Symptoms include fever, headache, muscular pains, vomiting, conjunctivitis, exhaustion, bleeding of nose and gums and, subsequently, internal bleeding and the *necrosis of various tissues. General therapy, in the absence of specific treatment, involves relief of dehydration and loss of blood; analgesics are given to alleviate pain.

kymograph *n.* an instrument for recording the flow and varying pressure of the blood within the blood vessels. —**kymography** *n.*

kypho- *combining form denoting* a hump.

kyphos *n.* a sharp posterior angulation of the spine due to localized collapse or wedging of one or more vertebrae. It results in the appearance of a hump on the back (a hunchback deformity). The cause may be a congenital defect, a fracture (which may or may not be pathological), or spinal tuberculosis.

kyphoscoliosis *n.* abnormal posterior and sideways curvature of the spine, i.e. *kyphosis combined with *scoliosis. The deformity may occur during growth for no apparent reason (**idiopathic kyphoscoliosis**) or may result from any of several diseases involving the vertebrae and spinal muscles. Special braces can reduce the extent of the deformity if this is mild. Severe deformity may require surgical correction by *fusion of the spine.

kyphosis *n.* outward curvature of the spine, which if excessive causes hunching of the back. A **mobile kyphosis** may be caused by bad posture or muscle weakness or may develop to compensate for another condition, such as hip deformity; it can be corrected by backward bending. A **fixed kyphosis** may be congenital; it may arise in adolescence (*see* SCHEUERMANN'S DISEASE); or it may result from collapse of the vertebrae, as in *osteoporosis, ankylosing *spondylitis, infections, or tumours. Treatment depends on the cause and may include physiotherapy, bracing, and surgery (spinal *osteotomy and fusion may be required in severe cases). *See also* KYPHOS, KYPHOSCOLIOSIS.

labelling index the proportion of cells in a sample of tissue that are producing DNA. Cells that are synthesizing DNA take up tritiated thymidine, which shows up on an autoradiograph (*see* AUTORADIOGRAPHY) of the sample.

labetalol *n.* a combined alpha- and beta-blocking drug, sometimes found to be more effective in the treatment of high blood pressure than beta blockers. It is administered by mouth or intravenously. Possible side-effects include faintness on standing up, scalp tingling, and difficulty with urination and ejaculation. Trade name: **Trandate**.

labia *pl. n. see* LABIUM.

labial *adj.* **1.** relating to the lips or to a labium. **2.** designating the surface of a tooth adjacent to the lips.

labio- *combining form denoting* the lip(s).

labiomancy *n.* lip-reading.

labioplasty (cheiloplasty) *n.* surgical repair of injury or deformity of the lips (*cleft lip).

labium *n.* (*pl.* **labia**) a lip-shaped structure, especially either of the two pairs of skin folds that enclose the *vulva. The larger outer pair are known as the **labia majora** and the smaller inner pair the **labia minora**.

labour *n.* the sequence of actions by which a baby and the afterbirth (placenta) are expelled from the uterus at childbirth. The process usually starts spontaneously about 280 days after conception, but it may be started by artificial means (*see* INDUCTION). In the first stage the muscular wall of the uterus begins contracting while the muscle fibres of the cervix relax so that the cervix expands. A portion of the membranous sac (amnion) surrounding the baby is pushed into the opening and ruptures under the pressure, releasing *amniotic fluid to the exterior. In the second stage the baby's head appears at the cervix and the contractions of the uterus strengthen. The passage of the infant through the vagina is assisted by contractions of the abdominal muscles and

conscious pushing by the mother. When the top of the baby's head appears at the vaginal opening the whole infant is eased clear of the vagina, and the umbilical cord is cut. If the emergence of the head is impeded an incision may be made in the surrounding tissue (*see* EPISIOTOMY). In the final stage the placenta and membranes are pushed out by the continuing contraction of the uterus, which eventually returns to its unexpanded state. The average duration of labour is about 12 hours in first pregnancies and about 8 hours in subsequent pregnancies. The pain of labour may be reduced if the mother trains her abdominal muscles during the prenatal period and by the use of drugs (**accelerated labour**). *See also* CAESAREAN SECTION.

labrum *n.* (*pl.* **labra**) a lip or liplike structure; occurring, for example, around the margins of the articulating socket (acetabulum) of the hip bone.

labyrinth (inner ear) *n.* a convoluted system of cavities and ducts comprising the organs of hearing and balance. The **membranous labyrinth** is a series of interconnected membranous canals and chambers consisting of the *semicircular canals, *utricle, and *saccule (concerned with balance) and the central cavity of the *cochlea (concerned with hearing). (See illustration.) It is filled with a fluid, **endolymph**. The **bony**

lateral semicircular canal
superior semicircular canal
ampulla of semicircular canal
endolymphatic duct
cochlear nerve
posterior semicircular canal
utricle
saccule
cochlea
spiral ganglion

Labyrinth. Membranous labyrinth of the right ear.

labyrinth is the system of the bony canals and chambers that surround the membranous labyrinth. It is embedded in the petrous part of the *temporal bone and is filled with fluid (**perilymph**).

labyrinthectomy *n.* a surgical procedure to ablate (*see* ABLATION) the structures of the *labyrinth, usually performed for cases of severe Ménière's disease.

labyrinthitis (otitis interna) *n.* inflammation of the inner ear (labyrinth). *See* OTITIS.

laceration *n.* a tear in the flesh caused by a blunt object producing a wound with irregular edges. A *gunshot wound is an example of a laceration caused by a high-velocity blunt object.

lacertus *n.* a band of fibres or a tendon-like structure.

lacrimal apparatus the structures that produce and drain away fluid from the eye (see illustration). The **lacrimal gland** secretes *tears, which drain away through small openings (**puncta**) at the inner corner of the eye into two **lacrimal canaliculi**. From there the tears pass into the nasal cavity via the **lacrimal sac** and the *nasolacrimal duct.

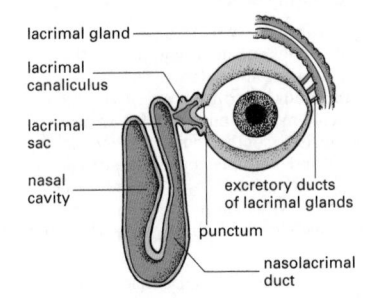

lacrimal gland
lacrimal canaliculus
lacrimal sac
nasal cavity
excretory ducts of lacrimal glands
punctum
nasolacrimal duct

The lacrimal apparatus of the left eye.

lacrimal bone the smallest bone of the face: either of a pair of rectangular bones that contribute to the orbits. *See* SKULL.

lacrimal nerve a branch of the *ophthalmic nerve that supplies the lacrimal gland (*see* LACRIMAL APPARATUS) and conjunctiva.

lacrimation *n.* the production of excess tears; crying. *See also* LACRIMAL APPARATUS.

lacrimator *n.* an agent that irritates the eyes, causing excessive secretion of tears.

lact- (lacti-, lacto-) *combining form denoting* **1.** milk. **2.** lactic acid.

lactalbumin *n.* a milk protein present in milk at a lower concentration than *casein. Unlike casein, it is not precipitated from milk under acid conditions; it is therefore a constituent of cheese made from whey rather than curd.

lactase *n.* an enzyme, secreted by the glands of the small intestine, that converts lactose (milk sugar) into glucose and galactose during digestion.

lactation *n.* the secretion of milk by the *mammary glands of the breasts, which begins normally at the end of pregnancy or may be pathological (*see* GALACTORRHOEA). A fluid called *colostrum is secreted before the milk is produced; both secretions are released in response to the sucking action of the infant on the nipple. Lactation is controlled by hormones (*see* PROLACTIN, OXYTOCIN); it stops when the baby is no longer fed at the breast.

lacteal *n.* a blind-ended lymphatic vessel that extends into a villus of the small *intestine. Digested fats are absorbed into the lacteals.

lactic acid a compound that forms in the cells as the end-product of glucose metabolism in the absence of oxygen (*see* GLYCOLYSIS). During strenuous exercise pyruvic acid is reduced to lactic acid, which may accumulate in the muscles and cause cramp. Lactic acid (owing to its low pH) is an important food preservative. The lactic acid produced by the fermentation of milk is responsible for the preservation and flavour of cheese, yoghurt, and other fermented milk products.

lactic acidosis excessive plasma acidity due to an accumulation of lactic acid. This may be caused by a variety of illnesses, including heart failure or severe dehydration. It can also be caused by the accumulation of *biguanide drugs used for treating type 2 *diabetes mellitus, particularly when kidney failure is present. Biguanides (*see* METFORMIN) should therefore not be used to treat patients who also have kidney disease or heart failure or who are dehydrated.

lactiferous *adj.* transporting or secreting milk, as the **lactiferous ducts** of the breast.

lactifuge *n.* a drug that reduces the secretion of milk. Some oestrogenic drugs have this effect and are used to suppress milk production in mothers not breastfeeding.

Lactobacillus *n.* a genus of Gram-positive nonmotile rodlike bacteria capable of growth in acid media and of producing lactic acid from the fermentation of carbohydrates. They are found in fermenting animal and plant products, especially dairy products, and in the alimentary tract and vagina. They are responsible for the souring of milk. The species *L. acidophilus* is found in milk and is associated with dental caries. It occurs in very high numbers in the faeces of breast- or bottle-fed infants.

lactogenic hormone *see* PROLACTIN.

lactose *n.* a sugar, consisting of one molecule of glucose and one of galactose, found only in milk. Lactose is split into its constituent sugars by the enzyme *lactase, which is secreted in the small intestine. This enzyme is missing or is of low activity in certain people of some Eastern and African races. This leads to the inability to absorb lactose, known as **lactose intolerance**.

lactosuria *n.* the presence of milk sugar (*lactose) in the urine. This often occurs during pregnancy and breastfeeding or if the milk flow is suppressed.

lactulose *n.* a disaccharide sugar that acts as a gentle but effective osmotic *laxative. It is administered by mouth but is not absorbed or broken down, remaining intact until it reaches the colon. There it is split by bacteria into simpler sugars that help to retain water, thereby softening the stools. Lactulose is also used as a bowel cleanser for treating *hepatic encephalopathy, being administered by mouth or enema. Trade names: **Lactugal, Regulose**.

lacuna *n.* (*pl.* **lacunae**) (in anatomy) a small cavity or depression; for example, one of the spaces in compact bone in which a bone cell lies.

laetrile *n.* a cyanide-containing compound extracted from peach stones. It has been used in *complementary medicine in the treatment of various forms of cancer.

laevo- *combining form. see* LEVO-.

laevocardia *n.* the normal position of the heart, in which its apex is directed towards the left. *Compare* DEXTROCARDIA.

lagaena (lagena) *n.* the closed end of the spiral *cochlea. This term is more commonly used to describe the structure homologous to the cochlea in primitive vertebrates.

lagophthalmos *n.* any condition in which the eye does not close completely. It may lead to corneal damage from undue exposure.

laking *n.* the physical or chemical treatment of blood to abolish the structure of the red cells and thus form a homogeneous solution. Laking is an important preliminary step in the analysis of haemoglobin or enzymes present in red cells.

-lalia *combining form denoting* a condition involving speech.

lambda *n.* the point on the skull at which the lambdoidal and sagittal *sutures meet.

lambda sign (twin-peak sign) an ultrasound diagnosis of dichorionicity at 10–14 weeks gestation: a peak of placental tissue protrudes into the base of the intertwin membrane. *See* CHORIONICITY.

lambdoidal suture *see* SUTURE.

lambliasis *n. see* GIARDIASIS.

lamella *n.* (*pl.* **lamellae**) 1. a thin layer, membrane, scale, or plate-like tissue or part. In *bone tissue, lamellae are thin bands of calcified matrix arranged concentrically around a Haversian canal. 2. a thin gelatinous medicated disc used to apply drugs to the eye. The disc is placed on the eyeball; the gelatinous material dissolves and the drug is absorbed. —**lamellar** *adj.*

lamellar bone mature *bone, in which the collagen fibres are arranged parallel to each other to form multiple layers (*lamellae) with the osteocytes lying between the lamellae. It exists in two structurally different forms: cortical (compact) and cancellous (spongy) bone. *See also* WOVEN BONE.

lamina *n.* (*pl.* **laminae**) 1. a thin membrane or layer of tissue. 2. the section of the posterior arch of a *vertebra located between the central spinous process and the transverse process on each side.

laminectomy *n.* surgical cutting into the backbone to obtain access to the vertebral (spinal) canal. The surgeon excises the rear part (the posterior arch) of one or more vertebrae. The operation is performed to remove tumours, to treat injuries to the spine, such as prolapsed intervertebral (slipped) disc (in which the affected disc is removed), or to relieve pressure on the spinal cord or roots.

laminotomy n. the surgical creation of a window-like opening in the posterior arch of a vertebra by removing a small piece of *lamina and adjacent *ligamentum flavum.

lamivudine n. a reverse transcriptase inhibitor (see REVERSE TRANSCRIPTASE).

lamotrigine n. an antiepileptic drug used in the control of partial seizures and tonic–clonic seizures. It is administered by mouth. Possible side-effects include nausea, headache, double vision, dizziness, *ataxia, and serious skin rashes. Trade name: **Lamictal**.

Lancefield classification a classification of the *Streptococcus bacteria based on the presence or absence of antigenic carbohydrate on the cell surface. Species are classified into the groups A–S. Most species causing disease in humans belong to groups A, B, and D. [R. C. Lancefield (1895–1981), US bacteriologist]

lancet n. a broad two-edged surgical knife with a sharp point.

lancinating adj. describing a sharp stabbing or cutting pain.

Landau reflex a reflex seen in normal babies from three months until one year, when it disappears. If the baby is held horizontally, face down, it will straighten its legs and back and try to lift up its head. The presence of this reflex beyond one year may be suggestive of a developmental disorder.

Langerhans cell histiocytosis overgrowth of cells of the *reticuloendothelial system. This includes disorders previously called **histiocytosis X**, including **eosinophilic granuloma**, **Hand-Schüller-Christian disease**, and **Letterer-Siwe disease**. [P. Langerhans (1847–88), German physician and anatomist]

Langer's lines normal permanent skin creases. Incisions parallel to Langer's lines heal well and are less visible. [C. R. von E. Langer (1819–87), Austrian anatomist]

lanreotide n. a somatostatin analogue (see SOMATOSTATIN).

lansoprazole n. see PROTON-PUMP INHIBITOR.

lanugo n. fine hair covering the body and limbs of the human fetus. It is most profuse at about the 28th week of gestation and is shed around 40 weeks.

laparo- combining form denoting the loins or abdomen.

laparoscope (peritoneoscope) n. a surgical instrument (a type of *endoscope) comprising an illuminated viewing tube generally connected to a camera, with the image viewed on a video screen. It is inserted through the abdominal wall to enable the surgeon to view the abdominal organs (see LAPAROSCOPY). It can be used as a means to allow surgical procedures to be carried out with special instruments without using a surgical incision. See also MINIMALLY INVASIVE SURGERY.

laparoscopic myolysis see FIBROID.

laparoscopy (peritoneoscopy) n. examination of the abdominal structures (which are contained within the peritoneum) by means of a (*laparoscope). This is passed through a small incision in the wall of the abdomen after insufflating carbon dioxide into the abdominal cavity (creating a pneumoperitoneum). In addition to being a diagnostic aid, it is used when taking a biopsy, aspirating cysts, and dividing adhesions. Surgery, including *cholecystectomy, *fundoplication, *prostatectomy, *colectomy, and *nephrectomy, and the occlusion of Fallopian tubes for sterilization, can also be performed through a laparoscope, using either a laser or diathermy to control bleeding (see also MINIMALLY INVASIVE SURGERY). The laparoscope is also used for collecting ova for *in vitro fertilization. —**laparoscopic** adj.

laparotomy n. a surgical incision into the abdominal cavity. The operation is done to examine the abdominal organs as a help to diagnosis; for example, to establish the spread of a tumour (**exploratory laparotomy**) or as a prelude to major surgery, for example in abdominal trauma.

lardaceous adj. resembling lard: often applied to tissue infiltrated with the starchlike substance amyloid (see AMYLOIDOSIS).

Lariam n. see MEFLOQUINE.

larva n. (pl. **larvae**) the preadult or immature stage hatching from the egg of some animal groups, e.g. insects and nematodes, which may be markedly different from the sexually mature adult and have a totally different way of life. For example, the larvae of some flies are parasites of animals and cause disease whereas the adults are free-living. —**larval** *adj*.

larva migrans *see* CREEPING ERUPTION.

laryng- (laryngo-) *combining form denoting* the larynx.

laryngeal mask an airway tube with an elliptical inflatable cuff at one end for insertion into the mouth of a patient requiring artificial ventilation. It is designed to fit snugly in the patient's throat over the top of the laryngeal opening. While it is relatively easy to insert and allows delivery of effective artificial ventilation, it does not provide the absolute protection of the airway from vomitus afforded by an endotracheal tube (*see* INTUBATION).

laryngeal reflex a cough produced by irritating the larynx.

laryngeal stroboscopy a method of studying the movements of the *vocal folds of the *larynx by using stroboscopic light (controlled intermittent flashes) to slow or freeze the movement.

laryngectomy *n*. surgical removal of the larynx in the treatment of laryngeal carcinoma. Postoperatively the patient breathes through a *tracheostomy. Speech is lost following the operation but can be restored by teaching the patient to swallow air and then belch it in a controlled fashion. Alternatively, a battery-powered vibrating device can be held in the mouth or underneath the chin to produce speech (*see* ELECTROLARYNX). Speech can also be facilitated by a one-way valve surgically implanted between the tracheostomy and the upper oesophagus, allowing the patient to divert air into the throat. **Partial laryngectomy** conserves part of the larynx and allows patients to breathe and speak normally. However, it is only suitable for a few patients with small tumours.

laryngismus *n*. closure of the vocal folds by sudden contraction of the laryngeal muscles, followed by a noisy indrawing of breath. It occurs in young children and was in the past associated with low-calcium rickets. Now it occurs when the larynx has been irritated following administration of anaesthetic, when a foreign body has lodged in the larynx, or in *croup.

laryngitis *n*. inflammation of the larynx and vocal folds, due to infection by bacteria or viruses or irritation by gases, chemicals, etc. The folds lose their vibrance (owing to swelling) and the voice becomes husky or is lost completely; breathing is harsh and difficult (*see* STRIDOR); and the cough is painful and honking. Obstruction of the airways may occasionally be serious, especially in children (*see* CROUP). The patient should rest his voice and remain in a warm moisture-laden atmosphere; steam inhalations for 15–20 minutes every 2–3 hours are traditionally beneficial.

laryngocele *n*. a condition in which an air sac communicates with the larynx. The sac forms a swelling in the neck that dilates on coughing or straining. The condition is probably congenital but is also noted in such people as glassblowers, who have chronically raised intralaryngeal pressure.

laryngofissure *n*. a surgical operation to open the larynx, enabling access for further procedures.

laryngology *n*. the study of diseases of the larynx and vocal folds.

laryngomalacia *n*. a condition characterized by paroxysmal attacks of breathing difficulty and *stridor. It occurs in small children and is caused by flaccidity of the structure of the larynx. It usually resolves spontaneously by the age of two years.

laryngopharynx *n*. *see* HYPOPHARYNX.

laryngoscope *n*. a device used to inspect the larynx. This can be for diagnostic purposes, to facilitate surgery on the laryngeal structures, or to aid insertion of an endotracheal tube (*see* INTUBATION). Diagnostic laryngoscopes for use on awake patients are generally fibreoptic devices that are introduced through the mouth or nose. Surgical laryngoscopes are hollow tubes that are passed through the mouth and pharynx and are often used in conjunction with an *operating microscope. Intubating or anaesthetic laryngoscopes consist of a handle and a curved blade, fitted with a light, for moving the tongue and epiglottis aside.

laryngoscopy *n*. examination of the larynx. This may be done indirectly using a small mirror or directly using a *laryngoscope.

laryngospasm *n*. involuntary closure of the larynx, obstructing the flow of air to the lungs.

laryngotomy *n.* surgical incision of the larynx. **Inferior laryngotomy**, in which an incision is made in the cricothyroid membrane beneath the larynx, is a life-saving operation for patients in whom there is obstruction to breathing at or above the larynx. *See* TRACHEOSTOMY.

laryngotracheobronchitis *n.* a severe and almost exclusively viral infection of the respiratory tract, especially of young children, in whom there may be a dangerous degree of obstruction either at the larynx (*see* CROUP) or main air passages (bronchi) due to the thickness and stickiness of the fluid (exudate) produced by the inflamed tissues. Symptoms normally start at night. Treatment is supportive until the condition resolves naturally. In mild and moderate cases the child may benefit from being kept in a humid atmosphere (e.g. a steamy room). Nebulized medications and oxygen can help in more severe cases. In extreme cases endotracheal *intubation may be necessary. The condition may recur.

larynx *n.* the organ responsible for the production of vocal sounds, also serving as an air passage conveying air from the pharynx to the lungs. It is situated in the front of the neck, above the trachea. It is made up of a framework of nine cartilages (see illustration) – the epiglottis, thyroid, cricoid, arytenoid (two), corniculate (two), and cuneiform (two) – bound together by ligaments and muscles and lined with mucous membrane. Within are a pair of *vocal folds, which function in the production of voice. —**laryngeal** *adj.*

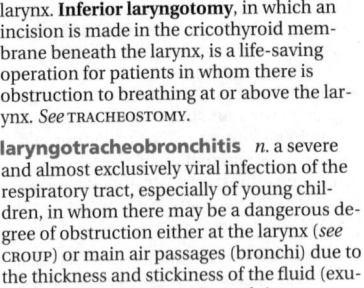

epiglottis
hyoid bone

thyroid cartilage

arytenoid cartilage

cricoid cartilage

trachea

The larynx.

LASEK *la*ser in *s*itu *e*pithelial *k*eratomileusis: a technique of laser refractive eye surgery used to correct both short sight (myopia) and long sight (hypermetropia). A flap of corneal epithelium is raised, the surface of the cornea is reshaped using an *excimer laser, and the epithelium is then replaced.

laser *n.* *l*ight *a*mplification by *s*timulated *e*mission of *r*adiation: a laser is a device that emits light through such a process; it can be used to operate on small areas of abnormality without damaging the delicate surrounding tissues. For example, lasers are used to unblock coronary arteries narrowed by atheroma and to remove certain types of birthmark (*see* NAEVUS). In ophthalmology different types of laser are used for operations on the cornea (*see* EXCIMER LASER), lens capsule (*see* YAG LASER), and retina (*see* ARGON LASER, DIODE LASER) and for glaucoma (*see* TRABECULOPLASTY). Lasers are also used in the treatment of *endometrial ablation (the **Nd:YAG laser**), *cervical intraepithelial neoplasia, and varicose veins (*endovenous laser treatment).

laser-assisted uvulopalatoplasty (LAUP) laser surgery to the palate, used in the treatment of *obstructive sleep apnoea.

laser Doppler flowmeter an instrument for measuring blood flow through tissue (e.g. skin) utilizing a laser beam.

laser laparoscopy *see* LAPAROSCOPY.

LASIK *la*ser in *s*itu *k*eratomileusis: laser refractive eye surgery used to correct both *myopia (short sight) and *hypermetropia (long sight). A thin corneal flap (epithelium and stroma) is raised using a keratome, the cornea is reshaped using an *excimer laser, and the flap is then replaced. *Compare* INTRASTROMAL KERATOMILEUSIS.

Lasix *n. see* FUROSEMIDE.

Lassa fever a serious virus disease confined to Central West Africa. After an incubation period of 3–21 days, headache, high fever, and severe muscular pains develop; difficulty in swallowing often arises. Death from kidney or heart failure occurs in over 50% of cases. Treatment with plasma from recovered patients is the best therapy, and the causative virus is susceptible to ribavirin.

lasting power of attorney a power of proxy given legal authority by the Mental Capacity Act 2005, which replaces the role of enduring power of attorney. Under the Act, anyone who has mental capacity may choose another person to make decisions (including decisions regarding health care) on their behalf if they subsequently lose capacity. Once the patient's loss of capacity is registered with the Public Guardian and the power of attorney is granted, the proxy becomes responsible for representing the patient's *best interests, but he or she can refuse life-sustaining treatment for the patient only if express written provision for such a decision was made by the patient in advance (*see* ADVANCE STATEMENT, DECISION, OR DIRECTIVE). The only circumstances in which the wishes of the proxy need not be followed is where clinicians believe that he or she is not acting in the patient's best interests. *See also* ADVOCACY, PROXY DECISION, SUBSTITUTED JUDGMENT.

latah *n.* a pattern of behaviour seen especially in certain cultures, such as that of Malaysia. After a psychological shock the affected individual becomes very anxious and very suggestible and shows excessive obedience and pathological imitation of the actions of another person (echopraxia).

latanoprost *n.* a *prostaglandin drug (an analogue of PGF₂) that both increases the drainage of aqueous humour from the eye and reduces the production of aqueous humour. It is used topically as a treatment for open-angle *glaucoma. Trade name: **Xalatan.**

late neonatal death death of a baby between 7 and 27 completed days of life.

latent period (in neurology) the pause of a few milliseconds between the time that a nerve impulse reaches a muscle fibre and the time that the fibre starts to contract.

late-onset schizophrenia a mental disorder characterized by systematic *delusions and commonly auditory *hallucinations, but without any other marked symptoms of *mental illness; it was formerly known as **paraphrenia**. The only loss of contact with reality is in areas affected by the delusions and hallucinations. It is typically seen in the elderly and can also occur in people with severe hearing impediments. Some people develop other symptoms of *schizophrenia over time but in many the personality remains intact over years. *Antipsychotic medication can be useful in some patients.

lateral *adj.* **1.** situated at or relating to the side of an organ or organism. **2.** (in anatomy) relating to the region or parts of the body that are furthest from the *median plane. *See* ANATOMICAL POSITION. **3.** (in radiology) in the *sagittal plane.

lathyrism *n.* a disease, characterized by muscular weakness and paralysis, found among people whose staple diet consists mostly of large quantites of *Lathyrus sativus*, a kind of chick pea, and/or vetches and pulses related to it. Except in mild cases complete recovery does not occur, despite administration of an adequate diet and physiotherapy.

laudanum *n.* a hydroalcoholic solution containing 1% morphine, prepared from macerated raw opium. It was formerly widely used as an opioid analgesic, taken by mouth.

laughing gas *see* NITROUS OXIDE.

LAUP *see* LASER-ASSISTED UVULOPALATO-PLASTY.

Laurence-Moon-Biedl syndrome an autosomal *recessive condition characterized by obesity, short stature, learning disabilities, *retinitis pigmentosa, *hypogonadism, and delayed puberty. [J. Z. Laurence (1830–74), British ophthalmologist; R. C. Moon (1844–1914), US ophthalmologist; A. Biedl (1869–1933), Austrian physician]

lavage *n.* washing out a body cavity, such as the colon or stomach, with water or a medicated solution. In cases of bowel obstruction the washing out can be done during the operation (**on-table lavage**). *See also* DIAGNOSTIC PERITONEAL LAVAGE.

laxative *n.* a drug used to stimulate or increase the frequency of bowel evacuation (also called a **cathartic** or **purgative**), or to encourage the passage of a softer or bulkier stool. The common laxatives are the stimulants (e.g. *bisacodyl, *senna and its derivatives); osmotic laxatives (e.g. magnesium salts, *lactulose); and *methylcellulose, *ispaghula husk, and other bulking agents.

lazy eye *see* AMBLYOPIA.

LBC *see* LIQUID-BASED CYTOLOGY.

LD₅₀ the dose of a toxic compound that causes death in 50% of a group of experimental animals to which it is administered: used as a measure of the toxicity of drugs.

LDL *see* LOW-DENSITY LIPOPROTEIN.

L-dopa *n. see* LEVODOPA.

lead¹ *n.* a soft bluish-grey metallic element that forms several poisonous compounds. Acute lead poisoning, which may follow inhalation of lead fumes or dust, causes abdominal pains, vomiting, and diarrhoea, with paralysis and convulsions and sometimes *encephalitis. In chronic poisoning a characteristic bluish marking of the gums ('lead line') is seen and the peripheral nerves are affected; there is also anaemia. Treatment is with *edetate. The use of lead in paints is now strictly controlled. Symbol: Pb.

lead² *n.* **1.** a portion of an electrocardiographic record that is obtained from a single electrode or a combination of electrodes placed on a particular part of the body (*see* ELECTROCARDIOGRAM, ELECTROCARDIOGRAPHY). In the conventional ECG, 12 leads are recorded. Each lead represents the electrical activity of the heart as 'viewed' from a different position on the body surface and may help to localize myocardial damage. **2.** a flexible steerable insulated wire introduced into the heart under X-ray control to allow electrical stimulation of the heart for the purpose of pacing (*see* PACEMAKER).

learning disability (learning difficulty) delayed or incomplete intellectual development (usually defined as an IQ of below 80) combined with some form of social malfunction, such as educational or occupational failure or inability of individuals to look after themselves. Good education alters the course of the disability, and a speciality of psychiatry provides treatment for patients who have a learning disability as well as a mental illness.

(🌐) SEE WEB LINKS

- Website of the British Institute of Learning Disabilities
- Website of Mencap, the UK's leading charity for those with learning disabilities

leather-bottle stomach *see* LINITIS PLASTICA.

Leber's congenital amaurosis a hereditary condition (inherited as an autosomal *recessive) causing severe visual loss in infants. The *fundus usually appears to be normal when examined with an *ophthalmoscope, but marked abnormalities are found on the ERG (*see* ELECTRORETINOGRAPHY), usually with extinguished wave

pattern. [T. Leber (1840–1917), German ophthalmologist]

Leber's optic atrophy a rare hereditary disorder, usually affecting young males, that is characterized by loss of central vision due to neuroretinal degeneration. Visual loss in one eye is rapid and usually followed by loss in the second eye. [T. Leber]

lecithin *n.* one of a group of *phospholipids that are important constituents of cell membranes and are involved in the metabolism of fat by the liver. An example is **phosphatidylcholine**. Lecithins are present in the *surfactant that occurs in fetal lung tissue. The **lecithin-sphingomyelin ratio (LS ratio)** is used as a measure of fetal lung maturity; an LS ratio below 2 indicates a higher risk of *respiratory distress syndrome (RDS). In such cases cortisone may be given to stimulate fetal lung maturity and hence reduce the risk of RDS in the newborn.

lecithinase *n.* an enzyme from the small intestine that breaks *lecithin down into glycerol, fatty acids, phosphoric acid, and choline.

leech *n.* a type of worm that possesses suckers at both ends of its body. Leeches occur in tropical forests and grasslands and in water. Certain parasitic species suck blood from animals and humans, and their bites cause irritation and, in some cases, infection. A leech can be detached from its host by applying salt. Formerly widely used for letting blood, the medicinal leech (*Hirudo medicinalis*) may now be used following microsurgery (e.g. to replace a severed finger) to restore patency to blocked or collapsed blood vessels and thus encourage the growth of new capillaries. The anticoagulants in the saliva of this and other species are now used for the treatment and prevention of thrombosis (*see* HIRUDIN).

leflunomide *n.* an *immunosuppressant drug used to treat rheumatoid and psoriatic arthritis that have not responded to methotrexate or other *disease-modifying antirheumatic drugs. Leflunomide is administered by mouth and side-effects, including blood disorders caused by impairment of bone-marrow function, may be severe. Trade name: **Arava**.

Le Fort classification a classification of fractures involving the *maxilla (upper jaw) and *orbit. Type I involves the maxilla only, type II the anterior orbit, and type III the posterior orbit. [R. Le Fort (19th century), French surgeon]

left ventricular failure *see* HEART FAIL-URE.

Legg-Calvé-Perthes disease (Perthes disease, pseudocoxalgia) necrosis of the head of the femur (thigh bone) due to interruption of its blood supply (*see* OSTEOCHONDRITIS). Of unknown cause, it occurs most commonly in boys between the ages of 5 and 10 and causes aching and a limp. The head of the femur can collapse and become deformed, resulting in a short leg and restricted hip movement. Affected boys are kept under observation and their activities are restricted; surgery may be required in more severe cases. [A. T. Legg (1874–1939), US surgeon; J. Calvé (1875–1954), French orthopaedist; G. C. Perthes (1869–1927), German surgeon]

legionnaires' disease an infection of the lungs caused by the bacterium *Legionella pneumophila*, named after an outbreak at the American Legion convention in Pennsylvania in 1976. *Legionella* organisms are widely found in water; outbreaks of the disease have been associated with defective central heating, air conditioning, and other ventilating systems. Symptoms appear after an incubation period of 2–10 days: malaise and muscle pain are succeeded by a fever, dry cough, chest pain, and breathlessness. X-ray of the lungs shows patchy consolidation. Erythromycin provides the most effective therapy.

Leigh syndrome a rare metabolic disorder that affects movement and development. Affected children are initially normal but lose coordination and balance as the disease progresses. There is no known cure at present. *See also* MITOCHONDRIAL DISORDERS. [D. Leigh (1915–98), British psychiatrist]

leio- *combining form denoting* smoothness. Example: **leiodermia** (abnormal smoothness of the skin).

leiomyoma *n.* a benign tumour of smooth muscle. Such tumours occur most commonly in the uterus (*see* FIBROID) but can also arise in the digestive tract, walls of blood vessels, etc. They may undergo malignant change (*see* LEIOMYOSARCOMA).

leiomyosarcoma *n.* a malignant tumour of smooth muscle, most commonly found in the uterus (it may arise in fibroids), stomach,

small bowel, and at the base of the bladder. It is the second most common *sarcoma of soft tissues. This tumour is rare in children, occurring most commonly in the bladder, prostate, and stomach.

Leishman-Donovan body *see* LEISHMANIA. [Sir W. B. Leishman (1865–1926), British surgeon; C. Donovan (1863–1951), Irish physician]

Leishmania *n.* a genus of parasitic flagellate protozoans, several species of which cause disease in humans (*see* LEISHMANIASIS). The parasite assumes a different form in each of its two hosts. In humans, especially in *kala-azar patients, it is a small rounded structure, with no flagellum, called a **Leishman-Donovan body**, which is found within the cells of the lymphatic system, spleen, and bone marrow. In the insect carrier it is long and flagellated.

leishmaniasis *n.* a disease, common in the tropics and subtropics, caused by parasitic protozoans of the genus *Leishmania*, which are transmitted by the bite of sandflies. There are two principal forms of the disease: **visceral leishmaniasis**, in which the cells of various internal organs are affected (*see* KALA-AZAR); and **cutaneous leishmaniasis**, which affects the tissues of the skin. Cutaneous leishmaniasis itself has several different forms, depending on the region in which it occurs and the species of *Leishmania* involved. In Asia it is common in the form of *oriental sore. In America there are several forms of leishmaniasis (*see* CHICLERO'S ULCER, ESPUNDIA). Leishmaniasis is treated with drugs containing antimony.

lemniscus *n.* a ribbon-like tract of nerve tissue conveying information from the spinal cord and brainstem upwards through the midbrain to the higher centres. On each side a **medial lemniscus** acts as a pathway from the spinal cord, while an outer **lateral lemniscus** commences higher up and is mainly concerned with hearing.

lemon sign *see* BANANA AND LEMON SIGNS.

lenalidomide *n.* a drug, related to *thalidomide, that affects the immune response and has activity against tumour cell formation and *angiogenesis. It is used to treat multiple myeloma and certain types of *myelodysplastic syndromes. It is taken by mouth; the most serious side-effects are deep vein thrombosis and neutropenia, and there is a risk of *teratogenesis (women capable of bearing children must practise contraception during treatment and for a month before and after it). Trade name: **Revlimid**.

lens *n*. **1**. (in anatomy) the transparent crystalline structure situated behind the pupil of the eye and enclosed in a thin transparent **capsule**. It helps to refract incoming light and focus it onto the *retina. *See also* ACCOMMODATION. **2**. (in optics) a piece of glass shaped to refract rays of light in a particular direction. **Convex lenses** converge the light, and **concave lenses** diverge it; they are worn to correct faulty eyesight. *See also* BIFOCAL LENS, CONTACT LENSES, TRIFOCAL LENSES.

lensectomy *n*. a surgical procedure in which the crystalline lens of the eye is removed.

lens implant *see* CATARACT.

lensmeter *n*. an instrument used to measure the refractive properties of an artificial lens, such as a spectacle lens.

lenticonus *n*. a condition in which the anterior surface (**anterior lenticonus**) or the posterior surface (**posterior lenticonus**) of the lens of the eye has a much steeper curvature than normal and bulges as a blunted cone. It is usually congenital.

lenticular nucleus (**lentiform nucleus**) *see* BASAL GANGLIA.

lentigo *n*. (*pl*. **lentigines**) a flat dark brown spot found mainly in the elderly on skin exposed to light. Lentigines have increased numbers of *melanocytes in the basal layer of the epidermis (freckles, by contrast, do not show an increase in these cells). **Lentigo maligna** (preinvasive or in-situ melanoma) occurs on the cheeks of the elderly and has variable pigmentation.

leontiasis *n*. a bilateral symmetrical hypertrophy of the bones of the face and cranium, said to resemble the appearance of a lion's head. It is a rare feature of untreated *Paget's disease; the cause is unknown. Medical name: **leontiasis ossea**.

lepirudin *n*. *see* HIRUDIN.

lepra reaction an aggravation of lumps on the skin caused by *leprosy, accompanied by fever and malaise.

leproma *n*. a lump on the skin characteristic of *leprosy.

lepromin *n*. a chemical prepared from

lumps on the skin caused by lepromatous *leprosy.

leprosy (**Hansen's disease**) *n*. a chronic disease, caused by the bacterium *Mycobacterium leprae*, that affects the skin, mucous membranes, and nerves. It is confined mainly to the tropics and is transmitted by direct contact. After an incubation period of 1–30 years, symptoms develop gradually and mainly involve the skin and nerves. **Lepromatous** (**multibacillary**) **leprosy** is a contagious steadily progressive form of the disease characterized by the development of widely distributed lumps on the skin, thickening of the skin and nerves, and in serious cases by severe numbness of the skin, muscle weakness, and paralysis, which leads to disfigurement and deformity. Tuberculosis is a common complication. **Tuberculoid leprosy** is a benign, often self-limiting, form of leprosy causing discoloration and disfiguration of patches of skin (sparsely distributed) associated with localized numbness. **Indeterminate leprosy** is a form of the disease in which skin manifestations represent a combination of the two main types; tuberculoid and indeterminate leprosy are known as **paucibacillary leprosy**.

Like tuberculosis, leprosy should be treated with a combination of antibacterial drugs, to overcome the problem of resistance developing to a single drug; the WHO advocates a combination of rifampicin and dapsone for six months to treat paucibacillary leprosy and these drugs with the addition of clofazimine for multibacillary leprosy, this **multidrug therapy** (**MDT**) to be continued for two years. Reconstructive surgery can repair some of the damage caused by the disease. A vaccine is being developed and tested.

lept- (**lepto-**) *combining form denoting* **1**. slender; thin. **2**. small. **3**. mild; slight.

leptin *n*. a protein that is produced and secreted by adipose tissue (especially white fat) and has a role in the regulation of eating (leptin receptors are concentrated in the hypothalamus). Increased amounts of adipose tissue result in higher concentrations of leptin and a reduction in appetite. A deficiency of leptin is responsible for a few cases of obesity.

leptocyte *n*. a red blood cell (*erythrocyte) that is wafer-thin, generally large in diameter, and displays a thin rim of haemoglobin at the periphery with a large area of central pallor. Leptocytes are seen in certain types of anaemia.

leptomeninges *pl. n.* the inner two *meninges: the arachnoid and pia mater.

leptomeningitis *n.* inflammation of the inner membranes (the *pia mater and *arachnoid) of the brain and spinal cord. *See also* MENINGITIS.

leptophonia *n.* weakness of the voice.

Leptospira *n.* a genus of spirochaete bacteria, commonly bearing hooked ends. They are not visible with ordinary light microscopy and are best seen using dark-ground microscopy. The parasitic species *L. icterohaemorrhagiae* is the main causative agent of Weil's disease (*see* LEPTOSPIROSIS), but many closely related species cause similar symptoms.

leptospirosis (Weil's disease) *n.* an infectious disease, caused by bacteria of the genus *Leptospira* (especially *L. icterohaemorrhagiae*), that occurs in rodents, dogs, and other mammals and may be transmitted to people whose work brings them into contact with these animals. The disease begins with a high fever and headache and may affect the liver (causing jaundice) or kidneys (resulting in renal failure); in some cases patients may go on to develop meningitis.

leptotene *n.* the first stage in the first prophase of *meiosis, in which the chromosomes become visible as single long threads.

Leriche's syndrome a condition in males characterized by absence of penile erection combined with absence of pulses in the femoral arteries and wasting of the buttock muscles. It is caused by occlusion of the abdominal aorta and iliac arteries. [R. Leriche (1879–1956), French surgeon]

Lesch-Nyhan disease a *sex-linked hereditary disease caused by an enzyme deficiency resulting in overproduction of uric acid. Affected boys are mentally retarded and suffer from *spasticity and gouty arthritis. They also have a compulsion for self-mutilation. [M. Lesch (1939–) and W. L. Nyhan Jr. (1926–), US physicians]

lesion *n.* a zone of tissue with impaired function as a result of damage by disease or wounding. Apart from direct physical injury, examples of primary lesions include abscesses, ulcers, and tumours; secondary lesions (such as crusts and scars) are derived from primary ones.

lethal gene a gene that, under certain conditions, causes the death of the individual carrying it. Lethal genes are usually *recessive: an individual will die only if he or she receives the gene from both parents.

lethargy *n.* mental and physical sluggishness: a degree of inactivity and unresponsiveness approaching or verging on the unconscious. The condition results from disease (such as sleeping sickness) or hypnosis.

letrozole *n. see* AROMATASE INHIBITOR.

Letterer-Siwe disease *see* LANGERHANS CELL HISTIOCYTOSIS. [E. Letterer (20th century) and S. A. Siwe (1897–1966), German physicians]

leuc- (leuco-, leuk-, leuko-) *combining form denoting* 1. lack of colour; white. 2. leucocytes.

leucapheresis *n.* a procedure for removing a quantity of white cells from the blood. Blood is withdrawn from the patient through a vein and passed through a machine (a cell separator). White cells are removed and the rest of the blood is returned to the patient through another vein. This method can be used to collect peripheral blood *stem cells from a patient.

leucine *n.* an *essential amino acid. *See also* AMINO ACID.

leucocidin *n.* a bacterial *exotoxin that selectively destroys white blood cells (leucocytes).

leucocyte (white blood cell) *n.* any blood cell that contains a nucleus. In health there are three major subdivisions: *granulocytes, *lymphocytes and *monocytes, which are part of the immune system, being involved in protecting the body against foreign substances and in antibody production. In disease, a variety of other types may appear in the blood, most notably immature forms of the normal red or white blood cells.

leucocytosis *n.* an increase in the number of white blood cells (leucocytes) in the blood. *See* BASOPHILIA, EOSINOPHILIA, LYMPHOCYTOSIS, MONOCYTOSIS.

leucocytospermia *n.* the presence of excess white blood cells (leucocytes) in the semen (more than 1 million/ml). It has an adverse effect on fertility.

leucoderma *n.* loss of pigment in areas of the skin, resulting in the appearance of white patches or bands and due to a variety of different causes.

leucolysin *n. see* LYSIN.

leucoma *n.* a white opacity occurring in the cornea. Most leucomas result from scarring after corneal inflammation or ulceration. Congenital types may be associated with other abnormalities of the eye.

leuconychia *n.* white discoloration of the nails, which may be total or partial. There are many causes.

leucopenia *n.* a reduction in the number of white blood cells (leucocytes) in the blood. *See* EOSINOPENIA, LYMPHOPENIA, NEUTROPENIA.

leucoplakia *n. see* LEUKOPLAKIA.

leucopoiesis *n.* the process of the production of white blood cells (leucocytes), which normally occurs in the blood-forming tissue of the *bone marrow. See also* GRANULOPOIESIS, HAEMOPOIESIS, LYMPHOPOIESIS, MONOBLAST.

leucorrhoea *n.* a whitish or yellowish discharge of mucus from the vaginal opening. It may occur normally, the quantity usually increasing before and after menstruation. An abnormally large discharge may indicate infection of the lower reproductive tract, e.g. by the protozoan *Trichomonas vaginalis* (*see* VAGINITIS).

leucotomy *n.* the surgical operation of interrupting the pathways of white nerve fibres within the brain: it was formerly the most common procedure in *psychosurgery. In the original form, **prefrontal leucotomy** (**lobotomy**), the operation involved cutting through the nerve fibres connecting the *frontal lobe with the *thalamus and the association fibres of the frontal lobe. This was often successful in reducing severe emotional tension. However, prefrontal leucotomy had serious side-effects and the procedure has now been abandoned.

Modern procedures use *stereotaxy and make selective lesions in smaller areas of the brain. Side-effects are uncommon and the operation is occasionally used for intractable pain, severe depression, obsessional neurosis, and chronic anxiety, where very severe emotional tension has not been relieved by other treatments.

leukaemia *n.* any of a group of malignant diseases in which the bone marrow and other blood-forming organs produce increased numbers of certain types of white blood cells (*leucocytes). Overproduction of these white cells, which are immature or abnormal forms, suppresses the production of normal white cells, red cells, and platelets. This leads to increased susceptibility to infection (due to *neutropenia), *anaemia, and bleeding (due to *thrombocytopenia). Other symptoms include enlargement of the spleen, liver, and lymph nodes.

Leukaemias are classified into **acute** or **chronic** varieties depending on the rate of progression of the disease. They are also classified according to the type of white cell that is proliferating abnormally; for example **acute lymphoblastic leukaemia** (*see* LYMPHOBLAST), **chronic lymphocytic leukaemia** (*see* LYMPHOCYTE), **acute myeloblastic leukaemia** (*see* MYELOBLAST), **hairy-cell leukaemia** (*see* HAIRY CELL), and **monocytic leukaemia** (*see* MONOCYTE). (*See also* MYELOID LEUKAEMIA.) Leukaemias can be treated with *cytotoxic drugs or *monoclonal antibodies, which suppress the production of the abnormal cells, or occasionally with radiotherapy.

⊕ SEE WEB LINKS
• Website of the Leukaemia Society

leukoplakia (**leucoplakia**) *n.* a thickened white patch on a mucous membrane, such as the mouth lining or vulva, that cannot be rubbed off. It is not a specific disease and is present in about 1% of the elderly. Occasionally leukoplakia can become malignant. **Hairy leukoplakia**, with a shaggy or hairy appearance, is a marker of AIDS. *See also* KHAT.

leukotaxine *n.* a chemical, present in inflammatory exudates, that attracts white blood cells (leucocytes) and increases the permeability of blood capillaries. It is probably produced by injured cells.

leukotriene *n.* one of a class of powerful chemical agents synthesized from arachidonic acid by mast cells, basophils, macrophages, and various other tissues. Leukotrienes are involved in inflammatory reactions and the immune response: they increase the permeability of small blood vessels, cause contraction of smooth muscle, and attract neutrophils to the site of an infection.

leukotriene receptor antagonist one

of a class of drugs that prevent the action of *leukotrienes by blocking their receptors on cell membranes, such as those in the airways. These drugs are used in the management of asthma for their effects in relaxing the smooth muscle of the airways and in reducing inflammation in the bronchial linings. Examples are **montelukast** (Singulair) and **zafirlukast** (Accolate), both of which are administered by mouth; side-effects may include headache and abdominal pain or gastrointestinal upsets.

leuprorelin *n. see* GONADORELIN ANALOGUE.

levamisole *n.* an *anthelmintic drug used to treat *ascariasis. It is administered by mouth; possible side-effects include nausea and vomiting.

levator *n.* **1.** a surgical instrument used for levering up displaced bone fragments in a depressed fracture of the skull. **2.** any muscle that lifts the structure into which it is inserted; for example, the **levator scapulis** helps to lift the shoulder blade.

Levitra *n. see* SILDENAFIL.

levo- (laevo-) *combining form denoting* **1.** the left side. **2.** (in chemistry) levorotation.

levobunolol *n.* a *beta blocker used as eye drops in the treatment of open-angle *glaucoma; it reduces intraocular pressure, probably by reducing the rate of production of aqueous humour. Side-effects may include local stinging and burning. Trade name: **Betagan**.

levodopa (L-dopa) *n.* a naturally occurring amino acid (*see* DOPA) used in the treatment of *parkinsonism. It is administered by mouth combined with benserazide in **co-beneldopa** (Madopar) or with carbidopa in **co-careldopa** (Sinemet). These drugs prevent the breakdown of levodopa to dopamine outside the brain, which reduces the severity of side-effects and enables lower doses of levodopa to be given. Side-effects may include nausea, vomiting, loss of appetite, faintness on standing up, and involuntary facial movements.

levodopa test a test of the ability of the pituitary to secrete growth hormone, in which levodopa is administered by mouth and plasma levels of growth hormone are subsequently measured (they should peak within the following hour). It is a safer alternative to the *insulin stress test but does not give information on cortisol production,

which is usually more clinically important to know.

levomepromazine (methotrimeprazine) *n.* a phenothiazine *antipsychotic drug used in the treatment of schizophrenia and to relieve tension, agitation, and pain in terminally ill patients. It is administered by mouth or injection; side-effects include drowsiness and weakness. Trade name: **Nozinan**.

levonorgestrel *n.* a synthetic female sex hormone – a *progestogen – used mainly in *oral contraceptives, either in combination with an oestrogen (in **Logynon**, **Ovranette**, etc.) or as a progestogen-only preparation (**Norgeston**). It is also used for emergency contraception (**Levonelle**: *see* POSTCOITAL CONTRACEPTION) and in the intrauterine system (**Mirena**: *see* IUS).

levothyroxine sodium *see* THYROXINE.

levulosuria *n. see* FRUCTOSURIA.

Lewy bodies *see* CORTICAL LEWY BODY DISEASE. [F. H. Lewy (1885–1950), German neurologist]

Leydig cells *see* INTERSTITIAL CELLS. [F. von Leydig (1821–1908), German anatomist]

Leydig tumour a tumour of the *interstitial (Leydig) cells of the testis. Such tumours often secrete testosterone, which in prepubertal boys causes *virilization.

LH *see* LUTEINIZING HORMONE.

Lhermitte's sign a tingling shocklike sensation passing down the arms or trunk when the neck is flexed. It is a nonspecific indication of disease in the cervical (neck) region of the spinal cord. Causes include multiple sclerosis, cervical *spondylosis, and deficiency of vitamin B_{12}. [J. Lhermitte (1877–1959), French neurologist]

LHRH analogue *see* GONADORELIN ANALOGUE.

liaison psychiatry the interface between medicine and psychiatry, recognized by the Royal College of Psychiatrists as a speciality of psychiatry. Liaison teams consist of psychiatric nurses, psychiatrists, and sometimes psychologists or social workers. They are usually located in general hospitals and see patients after *deliberate self-harm. They also see other patients in the general hospitals when a mental illness is suspected in order to diagnose and advise on treatment.

libido *n.* **1.** (in psychoanalytic theory) the

life instinct or, specifically, the sexual instinct. The libido (like the death instinct) is said to be one of the fundamental sources of energy for all mental life. **2.** sexual desire. Reduced or low libido may be caused by psychological or physical factors.

Librium *n. see* CHLORDIAZEPOXIDE.

lice *pl. n. see* LOUSE, PEDICULOSIS.

licence *n.* **1.** (in pharmaceutics) a document that allows a pharmaceutical company to market a particular drug. The company must apply for a licence to the regulatory body that issues them: in the UK this is the *Medicines and Healthcare products Regulatory Agency. A drug is licensed only for defined uses (indications), which the healthcare professional prescribing it should adhere to. **2.** (**licence to practice**) (in general practice) *see* LICENSING.

licensing *n.* a system to be introduced by the General Medical Council in November 2009, from which time the medical register will show whether a doctor is a licensed medical practitioner or holds registration only. It will be the **licence to practise** rather than registration that will signify to patients that a doctor has the legal authority to hold a post as a doctor, write prescriptions, sign death certificates, and exercise various other legal privileges. Once *revalidation is introduced, the licence will be subject to periodic renewal.

lichenification *n.* thickening of the epidermis of the skin with exaggeration of the normal creases, thought to resemble tree bark. The cause is abnormal scratching or rubbing of the skin. It is one of the cardinal features of chronic eczema.

lichenoid *adj.* describing any skin disease that resembles *lichen planus.

lichen planus an extremely itchy skin disease of unknown cause. Shiny flat-topped pink/purple spots may occur anywhere but are characteristically found on the inside of the wrists. It may take the form of a white lacy pattern in the mouth, which usually produces no symptoms. Trauma, such as a scratch, may induce a linear form of the disease (*see* KOEBNER PHENOMENON). Treatment with potent topical corticosteroids gives symptomatic relief. Tablet treatments may be necessary for generalized disease.

lichen sclerosus a chronic skin disease affecting the anogenital area (and rarely

other sites), especially the vulva in women and foreskin in men. It is characterized by sheets of thin ivory-white skin and may be caused by chronic irritation by urine. There is a risk of *squamous cell carcinoma. In women, the condition causes intense itching, and atrophy of the labia minora often occurs. Potent topical corticosteroids are helpful for women. In men, normal penile architecture is progressively lost and a constricting band around the foreskin may appear (causing sexual dysfunction and sometimes *paraphimosis) or sometimes narrowing of the urethral meatus may occur. This sometimes necessitates circumcision.

lichen simplex chronicus (neurodermatitis) thickened eczematous skin that develops at the site of constant rubbing in susceptible individuals. Common sites are the nape of the neck in women and the lower legs or scrotum in men. Stress may be a relevant factor.

Liddle's syndrome a rare autosomal *dominant condition characterized by hypertension associated with hypokalaemia, metabolic alkalosis, and low levels of plasma *renin and *aldosterone. The hypertension often starts in infancy and is due to excess resorption of sodium and excretion of potassium by the renal tubules. The syndrome is caused by a single genetic mutation on chromosome 16, which results in dysregulation of a sodium channel in the distal convoluted tubule. Treatment is with a low salt diet and a potassium-sparing diuretic that directly blocks the sodium channel, such as amiloride or triamterene. [G. G. Liddle (1921–89), US endocrinologist]

lidocaine (lignocaine) *n.* a widely used local *anaesthetic administered by injection for minor surgery and dental procedures. For the latter it is normally used in combination with adrenaline to achieve better and longer anaesthesia. Alone or in combination with other agents, it can also be applied directly to the eye, throat, and mouth, as it is absorbed through mucous membranes, and to the skin. Lidocaine is also injected to treat conditions involving abnormal heart rhythm (ventricular arrhythmias), particularly following myocardial infarction. When used as a local anaesthetic, side-effects are uncommon. Trade names: **Laryngojet, LMX 4, Xylocaine**.

lie *n.* the long axis of the fetus in relation to

that of the mother. It may be longitudinal, transverse, or oblique.

Lieberkühn's glands (crypts of Lieberkühn) simple tubular glands in the mucous membrane of the *intestine. In the small intestine they lie between the villi. They are lined with columnar *epithelium in which various types of secretory cells are found. In the large intestine Lieberkühn's glands are longer and contain more mucus-secreting cells. [J. N. Lieberkühn (1711–56), German anatomist]

lien *n. see* SPLEEN.

lien- (lieno-) *combining form denoting* the spleen. Example: **lienopathy** (disease of).

life table an actuarial presentation of the ages at which a group of males and/or females are expected to die and from which mean **life expectancy** at any age can be estimated, based on the assumption that mortality patterns current at the time of preparation of the table will continue to apply.

ligament *n.* **1.** a tough band of white fibrous connective tissue that links two bones together at a joint. Ligaments are inelastic but flexible; they both strengthen the joint and limit its movements to certain directions. **2.** a sheet of peritoneum that supports or links together abdominal organs.

ligamentum flavum an important posterior ligament of the spine, which is thickened and yellowish in colour and joins the *laminae of adjacent vertebrae.

ligand *n.* a molecule that binds to another molecule, as in antigen–antibody and hormone–receptor bondings.

ligation *n.* the application of a *ligature.

ligature *n.* any material – for example, nylon, silk, catgut, or wire – that is tied firmly round a blood vessel to stop it bleeding or around the base of a structure (such as the *pedicle of a growth) to constrict it.

light adaptation reflex changes in the eye to enable vision either in normal light after being in darkness or in very bright light after being in normal light. The pupil contracts (*see* PUPILLARY REFLEX) and the pigment in the *rods is bleached. *Compare* DARK ADAPTATION.

lightening *n.* the sensation experienced, usually after the 36th week of gestation, by many pregnant women, particularly those carrying their first child, as the presenting part of the fetus enters the pelvis. This reduces the pressure on the diaphragm and the woman notices that it is easier to breathe. *Compare* ENGAGEMENT.

light reflex *see* PUPILLARY REFLEX.

lignocaine *n. see* LIDOCAINE.

limbic system a complex system of nerve pathways and networks in the brain, involving several different nuclei, that is involved in the expression of instinct and mood in activities of the endocrine and motor systems of the body. Among the brain regions involved are the *amygdala, *hippocampal formation, and *hypothalamus. The activities of the body that are governed are those concerned with self-preservation (e.g. searching for food, fighting) and preservation of the species (e.g. reproduction and the care of offspring), the expression of fear, rage, and pleasure, and the establishment of memory patterns. *See also* RETICULAR ACTIVATING SYSTEM.

limb lengthening an orthopaedic procedure for increasing the length of a limb (usually the leg). An *external fixator is attached to the bone. This can be a circular frame surrounding the bone, which was invented by the Russian surgeon Ilizarov, or a bar down one side of the limb. The bone is divided, and the gap produced is slowly widened by moving the two ends of the frame apart; if a bar fixator is used, its body has a screw thread that is turned to increase the distance between the two ends. New bone is produced in the widening gap as the bone is stretched (*see* CALLOTASIS). Limb lengthening is undertaken when there is inequality in the length of the legs; for example, following trauma or resulting from paralysis in childhood. Both legs can be lengthened to increase the height of a person of excessively short stature.

limbus *n.* (in anatomy) an edge or border; for example, the **limbus sclerae** is the junction of the cornea and sclera of the eye.

limen *n.* (in anatomy) a border or boundary. The **limen nasi** is the boundary between the bony and cartilaginous parts of the nasal cavity.

liminal *adj.* (in physiology) relating to the threshold of perception.

limosis *n.* abnormal hunger or an excessive desire for food.

linac *n. see* LINEAR ACCELERATOR.

linctus *n.* a syrupy liquid medicine, particularly one used in the treatment of irritating coughs.

Lindau's tumour *see* HAEMANGIOBLASTOMA. [A. Lindau (1892–1958), Swedish pathologist]

linea *n.* (*pl.* **lineae**) (in anatomy) a line, narrow streak, or stripe. The **linea alba** is a tendinous line, extending from the xiphoid process to the pubic symphysis, where the flat abdominal muscles are attached.

linea nigra a dark line down the centre of the abdomen caused by increased pigmentation in pregnancy.

linear accelerator (**linac**) a machine that accelerates particles to produce high-energy radiation, used in the treatment (radiotherapy) of malignant disease.

linezolid *n.* a member of a class of antibiotics – the **oxazolidinones** – that are active against Gram-positive bacteria, including *MRSA. Linezolid is used to treat pneumonia and soft-tissue infections caused by these organisms when they have not responded to other antibacterials. It is administered by mouth or intravenous infusion; the most common side-effects are headache, a metallic taste in the mouth, diarrhoea, and nausea. Trade name: **Zyvox**.

lingual *adj.* relating to, situated close to, or resembling the tongue (lingua). The lingual surface of a tooth is the surface adjacent to the tongue.

lingula *n.* **1.** the thin forward-projecting portion of the anterior lobe of the cerebellum, in the midline. **2.** a small section of the upper lobe of the left lung, extending downwards in front of the heart. **3.** a bony spur on the inside of the mandible, above the angle of the jaw. **4.** a small backward-pointing projection on each side of the sphenoid bone.

liniment *n.* a medicinal preparation that is rubbed onto the skin or applied on a surgical dressing. Liniments often contain camphor.

lining *n.* (in dentistry) a protective layer placed in a prepared tooth cavity before a *filling is inserted.

linitis plastica (**leather-bottle stomach**) diffuse infiltration of the stomach submucosa with malignant tissue, producing rigidity and narrowing. Diagnosis by endoscopy may be difficult but radiological changes are more marked.

linkage *n.* (in genetics) the situation in which two or more genes lie close to each other on a chromosome and are therefore very likely to be inherited together. The further two genes are apart the more likely they are to be separated by *crossing over during meiosis.

LINKs *see* LOCAL INVOLVEMENT NETWORKS.

linoleic acid *see* ESSENTIAL FATTY ACID.

linolenic acid *see* ESSENTIAL FATTY ACID.

lint *n.* a material used in surgical dressings, made of scraped linen or a cotton substitute. It is usually fluffy one side and smooth the other.

liothyronine *n.* a preparation of the hormone *triiodothyronine, produced by the thyroid gland, that is used to treat conditions of severe thyroid deficiency. It is administered by mouth or injection and has a rapid but short-lived effect. Trade name: **Tertroxin**.

lip- (**lipo-**) *combining form denoting* **1.** fat. **2.** lipid.

lipaemia *n.* the presence in the blood of an abnormally large amount of fat.

lipase (**steapsin**) *n.* an enzyme, produced by the pancreas and the glands of the small intestine, that breaks down fats into glycerol and fatty acids during digestion.

lipid *n.* one of a group of naturally occurring compounds that are soluble in solvents such as chloroform or alcohol, but insoluble in water. Lipids are important dietary constituents, not only because of their high energy value but also because certain vitamins and essential fatty acids are associated with them. The group includes *fats, the *steroids, *phospholipids, and *glycolipids.

lipidosis (**lipoidosis**) *n.* (*pl.* **lipidoses**) any disorder of lipid metabolism within the cells of the body. The **brain lipidoses** (*see* GAUCHER'S DISEASE, HUNTER'S SYNDROME, HURLER'S SYNDROME, TAY-SACHS DISEASE) are inborn defects causing the accumulation of lipids within the brain.

lipoatrophy *n.* an immune reaction to insulin injections close to the site of injection, resulting in localized hollowing of the fat tissue, which is unsightly. It is rarely seen with more modern, highly purified, insulins.

lipochondrodystrophy *n.* multiple congenital defects affecting lipid (fat) metabolism, cartilage and bone, skin, and the major internal organs, leading to mental retardation, dwarfism, and deformities of the bones.

lipochrome *n.* a pigment that is soluble in fat and therefore gives colour to fatty materials. An example is *carotene, the pigment responsible for the colour of egg yolks and butter.

lipodystrophy *n.* any condition resulting in the loss and/or redistribution of fat tissue in part or all of the body. It may be congenital or acquired (for example, as an adverse effect of antiretroviral drug treatment). Congenital lipodystrophies include **Kobberling-Dunnigan syndrome**, an autosomal *dominant condition more common in women, who lose fat tissue from their limbs and lower bodies and often also suffer with *polycystic ovary syndrome; and **Seip-Beradinelli syndrome**, which is autosomal *recessive and involves more generalized fat-tissue loss. Acquired forms usually follow an acute illness in childhood and may involve all or part of the body.

lipofuscin *n.* a brownish pigment staining with certain fat stains. It is most common in the cells of heart muscle, nerves, and liver and is normally contained within the *lysosomes.

lipogenesis *n.* the process by which glucose and other substances, derived from carbohydrate in the diet, are converted to *fatty acids in the body.

lipogranulomatosis *n.* an abnormality of lipid metabolism causing deposition of yellowish nodules in the skin.

lipohypertrophy *n.* a local build-up of fat tissue at the site of repeated insulin injections, which tends to alter the rate of absorption of further injections. It is caused by the local action of the insulin, which (among other things) promotes fat storage.

lipoic acid a sulphur-containing compound that can be readily interconverted to and from its reduced form, **dihydrolipoic acid**. Lipoic acid functions in carbohydrate metabolism as one of the *coenzymes in the oxidative decarboxylation of pyruvate and other α-keto acids.

lipoidosis *n. see* LIPIDOSIS.

lipolysis *n.* the process by which lipids, particularly triglycerides in fat, are broken down into their constituent fatty acids in the body by the enzyme *lipase. —**lipolytic** *adj.*

lipoma *n.* (*pl.* **lipomas** or **lipomata**) a common benign tumour composed of well-differentiated fat cells.

lipomatosis *n.* **1.** the presence of an abnormally large amount of fat occurring in the tissues. **2.** the presence of multiple *lipomas.

lipopolysaccharide *n.* a complex molecule containing both a lipid component and a polysaccharide component. Lipopolysaccharides are constituents of the cell walls of Gram-negative bacteria and are important in determining the antigenic properties of these bacteria.

lipoprotein *n.* one of a group of compounds, found in blood plasma and lymph, each consisting of a protein (*see* APOLIPOPROTEIN) combined with a lipid (which may be cholesterol, a triglyceride, or a phospholipid). Lipoproteins are important for the transport of lipids in the blood and lymph (*see also* LIPOPROTEIN LIPASE). *See* CHYLOMICRON, HIGH-DENSITY LIPOPROTEIN, LOW-DENSITY LIPOPROTEIN, VERY LOW-DENSITY LIPOPROTEIN. *See also* HYPERLIPIDAEMIA.

lipoprotein lipase an enzyme that catalyses the hydrolysis of triglycerides in *chylomicrons and *very low-density lipoproteins to free fatty acids, which are absorbed from the capillaries into local tissues. Deficiency of this enzyme results in severe *hypertriglyceridaemia.

liposarcoma *n.* a rare malignant tumour of fat cells. It is most commonly found in the thigh and is rare under the age of 30 years. There are four main histological types: **well-differentiated**, **myxoid**, **pleomorphic**, and **round-cell liposarcomas**. Treatment is usually by surgery.

liposome *n.* a microscopic spherical membrane-enclosed vesicle or sac (20–30 nm in diameter) made artificially in the laboratory by the addition of an aqueous solution to a phospholipid gel. The membrane resembles a cell membrane and the whole vesicle is similar to a cell organelle. Liposomes can be incorporated into living cells and may be used to transport relatively toxic drugs into cancer cells, where they can exert their maximum effects. The cancerous organ is at a higher temperature than normal body temperature, so that when the liposome passes through its blood vessels the membrane melts and the drug (e.g. *doxorubicin) is released. Liposomes are also undergoing clinical trials as vehicles in *gene therapy for cystic fibrosis.

liposuction *n.* a technique for removing unwanted collections of subcutaneous fat by using a powerful suction tube passed through the skin at different locations.

lipotrophin *n.* a hormone-like substance from the anterior pituitary gland that stimulates the transfer of fat from the body stores to the bloodstream.

lipotropic *adj.* describing a substance that promotes the transport of fatty acids from the liver to the tissues or accelerates the utilization of fat in the liver itself. An example of such a substance is the amino acid methionine.

lipping *n.* overgrowth of bone around a joint as seen on X-ray. This is a characteristic sign of degenerative joint disease and occurs most frequently and prominently in osteoarthritis. *See also* OSTEOPHYTE.

Lipsitz score a scoring system used for newborn babies who may be withdrawing from maternal opioids or other (usually nonprescription) drugs. *See* NEONATAL ABSTINENCE SYNDROME.

lipuria *n.* the presence of fat or oil droplets in the urine.

liquid-based cytology (LBC) a relatively new technology intended to improve the detection of cytological abnormalities, which has been heralded as a way forward for *cervical screening. It involves thin-layer cytology based on a liquid sample and lends itself to automation. LBC provides uniformly well-fixed preparations that are free of inflammatory exudate and blood and seem easier to screen than conventional (Pap) *cervical smears. However, it is expensive in terms of equipment, capital costs, maintenance, consumables, training, technical preparation time, transportation, and disposal of liquid media.

liquor *n.* 1. (in pharmacy) any solution, usually an aqueous solution. 2. the amniotic fluid surrounding a fetus.

Lisch nodules pigmented *hamartomas of the iris of the eye seen in *neurofibromatosis type I. [K. Lisch (1907–99), Austrian ophthalmologist]

lissencephaly (smooth brain) *n.* a condition in which the brain develops abnormally – it has no grooves on the outside, large ventricles, and generally is smaller than it should be. Lissencephaly causes severe mental retardation and *failure to thrive. *See also* MILLER-DEIKER SYNDROME.

Listeria *n.* a genus of Gram-positive aerobic motile rodlike bacteria that are parasites of warm-blooded animals. The single species, *L. monocytogenes*, infects many domestic and wild animals. If it is transmitted to humans, by eating infected animals or animal products, it may cause disease (**listeriosis**), especially in the frail, ranging from influenza-like symptoms to meningoencephalitis. In pregnant women it may cause a miscarriage or damage the fetus.

lith- (litho-) *combining form denoting* a calculus (stone). Example: **lithogenesis** (formation of).

-lith *combining form denoting* a calculus (stone). Example: **faecalith** (a stony mass of faeces).

lithaemia *n. see* HYPERURICAEMIA.

lithiasis *n.* formation of stones (*see* CALCULUS) in an internal organ, such as the gall bladder (*see* GALLSTONE), urinary system, pancreas, or appendix.

lithium *n.* a metallic element used in the form of its salts (lithium carbonate and lithium citrate) to prevent and treat episodes of mania or depression in patients with *bipolar affective disorder. It is given by mouth; side-effects include tremor, weakness, nausea, thirst, and excessive urination. Thyroid function can be impaired after many years of use and regular thyroid function tests are compulsory. Reversible changes in the kidney can appear after long-term lithium treatment. The range of plasma levels within which lithium is most effective is small, therefore levels of lithium in the blood are regularly checked during long-term therapy. Trade names: **Priadel**, etc.

litholapaxy (lithotripsy) *n.* the operation of crushing a stone in the bladder, using an instrument called a **lithotrite**. The small fragments of stone can then be removed by irrigation and suction.

lithonephrotomy *n.* surgical removal of a stone from the kidney. *See* NEPHROLITHOT-OMY, PYELOLITHOTOMY.

lithopaedion *n.* a fetus that has died in the uterus or abdominal cavity and has become calcified.

lithotomy *n.* the surgical removal of a stone (calculus) from the urinary tract. *See* NEPHROLITHOTOMY, PYELOLITHOTOMY, URETEROLITHOTOMY.

lithotripsy *n.* **1.** the destruction of calculi (stones) by the application of shock waves. In **extracorporeal shock-wave lithotripsy (ESWL)**, used for destroying calculi in the upper urinary tract, the shock waves are generated and transmitted by an external power source. The specialized machine (a **lithotripter**) consists of a sophisticated radiological system to localize the stone accurately by biplanar X-ray or ultrasound and a shock head or transducer to produce and focus the energy source. The prototype machines required the patient to be anaesthetized and immersed in a water bath for treatment, but modern machines require neither water bath nor general anaesthesia. In **electrohydraulic lithotripsy (EHL)**, used for destroying urinary calculi, an electrically generated shock wave is transmitted to the stone by a contact probe delivered via a *nephroscope or *ureteroscope. **2.** *see* LITHOLAPAXY.

lithotrite *n.* a surgical instrument used for crushing a stone in the bladder. *See* LITHOLA-PAXY.

lithotrophic *adj. see* AUTOTROPHIC.

lithuresis *n.* the passage of small stones or *gravel in the urine.

lithuria *n. see* HYPERURICURIA.

litre *n.* a unit of volume equal to the volume occupied by 1 kilogram of pure water at 4°C and 760 mmHg pressure. In *SI units the litre is treated as a special name for the cubic decimetre, but is not used when a high degree of accuracy is required (1 litre = 1.0000028 dm^3). For approximate purposes 1 litre is assumed to be equal to 1000 cubic centimetres (cm^3), therefore 1 millilitre (ml) is often taken to be equal to 1 cm^3. This practice is now deprecated.

Little's area   the anterior region of the nasal septum (*see* NOSE). It has a rich capillary supply, called *Kiesselbach's plexus, and is a common site from which nosebleeds arise. *See* EPISTAXIS. [J. L. Little (1836–85), US surgeon]

Little's disease   a form of *cerebral palsy involving both sides of the body and affecting the legs more severely than the arms. [W. J. Little (1810–94), British surgeon]

Litzmann's obliquity   *see* ASYNCLITISM. [K. C. T. Litzmann (1815–90), German obstetrician]

livedo *n.* a discoloured area or spot on the skin, often caused by local congestion of the circulation.

liver *n.* the largest gland of the body, weighing 1200–1600 g. Situated in the top right portion of the abdominal cavity, the liver is divided by fissures (**fossae**) into four lobes: the **right** (the largest lobe), **left**, **quadrate**, and **caudate lobes**. It is connected to the diaphragm and abdominal walls by five ligaments: the membranous **falciform** (which separates the right and left lobes), **coronary**, and **right** and **left triangular ligaments** and the fibrous **round ligament**, which is derived from the embryonic umbilical vein. Venous blood containing digested food is brought to the liver in the **hepatic portal vein** (*see* PORTAL SYSTEM). Branches of this vein pass in between the lobules and terminate in the **sinusoids** (see illustration).

Oxygenated blood is supplied in the **hepatic artery**. The blood leaves the liver via a central vein in each lobule, which drains into the *hepatic vein. The liver is supplied by parasympathetic nerve fibres from the vagus nerve, and by sympathetic fibres from the solar plexus. The liver has a number of important functions. It synthesizes *bile, which drains into the *gall bladder before being released into the duodenum. The liver is an important site of metabolism of carbohydrates, proteins, and fats. It regulates the amount of blood sugar, converting excess glucose to *glycogen; it removes excess amino acids by breaking them down into ammonia and finally *urea; and it stores and metabolizes fats. The liver also synthesizes *fibrinogen and *prothrombin (essential blood-clotting substances) and *heparin, an anticoagulant. It forms red blood cells in the fetus and is the site of production of plasma proteins. It has an important role in the detoxification of poisonous substances and it breaks down worn out red cells and other unwanted substances, such as excess oestrogen in the male (*see also* KUPFFER CELLS). The liver is also the site of *vitamin A synthesis; this vitamin is stored in the liver, together with vitamins B$_{12}$, D, and K.

The liver is the site of many important diseases, including *hepatitis, *cirrhosis, amoebic *dysentery, *hydatid disease, and *hepatomas.

SEE WEB LINKS

• Website of the British Liver Trust: information on the liver, liver care, and liver conditions

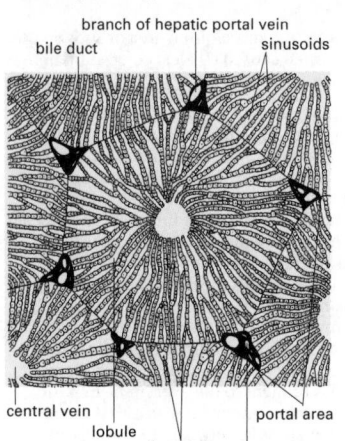

branch of hepatic portal vein
bile duct
sinusoids

central vein
lobule
liver cells
portal area

branch of hepatic artery

The liver (microscopic structure).

livid *adj.* denoting a bluish colour of the skin, such as that produced locally by a bruise or of the general complexion in *cyanosis.

lividity *n. see* HYPOSTASIS.

living will a colloquial term describing an *advance statement, decision, or directive in which a person expresses a preference or refuses treatment ahead of the point at which he or she loses capacity.

LLETZ large loop excision of the *transformation zone: a procedure for treating premalignant conditions of the cervix, including carcinoma in situ (CIN3; *see* CERVICAL INTRA-EPITHELIAL NEOPLASIA), that is performed under colposcopic control (*see* COLPOSCOPY) after application of local anaesthetic to the cervix. The transformation zone is removed using a thin loop of wire heated by electric current (*see* DIATHERMY).

LMC *see* LOCAL MEDICAL COMMITTEE.

Loa *n.* a genus of parasitic nematode worms (*see* FILARIA). The adult eye worm, *L. loa*, lives within the tissues beneath the skin, where it causes inflammation and swelling (*see* LOIASIS). The motile embryos, present in the blood during the day, may be taken up by bloodsucking *Chrysops* flies. Here they develop into infective larvae, ready for transmission to a new human host.

lobe *n.* a major division of an organ or part of an organ, especially one having a rounded form and often separated from other lobes by fissures or bands of connective tissue. For example, the brain, liver, and lung are divided into lobes. —**lobar** *adj.*

lobectomy *n.* the surgical removal of a lobe of an organ or gland, such as the lung, thyroid, or brain. Lobectomy of the lung may be performed for cancer or other disease of the lung; in some cases the operation can be done through an endoscope.

lobotomy (prefrontal leucotomy) *n. see* LEUCOTOMY.

lobular carcinoma cancer that arises in the lobules (rather than the ducts) of the breast. Like ductal carcinoma, it may be confined to its site of origin but can invade other tissues; however, it has a greater tendency than ductal carcinoma to affect both breasts.

lobule *n.* a subdivision of a part or organ that can be distinguished from the whole by boundaries, such as septa, that are visible with or without a microscope. For example, the **lobule of the liver** is a structural and functional unit seen in cross-section under a microscope as a column of cells drained by a central vein and bounded by a branch of the portal vein. The **lung lobule** is a practical subdivision of the lung tissue seen macroscopically in lung slices as outlined by incomplete septa of fibrous tissue. It is made up of three to five lung *acini.

local involvement networks (LINks) groups set up to help local people get involved in the development and delivery of health and social care services; they replaced **PPI forums** in 2008. LINks are funded via local authorities, and members may include patients and service users, local residents, charities, community groups, and local businesses.

local medical committee (LMC) a

group of representatives of the general practitioners working in a defined geographical area. There are separate LMCs for each area, and the members speak on behalf of the local practitioners by whom they are elected. Similar arrangements and responsibilities apply for dentists, pharmacists, and optometrists practising in the NHS outside hospitals.

lochia *n.* the material eliminated from the uterus through the vagina after the completion of labour. The first discharge, **lochia rubra** (**lochia cruenta**), consists largely of blood. This is followed by **lochia serosa**, a brownish mixture of blood and mucus, and finally **lochia alba** (**lochia purulenta**), a yellowish or whitish discharge containing microorganisms and cell fragments. Each stage may last for several days. —**lochial** *adj.*

locked-in syndrome *see* VEGETATIVE STATE.

lockjaw *n. see* TETANUS.

locomotor ataxia *see* TABES DORSALIS.

loculation *n.* the compartmentalization of a fluid-filled cavity into smaller spaces (locules) by fibrous septa. Loculation may occur in patients with long-standing pleural effusions, ascites, and in some cysts.

loculus *n.* (in anatomy) a small space or cavity.

locum tenens a doctor who stands in temporarily for a colleague who is absent or ill and looks after the patients in his practice. Often shortened to **locum**.

locus *n.* **1.** (in anatomy) a region or site. The **locus caeruleus** is a small pigmented *nucleus in the floor of the fourth ventricle of the brain. **2.** (in genetics) the region of a chromosome occupied by a particular gene.

lofepramine *n.* a tricyclic *antidepressant that is administered by mouth. It is less sedating than amitriptyline and has a lower incidence of *antimuscarinic side-effects.

log- (**logo-**) *combining form denoting* words; speech.

logopaedics *n.* the scientific study of defects and disabilities of speech and of the methods used to treat them. *See also* SPEECH AND LANGUAGE THERAPY.

logorrhoea *n.* a rapid flow of voluble speech, often with incoherence, such as is encountered in *mania.

-logy (**-ology**) *combining form denoting* field of study. Example: **cytology** (study of cells).

loiasis *n.* a disease, occurring in West and Central Africa, caused by the eye worm *Loa loa*. The adult worms live and migrate within the skin tissues, causing the appearance of transitory **calabar** swellings. These are probably an allergic reaction to the worms' waste products, and they sometimes lead to fever and itching. Worms often migrate across the eyeball just beneath the conjunctiva, where they cause irritation and congestion. Loiasis is treated with *diethylcarbamazine, which kills both the adults and larval forms.

loin *n.* the region of the back and side of the body between the lowest rib and the pelvis.

Lomotil *n. see* CO-PHENOTROPE.

longitudinal study *see* COHORT STUDY.

long QT syndrome prolongation of the *Q–T interval on the electrocardiogram. It indicates susceptibility to ventricular tachycardia (especially *torsades de pointes), ventricular fibrillation, and sudden death. It may be familial or caused by certain drugs (e.g. sotalol, amiodarone, certain antipsychotic drugs).

long-sightedness *n. see* HYPERMETROPIA.

loop *n.* **1.** a bend in a tubular organ, e.g. *Henle's loop in a kidney tubule. **2.** one of the patterns of dermal ridges in *fingerprints.

loop system *see* INDUCTION LOOP SYSTEM.

loosening of associations *see* ASSOCIATION OF IDEAS.

Looser zone *see* OSTEOMALACIA. [E. Looser (1877–1936), Swiss surgeon]

loperamide *n.* a drug used in the treatment of diarrhoea. It acts by reducing *peristalsis of the digestive tract and is administered by mouth; side-effects are rare, but include abdominal distension, drowsiness, and skin rash. Trade name: **Imodium**.

lopinavir *n. see* PROTEASE INHIBITOR.

loprazolam *n.* a short-acting benzodiazepine drug administered by mouth for the short-term treatment of insomnia (*see* HYPNOTIC). Possible side-effects include drowsiness and confusion.

loratidine *n. see* ANTIHISTAMINE.

lorazepam *n.* a *benzodiazepine used to relieve moderate or severe anxiety and tension, including that associated with insomnia. It is also used for premedication and for treating status epilepticus. It is administered by mouth or injection and may cause drowsiness, dizziness, blurred vision, and nausea. Trade name: **Ativan**.

lordosis *n.* inward curvature of the spine, which appears as a forward curvature when viewed from the side. A certain degree of lordosis is normal in the lumbar and cervical regions of the spine: loss of this may occur in ankylosing *spondylitis. Exaggerated lordosis may occur through faulty posture or as a result of disorders of vertebral development and spinal muscles. *Compare* KYPHOSIS.

losartan *n. see* ANGIOTENSIN II ANTAGONIST.

lotion *n.* a medicinal solution for washing or bathing the external parts of the body. Lotions usually have a cooling, soothing, or antiseptic action.

Lou Gehrig's disease amyotrophic lateral *sclerosis. *See also* MOTOR NEURON DISEASE. [Lou Gehrig (1903–41), US baseball player who suffered from it]

loupe *n.* **1.** a small magnifying hand lens used for examining the front part of the eye, usually with a pocket torch to provide illumination. In modern practice a slit-lamp microscope is used. **2. (loupes)** a binocular telescope system of variable magnification range mounted on a spectacle frame or a headband and used in microsurgical procedures, such as nerve repair or anastomosis of fine vessels.

louse *n.* (*pl.* **lice**) a small wingless insect that is an external parasite of humans. Lice attach themselves to hair and clothing using their well-developed legs and claws. Their flattened leathery bodies are resistant to crushing and their mouthparts are adapted for sucking blood. Lice thrive in overcrowded and unhygienic conditions; they can infest humans (*see* PEDICULOSIS) and they may transmit disease. *See also* PEDICULUS, PHTHIRUS.

Løvset's manoeuvre rotation of the trunk of the fetus during a breech birth to facilitate delivery of the arms and the shoulders. This procedure is used when the fetal arms are extended due to previous inappropriate traction. [J. Løvset (20th century), Norwegian obstetrician]

low-density lipoprotein (LDL) a *lipoprotein that is the principal form in which *cholesterol is transported in the bloodstream: it accounts for approximately 70% of the circulating cholesterol in an individual. LDL is derived from *very low-density lipoprotein and is eventually cleared from the circulation by the liver. LDL may be deposited within the lining of arteries, thus causing *atheroma; the higher the circulating concentration of LDL, the higher the likelihood of atheroma developing (*see also* HYPERCHOLESTEROLAEMIA). *Statins are effective in lowering circulating LDL levels.

lower urinary tract symptoms (LUTS) symptoms occuring during urine storage, voiding, or immediately after. These include *frequency, *urgency, *nocturia, *incontinence, *hesitation, *intermittency, *terminal dribble, *dysuria, and *postmicturition dribble. These symptoms used to be known as **prostatism**. Sometimes they are due to benign prostatic hyperplasia (*see* PROSTATE GLAND), but they may be due to *detrusor overactivity, excessive drinking, diuresis due to poorly controlled diabetes, or a urethral stricture.

lower uterine segment the lower portion of uterus, lying below the loose fold of peritoneum that lies between the uterus and bladder. It does not form until later in pregnancy and is less contractile than the rest of the uterus. A *Caesarean section is performed through the lower segment.

Lowe's syndrome *see* DENT'S DISEASE.

low-molecular-weight heparin a type of *heparin that is more readily absorbed and requires less frequent administration than standard heparin preparations used as *parenteral anticoagulant therapy to prevent and treat deep vein thrombosis following surgery or during kidney dialysis. Preparations in use include **bemiparin sodium** (Zibor), **dalteparin sodium** (Fragmin), **enoxaparin sodium** (Clexane), and **tinzaparin sodium** (Innohep).

lozenge *n.* a medicated tablet containing sugar. Lozenges should dissolve slowly in the mouth so that the medication is applied to the mouth and throat.

LSD *see* LYSERGIC ACID DIETHYLAMIDE.

lubb-dupp *n.* a representation of the normal heart sounds as heard through the stethoscope. Lubb (the first heart sound) coincides with closure of the mitral and tricuspid valves; dupp (the second heart sound) is due to closure of the aortic and pulmonary valves.

Lucentis *n. see* RANIBIZUMAB.

lucid interval temporary recovery of consciousness after a blow to the head, before relapse into coma. It is a sign of intracranial arterial bleeding (extradural *haematoma).

Ludwig's angina severe inflammation caused by infection of both sides of the floor of the mouth, resulting in massive swelling of the neck. If untreated, it may obstruct the airways, necessitating tracheostomy. [W. F. von Ludwig (1770–1865), German surgeon]

lues *n.* a serious infectious disease such as syphilis.

Lugol's iodine a solution of 5% iodine and 10% potassium iodide, used in the treatment of thyrotoxicosis in emergencies, such as *thyroid crisis, or when surgery cannot wait for more conventional treatments. For its mode of action it utilizes the abnormal *Wolff-Chaikoff effect, seen in cases of thyroiditis. [J. G. A. Lugol (1786–1851), French physician]

lumbago *n.* pain in the lumbar or loin region, of any cause or description. Severe lumbago, of sudden onset while bending or lifting, can be due either to a slipped disc or to a strained muscle or ligament. When associated with *sciatica it is often due to a prolapsed intervertebral disc.

lumbar *adj.* relating to the loin.

lumbar puncture a procedure performed under local anaesthetic in which cerebrospinal fluid is withdrawn by means of a hollow needle inserted into the *subarachnoid space in the region of the lower back (usually between the third and fourth lumbar vertebrae). The fluid obtained is examined for diagnosis of meningitis, multiple sclerosis, and various other disorders of the brain and spinal cord. Lumbar puncture may also be perfomed to inject agents into the subarachnoid space. The procedure is usually without risk to the patient, but in patients with raised intracranial pressure it may be hazardous. CT and MRI scanning prior to lumbar puncture have greatly reduced the risk of performing the test in patients with unsuspected raised intracranial pressure. The commonest side-effect of the procedure is a headache that is worse on standing and reduces on lying down (*intracranial hypotension headache). *See also* QUECKENSTEDT TEST.

lumbar triangle a weak area in the abdomen bounded by the iliac crest (below), the external oblique muscle (in front), and the erector spinae muscle (behind). It can be the site of a **lumbar hernia**.

lumbar vertebrae the five bones of the *backbone that are situated between the thoracic vertebrae and the sacrum, in the lower part of the back. They are the largest of the unfused vertebrae and have stout processes for attachment of the strong muscles of the lower back. *See also* VERTEBRA.

lumbo- *combining form denoting* the loin; lumbar region.

lumbosacral *adj.* relating to part of the spine composed of the lumbar vertebrae and the sacrum.

lumen *n.* **1.** the space within a tubular or sac-like part, such as a blood vessel, the intestine, or the stomach. **2.** the *SI unit of luminous flux, equal to the amount of light emitted per second in unit solid angle of 1 steradian by a point source of 1 candela. Symbol: lm.

luminescence *n.* the emission of light from a substance after it has been irradiated. *Fluorescence is a type of luminescence. This phenomenon is used in a *fluoroscope, a *gamma camera, an X-ray *cassette, and some types of *dosimeter.

lumpectomy *n.* an operation for *breast cancer in which the tumour and surrounding breast tissue are removed: muscles, skin, and lymph nodes are left intact (*compare* MASTECTOMY). The procedure, usually followed by radiation, is indicated for patients with a tumour less than 2 cm in diameter and who have no metastases to local lymph nodes or to distant organs.

LUNA laparoscopic uterine nerve ablation: a surgical technique for the treatment of endometriosis, in combination with division of adhesions and laser ablation. It involves dividing the parasympathetic sensory fibres to the cervix and sympathetic sensory fibres to the uterus.

lunate bone a bone of the wrist (*see* CARPUS). It articulates with the capitate and hamate bones in front, with the radius behind, and with the triquetral and scaphoid at the sides.

lung *n.* one of the pair of organs of *respiration, situated in the chest cavity on either side of the heart and enclosed by a serous membrane (*see* PLEURA). The lungs are fibrous elastic sacs that are expanded and compressed by movements of the rib cage and diaphragm during *breathing. They communicate with the atmosphere through the *trachea, which opens into the pharynx. The trachea divides into two bronchi (*see* BRONCHUS), which enter the lungs and branch into *bronchioles. These divide further and terminate in minute air sacs (*see* ALVEOLUS), the sites of gaseous exchange. (See illustration.) Atmospheric oxygen is absorbed and carbon dioxide from the blood of the pulmonary capillaries is released into the lungs; in each case down a concentration gradient (*see* PULMONARY CIRCULATION). The total capacity of the lungs in an adult male is about 5.5 litres, but during normal breathing only about 500 ml of air is exchanged (*see also* RESIDUAL VOLUME). Other functions of the lung include water evaporation: an important factor in the fluid balance and heat regulation of the body.

⊕ SEE WEB LINKS
• British Lung Foundation: basic information on the lungs and some common lung conditions

lung cancer cancer arising in the epithelium of the air passages (**bronchial cancer**) or lung (*see also* NON-SMALL-CELL LUNG CANCER, SMALL-CELL LUNG CANCER). It is a very common form of cancer, particularly in Britain, and is strongly associated with cigarette smoking and exposure to industrial air pollutants (including asbestos). There are often no symptoms in the early stages of the disease, when diagnosis is made on X-ray examination. Treatment includes surgical removal of the affected lobe or lung (less than 20% of cases are suitable for surgery), radiotherapy, and chemotherapy.

lunula *n.* the whitish crescent-shaped area at the base of a *nail.

lupus *n.* any of several chronic skin diseases. *See* LUPUS ERYTHEMATOSUS, LUPUS VERRUCOSUS, LUPUS VULGARIS.

lupus erythematosus (LE) a chronic inflammatory autoimmune disease of connective tissue, affecting the skin and various internal organs (**systemic LE, SLE**). Typically, there is a red scaly butterfly-shaped rash on the face, over the cheek and bridge of the nose (**butterfly rash**); arthritis; and progressive damage to the kidneys (*see* LUPUS NEPHRITIS). Often the heart, lungs, and brain are also affected by progressive attacks of inflammation followed by the formation of scar tissue (fibrosis). In a milder form, known as **discoid LE** (**DLE**), only the skin is affected. LE is an *autoimmune disease and

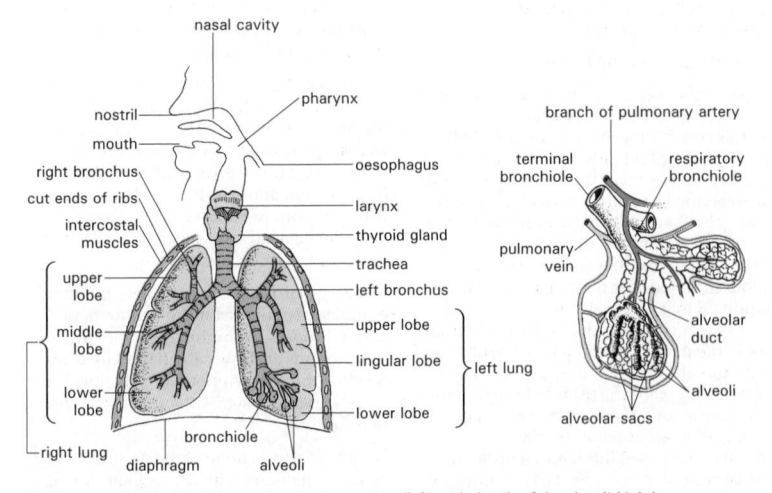

The lungs. Showing the lobes and main air passages (left) with details of the alveoli (right).

can be diagnosed by the presence of abnormal antibodies in the bloodstream. The disease is treated with corticosteroids or immunosuppressant drugs.

lupus nephritis a frequent and serious complication of systemic *lupus erythematosus (SLE). The 2002 WHO/ISN/RPS classification of lupus nephritis recognizes six classes: class I is the presence of mesangial deposits (*see* JUXTAGLOMERULAR APPARATUS) seen on immunofluorescence and/or electron microscopy; class II is the presence of mesangial deposits and mesangial hypercellularity; class III is focal and segmental *glomerulonephritis; class IV is diffuse segmental or global nephritis; class V is *membranous nephropathy; and class VI is advanced sclerotic glomerulonephritis. Untreated, outcomes are poor in classes III and IV, but much improved with immunosuppressant treatment.

lupus verrucosus a rare tuberculous infection of the skin – commonly the arm or hand – typified by warty lesions. It occurs in those who have been reinfected with tuberculosis.

lupus vulgaris tuberculous infection of the skin, usually due to direct inoculation of the tuberculosis bacillus into the skin. It is no longer common in the developed world. This type of lupus often starts in childhood, with dark red patches on the nose or cheek. Unless treated, lupus vulgaris may spread, ulcerate, and cause extensive scarring. Treatment is with antituberculous drugs.

lute *n.* (in dentistry) a thin layer of cement inserted into the minute space between a prepared tooth and a crown or inlay to hold and seal it permanently in place.

luteal cyst *see* OVARIAN CYST.

lutein *n.* **1.** *see* XANTHOPHYLL. **2.** the yellow pigment of the corpus luteum.

luteinizing hormone (LH) a hormone (*see* GONADOTROPHIN), synthesized and released by the anterior pituitary gland, that stimulates ovulation, *corpus luteum formation, progesterone synthesis by the ovary (*see also* MENSTRUAL CYCLE), and androgen synthesis by the interstitial cells of the testes. Also called: **interstitial cell stimulating hormone (ICSH).**

luteo- *combining form denoting* **1.** yellow. **2.** the corpus luteum.

luteotrophic hormone (luteotrophin) *see* PROLACTIN.

LUTS *see* LOWER URINARY TRACT SYMPTOMS.

lux *n.* the *SI unit of intensity of illumination, equal to 1 lumen per square metre. This unit was formerly called the metre candle. Symbol: lx.

luxation *n. see* DISLOCATION.

lyase *n.* one of a group of enzymes that catalyse the linking of groups by double bonds.

Lyell's syndrome *see* TOXIC EPIDERMAL NECROLYSIS. [A. Lyell (20th century), British dermatologist]

Lyme disease a disease caused by a spirochaete, *Borrelia burgdorferi*, and transmitted by certain ticks of the genus *Ixodes*. Following a 3–32-day incubation period, a slowly extending red rash develops in approximately 75% of cases; intermittent systemic symptoms include fever, malaise, headache and neck stiffness, and muscle and joint pains. Later, 60% of patients suffer intermittent attacks of arthritis, especially of the knees, each attack lasting months and recurring over several years. The spirochaete has been identified in synovium and synovial fluid. Neurological and cardiac involvement occurs in a smaller percentage of cases. Treatment is with doxycycline or a penicillin.

lymph *n.* the fluid present within the vessels of the *lymphatic system. It consists of the fluid that bathes the tissues, which is derived from the blood and is drained by the lymphatic vessels. Lymph passes through a series of filters (*lymph nodes) and is ultimately returned to the bloodstream via the *thoracic duct. It is similar in composition to plasma, but contains less protein and some cells, mainly *lymphocytes.

lymphaden- (lymphadeno-) *combining form denoting* lymph node(s).

lymphadenectomy *n.* surgical removal of lymph nodes, an operation commonly performed when a cancer has invaded nodes in the drainage area of an organ infiltrated by a malignant growth.

lymphadenitis *n.* inflammation of lymph nodes, which become swollen, painful, and tender. Some cases may be chronic (e.g. tuberculous lymphadenitis) but most are acute and localized adjacent to an area of infection. The most commonly affected lymph nodes are those in the neck, in association with tonsillitis. The lymph nodes help to contain and combat the infection. Occasionally generalized lymphadenitis occurs as a result of virus infections. The treatment is that of the cause.

lymphadenopathy *n.* enlargement of the lymph nodes. This is usually due to infection (e.g. viral or bacterial), when the nodes are painful and tender, but may alternatively be caused by malignancy (e.g. leukaemias, lymphomas), autoimmune disease (e.g. systemic lupus erythematosis), or adverse drug reactions.

lymphangi- (lymphangio-) *combining form denoting* a lymphatic vessel.

lymphangiectasis *n.* dilatation of the lymphatic vessels, which is usually congenital and produces enlargement of various parts of the body (e.g. the leg in Milroy's disease). It may also be caused by obstruction of the lymphatic vessels. *See* LYMPHOEDEMA.

lymphangiography (lymphography) *n.* X-ray examination of the lymphatic vessels and lymph nodes after a contrast medium has been injected into them (*see* ANGIOGRAPHY). Its main uses are in the investigation of the extent and spread of cancer of the lymphatic system and in the investigation of lymphoedema. Alternatively, the lymphatic system can be imaged using a gamma camera following the injection of a radioactive tracer. This examination has now largely been replaced by other *cross-sectional imaging techniques.

lymphangioma *n.* a localized collection of distended lymphatic vessels, which may result in a large cyst in the neck or armpit. This can be removed surgically.

lymphangiosarcoma *n.* a rare malignant tumour of the lymphatic vessels. It is most commonly seen in the chronically swollen (oedematous) arms of women who have had a mastectomy for breast cancer and may be induced by radiation.

lymphangitis *n.* inflammation of the lymphatic vessels, which can be seen most commonly as red streaks in the skin adjacent to a focus of streptococcal infection. Occasionally a more chronic form results in *lymphoedema. The infected part is rested and the infection can be eliminated by an antibiotic (e.g. penicillin).

lymphatic 1. *n.* a lymphatic vessel. *See* LYMPHATIC SYSTEM. 2. *adj.* relating to or transporting lymph.

lymphatic system a network of vessels that conveys electrolytes, water, proteins, etc. – in the form of *lymph – from the tissue fluids to the bloodstream (see illustration). It consists of fine blind-ended lymphatic capillaries, which unite to form lymphatic vessels. At various points along the lymphatic vessels are *lymph nodes. Lymph drains into the capillaries and passes into the lymphatic vessels, which have valves to prevent backflow of lymph. The lymphatics lead to two large channels – the **thoracic duct** and the **right lymphatic duct** – which return the lymph to the bloodstream via the innominate veins.

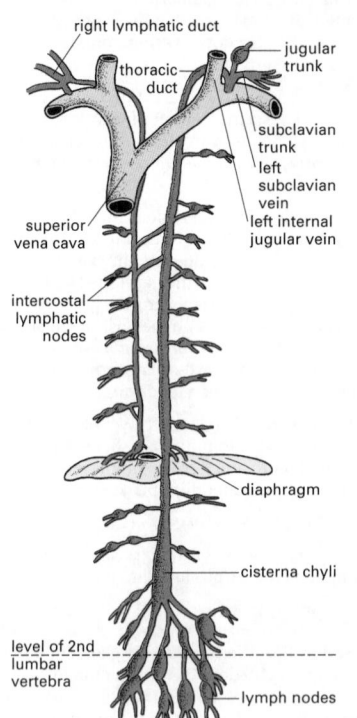

The lymphatic system.

lymph node one of a number of small swellings found at intervals along the lymphatic system. Groups of nodes are found in many parts of the body; for example, in the groin and armpit and behind the ear. They are composed of lymphoid tissue and act as filters for the lymph, preventing foreign particles from entering the bloodstream; they also produce lymphocytes.

lympho- *combining form denoting* lymph or the lymphatic system.

lymphoblast *n.* an abnormal cell present in the blood and the blood-forming organs in one type of leukaemia (**lymphoblastic leukaemia**). It has a large nucleus with very scanty cytoplasm and is thought to be the precursor of the lymphocyte. —**lymphoblastic** *adj.*

lymphocele *n.* a collection of lymph in the tissues, which follows injury to, or operations upon, lymph nodes or ducts.

lymphocyte *n.* a variety of white blood cell (leucocyte), present also in the lymph nodes, spleen, thymus gland, gut wall, and bone marrow. With *Romanowsky stains, lymphocytes can be seen to have dense nuclei with clear pale-blue cytoplasm. Lymphocytes with scanty cytoplasm are **small lymphocytes**; those with abundant cytoplasm are **large lymphocytes.** There are normally $1.5–4.0 \times 10^9$ lymphocytes per litre of blood. They are involved in *immunity and can be subdivided into **B lymphocytes** (or **B cells**), which produce circulating antibodies, and **T lymphocytes** (or **T cells**), which are primarily responsible for cell-mediated immunity. T lymphocytes can differentiate into *helper T cells or *cytotoxic T cells. There is an increase in the number of lymphocytes in the blood and bone marrow in chronic lymphocytic *leukaemia. —**lymphocytic** *adj.*

lymphocytopenia *n. see* LYMPHOPENIA.

lymphocytosis *n.* an increase in the number of *lymphocytes in the blood. Lymphocytosis may occur in a wide variety of diseases, including chronic lymphocytic *leukaemia and infections due to viruses.

lymphoedema *n.* an accumulation of lymph in the tissues, producing swelling; the legs are most often affected. It may be due to a congenital abnormality of the lymphatic vessels (as in **Milroy's disease**, congenital lymphoedema of the legs) or result from obstruction of the lymphatic vessels by a tumour, parasites, inflammation, or injury. Treatment consists of elastic support, by stockings or bandages, and diuretic drugs. A variety of surgical procedures has been devised but with little success.

lymphogranuloma venereum a sexually transmitted disease that is caused by *Chlamydia* and is most common in tropical regions. An initial lesion on the genitals is followed by swelling and inflammation of the lymph nodes in the groin; the lymph vessels in the genital region may become blocked, causing thickening of the skin of that area. Early treatment with sulphonamides or tetracyclines is usually effective.

lymphography *n. see* LYMPHANGIOGRAPHY.

lymphoid tissue a tissue responsible for the production of lymphocytes and antibodies. It occurs as discrete organs, in the form of the lymph nodes, tonsils, thymus, and spleen, and also as diffuse groups of cells not separated from surrounding tissue. *See also* IMMUNE SYSTEM.

lymphokine *n.* a substance produced by lymphocytes that has effects on other cells involved in the immune system (*see* CYTOKINES). An example is *interleukin 2 (IL-2).

lymphoma *n.* cancer of the lymph nodes, including *Hodgkin's disease and **non-Hodgkin's lymphomas**. There is a broad spectrum of malignancy, with prognosis ranging from a few months to many years. The patient usually shows evidence of multiple enlarged lymph nodes and may have constitutional symptoms such as weight loss, fever, and sweating (the so-called 'B symptoms'). Disease may be widespread, but in some cases is confined to a single area, which may be extranodal (such as the tonsil). Treatment is with drugs such as chlorambucil or combinations of cyclophosphamide, vincristine, and prednisolone, sometimes with the addition of doxorubicin and/or bleomycin; response to these drugs is often dramatic. New *targeted agents are used depending on the expression of cell surface molecules, particularly *rituximab against CD20 in diffuse B-cell lymphoma. Localized disease may be treated with radiotherapy followed by drugs. Patients with non-Hodgkin's lymphoma who do not respond to chemotherapy may be considered for a bone-marrow transplant.

lymphopenia (**lymphocytopenia**) *n.* a decrease in the number of *lymphocytes in the blood, which may occur in a wide variety of diseases.

lymphoplasmacytic lymphoma *see* WALDENSTROM'S MACROGLOBULINAEMIA.

lymphopoiesis *n.* the process of the production of *lymphocytes, which occurs in the *bone marrow as well as in the lymph nodes, spleen, thymus gland, and gut wall. The precursor cell from which lymphocytes are derived has not yet been identified.

lymphorrhagia *n.* the escape of the lymph from lymphatic vessels that have been injured.

lymphosarcoma *n.* a former name for non-Hodgkin's *lymphoma.

lymphuria *n.* the presence in the urine of lymph.

Lynch syndrome *see* HEREDITARY NON-POLYPOSIS COLORECTAL CANCER.

Lyon hypothesis the hypothesis that gene dosage imbalance between males and females, because of the presence of two X chromosomes in females (XX) as opposed to only one in males (XY), is compensated for by random inactivation of one of the X chromosomes in the somatic cells of females. The inactivated X chromosome becomes the Barr body (*see* SEX CHROMATIN). [M. F. Lyon (1925–), British geneticist]

lys- (lysi-, lyso-) *combining form denoting* lysis; dissolution.

lysergic acid diethylamide (LSD) an illegal hallucinogenic drug that was formerly used to aid treatment of certain psychological disorders. Side-effects include digestive upsets, dizziness, tingling, anxiety, sweating, dilated pupils, muscle incoordination and tremor. Alterations in sight, hearing, and other senses occur, psychotic effects, depression, and confusion are common, and tolerance to the drug develops rapidly. Because of these toxic effects, LSD is no longer used clinically.

lysin *n.* a specific *complement-fixing anti-body that is capable of bringing about the destruction (lysis) of whole cells. Names are given to varieties of lysin with different targets; for example, **haemolysin** attacks red blood cells; **leucolysin** attacks white cells; and a **bacteriolysin** targets bacterial cells.

lysine *n.* an *essential amino acid. *See also* AMINO ACID.

lysis *n.* the destruction of cells through damage or rupture of the plasma membrane, allowing escape of the cell contents. *See also* AUTOLYSIS, LYSOZYME.

-lysis *combining form denoting* 1. lysis; dissolution. 2. remission of symptoms.

lysogenic *adj.* producing *lysis.

lysogeny *n.* an interaction between a *bacteriophage and its host in which a latent form of the phage (**prophage**) exists within the bacterial cell, which is not destroyed. Under certain conditions (e.g. irradiation of the bacterium) the phage can develop into an active form, which reproduces itself and eventually destroys the bacterial cell.

lysosome *n.* a particle in the cytoplasm of cells that contains enzymes responsible for breaking down substances in the cell and is bounded by a single membrane. Lysosomes are especially abundant in liver and kidney cells. Foreign particles (e.g. bacteria) taken into the cell are broken down by the enzymes of the lysosomes. When the cell dies, these enzymes are released to break down the cell's components.

lysozyme *n.* an enzyme found in tears and egg white. It catalyses the destruction of the cell walls of certain bacteria. Bacterial cells that are attacked by lysozyme are said to have been **lysed**.

lytic *adj.* of, relating to, or causing *lysis. For example, bone metastases that involve lysis (destruction) of normal bone, typically seen in multiple *myeloma, are described as lytic.

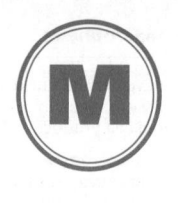

mA *symbol for* *milliamp.

MabThera *n. see* RITUXIMAB.

maceration *n.* **1.** the softening of a solid by leaving it immersed in a liquid. **2.** (in obstetrics) the natural breakdown of a dead fetus within the uterus.

machinery murmur a continuous heart *murmur that indicates patent *ductus arteriosus or arteriovenous *fistula.

Macleod's syndrome (Swyer-James syndrome) pulmonary *emphysema affecting only one lung and beginning in childhood or in adolescence; it occurs secondarily to necrotising bronchitis, probably caused by a virus. [W. M. Macleod (1911–77), British physician]

macr- (macro-) *combining form denoting* large size. Example: **macrencephaly** (abnormally enlarged brain).

macrocephaly (megalocephaly) *n.* abnormal largeness of the head in relation to the rest of the body. *Compare* MICROCEPHALY.

macrocheilia *n.* hypertrophy of the lips: a congenital condition in which the lips are abnormally large. *Compare* MICROCHEILIA.

macrocyte (megalocyte) *n.* an abnormally large red blood cell (*erythrocyte), seen in certain anaemias. *See also* MACROCYTOSIS. —**macrocytic** *adj.*

macrocytosis *n.* the presence of abnormally large red cells (**macrocytes**) in the blood. Macrocytosis is a feature of certain anaemias (**macrocytic anaemias**), including those due to deficiency of vitamin B_{12} or folate, and also of anaemias in which there is an increase in the rate of red cell production.

macrodactyly *n.* abnormally large size of one or more of the fingers or toes.

macrodontia *n.* a condition in which the teeth are unusually large.

macrogamete *n.* the nonmotile female sex cell of the malarial parasite (*Plasmodium*) and other protozoans. The macrogamete is similar to the ovum of ani-

mals and larger than the male sex cell (*see* MICROGAMETE).

macrogametocyte *n.* a cell that undergoes meiosis to form mature female sex cells (macrogametes) of the malarial parasite (*see* PLASMODIUM). Macrogametocytes are found in human blood but must be ingested by a mosquito before developing into macrogametes.

macrogenitosoma *n.* excessive bodily growth with marked enlargement of the genitalia. **Macrogenitosoma praecox** is a variant occurring in early childhood.

macroglia *n.* one of the two basic classes of *glia (the non-nervous cells of the central nervous system), divided into *astrocytes and *oligodendrocytes. *Compare* MICROGLIA.

macroglobulin *n.* **1.** (immunoglobulin M, IgM) a protein of the globulin series that is present in the blood and functions as an antibody, forming an effective first-line defence against bacteria in the bloodstream. *See also* IMMUNOGLOBULIN. **2.** an abnormal form of IgM (*see* PARAPROTEIN) produced by *lymphoma cells or in other plasma-cell disorders, such as multiple *myeloma.

macroglobulinaemia *n.* the presence in the blood of excessive amounts of *macroglobulin (IgM), produced by a malignant proliferation of the lymphocytes in certain *lymphomas. *See* WALDENSTROM'S MACROGLOBULINAEMIA.

macroglossia *n.* an abnormally large tongue. It may be due to a congenital defect, such as thyroid deficiency (cretinism); to infiltration of the tongue with *amyloid or a tumour; or to obstruction of the lymph vessels.

macrognathia *n.* a condition in which one or both jaws are unusually large.

macromelia *n.* abnormally large size of the arms or legs. *Compare* MICROMELIA.

macronormoblast *n.* an abnormal form of any of the cells (*normoblasts) that form a series of precursors of red blood cells. Macronormoblasts are unusually large but have normal nuclei (*compare* MEGALOBLAST); they are seen in certain anaemias in which red cell production is impaired.

macrophage *n.* a large scavenger cell (a *phagocyte) present in connective tissue and many major organs and tissues, including the bone marrow, spleen, *lymph nodes, liver (*see* KUPFFER CELLS), and the central nervous system (*see* MICROGLIA). They are closely related to *monocytes. **Fixed macrophages** (**histiocytes**) are stationary within connective tissue; **free macrophages** wander between cells and aggregate at focal sites of infection, where they remove bacteria or other foreign bodies from blood or tissues. *See also* RETICULOENDOTHELIAL SYSTEM.

macropsia *n.* a condition in which objects appear larger than they really are. It is usually due to disease of the retina affecting the *macula but may also occur in spasm of *accommodation.

macroscopic *adj.* visible to the naked eye. *Compare* MICROSCOPIC.

macrosomia *n.* abnormally large size. In **fetal macrosomia** the baby is large for its gestational age. This condition is associated with poorly controlled maternal diabetes, the increased size being due to excessive production of fetal insulin and thence to increased deposition of glycogen in the fetus.

macrotia *n.* a congenital deformity of the external ear in which the *pinna is larger than normal.

Macugen *n.* trade name for pegaptanib. *See* RANIBIZUMAB.

macula *n.* (*pl.* **maculae**) a small anatomical area that is distinguishable from the surrounding tissue. The **macula lutea** is the yellow spot on the retina at the back of the eye, which surrounds the greatest concentration of cones (*see* FOVEA). Maculae occur in the saccule and utricle of the inner ear (see illustration). Tilting of the head causes the otoliths to bend the hair cells, which send impulses to the brain via the vestibular nerve. *See also* LABYRINTH.

macular degeneration a group of conditions affecting the *macula lutea of the eye, resulting in a reduction or loss of central vision. **Age-related macular degeneration** (**AMD, ARMD**) is the most common cause of poor vision in the elderly. Two types are commonly recognized. **Atrophic** (or **dry**) **AMD** results from chronic choroidal ischaemia: small blood vessels of the choroid, which lies beneath the retina, become constricted, reducing the blood supply to the macula. This gives rise to degenerative changes in the retinal pigment epithelium (RPE; *see* RETINA), clinically recognized by macular pigmentation and the deposition of *drusen. **Wet AMD** is associated with the growth of abnormal new blood vessels underneath the retina, derived from the choroid (*see* (CHOROIDAL) NEOVASCULARIZATION). These can leak fluid and blood beneath the retina, which further reduces the macular function. Nutritional supplements, laser surgery (*see* PHOTOCOAGULATION, PHOTODYNAMIC THERAPY), and anti-VEGF therapy (*see* VASCULAR ENDOTHELIAL GROWTH FACTOR) can delay the progression of AMD in a few selected cases.

macule *n.* a flat (impalpable) circumscribed area of skin or an area of altered skin colour (e.g. a freckle). *Compare* PAPULE.

maculopapular *adj.* describing a rash that consists of both *macules and *papules.

maculopathy *n.* any abnormality of the *macula of the eye. For example, **bull's-eye maculopathy** describes the appearance of the macula in some toxic conditions (e.g. chloroquine toxicity) and in some hereditary disorders of the macula. *See also* EPIRETINAL MEMBRANE (CELLOPHANE MACULOPATHY).

madarosis *n.* **1.** a congenital deficiency of the eyelashes and eyebrows, which are sometimes absent altogether. **2.** a deficiency of the eyelashes alone, caused by chronic *blepharitis.

Maddox rod a series of transparent cylinders that change a point source of light into a linear streak perpendicular to the axis of the rods, used in the assessment of binocular

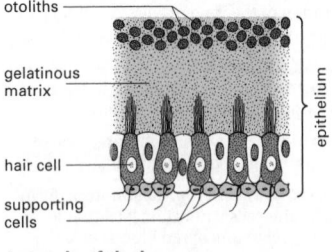

A macula of the inner ear.

visual functions. [E. E. Maddox (1860–1933), British ophthalmologist]

Madopar *n. see* LEVODOPA.

Madura foot an infection of the tissues and bones of the foot producing chronic inflammation (mycetoma), occurring in the tropics. It is caused by various filamentous fungi (including *Madurella*) and certain bacteria of the genera *Nocardia* and *Streptomyces*. Medical name: **maduromycosis**.

Madurella *n.* a genus of widely distributed fungi. The species *M. grisea* and *M. mycetomi* cause the tropical infection *Madura foot.

maduromycosis *n. see* MADURA FOOT.

MAG3 *m*ercapto*a*cetyltri*g*lycine: a tracer used in nuclear medicine, during *renography, when labelled with technetium-99m. This agent is both filtered and excreted by the kidneys and gives similar results to *DTPA with a lower dose of ionizing radiation. It enables the function and drainage of each kidney to be assessed.

magenta *n. see* FUCHSIN.

maggot *n.* the wormlike larva of a fly, which occasionally infests human tissues (*see* MYIASIS). Disinfected maggots may be used to assist in the cleaning and healing of serious wounds by feeding on dead tissue.

magic bullet a colloquial name for any drug treatment that is designed to target diseased tissue without adversely affecting healthy tissue. The term has been used especially in reference to new treatments for cancer.

Magill's forceps long angled forceps for use with a *laryngoscope in removing foreign bodies from the mouth and throat of an unconscious patient. [Sir I. V. Magill (1888–1975), British anaesthetist]

magnesium *n.* a metallic element essential to life. The body of an average adult contains about 25 g of magnesium, concentrated mostly in the bones. Magnesium is necessary for the proper functioning of muscle and nervous tissue. It is required as a *cofactor for approximately 90 enzymes. A good source of magnesium is green leafy vegetables. Symbol: Mg.

magnesium carbonate a weak *antacid used to relieve indigestion. It is usually com-

bined with other compounds in mixtures, powders, and tablets.

magnesium hydroxide a magnesium salt used as an osmotic *laxative to treat constipation. It is also combined with *aluminium hydroxide in antacid preparations.

magnesium sulphate a magnesium salt used in the form of mixtures or powders as an osmotic *laxative for rapid evacuation of the bowel. It is also administered intravenously to treat magnesium deficiency and serious *arrhythmias and to prevent the recurrence of convulsions in *eclampsia.

magnesium trisilicate a compound of magnesium with antacid and absorbent properties, used in the form of tablets or a mixture for the treatment of indigestion.

magnetic imager *see* 3-D MAGNETIC IMAGER.

magnetic resonance imaging (MRI) a diagnostic imaging technique based on the emission of electromagnetic waves from the body when the patient is placed in a strong magnetic field and exposed to radiofrequency radiation (*see* NUCLEAR MAGNETIC RESONANCE). The strength of the magnetic field is measured in *teslas. Most images rely on the signal from hydrogen in water, which is particularly strong, although other elements can be used (*see* MAGNETIC RESONANCE SPECTROSCOPY). A major advantage over *computerized tomography is the lack of X-rays, which reduces exposure to ionizing radiation. MRI is used for the noninvasive diagnosis and treatment planning of a wide range of diseases and also to guide interventional radiological procedures. *See also* FUNCTIONAL MAGNETIC RESONANCE IMAGING.

magnetic resonance spectroscopy (MRS) a diagnostic technique that utilizes the phenomenon of *nuclear magnetic resonance to obtain a biochemical profile of tissues by exciting elements other than hydrogen in water and other body components. It is particularly useful for biochemical analysis of tissues in the living body. The technique is still largely at the research level.

MAGPI operation *m*eatal *a*dvancement and *g*lanulo*p*lasty operation: a simple surgical procedure designed to correct minor to moderate degrees of coronal or subcoronal *hypospadias. This single-stage operation corrects any associated minor degrees of *chordee and transfers the urethral opening to the glans.

MAI complex a group of bacteria comprising *Mycobacterium avium* and *M. intracellulare*, which are responsible for *opportunistic infections of the lung. *See* MYCOBACTERIUM.

main d'accoucheur (obstetrician's hand) the appearance of the hand in a carpopedal *spasm (*see also* TETANY). The wrist is flexed, the fingers are tightly adducted, and the thumb is apposed across the palm.

major histocompatibility complex *see* MHC.

mal *n.* illness or disease.

mal- *combining form denoting* disease, disorder, or abnormality.

malabsorption *n.* a state in which absorption of one or more substances by the small intestine is reduced. It most commonly affects fat (causing *steatorrhoea), some vitamins (such as B$_{12}$, folate, vitamin D, and vitamin K), *electrolytes (such as calcium, potassium), iron, and amino acids. Symptoms (depending on the substances involved) include weight loss, diarrhoea, anaemia, *paraesthesia, swelling (oedema), and vitamin deficiencies. The commonest causes are *coeliac disease, *pancreatitis, *cystic fibrosis, *blind loop syndrome, chronic infection (e.g. giardiasis), or surgical removal of a length of small intestine.

malacia *n.* abnormal softening of a part, organ, or tissue, such as bone (*see* OSTEOMALACIA).

-malacia *combining form denoting* abnormal softening of a tissue. Example: **keratomalacia** (of the cornea).

maladie de Roger (Roger's disease) a form of congenital heart disease in which there is a small *ventricular septal defect that produces a loud heart *murmur. It usually causes no symptoms. [H. L. Roger (1809–91), French physician]

malaise *n.* a general feeling of being unwell. The feeling may be accompanied by identifiable physical discomfort and may indicate the presence of disease.

malakoplakia *n.* a rare form of chronic inflammatory disorder due to the defective destruction of phagocytosed bacteria. It is characterized by the formation of soft yellow plaques and nodules composed of foamy macrophages containing basophilic cytoplasmic inclusions (**Michaelis-Gutmann bodies**). Malakoplakia occurs most commonly in the urinary tract but can also occur in the skin.

malar bone *see* ZYGOMATIC BONE.

malaria (ague, marsh fever, periodic fever, paludism) *n.* an infectious disease due to the presence of parasitic protozoa of the genus *Plasmodium (*P. falciparum, P. malariae, P. ovale*, or *P. vivax*) within the red blood cells. The disease is transmitted by the *Anopheles* mosquito and is confined mainly to tropical and subtropical areas.

Parasites in the blood of an infected person are taken into the stomach of the mosquito as it feeds. Here they multiply and then invade the salivary glands. When the mosquito bites an individual, parasites are injected into the bloodstream and migrate to the liver and other organs, where they multiply. After an incubation period varying from 12 days (*P. falciparum*) to 10 months (some varieties of *P. vivax*), parasites return to the bloodstream and invade the red blood cells. Rapid multiplication of the parasites results in destruction of the red cells and the release of more parasites capable of infecting other red cells. This causes a short bout of shivering, fever, and sweating, and the loss of healthy red cells results in anaemia. When the next batch of parasites is released symptoms reappear. The interval between fever attacks varies in different types of malaria: in **quartan malaria** (or **fever**), caused by *P. malariae*, it is three days; in **tertian malaria** (*P. ovale* or *P. vivax*) it is two days (these two types are known as **benign malarias**). In **malignant** (or **falciparum**) **malaria** (caused by *P. falciparum*) – the most severe kind – the interval between attacks varies from a few hours to two days (*see also* BLACKWATER FEVER). Preventive and curative treatment includes such drugs as *chloroquine, *proguanil, *mefloquine, and *pyrimethamine.

Malarone *n. see* PROGUANIL.

Malassezia (Pityrosporum) *n.* a genus of yeasts producing superficial infections of the skin. The species *M. furfur* (including *P. orbiculare* and *P. ovale*) causes *pityriasis versicolor and other conditions.

malathion *n.* an organophosphorous insecticide used to treat head and pubic lice and scabies. It is applied externally in the form of a liquid or shampoo; side-effects include skin irritation and allergic reactions. Trade names: **Derbac-M**, **Prioderm**, **Quellada M**.

malformation *n.* any variation from the normal physical structure, due either to congenital or developmental defects or to disease or injury.

malignant *adj.* **1.** describing a tumour that invades and destroys the tissue in which it originates and has the potential to spread to other sites in the body via the bloodstream and lymphatic system. *See* CANCER, METASTASIS. **2.** describing any disorder that becomes life-threatening if untreated (e.g. *malignant hypertension). *Compare* BENIGN.

malignant hypertension dangerously high blood pressure (diastolic pressure >130 mmHg) associated with necrosis of small arteries and arterioles. Retinal haemorrhage and *papilloedema are present. Untreated, malignant hypertension causes severe organ damage, targeting the central nervous and cardiovascular systems and the kidneys (malignant *nephrosclerosis). Causes include complications of essential and secondary *hypertension and pregnancy and the use of certain drugs (e.g. MAO inhibitors).

malignant melanoma *see* MELANOMA.

malignant vasovagal syndrome *see* NEUROCARDIOGENIC SYNCOPE.

malingering *n.* pretending to be ill, usually in order to avoid work or gain attention. It may be a sign of mental disorder (*see also* MUNCHAUSEN'S SYNDROME).

malleolus *n.* either of the two protuberances on each side of the ankle: the **lateral malleolus** at the lower end of the *fibula or the **medial malleolus** at the lower end of the *tibia.

mallet finger a condition in which a finger (usually the index finger) is bent downwards at the tip, due to *avulsion of the long extensor tendon from the bone. Treatment is to hold the tip of the finger straight with a splint for at least six weeks.

malleus *n.* a hammer-shaped bone in the middle *ear that articulates with the incus and is attached to the eardrum. *See* OSSICLE.

Mallory bodies large irregular masses abnormally located in the hepatocytes of the liver. They are found in patients with alco-

holic hepatitis, Wilson's disease, primary biliary cirrhosis, severe obesity, and hepatoma. [F. B. Mallory (1862–1941), US pathologist]

Mallory's triple stain a histological stain consisting of water-soluble aniline blue or methyl blue, orange G, and oxalic acid. Before the stain is applied the tissue is mordanted, then treated with acid fuchsin and phosphomolybdic acid. Nuclei stain red, muscle red to orange, nervous tissue lilac, collagen dark blue, and mucus and connective tissue become blue. [F. B. Mallory]

Mallory-Weiss syndrome tearing of the lining (mucosa) around the junction of the oesophagus (gullet) and stomach as a result of violent vomiting or straining to vomit. It is associated with *haematemesis and rarely perforation of the oesophagus. [G. K. Mallory (1926–), US pathologist; S. Weiss (1899–1942), US physician]

malnutrition *n.* the condition caused by an improper balance between what an individual eats and what he or she requires to maintain health. This can result from eating too little (**subnutrition** or **starvation**) but may also result from dietary excess or an incorrect balance of basic foodstuffs such as protein, fat, and carbohydrate. A deficiency (or excess) of one or more minerals, vitamins, or other essential ingredients may arise from *malabsorption of digested food or metabolic malfunction of one or more parts of the body.

malocclusion *n.* a condition in which there is an abnormal arrangement of the teeth or discrepancy in the relationship of the jaws. It is usually treated by orthodontics. If jaw discrepancy is severe, it may require *orthognathic surgery.

Malpighian body the part of a *nephron comprising the blood capillaries of the glomerulus and its surrounding Bowman's capsule. [M. Malpighi (1628–94), Italian anatomist]

Malpighian layer the stratum germinativum: one of the layers of the *epidermis.

malposition *n.* (in obstetrics) an abnormal position of the fetal head when this is the presenting part in labour (*see* PRESENTATION). The head is in such a position that the diameter of the skull in relation to the pelvic opening is greater than normal (e.g. occipital transverse, occipital posterior: *see* OCCIPUT).

This is likely to result in a prolonged and complicated labour.

malpractice *n.* professional misconduct: treatment falling short of the standards of skill and care that can reasonably be expected from a qualified medical practitioner.

malpresentation *n.* the condition in which the presenting part of the fetus (*see* PRESENTATION) is other than the back of the head (e.g. the brow, face, shoulder, or buttocks). Malpresentation is likely to complicate labour and may necessitate delivery by *Caesarean section. Placenta praevia, fibroids, ovarian cysts, fetal malformations, multiple pregnancy, and abnormal uterus should be excluded as a cause of the malpresentation.

malt *n.* a mixture of carbohydrates, predominantly maltose, produced by the breakdown of starch contained in barley or wheat grains. The cereal grain is allowed to germinate and the malt is extracted with hot water. Malt is used for brewing and distilling; it has been used as a source of nutrients in wasting diseases.

MALT mucosa-associated lymphoid tissue: an important part of the peripheral lymphoid system with special features of immune cell production. It is associated with the digestive tract and is concentrated in such areas as the *tonsils and *Peyer's patches.

Malta fever *see* BRUCELLOSIS.

maltase *n.* an enzyme, present in saliva and pancreatic juice, that converts maltose into glucose during digestion.

maltoma *n.* a *m*ucosal *a*ssociated *l*ymphoid *t*issue tumour of low-grade malignancy, treated by chemotherapeutic agents.

maltose *n.* a sugar that consists of two molecules of glucose. Maltose is formed from the digestion of starch and glycogen and is found in germinating cereal seeds.

malt-worker's lung a form of extrinsic allergic *alveolitis seen in people who work with barley.

malunion *n.* *union of the fragments of a fracture in an unsatisfactory position. It occurs if fracture *reduction is inadequate or the splintage is inadequate to maintain the bone fragments in the correct position until healing occurs. Malunion may require surgical correction with *osteotomy.

mamilla *n. see* NIPPLE.

mamillary bodies two paired rounded swellings in the floor of the *hypothalamus, immediately behind the pituitary gland.

mamma *n. see* BREAST.

mammary gland the milk-producing gland of female mammals. *See* BREAST.

mammography *n.* the study of the breast by imaging techniques, most commonly X-rays. The breast is usually compressed between radiolucent plates before being exposed to relatively low-energy X-rays to emphasize differences in the soft tissues. Mammography is mainly concerned with the detection and diagnosis of breast cancer.

mammoplasty *n.* plastic surgery of the breasts, in order to alter their shape or increase or decrease their size. In the case of sagging breasts skin and glandular tissue are removed and the remaining breast tissue is fixed in the normal position. After a mastectomy, or when the breasts are too small, a prosthesis (*see* BREAST IMPLANT) may be inserted to improve the contour.

mammothermography *n.* the technique of examining the breasts for the presence of abnormalities by *thermography.

mancinism *n.* the condition of being left-handed.

mandible *n.* the lower jawbone. It consists of a horseshoe-shaped **body**, the upper surface of which bears the lower teeth (*see* ALVEOLUS), and two vertical parts (**rami**). Each ramus divides into a **condyle** and a *coronoid process. The condyle articulates with the temporal bone of the cranium to form the **temporomandibular joint** (a hinge joint). *See also* MAXILLA, SKULL. —**mandibular** *adj.*

mandibular advancement splint (MAS) an orthodontic device used to advance the mandible to improve the airway in the pharynx during sleep in the treatment of *obstructive sleep apnoea.

manganese *n.* a greyish metallic element, the oxide of which, when inhaled by miners in underventilated mines, causes brain damage and symptoms very similar to those of *parkinsonism. Minute quantities of the element are required by the body (*see* TRACE ELEMENT). Symbol: Mn.

mania *n.* a state of mind characterized by

excessive cheerfulness and increased activity. The mood is euphoric and can change rapidly to irritability. Thought and speech are pressured and rapid to the point of incoherence and the connections between ideas may be impossible to follow (loosening of associations: *see* ASSOCIATION OF IDEAS). Behaviour is overactive, extravagant, overbearing, and sometimes violent. Judgment is impaired, and therefore the patient may damage his or her own interests. There may be grandiose delusions. *Mixed affective states (such as low mood with pressured speech and irritability) are common. Treatment is usually with drugs, such as lithium, *benzodiazepines, or *antipsychotics, and hospital admission is frequently necessary. *See also* BIPOLAR AFFECTIVE DISORDER. —**manic** *adj.*

-mania *combining form denoting* obsession, compulsion, or exaggerated feeling for. Example: **pyromania** (for starting fires).

manic depression a former (but still quite commonly used) name for *bipolar affective disorder.

manikin *n. see* HOMUNCULUS.

manipulation *n.* the use of the hands to produce a desired movement or therapeutic effect in part of the body. Both physiotherapists and osteopaths use manipulation to restore normal working to stiff joints.

mannitol *n.* an osmotic *diuretic administered by intravenous infusion mainly to reduce intracranial pressure in brain injuries and also in the emergency treatment of glaucoma. Side-effects include fever and chills.

Mann-Whitney U test *see* SIGNIFICANCE.

manometer *n.* a device for measuring pressure in a liquid or gas. A manometer often consists of a U-tube containing mercury, water, or other liquid, open at one end and exposed to the fluid under pressure at the other end. The pressure can be read directly from a graduated scale. *See also* SPHYGMOMANOMETER.

manometry *n.* measurement of pressures within organs of the body. The technique is used to record changes within fluid-filled chambers (e.g. cerebral ventricles) or to indicate muscular activity in motile tubes, such as the oesophagus, rectum, or bile duct.

mantle *adj.* (in radiotherapy) *see* TREATMENT FIELD.

Mantoux test *see* TUBERCULIN. [C. Mantoux (1877–1947), French physician]

manubrium *n.* (*pl.* **manubria**) **1.** the upper section of the breastbone (*see* STERNUM). It articulates with the clavicles and the first costal cartilage; the second costal cartilage articulates at the junction between the manubrium and body of the sternum. **2.** the handle-like part of the *malleus (an ear ossicle), attached to the eardrum. —**manubrial** *adj.*

MAO *see* MONOAMINE OXIDASE.

MAO inhibitor a drug that prevents the activity of the enzyme *monoamine oxidase (MAO). MAO inhibitors include *phenelzine, **isocarboxazid**, and **tranylcypromine**. These drugs are irreversible inhibitors of monoamine oxidase A, whose use as antidepressants is now restricted because of the severity of their side-effects. These include interactions with other drugs (e.g. ephedrine, phenylephrine) and with foods containing *tyramine (e.g. cheese) to produce a sudden and dangerous increase in blood pressure. *Moclobemide is a reversible inhibitor of monoamine oxidase A (RIMA), with less severe side-effects. *See also* SELEGILINE.

maple syrup urine disease (aminoacidopathy) an inborn defect of amino acid metabolism causing an excess of valine, leucine, isoleucine, and alloisoleucine in the urine, which has an odour like maple syrup. Treatment is dietary; if untreated, the condition leads to mental retardation and death in infancy.

marasmus *n.* mixed deficiency of both protein and calories, resulting in severe wasting in infants. Body weight is below 60% of that expected for age, the infant looks 'old', has thin sparse hair, is pallid and apathetic, lacks skin fat, and has subnormal temperature. The condition may be due to *malabsorption, wrong feeding, metabolic disorders, repeated vomiting, diarrhoea, severe disease of the heart, lungs, kidneys, or urinary tract, or chronic bacterial or parasitic disease (especially in tropical climates). Maternal rejection of an infant may cause marasmus through undereating. Acute infection may precipitate death. Treatment depends on the underlying cause, but initially very gentle nursing and the provision of nourishment and fluids by gradual steps is appropriate for all.

maraviroc *n.* an *antiretroviral (ARV) drug used, in combination with other ARVs, for treating refractory HIV infection. It acts by binding to and antagonizing CCR5, a receptor for a class of *chemokines on the host cell needed by some HIV viruses to enter the cell. It is administered orally; side-effects include gastrointestinal upsets, cough, and dizziness. Trade name: **Celsentri**.

marble-bone disease *see* OSTEOPETROSIS.

Marburg disease (green monkey disease) a virus disease of vervet (green) monkeys transmitted to humans by contact (usually in laboratories) with blood or tissues from an infected animal. It was first described in Marburg, Germany. Symptoms include fever, malaise, severe headache, vomiting, diarrhoea and bleeding from mucous membranes in the mouth and elsewhere. Treatment with antiserum and measures to reduce the bleeding are sometimes effective.

march fracture a *stress fracture occurring in the distal section of the second or third metatarsal bone, associated with excessive walking or marching.

Marcus Gunn jaw-winking syndrome a congenital condition characterized by drooping (*ptosis) of one eyelid. On opening or moving the mouth, the droopy lid elevates momentarily, resembling a wink. It is believed to be due to an abnormal innervation of the levator muscle by the trigeminal nerve. [R. Marcus Gunn (1850–1909), British ophthalmologist]

Marfan's syndrome an inherited disorder of connective tissue characterized by excessive tallness, abnormally long and slender fingers and toes (**arachnodactyly**), heart defects, and partial dislocation of the lenses of the eyes. [B. J. A. Marfan (1858–1942), French physician]

marijuana *n. see* CANNABIS.

Marion's disease obstruction of the outlet of the bladder caused by enlargement of the muscle cells in the neck of the bladder. [J. B. C. G. Marion (1869–1960), French surgeon]

Marjolin's ulcer a carcinoma that develops at the edge of a chronic *ulcer of the skin, usually a venous ulcer in the ankle region. [J. N. Marjolin (1780–1850), French surgeon]

marrow *n. see* BONE MARROW.

marsupialization *n.* an operative technique for curing a cyst. The cyst is opened, its contents removed, and the edges then stitched to the skin incision. The wound is kept open until it has healed by *granulation.

MAS *see* MANDIBULAR ADVANCEMENT SPLINT.

masculinization *n.* development of excess body and facial hair, deepening of the voice, and increase in muscle bulk (secondary male sexual characteristics) in a female due to a hormone disorder or to hormone therapy. *See also* VIRILISM, VIRILIZATION.

massage *n.* manipulation of the soft tissues of the body with the hands. Massage is used to improve circulation, reduce oedema where present, prevent *adhesions in tissues after injury, reduce muscular spasm, and improve the tone of muscles. *See also* EFFLEURAGE, PETRISSAGE, TAPOTEMENT.

masseter *n.* a thick muscle in the cheek extending from the zygomatic arch to the outer corner of the mandible. It is important for mastication and acts by closing the jaws.

mast- (**masto-**) *combining form denoting* the breast.

mastalgia *n.* pain in the breast.

mast cell a large cell in *connective tissue with many coarse cytoplasmic granules. These granules contain the chemicals *heparin, *histamine, and *serotonin, which are released during inflammation and allergic responses.

mastectomy *n.* surgical removal of a breast. **Simple mastectomy**, performed for extensive but not necessarily invasive tumours, involves simple removal of the breast; the skin and if possible the nipple may be retained and a prosthesis (*see* BREAST IMPLANT) may be inserted under the skin to give the appearance of normality. When breast cancer has spread to involve the lymph nodes, **radical mastectomy** may be performed. This classically involves removal of the breast with the skin and underlying pectoral muscles together with all the lymphatic tissue of the armpit. This treatment may be followed up with radiotherapy and/or chemotherapy. In modern surgical practice a modified radical mastectomy, preserving the pectoral muscles, is more usual than the classical technique. *See also* LUMPECTOMY.

mastication *n.* the process of chewing food.

mastitis *n.* inflammation of the breast, usually caused by bacterial infection via damaged nipples. It most often occurs as acute **puerperal mastitis**, which develops during the period of breast-feeding, about a month after childbirth, and sometimes involves the discharge of pus. Chronic **cystic mastitis** has a different cause and does not involve inflammation. The breast feels lumpy due to the presence of cysts, and the condition is thought to be caused by hormone imbalance.

mastocytosis *n.* a condition caused by *mast cell proliferation due to *KIT* *proto-oncogene mutations. It most commonly manifests in the skin but also affects other organs. Maculopapular variants were formerly known as **urticaria pigmentosa**. Systemic involvement is common in adult cases, with bone marrow examination essential for accurate diagnosis. It may be associated with haematological abnormalities, including leukaemias. Resolution is common in children with skin involvement only. Treatment includes antihistamines, mast-cell stabilizers (such as sodium *cromoglicate), and *tyrosine kinase inhibitors.

mastoid *n.* the *mastoid process of the temporal bone. *See also* MASTOIDITIS.

mastoidectomy *n.* an operation to remove some or all of the air cells in the bone behind the ear (the *mastoid process of the temporal bone) when they have become infected (*see* MASTOIDITIS) or invaded by *cholesteatoma. *See also* ATTICOTOMY.

mastoiditis *n.* inflammation of the *mastoid process behind the ear and of the air space (**mastoid antrum**) connecting it to the cavity of the middle ear. It is usually caused by bacterial infection that spreads from the middle ear (*see* OTITIS (MEDIA)). Usually the infection responds to antibiotics, but surgery (*see* MASTOIDECTOMY) may be required in severe cases.

mastoid process a nipple-shaped process on the *temporal bone that extends downward and forward behind the ear canal and is the point of attachment of several neck muscles. It contains many air spaces (**mastoid cells**), which communicate with

the cavity of the middle ear via an air-filled channel, the **mastoid antrum**. This provides a possible route for the spread of infection from the middle ear (*see* MASTOIDITIS).

masturbation *n.* physical self-stimulation of the genitalia in order to produce sexual pleasure, often resulting in orgasm.

matched pair study *see* CASE CONTROL STUDY.

materia medica the study of drugs used in medicine and dentistry, including *pharmacognosy, *pharmacy, *pharmacology, and therapeutics.

maternal death deaths of women while pregnant or within 42 days of the end of the pregnancy from any cause related to, or aggravated by, the pregnancy or its management, but not from accidental or incidental causes. These deaths can be subdivided into four main categories:
(1) direct deaths: directly related to pregnancy;
(2) indirect deaths: due to pre-existing maternal disease aggravated by pregnancy;
(3) coincidental: unrelated to pregnancy;
(4) late deaths: occurring between six weeks and one year following delivery.
See also MATERNAL MORTALITY RATE.

maternal mortality rate the number of deaths due to complications of pregnancy, childbirth, and the puerperium per 100,000 live births (*see also* STILLBIRTH). In 1952 concern about maternal mortality resulted in Britain in the setting up of a triennial *confidential enquiry (CEMACH) into every such death to identify any shortfall in resources or care. A triennial report has been published since 1985. Levels of *maternal deaths are currently low: the seventh triennial CEMACH report (Dec 2007) counted 149 obstetric-related deaths (7 per 100,000). *Venous thromboembolism remained the commonest direct cause of death (41 deaths, 1.94 per 100,000), while heart disease was the commonest indirect cause of death. In contrast to the global figures (400 deaths per 100,000 live births), where the vast majority of women die from obstetric bleeding, obstructed labour, infection, eclampsia, and the consequences of illegal abortion, these conditions combined only totalled 14% of the maternal deaths in the UK for 2003–05.

matrix *n.* 1. (in histology) the substance of a tissue or organ in which more specialized structures are embedded; for example, the ground substance (**extracellular matrix**) of connective tissue. **2.** (in radiology) the division of an image into rows and columns with equally sized elements (*pixels). The final image is completed by assigning a density to each of these elements. Increasing the number of pixels in the matrix improves the resolution of the final image. A typical value could be 256 rows × 256 columns.

matrix band a flexible strip that is placed round a tooth to restore a wall, thus simplifying insertion of a dental filling.

matrix metalloproteinase (MMP) any one of a group of zinc-containing proteases capable of digesting the extracellular tissue matrix. These enzymes play an important role in cell division, cell migration, inflammation, neoplastic invasion (*metastasis), and *angiogenesis.

maturation *n.* the process of attaining full development. The term is applied particularly to the development of mature germ cells (ova and sperm).

maturity-onset diabetes of the young (MODY) a rare form of *diabetes mellitus caused by a number of identified genetic disorders and resulting in type 2 diabetes in people under 25 years old. Insulin is not required to treat the condition.

Mauriceau-Smellie-Viet manoeuvre (MSV manoeuvre) a technique used in breech delivery to promote flexion of, and safely deliver, the fetal head.

maxilla *n.* (*pl.* **maxillae**) loosely, the upper jaw, which bears the upper teeth. Strictly, the maxilla is one of a pair of bones that partly form the upper jaw, the outer walls of the maxillary sinus, and the floor of the orbit. *See also* MANDIBLE, SKULL. —**maxillary** *adj.*

maxillary sinus (maxillary antrum) *see* PARANASAL SINUSES.

maxillofacial *adj.* describing or relating to the region of the face, jaws, and related structures.

maximin principle *see* VEIL OF IGNORANCE.

maxwell *n.* a unit of magnetic flux equal to a flux of 1 gauss per square centimetre.

Mayer-Rokitansky-Küster-Hauser syndrome (Rokitansky-Küster-Hauser syndrome, Müllerian agenesis) congenital absence of the uterus and upper part of the vagina due to failure of development of the *Müllerian duct. It may be associated with skeletal, renal, and auditory abnormalities, but usually presents with amenorrhoea in a patient with otherwise normal secondary sexual characteristics. There is a multidisciplinary approach to treatment, with psychological support, counselling, discussion of creation of a neovagina (artificial vagina) with gradual use of vaginal dilators, and/or surgical vaginal reconstruction. Surrogacy is the only option for childbearing, although oocyte donation from the mother to a surrogate can be discussed. [K. W. Mayer (1795–1868), German gynaecologist; K. von Rokitansky (1804–78), Austrian pathologist; H. Küster and G. A. Hauser (20th century), German gynaecologists]

Mayo operation an overlapping repair of an umbilical hernia. [W. J. Mayo (1861–1939), US surgeon]

McArdle's disease an *inborn error of metabolism in which a deficiency of the enzyme myophosphorylase prevents the breakdown of glycogen to lactate in exercising muscle. This results in fatigue, pain, and cramps in exercising muscles. The only treatment is avoidance of sustained or excessive exercise. [B. McArdle (20th century), British biochemist]

McBurney's point the point on the abdomen that overlies the anatomical position of the appendix and is the site of maximum tenderness in acute appendicitis. It lies one-third of the way along a line drawn from the anterior superior iliac spine (the projecting part of the hipbone) to the umbilicus. [C. McBurney (1845–1913), US surgeon]

McCormick toy test a hearing test used in preschool children in which the child must discriminate between similar speech sounds. The test consists of 14 toys that are paired because their names sound similar; for example, tree and key, plane and plate. Having first identified all the objects, the child is then asked in a quiet voice to indicate a particular toy (e.g. Can you find the key?).

McCune-Albright syndrome polyostotic *fibrous dysplasia of long bones coupled with *café au lait spots and precocious puberty, occurring in both males and females. [D. J. McCune (1902–76), US paediatrician; F. Albright (1900–69), US physician]

McRobert's manoeuvre a manoeuvre

that overcomes most cases of *shoulder dystocia when the fetal shoulders are unable to pass through the mother's pelvis. The maternal hips are sharply flexed against her abdomen: this rotates the maternal pelvis to encourage delivery.

MCU micturating cystourethrogram. *See* URETHROGRAPHY.

MDCT *see* MULTIDETECTOR COMPUTERIZED TOMOGRAPHY.

MDRD eGFR *see* EGFR.

MDS *see* MYELODYSPLASTIC SYNDROMES.

MDT *see* MULTIDISCIPLINARY TEAM.

ME myalgic encephalomyelitis. *See* CFS/ME/PVF.

MEA microwave *endometrial ablation.

meals on wheels *see* SOCIAL SERVICES.

mean (arithmetic mean) *n.* the average of a group of observations calculated by adding their values and dividing by the number in the group. When one or more observations are substantially different from the rest, which can influence the arithmetic mean unduly, it is preferable to use the **geometric mean** (a similar calculation based on the logarithmic values of the observations) or – more commonly – the **median** (the middle observation of the series arranged in ascending order). A further method of obtaining an average or summary value for a group is to identify the **mode** – the observation (or group of observations when these occur as a continuous quantitative *variable) that occurs most often in the series.

measles *n.* a highly infectious virus disease that tends to appear in epidemics every 2–3 years and mainly affects children. After an incubation period of 8–15 days, symptoms resembling those of a cold develop accompanied by a high fever. Small red spots with white centres (**Koplik's spots**) may appear on the inside of the cheeks. On the third to fifth day a blotchy slightly elevated pink rash develops, first behind the ears then on the face and elsewhere; it lasts 3–5 days. The patient is infectious throughout this period. In most cases the symptoms soon subside but patients are susceptible to pneumonia and middle ear infections. Complete recovery may take 2–4 weeks. Severe complications include encephalitis (one in 1000 cases) and *subacute sclerosing panencephalitis. Measles is a common cause of childhood

mortality in malnourished children, particularly in the developing world. Vaccination against measles provides effective immunity (*see* MMR VACCINE). Medical names: **rubeola, morbilli**.

meat- (**meato-**) *combining form denoting* a meatus. Example: **meatotomy** (incision into the urethral meatus).

meatus *n.* (in anatomy) a passage or opening. The **auditory meatus** is the passage leading from the pinna of the outer *ear to the eardrum. A **nasal meatus** is one of three groovelike parts of the nasal cavity beneath each of the nasal conchae. The **urethral meatus** is the external opening of the urethra.

mebendazole *n.* an *anthelmintic drug used to get rid of roundworms, hookworms, threadworms, and whipworms. Side-effects may include stomach upsets. Trade name: **Vermox**. *See also* IMIDAZOLE.

mebeverine *n. see* ANTISPASMODIC.

mechanoreceptor *n.* a group of cells that respond to mechanical distortion, such as that caused by stretching or compressing a tissue, by generating a nerve impulse in a sensory nerve (*see* RECEPTOR). Touch receptors, *proprioceptors, and the receptors for hearing and balance all belong to this class.

mechanotherapy *n.* the use of mechanical equipment during physiotherapy to produce regularly repeated movements in part of the body. This is done to improve the functioning of muscles and joints.

Meckel's cartilage a cartilaginous bar in the fetus around which the *mandible develops. Part of Meckel's cartilage develops into the malleus (an ear ossicle) in the adult. [J. F. Meckel, the Younger (1781–1833), German anatomist]

Meckel's diverticulum *see* DIVERTICULUM.

meconism *n.* poisoning from the effects of eating or smoking *opium or the products derived from it, especially *morphine.

meconium *n.* the first stools of a newborn baby, which are sticky and dark green and composed of cellular debris, mucus, and bile pigments. The presence of meconium in the amniotic fluid during labour indicates fetal distress. *See also* (MECONIUM) ILEUS, (MECONIUM) PERITONITIS.

meconium aspiration a condition occurring during childbirth in which the baby inhales meconium into the lungs during delivery. This can cause plugs in the airways and the baby may become short of oxygen (hypoxic). Treatment is to assist breathing if necessary, with physiotherapy and antibiotics.

media (tunica media) *n.* **1.** the middle layer of the wall of a *vein or *artery. It is the thickest of the three layers, being composed of elastic fibres and smooth muscle fibres in alternating layers. **2.** the middle layer of various other organs or parts.

medial *adj.* **1.** relating to or denoting the parts of the body that are closest to the *median plane of the body. **2.** relating to or situated in the central region of an organ, tissue, or the body.

median *adj.* **1.** (in anatomy) situated in or denoting the **median plane**, which divides the body into right and left halves. *See* ANATOMICAL POSITION. **2.** (in statistics) *see* MEAN.

mediastinitis *n.* inflammation of the midline partition of the chest cavity (mediastinum), usually complicating a rupture of the oesophagus (gullet). **Sclerosing mediastinitis** often leads to *fibrosis, which may cause compression of other structures in the thorax, such as the superior vena cava, the bronchial tree, or the oesophagus.

mediastinoscopy *n.* examination of the *mediastinum, usually by means of an endoscope inserted through a small incision in the neck region. It can be used to assess the spread of intrathoracic tumours and for lymph node biopsy.

mediastinum *n.* the space in the thorax (chest cavity) between the two pleural sacs. The mediastinum contains the heart, aorta, trachea, oesophagus, and thymus gland and is divided into anterior, middle, posterior, and superior regions.

medical *adj.* **1.** of or relating to medicine, the diagnosis, treatment and prevention of disease. **2.** of or relating to conditions that require the attention of a physician rather than a surgeon. For example, a **medical ward** of a hospital accommodates patients with such conditions.

medical assistant a health service worker who is not a registered medical practitioner (often in the armed forces) working in association with a doctor to undertake minor treatments and preliminary assessments. In poorer countries, particularly in rural areas where qualified resources are short (e.g. China), agricultural workers receive limited training in health care and continue in a dual role as **barefoot doctors**; elsewhere, limited training concentrates more on environmental issues: the workers so trained are known as **sanitarians**.

medical audit *see* CLINICAL AUDIT.

medical certificate a certificate stating a doctor's diagnosis of a patient's medical condition, disability, or fitness to work. See Appendix 8.

medical committee *see* LOCAL MEDICAL COMMITTEE.

medical emergency team (MET) a team, usually consisting of a group of physicians, anaesthetists, and senior nurses, who can be summoned urgently to attend to patients with deteriorating medical conditions. The aim is to prevent further deterioration and to decide if enhanced levels of care are appropriate (e.g. on the high-dependency or intensive care units). The team will also assume the role of the *cardiac-arrest team.

medical ethics the branch of applied *ethics relating to moral behaviour and judgments in medical practice and clinical research. History suggests that healers have always been concerned with ethical questions: evidence can be seen in the *Hippocratic oath and other ancient codes. In the 19th century, medical ethics and professional codes were largely preoccupied with matters of etiquette rather than great moral questions. Currently medical ethics is seen to involve both discussion of complex moral issues in medicine and the negotiation of professional standards. Some commentators believe that medical ethics should cease to be treated as a separate discipline, preferring instead the term 'health-care ethics' as a better reflection of multidisciplinary-team-based clinical care in the 21st century NHS. Medical ethics remains to many a subspecialty of *bioethics and is taught in all medical schools in the UK as an essential part of a professional training. *See also* CLINICAL ETHICS, FEMINIST ETHICS, PUBLIC HEALTH ETHICS, PUBLICATION ETHICS, VIRTUE ETHICS.

(((●))) SEE WEB LINKS
• A–Z of ethical guidance from the website of the General Medical Council

medical jurisprudence the study or practice of the legal aspects of medicine. *See* FORENSIC MEDICINE.

medical negligence *see* NEGLIGENCE.

Medical Research Council (MRC) a government-supported body that is an important source of funds for medical research.

(((⊕)) SEE WEB LINKS)

• MRC website

medicated *adj.* containing a medicinal drug: applied to lotions, soaps, sweets, etc. Medicated dressings are applied to wounds to prevent infection and allow normal healing.

medication *n.* **1.** a substance administered by mouth, applied to the body, or introduced into the body for the purpose of treatment. *See also* PREMEDICATION. **2.** treatment of a patient using drugs.

medicine *n.* **1.** the science or practice of the diagnosis, treatment, and prevention of disease. **2.** the science or practice of nonsurgical methods of treating disease. **3.** any drug or preparation used for the treatment or prevention of disease, particularly a drug that is taken by mouth.

Medicines and Healthcare products Regulatory Agency (MHRA) a UK government agency that regulates the use of medicinal drugs and medical devices. The agency regulates and issues *licences for the clinical trial, manufacture, and marketing of new products. It also applies the regulations governing the collection, storage, and use of human blood and blood products.

(((⊕)) SEE WEB LINKS)

• Website of the MHRA

medicochirurgical *adj.* of or describing matters that are related to both medicine and surgery. A medicochirurgical disorder is one that calls for treatment by both a physician and a surgeon.

medicolegal *adj.* relating to the legal aspects of the practice of medicine. There has been rapid expansion of the branch of the law relating to medicine due to the increasing number of court actions for accidents and injuries, many of them seeking compensation for negligence by doctors or hospitals.

Mediterranean fever **1.** *see* BRUCELLOSIS. **2.** *see* POLYSEROSITIS.

medium *n.* **1.** any substance, usually a broth, agar, or gelatin, used for the *culture of microorganisms or tissue cells. An **assay medium** is used to determine the concentration of a growth factor or chemical by measuring the amount of growth it produces in a particular microorganism; all other nutrients are present in amounts adequate for growth. **2.** *see* CONTRAST MEDIUM.

medroxyprogesterone *n.* a synthetic female sex hormone (*see* PROGESTOGEN) used to treat menstrual disorders (including endometriosis) and certain cancers (especially breast and endometrial cancer) and in *hormone replacement therapy; it is administered by mouth. It is also used as a long-term contraceptive administered by *depot injection. Trade names: **Climanor**, **Depo-Provera**, **Provera**.

medulla *n.* **1.** the inner region of any organ or tissue when it is distinguishable from the outer region (the cortex), particularly the inner part of the kidney, adrenal glands, or lymph nodes. **2.** *see* MEDULLA OBLONGATA. **3.** the *myelin layer of certain nerve fibres. —**medullary** *adj.*

medulla oblongata (myelencephalon) the extension within the skull of the upper end of the spinal cord, forming the lowest part of the *brainstem. Besides forming the major pathway for nerve impulses entering and leaving the skull, the medulla contains centres that are responsible for the regulation of the heart and blood vessels, respiration, salivation, and swallowing. *Cranial nerves VI–XII leave the brain in this region.

medullary carcinoma a tumour whose consistency was thought to resemble that of bone marrow. **Medullary carcinoma of the thyroid** has associations with tumours of other organs (multiple endocrine neoplasia; *see* MENS) and is often familial: it arises from the *C cells of the thyroid and produces calcitonin, which can often be used as a *tumour marker.

medullated nerve fibre (myelinated nerve fibre) *see* MYELIN.

medulloblastoma *n.* a malignant brain tumour (*see* CEREBRAL TUMOUR) that occurs during childhood. It is derived from cells that have the apparent potential to mature into neurons and develops in the cerebellum, the part of the brain that is predominantly involved in the control of balance. The flow of cerebrospinal fluid (CSF) may become obstructed, causing *hydrocephalus. Symptoms include headaches, dizziness, and unsteadiness. Treatment involves surgery to remove most of the tumour and restore CSF flow, followed by radiotherapy directed using *stereotactic localization. Medulloblastoma is the second most common form of cancer of childhood (after leukaemia); recent advances have improved the survival rate so that 40% of affected children live for more than five years.

mefenamic acid an anti-inflammatory drug (see NSAID) used to treat headache, toothache, rheumatic pain, and similar conditions. It is administered by mouth; side-effects include digestive upsets, drowsiness, and skin rashes. Trade name: **Ponstan**.

mefloquine n. a drug used mainly in the prevention of malaria that is resistant to chloroquine. It is administered by mouth; side-effects can include dizziness, rash, gastrointestinal problems, and psychiatric disturbances (e.g. depression, psychosis), and the drug should not be taken during pregnancy, by psychiatric patients, or with beta blockers. Trade name: **Lariam**.

mega- combining form denoting 1. large size, or abnormal enlargement or distension. Example: **megacaecum** (of the caecum). 2. a million. Example: **megavolt** (a million volts).

megacolon n. dilatation, and sometimes lengthening, of the colon. It is caused by chronic obstruction of the colon (e.g. due to *Hirschsprung's disease) or longstanding constipation, or it may occur as a complication of ulcerative *colitis (**toxic megacolon**).

megakaryoblast n. a cell that gives rise to the platelet-forming cell *megakaryocyte, found in the blood-forming tissue of the bone marrow. It is derived from a *haemopoietic stem cell and matures via an intermediate stage (**promegakaryocyte**) into a megakaryocyte.

megakaryocyte n. a cell in the bone marrow that produces *platelets. It is large (35–160 μm in diameter), with an irregular multilobed nucleus, and with *Romanowsky stains its abundant cytoplasm appears pale blue with fine reddish granules. See also THROMBOPOIESIS.

megal- (megalo-) combining form denoting abnormal enlargement. Example: **megalomelia** (of limbs).

megaloblast n. an abnormal form of any of the cells that are precursors of red blood cells (see ERYTHROBLAST). Megaloblasts are unusually large and their nuclei fail to mature in the normal way; they are seen in the bone marrow in certain anaemias (**megaloblastic anaemias**) due to deficiency of vitamin B$_{12}$ or folate. —**megaloblastic** adj.

megalocephaly n. 1. see MACROCEPHALY. 2. overgrowth and distortion of skull bones (see LEONTIASIS).

megalocyte n. see MACROCYTE.

megalomania n. an obsolete word for delusions of grandeur, such as being God, royalty, etc. It may be a feature of a schizophrenic or manic illness or of cerebral syphilis.

-megaly combining form denoting abnormal enlargement. Example: **splenomegaly** (of spleen).

megaureter n. gross dilatation of the *ureter. This occurs above the site of a longstanding obstruction in the ureter, which blocks the free flow of urine from the kidney. A common cause of megaureter is reflux of urine from the bladder into the ureters (see VESICOURETERIC REFLUX), but some of the most striking examples are found in so-called **idiopathic megaureter**. In this condition, which may affect one or both ureters, there is a segment of normal ureter of varying length at the extreme lower end of the bladder, above which the ureter is enormously dilated. Both reflux and idiopathic megaureter can be complicated by urinary infection and/or renal impairment. Treatment of megaureter is by corrective surgery if functional obstruction can be demonstrated. Surgery for reflux is normally reserved for children with gross reflux distending the renal pelvis and is usually carried out in the first few months of life.

megestrol n. a synthetic female sex hormone (see PROGESTOGEN) that is administered by mouth in the treatment of metastatic breast cancer and metastatic endometrial cancer. Trade name: **Megace**.

meglitinides pl. n. a group of *oral hypoglycaemic drugs, including **repaglinide** (Prandin) and **nateglinide** (Starlix), used for treating type 2 *diabetes mellitus. They act by stimulating insulin release from the pancreas and should be taken before each meal.

megophthalmia n. an abnormally large eyeball.

meibomian cyst *n. see* CHALAZION.

meibomian glands (tarsal glands) small sebaceous glands that lie under the conjunctiva of the eyelids.

meibomianitis *n.* inflammation of the *meibomian glands of the eyelids.

Meigs syndrome the rare combination of a benign ovarian *fibroma with *ascites and a right-sided pleural effusion. [J. V. Meigs (1892–1963), US gynaecologist]

meiosis (reduction division) *n.* a type of cell division that produces four daughter cells, each having half the number of chromosomes of the original cell. It occurs before the formation of sperm and ova and the normal (*diploid) number of chromosomes is restored after fertilization. Meiosis also produces genetic variation in the daughter cells, brought about by the process of *crossing over. Meiosis consists of two successive divisions, each divided into four stages (*see* PROPHASE, METAPHASE, ANAPHASE, TELOPHASE). (See illustration.) *Compare* MITOSIS. —**meiotic** *adj.*

Meissner's plexus (submucous plexus) a fine network of parasympathetic nerve fibres in the wall of the alimentary canal, supplying the muscles and mucous membrane. [G. Meissner (1829–1905), German physiologist]

melaena *n.* black tarry faeces due to the presence of partly digested blood from the upper part of the digestive tract. Melaena is not apparent unless at least 500 ml of blood has entered the gut; therefore it is usually a sign of significant internal bleeding. It often occurs after vomiting blood (*see* HAEMATEMESIS), having the same causes, but may be due to disease in the small intestine or proximal large bowel, such as carcinoma or *angiodysplasia. *See also* HAEMORRHAGIC DISEASE OF THE NEWBORN (MELAENA NEONATORUM).

melan- (melano-) *combining form denoting* **1.** black coloration. **2.** melanin. Example: **melanaemia** (the presence in the blood of melanin).

melancholia *n.* an obsolete name for *depression not triggered by any stressor. *See also* ENDOGENOUS.

melanin *n.* a dark-brown to black pigment occurring in the hair, the skin, and in the iris and choroid layer of the eyes. Melanin is contained within special cells (**chromato-**

Prophase I leptotene

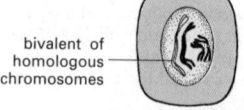

cytoplasm
chromosome — centriole
cell membrane — nuclear membrane

zygotene to pachytene

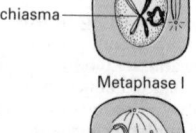

bivalent of homologous chromosomes

diplotene to diakinesis

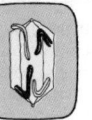

chiasma

Metaphase I

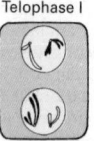

one chromosome of each pair goes to each pole

Anaphase I

Telophase I

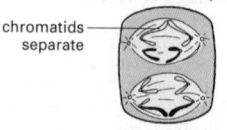

Metaphase II to Anaphase II

chromatids separate

Telophase II

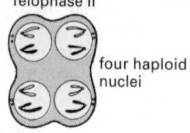

four haploid nuclei

Stages in meiosis.

phores or **melanophores**) and is produced by the metabolism of the amino acid tyrosine. Production of melanin by **melanocytes** in the epidermis of the skin is increased by the action of sunlight (producing tanning), which protects the underlying skin layers from the sun's radiation.

melanism (melanosis) *n.* an unusually pronounced darkening of body tissues caused by excessive production of the pigment *melanin. For example, melanism may affect the hair, the skin (after sunburn, during pregnancy, or in *Addison's disease), or the eye.

melanocyte *n.* any one of the cells, concentrated within the epidermis of skin, that produces the dark brown pigment *melanin.

melanocyte-stimulating hormone (MSH) a peptide hormone produced and secreted by the anterior pituitary gland. In humans it stimulates production and dispersal of melanin in the melanocytes. **Alpha-melanocyte-stimulating hormone (α-MSH)**, which is released by neurons in the hypothalamus, suppresses appetite and regulates energy balance. It also stimulates sexual activity and is involved in regulation of heart rate and blood pressure.

melanoma (malignant melanoma) *n.* a highly malignant tumour of melanin-forming cells, the *melanocytes. Such tumours usually occur in the skin (pale skin, genetic predisposition, and excessive exposure to sunlight, particularly repeated sunburn, are the most important factors); it may arise from a pre-existing mole or naevus or from apparently normal skin. It can rarely occur at other sites than the skin. Melanomas are usually dark, but may also be free of pigment (**amelanotic melanomas**). Spread of this cancer to other parts of the body, especially to the lymph nodes and liver, is common if the original melanoma is thick. The prognosis is inversely related to the thickness of the tumour; almost all patients with tumours less than 0.76 mm survive following surgical excision. The mainstay of treatment is surgery, but melanoma can be responsive to *immunotherapy and is currently the subject of investigational treatments using melanoma vaccines; the response rate to conventional chemotherapy is poor. Primary prevention programmes reducing episodes of sunburn are advanced in some parts of the world, such as Australia.

melanonychia *n.* blackening of the nails with the pigment *melanin.

melanophore *n. see* MELANIN.

melanoplakia *n.* pigmented areas of *melanin in the mucous membrane lining the inside of the cheeks.

melanosis *n.* **1.** *see* MELANISM. **2.** a disorder in the body's production of the pigment melanin. **3.** *cachexia associated with the spread of the skin cancer *melanoma. —**melanotic** *adj.*

melanuria *n.* the presence of dark pigment in the urine. This may be caused by the presence of melanin or its precursors, in some cases of *melanoma; it may alternatively be caused by metabolic disease, such as *porphyria.

MELAS mitochondrial encephalopathy lactic acidosis and stroke-like episodes: a rare metabolic disorder, usually inherited from the mother, that results in short stature and high levels of lactic acid in the blood (*see* LACTIC ACIDOSIS). Affected individuals are usually diagnosed in late childhood and early adult life. *See also* MITOCHONDRIAL DISORDERS.

melasma *n. see* CHLOASMA.

melatonin *n.* a hormone produced by the *pineal gland in darkness but not in bright light. Melatonin receptors in the brain, in a nucleus immediately above the *optic chiasm, react to this hormone and synchronize the nucleus to the 24-hour day/night rhythm, thus informing the brain when it is day and when it is night. Melatonin is a derivative of *serotonin, with which it works to regulate the sleep cycle, and is being used experimentally to treat jet lag, *SAD, and insomnia in shift workers and the elderly.

melioidosis *n.* a disease of wild rodents caused by the bacterium *Pseudomonas pseudomallei*. It can be transmitted to humans, possibly by rat fleas, causing pneumonia, multiple abscesses, and septicaemia. It is often fatal.

Melkersson-Rosenthal syndrome a rare disorder characterized by the occurrence together of facial paralysis, enlargement of the glottis, and swollen lips, which is due to lymphatic *stasis and the consequent build-up of protein in the facial tissues. [E. Melkersson (1898–1932), Swedish physician;

C. Rosenthal (20th century), German neurologist]

melomelus *n.* a fetus with one or more pairs of supernumerary limbs.

melphalan *n.* a drug (an *alkylating agent) used to treat various types of cancer, particularly myeloma. It is administered by mouth or intravenous injection or infusion. Side-effects include digestive upsets, mouth ulcers, and temporary hair loss. Trade name: **Alkeran**.

memantine hydrochloride an *NMDA-receptor antagonist drug indicated for treatment of moderate to severe Alzheimer's-type dementia. It is administered orally; its most common side-effects are dizziness, headache, and constipation. Trade name: **Ebixa**.

membrane *n.* **1.** a thin layer of tissue surrounding the whole or part of an organ or tissue lining a cavity, or separating adjacent structures or cavities. *See also* BASEMENT MEMBRANE, MUCOUS MEMBRANE, SEROUS MEMBRANE. **2.** the lipoprotein envelope surrounding a cell (**plasma** or **cell membrane**). —**membranous** *adj.*

membrane bone a bone that develops in connective tissue by direct *ossification, without cartilage being formed first. The bones of the face and skull are membrane bones.

membranous labyrinth *see* LABYRINTH.

membranous nephropathy a common cause of the *nephrotic syndrome in adults. The diagnosis is established by renal biopsy, which shows diffuse global subepithelial deposits within the glomerulus. Most cases of membranous nephropathy are idiopathic, but there are associations with infection (e.g. hepatitis B), malignancy (especially lung cancer), autoimmune disease (e.g. SLE, Hashimoto's disease), and drugs (e.g. gold and penicillamine). Recent studies suggest that idiopathic membranous nephropathy is an autoimmune disease with antibodies directed against an antigen (PLA$_2$R, a phospholipase A$_2$ receptor) on the *podocyte cell membrane. Without treatment, outcome is very variable: some patients will make a full recovery, while others will progress to end-stage kidney failure. Immunosuppressant treatment is often tried when there is evidence of declining renal function.

Memokath *n.* trade name for a prostatic *stent used as a minimally invasive treatment for men with *lower urinary tract symptoms due to benign prostatic hyperplasia (*see* PROSTATE GLAND) who are unfit for surgery. The stent is placed in the prostatic section of the urethra and bladder neck using a flexible cystoscope. The stent expands when warm water is passed through it; cold water causes contraction and allows removal.

MEN multiple endocrine neoplasia. *See* MENS.

men- (**meno-**) *combining form denoting* menstruation.

menarche *n.* the start of the menstrual periods and other physical and mental changes associated with puberty. The menarche occurs when the reproductive organs become functionally active and may take place at any time between 10 and 18 years of age. *Compare* GONADARCHE.

Mencap *n.* a British voluntary association that promotes the welfare of those with *learning disabilities and their families, through education, campaigning, and the provision of resources for projects.

mendelism *n.* the theory of inheritance based on *Mendel's laws.

Mendel's laws rules of inheritance based on the breeding experiments of the Austrian monk Gregor Mendel (1822–84), which showed that the inheritance of characteristics is controlled by particles now known as *genes. In modern terms they are as follows. (1) Each body (somatic) cell of an individual carries two factors (genes) for every characteristic and each gamete carries only one. It is now known that the genes are arranged on chromosomes, which are present in pairs in somatic cells and separate during gamete formation by the process of *meiosis. (2) Each pair of factors segregates independently of all other pairs at meiosis, so that the gametes show all possible combinations of factors. This law applies only to genes on different chromosomes; those on the same chromosome are affected by *linkage. *See also* DOMINANT, RECESSIVE.

Mendelson's syndrome inhalation of regurgitated stomach contents by an anaesthetized patient, which may result in death from anoxia or cause extensive lung damage or pulmonary *oedema with severe *bronchospasm. It is a well-recognized hazard of general anaesthesia in obstetrics and may be prevented by giving gastric-acid inhibitors (e.g. *cimetidine or *ranitidine) or sodium citrate before inducing anaesthesia. [C. L. Mendelson (1913–), US obstetrician]

Ménétrier's disease a disorder in which gross enlargement (*see* HYPERTROPHY) of the cells of the mucous membrane lining the stomach is associated with anaemia. Prominent gastric folds are seen at endoscopy or on barium studies. [P. Ménétrier (1859–1935), French physician]

Ménière's disease a disease of the inner ear characterized by episodes of deafness, buzzing in the ears (*tinnitus), and *vertigo. Typically the attacks are preceded by a sensation of fullness in the ear. Symptoms last for several hours and between attacks the affected ear may return to normal, although hearing does tend to deteriorate gradually with repeated attacks. It is thought to be caused by the build-up of fluid in the inner ear. Drug treatments include *prochlorperazine to reduce vertigo in acute attacks and *betahistine as prophylactic treatment. Ototoxic drugs, such as *gentamicin, can be injected through the eardrum into the middle ear to reduce activity in the inner ear. Surgical procedures used include decompression or drainage of the *endolymphatic sac, *vestibular nerve section, and *labyrinthectomy. Medical name: **endolymphatic hydrops**. [P. Ménière (1799–1862), French physician]

mening- (meningo-) *combining form denoting* the meninges.

meninges *pl. n.* (*sing.* **meninx**) the three connective tissue membranes that line the skull and vertebral canal and enclose the brain and spinal cord (see illustration). The outermost layer – the *dura mater (pachymeninx) – is inelastic, tough, and thicker than the middle layer (the *arachnoid mater) and the innermost layer (the *pia mater). The inner two membranes are together called the **leptomeninges**; between them circulates the *cerebrospinal fluid.

meningioma *n.* a benign tumour arising from the fibrous coverings of the brain and spinal cord (*meninges). It is usually slow-growing and produces symptoms by pressure on the underlying nervous tissue. In the brain the tumour may cause focal *epilepsy and gradually progressive neurological disability. In the spinal cord it may cause para-

plegia and the *Brown-Séquard syndrome. Rarely, meningiomas may behave in a malignant fashion and can invade neighbouring tissues. Treatment of the majority of cases is by surgical removal if the tumour is accessible. The histological classification of malignancy is controversial, but some tumours may also require additional radiotherapy. Some patients have been known to have symptoms for as long as 30 years before the tumour has been discovered.

meningism *n.* stiffness of the neck that is found in *meningitis.

meningitis *n.* an inflammation of the *meninges due to infection by viruses or bacteria or fungi. Meningitis causes an intense headache, fever, loss of appetite, intolerance to light (photophobia) and sound (phonophobia), rigidity of muscles, especially those in the neck (*see also* KERNIG'S SIGN), and in severe cases convulsions, vomiting, and delirium leading to death. The most important causes of bacterial meningitis are *Haemophilus influenzae* (especially in young children); two strains of *Neisseria meningitidis* (the meningococcus), B and C; and *Streptococcus pneumoniae* (**pneumococcal meningitis**). Immunization against *Haemophilus, Neisseria meningitidis* C, and pneumococcal meningitis is now routine for children (*see* HIB VACCINE, MENINGITIS C VACCINE, PNEUMOCOCCAL VACCINE); there is at present no vaccine available for meningitis

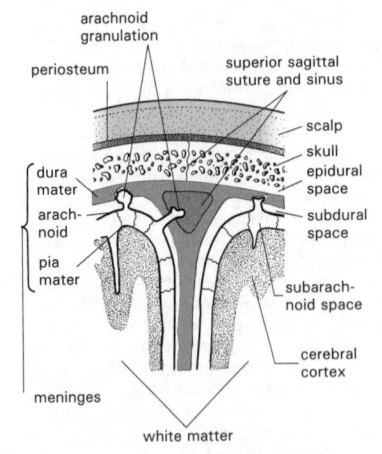

The meninges (in a section through the skull and brain).

B. In **meningococcal meningitis** (meningitis B and C, previously known as **cerebrospinal fever** and **spotted fever**) the symptoms appear suddenly and the bacteria can cause widespread meningococcal infection, which may be associated with **meningococcal septicaemia**, with its characteristic purple haemorrhagic rash anywhere on the body. The rash does not disappear on pressure (if a glass is pressed on the rash, it is still visible through the glass). Unless quickly diagnosed and treated, death can occur within a few hours.

Bacterial meningitis is treated with antibiotics administered as soon as possible after diagnosis. With the exception of herpes simplex *encephalitis (which is treated with aciclovir), viral meningitis does not respond to drugs but normally has a relatively benign prognosis. *See also* LEPTOMENINGITIS, PACHY-MENINGITIS.

(SEE WEB LINKS)

• Website of the Meningitis Trust: includes information on signs and symptoms of meningitis

meningitis C vaccine (MenC) a vaccine that provides protection against the C strain of the bacterium *Neisseria meningitidis* (the meningococcus), which accounts for approximately 50% of all cases of meningococcal meningitis and tends to occur in clusters. The vaccine is given at present to all babies with their primary *immunizations at 3 and 4 months of age and as a booster at 12 months. It can also be given as a single vaccine and is currently offered to everyone under the age of 24.

meningocele *n. see* NEURAL TUBE DEFECTS.

meningococcaemia *n.* the presence of meningococci (bacteria of the species *Neisseria meningitidis*) in the bloodstream. *See* MENINGITIS.

meningococcus *n.* (*pl.* **meningococci**) the bacterium *Neisseria meningitidis*, which can cause a serious form of septicaemia and is a common cause of *meningitis. —**meningococcal** *adj.*

meningoencephalitis *n.* inflammation of the brain and its membranous coverings (the meninges) caused by bacterial, viral, fungal, or amoebic infection. The disease may also involve the spinal cord, producing *myelitis with paralysis of both legs, sometimes called **meningoencephalomyelitis**.

meningoencephalocele *n. see* NEURAL TUBE DEFECTS.

meningoencephalomyelitis *n. see* MENINGOENCEPHALITIS.

meningomyelocele *n. see* NEURAL TUBE DEFECTS.

meningovascular *adj.* relating to or affecting the meninges covering the brain and spinal cord and the blood vessels that penetrate them to supply the underlying neural tissues. The term is also used to describe tertiary syphilitic infection of the nervous system.

meninx *n.* **1.** the thin layer of mesoderm that surrounds the brain of the embryo. It gives rise to most of the skull and the membranes that surround the brain. *See also* CHONDROCRANIUM. **2.** *see* MENINGES.

meniscectomy *n.* surgical removal of a cartilage (meniscus) in the knee. This is carried out when the meniscus has been torn or is diseased and is causing symptoms, such as pain, swelling, and 'locking' of the knee joint. The operation is now routinely performed using an *arthroscope.

meniscus *n.* (in anatomy) a crescent-shaped structure, such as the fibrocartilaginous disc that divides the cavity of a synovial joint.

Menkes kinky-hair disease a genetic disorder characterized by severe mental retardation, seizures, poor vision, colourless fragile hair, and chubby red cheeks. There is no treatment and affected infants usually die before the age of three. [J. H. Menkes (1928–), US neurologist]

menopause (climacteric) *n.* the time in a woman's life when the ovaries cease to produce an egg cell every four weeks: menstruation ceases and the woman is no longer able to bear children. The menopause can occur at any age between the middle thirties and the middle fifties, most commonly between 45 and 55 (the median age is 51). Natural menopause can only be established in retrospect after 12 consecutive months of *amenorrhoea. Around the time of the menopause (the **perimenopause**) there are marked changes in the menstrual cycle. Menstruation may decrease gradually in successive periods or the intervals between the periods may lengthen; alternatively there may be a sudden and complete stoppage of the periods. There is a change in the balance of sex hormones in the body, which sometimes leads to hot flushes and other *vasomotor symptoms, palpitations, and dryness of the mucous membrane lining the vagina. Some women may also experience emotional disturbances. Some of these symptoms may be alleviated by *hormone replacement therapy. The term 'menopause' is also used for the postmenopausal period. —**menopausal** *adj.*

menorrhagia *n.* abnormally heavy bleeding at menstruation, which may or may not be associated with abnormally long periods. Menorrhagia may be associated with pelvic inflammatory disease, tumours (especially fibroids) in the pelvic cavity, endometriosis, or the presence of an IUCD. In some cases no obvious pathology can be demonstrated; heavy, prolonged, or frequent uterine bleeding not associated with pelvic or systemic disease is known as **dysfunctional uterine bleeding**. Medical treatment for menorrhagia includes *NSAIDs, *antifibrinolytic drugs, and hormonal therapy. Surgical treatments include *endometrial ablation and hysterectomy.

menotrophin *n. see* HUMAN MENOPAUSAL GONADOTROPHINS.

MENS multiple endocrine neoplasia syndromes, designated as type 1 (**Wermer's syndrome**), type 2A (**Sipple's syndrome**), and type 2B. These involve tumour formation or hyperplasia in various combinations of endocrine glands. Type 1 involves the parathyroid, pituitary, and pancreas, whereas type 2A involves the thyroid medullary cells, the adrenal medulla (*phaeochromocytoma),

and the parathyroids. Type 2B is similar to 2A, but patients tend to resemble people with *Marfan's syndrome and have multiple *neuromas on their mucous membranes.

menses *n.* 1. the blood and other materials discharged from the uterus at menstruation. 2. *see* MENSTRUATION.

menstrual cycle the periodic sequence of events in sexually mature nonpregnant women by which an egg cell (ovum) is released from the ovary at four-weekly intervals until *menopause. The stages of the menstrual cycle are shown in the diagram. An ovum develops within a *Graafian follicle in the ovary. When mature, it bursts from the follicle and travels along the Fallopian tube to the uterus. A temporary endocrine gland – the corpus luteum – develops in the ruptured follicle and secretes the hormone *progesterone, which causes the lining of the uterus (endometrium) to become thicker and richly supplied with blood in preparation for pregnancy. If the ovum is not fertilized the cycle continues: the corpus luteum shrinks and the endometrium is shed at *menstruation. If fertilization does take place the fertilized ovum becomes attached to the endometrium and the corpus luteum continues to secrete progesterone, i.e. pregnancy begins.

menstruation (menses) *n.* the discharge of blood and of fragments of *endometrium from the vagina at intervals of about one month in women of child-bearing age (*see* MENARCHE, MENOPAUSE). Menstruation is that stage of the *menstrual cycle during which the endometrium, thickened in readi-

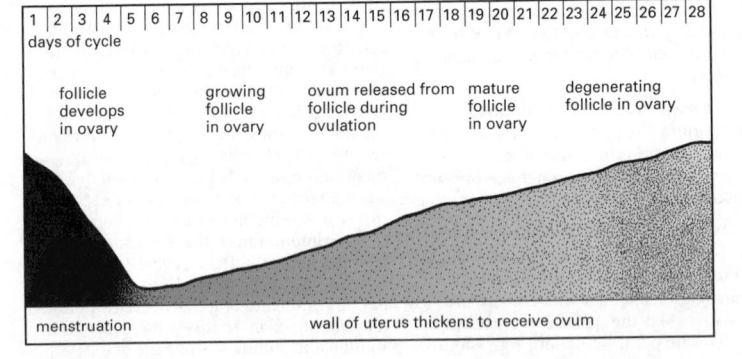

| 1 | 2 | 3 | 4 | 5 | 6 | 7 | 8 | 9 | 10 | 11 | 12 | 13 | 14 | 15 | 16 | 17 | 18 | 19 | 20 | 21 | 22 | 23 | 24 | 25 | 26 | 27 | 28 |

days of cycle

follicle develops in ovary

growing follicle in ovary

ovum released from follicle during ovulation

mature follicle in ovary

degenerating follicle in ovary

menstruation   wall of uterus thickens to receive ovum

The menstrual cycle.

ness to receive a fertilized egg cell (ovum), is shed because fertilization has not occurred. The normal duration of discharge varies from three to seven days. In **anovular menstruation**, discharge takes place without previous release of an egg cell from the ovary. **Vicarious menstruation** is bleeding from a mucous membrane other than the endometrium when normal menstruation is due. **Retrograde menstruation** is the backflow of blood and endometrial cells through the Fallopian tubes (*see* ENDOMETRIOSIS). *See also* AMENORRHOEA, DYSMENORRHOEA, MENORRHAGIA, OLIGOMENORRHOEA.

mental[1] *adj.* relating to or affecting the mind.

mental[2] *adj.* relating to the chin.

mental age a measure of the intellectual level at which an individual functions; for example, someone described as having a mental age of 6 years would be functioning at the level of an average 6-year-old child. This measure has largely been replaced by a comparison of the functioning of persons of the same age group (*see* INTELLIGENCE QUOTIENT, INTELLIGENCE TEST).

Mental Capacity Act 2005 legislation for England and Wales, which came into force in October 2007, to govern the treatment of people who lack *capacity to make decisions. It gives legal force to the importance of *autonomy in health care and to *advance statements, decisions, or directives. It also provides statutory legislation for medical and social decision-makers to act in the patient's best interests should he or she lose capacity (*see* INDEPENDENT MENTAL CAPACITY ADVOCATE). It allows proportionate force to implement decisions made in a patient's best interests. For Scotland the current legislation is the Adults with Incapacity (Scotland) Act 2000.

mental deficiency an obsolete term for *mental retardation.

mental handicap a former term for *learning disability.

Mental Health Act an Act of Parliament to govern the treatment of people with a mental disorder, which is defined as including *mental illness, *personality disorder, and *learning disability. For England and Wales the Mental Health Act 1983 has been amended by the Mental Health Act 2007. The legislation provides for the voluntary and

compulsory (involuntary) assessment and treatment of the mentally disordered. The purposes of involuntary admission are both to act in patients' best interests, providing treatment for them when they have lost *insight into their illness, and to manage the risk that may arise from a mental disorder to the patients themselves or to others. One of the principal and most controversial amendments in the 2007 Act is the introduction of **Community Treatment Orders**, which provide for the involuntary treatment of patients who have left hospital. Further controversy surrounds the introduction of sexual deviancy as a mental disorder to which the Act applies. In Scotland the current legislation is the Mental Health (Care and Treatment) (Scotland) Act 2003, which came into effect in April 2005.

Mental Health Act Commission a regulating body in England and Wales, governed by the Mental Health Act 2007, that was responsible for regularly visiting psychiatric hospitals, reviewing psychiatric care, giving second opinions on the need for certain psychiatric treatments, and acting as a forum for the discussion of psychiatric issues. It was subsumed under the *Care Quality Commission in April 2009.

Mental Health Review Tribunal (MHRT) a tribunal, established under the Mental Health Act 1959 and now operating under the Mental Health Act 2007, to which applications may be made for the discharge from hospital of a person compulsorily detained there under provisions of the Act (*see* COMPULSORY ADMISSION). When a patient is subject to a restriction order an application may only be made after his or her first six months of detention. The powers of the tribunal, which comprises both legally and medically qualified members, include reclassifying unrestricted patients, recommending leave of absence for a patient, delaying discharge, and transferring patients to other hospitals. Detained patients may also apply to have a **managers' hearing** to review their detention. The powers of the managers' hearing are slightly different from those of the MHRT, but both are defined in the Mental Health Act 2007 and both can discharge a patient from a section of the Mental Health Act.

mental illness a disorder of one or more of the functions of the mind (such as emotion, perception, memory, or thought), which causes suffering to the patient or others. If the sole problem is that the individual's behaviour as a whole is out of line with society's expectations, then the term 'illness' is not appropriate.

Mental illness should be distinguished from *mental retardation, in which an individual has a general failure of development of the normal intellectual capacities. Mental illnesses are broadly divided into disorders in which the capacity for appreciating reality is lost (*see* PSYCHOSIS) and those in which insight is retained (*see* NEUROSIS).

(⊕) SEE WEB LINKS

- Website of the Mental Health Foundation
- Website of MIND (National Association for Mental Health)
- Website of Rethink: provides an information and advice service for people living with mental illness

mental impairment (mostly in legal usage) the condition of significant or severe impairment of intellectual and social functioning.

mental retardation the state of those whose intellectual powers have failed to develop to such an extent that they are in need of care and protection and require special education. The handicap may be classified according to the *intelligence quotient (IQ) as mild (IQ 50–70), moderate to severe (IQ 20–50), and profound (IQ less than 20). Mildly handicapped people often make a good adjustment to life after special help with education. The moderately and severely handicapped usually need much more help and most are permanently dependent on other people, while the profoundly handicapped usually need constant attention. There are very many causes of mental retardation, including *Down's syndrome, *autism, inherited metabolic disorders, brain injury, and gross psychological deprivation; some are preventable or treatable. Individuals with mental retardation are at greater risk of developing mental illnesses, such as schizophrenia and dementia. Most European countries have specialist services to cater for this group of people.

mental state examination (MSE) a full psychiatric examination of signs and symptoms, which takes place during a psychiatric interview and should apply only to signs and symptoms elicited at that time; it should not take into account historical information. The examination is usually divided into the following subheadings: appearance and behaviour, speech, mood, *affect, thought and perception, *insight, and orientation. Usually it also includes a *risk assessment.

mento- *combining form denoting* the chin.

mentum *n.* the chin.

mepacrine *n.* a drug sometimes used to treat giardiasis. It is administered by mouth. Digestive upsets and headache may occur and the skin often turns yellow.

meralgia paraesthetica painful tingling and numbness felt over the lateral surface of the thigh when the lateral cutaneous nerve is trapped as it passes through the fibrous and muscular tissues of the groin. It is usually found in pregnant women.

mercaptoacetyltriglycine *n. see* MAG3.

mercaptopurine *n.* a drug that prevents the growth of cancer cells and is administered by mouth, chiefly in the treatment of acute leukaemias (*see* ANTIMETABOLITE). It commonly reduces the numbers of white blood cells; mouth ulcers and digestive upsets may also occur. Trade name: **Puri-Nethol**.

mercurialism (hydrargyria) *n.* mercury poisoning. Metallic mercury is absorbed through the skin and alimentary canal, and its vapour is taken in through the lungs. Acute poisoning causes vomiting, severe abdominal pains, bloody diarrhoea, and kidney damage, with failure to produce urine. Treatment is with *dimercaprol. Chronic poisoning causes mouth ulceration, loose teeth, loss of appetite, and intestinal and renal disturbances, with anaemia and nervous irritability. Treatment is removing the patient from further exposure.

mercury *n.* a silvery metallic element that is liquid at room temperature. Its toxicity caused a decline in the use of its compounds in medicine during the 20th century; mercurial compounds were formerly used in the treatment of syphilis and as purgatives, teething pastes and powders, fungicides, and antiparasitic agents. Mercury is still widely used in dentistry as a component of *amalgam fillings; when the mercury is combined with the filling alloy, it is nontoxic. Symbol: Hg. *See also* MERCURIALISM, PINK DISEASE.

merocrine (eccrine) *adj.* describing a type of *secretion in which the glandular cells remain intact during the process of secretion.

merozoite *n.* a stage in the life cycle of the malaria parasite (*Plasmodium*). Many merozoites are formed during the asexual division of the schizont (*see* SCHIZOGONY). The released merozoites may invade new red blood cells or new liver cells, and continue the asexual phase with the production of yet more merozoites, effectively spreading the infection. Alternatively, merozoites invade red blood cells and begin the sexual cycle with the formation of male and female sex cells (*see* MICROGAMETOCYTE, MACROGAMETOCYTE).

mes- (meso-) *combining form denoting* middle or medial.

MESA (microsurgical epididymal sperm aspiration) the removal of spermatozoa from the epididymis by needle *aspiration. This procedure, performed under anaesthetic, may be undertaken to assist conception in cases where the normal passage of sperm from the testis is obstructed, for example by blockage (through infection) of the ducts or by vasectomy. The extracted sperm are subjected to special treatment to select the strongest and most motile; these are then chemically treated to activate them and used for in vitro fertilization (*see* ICSI).

mesalazine *n. see* AMINOSALICYLATES.

mesangial cells *see* JUXTAGLOMERULAR APPARATUS.

mesangiocapillary glomerulonephritis (membranoproliferative glomerulonephritis) a renal disease characterized by changes in the glomeruli with mesangial cell proliferation and thickening of the capillary wall (*see* JUXTAGLOMERULAR APPARATUS). Three types are distinguished. Type 1 is associated with immune deposits in the subendothelial space and the mesangial cells, and may sometimes be associated with cryoglobulinaemia (*see* CRYOGLOBULIN) and infection with the hepatitis C virus. Type 2, also known as **dense deposit disease**, is associated with a ribbon of electron-dense material within the glomerular basement membrane. Type 3 is associated with immune deposits in the subendothelium, the basement membrane, and the subepithelial spaces. All three types have a variable presentation, ranging from asymptomatic abnormalities of the urinary sediment through *nephrotic syndrome to subacute renal failure. Apart from treatment of any coexisting

hepatitis C, there is no consensus regarding specific treatment of these conditions.

mesaortitis *n.* inflammation of the middle layer (media) of the wall of the aorta, generally the result of late syphilis. Aneurysm formation may result. The infection can be eradicated with penicillin.

mesarteritis *n.* inflammation of the middle layer (media) of an artery, which is often combined with inflammation in all layers of the artery wall. It is seen in syphilis, polyarteritis, temporal arteritis, and Buerger's disease.

mescaline *n.* an alkaloid present in **mescal buttons** (the dried tops of the Mexican cactus *Lophophora williamsii*) that produces inebriation and vivid colourful hallucinations when ingested.

mesencephalon *n. see* MIDBRAIN.

mesenchyme *n.* the undifferentiated tissue of the early embryo that forms almost entirely from *mesoderm. It is loosely organized and the individual cells migrate to different parts of the body where they form most of the skeletal and connective tissue, the blood and blood system, and the visceral (smooth) muscles.

mesentery *n.* a double layer of *peritoneum attaching the stomach, small intestine, pancreas, spleen, and other abdominal organs to the posterior wall of the abdomen. It contains blood and lymph vessels and nerves supplying these organs. —**mesenteric** *adj.*

mesial *adj.* 1. medial. 2. relating to or situated in the *median line or plane. 3. designating the surface of a tooth towards the midline of the jaw.

mesiodens *n.* an extra tooth that may occur in the midline of the palate, between the central incisors, and may interfere with their eruption.

mesmerism *n.* *hypnosis based on the ideas of the 18th-century physician Franz Mesmer, sometimes employing magnets and a variety of other equipment.

mesna *n.* a drug administered by mouth or intravenous injection to prevent the toxic effects of *alkylating agents, particularly *ifosfamide and *cyclophosphamide, on the bladder. It binds with the toxic metabolite acrolein in the urine. Trade name: **Uromitexan**.

mesoappendix *n.* the *mesentery of the appendix.

mesocolon *n.* the fold of peritoneum by which the colon is fixed to the posterior abdominal wall. Usually only the **transverse** and **sigmoid mesocolons** persist in the adult, attached to the transverse and sigmoid colon, respectively.

mesoderm *n.* the middle *germ layer of the early embryo. It gives rise to cartilage, muscle, bone, blood, kidneys, gonads and their ducts, and connective tissue. It separates into two layers – an outer **somatic** and an inner **splanchnic mesoderm**, separated by a cavity (**coelom**) that becomes the body cavity. The dorsal somatic mesoderm becomes segmented into a number of *somites. *See also* MESENCHYME. —**mesodermal** *adj.*

mesometrium *n.* the broad ligament of the uterus: a sheet of connective tissue that carries blood vessels to the uterus and attaches it to the abdominal wall.

mesomorphic *adj.* describing a *body type that has a well developed skeletal and muscular structure and a sturdy upright posture. —**mesomorph** *n.* —**mesomorphy** *n.*

mesonephros (Wolffian body) *n.* the second area of kidney tissue to develop in the embryo. Its excretory function only lasts for a very brief period before it degenerates. However, parts of it become incorporated into the male reproductive structures. Its duct – the **Wolffian** (or **mesonephric) duct** – persists in males as the epididymis and vas deferens, which conduct sperm from the testis. —**mesonephric** *adj.*

mesophilic *adj.* describing organisms, especially bacteria, that grow best at temperatures of about 25–45°C. *Compare* PSYCHROPHILIC, THERMOPHILIC.

mesosalpinx *n.* a fold of peritoneum that surrounds the Fallopian tubes. It is the upper part of the broad ligament that surrounds the uterus.

mesosome *n.* a structure occurring in some bacterial cells, formed by infolding of the cell membrane. Mesosomes are associated with the DNA and play a part in cell division.

mesotendon *n.* the delicate connective tissue membrane that surrounds a tendon.

mesothelioma *n.* a tumour of the pleura, peritoneum, or pericardium. The occurrence of pleural mesothelioma is often due to exposure to asbestos dust (*see* ASBESTOSIS), and workers in the asbestos industry who develop such tumours are entitled to industrial compensation. In other cases there is no history of direct exposure to asbestos at work but the patients had been exposed to asbestos via the clothes of relatives who had had direct contact with asbestos, or they themselves had lived very close to an asbestos factory. There is no curative treatment for the disease, but moderately good results have occasionally been obtained from radical surgery for limited disease, from radiotherapy, and more recently from chemotherapy.

mesothelium *n.* the single layer of cells that lines *serous membranes. It is derived from embryonic mesoderm. *Compare* EPITHELIUM.

mesovarium *n.* the *mesentery of the ovaries.

messenger RNA a type of RNA that carries the information of the *genetic code of the DNA from the cell nucleus to the ribosomes, where the code is translated into protein. *See* TRANSCRIPTION, TRANSLATION.

mestranol *n.* a synthetic female sex hormone (*see* OESTROGEN) used in combination with a progestogen (*norethisterone) as an *oral contraceptive. Trade name: **Norinyl-1**.

MET *see* MEDICAL EMERGENCY TEAM.

met- (meta-) *prefix denoting* **1.** distal to; beyond; behind. **2.** change; transformation.

meta-analysis *n.* a statistical technique for combining and analysing the results of a number of different studies on the same topic to enable identification of trends and patterns and more accurate estimation of significant effects.

metabolic syndrome (dysmetabolic syndrome, insulin resistance syndrome, syndrome X) a common combination of *insulin resistance and type 2 diabetes with central obesity (i.e. with fat distribution mainly around the waist), high blood pressure, and *hyperlipidaemia. It is associated with a risk of early atherosclerosis.

metabolism *n.* **1.** the sum of all the chemical and physical changes that take place within the body and enable its continued growth and functioning. Metabolism involves the breakdown of complex organic constituents of the body with the liberation of energy, which is required for other processes (*see* CATABOLISM) and the building up of complex substances, which form the material of the tissues and organs, from simple ones (*see* ANABOLISM). *See also* BASAL METABOLISM. **2.** the sum of the biochemical changes undergone by a particular constituent of the body; for example, protein metabolism. —**metabolic** *adj.*

metabolite *n.* a substance that takes part in the process of *metabolism. Metabolites are either produced during metabolism or are constituents of food taken into the body.

metacarpal 1. *adj.* relating to the bones of the hand (*metacarpus). **2.** *n.* any of the bones forming the metacarpus.

metacarpus *n.* the five bones of the hand that connect the *carpus (wrist) to the *phalanges (digits).

metacentric *n.* a chromosome in which the centromere is at or near the centre of the chromosome. —**metacentric** *adj.*

metacercaria *n.* (*pl.* **metacercariae**) a mature form of the *cercaria larva of a fluke. Liver fluke metacercariae are enveloped by thin cysts and develop on various kinds of vegetation.

metachromasia (metachromatism) *n.* **1.** the property of a dye of staining certain tissues or cells a colour that is different from that of the stain itself. **2.** the variation in colour produced in certain tissue elements that are stained with the same dye. **3.** abnormal coloration of a tissue produced by a particular stain. —**metachromatic** *adj.*

metaethics *n.* the study of moral rules, principles, problems, attitudes, and behaviour. *See also* ETHICS.

Metagonimus *n.* a genus of small flukes, usually less than 3 mm in length, that are common as parasites of dogs and cats in the Far East, N Siberia, and the Balkan States. Adult flukes of *M. yokogawai* occasionally infect the human duodenum if undercooked fish (the intermediate host) is eaten. They may cause inflammation and some ulceration of the intestinal lining, which produces a mild diarrhoea. Flukes can be easily removed with tetrachloroethylene.

metamorphopsia *n.* a condition in which objects appear distorted. It is usually due to a disorder of the retina affecting the *macula (the most sensitive part).

metamyelocyte *n.* an immature *granulocyte (a type of white blood cell), having a kidney-shaped nucleus (*compare* MYELOCYTE) and cytoplasm containing neutrophil, eosinophil, or basophil granules. It is normally found in the blood-forming tissue of the bone marrow but may appear in the blood in a wide variety of diseases, including acute infections and chronic *myeloid leukaemia. *See also* GRANULOPOIESIS.

metanephros *n.* the excretory organ of the fetus, which develops into the kidney and is formed from the rear portion of the *nephrogenic cord. It does not become functional until birth, since urea is transferred across the placenta to the mother.

metaphase *n.* the second stage of *mitosis and of each division of *meiosis, in which the chromosomes line up at the centre of the *spindle, with their centromeres attached to the spindle fibres.

metaphysis *n.* the growing portion of a long bone that lies between the *epiphyses (the ends) and the *diaphysis (the shaft).

metaplasia *n.* an abnormal change in the nature of a tissue, usually in response to an environmental factor. For instance, columnar epithelium lining the bronchi may be converted to squamous epithelium (**squamous metaplasia**) following exposure to cigarette smoke. Prolonged exposure to gastric acid may result in the squamous epithelium of the oesophagus being converted to glandular epithelium (**glandular metaplasia**). **Myeloid metaplasia** is the development of bone marrow elements, normally found only within the marrow cavities of the bones, in organs such as the spleen and liver. This may occur after bone marrow failure. Metaplasia is not itself a premalignant condition, but neoplasms (abnormal new growths) may arise in metaplastic tissues if the initiating stimulus is not removed. —**metaplastic** *adj.*

metaraminol *n.* a *sympathomimetic drug that stimulates alpha receptors and is used as a *vasoconstrictor to treat acute *hypotension. It is administered by intravenous injection or infusion.

metastasis *n.* the spread of a malignant tumour from its site of origin. This occurs by three main routes: (1) through the bloodstream (haematogenous); (2) through the

m

lymphatic system; (3) across body cavities, e.g. through the peritoneum (*see* TRANSCOE-LOMIC SPREAD). Highly malignant tumours have a greater potential for metastasis. Individual tumours may spread by one or all of the above routes, although *carcinoma is said classically to metastasize via the lymphatics and *sarcoma via the bloodstream. —**metastatic** *adj.*

metastasize *vb.* (of a malignant tumour) to spread by *metastasis.

metastatic calcification the calcification of otherwise normal tissues in patients with *hypercalcaemia. *Compare* DYSTROPHIC CALCIFICATION.

metatarsal 1. *adj.* relating to the bones of the foot (*metatarsus). 2. *n.* any of the bones forming the metatarsus.

metatarsalgia *n.* aching pain in the metatarsal bones of the foot. It usually arises beneath the metatarsal heads in the transverse plantar arch. Repeated injury, arthritis, and deformities of the foot are common causes, and corrective footwear and insoles may be prescribed.

metatarsus *n.* the five bones of the foot that connect the *tarsus (ankle) to the *phalanges (toes).

metathalamus *n.* a part of the *thalamus consisting of two nuclei through which impulses pass from the eyes and ears to be distributed to the cerebral cortex.

metencephalon *n.* part of the hindbrain, formed by the pons and the cerebellum and continuous below with the medulla oblongata. *See* BRAIN.

meteorism *n. see* TYMPANITES.

-meter *combining form denoting* an instrument for measuring. Example: **perimeter** (instrument for measuring the field of vision).

metformin *n.* a *biguanide drug that is used to treat type 2 diabetes. It is administered by mouth and may cause loss of appetite and minor digestive upsets; it should not be used in patients with kidney disease, in whom it may cause *lactic acidosis. Trade names: **Bolamyn SR**, **Glucophage**. *See also* ORAL HYPOGLYCAEMIC DRUG.

methadone *n.* a potent opioid (*see* OPIATE) administered by mouth or injection to relieve severe pain and as a linctus to suppress coughs in terminal illness. An opioid agonist, it can also be substituted for heroin to prevent withdrawal symptoms in heroin dependence. Digestive upsets, drowsiness, and dizziness may occur, and prolonged use may lead to dependence. Trade names: **Methadose**, **Physeptone**, **Synastone**.

methaemalbumin *n.* a chemical complex of the pigment portion of haemoglobin (**haem**) with the plasma protein *albumin. It is formed in the blood in such conditions as *blackwater fever or paroxysmal nocturnal haemoglobinuria, in which red blood cells are destroyed and free haemoglobin is released into the plasma. In such conditions methaemalbumin can be detected in both the blood and urine.

methaemoglobin *n.* a substance formed when the iron atoms of the blood pigment *haemoglobin have been oxidized from the ferrous to the ferric form (*compare* OXY-HAEMOGLOBIN). The methaemoglobin cannot bind molecular oxygen and therefore it cannot transport oxygen round the body. The presence of methaemoglobin in the blood (**methaemoglobinaemia**) may result from the ingestion of oxidizing drugs or from an inherited abnormality of the haemoglobin molecule. Symptoms include fatigue, headache, dizziness and *cyanosis.

methanol *n. see* METHYL ALCOHOL.

methenamine (**hexamine**) *n.* a drug used for the prevention and treatment of chronic or recurrent lower urinary tract infections. It is taken by mouth; high doses may cause irritation of the stomach or bladder. Trade name: **Hiprex**.

methicillin *n. see* METICILLIN.

methimazole *n. see* CARBIMAZOLE.

methionine *n.* a sulphur-containing *essential amino acid. *See also* AMINO ACID.

methotrexate *n.* a drug that interferes with cell growth and is used to treat many types of cancer, including leukaemia in children and various solid tumours (*see* ANTI-METABOLITE, DIHYDROFOLATE REDUCTASE INHIBITOR). It also affects the immune response and may be used in the treatment of rheumatoid arthritis, Crohn's disease, and severe psoriasis (*see* DISEASE-MODIFYING AN-TIRHEUMATIC DRUG). Methotrexate is administered by mouth or injection; common side-effects include mouth sores, digestive upsets, skin rashes, and hair loss. Trade name: **Metoject**.

methotrimeprazine *n. see* LEVOMEPRO-MAZINE.

methyl alcohol (methanol) wood alcohol: an alcohol that is oxidized in the body much more slowly than ethyl alcohol and forms poisonous products. As little as 10 ml of pure methyl alcohol can produce permanent blindness, and 100 ml is likely to be fatal. The breakdown product formaldehyde is responsible for damage to the eyes; it is itself converted to formic acid, which causes acidosis and death from respiratory failure. *See also* METHYLATED SPIRITS.

methylated spirits a mixture consisting mainly of ethyl alcohol with *methyl alcohol and petroleum hydrocarbons. The addition of pyridine gives it an objectionable smell, and the dye methyl violet is added to make it recognizable as unfit to drink. It is used as a solvent, cleaning fluid, and fuel.

methylcellulose *n.* a compound that absorbs water and is used as a bulk *laxative to treat constipation, to control diarrhoea, and in patients with a *colostomy. It is administered by mouth and usually has no side-effects. Trade name: **Celevac**.

methyldopa *n.* a drug that acts on receptors in the brain to reduce blood pressure. It is administered by mouth or injection, and drowsiness commonly occurs during the first days of treatment. Trade name: **Aldomet**.

methylene blue a blue dye used to stain bacterial cells for microscopic examination.

methyl green a basic dye used for colouring the stainable part of the cell nucleus (chromatin) and – with pyronin – for the differential staining of RNA and DNA, which give a red and a green colour respectively.

methylmalonic aciduria (methylmalonic acidaemia, aminoacidopathy) a defect of amino acid metabolism causing an excess of methylmalonic acid in the urine and blood. There are two types: one is an *inborn error of metabolism due to a deficiency of the enzyme methylmalonyl-CoA mutase; the other is an acquired type due to deficiency of vitamin B_{12}, which results in defective synthesis of adenosylcobalamin (a cofactor in this metabolic process).

methylphenidate *n.* a drug that stimulates the central nervous system. Adminis-

tered by mouth, it is used to treat attention-deficit/hyperactivity disorder in children; side-effects such as nervousness and insomnia may occur. Trade names: **Concerta XL**, **Equasym XL**, **Medikinet XL**, **Ritalin**.

methylprednisolone *n.* a glucocorticoid (*see* CORTICOSTEROID) used in the treatment of inflammatory conditions and allergic states. It is administered by mouth or by intravenous, intramuscular, or intra-articular injection; side-effects include *electrolyte imbalance, muscle weakness, and abdominal distension. Trade names: **Depo-Medrone**, **Medrone**, **Solu-Medrone**.

methyl salicylate oil of wintergreen: a liquid with *counterirritant and *analgesic properties, applied to the skin as an ingredient in preparations to relieve pain in lumbago, sciatica, and rheumatic conditions.

methyl violet (gentian violet) a dye used mainly for staining protozoans.

methysergide *n.* a drug used to prevent severe migraine attacks and cluster headaches and to control diarrhoea associated with *carcinoid syndrome. Taken by mouth, it is administered under supervision in hospital because it carries a risk of dangerous fibrotic reactions (*see* FIBROSIS); other, more common, side-effects are digestive upsets, dizziness, and drowsiness. Trade name: **Deseril**.

meticillin (methicillin) *n.* a semisynthetic penicillin that was originally used to treat infections by penicillin-resistant staphylococci. It has been superseded for this purpose by *flucloxacillin but continues to be used to test the drug sensitivity of staphylococci. **Meticillin-resistant staphylococci** (MRS) can be responsible for increasing rates of infection in hospitals. Until recently, such infections have responded to *vancomycin, but strains of bacilli have emerged that are resistant to vancomycin, giving rise to infections that are very difficult to treat. *See also* SUPERINFECTION.

metoclopramide *n.* a drug that antagonizes the actions of *dopamine; it is used to treat nausea and vomiting, particularly when associated with gastrointestinal disorders. It is administered by mouth or injection; high doses may cause drowsiness and muscle spasms. Trade name: **Maxolon**.

metolazone *n.* a *diuretic used to treat fluid retention (oedema) and high blood pressure. It is administered by mouth; side-effects include headache, loss of appetite, and digestive upsets, and blood potassium levels may be reduced. Trade name: **Metenix 5**.

metoprolol *n.* a drug that controls the activity of the heart (*see* BETA BLOCKER) and is used to treat high blood pressure, angina, and abnormal heart rhythms. It is administered by mouth or injection; the commonest side-effects are tiredness and digestive upsets. Trade names: **Betaloc**, **Lopresor**.

metr- (metro-) *combining form denoting* the uterus.

metre *n.* the *SI unit of length that is equal to 39.37 inches. It is formally defined as the length of the path travelled by light in a vacuum during a time interval of 1/299 792 458 of a second. Symbol: m.

metritis *n.* inflammation of the uterus. *See also* ENDOMETRITIS, MYOMETRITIS.

metronidazole *n.* a drug used to treat infections of the urinary, genital, and digestive systems (such as trichomoniasis, *Helicobacter pylori* infection, amoebic dysentery, and giardiasis), acute ulcerative gingivitis, fungating wounds, and rosacea. It is administered by mouth, in suppositories, by infusion, or topically; side-effects include digestive upsets and an unpleasant taste in the mouth. Trade names: **Anabact**, **Flagyl**, **Metrogel**, **Metrolyl**, **Metrosa**, **Metrotop**, **Noritate**, **Rosiced**, **Rozex**, **Zyomet**.

-metry *combining form denoting* measuring or measurement.

metyrapone *n.* a drug that interferes with the production of the hormones *cortisol and *aldosterone and is used in the diagnosis and treatment of *Cushing's syndrome. It is administered by mouth. Side-effects may include nausea, vomiting, low blood pressure, and allergic reactions. Trade name: **Metopirone**.

MHC major histocompatibility complex: a series of genes located on chromosome no. 6 that code for antigens, including the *HLA antigens, that are important in the determination of histocompatibility.

MHRA *see* MEDICINES AND HEALTHCARE PRODUCTS REGULATORY AGENCY.

MHRT *see* MENTAL HEALTH REVIEW TRIBUNAL.

mianserin *n.* a drug related to the tricyclic *antidepressants, that is used to relieve moderate or severe depression associated with anxiety. It is administered by mouth; side-effects are milder than with tricyclic antidepressants, the commonest being drowsiness.

MIBG Meta-IodoBenzylGuanidine: a radioactive *tracer, labelled with iodine-123 or iodine-131, which binds to adrenergic nerve tissue. With the aid of a gamma camera, it can be used to detect the presence of a range of adrenergic tumours, including *neuroblastoma and *phaeochromocytoma.

micelle *n.* one of the microscopic particles into which the products of fat digestion (i.e. fatty acids and monoglycerides), present in the gut, are dispersed by the action of *bile salts. Fatty material in this finely dispersed form is more easily absorbed by the small intestine.

Michaelis-Gutmann bodies *see* MALAKOPLAKIA.

miconazole *n.* a drug used to treat fungal skin infections, such as *ringworm of the scalp, body, and feet, and oral and vaginal candidiasis (*see* IMIDAZOLE). It is administered by mouth, intravaginally, or topically; side-effects include itching, skin rash, and nausea and vomiting. Trade names: **Daktarin**, **Gyno-Daktarin**.

micr- (micro-) *combining form denoting* 1. small size. 2. one millionth part.

microaerophilic *adj.* describing microorganisms that grow best at very low oxygen concentrations (i.e. below the atmospheric level).

microalbuminuria *n.* the presence of albumin in the urine at levels that are higher than normal but lower than those detected by standard protein dipsticks. The measured cut-offs are 30–300 mg/24 hours. Microalbuminuria is an important risk factor for the development of cardiac disease among diabetics. Its presence can be reversed by medication and careful control of blood pressure.

microaneurysm *n.* a minute localized swelling of a capillary wall, which is found in the retina of patients with diabetic *retinopathy. It is recognized as a small red dot when the interior of the eye is examined with an *ophthalmoscope.

microangiopathy *n.* damage to the walls of the smallest blood vessels. It may result from a variety of diseases, including diabetes mellitus, connective-tissue diseases, infections, and cancer. Some common manifestations of microangiopathy are kidney failure, haemolysis (damage to red blood cells), and purpura (bleeding into the skin). The treatment is that of the underlying cause.

microbe *n. see* MICROORGANISM.

microbiology *n.* the science of *microorganisms. Microbiology in relation to medicine is concerned mainly with the isolation and identification of the microorganisms that cause disease. —**microbiological** *adj.* —**microbiologist** *n.*

microblepharon (microblepharism) *n.* the condition of having abnormally small eyelids.

microbubbles *pl. n.* (in radiology) an ultrasound *contrast medium consisting of small bubbles containing gas that are introduced into the vascular system or the Fallopian tubes in order to enhance ultrasound images.

microcephaly *n.* abnormal smallness of the head in relation to the size of the rest of the body: a congenital condition in which the brain is not fully developed. *Compare* MACROCEPHALY.

microcheilia *n.* abnormally small size of the lips. *Compare* MACROCHEILIA.

Micrococcus *n.* a genus of spherical Gram-positive bacteria occurring in colonies. They are saprophytes or parasites. The species *M. tetragenus* (formerly *Gaffkya tetragena*) is normally a harmless parasite in humans but it can become pathogenic, causing arthritis, endocarditis, meningitis, or abscesses in tissues. It occurs in groups of four.

microcyte *n.* an abnormally small red blood cell (*erythrocyte). *See also* MICROCYTOSIS. —**microcytic** *adj.*

microcytosis *n.* the presence of abnormally small red cells (**microcytes**) in the blood. Microcytosis is a feature of certain anaemias (**microcytic anaemias**), including iron-deficiency anaemias, certain *haemoglobinopathies, anaemias associated with chronic infections, etc.

microdactyly *n.* abnormal smallness or shortness of the fingers.

microdiscectomy *n.* surgical removal of all or part of a *prolapsed intervertebral disc

using an *operating microscope, a very short incision, and very fine instruments that can be inserted between the individual vertebrae of the backbone. The procedure is used to relieve pressure on spinal nerve roots or on the spinal cord caused by protrusion of the pulpy matter of the disc (**nucleus pulposus**). This is a form of *minimally invasive surgery.

microdissection *n.* the process of dissecting minute structures under the microscope. Miniature surgical instruments, such as knives made of glass, are manipulated by means of geared connections that reduce the relatively coarse movements of the operator's fingers into microscopic movements. Using this technique it is possible to dissect the nuclei of cells and even to separate individual chromosomes. *See also* MICROSURGERY.

microdochectomy *n.* an exploratory operation on the mammary ducts, usually to detect (or exclude) the presence of a suspected tumour (adenoma).

microdontia *n.* a condition in which the teeth are unusually small.

microelectrode *n.* an extremely fine wire used as an electrode to measure the electrical activity in small areas of tissue. Microelectrodes can be used for recording the electrical changes that occur in the membranes of cells, such as those of nerve and muscle.

microfilaria *n.* (*pl.* **microfilariae**) the motile embryo of certain nematodes (*see* FILARIA). The slender microfilariae, 150–300 μm in length, are commonly found in the circulating blood or lymph of patients suffering an infection with any of the filarial worms, e.g. *Wuchereria*. They mature into larvae, which are infective, within the body of a bloodsucking insect, such as a mosquito.

microgamete *n.* the motile flagellate male sex cell of the malarial parasite (*Plasmodium*) and other protozoans. The microgamete is similar to the sperm cell of animals and smaller than the female sex cell (*see* MACROGAMETE).

microgametocyte *n.* a cell that undergoes meiosis to form 6–8 mature male sex cells (microgametes) of the malarial parasite (*see* PLASMODIUM). Microgametocytes are found in human blood but must be ingested by a mosquito before developing into microgametes.

microglia *n.* one of the two basic classes of *glia (the non-nervous cells of the central nervous system), having a mainly scavenging function (*see* MACROPHAGE). *Compare* MACROGLIA.

microglossia *n.* abnormally small size of the tongue.

micrognathia *n.* a condition in which one or both jaws are unusually small.

microgram *n.* one millionth of a gram. Symbol: μg.

micrograph (photomicrograph) *n.* a photograph of an object as viewed through a microscope. An **electron micrograph** is photographed through an electron microscope; a **light micrograph** through a light microscope.

microgyria *n.* a developmental disorder of the brain in which the folds (convolutions) in its surface are small and its surface layer (cortex) is structurally abnormal. It is associated with mental and physical retardation.

microhaematocrit *n.* a measurement of the proportion of red blood cells in a volume of circulating blood. It is determined by taking a sample of the patient's blood in a fine tube and spinning it in a centrifuge until settling is complete. *See* PACKED CELL VOLUME.

micromanipulation *n.* the manipulation of extremely small structures under the microscope, as in *microdissection, or *microsurgery.

micromelia *n.* abnormally small size of the arms or legs. *Compare* MACROMELIA.

micrometastasis *n.* a secondary tumour that is undetectable by clinical examination or diagnostic tests but is visible under the microscope.

micrometer *n.* an instrument for making extremely fine measurements of thickness or length, often relying upon the movement of a screw thread and the principle of the *vernier.

micrometre *n.* one millionth of a metre (10^{-6} m). Symbol: μm.

microorganism (microbe) *n.* any organism too small to be visible to the naked eye. Microorganisms include *bacteria (including *mycoplasmas and *rickettsiae), some *fungi, *protozoa, and *viruses.

microphotograph *n.* 1. a photograph reduced to microscopic proportions. 2. (loosely) a *photomicrograph.

microphthalmos *n.* a congenitally small eye, usually associated with a small eye socket.

micropipette *n.* an extremely fine tube from which minute volumes of liquid can be delivered. It can also be used to draw up minute quantities of liquid for examination. Using a micropipette it is possible to add or take away material from individual cells under the microscope.

micropsia *n.* a condition in which objects appear smaller than they really are. It is usually due to disease of the retina affecting the *macula but may occur in paralysis of *accommodation.

microscope *n.* an instrument for producing a greatly magnified image of an object, which may be so small as to be invisible to the naked eye. **Light** or **optical microscopes** use light as a radiation source for viewing the specimen and combinations of lenses to magnify the image; these are usually an *objective and an *eyepiece. *See also* ELECTRON MICROSCOPE, OPERATING MICROSCOPE, ULTRAMICROSCOPE. —**microscopical** *adj.* —**microscopy** *n.*

microscopic *adj.* 1. too small to be seen clearly without the use of a microscope. 2. of, relating to, or using a microscope.

microsome *n.* a small particle consisting of a piece of *endoplasmic reticulum to which ribosomes are attached. Microsomes are formed when homogenized cells are centrifuged. —**microsomal** *adj.*

Microsporum *n.* a genus of fungi causing *ringworm. *See also* DERMATOPHYTE.

microsurgery *n.* the branch of surgery in which extremely intricate operations are performed through highly refined *operating microscopes using miniaturized precision instruments (forceps, scissors, needles, etc.). The technique enables surgery of previously inaccessible parts of the eye, inner ear, spinal cord, and brain (e.g. for the removal of tumours and repair of cerebral aneurysms), as well as the reattachment of amputated fingers (necessitating the suturing of minute nerves and blood vessels) and the reversal of vasectomies.

microsurgical epididymal sperm aspiration *see* MESA.

microtia *n.* a congenital deformity of the external ear in which the *pinna is small or absent. The ear canal may also be absent, giving a conductive *deafness. Microtia may be associated with other congenital deformities.

microtome *n.* an instrument for cutting extremely thin slices of material that can be examined under a microscope. The material is usually embedded in a suitable medium, such as paraffin wax. A common type of microtome is a steel knife.

microvascular *adj.* involving small vessels. The term is often applied to techniques of *microsurgery for reuniting small blood vessels (the same techniques are applied frequently to nerve suture).

microvillus *n.* (*pl.* **microvilli**) one of a number of microscopic hairlike structures (about 5 µm long) projecting from the surface of epithelial cells (*see* EPITHELIUM). They serve to increase the surface area of the cell and are seen on absorptive and secretory cells. In some regions (particularly the intestinal tract) microvilli form a dense covering on the free surface of the cells: this is called a **brush border**.

microwave endometrial ablation *see* ENDOMETRIAL ABLATION.

microwave therapy a form of *diathermy using electromagnetic waves of extremely short wavelength. In modern apparatus the electric currents induced in the tissues have frequencies of up to 25,000 million cycles per second.

micturating cystourethrogram (MCU) *see* URETHROGRAPHY.

micturition *n. see* URINATION.

midazolam *n.* a *benzodiazepine drug used as a sedative before and after surgery and to induce general anaesthesia. It is administered by injection. Possible side-effects include headache, dizziness, and difficulty in breathing. Trade name: **Hypnovel**.

midbrain (mesencephalon) *n.* the small portion of the *brainstem, excluding the pons and the medulla, that joins the hindbrain to the forebrain.

middle ear (tympanic cavity) the part of the *ear that consists of an air-filled space within the petrous part of the temporal bone. It is lined with mucous membrane and is connected to the pharynx by the *Eustachian tube and to the outer ear by the eardrum (*tympanic membrane). Within the middle ear are three bones – the auditory *ossicles – which transmit sound vibrations from the outer ear to the inner ear (*see* LABYRINTH).

midgut *n.* the middle portion of the embryonic gut, which gives rise to most of the small intestine and part of the large intestine. Early in development it is connected with the *yolk sac outside the embryo via the *umbilicus.

midstream specimen of urine (MSU) a specimen of urine that is subjected to examination for the presence of microorganisms. In order to obtain a specimen that is free of contamination, the periurethral area is cleansed and the patient is requested to discard the initial flow of urine before collecting the specimen in a sterile container.

midwifery *n.* the profession of providing assistance and medical care to women undergoing labour and childbirth during the antenatal, perinatal, and postnatal periods. *See also* COMMUNITY MIDWIFE, OBSTETRICS. —**midwife** *n.*

mifepristone *n.* a drug used to produce a medical abortion; it acts by blocking the action of *progesterone, which is essential for maintaining pregnancy. It is taken by mouth, followed after 36–48 hours by *gemeprost or *misoprostol intravaginally. Side-effects include faintness, headache, and vaginal bleeding. Trade name: **Mifegyne**.

migraine *n.* a neurovascular disorder in a genetically predisposed individual. There is an instability within the brainstem that is triggered by a variety of stimuli (e.g. foods, light, stress) and results in a recurrent throbbing headache that characteristically affects one side of the head. The patient sometimes has forewarning of an attack (an **aura**) consisting of visual disturbance or tingling and/or weakness of the limbs, which clear up as the headache develops. It is often accompanied by prostration, nausea and vomiting, and *photophobia. Effective preventive medication (e.g. beta blockers and some antiepileptic drugs) is available for patients with frequent migraine attacks, and *$5HT_1$ agonists may be used to treat acute attacks. *See also* CLUSTER HEADACHE.

Mikulicz's disease swelling of the lacrimal and salivary glands as a result of infiltration with *lymphoid tissue. [J. von

Mikulicz Radecki (1850–1905), Polish surgeon]

miliaria rubra *see* PRICKLY HEAT.

miliary *adj.* describing or characterized by very small nodules or lesions, resembling millet seed.

miliary tuberculosis acute generalized *tuberculosis characterized by lesions in affected organs, which resemble millet seeds.

milium *n.* (*pl.* **milia**) a white nodule in the skin, particularly on the face. Up to 2 mm in diameter, milia are tiny *keratin cysts occurring just beneath the outer layer (epidermis) of the skin. Milia are commonly seen in newborn babies around the nose; they may disappear without active treatment. In adults they may be lifted out with a needle or removed by an abrasive sponge.

milk *n.* the liquid food secreted by female mammals from the mammary gland. It is the sole source of food for the young of most mammals at the start of life. Milk is a complete food in that it has most of the nutrients necessary for life: protein, carbohydrate, fat, minerals, and vitamins. The composition of milk varies very much from mammal to mammal. Cows' milk contains nearly all the essential nutrients but is comparatively deficient in vitamins C and D. Human milk contains more sugar (lactose) and less protein than cows' milk.

milk formulas See Appendix 9.

milk rash a spotty red facial rash that is common during the first few months of life; it disappears without treatment.

milk teeth *Colloquial.* the primary teeth of children. *See* DENTITION.

Miller-Deiker syndrome a chromosomal abnormality resulting in a characteristic facial appearance and the absence of the grooves on the surface of the brain (*see* LISSENCEPHALY). Affected individuals have severe mental retardation.

milli- *prefix denoting* one thousandth part.

milliamp *n.* short for **milliampere**: one thousandth of an *ampere (10^{-3} A; symbol: mA). In radiography, the mA setting on an X-ray machine determines the number of X-ray photons produced per second. The setting is important to obtain appropriate exposure and varies with body size (among other factors). *See also* KILOVOLT.

milligram *n.* one thousandth of a gram. Symbol: mg.

millilitre *n.* one thousandth of a litre. Symbol: ml. *See* LITRE.

millimetre *n.* one thousandth of a metre (10^{-3} m). Symbol: mm.

millimole *n.* one thousandth of a mole (*see* MOLE[1]). The concentration of a solution is expressed in millimoles per litre. Symbol: mmol.

milnacipran *n. see* SNRI.

Milroy's disease *see* LYMPHOEDEMA. [W. F. Milroy (1855–1942), US physician]

Minamata disease a form of mercury poisoning (from ingesting methyl mercury in contaminated fish) that caused 43 deaths in the Japanese coastal town of Minamata during 1953–56. The source of mercury was traced to an effluent containing mercuric sulphate from a local PVC factory. Symptoms include numbness, difficulty in controlling the limbs, and impaired speech and hearing.

MIND the National Association for Mental Health. It is a voluntary association, registered as a charity that promotes the welfare of those with *mental illness through advice, education, campaigning, and the provision of resources.

mineralocorticoid *n. see* CORTICO-STEROID.

minim *n.* a unit of volume used in pharmacy, equivalent to one sixtieth part of a fluid *drachm.

minimal change nephropathy the commonest cause of *nephrotic syndrome in children and an important cause of this syndrome in adults. The condition is so named because of the apparent lack of abnormalities seen on light microscopy of biopsy samples. Changes can, however, be seen on electron microscopy, with effacement of the *podocyte foot processes along the glomerular basement membrane. It is postulated that minimal change disease is a T-cell disease and that *cytokine damage to the podocytes leads to loss of the selective filtering characteristics of the glomerulus. The condition usually responds to corticosteroids and has a good prognosis, but there is clinical overlap with primary *focal segmental glomerulosclerosis, which may have similar histological appearances in its early stages, tends not to respond to steroids, and is associated with a poor renal prognosis.

minimally invasive surgery (minimal-access surgery) surgical intervention involving the least possible physical trauma to the patient, particularly surgery performed using an operating laparoscope or other endoscope (*see* LAPAROSCOPY) passed through a tiny incision; it is known popularly as **keyhole surgery**. Several types of abdominal surgery, including gall bladder removal (*see* CHOLECYSTECTOMY) and extracorporeal shock-wave *lithotripsy for stones in the urinary or bile drainage system, are commonly performed in this way. Such methods usually allow the patient to resume normal activity much sooner than would be possible after more conventional procedures. *See also* INTERVENTIONAL RADIOLOGY.

minitracheostomy *n.* temporary *tracheostomy using a needle or fine-bore tube inserted through the skin.

minocycline *n.* a *tetracycline antibiotic active against a wide range of bacteria, including *Chlamydia*, *Borrelia*, rickettsiae, and mycoplasmas. It is administered by mouth; side-effects include loss of appetite, skin rash, and dizziness. Trade names: **Acnamino MR**, **Minocin MR**, **Sebomin MR**.

minoxidil *n.* a peripheral vasodilator used in the treatment of high blood pressure (hypertension) when other drugs are not effective; it is administered by mouth in conjunction with a diuretic and a beta blocker. Side-effects include ECG changes and transient oedema. It is also applied to the scalp, in the form of a solution, to restore hair growth. Trade names: **Loniten**, **Regaine**.

mio- *combining form denoting* 1. reduction or diminution. 2. rudimentary.

miosis (myosis) *n.* constriction of the pupil. This occurs normally in bright light. It is also seen in *Horner's syndrome, but persistent miosis is most commonly caused by certain types of eye drops used to treat glaucoma. *See also* MIOTIC. *Compare* MYDRIASIS. —**miotic** *adj.*

miotic 1. *n.* a drug that causes the pupil of the eye to contract by constricting the ciliary muscle (*see* CILIARY BODY). Miotics, such as *pilocarpine, are used to reduce the pressure in the eye in the treatment of glaucoma: contraction of the ciliary muscle increases the angle between the iris and cornea through

which aqueous humour drains from the eye. 2. *adj.* showing *miosis.

miracidium *n.* (*pl.* **miracidia**) the first-stage larva of a parasitic *fluke. Miracidia hatch from eggs released into water with the host's excreta. They have *cilia and swim about until they reach a snail. The miracidia then bore into the snail's soft tissues and there continue their development as *sporocysts.

Mirena *n. see* IUS.

miscarriage *n.* spontaneous loss of pregnancy before 24 weeks, formerly known as **spontaneous abortion**. In **threatened miscarriage** there is vaginal bleeding (often minimal) associated with mild period-type pains; the cervix is closed and ultrasound confirms a viable pregnancy. In **inevitable miscarriage**, vaginal bleeding is associated with crampy pelvic pains and an open cervix; the pregnancy has not yet been expelled, but eventually will be. The miscarriage is **incomplete** if the cervix remains open and the uterus still contains some fetal tissue (which may need to be removed to prevent further haemorrhage). The miscarriage is **complete** if the cervix has closed and ultrasound scanning shows an empty uterus. Failure of a nonviable fetus to be expelled from the uterus is called a **silent** (or **missed**) **miscarriage**. A **late miscarriage** is one occurring after 20–24 weeks when the fetus has shown no signs of life after delivery. **Recurrent miscarriage** is the loss of three or more pregnancies consecutively; there are many possible causes, including *antiphospholipid antibody syndrome.

miso- *combining form denoting* hatred. Example: **misopedia** (of children).

misophonia *n.* dislike of or aversion to sound. *See* HYPERACUSIS; PHONOPHOBIA.

misoprostol *n.* a *prostaglandin drug administered by mouth in the prevention and treatment of peptic ulcer, especially when caused by nonsteroidal anti-inflammatory drugs (*see* NSAID), in which case it is given in conjunction with the NSAID (*see* DICLOFENAC, NAPROXEN). It is also used to terminate a pregnancy, being administered vaginally following *mifepristone. Possible side-effects include diarrhoea. Trade name: **Cytotec**.

Misuse of Drugs Act 1971 (in the UK) an Act of Parliament restricting the use of dangerous drugs. These **controlled drugs** are divided into three classes: class A drugs (e.g. heroin, morphine and other potent opioid analgesics, cocaine, LSD) cause the most harm when misused; class B drugs include amphetamines, barbiturates, and cannabis, and class C drugs include most benzodiazepines and anabolic steroids. The Act specifies certain requirements for writing prescriptions for these drugs. The Misuse of Drugs (Supply to Addicts) Regulations 1997 and the Misuse of Drugs Regulations 2001 lay down who may supply controlled drugs and the rules governing their supply, prescription, etc.

mite *n.* a free-living or parasitic arthropod belonging to a group (Acarina) that also includes the *ticks. Most mites are small, averaging 1 mm or less in length. A mite has no antennae or wings, and its body is not divided into a distinct head, thorax, and abdomen. Medically important mites include the many species causing dermatitis (e.g. *Dermatophagoides*) and the harvest mite (*see* TROMBICULA), which transmits scrub typhus.

mitochondrial disorders a group of inherited conditions transmitted through mitochondrial DNA (*see* MITOCHONDRION), which can affect any organ and can present at any age. Most of these conditions are very rare; examples of those that are less rare include *Leigh syndrome, congenital *lactic acidosis, *MELAS, and Pearson syndrome.

mitochondrion (chondriosome) *n.* (*pl.* **mitochondria**) a structure, occurring in varying numbers in the cytoplasm of every cell, that is the site of the cell's energy production. Mitochondria contain *ATP and the enzymes involved in the cell's metabolic activities, and also their own DNA; mitochondrial genes (which in humans encode 13 proteins) are inherited through the female line. Each mitochondrion is bounded by a double membrane, the inner being folded inwards to form projections (**cristae**). —**mitochondrial** *adj.*

mitogen *n.* any substance that can cause cells to begin division (*mitosis).

mitomycin an *anthracycline antibiotic that inhibits the growth of cancer cells. Administered intravenously or by bladder instillation, it causes severe marrow suppression but is of use in the treatment of stomach, breast, and bladder cancers. Trade name: **Mitomycin C Kyowa**.

mitosis *n.* a type of cell division in which a single cell produces two genetically identical daughter cells. It is the way in which new body cells are produced for both growth and repair. Division of the nucleus (**karyokinesis**) takes place in four stages (*see* PROPHASE, METAPHASE, ANAPHASE, TELOPHASE) and is followed by division of the cytoplasm (**cytokinesis**) to form the two daughter cells (see illustration). *Compare* MEIOSIS. —**mitotic** *adj.*

mitotic index the proportion of cells in a tissue that are dividing at a given time.

mitoxantrone *n.* an *anthracycline antibiotic used in the treatment of certain cancers, including prostate cancer and non-Hodgkin's lymphoma. It is given intravenously; side-effects are usually mild. Trade name: **Onkotrone**.

mitral regurgitation (mitral incompetence) failure of the *mitral valve to close, allowing a reflux of blood from the left ventricle of the heart to the left atrium. It may be due to **mitral valve prolapse** (**MVP**) in which one or both valve leaflets flop back into the left atrium (also known as 'floppy mitral valve'). It also results from chronic rheumatic scarring of the valve, or is secondary to left ventricular muscle damage. Its manifestations include breathlessness, atrial *fibrillation, embolism, enlargement of the left ventricle, and a systolic *murmur. Mild cases are symptomless and require no treatment, but in severe cases the affected valve should be repaired or replaced with an artificial one (**mitral prosthesis**).

mitral stenosis narrowing of the opening of the mitral valve: a result of chronic scarring that follows rheumatic fever. It may be seen alone or combined with *mitral regurgitation. The symptoms are similar to those of mitral regurgitation except that the patient has a diastolic *murmur. Mild cases need no treatment, but severe cases are treated by reopening the stenosis with an Inoue balloon passed to the heart through the venous system under X-ray control (**percutaneous balloon mitral valvuloplasty**) or surgically by inserting an artificial valve (**mitral prosthesis**).

mitral valve (bicuspid valve) a valve in the heart consisting of two flaps (cusps) attached to the walls at the opening between the left atrium and left ventricle. It allows

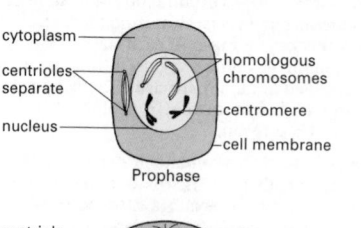

Prophase

- cytoplasm
- centrioles separate
- nucleus
- homologous chromosomes
- centromere
- cell membrane

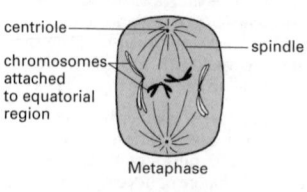

Metaphase

- centriole
- chromosomes attached to equatorial region
- spindle

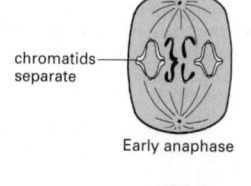

Early anaphase

- chromatids separate

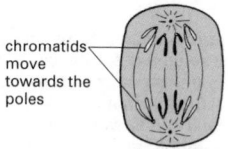

Anaphase

- chromatids move towards the poles

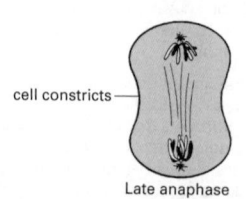

Late anaphase

- cell constricts

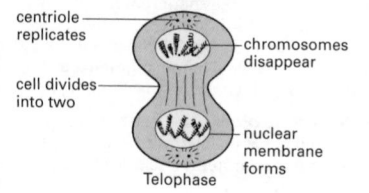

Telophase

- centriole replicates
- cell divides into two
- chromosomes disappear
- nuclear membrane forms

Stages in mitosis.

blood to pass from the atrium to the ventricle, but prevents any backward flow.

mittelschmerz *n.* pain in the lower abdomen experienced about midway between successive menstrual periods, i.e. when the egg cell is being released from the ovary. *See also* MENSTRUAL CYCLE.

mixed affective state a state of disordered mood that combines elements of *mania and *depression; it is a common feature of *bipolar affective disorder. Symptoms include overactivity, flight of ideas, depressed mood, and suicidal *ideation.

mixed connective tissue disease a disease with features in common with systemic *lupus erythematosus, *polymyositis, and *scleroderma. It is characterized by high levels of antibodies to ribonucleoprotein and most commonly affects women between 20 and 40 years of age.

ml *symbol for* *millilitre.

MLC *see* MLR.

MLD minimal lethal dose: the smallest quantity of a toxic compound that is recorded as having caused death. *See also* LD_{50}.

MLR (MLC) mixed lymphocyte reaction (or culture): a test in which lymphocytes from prospective donor and recipient are cultured together in a test tube to assess the suitability of transplanting organs or bone marrow cells.

mmHg a unit of pressure equal to 1 millimetre of mercury. 1 mmHg = 133.3224 pascals.

MMR vaccine a combined vaccine against *m*easles, *m*umps, and German measles (*r*ubella). It is currently recommended that this vaccine is given to all children at 13 months of age with a booster dose at 3½–5 years (*see* IMMUNIZATION). Specific contraindications include immunosuppression and allergy to eggs. Links between the vaccine and autism and Crohn's disease have been suggested, but these are as yet unsubstantiated.

MND *see* MOTOR NEURON DISEASE.

Mobitz type I and type II types of abnormality on an *electrocardiogram (ECG) tracing that indicate forms of *heart block, in which the communication between the upper and lower chambers of the heart is impaired. [W. Mobitz (20th century), German cardiologist]

moclobemide *n.* an antidepressant drug that reversibly inhibits the enzyme *monoamine oxidase A. The adverse effects of irreversible *MAO inhibitors, which include severe hypertensive reactions when cheese or other tyramine-containing foods are eaten by patients taking them, are less likely with reversible inhibitors. Moclobemide is used to treat major depression and social anxiety disorder; it is taken by mouth. Trade name: **Manerix**.

modality *n.* **1.** a form of sensation, such as smell, hearing, tasting, or detecting temperature. Differences in modality are not due to differences in the structure of the nerves concerned, but to differences in the working of the sensory receptors and the areas of brain that receive the messages. **2.** one form of therapy as opposed to another, such as the modality of physiotherapy contrasted with that of radiotherapy.

mode *n. see* MEAN.

Modecate *n. see* FLUPHENAZINE.

modelling *n.* **1.** a technique used in *behaviour modification, whereby an individual learns a behaviour by observing someone else doing it. Together with *prompting, it is useful for introducing new behaviours to the individual. **2.** An element of normal social learning and development whereby children learn through emulating other people's behaviour (often that of parents, other adults, or other children).

modified release (sustained release) describing an oral drug formulation that releases the active component slowly over a long period.

modiolus *n.* the conical central pillar of the *cochlea in the inner ear.

MODS *see* MULTIPLE ORGAN DYSFUNCTION SYNDROME.

Moduretic *n. see* AMILORIDE.

MODY *see* MATURITY-ONSET DIABETES OF THE YOUNG.

MOF multi-organ failure. *See* MULTIPLE ORGAN DYSFUNCTION SYNDROME.

Mohs' micrographic surgery a surgical technique used for removing primarily high-risk nonmelanoma skin cancers, particularly basal cell carcinoma. The technique allows the surgeon to see beyond the visible tumour as the specimen is removed and the histology checked in stages. At each stage, if the tumour involves the margins, further tissue is resected until they are clear. There is an extremely high cure rate. [F. E. Mohs (1910–2002), US surgeon]

molar *n.* in the permanent *dentition, the sixth, seventh, or eighth tooth from the midline on each side in each jaw (*see* WISDOM TOOTH). Permanent molars do not replace primary teeth. In the primary dentition, molars are the fourth and fifth teeth from the midline on each side in each jaw.

molar–incisor hypomineralization a deficiency in the mineralization of permanent first molar and incisor teeth, thought to be due to a disturbance of development around the time of birth.

molarity *n.* the strength of a solution, expressed as the weight of dissolved substance in grams per litre divided by its molecular weight, i.e. the number of moles per litre. Molarity is indicated as 0.1 M, 1 M, 2 M, etc.

molar solution a solution in which the number of grams of dissolved substance per litre equals its molecular weight, i.e. a solution of molarity 1 M.

mole[1] *n.* the *SI unit of amount of substance, equal to the amount of substance that contains as many elementary units as there are atoms in 0.012 kilograms of carbon-12. The elementary units, which must be specified, may be atoms, molecules, ions, electrons, etc., or a specified group of such entities. One mole of a compound has a mass equal to its molecular weight expressed in grams. Symbol: mol.

mole[2] *n.* a nonmalignant collection of pigmented cells in the skin. Moles are rare in infancy, increase in numbers during childhood and especially in adolescence, but decline in numbers in old age. They vary widely in appearance, being flat or raised, smooth or hairy. Changes in the shape, colour, etc., of moles in adult life should be investigated as this may be an early sign of malignant *melanoma. Medical name: **pigmented naevus**. *See also* ATYPICAL MOLE SYNDROME.

molecular biology the study of the molecules that are associated with living organisms, especially proteins and nucleic acids.

molecular imaging an emerging area of imaging that exploits recent developments of molecular and cell biology to create new markers. Most molecular imaging uses versions of these markers labelled with radioactive isotopes, which – after administration – are localized in the body and can be detected using such techniques as *positron emission tomography, *SPECT scanning, and *magnetic resonance spectroscopy.

molluscum contagiosum a common disease of the skin, mainly affecting children. Characterized by papules less than 5 mm in diameter, each with a central depression, the disease is caused by a *poxvirus and is spread by direct contact. Untreated, the papules generally disappear in 6–9 months. Widespread molluscum contagiosum in an adult may be a sign of HIV infection.

Molteno implant a valved device used in the surgical treatment of some types of glaucoma to control intraocular pressure by allowing fluid to drain from the anterior chamber into the subconjunctival space.

mon- (mono-) *combining form denoting* one, single, or alone.

MONA morphine, oxygen, nitrates, aspirin: the standard treatments for *acute coronary syndromes.

Mongolian blue spots blue-black pigmented areas seen at the base of the back and on the buttocks of babies. They are more common in dark-skinned babies and usually fade during the first year of life. The spots are sometimes mistaken for bruising.

mongolism *n. see* DOWN'S SYNDROME.

Monilia *n.* the former name of the genus of yeasts now known as *Candida.

moniliasis *n.* an obsolete name for *candidiasis.

Monitor an independent body set up under the Health and Social Care Act 2003 to authorize, monitor, and regulate *foundation trusts.

monoamine oxidase (MAO) an enzyme that catalyses the oxidation of a large variety of monoamines, including adrenaline, noradrenaline, and serotonin. Monoamine oxidase is found in most tissues, particularly the gastrointestinal tract and nervous system, and exists in two forms in humans: monoamine oxidase A primarily breaks down noradrenaline and serotonin, whereas monoamine oxidase B primarily degrades dopamine. Drugs that act as inhibitors of monoamine oxidase A may be used in the treatment of depression (*see* MAO INHIBITOR); monoamine oxidase B inhibitors are used to treat Parkinson's disease.

monoarthritis *n. see* ARTHRITIS.

monoblast *n.* the earliest identifiable cell that gives rise to a *monocyte. It is probably identical with the *myeloblast and matures via an intermediate stage (**promonocyte**). It is normally found in the blood-forming tissue of the *bone marrow but may appear in the blood in certain diseases, most notably in acute monoblastic *leukaemia.

monochorionicity *n. see* CHORIONICITY, TWINS. —**monochorionic** *adj.*

monochromat *n.* a person who is completely colour-blind. There are two types. The **rod monochromat** appears to have totally defective *cones: he has very poor visual acuity as well as the inability to discriminate colours. The **cone monochromat** has normal visual acuity: his cones appear to respond normally to light but to be completely unable to discriminate colours. It is possible in this case that the defect does not lie in the cones themselves but in the integration of the nerve impulses as they pass from the cones to the brain. Both types of colour blindness are probably inherited.

monochromatic *adj.* denoting radiation, especially light, of the same frequency or wavelength.

monoclonal antibody an antibody produced artificially from a cell *clone and therefore consisting of a single type of immunoglobulin. Monoclonal antibodies are produced by fusing antibody-forming lymphocytes from mouse spleen with mouse myeloma cells. The resulting hybrid cells multiply rapidly (like cancer cells) and produce the same antibody as their parent lymphocytes. In addition to their use in research, monoclonal antibodies are valuable diagnostic tools and have also been developed as pharmaceutical agents for treating a variety of conditions. For example, they are used in the detection and treatment of cancer, as each one recognizes different proteins on the surface of both malignant and benign cells. They can be used alone as monotherapy or to deliver drugs or radioactive materials (e.g. yttrium-90) directly to tumour cells.

monocular *adj.* relating to or used by one eye only. *Compare* BINOCULAR.

monocyte *n.* a variety of white blood cell, 16–20 μm in diameter, that has a kidney-shaped nucleus and greyish-blue cytoplasm (when treated with *Romanowsky stains). Its function is the ingestion of foreign particles, such as bacteria and tissue debris. There are normally $0.2–0.8 \times 10^9$ monocytes per litre of blood. —**monocytic** *adj.*

monocytosis *n.* an increase in the number of *monocytes in the blood. It occurs in a variety of diseases, including monocytic *leukaemia and infections due to some bacteria and protozoa.

monodactylism *n.* the congenital absence of all but one digit on each hand and foot.

monodelusional disorder a condition marked by a persistent delusion not associated with any other *mental illness. It is often of a *paranoid or persecutory nature, but in theory can have any delusional content. Treatment is often difficult because patients often lack insight and refuse to try medication. When compliance can be achieved, the majority of patients respond well to antipsychotic medication.

monoiodotyrosine *n.* an iodine-containing substance produced in the thyroid gland from which the *thyroid hormones are derived.

mononeuritis *n.* disease affecting a single peripheral nerve. **Mononeuritis multiplex** is the separate involvement of two or more nerves. *See also* PERIPHERAL NEUROPATHY.

mononucleosis *n.* the condition in which the blood contains an abnormally high number of mononuclear leucocytes (*monocytes and *lymphocytes). *See* GLANDULAR FEVER (INFECTIOUS MONONUCLEOSIS).

monophasic defibrillator *see* DEFIBRILLATOR.

monophyletic *adj.* describing a number of individuals, species, etc., that have evolved from a single ancestral group. *Compare* POLYPHYLETIC.

monoplegia *n.* paralysis of one limb. —**monoplegic** *adj.*

monoploid *adj. see* HAPLOID.

monorchism *n.* absence of one testis. This is usually due to failure of one testicle to descend into the scrotum before birth. The term is sometimes used for the condition in which one testicle has been removed surgically or destroyed by injury or disease. If the single testis is normal, no adverse effects result from the absence of the other.

monosaccharide *n.* a simple sugar having the general formula $(CH_2O)_n$. Monosaccharides may have between three and nine carbon atoms, but the most common number is five or six. Monosaccharides are classified according to the number of carbon atoms they possess. Thus **trioses** have three carbon atoms, **tetroses** four, **pentoses** five, and **hexoses** six. The most abundant monosaccharide is glucose (a hexose).

monosomy *n.* a condition in which there is one chromosome missing from the normal (*diploid) set. *Compare* TRISOMY. —**monosomic** *adj.*

monozygotic twins *see* TWINS.

mons *n.* (in anatomy) a rounded eminence. The **mons pubis** is the mound of fatty tissue lying over the pubic symphysis.

montelukast *n. see* LEUKOTRIENE RECEPTOR ANTAGONIST.

mood disorder *see* AFFECTIVE DISORDER.

mood stabilizer a drug used in the treatment of bipolar affective disorder to reduce the severity of manic and depressive episodes. Mood stabilizers include *lithium and *carbamazepine.

moon face the classical facial appearance of a patient with *Cushing's syndrome. The face is rounded and free of wrinkles, and the hair is often thin.

Mooren's ulcer a severe ulceration at the periphery of the cornea, characterized by an overhanging advancing edge and vascularization of the ulcer bed. It is usually very painful, progressive, and difficult to control. [A. Mooren (1829–99), German ophthalmologist]

moral agency the state of being able to make ethical or moral judgements and to take responsibility for choices and actions.

morality *n.* a system of values, normative rules, or principles according to which intentions or behaviours are judged to be *good or bad, *right or wrong. Such judgment can arise from cultural, religious, or philosophical beliefs. *See* ETHICS.

Moraxella *n.* a genus of short rodlike Gram-negative aerobic bacteria, usually occurring in pairs. They exist as parasites in many warm-blooded animals. The species *M. lacunata* causes conjunctivitis.

morbid *adj.* diseased or abnormal; pathological.

morbidity *n.* the state of being ill or having a disease. *See also* INCIDENCE RATE, PREVALENCE.

morbilli *n. see* MEASLES.

morbilliform *adj.* describing a *maculopapular skin rash resembling that of measles.

morbus *n.* disease. The term is usually used as part of the medical name of a specific disease.

mordant *n.* (in microscopy) a substance, such as alum or phenol, used to fix a *stain in a tissue.

moribund *adj.* dying.

morning sickness nausea and vomiting occurring during early pregnancy. In some women the symptoms disappear if a small amount of food is eaten before rising in the morning. *Compare* HYPEREMESIS GRAVIDARUM.

Moro reflex (startle reflex) a primitive reflex seen in newborn babies in response to the stimulus of a sudden noise or movement: the baby will fling its arms and legs wide and will appear to stiffen; the arms and legs are then drawn back into flexion. The Moro reflex should disappear spontaneously by four months. Its presence beyond this age is suggestive of an underlying neurological disorder, such as cerebral palsy. [E. Moro (1874–1951), German paediatrician]

morphine *n.* a potent opioid analgesic (*see* OPIATE) used mainly to relieve severe and persistent pain, particularly in terminally ill patients; it also induces feelings of euphoria. It is administered by mouth, injection, or in suppositories; common side-effects are nausea and vomiting, constipation, and drowsiness. With regular use, *tolerance develops and *dependence may occur. Trade names: **Morphgesic SR, MST Continus, MXL, Oramorph, Sevredol, Zomorph.**

morpho- *combining form denoting* form or structure.

morphoea *n.* a localized form of *scleroderma characterized by firm ivory-coloured waxy plaques in the skin without any internal sclerosis. The plaques may often disappear spontaneously but resolution is slow.

morphogenesis *n.* the development of form and structure of the body and its parts.

morphology *n. see* ANATOMY.

-morphous *combining form denoting* form or structure (of a specified kind).

Morquio-Brailsford disease a defect of *mucopolysaccharide metabolism (*see* INBORN ERROR OF METABOLISM) that causes dwarfism with a *kyphosis, a short neck, *knock-knee, and an angulated sternum in affected children. Intelligence is normal. [L. Morquio (1865–1935), Uruguayan physician; J. F. Brailsford (1888–1961), British radiologist]

mortality rate the incidence of death in the population in a given period. The **annual mortality rate** is the number of registered deaths in a year, multiplied by 1000 and divided by the population at the middle of the year. *See also* INFANT MORTALITY RATE, MATERNAL MORTALITY RATE.

mortification *n. see* NECROSIS.

morula *n.* an early stage of embryonic development formed by *cleavage of the fertilized ovum. It consists of a solid ball of cells and is an intermediate stage between the zygote and *blastocyst.

mosaicism *n.* a condition in which the cells of an individual do not all contain identical chromosomes; there may be two or more genetically different populations of cells. Often one of the cell populations is normal and the other carries a chromosome defect such as *Down's syndrome or *Turner's syndrome. In affected individuals the chromosome defect is usually not fully expressed. —**mosaic** *adj.*

mosquito *n.* a small winged bloodsucking insect belonging to a large group – the *Diptera (two-winged flies). Its mouthparts are formed into a long proboscis for piercing the skin and sucking blood. Female mosquitoes transmit the parasites responsible for several major infectious diseases, such as *malaria. *See* ANOPHELES, AËDES, CULEX.

motile *adj.* being able to move spontaneously, without external aid: usually applied to a *microorganism or a cell (e.g. a sperm cell).

motion sickness (**travel sickness**) nausea, vomiting, and headache caused by motion during travel by sea, road, or air. The symptoms are due to overstimulation of the balance organs in the inner ear by repeated small changes in the position of the body and are aggravated by movements of the horizon. Sedative antihistamine drugs (*see* ANTIEMETIC) are effective in preventing motion sickness.

motivational interviewing a technique that combines psychiatric assessment with elements of problem-solving *psychotherapy. It is mostly used with patients who have substance abuse problems. The interviewer elicits the psychiatric history and the extent of the patient's difficulties, gives educational information, and tries to motivate the patient to change his or her habits.

motor cortex the region of the *cerebral cortex that is responsible for initiating nerve impulses that bring about voluntary activity in the muscles of the body. It is possible to map out the cortex to show which of its areas is responsible for which particular part of the body. The motor cortex of the left cerebral hemisphere is responsible for muscular activity in the right side of the body.

motor nerve one of the nerves that carry impulses outwards from the central nervous system to bring about activity in a muscle or gland. *Compare* SENSORY NERVE.

motor neuron one of the units (*neurons) that goes to make up the nerve pathway between the brain and an effector organ, such as a skeletal muscle. An **upper motor neuron** has a cell body in the brain and an axon that extends into the spinal cord, where it ends in synapses. It is thus entirely within the central nervous system. A **lower motor neuron**, on the other hand, has a cell body in the spinal cord or brainstem and an axon that extends outwards in a cranial or spinal motor nerve to reach an effector.

motor neuron disease (**motor neurone disease,, MND**) a progressive degenerative disease of the motor system occurring in middle age and causing muscle weakness and wasting. It primarily affects the cells of the anterior horn of the spinal cord, the motor nuclei in the brainstem, and the corticospinal fibres. There are three clinically distinct forms: **amyotrophic lateral sclerosis** (**ALS**, **Lou Gehrig's disease**), **progressive muscular atrophy**, and **progressive bulbar palsy**. Some forms of MND (5%) are familial (inherited). The drug *riluzole has been licensed for the treatment of MND with upper motor neuron involvement, but its benefits are limited.

(((⊕))) SEE WEB LINKS
- Website of the Motor Neurone Disease Association: information for patients, carers, and professionals

mould *n.* any multicellular filamentous fungus that commonly forms a rough furry coating on decaying matter.

moulding *n.* the changing of the shape of an infant's head during labour, due to movement of the bones of the skull, brought about by the pressures to which it is subjected when passing through the birth canal.

mountain sickness *see* ALTITUDE SICKNESS.

mouth-to-mouth resuscitation a form of *artificial respiration (known informally as the 'kiss of life') performed on an individual who has stopped breathing. The nostrils are pinched shut, the head is placed in the *head-tilt, chin-lift position, a seal is formed between the mouths of the casualty and rescuer, and air is blown firmly and steadily into the lungs for intervals of around three seconds. The small but definite infection risk with this technique can be avoided by using a *pocket resuscitation mask. **Mouth-to-nose resuscitation** is a similar technique in which the breaths are delivered through the casualty's nose.

mouthwash *n.* an aqueous solution used for rinsing of the mouth and teeth. Mouthwashes are used to prevent dental caries and gingivitis (*see also* CHLORHEXIDINE), to strengthen teeth against decay (*see* FLUORIDE), and to treat mild throat infections.

mouthwash test a simple noninvasive procedure that enables the detection of *carriers for single gene defects, e.g. *cystic fibrosis. Epithelial cells from the buccal cavity are obtained from a saline mouthwash: from these it is possible to isolate DNA, which is amplified by the *polymerase chain reaction to enable gene analysis.

moxibustion *n.* a form of treatment favoured in Japan, in which cones of sunflower pith or down from the leaves of the plant *Artemisia moxa* are stuck to the skin and ignited. The heat produced by the smouldering cones acts as a counterirritant and is reputed to cure a variety of disorders.

MPR *see* MULTIPLANAR RECONSTRUCTION.

MR magnetic resonance: relating to *mag-netic resonance imaging, as in **MR scan**.

MRC *see* MEDICAL RESEARCH COUNCIL.

MRCP magnetic resonance cholangiopan-creatography. *See* CHOLANGIOGRAPHY.

MRI *see* MAGNETIC RESONANCE IMAGING.

MRS *see* MAGNETIC RESONANCE SPECTROS-COPY.

MRSA meticillin- (or multiple-)resistant *Staphylococcus aureus*: an increasingly com-mon dangerous bacterium that is resistant to many antibiotics. It is responsible for many infections in already ill people in hospitals and is now also seen more widely in the gen-eral community (**community-associated MRSA; CA-MSRA**), usually in the form of skin infections. *See* METICILLIN.

MS *see* MULTIPLE SCLEROSIS.

MSA *see* MULTIPLE SYSTEM ATROPHY.

MSE *see* MENTAL STATE EXAMINATION.

MSH *see* MELANOCYTE-STIMULATING HOR-MONE.

MSU *see* MIDSTREAM SPECIMEN OF URINE.

MSV manoeuvre *see* MAURICEAU-SMELLIE-VIET MANOEUVRE.

mucilage *n.* (in pharmacy) a thick aque-ous solution of a gum used as a lubricant in skin preparations (*see also* GLYCERIN), for the production of pills, and for the suspension of insoluble substances. The most important mucilages are of acacia, tragacanth, and starch.

mucin *n.* the principal constituent of *mucus. Mucin is a *glycoprotein.

muco- *combining form denoting* 1. mucus. 2. mucous membrane.

mucociliary transport the process by which cilia (*see* CILIUM) move a thin film of *mucus from the upper and lower respira-tory tracts towards the digestive tract. Parti-cles of dust and microorganisms are trapped on the mucus and thereby removed from the respiratory tract.

mucocoele *n.* a space or organ distended with mucus. For example, it may occur in the gall bladder when the exit duct becomes ob-structed so that the mucus secretions are re-tained and dilate the cavity of the organ. A mucocoele in the soft tissues arising from a salivary gland occurs when the duct is blocked or ruptured.

mucolytic *n.* an agent that dissolves or breaks down mucus. Mucolytics such as **car-bocisteine** and dornase alfa (*see* DNASE) break down mucus in sputum and thus facil-itate its expectoration; they are used to treat chest conditions involving excessive or thickened mucus secretions.

mucopolysaccharide *n.* one of a group of complex carbohydrates functioning mainly as structural components in connective tis-sue. Mucopolysaccharide molecules are usu-ally built up of two repeating sugar units, one of which is an amino sugar. An example of a mucopolysaccharide is *chondroitin sul-phate, occurring in cartilage.

mucopolysaccharidosis *n.* any one of a group of several rare genetic diseases that are *inborn errors of metabolism in which the storage of complex carbohydrates is dis-ordered. The two most common are *Hunter's syndrome and *Hurler's syn-drome.

mucoprotein *n.* one of a group of proteins found in the *globulin fraction of blood plasma. Mucoproteins are globulins com-bined with a carbohydrate group (an amino sugar). They are similar to *glycoproteins but contain a greater proportion of carbohy-drate.

mucopurulent *adj.* containing mucus and pus. *See* MUCOPUS.

mucopus *n.* a mixture of *mucus and *pus.

Mucor *n.* a genus of mould fungi com-monly seen on dead and decaying organic matter. They can be pathogenic in humans.

mucormycosis *n.* infection caused by fungi of the genus *Mucor*. It most com-monly affects the sinuses, lungs, or brain in immunocompromised patients.

mucosa *n. see* MUCOUS MEMBRANE. —**mu-cosal** *adj.*

mucous membrane (mucosa) the moist membrane lining many tubular structures and cavities, including the nasal sinuses, res-piratory tract, gastrointestinal tract, biliary, and pancreatic systems. The surface of the mouth is lined by mucous membrane, the nature of which varies according to its site.

The mucous membrane consists of a surface layer of *epithelium, which contains glands secreting *mucus, with underlying layers of connective tissue (lamina propria) and muscularis mucosae, which forms the inner boundary of the mucous membrane.

mucoviscidosis *n. see* CYSTIC FIBROSIS.

mucus *n.* a viscous fluid secreted by *mucous membranes. Mucus acts as a protective barrier over the membranes, a lubricant, and a carrier of enzymes. It consists chiefly of *glycoproteins, particularly **mucin**. —**mucous**, **mucoid** *adj.*

MUGA scan (multiple-gated acquisition scan) a technique used in *nuclear medicine for studying the left-ventricular function and wall motion of the heart. The patient's red cells are labelled with radioactive technetium-99m. A gamma camera, connected to an ECG, collects information over a prolonged period for each phase of heart movement (**ECG gating**) to form an image of the blood pool within the heart at specific points in the cardiac cycle. Tomographic reconstructions can be made to give cross-sectional images of the heart in different phases of the cardiac cycle, using reconstruction *algorithms comparable to CT scanning (*see* SPECT SCANNING).

Müllerian duct (paramesonephric duct) either of the paired ducts that form adjacent to the Wolffian ducts (*see* MESONEPHROS) in the embryo. In the female these ducts develop into the Fallopian tubes, uterus, and part of the vagina. In the male **anti-Müllerian hormone**, produced by the fetal testis, arrests their development and by the tenth week of fetal life they have degenerated almost completely. [J. P. Müller (1801–58), German physiologist]

multidetector computerized tomography (MDCT) a development of *spiral CT scanning that uses more than one array of detectors opposite the X-ray tube, so that more tissue can be included, with thinner cuts, in a single rotation of the machine. This is particularly important for three-dimensional reconstruction of tissues. It also allows *multiplanar reconstruction, which is best achieved when the thickness of the slice is similar to the size resolution of the detectors in the other two planes. This is known as *isotropic imaging and occurs with slice thicknesses around 1 mm. Modern CT scanners are now usually equipped with between 16 and 256 detector arrays. The technique is particularly valuable for imaging fast-moving structures, such as the heart.

multidisciplinary team (MDT) a group of health-care professionals with different areas of expertise who unite to plan and carry out treatment of complex medical conditions.

multifactorial *adj.* describing a condition that is believed to have resulted from the interaction of genetic factors, usually polygenes, with an environmental factor or factors. Many disorders, e.g. spina bifida and anencephaly, are thought to be multifactorial.

multifocal lenses lenses containing more than one segment made to different prescriptions for visual correction. *See* BIFOCAL LENS, TRIFOCAL LENSES.

multigravida *n.* a woman who has been pregnant at least twice.

multi-organ failure (MOF) *see* MULTIPLE ORGAN DYSFUNCTION SYNDROME.

multipara *n.* a woman who has given birth to a live child after each of at least two pregnancies. *See also* GRAND MULTIPARITY.

multiplanar reconstruction (MPR) a computer technique that allows images to be created, after the information has been collected (*see* POST-PROCESSING), in any of the three named planes – *axial, *sagittal, or *coronal – or variations of these, such as oblique or curved planes. The effect is similar to allowing parts of the body to be sliced away, revealing the tissues inside so that they can be studied.

multiple organ dysfunction syndrome (MODS, multi-organ failure, multiple organ failure, MOF) a common cause of death following severe injury, overwhelming infection, or immune deficiency states.

multiple personality disorder a supposed psychiatric disorder in which the affected person has two or more distinct, and often contrasting, personalities. As each personality assumes dominance, it determines attitudes and behaviour and usually appears to be unaware of the other personality (or personalities). Transition is sudden and the mental states of the different personalities are normal. The vast majority of psychiatrists deny its existence, and many other explanatory models exist for persons who occasionally show symptoms similar to those described above.

multiple sclerosis (MS, disseminated sclerosis) a chronic disease of the nervous system affecting young and middle-aged adults. The *myelin sheaths surrounding nerves in the brain and spinal cord are damaged, which affects the function of the nerves involved. The course of the illness is usually characterized by recurrent relapses followed by remissions, but a proportion of patients run a chronic progressive course. The disease affects different parts of the brain and spinal cord, resulting in typically scattered symptoms. These include unsteady gait and shaky movements of the limbs (ataxia), abnormal eye movements (e.g. *nystagmus and internuclear *ophthalmoplegia), defects in speech pronunciation (dysarthria), spastic weakness, and *retrobulbar neuritis. The underlying cause of the nerve damage remains unknown, but an autoimmune process may be involved. Steroid treatment may be used in an acute relapses. *Interferon beta and *glatiramer acetate given by regular self-administered injections reduce the relapse rate by 30% in some patients. Newer monoclonal antibody treatments are also available.

(((⊕))) SEE WEB LINKS

• Website of the Multiple Sclerosis Society

multiple system atrophy (MSA) a condition that results from degeneration of brain cells in the *basal ganglia (resulting in *parkinsonism), the *cerebellum (resulting in *ataxia), and the *pyramidal system and degeneration of cells in the *autonomic nervous system.

multipotent *adj. see* STEM CELL.

multisystem *adj.* describing a disease that affects many systems of the body.

multivariate analysis *see* CORRELATION.

mummification *n.* **1.** the conversion of dead tissue into a hard shrunken mass, chiefly by dehydration. **2.** (in dentistry) the application of a fixative to the dental pulp to prevent decomposition.

mumps *n.* a common virus infection mainly affecting school-age children. Symptoms appear 2–3 weeks after exposure: fever, headache, and vomiting may precede a typical swelling of the *parotid salivary glands. The gland on one side of the face often swells up days before the other but some-

times only one side is affected. The symptoms usually vanish within three days, the patient remaining infectious until the swelling has completely disappeared, but the infection may spread to other salivary glands and to the pancreas, brain (causing an aseptic meningitis), and testicles (after puberty mumps affecting the testicles can cause sterility). Vaccination against mumps provides effective immunity (*see* MMR VACCINE). Medical name: **infectious parotitis**.

Munchausen's syndrome (Münchhausen's syndrome) a mental disorder in which the patient persistently tries to obtain invasive hospital treatment, especially surgery, for an illness that is nonexistent. The disease may be described in vivid detail, and in some cases injury may be deliberately self-inflicted in an attempt to give the appearance of authenticity to the claims being made. In **Munchausen's syndrome by proxy**, the patient (usually a mother) presents false health information about someone (usually her child) or inflicts harm on the child in order to attract medical attention. [Baron von Münchhausen, a fictional character in German literature who told exaggerated stories]

murmur *n.* a noise, heard with the aid of a stethoscope, that is generated by turbulent blood flow within the heart or blood vessels. Turbulent flow is produced by damaged valves, *septal defects, narrowed arteries, or arteriovenous communications. Heart murmurs can also be heard in normal individuals, especially those who have hyperactive circulation, and frequently in normal children (**innocent murmurs**). Murmurs are classified as **systolic** or **diastolic** (heard in ventricular *systole or *diastole respectively); **continuous murmurs** are heard throughout systole and diastole.

Murphy's sign a sign of inflammation of the gall bladder: continuous pressure over the gall bladder while the patient is taking a deep breath will cause a catch in the breath at the point of maximum inhalation. [J. B. Murphy (1857–1916), US surgeon]

muscae volitantes *see* FLOATERS.

muscle *n.* a tissue whose cells have the ability to contract, producing movement or force (see illustration). Muscles possess mechanisms for converting energy derived from chemical reactions into mechanical energy. The major functions of muscles are to

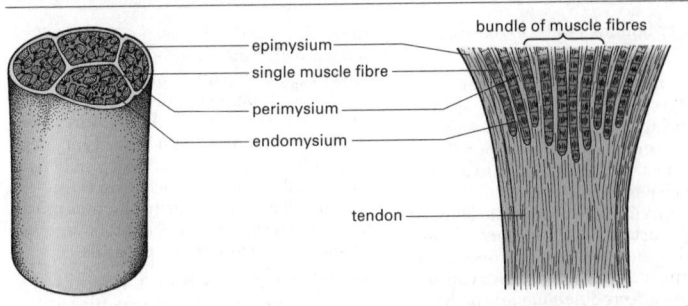

epimysium
single muscle fibre
perimysium
endomysium

bundle of muscle fibres

tendon

Muscle. A voluntary muscle in transverse section (left) and in longitudinal section at its junction with a tendon (right).

produce movements of the body, to maintain the position of the body against the force of gravity, to produce movements of structures inside the body, and to alter pressures or tensions of structures in the body. There are three types of muscle: *striated muscle, attached to the skeleton; *smooth muscle, which is found in such tissues as the stomach, gut, and blood vessels; and *cardiac muscle, which forms the walls of the heart.

muscle relaxant an agent that reduces tension in voluntary muscles. Drugs such as *baclofen, *dantrolene, and *diazepam are used to relieve skeletal muscular spasms in various spastic conditions, parkinsonism, and tetanus. The drugs used to relax voluntary muscles during the administration of anaesthetics in surgical operations act by blocking the transmission of impulses at neuromuscular junctions. Nondepolarizing muscle relaxants, e.g. *atracurium besilate, **cisatracurium** (Nimbex), **pancuronium**, and **rocuronium** (Esmeron), bind to receptor sites normally occupied by acetylcholine; depolarizing muscle relaxants, e.g. *suxamethonium, mimic the action of acetylcholine but *depolarization is prolonged.

muscle spindle a specialized receptor, sensitive to stretch, that is embedded between and parallel to the fibres of striated muscles. These receptors are important for coordinated muscular movement. *See also* STRETCH RECEPTOR.

muscular dystrophy a group of muscle diseases, marked by weakness and wasting of selected muscles, in which there is a recognizable pattern of inheritance. The affected muscle fibres degenerate and are replaced by fatty tissue. The muscular dys-

trophies are classified according to the patient's age at onset, distribution of the weakness, the progression of the disease, and the mode of inheritance. Isolated cases may occur as a result of gene mutation. Confirmation of the diagnosis is based upon *electromyography and muscle biopsy.

One common form is **Duchenne's muscular dystrophy**, which is inherited as a *sex-linked recessive character and is nearly always restricted to boys. It usually begins before the age of four, with selective weakness and wasting of the muscles of the pelvic girdle and back. The child has a waddling gait and *lordosis of the lumbar spine. The calf muscles – and later the shoulders and upper limbs – often become firm and bulky. Although the disease cannot be cured, physiotherapy and orthopaedic measures can relieve the disability. The identification of the gene abnormality raises the possibility of *gene therapy in the future. *See also* BECKER MUSCULAR DYSTROPHY, DYSTROPHIA MYOTONICA (MYOTONIC DYSTROPHY).

(⊕) SEE WEB LINKS

• Website of the Muscular Dystrophy Campaign

muscularis *n.* a muscular layer of the wall of a hollow organ (such as the stomach) or a tubular structure (such as the intestine or the ureter). The **muscularis mucosae** is the muscular layer of a mucous membrane complex, especially that of the stomach or intestine.

muscular rheumatism any aching pain in the muscles and joints. Commonly the symptoms are due to *fibrositis; wear and tear of the joints (*osteoarthritis); or to inflammation of the muscles associated with abnormal immune reactions (*polymyalgia rheumatica).

musculo- *combining form denoting* muscle.

musculocutaneous nerve a nerve of the *brachial plexus that supplies some muscles of the arm and the skin of the lateral part of the forearm.

mushroom *n.* the aerial fruiting (spore-producing) body of various fungi. Edible species include field mushrooms and cultivated mushrooms (*Agaricus campestris* and *A. bisporus*), the chanterelle (*Cantherellus cibarius*), and the parasol (*Lepiota procera*). However, great care must be taken in identifying edible fungi. Many species are poisonous, especially the death cap and panther cap (*see* AMANITA).

mutagen *n.* an external agent that, when applied to cells or organisms, can increase the rate of *mutation. Mutagens usually only increase the number of mutants formed and do not cause mutations not found under natural conditions. Several kinds of radiation, many chemicals, and certain viruses can act as mutagens. *Compare* ANTI-MUTAGEN.

mutant *adj.* affected by or showing the effects of a mutation. —**mutant** *n.*

mutation *n.* a change in the genetic material (*DNA) of a cell, or the change this causes in a characteristic of the individual, which is not caused by normal genetic processes. In a **point** (or **gene**) **mutation** there is a change in a single gene; in a **chromosome mutation** there is a change in the structure or number of the chromosomes. All mutations are rare events and may occur spontaneously or be caused by external agents (*mutagens). If a mutation occurs in developing sex cells (gametes) it may be inherited. Mutations in any other cells (**somatic mutations**) are not inherited.

mutism *n.* inability or refusal to speak. Innate speechlessness most commonly occurs in those who have been totally deaf since birth (**deaf-mutism**). Inability to speak may result from brain damage (*see* APHASIA). It may also be caused by depression, psychosis, or psychological trauma, in which case the patient either does not speak at all or speaks only to particular persons or in particular situations. This latter condition is called **selective** (or **elective**) **mutism**.
    Treatment of mutism due to psychological causes is now increasingly by behavioural means, such as *prompting: people that the patient does not address are slowly introduced into the situation where the patient does speak. This may be done either alone or in combination with more traditional psychotherapy. Psychotic or depressive mutism or *catatonia are addressed by treating the underlying condition. —**mute** *adj., n.*

mutualism *n.* the intimate but not necessarily obligatory association between two different species of organism in which there is mutual aid and benefit. *Compare* SYMBIOSIS.

my- (**myo-**) *combining form denoting* muscle.

myalgia *n.* pain in the muscles. —**myalgic** *adj.*

myalgic encephalomyelitis (myalgic encephalopathy) *see* CFS/ME/PVF.

myasthenia gravis a chronic disease marked by abnormal fatigability and weakness of selected muscles, which is relieved by rest. The degree of fatigue is so extreme that these muscles are temporarily paralysed. The muscles initially affected are those around the eyes, mouth, and throat, resulting in drooping of the upper eyelids (*ptosis), double vision, *dysarthria, and *dysphagia. Myasthenia gravis is an *autoimmune disease in which acetylcholine-receptor autoantibodies bind to cholinergic receptors on muscle cells, which impairs the ability of the neurotransmitter acetylcholine to induce muscular contraction. Treatment with *anticholinesterase drugs and surgical removal of the thymus in younger patients (under the age of 45 years) lessen the severity of the symptoms. Steroid therapy, intravenous immunoglobulin treatment, and plasma exchange may be used to treat the more severely affected patients.

myc- (**myco-, mycet(o)-**) *combining form denoting* a fungus.

mycelium *n.* (*pl.* **mycelia**) the tangled mass of fine branching threads that make up the feeding and growing part of a *fungus.

mycetoma *n.* a chronic inflammation of tissues caused by a fungus. *See* MADURA FOOT.

Mycobacterium *n.* a genus of rodlike Gram-positive aerobic bacteria that can form filamentous branching structures. Some species are pathogenic to animals and humans: *M. leprae* (**Hansen's bacillus**) causes *leprosy; *M. tuberculosis* (**Koch's bacillus**) causes *tuberculosis. *M. bovis* causes tuberculosis in cattle but can also infect the human lungs, joints, and intestines. *M. paratuberculosis*, which causes Johne's disease in cattle, can also be transmitted in milk and is suspected of being a cause of Crohn's disease.

M. tuberculosis is by far the most common species responsible for infections of the lung. Other mycobacteria that infect the lung are variously described as atypical, anonymous, or *opportunistic – the favoured term since they usually require pre-existing lung damage or a defect in the patient's immunity before they can give rise to infection. The opportunistic mycobacteria that most commonly cause lung infections are *M. kansacii*, *M. xenopi*, *M. malmoense*, and a group known as the **MAI complex** (*M. avium*, *M. intracellulare*). Infections caused by all these organisms can mimic pulmonary tuberculosis but are much more difficult to treat since they are resistant to many of the antituberculosis drugs. The MAI organisms are particularly likely to cause superimposed infection in cases of AIDS.

mycology *n.* the science of fungi. *See also* MICROBIOLOGY. —**mycologist** *n.*

mycophenolate mofetil (MMF) an immunosuppressant drug used to prevent rejection in organ transplantation and also in the treatment of a range of autoimmune diseases. It is derived from the fungus *Penicillium stoloniferum* and acts by blocking purine synthesis in lymphocytes. It is administered by mouth or intravenous infusion; neutropenia and gastrointestinal side-effects may limit its use. Trade name: **CellCept**.

mycoplasma *n.* one of a group of minute nonmotile bacteria that lack a rigid cell wall and hence display a variety of forms. The group includes some species that cause severe respiratory disease in cattle, sheep, and goats; one of these, *Mycoplasma pneumoniae*, causes *atypical pneumonia in humans.

mycosis *n.* any disease caused by a fungus, including actinomycosis, aspergillosis, cryptococcosis, rhinosporidiosis, ringworm, and sporotrichosis.

mycosis fungoides the most common form of *cutaneous T-cell lymphoma, with patches, plaques, and later nodules on the skin. It typically progresses very slowly and

can be treated with topical corticosteroids, phototherapy, radiotherapy, or other agents.

Mycota *n. see* UNDECENOIC ACID.

mydriasis *n.* widening of the pupil, which occurs normally in dim light. The commonest cause of prolonged mydriasis is drug therapy (*see* MYDRIATIC) or injury to the eye. *See also* CYCLOPLEGIA. *Compare* MIOSIS.

mydriatic *n.* a drug that causes the pupil of the eye to dilate. Examples are *atropine, *cyclopentolate, and *phenylephrine. Mydriatics in the form of eye drops or ointments are used to aid examination of the eye and to treat some eye inflammations such as iritis and cyclitis.

myectomy *n.* a surgical operation to remove part of a muscle.

myel- (myelo-) *combining form denoting* 1. the spinal cord. 2. bone marrow. 3. myelin.

myelencephalon *n. see* MEDULLA OBLONGATA.

myelin *n.* a complex material formed of protein and *phospholipid that is laid down

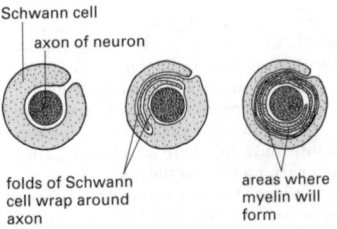

Myelin. Formation of a myelin sheath by a Schwann cell.

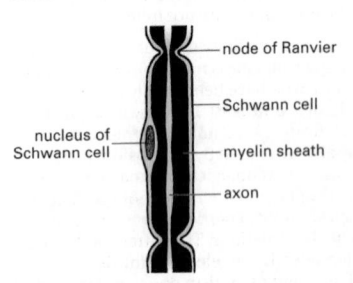

Myelin. Longitudinal section through a myelinated nerve fibre.

as a sheath surrounding and insulating the *axons of certain neurons, known as **myelinated** (or **medullated**) **nerve fibres**. The material is produced and laid down in concentric layers by *Schwann cells at regular intervals along the nerve fibre (see illustrations). Myelinated nerves conduct impulses more rapidly than nonmyelinated nerves.

myelination *n.* the process in which *myelin is laid down as an insulating layer around the axons of certain nerves. Myelination of nerve tracts in the central nervous system is completed by the second year of life.

myelitis *n.* 1. an inflammatory disease of the spinal cord. The most usual kind (**transverse myelitis**) most often occurs during the development of multiple sclerosis, but it is sometimes a manifestation of *encephalomyelitis, when it can occur as an isolated attack. The inflammation spreads more or less completely across the tissue of the spinal cord, resulting in a loss of its normal function to transmit nerve impulses up and down. It is as though the spinal cord had been severed: paralysis and numbness affects the legs and trunk below the level of the diseased tissue. 2. inflammation of the bone marrow. *See* OSTEOMYELITIS.

myeloblast *n.* the earliest identifiable cell that gives rise to a *granulocyte, having a large nucleus and scanty cytoplasm. It is normally found in the blood-forming tissue of the bone marrow, but may appear in the blood in a variety of diseases, most notably in acute myeloblastic *leukaemia. *See also* GRANULOPOIESIS. —**myeloblastic** *adj.*

myelocele *n. see* NEURAL TUBE DEFECTS.

myelocyte *n.* an immature form of *granulocyte having an oval nucleus (*compare* METAMYELOCYTE) and neutrophil, eosinophil, or basophil granules within its cytoplasm (*compare* PROMYELOCYTE). It is normally found in the blood-forming tissue of the bone marrow, but may appear in the blood in a variety of diseases, including infections, infiltrations of the bone marrow, and certain leukaemias. *See also* GRANULOPOIESIS.

myelodysplastic syndromes (MDS) a group of diseases in which the production of any one or all types of blood cells by the bone marrow is disrupted. Although myelodysplastic syndromes were previously referred to as **preleukaemia**, only a minority of patients with myelodysplastic syndromes develop leukaemia.

myelofibrosis *n.* a chronic but progressive disease characterized by *fibrosis of the bone marrow, which leads to anaemia and the presence of immature red and white blood cells in the circulation. Other features include enlargement of the spleen and the presence of blood-forming (myeloid) tissue in abnormal sites, such as the spleen and liver (extramedullary *haemopoiesis). Its cause is unknown.

myelography *n.* a specialized method of X-ray examination to demonstrate the spinal canal that involves injection of a radiopaque contrast medium into the subarachnoid space by *lumbar puncture. The X-rays obtained are called **myelograms**. It is of importance in the recognition of tumours of the spinal cord and other conditions compressing the cord or the nerve roots. The former use of oil-based dyes in myelography was an occasional cause of *arachnoiditis. This complication is now avoided by the use of water-soluble contrast media. Myelography is now often combined with simultaneous CT scanning but is becoming increasingly superseded by *magnetic resonance imaging.

myeloid *adj.* 1. like, derived from, or relating to bone marrow. 2. resembling a *myelocyte. 3. relating to the spinal cord.

myeloid leukaemia a variety of *leukaemia in which the type of blood cell that proliferates abnormally originates in the blood-forming (myeloid) tissue of the bone marrow. Myeloid leukaemias may be acute or chronic and may involve any one of the cells produced by the marrow. Blood cells in patients with chronic myeloid leukaemia contain a reciprocal *translocation between chromosomes 9 and 22 (*see* PHILADELPHIA CHROMOSOME); molecular characterization of the translocation has led to the development of specific drugs to block the effects of this abnormality (*see* TYROSINE KINASE INHIBITOR).

myeloid tissue a tissue in the *bone marrow in which the various classes of blood cells are produced. *See also* HAEMOPOIESIS.

myeloma (multiple myeloma, myelomatosis) *n.* a malignant disease of the bone marrow, characterized by two or more of the following criteria: (1) the presence of an excess of abnormal malignant plasma cells in the bone marrow; (2) typical *lytic deposits in the bones on X-ray, giving the appearance of holes; (3) the presence in the serum of an abnormal gammaglobulin, usually IgG (an immunoglobulin; *see* PARAPROTEIN). *Bence-Jones protein may also be found in the serum or urine. The patient may complain of tiredness due to anaemia and of bone pain and may develop pathological fractures. Treatment is usually with such drugs as steroids, melphalan, cyclophosphamide, or thalidomide with local radiotherapy to particular areas of pain. *See also* PLASMACYTOMA.

myeloma kidney *see* CAST NEPHROPATHY.

myelomalacia *n.* softening of the tissues of the spinal cord, most often caused by an impaired blood supply.

myelomatosis *n. see* MYELOMA.

myelomeningocele *n. see* NEURAL TUBE DEFECTS.

myeloproliferative disorders (MPD) a group of diseases in which there is excessive production of blood cells in the bone marrow. Myeloproliferative disorders include *polycythaemia vera, essential *thrombocythaemia, idiopathic *myelofibrosis, and chronic *myeloid leukaemia.

myelosuppression *n.* a reduction in blood-cell production by the bone marrow. It commonly occurs after chemotherapy and may result in anaemia, infection, and abnormal bleeding (*see* THROMBOCYTOPENIA, NEUTROPENIA). —**myelosuppressive** *adj.*

myenteric reflex a reflex action of the intestine in which a physical stimulus causes the intestine to contract above and relax below the point of stimulation.

myenteron *n.* the muscular layer of the *intestine, consisting of a layer of circular muscle inside a layer of longitudinal muscle. These muscles are used in *peristalsis. —**myenteric** *adj.*

myiasis *n.* an infestation of a living organ or tissue by maggots. The flies normally breed in decaying animal and vegetable matter; myiasis therefore generally occurs only in regions of poor hygiene, and in most cases the infestations are accidental. Various genera may infect humans. *Gasterophilus, *Hypoderma, *Dermatobia, and *Cordylobia affect the skin; *Fannia* invades the alimentary canal and the urinary system; *Phormia and *Wohlfahrtia can infest open wounds and ulcers; *Oestrus attacks the eyes; and

Cochliomyia invades the nasal passages. Treatment of external myiases involves the destruction and removal of maggots followed by the application of antibiotics to wounds and lesions.

mylohyoid *n.* a muscle in the floor of the mouth, attached at one end to the mandible and at the other to the hyoid bone.

myo- *combining form. see* MY-.

myoblast *n.* a cell that develops into a muscle fibre. —**myoblastic** *adj.*

myocardial infarction death of a segment of heart muscle, which follows interruption of its blood supply (*see* CORONARY THROMBOSIS). Myocardial infarction is usually confined to the left ventricle. The patient experiences a 'heart attack': sudden severe chest pain, which may spread to the arms and throat. Although severe chest pain is the most widely recognized symptom of myocardial infarction, many patients – especially women – do not have chest pain. Other presenting symptoms include abdominal pain, nausea, vomiting, sweating, shortness of breath, and dizziness. The main danger is that of ventricular *fibrillation, which accounts for most of the fatalities. Other *arrhythmias are also frequent. Other complications include heart failure, rupture of the heart, phlebothrombosis, pulmonary embolism, pericarditis, shock, mitral regurgitation, and perforation of the septum between the ventricles.

Patients with myocardial infarction are best cared for in a specialized coronary care unit with facilities for the early detection, prevention, and treatment of arrhythmias and *cardiac arrest. Blockage of a major coronary artery is detected by elevation of the *S–T segment on the *electrocardiogram (**STEMI** or **S–T elevation myocardial infarction**) and is relieved by the intravenous infusion of a drug to dissolve thrombus (*thrombolysis) or by emergency *coronary angioplasty (commonly called primary *percutaneous coronary intervention). Most survivors of myocardial infarction are able to return to a full and active life, including those who have been successfully resuscitated from cardiac arrest. Lesser degrees of coronary obstruction may not be seen on the electrocardiogram but are revealed by the detection of raised *troponin levels in the blood (**NSTEMI** or **non-S–T elevation myocardial infarction**). Treatment is with *antiplatelet drugs and early percutaneous coronary intervention.

myocarditis *n.* acute or chronic inflammation of the heart muscle. It may be seen alone or as part of pancarditis (*see* ENDO-MYOCARDITIS).

myocardium *n.* the middle of the three layers forming the wall of the heart (*see also* ENDOCARDIUM, EPICARDIUM). It is composed of *cardiac muscle and forms the greater part of the heart wall, being thicker in the ventricles than in the atria. —**myocardial** *adj.*

myoclonus *n.* a sudden spasm of the muscles. Occasional **myoclonic jerks** occur between seizures in patients with idiopathic *epilepsy, and myoclonus is a major feature of some progressive neurological illnesses with extensive degeneration of the brain cells (including the *spongiform encephalopathies). Myoclonic jerks on falling asleep (**nocturnal myoclonus**) occur in normal individuals. —**myoclonic** *adj.*

myocyte *n.* a muscle cell.

myoepithelium *n.* a tissue consisting of cells of epithelial origin having a contractile cytoplasm. Myoepithelial cells play an important role in encouraging the secretion of substances into ducts.

myofibril *n.* one of numerous contractile filaments found within the cytoplasm of *striated muscle cells. When viewed under a microscope myofibrils show alternating bands of high and low refractive index, which give striated muscle its characteristic appearance.

myogenic *adj.* originating in muscle: applied to the inherent rhythmicity of contraction of some muscles (e.g. cardiac muscle), which does not depend on neural influences.

myoglobin (myohaemoglobin *n.* an iron-containing protein, resembling *haemoglobin, found in muscle cells. Like haemoglobin it contains a haem group, which binds reversibly with oxygen, and so acts as an oxygen reservoir within the muscle fibres.

myoglobinuria (myohaemoglobinuria *n.* the presence in the urine of the pigment myoglobin.

myoglobinuric acute renal failure acute kidney injury caused by myoglobin that is released from damaged skeletal mus-

cle (*rhabdomyolysis). This is usually the result of trauma and the condition was first recognized in victims trapped and crushed during the London Blitz. Muscle injury can also occur with pressure necrosis, particularly in the unconscious or immobile patient, or with a *compartment syndrome. Rarely it may complicate intensive muscular exercise or extensive viral myositis and it is a recognized complication of modest overexertion in some inherited disorders of muscle metabolism, such as *McArdle's disease.

myogram *n.* a recording of the activity of a muscle. *See* ELECTROMYOGRAPHY.

myograph *n.* an instrument for recording the activity of muscular tissues. *See* ELECTRO-MYOGRAPHY.

myohaemoglobin *n. see* MYOGLOBIN.

myohaemoglobinuria *n. see* MYOGLOBIN-URIA.

myokymia *n.* prominent quivering of a few muscle fibres, not associated with any other abnormal features. It is usually a benign condition. *See also* FASCICULATION.

myology *n.* the study of the structure, function, and diseases of the muscles.

myolysis *n. see* FIBROID.

myoma *n.* a benign tumour of muscle. It may originate in smooth muscle (*see* LEIOMY-OMA) or in striated muscle (*see* RHABDOMY-OMA).

myomectomy *n.* surgical removal of a fibroid (myoma) from the uterus.

myometritis *n.* inflammation of the muscular wall (myometrium) of the uterus.

myometrium *n.* the muscular tissue of the uterus, which surrounds the *endometrium. It is composed of smooth muscle that undergoes small regular spontaneous contractions. The frequency and amplitude of these contractions alter in response to the hormones *oestrogen, *progesterone, and *oxytocin, which are present at particular stages of the menstrual cycle and pregnancy.

myoneural junction *see* NEUROMUSCULAR JUNCTION.

myopathy *n.* any disease of the muscles. The myopathies are usually subdivided into those that are inherited (*see* MUSCULAR DYS-TROPHY) and those that are acquired. The acquired myopathies include *polymyositis and muscular diseases complicating endocrine disorders, carcinoma, or drug therapy. All are typified by weakness and wasting of the muscles, which may be associated with pain and tenderness.

myopia (short-sightedness) *n.* the condition in which parallel light rays are brought to a focus in front of the retina (see illustration). Closer objects are clearer as compared to distant objects. Myopia is corrected by wearing spectacles with concave lenses; contact lenses and surgery can also be used to correct myopia (*see* EXCIMER LASER, LASEK, LASIK). *Compare* EMMETROPIA, HYPERMETROPIA. —**myopic** *adj.*

focusing point falls short of retina

Uncorrected

Corrected

concave lens diverges light rays falling on the eye

Myopia (short-sightedness).

myoplasm *n. see* SARCOPLASM.

myoplasty *n.* the plastic surgery of muscle, in which part of a muscle is partly detached and used to repair tissue defects or deformities in the vicinity of the muscle. It is frequently used in *flap surgery and anal operations (*anoplasty).

myosarcoma *n.* a malignant tumour of muscle. *See also* LEIOMYOSARCOMA, RHABDOMYOSARCOMA.

myosin *n.* the most abundant protein in muscle fibrils, having the important properties of elasticity and contractility. With actin, it comprises the principal contractile element of muscles. *See* STRIATED MUSCLE.

myosis *n. see* MIOSIS.

myositis *n.* any of a group of muscle diseases in which inflammation and degenerative changes occur. *Polymyositis is the most commonly occurring example, but myositis may be found in relation to systemic *connective-tissue diseases and a minority are caused by bacterial or parasitic infections.

myositis ossificans the formation of bone within a *muscle, which most commonly occurs after dislocations or severe muscle bruising, especially around the elbow, shoulder, hip, or knee. Initial symptoms of pain, swelling, and tenderness are followed by joint stiffness; if this persists, surgery may be required to remove the bone once it has stopped growing.

myotactic *adj.* relating to the sense of touch in muscles.

myotatic reflex *see* STRETCH REFLEX.

myotome *n.* that part of the segmented mesoderm in the early embryo that gives rise to all the skeletal muscle of the body. Visceral (smooth) muscles develop from unsegmented mesoderm (*see* MESENCHYME). *See also* SOMITE.

myotomy *n.* the dissection or surgical division of a muscle. For example, **cardiomyotomy** is division of the *sphincter muscle of the gastro-oesophageal junction (*see* ACHALASIA).

myotonia *n.* a disorder of the muscle fibres that results in abnormally prolonged contractions. The patient has difficulty in relaxing a movement (e.g. his grip) after any vigorous effort. It is a feature of a hereditary condition starting in infancy or early childhood (**myotonia congenita**) and of a form of muscular dystrophy (*dystrophia myotonica).

myotonic *adj.* **1.** relating to muscle tone. **2.** relating to *myotonia.

myotonus *n.* **1.** a tonic muscular spasm. **2.** muscle tone.

myringa *n.* the eardrum (*see* TYMPANIC MEMBRANE).

myringitis *n.* inflammation of the eardrum. *See* OTITIS.

myringoplasty (tympanoplasty) *n.* surgical repair of a perforated eardrum by grafting.

myringotomy *n.* incision of the eardrum to create an artificial opening, either to allow infected fluid to drain from the middle ear in acute *otitis media or to remove fluid in *glue ear and permit the insertion of a *grommet.

myx- (myxo-) *combining form denoting* mucus.

myxoedema *n.* **1.** a dry firm waxy swelling of the skin and subcutaneous tissues found in patients with underactive thyroid glands (*see* HYPOTHYROIDISM). **2.** the clinical syndrome due to hypothyroidism in adult life, including coarsening of the skin, intolerance to cold, weight gain, and mental dullness. The symptoms are abolished with thyroxine treatment. —**myxoedematous** *adj.*

myxoedema coma a life-threatening condition due to severe *hypothyroidism, which is often precipitated by an acute event, such as surgery, prolonged exposure to cold, infection, trauma, other severe illness, or sedative drugs. It manifests as hypothermia, slowing of the heart rate with a reduction in blood pressure and sometimes heart failure, pleural and peritoneal effusions, urinary retention, and a gradually reduced conscious state resulting in coma. Blood tests show hypothyroidism, *hyponatraemia, hypercholesterolaemia, retention of carbon dioxide, and anaemia. Treatment is with intravenous *thyroxine at a high dosage until the patient wakes up, when tablets can be administered. Support on a ventilator and intravenous fluids may be needed. Active slow rewarming should be undertaken.

myxofibroma *n.* a benign tumour of fibrous tissue that contains myxomatous elements (*see* MYXOMA) or has undergone mucoid degeneration.

myxoid cyst a small (and often painful) cyst containing a thick sticky fluid that develops over the end joint of a finger or toe. It may be in communication with the underlying joint.

myxoma *n.* a benign gelatinous tumour of connective tissue. **Atrial myxoma** is a tumour of the heart, usually of the left side, arising from the septum dividing the two upper chambers. Symptoms may include fever, lassitude, joint pains, and sudden loss of consciousness due to obstruction of the bloodflow. The tumour may be wrongly diagnosed as stenosis of the mitral valve as it can produce a similar murmur. Treatment requires surgical removal. —**myxomatous** *adj.*

myxosarcoma *n.* a *sarcoma containing mucoid material, such as a *liposarcoma or a *fibrosarcoma.

myxovirus *n.* one of a group of RNA-containing viruses that are associated with various diseases in animals and humans. The **orthomyxoviruses** cause diseases of the respiratory tract, most notably influenza. The related **paramyxoviruses** include the *respiratory syncytial virus (RSV) and the agents that cause measles, mumps, and parainfluenza.

nabilone *n.* a drug related to cannabis, used to control severe nausea and vomiting caused by anticancer drugs, when this has not responded to other antiemetics. Administered by mouth, it can cause drowsiness, vertigo, dry mouth, hallucinations, and mood changes.

nabothian follicle (**nabothian cyst**, **nabothian gland**) one of a number of retention *cysts on the neck (cervix) of the uterus, near its opening to the vagina. The sacs, which contain mucus, form when the ducts of the glands in the cervix are blocked by a new growth of surface cells (epithelium) over an area damaged because of infection.

NAD (**nicotinamide adenine dinucleotide**) a *coenzyme that acts as a hydrogen acceptor in oxidation-reduction reactions, particularly in the *electron transport chain in cellular respiration. NAD and the closely related coenzyme **NADP** (**nicotinamide adenine dinucleotide phosphate**) are derived from nicotinic acid; they are reduced to **NADH** and **NADPH**, respectively.

nadolol *n.* a *beta blocker used mainly in the treatment of angina pectoris and *arrhythmias and to prevent migraine attacks. It is administered by mouth; side-effects include decreased heart rate, dizziness, and low blood pressure. Trade name: **Corgard**.

NADP (**nicotinamide adenine dinucleotide phosphate**) *see* NAD.

Naegele rule a method used to calculate the estimated date of delivery: nine months and seven days are added to the date of the start of the last menstrual period. A correction is required if the woman does not have 28-day menstrual cycles. [F. K. Naegele (1777–1851), German obstetrician]

Naegele's obliquity *see* ASYNCLITISM.

Naegleria *n.* a genus of *amoebae that normally live in damp soil or mud. *Naegleria* species can, however, live as parasites in humans: *N. fowleri* is responsible for primary amoebic *meningoencephalitis, a very rare, but fatal, infection of the brain.

naevus *n.* (*pl.* **naevi**) a birthmark: a clearly defined malformation of the skin, present at birth. There are many different types of naevi. Some, including the strawberry naevus and port-wine stain, are composed of small blood vessels (*see* HAEMANGIOMA). The **strawberry naevus** (or **strawberry mark**) is a raised red lump usually appearing on the face and growing rapidly in the first month of life. These birthmarks slowly resolve and spontaneously disappear between the ages of five and ten. The **port-wine stain** (or **capillary naevus**) is a permanent purplish discoloration that may occur anywhere but usually appears on the upper half of the body. Laser treatment can reduce the discoloration. Occasionally a port-wine stain may be associated with a malformation of blood vessels over the brain, for example in the Sturge-Weber syndrome (*see* ANGIOMA).

It is not uncommon for a pale or white halo to develop around an ordinary pigmented naevus, especially on the trunk, forming a **halo naevus**. The pigmented naevus disappears over the course of a few months; this is followed by resolution of the pale area. A **blue naevus** is a small blue-grey papule appearing at birth or later in life, mainly on the extremities. Progression to malignant melanoma is very rare. A **naevus of Ota** is a blue-grey pigmented area on the cheek, eyelid, or forehead with similar pigmentation of the sclera of an eye. It is associated with melanomas of the uvea, orbit, and brain as well as with glaucoma of the affected eye. *See also* MOLE² (PIGMENTED NAEVUS).

NAFLD *see* NONALCOHOLIC FATTY LIVER DISEASE.

Naga sore *see* TROPICAL ULCER.

NAI *see* NONACCIDENTAL INJURY.

nail *n.* a horny structure, composed of keratin, formed from the epidermis on the dorsal surface of each finger and toe (see illustration). The exposed part of the nail is the **body**, behind which is the **root**. The whitish crescent-shaped area at the base of the body is called the **lunula**. Growth of the

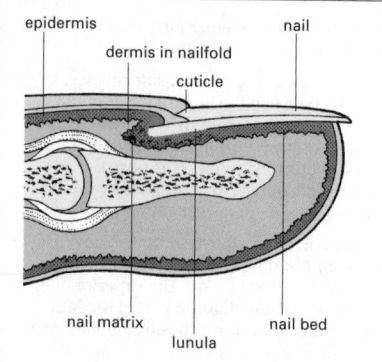

epidermis   nail
    dermis in nailfold
         cuticle

    nail matrix   nail bed
         lunula

Nail. Longitudinal section through the fingertip and nail.

nail occurs at the end of the nail root by division of the germinative layer of the underlying *epidermis (which forms part of the **matrix**). The growing nail slides forward over the **nail bed**. The fold of skin that lies above the root is the **nail fold**; folds of skin on either side of the nail are the **nail walls**. The epidermis of the nail fold that lies next to the nail root is called the **eponychium** (forming the 'cuticle' at the base of the nail). Anatomical name: **unguis**.

nalidixic acid a *quinolone antibiotic active against various bacteria and used to treat infections of the urinary tract. It is administered by mouth; common side-effects are nausea, vomiting, and skin reactions. Trade name: **Uriben**.

naloxone *n.* a drug that is a specific antidote to morphine and other opioids. Administered by intravenous injection, it is used in the emergency treatment of opioid overdosage and to reverse the respiratory depression induced by opioid analgesics used during surgery. As it is short-acting, repeated doses may be necessary.

naltrexone *n.* an opioid antagonist drug that is used to prevent relapse in formerly heroin- and other opioid-dependent patients. It is administered by mouth. Possible side-effects include abdominal cramps, nausea and vomiting, sleep difficulties, and dizziness. Trade names: **Nalorex, Opizone**.

nandrolone *n.* a synthetic male sex hormone with *anabolic effects. It is administered by deep intramuscular injection in the treatment of aplastic *anaemia and high

doses may cause signs of *virilization in women. Trade name: **Deca-Durabolin**.

nano- *combining form denoting* **1.** extremely small size. **2.** one-thousand-millionth part (10^{-9}).

nanometre *n.* one thousand-millionth of a metre (10^{-9} m). One nanometre is equal to 10 angstrom. Symbol: nm.

nanophthalmos *n.* a congenitally small eye in which all the structures are proportionally reduced.

nanotechnology *n.* a field of science focused on matter 100 nm or smaller (a DNA double helix has a diameter around 2 nm). Such substances (e.g. **nanoparticles, nanostructures, nanocrystals**) include those at the molecular and atomic levels. **Nanomedicine** is the use of nanotechnology to deliver diagnostic or treatment modalities (e.g. drugs) directly to the relevant cells (e.g. cancer cells) in the human body.

napkin rash (**nappy rash**) a red skin rash within the napkin area, usually caused by chemical irritation (ammoniacal *dermatitis) or infection with *Candida. Ammoniacal dermatitis is caused by skin contact with wet soiled nappies, the stool bacteria reacting with urine to form irritant ammonia. Treatment involves exposure to air, application of barrier creams, and frequent nappy changes. Candidal nappy rash is treated with antifungal creams. Other causes of napkin rash include eczema and psoriasis.

naprapathy *n.* a system of medicine based on the belief that a great many diseases are attributable to displacement of ligaments, tendons, and other connective tissues and that cure can be brought about only by manipulation to correct these displacements.

naproxen *n.* an analgesic drug that also reduces inflammation and fever (*see* NSAID). It is used to treat rheumatoid arthritis, dysmenorrhoea, and gout. It is administered by mouth; side-effects may include digestive upsets and rashes: gastric bleeding can be prevented by administering naproxen in combination with *misoprostol (as **Napratec**). Trade names: **Naprosyn, Synflex**.

naratriptan *n. see* $5HT_1$ AGONIST.

narcissism *n.* an excessive involvement with oneself and one's self-importance, often to cover insecurity. In Freudian terms it is a state in which the *ego has taken itself as a love object. Some degree of narcissism is present in most individuals, but when it is shown to an extreme degree it may become a *personality disorder. —**narcissistic** *adj.*

narco- *combining form denoting* narcosis; stupor.

narcolepsy *n.* an extreme tendency to fall asleep in quiet surroundings or when engaged in monotonous activities. The patient can be woken easily and is immediately alert. It is often associated with *cataplexy, *sleep paralysis, and *hypnagogic hallucinations. One in 2000 individuals may be affected. Narcolepsy is strongly associated with reduced levels of *hypocretin in the cerebrospinal fluid. —**narcoleptic** *adj., n.*

narcosis *n.* a state of diminished consciousness or complete unconsciousness caused by the use of narcotic (i.e. opioid) drugs, which have a depressant action on the nervous system. The body's normal reactions to stimuli are diminished and the body may become sedated or completely anaesthetized.

narcotic *n.* a drug that induces stupor and insensibility and relieves pain. Now largely obsolete in medical contexts, the term was used particularly for morphine and other derivatives of opium (*see* OPIATE) but also referred to other drugs that depress brain function (e.g. general anaesthetics and hypnotics). In legal terms a narcotic is any addictive drug subject to illegal use.

nares *pl. n.* (*sing.* **naris**) openings of the nose. The two **external** (or **anterior**) **nares** are the nostrils, leading from the nasal cavity to the outside. The two **internal** (or **posterior**) **nares** (**choanae**) are the openings leading from the nasal cavity into the pharynx.

narrative ethics an approach to ethical problems and practice that involves listening to and interpreting people's stories rather than applying principles or rules to particular situations. This context-specific empathetic approach to patient and professional life stories is often contrasted with the universalizing rationalist approach of *Kantian ethics. Narrative ethics has an obvious relevance to the doctor–patient relationship and mirrors the clinical context in which moral choices are made.

NAS *see* NEONATAL ABSTINENCE SYNDROME.

nasal bone either of a pair of narrow ob-

long bones that together form the bridge and root of the nose. *See* SKULL.

nasal cavity the space inside the nose that lies between the floor of the cranium and the roof of the mouth. It is divided into two halves by a septum: each half communicates with the outside via the nostrils and with the nasopharynx through the posterior nares.

nasal concha (**turbinate bone**) any of three thin scroll-like bones that form the sides of the *nasal cavity. The **superior** and **middle nasal conchae** are part of the *ethmoid bone; the **inferior nasal conchae** are a separate pair of bones of the face. *See* SKULL.

NASH nonalcoholic steatohepatitis. *See* NONALCOHOLIC FATTY LIVER DISEASE.

nasion *n.* the point on the bridge of the nose at the centre of the suture between the nasal and frontal bones.

naso- *combining form denoting* the nose.

nasogastric tube a tube passed through the nose into the stomach, used to aspirate fluid from, or introduce material into, the stomach (*see* RYLE'S TUBE).

nasolacrimal *adj.* relating to the nose and the lacrimal (tear-producing) apparatus.

nasolacrimal duct the duct that passes through the hole (**nasolacrimal canal**) in the palatine bone of the skull. It drains the tears away from the *lacrimal apparatus into the inferior meatus of the nose.

nasopharyngeal airway a curved tube to be slotted down one nostril of an unconscious patient, to sit behind the tongue, to create a patent airway. *See also* OROPHARYNGEAL AIRWAY.

nasopharynx (**postnasal space, rhino-pharynx**) *n.* the part of the *pharynx that lies above the level of the junction of the hard and soft palates. It connects the *nasal cavity to the *oropharynx. —**nasopharyngeal** *adj.*

natalizumab *n.* a monoclonal antibody used for the treatment of severe relapsing-remitting multiple sclerosis: it reduces demyelination and inflammation by inhibiting migration of leucocytes into the central nervous system. It is administered by intravenous infusion; side-effects include an increased risk of neurological damage and opportunistic infections. Trade name: **Tysabri**.

natal teeth teeth that are present at the time of birth.

nateglinide *n. see* MEGLITINIDES.

nates *pl. n.* the buttocks. —**natal** *adj.*

national census *see* CENSUS, OFFICE FOR NATIONAL STATISTICS.

National Clinical Assessment Service (NCAS) part of the *National Patient Safety Agency providing advice and support to NHS trusts and health authorities in England, Wales, and Northern Ireland on managing poor clinical performance of individual doctors, dentists, and pharmacists. The emphasis of the service is on local resolution.

(⊕) **SEE WEB LINKS**
• NCAS website

National Health Service (NHS) (in Britain) a comprehensive service offering therapeutic and preventive medical and surgical care, including the prescription and dispensing of medicines, spectacles, and medical and dental appliances. Exchequer funds pay for the services of doctors, nurses, and other professionals, as well as residential costs in NHS hospitals, and meet a substantial part of the cost of the medicines and appliances. Legislation enacted in 1946 was implemented in 1948 and the services were subjected to substantial reorganization in 1974 and again in 1982, 1991, and 1999. In England overall responsibility is vested in the Secretary of State for Health assisted by a comprehensive department (*see* DEPARTMENT OF HEALTH). Administration was based on a system of delegation downwards and accountability upwards through a hierarchy of regions, each subdivided into a number of districts. In 1991 district health authorities (DHAs) developed a new role as purchasers of health care, assessing the health needs of local populations and negotiating contracts with a range of health-care providers to meet those needs. Family health service authorities (FHSAs) were responsible for the regulation, management, and funding of general practitioners, pharmacists, opticians, and dentists. In 1999 *primary care trusts were established to take responsibility for most of the functions originally carried out by DHAs and FHSAs and subsequently (from 1996) by health authorities. In 2002 the government merged and renamed the health authorities to form 28 *strategic health authorities. In 2006 there was a further programme of reor-

ganization and mergers, resulting in 10 strategic health authorities and 152 primary care trusts. Some specialist resources for patients with rarer complaints are shared on a regional or supraregional basis (*see* SPECIALIZED COMMISSIONING GROUP).

Different arrangements apply in Northern Ireland, Wales, and Scotland.

(⊕) **SEE WEB LINKS**
• NHS Choices: provides basic medical advice and a guide to local services

National Institute for Health and Clinical Excellence (NICE) a special health authority covering England and Wales, set up in April 1999 and originally called the **National Institute for Clinical Excellence**. It consists of policy makers, clinicians working in the NHS, academics, and patients. NICE is responsible for examining the evidence for treatments and services and using that evidence to maximize cost-effectiveness. It issues guidance and advice on best clinical practice and seeks to reduce geographical variations in care. In 2005 NICE took over the functions of the **Health Development Agency**, including providing guidance on preventing disease and promoting health. *See* CLINICAL GOVERNANCE.

(⊕) **SEE WEB LINKS**
• NICE website

National Insurance (in Britain) a compulsory scheme of insurance under the terms of which employers and employees make joint contributions so that those who have contributed for a qualifying period may claim national insurance benefits in times of sickness, injury, maternity leave, unemployment, and retirement; self-employed persons pay all their own contributions. Those who do not qualify under the terms of this insurance scheme may also receive financial payments in times of need, but only subject to a means test.

National Patient Safety Agency (NPSA) a special health authority that leads and coordinates work to improve all aspects of patient safety in England. The NPSA comprises three divisions: the **National Reporting and Learning Service**, the **National Research Ethics Service**, and the **National Clinical Assessment Service**. The National Reporting and Learning Service is a confidential reporting system of adverse events and near misses involving NHS patients. It is particularly concerned with dissemination of learning to prevent recurrences. The National Research Ethics Service (formerly the Central Office for Research Ethics Committees) leads the national network of NHS research ethics committees, working to protect the safety and wellbeing of participants in research (*see* ETHICS COMMITTEE). The National Clinical Assessment Service addresses concerns about the performance of individual doctors, dentists, and pharmacists. The NPSA is also responsible for wider aspects of patient safety, including hospital design, cleanliness, and food (formerly the responsibility of NHS Estates), and for commissioning the *confidential enquiries.

(((()))) SEE WEB LINKS

• Website of the NPSA

national service frameworks (NSFs) national standards of care published for a variety of conditions and patient groups (the first were for coronary heart disease and mental health). The NSFs are designed to improve, and reduce variations in, the quality of care by defining long-term strategies for delivery of the standards and by setting specific goals.

National Statistics Socio-economic Classification (NS-SEC) an occupational classification of the national population that was developed to replace older systems based on **social classes** and **socio-economic groups**. The groupings are intended to stratify the population according to different forms of employment: households are classified according to the occupation of the household reference person (the person renting, owning, or otherwise responsible for accommodation). The NS-SEC is used for official surveys and statistics, including the *census. The analytic version of the classification has eight classes and is the version used for most analyses.

natriuresis *n.* the excretion of sodium in the urine, especially in greater than normal amounts.

natriuretic *n.* an agent that promotes the excretion of sodium salts in the urine. Most *diuretics are natriuretics.

natriuretic peptide any of several peptides that stimulate diuresis (increased urine production) and vasodilatation (widening of blood vessels). They act on the kidney tubules to promote excretion of sodium (natriuresis) and water. **Atrial natriuretic pep-**

tide (ANP) is produced in the atria of the heart in response to a rise in atrial pressure. **Brain natriuretic peptide** (BNP) is produced in the brain and the ventricles of the heart, mainly in response to stretching of the ventricular muscle (as occurs in congestive heart failure). Measurement of blood levels of BNP is used as a screening test (the **BNP test**) for the detection of heart failure; levels >99 ng/l indicate a positive result.

natural killer cell (NK cell) a type of *lymphocyte that is able to kill virus-infected cells and cancerous cells and mediates rejection of bone-marrow grafts. NK cells are a part of natural (or innate) *immunity. Their function is regulated by a balance between activating receptors, which recognize proteins on cancerous or virus-infected cells, and inhibitory receptors specific for certain molecules encoded by the *HLA system.

naturopathy *n.* a system of medicine that relies upon the use of only 'natural' substances for the treatment of disease, rather than drugs. Herbs, food grown without artificial fertilizers and prepared without the use of preservatives or colouring material, pure water, sunlight, and fresh air are all employed in an effort to rid the body of 'unnatural' substances, which are said to be at the root of most illnesses.

nausea *n.* the feeling that one is about to vomit, as experienced in seasickness and in morning sickness of early pregnancy. Actual vomiting often occurs subsequently.

navel *n. see* UMBILICUS.

navicular bone a boat-shaped bone of the ankle (*see* TARSUS) that articulates with the three cuneiform bones in front and with the talus behind.

NCAS *see* NATIONAL CLINICAL ASSESSMENT SERVICE.

nearthrosis *n. see* PSEUDARTHROSIS.

nebula *n.* a faint opacity of the cornea that remains after an ulcer has healed.

nebulizer *n.* an instrument used for applying a liquid in the form of a fine spray.

NEC *see* NECROTIZING ENTEROCOLITIS.

Necator *n.* a genus of *hookworms that live in the small intestine. The human hookworm, *N. americanus*, occurs in tropical Africa, Central and South America, India, and the Pacific Islands. The worm possesses two pairs of sharp cutting plates inside its mouth cavity, which enable it to feed on the blood and tissues of the gut wall. *Compare* Ancylostoma.

necatoriasis *n.* an infestation of the small intestine by the parasitic hookworm *Necator americanus. See also* HOOKWORM DISEASE.

neck *n.* **1.** the part of the body that connects the head and the trunk. It is the region supported by the *cervical vertebrae. **2.** *see* CERVIX.

necro- *combining form denoting* death or dissolution.

necrobiosis *n.* a gradual process by which cells lose their function and die. **Necrobiosis lipoidica** is a disease in which degeneration of collagen produces sharply demarcated yellowish-brown plaques, especially on the shins of women. The association with diabetes mellitus is controversial.

necrology *n.* the study of the phenomena of death, involving determination of the moment of death and the different changes that occur in the tissues of the body after death.

necropsy *n. see* AUTOPSY.

necrosis (**mortification**) *n.* the death of some or all of the cells in an organ or tissue, caused by disease, physical or chemical injury, or interference with the blood supply (*see* GANGRENE). **Caseous necrosis** occurs in pulmonary tuberculosis, the lung tissue becoming soft, dry, and cheeselike. **Coagulative necrosis** – the commonest form of necrosis – occurs in almost all organs (except the brain) and results in a solid mass of dead tissue. **Colliquative necrosis** occurs in the brain, where the absence of stroma (connective tissue) results in total liquefaction of necrotic tissue. —**necrotic** *adj.*

necrospermia *n.* the presence of either dead or motionless spermatozoa in the semen. *See* INFERTILITY.

necrotizing enterocolitis (**NEC**) a serious disease affecting the bowel during the first three weeks of life; it is much more common in preterm babies. The abdomen distends and blood and mucus appear in the stools; the bowel may perforate. Treatment is to rest the bowel and administer antibiotics. If the bowel becomes necrotic, surgery may be necessary. The cause is unknown but the disease may be the result of a reduced supply of oxygen to the bowel or infection.

necrotizing fasciitis a life-threatening bacterial infection of the layer of *fascia beneath the skin, usually by *Streptococcus* Type A. Symptoms appear rapidly after initial infection; they include a rash with blistering and discoloration of the skin, pain and inflammation of lymph nodes, fever, drowsiness, diarrhoea, and vomiting. Tissue necrosis and toxin production can result in shock and possible multi-organ failure. Necrotizing fasciitis is often associated with vascular disease, especially in diabetics, and the elderly and those who have recently undergone surgery are also vulnerable to the infection, which requires prompt treatment with intravenous antibiotics and excision of the involved tissue.

nedocromil *n.* a drug, related to sodium *cromoglicate, used to prevent asthma attacks and to treat allergic conjunctivitis. It is administered by metered-dose aerosol inhaler or as eye drops; possible side-effects include local irritation. Trade names: **Rapitil**, **Tilade CFC-free Inhaler**.

need *n.* requirement or necessity. In the context of health care and medical ethics, a distinction is often made between needs and wants. As such, for the purpose of allocating limited health-care resources, clinical need is often defined as the capacity to benefit from an intervention, as opposed to merely the lack of it, and assessed on a utilitarian basis (*see* QUALITY OF LIFE). However, there are other conceptions of need, such as the state of requiring rescue from a life-threatening situation.

needle *n.* a slender sharp-pointed instrument used for a variety of purposes. The size and shape of needles used in surgery for stitching tissue depend on the type of surgery. Most surgical needles have suture material fused onto them (so-called **atraumatic needles**). Hollow needles are used to inject substances into the body (in hypodermic syringes), to obtain specimens of tissue (*see* PUNCTURE), or to withdraw fluid from a cavity (*see* ASPIRATION, BIOPSY). *See also* STOP NEEDLE.

needle-stick injury a common accidental injury to the fingers and hands of nurses and doctors by contaminated injection needles. It can result in transmitted infections (e.g. hepatitis, AIDS).

needling *n.* the use of a sharp needle to make a hole in the lens capsule, usually to deal with the haze developing in the posterior capsule after cararact. This technique has now largely been replaced by use of the *YAG laser.

negative feedback loop a physiological loop for the control of hormone production by a gland. High levels of a circulating hormone act to reduce production of the releasing factors triggering its own production, i.e. they have a negative *feedback on these trigger factors. As circulating levels of the hormone fall, the negative feedback is reduced and the releasing factor starts to be produced again, allowing the hormone level to rise again.

negative symptoms (in psychiatry) symptoms of schizophrenia characterized by a deficiency in or absence of some aspect of functioning, such as social withdrawal, loss of initiative, and blunted affect. *Compare* POSITIVE SYMPTOMS.

negativism *n.* behaviour that is the opposite of that suggested by others. In **active negativism** the individual does the opposite of what is asked for (for example, screws the eyes up when asked to open them). In *psychosis it is usually associated with other features of *catatonia. In **passive negativism** the person fails to cooperate (for example, stops eating). This occurs in *schizophrenia and *depression.

negligence *n.* failure by a health-care professional to exercise a reasonable standard of care, as defined in the UK by the *Bolam test (as amended by the *Bolitho amendment), which asks whether the care provided fell short of that of a reasonable body of professional opinion and whether actions or omissions withstand logical analysis (the determination of which falls to the court). In order to establish negligence a claimant must show that a doctor had a *duty of care, that he or she breached this duty by falling below the expected standard of care, and that foreseeable harm was caused as a result of the professional's conduct. The standard of proof in negligence actions is that of the civil law (i.e. on the balance of probabilities). Payment of *compensation to the claimant upon proving negligence is required by the UK civil law. Rarely, doctors may be charged with the criminal offence of manslaughter by gross negligence, which must be proved according to the standards of the criminal law (beyond reasonable doubt). If convicted, the sentence for gross negligence cases is likely to be custodial.

(⊕) SEE WEB LINKS
• Website of the NHS Litigation Authority

Neisseria *n.* a genus of spherical Gram-negative aerobic nonmotile bacteria characteristically grouped in pairs. They are parasites of animals, and some species are normal inhabitants of the human respiratory tract. The species *N. gonorrhoeae* (the **gonococcus**) causes *gonorrhoea. Gonococci are found within pus cells of urethral and vaginal discharge; they can be cultured only on serum or blood agar. *N. meningitidis* (the **meningococcus**) causes meningococcal *meningitis. Meningococci are found within pus cells of infected cerebrospinal fluid and blood or in the nasal passages of carriers. They too can only be cultured on serum or blood agar.

nelfinavir *n. see* PROTEASE INHIBITOR.

Nelson's syndrome a condition in which an *ACTH-producing pituitary tumour develops after loss of negative *feedback following bilateral adrenalectomy, usually for *Cushing's syndrome. [D. H. Nelson (1925–), US physician]

nematode (roundworm) *n.* any one of a large group of worms having an unsegmented cylindrical body, tapering at both ends. This distinguishes nematodes from other *helminths. Nematodes occur either as free-living forms in the sea, fresh water, and soil or as parasites of plants, animals, and humans. *Hookworms and *threadworms infest the alimentary canal. *Filariae are found in the lymphatic tissues. The *guinea worm and *Onchocerca affect connective tissue. Some nematodes (e.g. threadworms) are transmitted from host to host by the ingestion of eggs; others (e.g. *Wuchereria*) by the bite of a bloodsucking insect.

neo- *combining form denoting* new or newly formed.

neoadjuvant chemotherapy chemotherapy that is given before the (usually) surgical treatment of a primary tumour with the aim of improving the results of surgery or radiotherapy and preventing the development of metastases. *Compare* ADJUVANT THERAPY.

neocerebellum *n.* the middle lobe of the *cerebellum, excluding the pyramid and uvula. In evolutionary terms it is the newest part, occurring only in mammals.

neointimal hyperplasia a pathological process involved in *atherosclerosis, arteriosclerosis induced by vein grafts, and *restenosis in response to angioplasty and stent placement. Damage to the endothelium of the artery exposes the underlying smooth muscle cells in the *media to cytokines, growth factors, and other plasma components in the circulation, which results in loss of their contractile characteristics. These abnormal muscle cells migrate to the *intima, where they proliferate and eventually form a thick layer of tissue (neointima), which occludes the artery.

neologism *n.* (in psychiatry) the invention of words that do not exist in one's language. It is common in childhood, but when it occurs in an adult it may be a symptom of a psychotic illness, such as *schizophrenia. It should be distinguished from *paraphasia, in which new meanings are attached to ordinary words.

neomycin *n.* an *aminoglycoside antibiotic used to treat infections caused by a wide range of bacteria, mainly those affecting the skin, ears, and eyes. Too toxic to be injected, it is usually applied in creams, ointments, or drops with other antibiotics, but can be given by mouth to sterilize the bowel before surgery.

neonatal abstinence syndrome (NAS) symptoms and signs exhibited by a newborn baby (neonate) due to drug withdrawal (*see* DEPENDENCE). This results when the fetus has been exposed to addictive drugs through maternal substance abuse or misuse. Symptoms tend to occur in the first few days of life (in the case of methadone, which is a long-acting opioid, symptom onset may be delayed). They include tremors and jerking, high-pitched crying, sneezing, sucking of fists, feeding difficulties, shortened periods of sleep between feeds, rapid breathing, sweating, loose stools, nasal stuffiness, and frequent yawning. Treatment includes swaddling or snugly wrapping in a blanket, as babies with NAS are often difficult to comfort. Other nonpharmacological measures include frequent small feeds using high-calorie formula and intravenous fluids if babies become dehydrated. Drug therapy may be used for seizures and withdrawal symptoms.

neonatal mortality rate *see* INFANT MORTALITY RATE.

neonatal screening *screening tests carried out on newborn babies to detect diseases that appear in the neonatal period, such as phenylketonuria (*see* GUTHRIE TEST). If these diseases are detected early enough, treatment may be instigated before any irreversible damage occurs to the baby.

neonatal teeth teeth that emerge through the gingiva (gums) during the first month of life.

neonate *n.* an infant at any time during the first 28 days of life. The word is particularly applied to infants just born or in the first week of life. —**neonatal** *adj.*

neopallium *n.* an enlargement of the wall of each cerebral hemisphere. In evolutionary terms it is the newest part of the cerebrum, formed by the development of new pathways for sight and hearing in mammals.

neoplasia *n.* a form of abnormal growth that is independent of the body's normal homeostatic growth-regulating mechanisms, continues after the initiating stimulus has been removed, and is purposeless. Neoplasia is always pathological. *See* CERVICAL INTRAEPITHELIAL NEOPLASIA (CIN), GESTATIONAL TROPHOBLASTIC NEOPLASIA, MENS (MULTIPLE ENDOCRINE NEOPLASIA SYNDROMES, PROSTATIC INTRAEPITHELIAL NEOPLASIA (PIN), VULVAL INTRAEPITHELIAL NEOPLASIA (VIN). *Compare* HYPERPLASIA. —**neoplastic** *adj.*

neoplasm *n.* any new and abnormal growth: any *benign or *malignant tumour. —**neoplastic** *adj.*

neosphincter *n.* a substituted muscle or an implant for an absent or ineffective sphincter (*see* ARTIFICIAL SPHINCTER).

neostigmine *n.* an *anticholinesterase drug used mainly to diagnose and treat *myasthenia gravis and to reverse the action of nondepolarizing *muscle-relaxant drugs used during surgery. It is administered by mouth or injection; side-effects include abdominal cramps, diarrhoea, increased salivation, and a slow heart rate (*bradycardia).

neovascularization *n.* the abnormal formation of new and fragile blood vessels, usually in response to ischaemia. In **choroidal neovascularization**, which occurs in such conditions as *macular degeneration, abnormal vessels, derived from the *choroid, form in the space between the retinal pigment epithelium (RPE) and the choroid (*see* RETINA).

nephr- (**nephro-**) *combining form denoting* the kidney(s).

nephralgia *n.* pain in the kidney. The pain is felt in the loin and can be caused by a variety of kidney complaints.

nephrectomy *n.* surgical removal of a kidney. When performed for cancer of the kidney, the entire organ is removed together with its surrounding fat and the adjacent adrenal gland (**radical nephrectomy**). Removal of either the upper or lower pole of the kidney is termed **partial nephrectomy**. The operation can be performed by *laparoscopy.

nephrin *n.* a transmembrane protein localized to the slit diaphragm of the *podocyte and necessary for the proper functioning of the renal filtration barrier. The latter consists of fenestrated endothelial cells, the basement membrane, and the epithelial podocyte. A defect in the gene coding for nephrin (*NPHS1*) on chromosome 19 results in congenital nephrotic syndrome of Finnish type (which is not exclusive to the Finnish population).

nephritic syndrome generalized inflammation of the glomeruli of the kidneys resulting in a reduction in *glomerular filtration rate, with mild oedema and hypertension resulting from renal salt and water retention. Urine analysis shows the presence of proteinuria and microscopic haematuria with red cell casts. Common and usually self-limiting causes are *Berger's nephropathy and poststreptococcal glomerulonephritis. Less common but more serious causes of the nephritic syndrome are the vasculitides (*see* VASCULITIS) and *Goodpasture's disease, which, untreated, usually prove fatal.

nephritis (Bright's disease) *n.* inflammation of the kidney. Nephritis is a nonspecific term used to describe a condition resulting from a variety of causes. *See* GLOMERULO-NEPHRITIS.

nephroblastoma (Wilms' tumour) *n.* a malignant tumour arising from the embryonic kidney and occurring in young children, usually below the age of three and rarely over the age of eight. In some cases it involves both kidneys. Treatment consists of removing the kidney (*see* NEPHRECTOMY)

and giving chemotherapy. Although almost half the cases have spread by the time diagnosis is made, this does not prevent a cure: the number of children that survive at least five years after diagnosis is improving, being currently around 75%. In some children the tumour is associated with an abnormality of chromosome number 13; in these cases other features, such as absence of the iris in the eye (*see* ANIRIDIA) and *hemihypertrophy, are present. In other cases there is an association with congenital nephropathy and intersex disorders (*see* DENYS-DRASH SYNDROME).

nephrocalcinosis *n.* the presence of calcium deposits in the kidneys. This can be caused by excess calcium in the blood, as caused by overactivity of the parathyroid glands, or it may result from an underlying abnormality of the kidney. The cause of nephrocalcinosis must be detected by full biochemical, radiological, and urological investigation so that appropriate treatment can be undertaken.

nephrogenic cord either of the paired ridges of tissue that run along the dorsal surface of the abdominal cavity of the embryo. Parts of it develop into the kidney, ovary, or testis and their associated ducts. Intermediate stages of these developments are the *pronephros, *mesonephros, and *metanephros.

nephrogenic diabetes insipidus (NDI) a condition characterized by *polyuria and *polydipsia and due to failure of the renal tubules to respond, or to respond fully, to *vasopressin. One form of congenital NDI is caused by an X-linked (*see* SEX-LINKED) dominant mutation of the gene encoding the vasopressin V2 receptor. A rarer form of congenital NDI is an autosomal recessive condition associated with genetic mutations in the gene encoding AQP-2 water channels (*see* AQUAPORIN). Acquired NDI is much commoner than the congenital form and usually less severe. It is present in most patients with advancing chronic renal failure, is a feature of certain electrolyte disorders (hypokalaemia, hypercalcaemia), and can complicate chronic lithium treatment.

nephrogenic systemic fibrosis (NSF, nephrogenic fibrosing dermopathy) a rare condition, first reported in 1997, that occurs exclusively in patients with chronic kidney disease (CKD), who develop large areas of hardened skin with fibrotic nodules and plaques. Flexion contractures with an accompanying limitation of range of motion can also occur. Exposure to gadolinium, used as a contrast agent in magnetic resonance imaging, has been identified as a causative factor, but many patients with severe CKD have been exposed to gadolinium without consequence. Linear gadolinium preparations (Omniscan, OptiMARK) appear to carry the highest risk of NSF. There is no cure for the condition.

nephrolithiasis *n*. the presence of stones in the kidney (*see* CALCULUS). Such stones can cause pain and blood in the urine, but they may produce no symptoms. Full investigation is undertaken to determine the underlying cause of stone formation. When stones are associated with urinary obstruction and infection they usually require surgical removal (*see* NEPHROLITHOTOMY, PYELOLITHOTOMY).

nephrolithotomy *n*. the surgical removal of a stone from the kidney by an incision into the kidney substance. It is normally performed in combination with an incision into the renal pelvis (*see* PYELOLITHOTOMY). *See also* PERCUTANEOUS NEPHROLITHOTOMY.

nephrology *n*. the branch of medicine concerned with the study, investigation, and management of diseases of the kidney. *See also* UROLOGY. —**nephrologist** *n*.

nephron *n*. the active unit of excretion in the kidney (see illustration). Blood, which is supplied by branches of the renal artery, is filtered through a knot of capillaries (**glomerulus**) into the cup-shaped **Bowman's capsule** so that water, nitrogenous waste, and many other substances (excluding colloids) pass into the **renal tubule**. Here most of the substances are reabsorbed back into the blood, the remaining fluid (*urine) passing into the collecting duct, which drains into the *ureter.

nephropathy *n*. disease of the kidney. *See also* BALKAN NEPHROPATHY, BERGER'S NEPHROPATHY, CAST NEPHROPATHY, CHINESE HERB NEPHROPATHY, DIABETIC NEPHROPATHY, HAN, HIVAN, HYPERCALCAEMIC NEPHROPATHY, HYPOKALAEMIC NEPHROPATHY, MEMBRANOUS NEPHROPATHY, MINIMAL CHANGE NEPHROPATHY, SICKLE-CELL NEPHROPATHY.

nephropexy *n*. an operation to fix a mobile kidney. The kidney is fixed to the twelfth rib and adjacent posterior abdominal wall to prevent descent of the kidney on standing (*see* NEPHROPTOSIS).

nephroptosis *n*. abnormal descent of a kidney into the pelvis on standing, which may occur if it is excessively mobile (for example, in thin women). If this is accompanied by pain and obstruction to free drainage of urine by the kidney, *nephropexy may be advised.

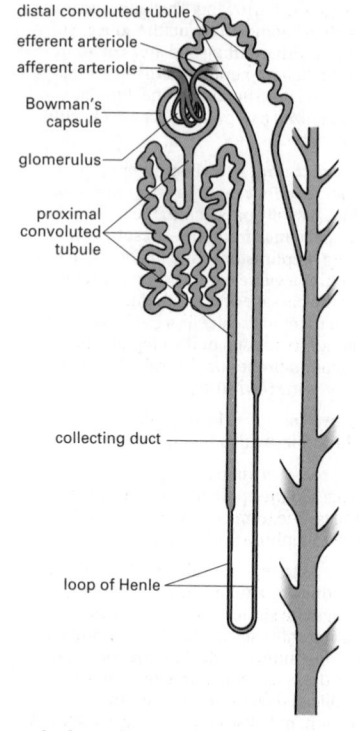

distal convoluted tubule
efferent arteriole
afferent arteriole
Bowman's capsule
glomerulus
proximal convoluted tubule
collecting duct
loop of Henle

A single nephron.

nephrosclerosis *n*. hardening of the arteries and arterioles of the kidneys. **Benign nephrosclerosis** is associated with essential hypertension. There is preferential involvement of the preglomerular arterial vessels, primarily the afferent arteriole and the interlobular artery. The classic arterial lesion, which is termed **arteriolosclerosis**, involves replacement of smooth muscle cells in the media of the vessel by connective tissue. There is often evidence of ischaemia in the glomerulus and *tubulointerstitium. Functionally there may be some degree of renal impairment. End-stage renal failure is uncommon, but more likely to occur in Afro-Caribbeans. **Malignant nephrosclerosis** is the hallmark of *malignant hypertension, with arterioles showing mucoid change, endothelial cell swelling, and fibrinoid necrosis. The lumen of the vessel is reduced and red cells fragmented in their passage through the narrowing. The kidney shows petechial haemorrhage on the subcapsular surface, with mottling and areas of infarction. Malignant nephrosclerosis can lead to a very rapid destruction of renal function and is recognized as a potential cause of acute renal failure.

nephroscope *n.* an instrument (*endoscope) used for examining the interior of the kidney, usually passed into the renal pelvis through a track from the skin surface after needle *nephrostomy and dilatation of the tract over a guide wire. The nephroscope allows the passage of instruments under direct vision to remove calculi (*see* PERCUTANEOUS NEPHROLITHOTOMY) or disintegrate them by ultrasound probes or electrohydraulic shock waves (*see* LITHOTRIPSY).

nephroscopy *n.* inspection of the interior of the kidney with a *nephroscope.

nephrosis *n.* (in pathology) degenerative changes in the epithelium of the kidney tubules. The term is sometimes used loosely for the *nephrotic syndrome.

nephrostomy *n.* drainage of urine from the kidney by a tube (catheter) passing through the kidney via the skin surface. This is commonly used as a temporary procedure after operations on the kidney. Long-term urine drainage by nephrostomy may be complicated by the attendant problems of infection and obstruction of the catheter by debris. Nephrostomy is also performed to enable the passage of a *nephroscope.

nephrotic syndrome (NS) a condition defined by the triad of peripheral oedema, heavy proteinuria (>3.5 g/day), and hypoalbuminaemia (serum albumin usually >25 g/l). In most cases there is hypercholesterolaemia and lipiduria. There are many causes of the nephrotic syndrome. In children, the main cause is *minimal change nephropathy, which is usually steroid-responsive. In adults, minimal change disease is still an important cause of NS, but is responsible for

only a minority of cases. Many of the other causes of NS in adults are unlikely to respond to steroids and it is therefore usual practice to perform a biopsy before considering specific treatment. The commonest causes of NS in adults are *diabetic nephropathy, *focal segmental glomerulosclerosis, and *membranous nephropathy. Pre-eclampsia is an important cause in late pregnancy.

nephrotomy *n.* surgical incision into the substance of the kidney. This is usually undertaken to remove a kidney stone (*see* NEPHROLITHOTOMY).

nephrotoxic *adj.* liable to cause damage to the kidneys. Nephrotoxic drugs include *aminoglycoside antibiotics, sulphonamides, and gold compounds. —**nephrotoxicity** *n.*

nephroureterectomy (ureteronephrectomy) *n.* the surgical removal of a kidney together with its ureter. This operation is performed for cancer of the kidney pelvis or ureter. It is also undertaken when the kidney has been destroyed by *vesicoureteric reflux, to prevent subsequent continuing reflux into the stump of the ureter that would occur if the kidney alone were removed.

nerve *n.* a bundle of conducting *nerve fibres (see illustration) that transmit im-

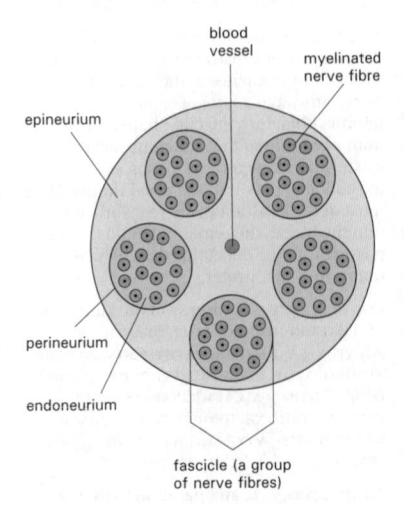

Nerve. Transverse section through a peripheral nerve with five fascicles.

pulses from the brain or spinal cord to the muscles and glands (**motor nerves**) or inwards from the sense organs to the brain and spinal cord (**sensory nerves**). Most large nerves are **mixed nerves**, containing both motor and sensory nerve fibres running to and from a particular region of the body.

nerve block a method of producing *anaesthesia in part of the body by blocking the passage of pain impulses in the sensory nerves supplying it. A local anaesthetic, such as lidocaine, is injected into the tissues in the region of a nerve. In this way anaesthesia can be localized, so that minor operations can be performed without the necessity of giving a general anaesthetic. A *ring block is a common technique used for anaesthetizing a digit.

nerve cell *see* NEURON.

nerve ending the final part (terminal) of one of the branches of a nerve fibre, where a *neuron makes contact either with another neuron at a synapse or with a muscle or gland cell at a neuromuscular or neuroglandular junction.

nerve entrapment syndrome any syndrome resulting from pressure on a nerve from surrounding structures. Examples include the *carpal tunnel syndrome and *meralgia paraesthetica.

nerve fibre the long fine process that extends from the cell body of a *neuron and carries nerve impulses. Bundles of nerve fibres running together form a *nerve. Each fibre has a sheath, which in medullated nerve fibres is a relatively thick layer containing the fatty insulating material *myelin.

nerve gas any gas that disrupts the normal functioning of nerves and thus of the muscles they supply. There are two groups, the **G agents** and the **V agents**. The latter are more than 300 times as deadly as mustard gas: one inhalation can kill by paralysing the respiratory muscles. V agents also act through the skin, therefore gas masks are ineffective protection against them.

nerve growth factor (NGF) a protein (*see* GROWTH FACTOR), consisting of two polypeptide chains, that is required for the development and longevity of some neurons, including those in the sympathetic nervous system and some central nervous system and sensory neurons. Nerve growth factor is necessary for axon growth and also

for initiating new neuronal connections with other cells. The role of NGFs in preventing the degeneration of brain cells is being explored in research into Alzheimer's disease.

nerve impulse the electrical activity in the membrane of a *neuron that – by its rapid spread from one region to the next – is the means by which information is transmitted within the nervous system along the axons of the neurons. The membrane of a resting nerve is charged (**polarized**) because of the different concentrations of ions inside and outside the cell. When a nerve impulse is triggered, a wave of *depolarization spreads, and ions flow across the membrane (*see* ACTION POTENTIAL). Until the nerve has undergone *repolarization no further nerve impulses can pass.

nerve regeneration the growth of new nerve tissue, which occurs at a very slow rate (1–2 mm per day) after a nerve has been severed and is often partially or totally incomplete. *Microsurgery has improved the results by facilitating primary repair in the immediate aftermath of injury. *See also* AXONOTMESIS, NEUROTMESIS.

nervous breakdown a nonmedical term applied to a range of emotional crises varying from a brief attack of 'hysterical' behaviour to a major *mental illness. The term is also sometimes used as a euphemism for a frank psychiatric illness, such as *schizophrenia.

nervous system the vast network of cells specialized to carry information (in the form of *nerve impulses) to and from all parts of the body in order to bring about bodily activity. The brain and spinal cord together form the *central nervous system; the remaining nervous tissue is known as the *peripheral nervous system and includes the *autonomic nervous system, which is itself divided into the sympathetic and parasympathetic nervous systems. The basic functional unit of the nervous system is the *neuron (nerve cell).

Nesbit's operation an operation devised to surgically straighten a congenitally curved penis but now more frequently employed to correct the penile curvature caused by *Peyronie's disease. [R. M. Nesbit (20th century), US surgeon]

nesidioblastosis *n.* a rare condition of childhood in which abnormal cells in the pancreas fail to mature properly and secrete a selection of hormones (including insulin) in an uncontrolled manner. This causes a variety of problems, including recurrent *hypoglycaemia. It can sometimes be treated with medication; if this fails, surgical removal of a portion of the pancreas may be necessary.

nettle rash *see* URTICARIA.

neur- (neuro-) *combining form denoting* nerves or the nervous system.

neural arch *see* VERTEBRA.

neural crest the two bands of ectodermal tissue that flank the *neural plate of the early embryo. Cells of the neural crest migrate throughout the embryo and develop into sensory nerve cells and peripheral nerve cells of the autonomic nervous system.

neuralgia *n.* a severe burning or stabbing pain often following the course of a nerve. **Postherpetic neuralgia** is an intense debilitating pain felt at the site of a previous attack of shingles. In **trigeminal neuralgia (tic douloureux)** there are brief paroxysms of searing pain felt in the distribution of one or more branches of the *trigeminal nerve in the face. Trigeminal neuralgia is managed principally by prescription of *carbamazepine. **Migrainous neuralgia** is characterized by severe unilateral pain around one eye (*see* CLUSTER HEADACHE).

neural plate the strip of ectoderm lying along the central axis of the early embryo that forms the *neural tube and subsequently the central nervous system.

neural spine the spinous process situated on the neural arch of a *vertebra.

neural tube the embryological structure from which the brain and spinal cord develop. It is a hollow tube of ectodermal tissue formed when two edges of a groove in a plate of primitive neural tissue (**neural plate**) come together and fuse. Failure of normal fusion results in a number of congenital defects (*see* NEURAL TUBE DEFECTS).

neural tube defects a group of congenital abnormalities caused by failure of the *neural tube to form normally. In *spina bifida the bony arches of the spine, which protect the spinal cord and its coverings (the meninges), fail to close. More severe defects of fusion of these bones will result in increasingly serious neurological conditions. A **meningocele** is the protrusion of the meninges through the gap in the spine, the skin covering being vestigial. There is a constant risk of damage to the meninges, with resulting infection. Urgent surgical treatment to protect the meninges is therefore required. In a **meningomyelocele (myelomeningocele, myelocele)** the spinal cord and the nerve roots are exposed, often adhering to the fine membrane that overlies them. There is a constant risk of infection and this condition is accompanied by paralysis and numbness of the legs and urinary incontinence. *Hydrocephalus and an *Arnold-Chiari malformation are usually present. A failure of fusion at the cranial end of the neural tube (**cranium bifidum**) gives rise to comparable disorders. The bone defect is most often in the occipital region of the skull but it may occur in the frontal or basal regions. A protrusion of the meninges alone is known as a **cranial meningocele**. The terms **meningoencephalocele, encephalocele**, and **cephalocele** are used for the protrusion of brain tissue through the skull defect. This is accompanied by severe mental and physical disorders.

neuraminidase (NA, N) *n.* a glycoprotein projecting from the surface layer of the lipid bilayer envelope of *influenza virions. It attacks sialic acid residues on host cells and may be involved in virus release. It is a key target for antibody attack and therefore is important in vaccination.

neurapraxia *n.* temporary loss of nerve function resulting in tingling, numbness, and weakness. It is usually caused by compression of the nerve and there is no structural damage involved. Complete recovery occurs. *Compare* AXONOTMESIS, NEUROTMESIS.

neurasthenia *n.* a set of psychological and physical symptoms, including fatigue, irritability, headache, dizziness, anxiety, and intolerance of noise. It can be caused by organic damage, such as a head injury, or it can be due to neurosis. —**neurasthenic** *adj., n.*

neurectasis *n.* the surgical procedure for stretching a peripheral nerve.

neurectomy *n.* the surgical removal of the whole or part of a nerve.

neurilemma (neurolemma) *n.* the sheath of the *axon of a nerve fibre. The neurilemma of a medullated fibre contains *myelin laid down by Schwann cells. —**neurilemmal** *adj.*

neurilemmoma (neurinoma) *n.* a benign slow-growing tumour that arises from the neurilemma of a nerve fibre.

neurinoma *n. see* NEURILEMMOMA.

neuritis *n.* a disease of the peripheral nerves showing the pathological changes of inflammation. The term is also used in a less precise sense as an alternative to *neuropathy. *See also* RETROBULBAR NEURITIS.

neuroanatomy *n.* the study of the structure of the nervous system, from the gross anatomy of the brain down to the microscopic details of neurons.

neurobiotaxis *n.* the predisposition of a nerve cell to move towards the source of its stimuli during development.

neuroblast *n.* any of the nerve cells of the embryo that give rise to functional nerve cells (neurons).

neuroblastoma *n.* a malignant tumour, usually of childhood, composed of embryonic nerve cells. It may originate in any part of the sympathetic nervous system, most commonly in the medulla of the adrenal gland, and secondary growths are often widespread in other organs and in bones. It can nevertheless be very responsive to systemic chemotherapy.

neurocardiogenic syncope (malignant vasovagal syndrome) recurrent loss of consciousness due to a drop in blood pressure mediated by *vasodilatation, *bradycardia, or a combination of the two. Attacks resemble a simple faint, but can be very disabling because they are much more frequent and severe. Treatment comprises increased fluid and salt intake together with training in postural manoeuvres that may prevent attacks. A variety of drug treatments is available, but these are commonly ineffective. Implantation of a permanent *pacemaker may be required if profound bradycardia is a feature.

neurocranium *n.* the part of the skull that encloses the brain.

neurodermatitis *n. see* LICHEN SIMPLEX CHRONICUS.

neuroendocrine system the system of dual control of certain activities of the body by means of both nerves and circulating hormones. The functioning of the autonomic nervous system is particularly closely linked to that of the pituitary and adrenal glands.

The system can give rise to **neuroendocrine tumours**, which have special structural features and often produce active hormones. *See also* NEUROHORMONE, NEUROSECRETION.

neuroepithelioma *n.* a malignant tumour of the retina of the eye. It is a form of *glioma and may spread into the brain if not treated early.

neuroepithelium *n.* a type of epithelium associated with organs of special sense. It contains sensory nerve endings and is found in the retina, the membranous labyrinth of the inner ear, the mucous membrane lining the nasal cavity, and the taste buds. —**neuroepithelial** *adj.*

neurofibril *n.* one of the microscopic threads of cytoplasm found in the cell body of a *neuron and also in the *axoplasm of peripheral nerves.

neurofibrillary tangles twisted filaments composed of an abnormal form of tau protein, which normally occurs in microtubules (structural elements) of cells. They are found in the brains of patients with *Alzheimer's disease.

neurofibroma *n.* a benign tumour growing from the fibrous coverings of a peripheral nerve: it arises from *Schwann cells, lacks a capsule (therefore it may incorporate nerve fibres), and is usually symptomless. When it develops from the sheath of a nerve root, it causes pain and may compress the spinal cord. A **schwannoma** is similar but encapsulated (sometimes the terms are used synonymously).

neurofibromatosis *n.* either of two hereditary conditions inherited as autosomal *dominant traits and characterized by benign tumours growing from the fibrous coverings of nerves (*see* NEUROFIBROMA). In **neurofibromatosis type I (von Recklinghausen's disease)**, in which the abnormal gene is found on chromosome 17, numerous tumours affect the peripheral nerves. The tumours can be felt beneath the skin along the course of the nerves; they may become large, causing disfigurement, and rarely they become malignant, giving rise to **neurofibrosarcomas**. Pigmented patches on the skin (*see* CAFÉ AU LAIT SPOTS) are commonly found and *Lisch nodules are present. **Neurofibromatosis type II** presents with bilateral *vestibular schwannomas (causing hearing loss) and *meningiomas. The abnormal gene is on chromosome 22.

neurogenesis *n.* the growth and development of nerve cells.

neurogenic *adj.* **1.** caused by disease or dysfunction of the nervous system. **2.** arising in nervous tissue. **3.** caused by nerve stimulation.

neuroglia *n. see* GLIA.

neurohormone *n.* a hormone that is produced within specialized nerve cells and is secreted from the nerve endings into the circulation. Examples are the hormones oxytocin and vasopressin, produced within the nerve cells of the hypothalamus and released into the circulation in the posterior pituitary gland, and noradrenaline, released from *chromaffin tissue in the adrenal medulla.

neurohumour *n.* a *neurohormone or a *neurotransmitter.

neurohypophysis *n.* the posterior lobe of the *pituitary gland.

neurolemma *n. see* NEURILEMMA.

neurology *n.* the study of the structure, functioning, and diseases of the nervous system (including the brain, spinal cord, the peripheral nerves, and muscles). —**neurological** *adj.* —**neurologist** *n.*

neuroma *n.* any tumour derived from cells of the nervous system. Such tumours are now usually categorized more specifically (e.g. *neurofibroma, *neurilemmoma). *See also* VESTIBULAR SCHWANNOMA.

neuromuscular junction (myoneural junction) the meeting point of a nerve fibre and the muscle fibre that it supplies. Between the enlarged end of the nerve fibre (**motor end-plate**) and the membrane of the muscle is a gap across which a *neurotransmitter must diffuse from the nerve to trigger contraction of the muscle.

neuromyelitis optica (Devic's disease) a condition that resembles multiple sclerosis. The diagnosis is confirmed by the finding of the antiaquaporin-4 antibody (NMO IgG antibody). Typically there is a transverse *myelitis, producing paralysis and numbness of the legs and trunk below the inflamed spinal cord, and *retrobulbar (optic) neuritis affecting both optic nerves. The attacks of myelitis and optic neuritis may coincide or they may be separated by days or weeks. Recovery from the initial attack is often incomplete, but relapses appear to be less common than in conventional multiple sclerosis.

neuron (neurone, nerve cell) *n.* one of the basic functional units of the nervous system: a cell specialized to transmit electrical *nerve impulses and so carry information from one part of the body to another (see illustration). Each neuron has an enlarged portion, the **cell body** (**perikaryon**), containing the nucleus; from the body extend several processes (**dendrites**) through which impulses enter from their branches. A longer process, the nerve fibre (*see* AXON), extends outwards and carries impulses away from the cell body. This is normally unbranched except at the *nerve ending. The point of contact of one neuron with another is known as a *synapse.

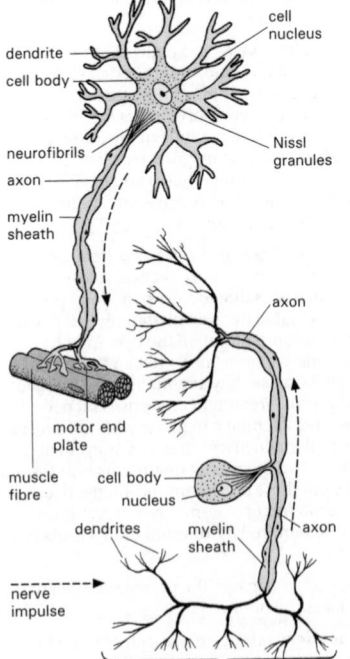

Neuron. A motor neuron (left) and a sensory neuron (right).

neuronophagia *n.* the process whereby damaged or degenerating nerve cells finally disintegrate and are removed by scavenger cells (*phagocytes).

neuronoplasty *n.* reconstructive surgery for damaged or severed peripheral nerves.

neuropathic arthritis (Charcot's joint) an extreme form of osteoarthritis resulting from damage to the sensory nerves that supply a joint. Causes include diabetes mellitus (*see* DIABETIC NEUROPATHY), *tabes dorsalis, *syringomyelia, leprosy, congenital insensitivity to pain, and other neurological problems. Patients develop an unstable painless swollen joint; treatment is focused on limitation of activity and bracing.

neuropathic bladder a malfunctioning bladder due to partial or complete interruption of its nerve supply. Causes include injury to the spinal cord, spina bifida, multiple sclerosis, and diabetic neuropathy.

neuropathy *n.* any disease of the peripheral nerves, usually causing weakness and numbness. In a **mononeuropathy** a single nerve is affected and the extent of the symptoms depends upon the distribution of that nerve. In a **polyneuropathy** (*see* PERIPHERAL NEUROPATHY) many or all of the nerves are involved and the symptoms are most profound at the extremities of the limbs. *See also* DIABETIC NEUROPATHY. —**neuropathic** *adj.*

neuropeptide Y a peptide, related to *pancreatic polypeptide, that is found in the central and peripheral nervous systems (it is particularly abundant in the hypothalamus). It has a variety of actions, including stimulation of appetite, gastrointestinal regulation, reproduction, memory, circadian rhythms, and cardiovascular functioning.

neurophysiology *n.* the study of the complex chemical and physical changes that are associated with the activity of the nervous system.

neuropil *n.* nerve tissue that is visible microscopically as a mass of interwoven and interconnected nerve endings, dendrites, and other neuron components, rather than an ordered array of axons.

neuroplasticity (neural plasticity) *n.* the ability of the brain to develop new neurons and/or new synapses in response to stimulation and learning. Recent research shows that the brain retains its plasticity throughout life, more or less, depending on the person's state of health, etc. Following injury to the brain, neuroplasticity may allow uninjured areas to take over the processes previously carried out by the injured areas.

neuropsychiatry *n.* the branch of medicine concerned with the psychiatric effects of disorders of neurological function or structure. Increasingly, the correlation is being drawn between demonstrable brain changes and the resulting effects on the mind. It is the function of the growing speciality of neuropsychiatry to investigate this relationship.

neuroretinitis *n.* combined inflammation of the optic nerve and the retina.

neurosecretion *n.* any substance produced within, and secreted by, a nerve cell. Important examples are the hormone-releasing factors produced by the cells of the *hypothalamus and released into blood vessels of the pituitary gland, on which they act.

neurosis *n.* (*pl.* **neuroses**) any long-term mental or behavioural disorder in which contact with reality is retained and the condition is recognized by the sufferer as abnormal: the term and concept were originated by Freud. A neurosis essentially features anxiety or behaviour exaggeratedly designed to avoid anxiety. Defence mechanisms against anxiety take various forms and may appear as phobias, obsessions, compulsions, or sexual dysfunctions. In recent classifications, the disorders formerly included under the neuroses have been renamed. The general term is now **anxiety disorder**; hysteria has become *conversion disorder; amnesia, fugue, and depersonalization are *dissociative disorders; obsessional neurosis is now known as **obsessive–compulsive disorder** (*see* OBSESSION); and depressive neurosis has become *dysthymia. Psychoanalysis has proved of little value in curing these conditions; *behaviour therapy and *SSRIs are effective in many cases. —**neurotic** *adj.*

neurosurgery *n.* the surgical or operative treatment of diseases of the brain and spinal cord. This includes the management of head injuries, the relief of raised intracranial pressure and compression of the spinal cord, the eradication of infection (e.g. cerebral *abscess), the control of intracranial haemorrhage, and the diagnosis and treatment of tumours. The development of neurosurgery has been supported by advances in anaesthetics, radiology, and scanning techniques.

neurosyphilis *n.* *syphilis affecting the nervous system.

neuroticism *n.* a dimension of personality derived from questionnaires and psychological tests. People with high scores in neuroticism are anxious and intense, emotionally unstable, and more prone to develop *neurosis.

neurotmesis *n.* the complete severance of a peripheral nerve, which is associated with degeneration of the nerve fibres distal to the point of severance and slow *nerve regeneration. *Compare* AXONOTMESIS, NEURAPRAXIA.

neurotomy *n.* the surgical procedure of severing a nerve.

neurotoxic *adj.* poisonous or harmful to nerve cells. —**neurotoxicity** *n.*

neurotransmitter *n.* a chemical substance released from nerve endings to transmit impulses across *synapses to other nerves and across the minute gaps between the nerves and the muscles or glands that they supply. Outside the central nervous system the chief neurotransmitter is *acetylcholine; *noradrenaline is released by nerve endings of the sympathetic system. In the central nervous system, as well as acetylcholine and noradrenaline, *dopamine, *serotonin, *gamma-aminobutyric acid, the amino acid glutamate, and several other substances act as transmitters.

neurotrophic *adj.* relating to the growth and nutrition of neural tissue in the body.

neurotropic *adj.* growing towards or having an affinity for neural tissue. The term may be applied to viruses, chemicals, or toxins.

neutropenia *n.* an abnormal decrease in the number of *neutrophils in peripheral blood. Neutropenia may occur in a wide variety of diseases, including certain hereditary defects, aplastic *anaemias, tumours of the bone marrow, *agranulocytosis, and acute leukaemias. In cancer patients it is often due to the deleterious effects of *cytotoxic drugs on bone marrow cells. Neutropenia results in an increased susceptibility to infections; if patients become unwell, due to infection, this can lead to neutropenic sepsis, which can be life-threatening. —**neutropenic** *adj.*

neutrophil *n.* a variety of *granulocyte (a type of white blood cell) distinguished by a lobed nucleus and the presence in its cytoplasm of fine granules that stain purple with *Romanowsky stains. It is capable of ingesting and killing bacteria and provides an im-

portant defence against infection. There are normally $2.0-7.5 \times 10^9$ neutrophils per litre of blood. *See also* POLYMORPH.

newton *n.* the *SI unit of force, equal to the force required to impart to 1 kilogram an acceleration of 1 metre per second per second. Symbol: N.

nexus *n.* (in anatomy) a connection or link.

NGF *see* NERVE GROWTH FACTOR.

NHS *see* NATIONAL HEALTH SERVICE.

NHS Direct a 24-hour nurse-led telephone helpline providing care advice and information on a variety of health problems, local health-care services, and self-help organizations. There is also an online service.

( ) SEE WEB LINKS
- NHS Direct Online: provides details of local hospitals and doctors as well as much useful information and advice.

NHS walk-in centre a medical centre offering free and fast access to health-care advice and treatment. The first centres were opened in 2000. They provide advice and treatment for minor injuries and illnesses as well as guidance on how to use NHS services.

niacin *n. see* NICOTINIC ACID.

nicardipine *n.* a *calcium-channel blocker used to prevent angina and treat hypertension. It is administered by mouth. Possible side-effects include nausea, dizziness, headache, flushing, and palpitations. Trade name: **Cardene**.

NICE *see* NATIONAL INSTITUTE FOR HEALTH AND CLINICAL EXCELLENCE.

niche *n.* (in anatomy) a recess or depression in a smooth surface.

niclosamide *n.* an *anthelmintic drug used to remove tapeworms. It is administered by mouth; unlike older treatments, side-effects are limited to gastrointestinal disturbance, itching, and lightheadedness.

nicorandil *n. see* POTASSIUM-CHANNEL ACTIVATOR.

nicotinamide *n.* a B vitamin: the amide of *nicotinic acid.

nicotinamide adenine dinucleotide *see* NAD.

nicotine *n.* a poisonous alkaloid derived from *tobacco, responsible for the dependence of regular smokers on cigarettes. In small doses nicotine has a stimulating effect on the autonomic nervous system, causing in regular smokers such effects as raised blood pressure and pulse rate and impaired appetite. Large doses cause paralysis of the autonomic ganglia. Nicotine replacement therapy (nicotine products formulated as chewing gum, skin patches, nasal sprays, etc.) is used as an aid to stop smoking.

nicotinic acid (niacin) a B vitamin. Nicotinic acid is a derivative of pyridine and is interchangeable with its amide, **nicotinamide**. Both forms of the vitamin are equally active. Nicotinamide is a component of the coenzymes *NAD (nicotinamide adenine dinucleotide) and NADP, its phosphate. Nicotinic acid is required in the diet but can also be formed in small amounts in the body from the essential amino acid tryptophan. A deficiency of the vitamin leads to *pellagra. Good sources of nicotinic acid are meat, yeast extracts, and pulses. The adult recommended intake is 18 mg equivalent per day (1 mg equivalent is equal to 1 mg of available nicotinic acid or 60 mg tryptophan).

Nicotinic acid is used clinically as a lipid-lowering drug. It is effective in reducing levels of triglycerides and low-density lipoproteins in the blood when these are not adequately controlled by *statins alone. It is administered by mouth; side-effects include vasodilatation, diarrhoea, nausea and vomiting, abdominal pain, and rash. Trade name: **Niaspan**.

nictitation *n.* exaggerated and frequent blinking or winking of the eyes.

nidation *n. see* IMPLANTATION.

nidus *n.* **1.** a place in which bacteria have settled and multiplied because of particularly suitable conditions: a focus of infection. **2.** the nucleus of a crystal.

Niemann-Pick disease an inherited (autosomal *recessive) disorder of lipid metabolism due to a defect in the enzyme sphingomyelinase and resulting in accumulation of sphingomyelin (a sphingolipid) and other phospholipids in the bone marrow, brain, liver, and spleen. Patients present with neurological problems, mental retardation, and enlargement of the liver and spleen at a young age. There are four known types of the disease. [A. Niemann (1880–1921), German paediatrician; L. Pick (1868–1944), German pathologist]

nifedipine *n.* a *calcium-channel blocker used in the prevention of angina and treatment of high blood pressure (hypertension) and Raynaud's phenomenon. It is administered by mouth; side-effects include dizziness, headache, and nausea. Trade names: **Adalat, Adipine MR, Coracten SR, Tensipine MR**, etc.

night blindness (nyctalopia) the inability to see in dim light or at night. It is due to a disorder of the cells in the retina that are responsible for vision in dim light (*see* ROD), and can result from dietary deficiency of *vitamin A. Vitamin A deficiency may progress to cause *xerophthalmia and *keratomalacia. Night blindness may be caused by other retinal diseases, e.g. *retinitis pigmentosa. **Congenital stationary night blindness** is characterized by poor night vision from early childhood that does not get worse, in association with *nystagmus. *Compare* DAY BLINDNESS.

night sweat copious sweating during sleep. Night sweats may be an early indication of tuberculosis, AIDS, or other disease.

night terror the condition in which a child (usually aged 2–7 years), soon after falling asleep, starts screaming and appears terrified. The child cannot be comforted because he or she remains mentally inaccessible; the attack ceases on fully wakening and is never remembered. Attacks sometimes follow a stressful experience.

Nile blue an oxazine chloride, used for staining lipids and lipid pigments. **Nile blue A** (**Nile blue sulphate**), which stains fatty acids, changes from blue to purplish at pH 10–11.

nilotinib *n. see* TYROSINE KINASE INHIBITOR.

ninhydrin reaction a histochemical test for proteins, in which ninhydrin (triketohydrindene hydrate) is boiled with the test solution and gives a blue colour in the presence of amino acids and proteins.

nipple (mamilla, papilla) *n.* the protuberance at the centre of the *breast. In females the milk ducts open at the nipple.

NIPPV noninvasive intermittent positive-pressure ventilation (*see* NONINVASIVE VENTILATION).

Nippy trade name for a brand of noninvasive positive-pressure ventilator that delivers air through a close-fitting nasal mask (*see*

NONINVASIVE VENTILATION). The Nippy was one of the early ventilators from the late 1980s and early 1990s, initially used in intensive care units. Although many others are now in use, the name is often used as a generic term for devices used on general wards for ventilatory support for patients with acute exacerbations of *chronic obstructive pulmonary disease.

Nissl granules collections of dark-staining material, containing RNA, seen in the cell bodies of neurons on microscopic examination. [F. Nissl (1860–1919), German neuropathologist]

nit *n.* the egg of a *louse. The eggs of head lice are firmly cemented to the hair, usually at the back of the head; those of body lice are fixed to the clothing. Nits, 0.8×0.3 mm, are visible as light white specks.

nitrates *pl. n.* a class of drugs used as coronary *vasodilators for the treatment and prevention of angina attacks. They include *glyceryl trinitrate, *isosorbide dinitrate, and isosorbide mononitrate.

nitrazepam *n.* a benzodiazepine drug administered by mouth for the short-term treatment of insomnia and sleep disturbances (*see* HYPNOTIC). Morning drowsiness, lightheadedness, and confusion may occur. Trade names: **Mogadon**, **Somnite**, etc.

nitric acid a strong corrosive mineral acid, HNO_3, the concentrated form of which is capable of producing severe burns of the skin. Swallowing the acid leads to intense burning pain and ulceration of the mouth and throat. Treatment is by immediate administration of alkaline solutions, followed by milk or olive oil.

nitric oxide an important member of the group of gaseous mediators, which – together with amine mediators (e.g. adrenaline, noradrenaline, histamine, acetylcholine) and lipid mediators (e.g. prostaglandins) – produce many physiological responses (e.g. smooth muscle relaxation). Nitric oxide is involved in the manifestations of sepsis and septic shock. Formula: NO.

nitrofurantoin *n.* a drug used to treat bacterial infections of the urinary system. It is administered by mouth and may cause nausea, vomiting, loss of appetite, diarrhoea, and skin rashes. Trade names: **Furadantin**, **Macrobid**, **Macrodantin**.

nitrogen *n.* a gaseous element and a major constituent of air (79 per cent). Nitrogen is an essential constituent of proteins and nucleic acids and is obtained by animals in the form of protein-containing foods (atmospheric nitrogen cannot be utilized directly). Nitrogenous waste is excreted as *urea. Liquid nitrogen is used to freeze some specimens before pathological examination. Symbol: N.

nitrogen balance the relationship between the nitrogen taken into the body and that excreted, denoting the balance between the manufacture and breakdown of the body mass. A negative nitrogen balance, when excretion exceeds intake, is usual after injury or operations as the energy requirements of the body are met disproportionately from endogenous sources.

nitroglycerin *n. see* GLYCERYL TRINITRATE.

nitroprusside (sodium nitroprusside) *n.* a cyanide-containing drug used in the emergency treatment of high blood pressure. Given by controlled infusion into a vein, it is the most effective known means of reducing dangerously high pressure, but its effects and level in the blood must be closely monitored. Possible side-effects include nausea, vomiting, headache, palpitations, sweating, and chest pain.

nitrous oxide a colourless gas used as an *anaesthetic with good analgesic properties. It is administered by inhalation, in conjunction with oxygen and other agents, for the maintenance of anaesthesia. A mixture of oxygen and nitrous oxide (**Entonox**, **Equanox**) provides effective analgesia for some dental procedures and in childbirth; such a state is known as *relative analgesia. Nitrous oxide was formerly referred to as **laughing gas** because of its tendency to excite the patient when used alone.

NIV *see* NONINVASIVE VENTILATION.

nizatidine *n.* an H_2-receptor antagonist (*see* ANTIHISTAMINE) used to treat gastric and duodenal ulcers and prevent their recurrence and to treat *gastro-oesophageal reflux disease. It is administered by mouth or intravenous infusion; side-effects include diarrhoea, dizziness, sweating, and headache. Trade name: **Axid**.

NK cell *see* NATURAL KILLER CELL.

nm *symbol for* *nanometre.

NMC *see* NURSING AND MIDWIFERY COUNCIL.

NMDA receptor a receptor on synapses that binds the *neurotransmitter glutamate and also binds its *agonist NMDA (*N*-methyl-*D*-*a*spartate). This receptor is involved in learning, memory, mood, and cognition; its overactivity is associated with chronic pain. **NMDA-receptor antagonists** (e.g. *amantadine, *memantine hydrochloride, *riluzole) are used in the treatment of (among other conditions) epilepsy, Alzheimer's disease, and chronic pain syndromes.

NMP22 nuclear matrix protein 22, which is involved in DNA replication and gene expression. Significantly elevated levels of NMP22 have been detected in the urine of patients with bladder cancer, which can aid the diagnosis of primary cancer or identify recurrent cancer.

NMR *see* NUCLEAR MAGNETIC RESONANCE.

Nocardia *n.* a genus of rodlike or filamentous Gram-positive nonmotile bacteria found in the soil. As cultures age, filaments form branches, but these soon break up into rodlike or spherical cells. Three or more spores may form in each cell; these germinate to form filaments. Some species are pathogenic: *N. asteroides* causes *nocardiosis and *N. madurae* is associated with the disease *Madura foot.

nocardiosis *n.* a disease caused by bacteria of the genus *Nocardia*, primarily affecting the lungs, skin, and brain, resulting in the formation of abscesses. Treatment involves antibiotics and sulphonamides.

noci- *combining form denoting* pain or injury.

nociceptive *adj.* describing nerve fibres, endings, or pathways that are concerned with the condition of pain.

nociceptor *n.* a *receptor that responds to the stimuli responsible for the sensation of pain. Nociceptors may be *interoceptors, responding to such stimuli as inflammation, or *exteroceptors, sensitive to heat, etc.

noct- (**nocti-**) *combining form denoting* night.

nocturia *n.* the passage of urine at night. In the absence of a high fluid intake, sleep is not normally interrupted by the need to pass urine. Nocturia usually occurs in elderly men or women. In younger men or women, less

urine is made at night than during the day, but this rhythm is lost with age in both sexes. Men may have additional problems arising from benign prostatic hyperplasia (*see* PROSTATE GLAND), but transurethral resection of the prostate often does not reduce nocturia.

node *n.* a small swelling or knot of tissue. *See* ATRIOVENTRICULAR NODE, LYMPH NODE, SINOATRIAL NODE.

node of Ranvier one of the gaps that occur at regular intervals in the *myelin sheath of medullated nerve fibres, between adjacent *Schwann cells.

nodule *n.* a small swelling or aggregation of cells.

noma *n.* a gangrenous infection of the mouth that spreads to involve the face: a severe form of *ulcerative gingivitis. It is rare in countries with working infrastructures and is usually found in debilitated or malnourished individuals.

nonaccidental injury (NAI) injury inflicted on babies and young children; the perpetrator is usually an adult – often a parent or step-parent. Most commonly seen in babies aged six months or less, it usually takes the form of bruising, particularly on the face; bite marks; burns or scalds, particularly cigarette burns; and bone injuries, especially spiral fractures of the long bones in the limbs and skull fractures. Internal injuries may be fatal. Careful examination often reveals several injuries of different ages, indicating long-term abuse. NAI usually has serious consequences for the child, including *failure to thrive and behavioural problems.

Known colloquially as the **battered baby** (or **child**) **syndrome**, it may be precipitated by many factors, including relationship difficulties, social problems, and ill health, and is more common if the child is handicapped. It is often found that abusers suffered similar abuse themselves when young. Many abused children suffer further injury if discharged into the same environment with no support (*see also* RISK REGISTER). A child at considerable risk may need to be removed from the family home.

nonadherence *n. see* ADHERENCE.

nonalcoholic fatty liver disease (NAFLD) a spectrum of conditions affecting the liver and not associated with excessive alcohol consumption: a common cause of referral with abnormal liver function tests. **Fatty liver** is excessive fat accumulation in the liver seen characteristically on ultrasound examination as a bright and often enlarged liver. This usually does not lead to any irreversible liver damage in the majority of cases. **Nonalcoholic steatohepatitis** (**NASH**) is inflammation in the liver with underlying fatty liver. It is often associated with insulin resistance, diabetes, hypertension, obesity, and *metabolic syndrome. Treatment usually involves dietary restriction, regular physical exercise, weight reduction, and management of underlying conditions (e.g. diabetes, hypertension, and hiperlipidaemia). NASH can lead to *cirrhosis requiring liver transplantation.

nondisjunction *n.* a condition in which pairs of homologous chromosomes fail to separate during meiosis or a chromosome fails to divide at *anaphase of mitosis or meiosis. It results in a cell with an abnormal number of chromosomes (*see* MONOSOMY, TRISOMY).

non-Hodgkin's lymphoma *see* LYMPHOMA.

noninvasive *adj.* 1. denoting techniques of investigation or treatment that do not involve penetration of the skin by needles or knives. 2. denoting tumours that do not spread into surrounding tissues (*see* BENIGN).

noninvasive ventilation (**NIV**) mechanical assistance with breathing that does not require the insertion of an endotracheal tube (*see* INTUBATION). In **noninvasive intermittent positive-pressure ventilation** (**NIPPV**) air is blown into the lungs through a close-fitting mask: designs range from helmet-like devices to nasal cushions and full-face or nasal masks (*see also* NIPPY). A ventilator then applies positive pressure to the mask in a cyclical fashion. The technique simplifies the process of ventilation in respiratory failure and reduces or eliminates the need for paralysis and anaesthesia, which are required for endotracheal intubation. *See also* BiPAP, CONTINUOUS POSITIVE AIRWAYS PRESSURE.

Negative-pressure ventilation involves the use of devices that draw air into and out of the lungs noninvasively by applying negative pressure in a cyclical way (*see* VENTILATOR).

nonmaleficence *n.* one of the *four principles and common to many theories of medical ethics: doctors should avoid causing harm to patients (*see* PRIMUM NON NOCERE). As almost all medical interventions carry some risk of harm, however small, in practice a doctor should avoid risking unnecessary harm or any harm that is disproportionate to the benefit intended. Consequently, risks should be minimized and considered along with the intended benefits when evaluating specific interventions. Harm can include psychological, emotional, or social harm as well as physical damage. *Compare* BENEFICENCE.

nonsecretor *n.* a person in whose body fluids it is not possible to detect soluble forms of the A, B, or O agglutinogens that determine blood group. *Compare* SECRETOR.

non-small-cell lung cancer (**NSCLC**) any type of lung cancer other than *small-cell lung cancer. Such cancers include *adenocarcinoma of the lung, large-cell carcinomas, and squamous-cell carcinoma of the lung.

nonspecific interstitial pneumonitis (**NSIP**) *see* INTERSTITIAL PNEUMONITIS.

nonsteroidal anti-inflammatory drug *see* NSAID.

Noonan's syndrome an autosomal *dominant condition of males who have all or some of the physical features of *Turner's syndrome in females but normal sex chromosomes. It is often associated with a low testosterone level and sometimes with reduced sperm production. Other features include cardiovascular defects and most affected individuals have short stature and mild mental retardation. [J. Noonan (1921–), US paediatrician]

noradrenaline (norepinephrine) *n.* a hormone, closely related to *adrenaline and with similar actions, secreted by the medulla of the *adrenal gland and also released as a *neurotransmitter by sympathetic nerve endings. Among its many actions are constriction of small blood vessels leading to an increase in blood pressure, increased blood flow through the coronary arteries and a slowing of the heart rate, increase in the rate and depth of breathing, and relaxation of the smooth muscle in intestinal walls.

norepinephrine *n. see* NORADRENALINE.

norethisterone *n.* a synthetic female sex hormone (*see* PROGESTOGEN) administered by mouth to treat menstrual disorders, including endometriosis. Its main use, however, is in oral contraceptives, often in combination with an oestrogen; it is also used in *hormone replacement therapy. Trade names: **Micronor**, **Primolut N**, **Utovlan**.

norfloxacin *n.* a *quinolone antibiotic used for treating urinary-tract infections. It is administered by mouth; side-effects are those of the other quinolones. Trade name: **Utinor**.

norma *n.* a view of the skull from one of several positions, from which it can be described or measured. For example the **norma lateralis** is a side view of the skull; the **norma verticalis** is the view of the top of the skull.

normal distribution *see* FREQUENCY DISTRIBUTION, SIGNIFICANCE.

normalization *n.* (in psychiatry) the process of making the living conditions of people with learning disabilities as similar as possible to those of people who are not handicapped. This includes moves to living outside institutions and encouragement to cope with work, pay, social life, sexuality, and civil rights.

normo- *combining form denoting* normality.

normoblast *n.* a nucleated cell that forms part of the series giving rise to the red blood cells and is normally found in the blood-forming tissue of the bone marrow. Normoblasts pass through three stages of maturation: **early** (or **basophilic**), **intermediate** (or **polychromatic**), and **late** (or **orthochromatic**) forms. *See also* ERYTHROBLAST, ERYTHROPOIESIS.

normocyte *n.* a red blood cell of normal size. A **normocytic anaemia** is one characterized by the presence of such cells. —**normocytic** *adj.*

normoglycaemia (**euglycaemia**) *n.* the state of having normal blood glucose levels, which – depending on when food was last eaten – are generally between 4 and 7 mmol/l.

normotensive *adj.* describing the state in which the arterial blood pressure is within the normal range. *Compare* HYPERTENSION, HYPOTENSION.

norovirus (**Norwalk virus**) *n.* a member of a group of RNA viruses that cause acute gastroenteritis in humans. The faecal–oral route is the usual mode of transmission and symptoms appear after an incubation period of between 24 and 48 hours. Noroviruses are highly contagious and are implicated in over 50% of all gastroenteritis outbreaks. Symptomatic treatment with fluid replacement and electrolyte correction remains the mainstay of treatment.

Northern blot analysis a technique for identifying a specific form of messenger RNA in cells. It uses a gene *probe known to match the RNA being sought. *Compare* SOUTHERN BLOT ANALYSIS, WESTERN BLOT ANALYSIS.

Northern Irish Sign Language (NISL) *see* SIGN LANGUAGE.

nortriptyline *n.* a tricyclic *antidepressant drug that is used to relieve depression and treat neuropathic pain. It is administered by mouth; side-effects may include dry mouth and drowsiness. Trade name: **Allegron**.

nose *n.* the organ of olfaction, which also acts as an air passage that warms, moistens, and filters the air on its way to the lungs. The **external nose** is a triangular projection in the front of the face that is composed of cartilage and covered with skin. It leads to the **nasal cavity** (**internal nose**), which is lined with mucous membrane containing olfactory cells and is divided into two chambers (**fossae**) by the **nasal septum**. The lateral wall of each chamber is formed by the three scroll-shaped *nasal conchae, below each of which is a groovelike passage (**meatus**). The *paranasal sinuses open into these meatuses.

nosebleed *n. see* EPISTAXIS.

noso- *combining form denoting* disease.

nosocomial infection (hospital infection) an infection that originates in a hospital. It may develop in a hospitalized patient or a member of the hospital staff, or it may be acquired in hospital but only develops after discharge. Such infections include those caused by fungi and opportunist bacteria. They are aggravated by factors favouring the spread of organisms (cross-contamination), such as insufficient hand washing among medical staff, and by reduced resistance of individual patients, as well as by antibiotic-resistant strains of bacteria (*see* CLOSTRIDIUM, ENTEROCOCCUS, MRSA).

nosology *n.* the naming and classification of diseases.

Nosopsyllus *n.* a genus of fleas. The common rat flea of temperate regions, *N. fasciatus*, will, in the absence of rats, bite humans and may therefore transmit plague or murine typhus from an infected rat population. The rat flea is also an intermediate host for the larval stage of two tapeworms, *Hymenolepis diminuta* and *H. nana*.

nostrils *n.* *see* NARES.

notch *n.* (in anatomy) an indentation, especially one in a bone.

NOTES (natural orifice transluminal endoscopic surgery) an emerging technique of performing abdominal operations with access to the abdominal cavity via natural orifices (e.g. the mouth, vagina, or rectum), thereby avoiding abdominal wall incisions.

notifiable disease a disease that must be reported to a proper officer of the local authority (usually a *Consultant in Communicable Disease Control) so that prompt control and preventive action may be undertaken if necessary. Such diseases include diphtheria, dysentery, food poisoning, infective jaundice, malaria, measles, poliomyelitis, tuberculosis, typhoid, and whooping cough. The list varies for different countries, and some diseases are internationally notifiable through the *World Health Organization; these include cholera, plague, relapsing fever, typhus, and yellow fever. The appropriate reporting of notifiable diseases is legally required by the Public Health (Control of Disease) Act 1984 and the Health and Social Care Act 2008.

notochord *n.* a strip of mesodermal tissue that develops along the dorsal surface of the early embryo, beneath the *neural tube. It becomes almost entirely obliterated by the development of the vertebrae, persisting only as part of the intervertebral discs.

NPSA *see* NATIONAL PATIENT SAFETY AGENCY.

NSAID (nonsteroidal anti-inflammatory drug) any one of a large group of drugs used for pain relief, particularly in rheumatic disease associated with inflammation but also in dysmenorrhoea and metastatic bone disease. NSAIDs act by inhibiting the cyclooxygenase enzymes (COX-1 and COX-2) responsible for controlling the formation of *prostaglandins, which are important mediators of inflammation. They include *aspirin, *ibuprofen, *ketoprofen, and *naproxen. Adverse effects include gastrointestinal bleeding and ulceration. Some NSAIDs act by selectively inhibiting COX-2 and are therefore less likely to cause gastric side-effects (*see* COX-2 INHIBITOR).

NSFs *see* NATIONAL SERVICE FRAMEWORKS.

NSIP nonspecific *interstitial pneumonitis.

NSTEMI non-S–T elevation *myocardial infarction.

nucha *n.* the nape of the neck. —**nuchal** *adj.*

nuchal translucency scanning (NT scanning) an ultrasound screening test performed during pregnancy at 11 weeks of gestation that measures the maximum thickness of the translucency between the skin and the soft tissue overlying the cervical (neck) region of the spine of the fetus. Increased NT is associated with an increased risk of chromosomal abnormalities and of a wide variety of structural abnormalities (e.g. heart defects). *See also* ULTRASOUND MARKER.

nuclear cardiology the study and diagnosis of heart disease by the intravenous injection of different types of *radionuclide. The radionuclide emits gamma rays, enabling a gamma camera and computer to form an image of the heart. *See* MUGA SCAN, SPECT SCANNING, THALLIUM SCAN.

nuclear magnetic resonance (NMR) the absorption and emission of high-frequency radio waves by the nuclei of certain elements when placed in a strong magnetic field. The strongest signal is obtained from hydrogen atoms, which are abundant in the water and organic molecules in the body. In clinical use for *magnetic resonance imaging, the signal is highly dependent on the concentration and mobility of water molecules within each tissue. NMR has important applications in noninvasive diagnostic techniques. *See also* MAGNETIC RESONANCE SPECTROSCOPY.

nuclear medicine the use of *radionuclides (especially *technetium-99m) as *tracers to study the structure and function of organs of the body. The radionuclide is attached to a compound suitable for the particular test and then injected, inhaled, or ingested. When concentrated in the organ under investigation, the tracer can be imaged using a *gamma camera, revealing the structure or demonstrating the function of the organ. Alternatively, blood or urine samples may be analysed. *See also* NUCLEAR CARDIOLOGY.

nuclease *n.* an enzyme that catalyses the breakdown of nucleic acids by cleaving the bonds between adjacent nucleotides. Examples are **ribonuclease**, which acts on RNA, and **deoxyribonuclease**, which acts on DNA.

nucleic acid either of two organic acids, *DNA or *RNA, present in the nucleus and in some cases the cytoplasm of all living cells. Their main functions are in heredity and protein synthesis.

nucleolus *n.* (*pl.* **nucleoli**) a dense spherical structure within the cell *nucleus that disappears during cell division. The nucleolus contains *RNA for the synthesis of *ribosomes and plays an important part in RNA and protein synthesis.

nucleoplasm (karyoplasm) *n.* the protoplasm making up the nucleus of a cell.

nucleoprotein *n.* a compound that occurs in cells and consists of nucleic acid and protein tightly bound together. *Ribosomes are nucleoproteins containing RNA; *chromosomes are nucleoproteins containing DNA.

nucleoside *n.* a compound consisting of a nitrogen-containing base (a *purine or *pyrimidine) linked to a sugar. Examples are *adenosine, *guanosine, *cytidine, *thymidine, and uridine.

nucleotide *n.* a compound consisting of a nitrogen-containing base (a *purine or *pyrimidine) linked to a sugar and a phosphate group. Nucleic acids (DNA and RNA) are long chains of linked nucleotides (**polynucleotide** chains), which in DNA contain the purine bases adenine and guanine and the pyrimidines thymine and cytosine; in RNA, thymine is replaced by uracil.

nucleus *n.* **1.** the part of a *cell that contains the genetic material, *DNA. The DNA, which is combined with protein, is normally dispersed throughout the nucleus as *chromatin. During cell division the chromatin becomes visible as *chromosomes. The nucleus also contains *RNA, most of which is located in the *nucleolus. The nucleus is separated from the cytoplasm by a double membrane, the **nuclear envelope**. **2.** an anatomically and functionally distinct mass of nerve cells within the brain or spinal cord.

3. the central part of the lens of the eye, which is harder than the outer cortex.

nude mouse a mouse born without a thymus and therefore no T lymphocytes. Human tumours will often grow in these mice. For unknown reasons these mice are also hairless, hence the name.

nuisance *n.* any noxious substance, accumulating in refuse or as dust or effluent, that is deemed by British law to be injurious to health or offensive. It can also include dwellings, work premises, animals, and noise.

null hypothesis *see* SIGNIFICANCE.

nullipara *n.* a woman who has never given birth. *See also* GRAVID.

nurse *n.* a person trained and experienced in nursing matters and entrusted with the care of the sick and the carrying out of medical and surgical routines. In Britain, student nurses gain a diploma or degree in nursing and must undertake a specified period of training in a hospital approved by the *Nursing and Midwifery Council before qualifying for registration as a **general nurse**. *See also* COMMUNITY MIDWIFE, DISTRICT NURSE, HEALTH VISITOR, NURSE PRACTITIONER, PRACTICE NURSE, SCHOOL NURSE.

nurse practitioner a registered nurse with advanced training and experience who assumes some of the duties and responsibilities formerly assumed only by a physician. Such nurses can practise in hospital or community settings within various domains of clinical activity, which may be condition-specific (e.g. diabetes, breast care), client-specific (e.g. children, the elderly, the homeless), or area-specific (e.g. general practice, dermatology).

Nursing and Midwifery Council (NMC) a statutory body that regulates the nursing and midwifery professions in the public interest. *See* NURSE.

nursing home a residential facility that provides nursing supervision and limited medical care to individuals who do not require hospitalization.

nutation *n.* the act of nodding the head.

nutrient *n.* a substance that must be consumed as part of the diet to provide a source of energy, material for growth, or a means of regulating growth or energy production. Nutrients include carbohydrates, fats, proteins, minerals, and vitamins. *See also* ESSENTIAL AMINO ACID, ESSENTIAL FATTY ACID, TRACE ELEMENT.

nutrition *n.* **1.** the study of food in relation to the physiological processes that depend on its absorption by the body (growth, energy production, repair of body tissues, etc.). The science of nutrition includes the study of diets and of deficiency diseases. **2.** the intake of nutrients and their subsequent absorption and assimilation by the tissues. Patients who cannot be fed in a normal way can be given nutrients by tubes into the intestines (**enteral feeding**) or by infusion into a vein (**intravenous feeding**).

nux vomica the seed of the tree *Strychnos nux-vomica*, which contains the poisonous alkaloid *strychnine.

nyct- (nycto-) *combining form denoting* night or darkness.

nyctalopia *n. see* NIGHT BLINDNESS.

nyctohemeral *adj.* denoting a cyclical event occurring both in the day and the night. *Compare* CIRCADIAN; ULTRADIAN.

nyctophobia *n.* extreme fear of the dark. It is common in children and not unusual in normal adults.

nymph *n.* **1.** an immature stage in the life history of certain insects, such as grasshoppers and *reduviid bugs. On emerging from the eggs, nymphs resemble the adult insects except that they are smaller, do not have fully developed wings, and are not sexually mature. **2.** the late larval stage of a tick.

nympho- *combining form denoting* **1.** the labia minora. **2.** female sexuality.

nystagmus *n.* rapid involuntary movements of the eyes, which may be from side to side, up and down, rotatory, or a mixture. Nystagmus may be congenital and associated with poor sight; it also occurs in disorders of the part of the brain responsible for eye movements and their coordination (e.g. multiple sclerosis) and in disorders of the organ of balance in the ear or the associated parts of the brain. Certain drugs, especially in excessive doses (e.g. phenytoin), also cause nystagmus. **Optokinetic nystagmus** occurs in normal people when they try to look at a succession of objects moving quickly across their line of sight. Jerking eye movements sometimes occur in normal people when tired, on concentrating their gaze in any direction. These are called **nystagmoid jerks** and they do not imply disease.

nystagmus block syndrome a type of squint (convergent *strabismus) that results from the use of the convergence mechanism to block or dampen down *nystagmus in an attempt to improve visual acuity.

nystatin *n.* an antifungal drug used especially to treat skin, oral, and intestinal infections caused by *Candida*. It is formulated, often in combination with other drugs, as a cream or ointment for skin infections and as a suspension for oral and intestinal infections. Side-effects include mild digestive upsets. Trade names: **Nystan**, **Nystaform**.

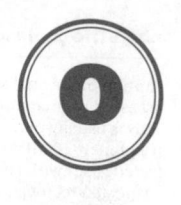

OAD *see* OBSCURE AUDITORY DYSFUNCTION.

OAE *see* OTOACOUSTIC EMISSIONS.

OASIS *see* OBSTETRIC ANAL SPHINCTER INJURY.

oat cell *see* SMALL-CELL LUNG CANCER.

obesity *n.* the condition in which excess fat has accumulated in the body, mostly in the subcutaneous tissues. Clinical obesity is considered to be present when a person has a *body mass index of 30 or over. The accumulation of fat is usually caused by the consumption of more food than is required for producing enough energy for daily activities. However, recent evidence indicates that a genetic element is involved. Hunger and satiety appear to be controlled by peptide messengers, encoded by specific genes and acting on the brain; an example is *leptin. Obesity is the most common nutritional disorder of recent years in Western societies: some patients may require surgical treatment to attain worthwhile weight reduction (*see* BARIATRIC SURGERY); drug treatments also exist (*see* ORLISTAT, SIBUTRAMINE). —**obese** *adj.*

obex *n.* the curved lower margin of the fourth *ventricle of the brain, between the medulla oblongata and the cerebellum.

objective *n.* (in microscopy) the lens or system of lenses in a light microscope that is nearest to the object under examination and furthest from the *eyepiece. In many types of microscope interchangeable objectives with different powers of magnification are provided.

objective structured clinical examination (OSCE) a type of examination used increasingly in the health sciences (medicine, dentistry, nursing, physiotherapy, pharmacy) to assess clinical skills in examination, communication, medical procedures, and interpretation of results. The examination usually takes the form of a circuit of stations around which each candidate moves after a specified time interval (5–10 minutes) at each station. Stations are a mixture of interactive and noninteractive tasks. Some have

an examiner and a simulated patient, either an actor for assessment of communication or history-taking skills or a manikin of a specific part of the body (e.g. to demonstrate how to use an auriscope). Other stations have investigation results with a list of questions that are to be completed on computer-marked examination papers. Each station has a different examiner and the stations are standardized with specific marking criteria, thus enabling fairer comparison with others.

obligate *adj.* describing an organism that is restricted to one particular way of life; for example, an **obligate parasite** cannot exist without a host. *Compare* FACULTATIVE.

obligation *n. see* DUTY.

obscure auditory dysfunction (OAD, King-Kopetzky syndrome) hearing difficulty, especially in noisy environments, in an individual with a normal *audiogram. Treatment includes *hearing therapy.

observer error *see* VALIDITY.

obsession *n.* a recurrent thought, feeling, or impulse that is unpleasant and provokes anxiety but cannot be got rid of. Although an obsession dominates the person, he (or she) realizes its senselessness and struggles to resist it: this resistance causes anxiety. The obsession may, for example, be a vivid image, a fear (e.g. of contamination), or an impulse (e.g. to wash the hands repetitively). It is a feature of **obsessive–compulsive disorder** (*see also* COMPULSION, NEUROSIS) and sometimes of depression and of organic states, such as encephalitis. It can be treated with behaviour therapy and *antidepressant medication, particularly clomipramine and SSRIs. —**obsessional** *adj.*

obsessive–compulsive disorder *see* OBSESSION.

obstetric anal sphincter injury (OASIS) a spectrum of injuries that encompasses both third- and fourth-degree *perineal tears. Injury to the anal sphincter mechanism during childbirth may arise secondarily to direct disruption of the sphincter muscles and/or traction of the pudendal nerves. Disruption of the anal sphincter muscles is best assessed by anal ultrasound examination. This is usually performed using a high-frequency (10 MHz) endoanal probe. In selected cases with complex injury and/or suspected rectovaginal *fistula, magnetic resonance imaging (MRI) may also be employed.

obstetric cholestasis a pregnancy-related condition characterized by intense *pruritus (itch) – and consequent sleep deprivation – in the absence of a skin rash, with abnormal liver function tests and elevated bile acids, all of which remit following delivery. The clinical importance of obstetric cholestasis lies in the potential fetal risks, which may include prematurity and intra-uterine death.

obstetrics n. the branch of medical science concerned with the care of women during pregnancy, childbirth, and the period of about six weeks following the birth, when the reproductive organs are recovering. *Compare* GYNAECOLOGY. —**obstetric** *adj.* —**obstetrician** n.

obstipation n. *Chiefly US.* severe or complete constipation.

obstructed labour failure of the presenting part to descend in spite of uterine contractions, which implies a mechanical cause. Obstruction is usually due to (1) an abnormality in the woman's pelvis (a contracted pelvis); (2) an abnormality in her baby (e.g. hydrocephaly); or (3) an abnormality in the relationship between them, either (a) an abnormal *lie (e.g. transverse) or *malpresentation, or (b) *cephalopelvic disproportion (CPD). CPD and impacted transverse lie are the most important causes. Much of the purpose of antenatal care is to screen mothers who are at risk from obstructed labour, which can be detected early by means of a *partogram. If undetected, it can lead to rupture of the uterus, death of the fetus, obstetric fistulae, or maternal death.

obstructive airways disease *see* BRONCHOSPASM.

obstructive sleep apnoea (OSA, obstructive sleep apnoea syndrome, OSAS) a serious condition in which airflow from the nose and mouth to the lungs is restricted during sleep, also called **sleep apnoea syndrome** (**SAS**). It is defined by the presence of more than five episodes of *apnoea per hour of sleep associated with significant daytime sleepiness. Snoring is a feature of the condition but it is not universal. There are significant medical complications of prolonged OSA, including heart failure and high blood pressure. Patients perform poorly on driving simulators, and driving licence authorities may impose limitations on possession of a driving licence. There are associated conditions in adults, the *hypopnoea syndrome and the upper airways resistance syndrome, with less apnoea but with daytime somnolence and prominent snoring. In children the cause is usually enlargement of the tonsils and adenoids and treatment is by removing these structures. In adults the tonsils may be implicated but there are often other abnormalities of the pharynx, and patients are often obese. Treatment may include weight reduction or nasal *continuous positive airways pressure (nCPAP) devices, *mandibular advancement splints, or noninvasive ventilation. Alternatively *tonsillectomy, *uvulo-palatopharyngoplasty, *laser-assisted uvulopalatoplasty, or *tracheostomy may be required.

obstructive sleep apnoea syndrome (OSAS) *see* OBSTRUCTIVE SLEEP APNOEA.

obtund *vb.* to blunt or deaden sensitivity; for example, by the application of a local anaesthetic, which reduces or causes complete loss of sensation in nearby nerves.

obturation n. obstruction of a body passage, usually by impaction of a foreign body, thickened secretions, or hard faeces.

obturator n. **1.** *see* OBTURATOR MUSCLE. **2.** a wire or rod within a cannula or hollow needle for piercing tissues or fitting aspirating needles. **3.** a removable form of denture that both closes a defect in the palate and also restores the dentition. The defect may result from removal of a tumour or, less commonly, be congenital, as in a cleft palate.

obturator foramen a large opening in the *hip bone, below and slightly in front of the acetabulum. *See also* PELVIS.

obturator muscle either of two muscles that cover the outer surface of the anterior wall of the pelvis (the **obturator externus** and **obturator internus**) and are responsible for lateral rotation of the thigh and movements of the hip.

obtusion n. the weakening or blunting of normal sensations. This may be associated with disease.

occipital bone a saucer-shaped bone of the *skull that forms the back and part of the base of the cranium. At the base of the occipital are two **occipital condyles**: rounded surfaces that articulate with the first (atlas) vertebra of the backbone. Between the condyles is the **foramen magnum**, the cavity through which the spinal cord passes.

occiput *n.* the back of the head. In obstetrics, the occiput is used as a *denominator when a fetus presents by the vertex (*see* PRESENTATION). The most favourable position for delivery is **occipitoanterior** (or **occipital anterior**), with the occiput of the fetus presenting towards the anterior aspect of the maternal pelvis as it enters the pelvic inlet. In the **occipitotransverse** (or **occipital transverse**) and **occipitoposterior** (or **occipital posterior**) positions, the occiput presents towards the lateral and posterior aspects, respectively, of the maternal pelvis; these are *malpositions. —**occipital** *adj.*

occlusal *adj.* (in dental anatomy) denoting or relating to the biting surface of a premolar or molar tooth.

occlusal rim the occlusal extension of a denture base to allow analysis of jaw relations and to record jaw relations for the construction of *dentures, bridges, and extensive crowning.

occlusion *n.* **1.** the closing or obstruction of a hollow organ or part. **2.** (in dentistry) the relation of the upper and lower teeth when they are in contact. Maximum contact between the teeth is known as **intercuspal** (or **centric**) **occlusion**. *See also* MALOCCLUSION.

occult *adj.* not apparent to the naked eye; not easily determined or detected. For example **occult blood** is blood present in such small quantities that it can only be detected microscopically or by chemical testing. *See* FAECAL OCCULT BLOOD TEST.

occupational disease a disease to which workers in certain occupations are particularly prone. **Industrial diseases**, associated with a particular industry or group of industries, fall within this category. Examples of such diseases include the various forms of *pneumoconiosis, which affect the lungs of workers continually exposed to dusty atmospheres; cataracts in glassblowers; decompression sickness in divers; poisoning from toxic metals in factory and other workers; and infectious diseases contracted from animals by farm workers, such as woolsorter's disease (*see* ANTHRAX). *See also* COSHH, PRESCRIBED DISEASE, INDUSTRIAL INJURIES DISABLEMENT BENEFIT.

occupational health service (OHS) a scheme by which employers provide a mainly preventive health service for employees. Specially trained doctors and nurses advise management on hazardous situations at work. Advice is also given to management to ensure that people with ill health or disability are not prevented from taking up employment and on the potential for rehabilitating employees with prolonged or repeated sickness absence. Instruction may be given to the workforce on simple first aid procedures, and *health promotion programmes may be offered in relation to nutrition, physical activity, and stress. With the approval of the *Health and Safety Executive, the OHS may conduct routine tests on employees working with potentially hazardous substances, such as lead. *See also* COSHH.

occupational mortality rates and causes of death in relation to different jobs, occupational and socioeconomic groups, or social class. Because some occupations have older incumbents than others (e.g. judges) allowance for age bias is made by comparing either *standardized mortality ratios for those aged 15–64 years or related but less familiar indices, such as **comparative mortality figures** or **proportional mortality ratios**.

occupational therapy the treatment of physical and psychiatric conditions by encouraging patients to undertake specific selected activities that will help them to reach their maximum level of function and independence in all aspects of daily life. These activities are designed to make the best use of the patient's capabilities and are based on individual requirements. They range from woodwork, metalwork, and printing to pottery and other artistic activities, household management, social skills (for psychiatric patients), and leisure activities (for geriatric patients). Occupational therapy also includes assessment for mechanical aids and adaptations in the home.

ochronosis *n.* the presence of brown-black pigment in the skin, cartilage, and other tissues due to the abnormal accumulation of homogentisic acid that occurs in the metabolic disease *alcaptonuria.

OCT *see* OPTICAL COHERENCE TOMOGRAPHY.

oct- (octa-, octi-, octo-) *combining form denoting* eight.

octreotide *n*. a somatostatin analogue (*see* SOMATOSTATIN).

ocular *adj*. of or concerned with the eye or vision.

oculist *n*. a former name for an *ophthalmologist.

oculo- *combining form denoting* the eye(s).

oculogyric *adj*. causing or concerned with movements of the eye.

oculogyric crisis a spasmodic deviation of the eyes upwards with head tilted backwards, which may last minutes or hours. It occurs in patients with postencephalitic *parkinsonism and in patients taking phenothiazine drugs. Treatment is with antimuscarinic drugs.

oculomotor *adj*. concerned with eye movements.

oculomotor nerve the third *cranial nerve (III), which is composed of motor fibres distributed to muscles in and around the eye. Fibres of the parasympathetic system are responsible for altering the size of the pupil and the lens of the eye. Fibres outside the eye run to the upper eyelid and to muscles that turn the eyeball in different directions.

oculonasal *adj*. concerned with the eye and nose.

oculoplastics *n*. a surgical specialty concerned with reconstructive and cosmetic surgery around the eye (including the orbit, eyelids, lacrimal apparatus, and other accessory structures).

oculoplethysmography *n*. measurement of the pressure inside the eyeball. A rising or above-normal pressure is an important indication of the presence of *glaucoma.

odont- (odonto-) *combining form denoting* a tooth. Example: **odontalgia** (toothache).

odontoblast *n*. a cell that forms dentine. Odontoblasts line the pulp and have small processes that extend into the dentine.

odontogenic tumour any one of a group of rare tumours composed of dental tissue; the most important example is the *ameloblastoma.

odontoid process a toothlike process from the upper surface of the axis vertebra. *See* CERVICAL VERTEBRAE.

odontology *n*. the study of the teeth.

odontome *n*. an abnormal mass of calcified dental tissue, which usually represents a developmental abnormality. *Compare* HAMARTOMA.

-odynia *combining form denoting* pain in (a specified part).

odynophagia *n*. painful swallowing. This can be due to severe inflammation of the gullet (oesophagus) due to oesophagitis from *gastro-oesophageal reflux disease or infective causes, such as cytomegalovirus, candidiasis, or herpes simplex virus. Other causes include neuromuscular problems, such as *achalasia, or foreign bodies, such fish bones or coins, as well as oesophageal malignancy.

oedema *n*. excessive accumulation of fluid in the body tissues: popularly known as **dropsy**. The resultant swelling may be local, as with an injury or inflammation, or more general, as in heart or kidney failure. In generalized oedema there may be collections of fluid within the chest cavity (**pleural effusions**), abdomen (*see* ASCITES), or within the air spaces of the lung (**pulmonary oedema**). It may result from heart or kidney failure, cirrhosis of the liver, acute nephritis, the nephrotic syndrome, starvation, allergy, or drugs (e.g. cortisone derivatives). In such cases the kidneys can usually be stimulated to get rid of the excess fluid by the administration of *diuretic drugs. **Subcutaneous oedema** commonly occurs in the legs and ankles due to the influence of gravity and (in women) before menstruation; the swelling subsides with rest and elevation of the legs. —**oedematous** *adj*.

Oedipus complex in *Freudian theory, repressed sexual feelings of a child for its opposite-sexed parent, combined with rivalry towards the same-sexed parent: said to be a normal stage of development. The end of the Oedipus complex in children is marked by a loss of sexual feelings towards the opposite-sexed parent and an increase in identification with the same-sexed parent. Arrest of development at the Oedipal stage is said to be responsible for sexual deviations and other neurotic behaviour.

oesophag- (oesophago-) *combining form*

denoting the oesophagus. Example: **oesophagectomy** (surgical removal of).

oesophageal ulcer *see* PEPTIC ULCER, OESOPHAGITIS.

oesophageal varices dilated veins in the lower oesophagus due to *portal hypertension. These may rupture and bleed, resulting in *haematemesis; bleeding is usually serious and life-threatening. Bleeding may be arrested by endoscopic therapy (either injection of sclerosants or application of rubber bands). If this fails to stop the bleeding, a compression balloon (e.g. a Sengstaken tube) may be inserted. Intravenous infusions (e.g. of terlipressin or octreotide) may be used as an additional measure.

oesophagitis *n.* inflammation of the oesophagus (gullet). Frequent regurgitation of acid and peptic juices from the stomach causes **reflux oesophagitis**, the commonest form, which may be associated with a hiatus *hernia. The main symptoms are heartburn, regurgitation of bitter fluid, *odynophagia, and sometimes difficulty in swallowing (dysphagia); complications include bleeding, narrowing (*stricture) of the oesophageal canal, ulceration, and *Barrett's oesophagus. It is treated by antacid medicines, drugs to reduce acid secretion, and weight reduction; in severe cases *fundoplication surgery may be required. **Corrosive oesophagitis** is caused by the ingestion of caustic acid or alkali. It is often severe and may lead to perforation of the oesophagus or to extensive stricture formation. Treatment includes avoidance of food and administration of antibiotics; later dilatation of the stricture is often needed. **Infective oesophagitis** is most commonly due to a fungus (*Candida*) infection in debilitated patients, especially those being treated with antibiotics, corticosteroids, and immunosuppressant drugs, but is occasionally due to viruses (such as cytomegalovirus or herpesvirus). All these infections are common in patients with AIDS. **Eosinophilic oesophagitis** is a poorly understood condition characterized by infiltration of the lining of the oesophagus by excess eosinophils. Autoimmune disease and food allergy are two commonly proposed causes. Treatment is directed towards exclusion of allergens and oral or inhaled steroids.

oesophagocele *n.* protrusion of the lining (mucosa) of the oesophagus (gullet) through a tear in its muscular wall.

oesophagogastroduodenoscopy (OGD) *n.* endoscopic examination of the upper alimentary tract using a fibreoptic or video instrument. *See also* GASTROSCOPE.

oesophagoscope *n.* an illuminated optical instrument used to inspect the interior of the oesophagus (gullet), dilate its canal (in cases of stricture), obtain material for biopsy, or remove a foreign body. It may be a rigid metal tube or a flexible fibreoptic or video-camera instrument (*see* GASTROSCOPE). —**oesophagoscopy** *n.*

Oesophagostomum *n.* a genus of parasitic nematodes occurring in Brazil, Africa, and Indonesia. It is a rare intestinal parasite of humans, producing symptoms of dysentery in cases of heavy infection. The worms may also invade the tissues of the gut wall, giving rise to abscesses. The worms can be eliminated with anthelmintics.

oesophagostomy *n.* a surgical operation in which the oesophagus (gullet) is opened onto the neck. It is usually performed after operations on the throat as a temporary measure to allow feeding.

oesophagotomy *n.* surgical opening of the oesophagus (gullet) in order to inspect its interior or to remove or insert something.

oesophagus *n.* the gullet: a muscular tube, about 23 cm long, that extends from the pharynx to the stomach. It is lined with mucous membrane, whose secretions lubricate food as it passes from the mouth to the stomach. Waves of *peristalsis assist the passage of food.
  Diseases of the oesophagus include *achalasia, carcinoma, hiatus hernia, *oesophageal varices, *oesophagitis, and *peptic ulcer. —**oesophageal** *adj.*

oestradiol *n.* the major female sex hormone produced by the ovary. *See* OESTROGEN.

oestriol *n.* one of the female sex hormones produced by the ovary. *See* OESTROGEN.

oestrogen *n.* one of a group of steroid hormones (including oestriol, oestrone, and oestradiol) that control female sexual development, promoting the growth and function of the female sex organs (*see* MENSTRUAL CYCLE) and female secondary sexual characteristics (such as breast development). Oestrogens are synthesized mainly by the ovary; small amounts are also produced by the adrenal cortex, testes, and placenta. In men excessive production of oestrogen gives rise to *feminization.

Naturally occurring and synthetic oestrogens, given by mouth or injection, are used to treat *amenorrhoea and menopausal symptoms (see HORMONE REPLACEMENT THERAPY), as well as androgen-dependent cancers (e.g. cancer of the prostate). Synthetic oestrogens are a major constituent of *oral contraceptives. Side-effects of oestrogen therapy may include nausea and vomiting, headache and dizziness, irregular vaginal bleeding, fluid and salt retention, and feminization in men. Oestrogens should not be used in patients with a history of cancer of the breast, uterus, or genital tract. —**oestrogenic** *adj.*

oestrogen receptor a specific site on the surface of a cell that binds to *oestrogen; the binding triggers responses of the cell to the hormone (see RECEPTOR). Oestrogen receptors occur on all target cells normally responsive to oestrogen (e.g. in the uterus) and are also found on some cancer cells, particularly in breast cancer. Oestrogen-receptor-positive cancer cells rely on oestrogen to grow and are therefore susceptible to *antioestrogen therapy, which prevents oestrogen from binding to these receptors. This type of cancer tends to have a better prognosis than oestrogen-receptor-negative breast cancer.

oestrogen-receptor antagonist see ANTI-OESTROGEN.

oestrone *n.* one of the female sex hormones produced by the ovary. See OESTROGEN.

Oestrus *n.* a genus of widely distributed nonbloodsucking flies, occurring wherever sheep and goats are raised. The parasitic larvae of *O. ovis*, the sheep nostril fly, may occasionally and accidentally infect humans. By means of large mouth hooks, it attaches itself to the conjunctiva of the eye, causing a painful *myiasis that may result in loss of sight. This is an occupational disease of shepherds. Larvae can be removed with forceps following anaesthesia.

Office for National Statistics (ONS) (in Britain) an executive agency of the Treasury that was formed in 1996. It is responsible for the compilation and publication of statistics relating to national and local populations, including their social and economic situation and contribution to the economy, and the demographic patterns of births, marriages, and deaths (including the medical cause of death). The ONS organizes a national *census at ten-yearly intervals.

ofloxacin *n.* a *quinolone antibiotic used to treat urinary-tract and sexually transmitted infections and also infections of the respiratory tract, skin, and eye. It is administered by mouth, intravenous infusion, or as eye drops; possible side-effects include nausea, vomiting, and skin rashes. Trade names: **Exocin, Tarivid**.

OGD *n. see* OESOPHAGOGASTRODUODENOSCOPY.

Ogilvie's syndrome *see* PSEUDO-OBSTRUCTION.

ohm *n.* the *SI unit of electrical resistance, equal to the resistance between two points on a conductor when a constant potential difference of 1 volt applied between these points produces a current of 1 ampere. Symbol: Ω.

-oid *suffix denoting* like; resembling. Example: **pemphigoid** (condition resembling pemphigus).

ointment *n.* a greasy preparation, which may or may not contain medication, for use on skin or mucous membranes. Although less pleasant to use than the equivalent *cream, it is more effective since it forms an impermeable layer in the outer layer of the skin, reducing evaporation from the surface.

olanzapine *n. see* ANTIPSYCHOTIC.

olaparib *n. see* PARP INHIBITOR.

olecranon process the large process of the *ulna that projects behind the elbow joint.

oleic acid *see* FATTY ACID.

oleo- *combining form denoting* oil.

oleothorax *n.* the procedure of introducing paraffin wax extrapleurally so that the lung is allowed to collapse. This was sometimes formerly undertaken to allow closure of tuberculous cavities within the lung.

oleum *n.* (in pharmacy) an oil.

olfaction *n.* **1.** the sense of smell. **2.** the process of smelling. Sensory cells in the mucous membrane that lines the nasal cavity are stimulated by the presence of chemical particles dissolved in the mucus. See NOSE. —**olfactory** *adj.*

olfactory nerve the first *cranial nerve

(I): the special sensory nerve of smell. Fibres of the nerve run upwards from smell receptors in the nasal mucosa high in the roof of the nose, through minute holes in the skull, join to form the olfactory tract, and pass back to reach the brain.

olig- (oligo-) *combining form denoting* **1.** few. **2.** a deficiency.

oligaemia *n. see* HYPOVOLAEMIA.

oligoarthritis *n. see* ARTHRITIS.

oligoclonal bands immunoglobulin bands found in the cerebrospinal fluid (CSF) taken at *lumbar puncture. Bands isolated only in the CSF and not in the serum indicate local synthesis and are seen in such conditions as multiple sclerosis.

oligodactylism *n.* the congenital absence of some of the fingers and toes.

oligodendrocyte *n.* one of the cells of the *glia, responsible for producing the *myelin sheaths of the neurons of the central nervous system and therefore equivalent to the *Schwann cells of the peripheral nerves.

oligodendroglioma *n.* a tumour of the central nervous system derived from a type of *glia (the supporting tissue) rather than from the nerve cells themselves. *See also* GLIOMA.

oligodipsia *n.* a condition in which thirst is diminished or absent.

oligodontia *n.* the congenital absence of some of the teeth.

oligohydramnios *n.* a decrease in the amount of amniotic fluid surrounding the fetus, which may occur in the second and third trimesters. It is usually associated with restricted fetal growth and may indicate serious fetal kidney abnormalities. *See* POTTER SYNDROME. *See also* ANHYDRAMNIOS.

oligomenorrhoea *n.* menstrual bleeding at intervals of between 35 days and 6 months.

oligo-ovulation *n.* infrequent occurrence of ovulation.

oligospermia *n.* a reduced number of spermatozoa in the semen (*see* SEMINAL ANALYSIS). In oligospermia there are less than 20 million spermatozoa per ml with poor motility (**asthenospermia**) and often including many bizarre and immature forms (**teratospermia**). Treatment is directed to any

underlying cause (such as *varicocele). *See also* ANDROLOGY, INFERTILITY.

oliguria *n.* the production of an abnormally small volume of urine. This may be a result of copious sweating associated with intense physical activity and/or hot weather. It can also be due to kidney disease, retention of water in the tissues (*see* OEDEMA), loss of blood, diarrhoea, or poisoning.

olive *n.* a smooth oval swelling in the upper part of the medulla oblongata on each side. It contains a mass of nerve cells, mainly grey matter (**olivary nucleus**). —**olivary** *adj.*

Ollier's disease *see* DYSCHONDROPLASIA. [L. L. X. E. Ollier (1830–1900), French surgeon]

-ology *combining form. see* -LOGY.

olsalazine *n.* a salicylate preparation used to treat mild ulcerative colitis. It is administered by mouth. Possible side-effects include nausea, vomiting, headache, joint pain, and skin rashes. Trade name: **Dipentum**.

om- (omo-) *combining form denoting* the shoulder.

-oma *combining form denoting* a tumour. Examples: **hepatoma** (of the liver); **lymphoma** (of the lymph nodes).

omalizumab *n.* a *monoclonal antibody used in the prevention of severe allergic asthma that has not responded to standard therapy. It acts by binding to IgE, an *immunoglobulin that mediates the allergic response. It is administered by subcutaneous injection. Trade name: **Xolair**.

omega fatty acid *see* ESSENTIAL FATTY ACID.

omentectomy *n.* the removal of all or part of the omentum (the fold of peritoneum between the stomach and other abdominal organs).

omentum (epiploon) *n.* a double layer of *peritoneum attached to the stomach and linking it with other abdominal organs, such as the liver, spleen, and intestine. The **great omentum** is a highly folded portion of the omentum, rich in fatty tissue, that covers the intestines in an apron-like fashion. It acts as a heat insulator and prevents friction between abdominal organs. The **lesser omentum** links the stomach with the liver. —**omental** *adj.*

omeprazole *n.* a *proton-pump inhibitor

used to treat gastric and duodenal ulcers, *gastro-oesophageal reflux disease, and the *Zollinger-Ellison syndrome. Omeprazole can be effective in cases that have failed to respond to H_2-receptor antagonists, such as *ranitidine. Administered by mouth or intravenously, it is long-acting and need only be taken once a day. Possible side-effects include nausea, diarrhoea, headache, constipation, and skin rashes. Trade name: **Losec**.

Ommaya reservoir a device inserted into the ventricles of the brain to enable the repeated injection of drugs into the cerebrospinal fluid. It is used, for example, in the treatment of malignant meningitis, particularly in children with leukaemia. It can also be used to allow aspiration of cystic gliomas.

omphal- (omphalo-) *combining form denoting* the navel or umbilical cord.

omphalitis *n.* inflammation of the navel, especially in newborn infants.

omphalocele *n.* an umbilical *hernia.

omphalus *n. see* UMBILICUS.

Onchocerca *n.* a genus of parasitic worms (*see* FILARIA) occurring in central Africa and central America. The adult worms are found in fibrous nodules within the connective tissues beneath the skin and their presence causes disease (*see* ONCHOCERCIASIS). Various species of black fly, in which *Onchocerca* undergoes part of its development, transmit the infective larvae to humans.

onchocerciasis *n.* a tropical disease of the skin and underlying connective tissue caused by the parasitic worm *Onchocerca volvulus*. Fibrous nodular tumours grow around the adult worms in the skin; these may take several months to appear, and if secondary bacterial infection occurs they may degenerate into abscesses. The skin also becomes inflamed and itches. The migration of the *microfilariae into the eye can cause total or partial blindness – called **river blindness** in Africa. Onchocerciasis occurs in Africa and Central and South America. *Ivermectin is used in treatment; if possible, the nodules are removed as and when they appear.

onco- *combining form denoting* **1.** a tumour. **2.** volume.

oncofetal antigen a protein normally produced only by fetal tissue but often produced by certain tumours. An example is *carcino-embryonic antigen (CEA), which has been used as a *tumour marker, especially in colorectal carcinomas.

oncogene *n.* a gene in viruses (*v-onc*) and mammalian cells (*c-onc*) that can cause cancer. It results from the mutation of a normal gene (a *proto-oncogene). An oncogene is capable of both initiation and continuation of malignant transformation of normal cells. It probably produces proteins (*growth factors) regulating cell division that, under certain conditions, become uncontrolled and may transform a normal cell to a malignant state.

oncogenesis *n.* the development of a new abnormal growth (a benign or malignant tumour).

oncogenic *adj.* describing a substance, organism, or environment that is known to be a causal factor in the production of a tumour. Some viruses are considered to be oncogenic; these include the *papovaviruses, the *retroviruses, certain *adenoviruses and *herpesviruses, and the *Epstein-Barr virus. *See also* CARCINOGEN.

oncology *n.* the study and practice of treating tumours. It is often subdivided into medical, surgical, clinical, and radiation oncology. —**oncologist** *n.*

oncolysis *n.* the destruction of tumours and tumour cells. This may occur spontaneously or, more usually, in response to treatment with drugs or by radiotherapy.

oncometer *n.* an instrument for measuring the volume of blood circulating in one of the limbs. *See* PLETHYSMOGRAPHY.

oncosphere (hexacanth) *n.* the six-hooked larva of a *tapeworm. If ingested by a suitable intermediate host, such as a pig or an ox, the larva will use its hooks to penetrate the wall of the intestine. The larva subsequently migrates to the muscles, where it develops into a *cysticercus.

oncotic *adj.* **1.** characterized by a tumour or swelling. **2.** relating to an increase in volume or pressure.

oncotic pressure a pressure represented by the pressure difference that exists between the osmotic pressure of blood and that of the lymph or tissue fluid. Oncotic pressure is important for regulating the flow of water between blood and tissue fluid. *See also* OSMOSIS.

ondansetron *n.* a drug used to control severe nausea and vomiting, especially when it results from chemotherapy and radiotherapy. Ondansetron works by opposing the action of the neurotransmitter *serotonin (5-hydroxytryptamine) at 5HT$_3$ receptors. It is administered by mouth, injection, or as rectal suppositories; side-effects include constipation, headache, and flushing. Related drugs with similar actions and effects include **dolasetron** (Anzemet) and **granisetron** (Kytril). Trade name: **Zofran**.

oneir- (oneiro-) *combining form denoting* dreams or dreaming.

on–off phenomenon the rapid alternation between jerky uncontrolled movements (on) and very limited or no movement (off) most often seen in patients with Parkinson's disease who have been undergoing long-term treatment with levodopa.

ONS *see* OFFICE FOR NATIONAL STATISTICS.

ontogeny *n.* the history of the development of an individual from the fertilized egg to maturity.

onych- (onycho-) *combining form denoting* the nail(s).

onychogryphosis *n.* gross thickening and hardening of a nail, which becomes elongated and deformed. It may be caused by poor blood supply, injury to the matrix, fungal infection, diabetes, and/or malnutrition.

onycholysis *n.* separation or loosening of part or all of a nail from its bed. The condition may occur due to *psoriasis, fungal infections of the skin/nail bed, trauma, or drugs. It is commoner in women and may return to normal spontaneously.

onychomycosis *n.* fungus infection of the nails caused by *dermatophytes or *Candida. The nails become discoloured, opaque, and thickened. *See also* RINGWORM.

O'nyong nyong fever (joint-breaker fever) a disease of Africa and Malaysia, caused by an *arbovirus and transmitted by mosquitoes of the genus *Anopheles. It is similar to *dengue and symptoms include rigor, severe headache, an irritating rash, fever, and pains in the joints. The patient is given drugs to relieve the pain and fever.

oo- *combining form denoting* an egg; ovum.

oocyst *n.* a spherical structure, 50–60 μm in diameter, that develops from the zygote (*see* OOKINETE) of the malarial parasite (*Plasmodium*) on the outer wall of the mosquito's stomach. The oocyst steadily grows in size and its contents divide repeatedly to form *sporozoites, which are released into the body cavity of the mosquito when the oocyst bursts.

oocyte *n.* a cell in the ovary that undergoes *meiosis to form an ovum. **Primary oocytes** develop from *oogonia in the fetal ovary as they enter the early stages of meiosis. Only a fraction of the primary oocytes survive until puberty, and even fewer will be ovulated. At ovulation the first meiotic division is completed and a **secondary oocyte** and a **polar body** are formed. Fertilization stimulates the completion of the second meiotic division, which produces a second polar body and an ovum.

oocyte donation (egg donation) the transfer of secondary *oocytes from one woman to another. Possible recipients include women with primary or secondary ovarian failure or severe genetic disorders, and women in whom ovulation has been suppressed as an incidental result of drug treatment for another condition (e.g. cancer). Pregnancy rates are higher than with *in vitro fertilization.

oogenesis *n.* the process by which mature ova (egg cells) are produced in the ovary (see illustration). Primordial germ cells multiply to form *oogonia, which start their first meiotic division to become *oocytes in the fetus.

Oogenesis.

This division is not completed until each oocyte is ovulated. The second division is only completed on fertilization. Each meiotic division is unequal, so that one large ovum is produced with a much smaller polar body.

oogonium *n.* (*pl.* **oogonia**) a cell produced at an early stage in the formation of an ovum (egg cell). Primordial germ cells that have migrated to the embryonic ovary multiply to form numerous small oogonia. After the fifth month of pregnancy they enter the early stages of the first meiotic division to form the *oocytes. *See also* OOGENESIS.

ookinete *n.* the motile elongated *zygote of the malarial parasite (*Plasmodium*), formed after fertilization of the *macrogamete. The ookinete bores through the lining of the mosquito's stomach and attaches itself to the outer wall, where it later forms an *oocyst.

oophor- (oophoro-) *combining form denoting* the ovary.

oophorectomy (ovariectomy) *n.* surgical removal of an ovary, performed, for example, when the ovary contains tumours or cysts or is otherwise diseased. *See also* OVARIOTOMY.

oophoritis (ovaritis) *n.* inflammation of an ovary, either on the surface or within the organ. Oophoritis may be associated with infection of the Fallopian tubes (*see* SALPINGITIS) or the lower part of the abdominal cavity. **Follicular oophoritis** is inflammation of the ovarian (Graafian) follicles. A bacterial infection usually responds to antibiotics.

oophoropexy *n.* the stitching of a displaced ovary to the wall of the pelvic cavity.

operant *adj.* describing a unit of behaviour that is defined by its effect on the environment. *See* CONDITIONING.

operating microscope a binocular microscope commonly in use for microsurgery. The field of operation is illuminated through the objective lens by a light source within the microscope (see illustration). Many models incorporate a beam splitter and a second set of eyepieces, to enable the surgeon's assistant to view the operation.

operculum *n.* (*pl.* **opercula**) 1. a plug of mucus that blocks the cervical canal of the uterus in a pregnant woman. When the cervix begins to dilate at the start of labour,

the operculum, slightly stained with blood, comes away as a discharge ('show'). 2. (in embryology) a plug of fibrin and blood cells that develops over the site at which a developing fertilized ovum has become embedded in the wall of the uterus. 3. (in neurology) one of the folded and overlapping regions of cerebral cortex that conceal the *insula on each side of the brain. 4. (in dentistry) a flap of gingival tissue that overlies the crown of a partially erupted tooth.

operon *n.* a group of closely linked genes that regulate the production of enzymes in bacteria. An operon is composed of one or more **structural genes**, which determine the nature of the enzymes made, and **operator** and **promoter genes**, which control the working of the structural genes. The operator is itself controlled by a **regulator gene**, which is not part of the operon.

ophthalm- (ophthalmo-) *combining form denoting* the eye or eyeball. Examples: **ophthalmectomy** (surgical removal of); **ophthalmorrhexis** (rupture of); **ophthalmotomy** (incision into).

ophthalmia *n.* inflammation of the eye, particularly the conjunctiva (*see* CONJUNCTIVITIS). **Sympathetic ophthalmia** is a granulomatous *uveitis affecting all parts of the uveal tract of both eyes that may develop after perforating trauma or (more rarely) after intraocular surgery.

ophthalmia neonatorum conjunctivitis occurring in newborn infants. The two most common infections are gonorrhoea and *Chlamydia* (*see* INCLUSION CONJUNCTIVITIS); the infection may be contracted as the baby passes through an infected birth canal. If left untreated, it may cause lasting damage to the eye. Diagnosis should be confirmed with microbiological studies, and both baby and mother treated with appropriate antibiotics.

ophthalmic *adj.* concerned with the eye.

ophthalmic nerve the smallest of the three branches of the *trigeminal nerve. It supplies sensory fibres to the eyeball, conjunctiva, and lacrimal gland, to a small region of the nasal mucous membrane, and to the skin of the nose, brows, and scalp.

ophthalmitis *n.* inflammation of the eye. *See* CONJUNCTIVITIS, UVEITIS.

ophthalmodynamometry *n.* measurement of the blood pressure in the vessels of the retina of the eye. A small instrument is pressed against the eye until the vessels are seen (through an *ophthalmoscope) to collapse. The pressure recorded by the instrument reflects the pressure within the vessels of the retina. In certain disorders of the blood circulation to the eye, the pressure in the vessels is reduced and the vessels can be made to collapse by a lower than normal pressure on the eyeball.

ophthalmologist *n.* a doctor who specializes in the diagnosis and treatment of eye diseases.

ophthalmology *n.* the branch of medicine that is devoted to the study and treatment of eye diseases. —**ophthalmological** *adj.*

ophthalmometer *n. see* KERATOMETER.

ophthalmoplegia *n.* paralysis of the muscles of the eye. **Internal ophthalmoplegia** affects the muscles inside the eye: the iris (which controls the size of the pupil) and also the ciliary muscle (which is responsible for *accommodation). **External ophthalmoplegia** affects the muscles moving the eye. **Chronic progressive external ophthalmoplegia** is a progressive disease of the extrinsic eye muscles leading to *ptosis and then paralysis of the muscles; eye movements become increasingly frozen in the primary position. Ophthalmoplegia may accompany *exophthalmos due to thyrotoxicosis. **Internuclear ophthalmoplegia** (INO), due to a le-

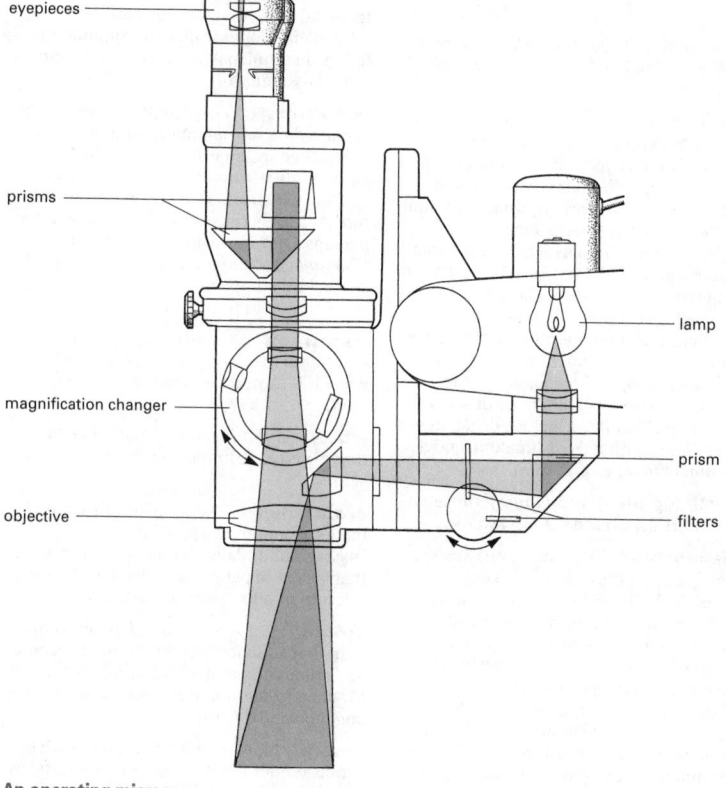

eyepieces

prisms

magnification changer

objective

lamp

prism

filters

An operating microscope.

sion in the brainstem, is seen, for example, in patients with multiple sclerosis or stroke.

ophthalmoscope *n.* an instrument for examining the interior of the eye. There are two types. The **direct ophthalmoscope** enables a fine beam of light to be directed into the eye and at the same time allows the examiner to see the spot where the beam falls inside the eye. Examiner and subject are very close together. In the **indirect ophthalmoscope** an image of the inside of the eye is formed between the subject and the examiner; it is this image that the examiner sees. The examiner and subject are almost an arm's length apart. A **scanning laser ophthalmoscope** uses a scanning camera, rather than a human observer, to view the inside of the eye. —**ophthalmoscopy** *n.*

ophthalmotonometer *n. see* TONOMETER.

-opia *combining form denoting* a defect of the eye or of vision. Example: **asthenopia** (eyestrain).

opiate *n.* strictly, one of a group of drugs derived from opium, including *morphine, *codeine, and *heroin (diacetylmorphine). The term may be used more loosely to include, in addition, synthetic drugs with similar effects, such as *methadone and *buprenorphine; in this case the term **opioid** is usually preferred. Opiates depress the central nervous system: they relieve pain, induce feelings of euphoria, suppress coughing, and stimulate vomiting. Because prolonged use can lead to *tolerance and *dependence, opioid *analgesics are reserved for the relief of moderate or severe pain; other side-effects include drowsiness, nausea and vomiting, constipation, and depression of breathing.

opisth- (opistho-) *combining form denoting* 1. dorsal; posterior. 2. backwards.

opisthorchiasis *n.* a condition caused by the presence of the parasitic fluke *Opisthorchis in the bile ducts. The infection is acquired through eating raw or undercooked fish that contains the larval stage of the parasite. Heavy infections can lead to considerable damage of the tissues of the bile duct and liver, progressing in advanced cases to *cirrhosis. Symptoms may include loss of weight, abdominal pain, indigestion, and sometimes diarrhoea. The disease is treated with praziquantel.

Opisthorchis *n.* a genus of parasitic flukes occurring in E Europe, Russia, India, Japan, and SE Asia. *O. felineus* is normally a parasite of fish-eating mammals but humans can become infected after eating raw or undercooked fish. The adult flukes, which live in the bile ducts, can cause *opisthorchiasis.

opisthotonos *n.* the position of the body in which the head, neck, and spine are arched backwards. It is assumed involuntarily by patients with tetanus and strychnine poisoning.

opium *n.* an extract from the poppy *Papaver somniferum*, which contains a number of alkaloids, principally morphine (which accounts for its analgesic, euphoric, and addictive effects: *see* OPIATE) with smaller amounts of codeine, papaverine, and others.

opponens *n.* one of a group of muscles in the hand that bring the digits opposite to other digits. For example, the **opponens pollicis** is the principal muscle causing opposition of the thumb.

opportunistic *adj.* denoting a disease that occurs when the patient's immune system is impaired by, for example, an infection, another disease, or drugs. The infecting organism, which is also described as opportunistic, rarely causes the disease in healthy persons. Opportunistic infections, such as *Pneumocystis pneumonia and that caused by the MAI complex (*see* MYCOBACTERIUM), are common in patients with AIDS.

opposition *n.* (in anatomy) the position of the thumb in relation to the other fingers when it is moved towards the palm of the hand.

-opsia *combining form denoting* a condition of vision. Example: **erythropsia** (red vision).

opsoclonus *n.* a series of erratic eye movements, resembling a large-amplitude fast *nystagmus and developing spontaneously, that is seen in people with disease of the cerebellum or other parts of the brain.

opsonin *n.* a serum *complement component that attaches itself to invading bacteria and apparently makes them more attractive to *phagocytes and thus more likely to be engulfed and destroyed.

opsonization *n.* the process by which opsonins render foreign organisms or particles more attractive to *phagocytes by attaching to their outer surfaces and changing their physical and chemical composition. Phagocytic leucocytes express receptors for these opsonins and thereby engulf and digest foreign organisms or particles.

opt- (opto-) *combining form denoting* vision or the eye.

optic *adj.* concerned with the eye or vision.

optical activity the property possessed by some substances of rotating the plane of polarization of polarized light. A compound that rotates the plane to the left is described as **laevorotatory** (or l-); one that rotates the plane to the right is described as **dextrorotatory** (or d-).

optical coherence tomography (OCT) a class of optical tomographic techniques that allows extremely high-quality micrometre-resolution three-dimensional images to be obtained from within optical scattering media (e.g. biological tissue). OCT is proving valuable in diverse areas, including diagnostic medicine (notably in ophthalmology, where it permits remarkable noninvasive images of the ocular structures).

optic atrophy degeneration of the optic nerve. It may be secondary to disease within the eye or it may follow damage to the nerve itself resulting from injury or inflammation. It is visible as pallor of the optic nerve as viewed inside the eye with an ophthalmoscope.

optic chiasm (optic commissure) the X-shaped structure formed by the two optic nerves, which pass backwards from the eyeballs to meet in the midline beneath the brain, near the pituitary gland (see illustration). Nerve fibres from the nasal side of the retina of each eye cross over to join fibres from the lateral side of the retina of the opposite eye. The optic tracts resulting from the junction pass backwards to the occipital lobes.

optic cup either of the paired cup-shaped outgrowths of the embryonic brain that form the retina and iris of the eyes.

optic disc (optic papilla) the start of the optic nerve, where nerve fibres from the rods and cones leave the eyeball. *See* BLIND SPOT.

optic foramen the groove in the top of the *orbit that contains the optic nerve and the ophthalmic artery.

optician (dispensing optician) *n.* a person who is trained to make and fit glasses. *Compare* OPTOMETRIST.

optic nerve the second *cranial nerve (II), which is responsible for vision. Each nerve contains about one million fibres that receive information from the rod and cone cells of the retina. It passes into the skull behind the eyeball to reach the *optic chiasm, after which the **visual** (or **optic**) **pathway** continues to the cortex of the occipital lobe of the brain on each side (see illustration).

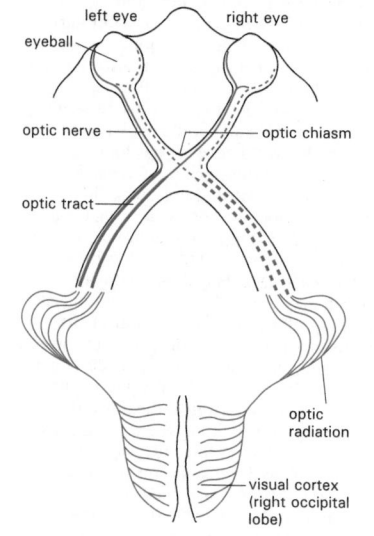

Optic nerve. The visual (or optic) pathway.

optic neuritis *see* RETROBULBAR NEURITIS.

opticokinetic *adj.* relating to the movements of the eye.

optometer (refractometer) *n.* an instrument for measuring the *refraction of the eye. An **autorefractor** calculates the required spectacle lens correction automatically. Because the design and use of optometers is very complex, errors of refraction are usually determined using a *retinoscope.

optometrist (ophthalmic optician) *n.* a health specialist qualified to examine the eyes for eye diseases and visual defects and prescribe corrective lenses. Optometrists must be registered with the General Optical

Council, having obtained a degree in optometry and one year's preregistration experience. *Compare* OPTICIAN.

oral *adj.* **1.** relating to the mouth. **2.** taken by mouth: applied to medicines, etc.

oral cavity the mouth.

oral contraceptive a tablet containing one or more synthetic female sex hormones, taken by women to prevent conception. Most oral contraceptives are combined pills, consisting of an *oestrogen, which blocks the normal process of ovulation, and a *progestogen, which acts on the pituitary gland to block the normal control of the menstrual cycle. Progestogens also alter the lining of the uterus and the viscosity of mucus in its outlet, the cervix, so that conception is less likely should ovulation occur. These pills are taken every day for three weeks and then stopped for a week, during which time menstruation occurs. Side-effects may include headache, weight gain, nausea, skin changes, and depression. There is also a small risk that blood clots may form in the veins, especially those of the legs (which may lead to *pulmonary embolism), or that prolonged use of hormonal contraceptives may reduce fertility. The unwanted pregnancy rate is less than 1 per 100 woman-years. With progestogen-only pills (sometimes known as **minipills**) the unwanted pregnancy rate is slightly higher (1–2 per 100 woman-years) but there are fewer side-effects (due to the absence of oestrogen).

Other hormonal contraceptives include injections and implants (*see* CONTRACEPTION). *See also* POSTCOITAL CONTRACEPTION.

oral hypoglycaemic drug (oral antidiabetic drug) one of the group of drugs that reduce the level of glucose in the blood and are taken by mouth for the treatment of non-insulin-dependent (type 2) *diabetes mellitus. They include the *sulphonylurea group (e.g. chlorpropamide, glibenclamide, tolbutamide), metformin (a *biguanide), *alpha-glucosidase inhibitors, *meglitinides, and *thiazolidinediones.

oral rehabilitation the procedure of rebuilding a dentition that has been mutilated as a result of disease, wear, or trauma.

oral rehydration therapy (ORT) the administration of an isotonic solution of various sodium salts, potassium chloride, glucose, and water to treat acute diarrhoea, particularly in children. In developing countries it is the mainstay of treatment for cholera. Once the diarrhoea has settled, normal feeding is gradually resumed. Preparations in clinical use include **Dioralyte** and **Electrolade**.

orbicularis *n.* either of two circular muscles of the face. The **orbicularis oris**, around the mouth, closes and compresses the lips. The **orbicularis oculi**, around each orbit, is responsible for closing the eye.

orbit *n.* the cavity in the skull that contains the eye. It is formed from parts of the frontal, sphenoid, zygomatic, lacrimal, ethmoid, palatine, and maxillary bones. —**orbital** *adj.*

orbitotomy *n.* surgical removal of part of the orbital bones to gain access to the orbital space.

orchi- (orchido-, orchio-) *combining form denoting* the testis or testicle. Example: **orchioplasty** (plastic surgery of).

orchidalgia *n.* pain in the testicle, often due to a *varicocele, *orchitis, or *torsion of the testis. The pain may also be caused by a hernia in the groin or the presence of a stone in the lower ureter.

orchidectomy *n.* surgical removal of a testis, usually to treat germ-cell tumours of the testis, such as *seminoma or *teratoma, which are malignant tumours of the testis. Removal of both testes (**bilateral orchidectomy**: *see* CASTRATION) causes sterility and reduces levels of testosterone by 90%, which is an effective treatment for prostate cancer.

orchidometer *n.* a calliper device for measuring the size of the testicles. The **Prader orchidometer** consists of a collection of testicle-shaped beads of different sizes, each of known volume, for direct comparison to and sizing of the testicles. It enables the precise charting of testicular growth.

orchidopexy *n.* the operation of mobilizing an undescended testis in the groin and fixing it in the scrotum. The operation should be performed well before puberty to allow the testis every chance of normal development (*see* CRYPTORCHIDISM).

orchidotomy *n.* an incision into the testis, usually done to obtain *biopsy material for histological examination, particularly in men with few or no sperm in their semen (*see* AZOOSPERMIA, OLIGOSPERMIA). *See also* TESA.

orchitis *n.* inflammation of the testis. This causes pain, redness, and swelling of the scrotum, and may be associated with inflammation of the epididymis (**epididymo-orchitis**). The condition may affect one or both testes; it is usually caused by infection spreading down the vas deferens but can develop in mumps. Mumps orchitis affecting both testes may result in sterility. Treatment of epididymo-orchitis is by local support and by administration of analgesics and antibiotics; mumps orchitis often responds to *corticosteroids.

orf *n.* an infectious disease of sheep and goats caused by a parapoxvirus. Those bottle-feeding infected lambs may develop a painful nodule, 2–3 cm across, on the fingers or hands; it resolves spontaneously.

organ *n.* a part of the body, composed of more than one tissue, that forms a structural unit responsible for a particular function (or functions). Examples are the heart, lungs, and liver.

organelle *n.* a structure within a cell that is specialized for a particular function. Examples of organelles are the nucleus, endoplasmic reticulum, Golgi apparatus, lysosomes, and mitochondria.

organic *adj.* **1.** relating to any or all of the organs of the body. **2.** describing chemical compounds containing carbon, found in all living systems.

organic disorder a disorder associated with changes in the structure of an organ or tissue. *Compare* FUNCTIONAL DISORDER.

organism *n.* any living thing, which may consist of a single cell (*see* MICROORGANISM) or a group of differentiated but interdependent cells.

organo- *combining form denoting* organ or organic. Examples: **organogenesis** (formation of); **organopathy** (disease of).

organ of Corti (spiral organ) the sense organ of the *cochlea of the inner ear, which converts sound signals into nerve impulses that are transmitted to the brain via the cochlear nerve. [A. Corti (1822–88), Italian anatomist]

organ of Jacobson (vomeronasal organ) a small blind sac in the wall of the nasal cavity. In humans it never develops properly and has no function, but in lower animals (e.g. snakes) it is one of the major organs of olfaction. [L. L. Jacobson (1783–1843), Danish anatomist]

organotrophic *adj. see* HETEROTROPHIC.

orgasm *n.* the climax of sexual excitement, which – in men – occurs simultaneously with *ejaculation. In women its occurrence is much more variable, being dependent upon a number of physiological and psychological factors.

oriental sore (Baghdad boil, Delhi boil, Aleppo boil) a skin disease, occurring in tropical and subtropical Africa and Asia, caused by the parasitic protozoan *Leishmania tropica* (*see* LEISHMANIASIS). The disease commonly affects children and takes the form of a slow-healing open sore or ulcer, which sometimes becomes secondarily infected with bacteria. Antibiotics are administered to combat the infection.

orientation *n.* (in psychology) awareness of oneself in time, space, and place. Orientation may be disturbed in such conditions as organic brain disease, toxic drug states, mental illness, and concussion.

origin *n.* (in anatomy) **1.** the point of attachment of a muscle that remains relatively fixed during contraction of the muscle. *Compare* INSERTION. **2.** the point at which a nerve or blood vessel branches from a main nerve or blood vessel.

orlistat *n.* a drug that reduces the absorption of fat in the stomach and small intestine by inhibiting the action of pancreatic *lipases. It is administered by mouth in the treatment of clinical *obesity, in conjunction with appropriate dietary measures. Side-effects include the production of copious oily stools and flatulence. Trade names: **Alli**, **Xenical**.

ornithine *n.* an *amino acid produced in the liver as a by-product during the conversion of ammonia to *urea.

Ornithodoros (Ornithodorus) *n.* a genus of soft *ticks, a number of species of which are important in various parts of the world in the transmission of *relapsing fever.

ornithosis *n. see* PSITTACOSIS.

oro- *combining form denoting* the mouth.

oroantral fistula a connection between the mouth and the maxillary sinus (antrum), usually as a sequel to tooth extraction. It may resolve or require surgical closure.

oropharyngeal airway a curved tube designed to be placed in the mouth of an unconscious patient, behind the tongue, to create a patent airway. *See also* NASOPHARYNGEAL AIRWAY.

oropharynx *n.* the part of the *pharynx that lies between the level of the junction of the hard and soft palates above, the hyoid bone below, and the arch of the soft palate in front. It contains the *tonsils and connects the oral cavity and *nasopharynx to the *hypopharynx. —**oropharyngeal** *adj.*

Oroya fever *see* BARTONELLOSIS.

orphenadrine *n.* an *antimuscarinic drug that relieves spasm in muscle, used to treat parkinsonism induced by antipsychotic drugs. It is administered by mouth; side-effects may include dry mouth, sight disturbances, and difficulty in urination. Trade names: **Biorphen**, **Disipal**.

ORT *see* ORAL REHYDRATION THERAPY.

ortho- *combining form denoting* **1.** straight. Example: **orthograde** (having straight posture). **2.** normal. Example: **orthocrasia** (normal reaction to drugs).

orthochromatic *adj.* describing or relating to a tissue specimen that stains normally.

orthodontic appliance an appliance used to move teeth as part of orthodontic treatment. A **fixed appliance** is fitted to the teeth by stainless steel bands or brackets that hold a special archwire, to perform complex tooth movements; it is used by dentists with specialist training (**orthodontists**). A **removable appliance** is a dental plate with appropriate retainers and springs to perform simple tooth movements; it is removed from the mouth for cleaning by the patient.

orthodontics *n.* the branch of dentistry concerned with the growth and development of the face and jaws and the treatment of irregularities of the teeth. *See* ORTHODONTIC APPLIANCE. —**orthodontic** *adj.*

orthognathic surgery surgical correction of severe *malocclusion, in which development of one or both jaws is abnormal, to improve facial appearance. It needs to be carried out in combination with orthodontic treatment and may involve surgery to one or both jaws.

orthokeratology *n.* the use of contact lenses designed to reshape the cornea in the treatment of refractive errors, such as myopia (short sight).

orthopaedics *n.* the science or practice of correcting deformities caused by disease of or damage to the bones and joints of the skeleton. This specialized branch of surgery may involve operation, manipulation, traction, *orthoses, or *prostheses. —**orthopaedic** *adj.*

orthophoria *n.* the condition of complete balance between the alignment of the two eyes, such that perfect alignment is maintained even when one eye is covered. This theoretically normal state is in fact rarely seen, since in most people there is a minimal tendency for the eyes to deviate (*see* HETEROPHORIA).

orthopnoea *n.* breathlessness that prevents the patient from lying down, so that he has to sleep propped up in bed or sitting in a chair. —**orthopnoeic** *adj.*

orthoptics *n.* the practice of using nonsurgical methods, particularly eye exercises, to treat abnormalities of vision and of coordination of eye movements (most commonly strabismus (squint) and amblyopia). Orthoptics also includes the detection and measurement of the degree of any such abnormalities. —**orthoptic** *adj.* —**orthoptist** *n.*

orthoptoscope *n. see* AMBLYOSCOPE.

orthosis *n.* (*pl.* **orthoses**) a surgical appliance that exerts external forces on part of the body to support joints or correct deformity. —**orthotic** *adj.*

orthostatic *adj.* relating to the upright position of the body: used when describing this posture or a condition caused by it. *See* HYPOTENSION.

orthotics *n.* the science and practice of fitting an *orthosis to improve the mechanical functioning of a limb, part of a limb, or the trunk.

Ortolani manoeuvre a test for *congenital dislocation of the hip in which, with the baby lying supine and the pelvis steadied with one hand, the examiner attempts to relocate a dislocated hip by gently abducting the hip while simultaneously pushing upwards on the greater trochanter. If the hip is dislocated, it will relocate with a detectable and sometimes audible clunk.

[M. Ortolani (20th century), Italian ortho-paedic surgeon]

os¹ *n.* (*pl.* **ossa**) a bone.

os² *n.* (*pl.* **ora**) the mouth or a mouthlike part.

OSA *see* OBSTRUCTIVE SLEEP APNOEA.

OSAS obstructive sleep apnoea syndrome (*see* OBSTRUCTIVE SLEEP APNOEA).

OSCE *see* OBJECTIVE STRUCTURED CLINICAL EXAMINATION.

osche- (**oscheo-**) *combining form denoting* the scrotum. Example: **oscheocele** (a scrotal hernia).

oscilloscope *n.* a cathode-ray tube de-signed to display electronically a wave form corresponding to the electrical data fed into it. Oscilloscopes are used to provide a con-tinuous record of many different measure-ments, such as the activity of the heart and brain. *See* ELECTROCARDIOGRAPHY, ELECTRO-ENCEPHALOGRAPHY.

osculum *n.* (in anatomy) a small aperture.

oseltamivir *n.* an antiviral drug that acts by inhibiting the action of the enzyme *neu-raminidase in viruses, which reduces their replication in host cells. Oseltamivir is ad-ministered orally for the prevention and treatment of influenza A and B. To be effec-tive, the drug must be taken within 48 hours of exposure to influenza (for prophylaxis) or onset of symptoms (for treatment). Trade name: **Tamiflu**.

Osgood-Schlatter disease inflamma-tion and swelling at the site of insertion of the patellar tendon at the tibial tuberosity, just below the knee (*see* APOPHYSITIS), result-ing in a prominent painful lump. It occurs in adolescence, as a result of excessive physical activity, and most cases resolve with time and rest. [R. B. Osgood (1873–1956), US or-thopaedist; C. Schlatter (1864–1934), Swiss surgeon]

-osis *suffix denoting* **1.** a diseased condi-tion. Examples: **nephrosis** (of the kidney); **leptospirosis** (caused by *Leptospira* species). **2.** any condition. Example: **narcosis** (of stu-por). **3.** an increase or excess. Example: **leu-cocytosis** (of leucocytes).

Osler-Rendu-Weber disease (**hereditary haemorrhagic telangiectasia**) a hereditary (autosomal *dominant) disorder character-ized by thinning of the blood vessel walls, re-sulting in abnormally wide and fragile blood vessels. Patients may develop telangiectasia (*see* TELANGIECTASIS), nosebleeds, and arte-riovenous malformations (*see* ANGIOMA). It is caused by mutations in the endoglin (*ENG*) gene or the activin receptor-like kinase (*ALK-1*) gene. [Sir W. Osler (1849–1919), Canadian physician; H. J. M. Rendu (1844–1902), French physician; F. P. Weber (1863–1962), British physician]

Osler's nodes purplish nodes on the finger pulp or the *thenar or *hypothenar eminence. They are usually tender and a sign of bacterial *endocarditis. [Sir W. Osler]

osm- (**osmo-**) *combining form denoting* **1.** smell or odour. **2.** osmosis or osmotic pressure.

osmic acid *see* OSMIUM TETROXIDE.

osmiophilic *adj.* describing a tissue that stains readily with osmium tetroxide.

osmium tetroxide (**osmic acid**) a colour-less or faintly yellowish compound used to stain fats or as a *fixative in the preparation of tissues for microscopical study. Osmium tetroxide evaporates readily, the vapour hav-ing a toxic action on the eyes, skin, and res-piratory tract.

osmolality *n.* the concentration of body fluids (e.g. plasma, urine) measured in terms of the amount of dissolved substances per unit mass of water. It is usually given in units of mOsm kg^{-1}.

osmolar gap the difference between the measured serum osmolality and the calcu-lated osmolality using the following formula:

calculated osmolality = 2[Na⁺ (in mmol/l) + glucose (in mmol/l) + urea (in mmol/l)]

It is an aid to the diagnosis of severe *anion gap acidoses. The normal range for the dif-ference is ± 10 mOsm/kg. A high osmolar gap is normally due to the presence of acetone, mannitol, or an alcohol.

osmole *n.* a unit of osmotic pressure equal to the molecular weight of a solute in grams divided by the number of ions or other parti-cles into which it dissociates in solution.

osmoreceptor *n.* a group of cells in the *hypothalamus that monitor blood concen-tration. Should this increase abnormally, as in dehydration, the osmoreceptors send nerve impulses to the hypothalamus, which then increases the rate of release of *vasopressin from the posterior pituitary gland. Loss of water from the body in the urine is thus restricted until the blood concentration returns to normal.

osmosis *n.* the passage of a solvent from a less concentrated to a more concentrated solution through a *semipermeable membrane. This tends to equalize the concentrations of the two solutions. In living organisms the solvent is water and cell membranes function as semipermeable membranes, and the process of osmosis plays an important role in controlling the distribution of water. The **osmotic pressure** of a solution is the pressure by which water is drawn into it through the semipermeable membrane; the more concentrated the solution (i.e. the more solute molecules it contains), the greater its osmotic pressure. —**osmotic** *adj.*

osseointegration *n.* the process by which certain materials, such as titanium, may be introduced into living bone without producing a foreign-body reaction. This allows a very tight and strong joint between the two structures. Osseointegration is used, for example, to fix certain types of dental *implants and *bone-anchored hearing aids.

osseous *adj.* bony: applied to the bony parts of the inner ear (cochlea, semicircular canals, labyrinth).

ossicle *n.* a small bone. The **auditory ossicles** are three small bones (the incus, malleus, and stapes) in the middle *ear. They transmit sound from the outer ear to the labyrinth (inner ear).

ossification (osteogenesis) *n.* the formation of *bone, which takes place in three stages by the action of special cells (osteoblasts). A meshwork of collagen fibres is deposited in connective tissue, followed by the production of a cementing polysaccharide. Finally the cement is impregnated with minute crystals of calcium salts. The osteoblasts become enclosed within the matrix as **osteocytes** (**bone cells**). In **intracartilaginous** (or **endochondral**) **ossification** the bone replaces cartilage. This process starts to occur soon after the end of the second month of embryonic life. **Intramembranous ossification** is the formation of a *membrane bone (e.g. a bone of the skull). This starts in the early embryo and is not complete at birth (*see* FONTANELLE).

ost- (oste-, osteo-) *combining form denot-*

ing bone. Examples: **ostalgia** (pain in); **osteocarcinoma** (carcinoma of); **osteonecrosis** (death of); **osteoplasty** (plastic surgery of).

ostectomy *n.* the surgical removal of a bone or a piece of bone. *See also* OSTEOTOMY.

osteitis *n.* inflammation of bone, due to infection, damage, or metabolic disorder. **Osteitis fibrosa cystica** refers to the characteristic cystic changes that occur in bones during long-standing *hyperparathyroidism. *See also* PAGET'S DISEASE (OSTEITIS DEFORMANS).

osteo- *combining form. see* OST-.

osteoarthritis (osteoarthrosis) *n.* a degenerative disease of joints resulting from wear of the articular cartilage, which may lead to secondary changes in the underlying bone. It can be primary or it can occur secondarily to abnormal load to the joint or damage to the cartilage from inflammation or trauma. The joints are painful and stiff with restricted movement. Osteoarthritis is recognized on X-ray by narrowing of the joint space (due to loss of cartilage) and the presence of *osteophytes, *osteosclerosis, and cysts in the bone. The condition is treated with analgesics, by reducing the load to the joint by weight loss or the use of a walking stick, or surgically by *osteotomy, *arthrodesis, or *arthroplasty.

osteoarthropathy *n.* any disease of the bone and cartilage adjoining a joint. **Hypertrophic osteoarthropathy** is characterized by the formation of new bony tissue and occurs as a complication of chronic diseases of the chest, including pulmonary abscess, mesothelioma, and lung cancer.

osteoarthrosis *n. see* OSTEOARTHRITIS.

osteoarthrotomy *n.* surgical excision of the bone adjoining a joint.

osteoblast *n.* a cell, originating in the mesoderm of the embryo, that is responsible for the formation of *bone. *See also* OSSIFICATION.

osteochondritis (osteochondrosis) *n.* any one of a group of conditions affecting areas of growth at the *epiphyses and *apophyses of bones before skeletal maturity. Symptoms of localized pain and swelling are most common during periods of rapid growth in early adolescence. There are three types of osteochondritis: **crushing** (*see* KÖHLER'S DISEASE, KIENBÖCK'S DISEASE, LEGG-

CALVÉ-PERTHES DISEASE, SCHEUERMANN'S DISEASE); **splitting** (*see* OSTEOCHONDRITIS DISSECANS); and **pulling** (*see* OSGOOD-SCHLATTER DISEASE, SEVER'S DISEASE).

osteochondritis dissecans the development of a small area of avascular bone on the surface of a joint, most commonly the knee, which typically occurs in males aged between 10 to 20 years. Sometimes the area with its overlying articular cartilage can become loose and may eventually detach. Symptoms include activity-related pain, localized tenderness, stiffness, and swelling. In children, spontaneous healing may occur, but adults usually require surgery to reattach or remove the fragment.

osteochondroma a bony protuberance covered by a cap of cartilage arising usually from the end of a long bone, most commonly around the knee or shoulder. It is due to overgrowth of cartilage at the edge of the *physis (growth plate) of growing bones. The protuberance may be flattened (**sessile**) or stalklike (*see* EXOSTOSIS) and usually appears before the age of 30, with patients complaining of either pain or a lump. There is a small incidence (1–2% in solitary lesions, higher if multiple) of malignant transformation of the cartilage cap into a *chondrosarcoma. If the lump causes symptoms or continues to grow in an adult, it should be excised.

osteochondrosis *n. see* OSTEOCHONDRITIS.

osteoclasia (osteoclasis) *n.* 1. (osteoclasty) the deliberate breaking of a malformed or malunited bone, carried out by a surgeon to correct deformity. 2. dissolution of bone through disease (*see* OSTEOLYSIS).

osteoclasis *n.* 1. remodelling of bone by *osteoclasts, during growth or the healing of a fracture. 2. *see* OSTEOCLASIA.

osteoclast *n.* 1. a large multinucleate cell that resorbs calcified bone. Osteoclasts are only found when bone is being resorbed and may be seen in small depressions on the bone surface. 2. a device for fracturing bone for therapeutic purposes.

osteoclastoma *n.* a rare tumour of bone, caused by proliferation of *osteoclast cells.

osteocyte *n.* a bone cell: an *osteoblast that has ceased activity and has become embedded in the bone matrix.

osteodystrophy *n.* any generalized bone disease resulting from a metabolic disorder.

In **renal osteodystrophy** chronic kidney failure leads to diffuse bone changes resulting from a number of factors, including osteomalacia, secondary *hyperparathyroidism stimulated by hypocalcaemia and hyperphosphataemia, acidosis from the renal failure, and metastatic calcification related to high levels of calcium and phosphate in the blood. *See also* ALBRIGHT'S HEREDITARY OSTEODYSTROPHY.

osteogenesis *n. see* OSSIFICATION.

osteogenesis imperfecta (fragilitas ossium) a congenital disorder of connective tissue formation that affects bone, teeth, and soft tissues. It has an incidence of 1 in 20,000 and there are four types, of varying severity, the worst being lethal at birth. In all types the bones are brittle and fracture easily; the *sclerae may be blue and teeth are often deformed.

osteogenic *adj.* arising in, derived from, or composed of any of the tissues that are concerned with the production of bone. An **osteogenic sarcoma** (*see* OSTEOSARCOMA) affects bone-producing cells.

osteology *n.* the study of the structure and function of bones and related structures.

osteolysis (osteoclasia) *n.* dissolution of bone through disease, commonly by infection or by loss of the blood supply (ischaemia) to the bone. In **acro-osteolysis** the terminal bones of the fingers or toes are affected: a common feature of some disorders involving blood vessels (including *Raynaud's disease), *scleroderma, and systemic *lupus erythematosus.

osteoma a benign bone tumour, of which there are two types. An **osteoid osteoma** most commonly occurs in the shaft of the femur or tibia. It is small, solitary, and relatively common; its characteristic feature is that it causes nocturnal pain that is relieved by aspirin. Treatment is by surgical excision. A **compact osteoma** (**ivory exostosis**) is a slow-growing tumour-like mass that usually causes no symptoms. Such tumours are relatively uncommon, occurring usually in the skull and facial bones. If they do cause symptoms, usually from local compression, they may be excised.

osteomalacia *n.* softening of the bones due to inadequate mineralization: it is the adult counterpart of *rickets. Causes include a significant calcium deficiency and lack of vitamin D, the latter resulting from poor diet, lack of sunshine, intestinal malabsorption, liver or kidney disease, or anticonvulsant medication. The most common symptoms are bone pain, backache, and muscle weakness. The characteristic X-ray finding is a thin transverse radiolucent band (a **Looser zone**) in an otherwise normal-looking bone. Treatment usually involves large doses of vitamin D.

osteomyelitis *n.* inflammation of bone due to infection. **Acute osteomyelitis** occurs when bacteria enter the bone via the bloodstream and is more common in children. There is severe pain, tenderness, and redness over the involved bone, accompanied by general illness and high fever. Treatment is by antibiotics, and surgical drainage and curettage are often required. **Chronic osteomyelitis** may develop from partially treated acute osteomyelitis or after open fractures or surgery during which the bone is contaminated; tuberculosis is an occasional cause. Osteomyelitis can cause fracture and deformity of the bone.

osteonecrosis *n.* death of bony tissue, usually adjacent to a joint surface where it is enclosed by avascular cartilage. It is usually caused by loss of blood supply (**avascular necrosis**) due to trauma and is a definitive feature in a variety of conditions, including *Legg-Calvé-Perthes disease, *sickle-cell disease, *Gaucher's disease, epiphyseal infection and fractures, alcohol abuse, and high-dosage corticosteroids. Sites that are particularly susceptible include the head of the femur, the scaphoid and lunate bones of the wrist, the *capitulum of the humerus, and the talus and navicular bones of the ankle. In its earliest stages there is localized pain without any changes visible on X-ray examination; a *bone scan or MRI will assist with diagnosis.

osteopathy *n.* a system of diagnosis and treatment based on the theory that many diseases are associated with disorders of the musculoskeletal system. Diagnosis and treatment of these disorders involve palpation, manipulation, and massage. Osteopathy provides relief for many disorders of bones and joints, especially those producing back pain. —**osteopath** *n.* —**osteopathic** *adj.*

osteopenia *n.* a degree of bone loss less severe than *osteoporosis. *See* T SCORE.

osteopetrosis (Albers-Schönberg disease, marble-bone disease) *n.* a congenital abnormality in which bones become abnormally dense and brittle and tend to fracture. Affected bones appear unusually opaque to X-rays. In severe forms the bone marrow is obliterated, causing anaemia and infections. Treatment is by bone marrow transplantation. *See also* OSTEOSCLEROSIS.

osteophyte *n.* a projection of bone, usually shaped like a rose thorn, that occurs at sites of cartilage degeneration or destruction near joints and intervertebral discs. Osteophyte formation is an X-ray sign of *osteoarthritis but is not a cause of symptoms in itself.

osteoporosis *n.* a reduction in bone mineral density, resulting in bones that are brittle and liable to fracture. Infection, injury, and *synovitis can cause localized osteoporosis of adjacent bone. Generalized osteoporosis is common in the elderly, and in women often follows the menopause. It is also a feature of *Cushing's syndrome and prolonged steroid therapy. Osteoporosis can be detected by *quantitative digital radiography and by *DEXA scans. A diet with adequate calcium, together with exercise, are preventative, and *bisphosphonates or *raloxifene can be used to reduce or halve further bone loss.

osteosarcoma (osteogenic sarcoma) *n.* a highly malignant tumour arising from within a bone, usually in the *metaphysis of the long bones of the body and especially around the knee and the proximal end of the humerus. It is usually seen in children and adolescents but can occur in adults of all ages, occasionally in association with *Paget's disease of bone. In children the usual site for the tumour is the leg, particularly the femur. Secondary growths (metastases) are common, most frequently in the lungs (though other sites, such as the liver, may also be involved). The symptoms are usually pain and swelling at the site of the tumour and there is often a history of preceding trauma, although it is doubtful whether this contributes to the cause. Treatment of disease localized to the primary site was traditionally by amputation of the limb; limb-sparing surgery is now possible after *neoadjuvant chemotherapy, with replacement of the diseased bone by a metal prosthesis. Many centres also give *adjuvant therapy in an attempt to kill any microscopic tumour that might have already spread. The drugs used include doxorubicin, cisplatin, vincristine, cyclophosphamide, and methotrexate.

osteosclerosis *n.* an abnormal increase in the density of bone, as a result of poor blood supply, chronic infection, or tumour. The affected bone is more opaque to X-rays than normal bone. *See also* OSTEOPETROSIS.

osteotome *n.* a surgical chisel designed to cut bone (see illustration).

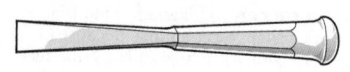

An osteotome.

osteotomy *n.* a surgical operation to cut a bone into two parts, followed by realignment of the ends to allow healing. The operation is performed to reduce pain and disability in an arthritic joint, by changing the biomechanics of the joint, for cases in which conservative treatment has failed. Osteotomy of the jaws is performed to improve severe discrepancies in jaw relation.

ostium *n.* (*pl.* **ostia**) (in anatomy) an opening. The **ostium abdominale** is the opening of the Fallopian tube into the abdominal cavity.

-ostomy *combining form. see* -STOMY.

ot- (oto-) *combining form denoting* the ear. Example: **ototomy** (surgical incision of).

otalgia *n.* pain in the ear. Apart from local causes it may be due to diseases of the jaw joints, neck, throat, or teeth.

OTC drug *see* OVER-THE-COUNTER DRUG.

otic *adj.* relating to the ear.

otic capsule the cup-shaped cartilage in the head of an embryo that later develops into the bony *labyrinth of the ear.

otitis *n.* inflammation of the ear. **Otitis externa** is inflammation of the canal between the eardrum and the external opening of the ear (the external auditory meatus). **Myringitis** is inflammation of the eardrum, often due to viral infection. **Acute otitis media** is inflammation, usually due to viral or bacterial infection, of the middle ear (the chamber lying behind the eardrum and containing the three bony ossicles that conduct sound to the inner ear). Symptoms include pain and a

high fever. Treatment is with antibiotics and sometimes also by surgical drainage (*myringotomy). **Secretory otitis media** (or **otitis media with effusion**) is a chronic accumulation of fluid in the middle ear, causing hearing loss (*see* GLUE EAR). **Chronic otitis media** (**COM**) is chronic inflammation of the middle ear associated with perforations of the eardrum and in some instances with *cholesteatoma. The treatment involves surgical repair of perforations (*myringoplasty) or removal of the air cells in the mastoid bone (*mastoidectomy). Chronic otitis media was previously known as **chronic suppurative otitis media** but the terminology was changed as the formation of pus is not an inevitable part of the condition. **Labyrinthitis** (**otitis interna**) is inflammation of the inner ear causing vertigo, vomiting, loss of balance, and deafness.

otoacoustic emissions (OAE, Kemp echoes) tiny sounds that emerge from the inner ear either spontaneously (**spontaneous otoacoustic emissions**, SOAE) or shortly after the ear is exposed to an external sound (**evoked otoacoustic emissions**, EOAE). An objective test of hearing has been developed using otoacoustic emissions. The test equipment creates a small sound and then detects any response from the ear. This can be done using a click stimulus (**transient otoacoustic emissions**, TOAE) or two separate tones (**distortion product otoacoustic emissions**, DPOAE). A normal response suggests that the ear is functioning and that hearing is satisfactory. All newborn children in the UK are now screened using this technique.

otoconium *n. see* OTOLITH.

otocyst *n.* a small cavity in the mesoderm of the head of an embryo that later develops into the membranous *labyrinth of the ear.

otolaryngology *n.* the study of diseases of the ears and larynx.

otolith (otoconium) *n.* one of the small particles of calcium carbonate associated with a macula in the *saccule or *utricle of the inner ear.

otology *n.* the study of diseases of the ear.

-otomy *combining form. see* -TOMY.

otomycosis *n.* a fungus infection of the ear, causing irritation and inflammation of the canal between the eardrum and the external opening of the ear (external auditory meatus). It is one of the causes of *otitis externa.

otoplasty (pinnaplasty) *n.* surgical repair or reconstruction of the ears after injury or in the correction of a congenital defect (such as 'bat ears').

otorhinolaryngology *n.* the study of ear, nose, and throat diseases (i.e. ENT disorders).

otorrhagia *n.* bleeding from the ear.

otorrhoea *n.* any discharge from the ear, commonly a purulent discharge in chronic middle ear infection (*otitis media).

otosclerosis (otospongiosis) *n.* a disorder causing deafness in adult life. An overgrowth of the bone of the inner ear leads to the third ear ossicle (the stapes) becoming fixed to the fenestra ovalis, which separates the middle and inner ears, so that sounds cannot be conducted to the inner ear. *Deafness is progressive and may become very severe, but treatment by surgery is highly effective (*see* FENESTRATION, STAPEDECTOMY). Nonsurgical treatments include fluoride tablets and the provision of suitable *hearing aids.

otoscope *n. see* AURISCOPE.

otospongiosis *n. see* OTOSCLEROSIS.

ototoxic *adj.* having a toxic effect on the organs of balance or hearing in the inner ear or on the vestibulocochlear nerve. Ototoxic drugs may be used in the treatment of *Ménière's disease. —**ototoxicity** *n.*

outbreeding *n.* the production of offspring by parents who are not closely related. *Compare* INBREEDING.

outer ear the pinna and the external auditory meatus of the *ear.

out-of-hours (in general practice) denoting the period from 6.30 pm to 8.00 am on weekdays and the whole of weekends, bank holidays, and public holidays. Most GPs use a deputizing service to provide health-care services during the out-of-hours period. *See* GENERAL PRACTITIONER.

out-of-body experience a form of *derealization in which there is a sensation of leaving one's body, sometimes accompanied by visions of travel. It typically occurs after anaesthesia or severe illness and is often attributed to *anoxia of the brain.

out-patient *n.* a patient who receives treatment at a hospital, either at a single attendance or at a series of attendances, but is not admitted to a bed in a hospital ward. Large hospitals have *clinics at which outpatients with various complaints can be given specialist treatment. *Compare* IN-PATIENT.

oval window *see* FENESTRA (OVALIS).

ovari- (ovario-) *combining form denoting* the ovary.

ovarian cancer a malignant tumour of the ovary, usually a carcinoma. Because of its wide-ranging pathology and an imperfect understanding of its causes, ovarian cancer is not readily detected in the early stages of development, when the tumour is small and produces few suspicious symptoms. Increased susceptibility to the disease is associated with raised serum levels of *CA125 (*see also* BRCA1 AND BRCA2). Diagnosis is based on the finding of a solid or cystic mass arising from the pelvis; there may be associated *ascites. The incidence of ovarian cancer reaches a peak in postmenopausal women; treatment involves surgery and most cases also require combined chemotherapy and/or radiotherapy.

ovarian cyst a benign tumour of the ovary, of which there are many varieties. The most common is a **follicular cyst**, resulting from growth of a *Graafian follicle that fails to ovulate or from involution of a mature follicle. It may rupture, causing pain. A **luteal cyst** occurs after an egg has been released from a follicle, which then becomes a *corpus luteum; instead of breaking down if a pregnancy does not occur, it fills with blood or fluid. It is usually found on only one side of the ovary and produces no symptoms. Although most ovarian cysts are not malignant, they may reach a very large size, causing gross swelling of the abdomen and pressure on surrounding organs. The cyst may rotate on its stalk, thus cutting off its blood supply and causing severe abdominal pain and vomiting. In this case the cyst requires urgent surgical removal. Ovarian cysts that do become malignant may not be recognized until the tumour has advanced to a stage where treatment may be unsuccessful in eradicating the cancer. Screening programmes, based on ultrasound techniques, and *CA125 estimation, have been introduced in some areas to assist with the early detection of ovarian cysts and tumours.

ovarian hyperstimulation syndrome
a potentially life-threatening condition classically associated with ovarian stimulation using gonadotrophins in assisted conception procedures, such as in vitro fertilization (*see* SUPEROVULATION). It is characterized by gross enlargement of the ovaries resulting in *haemoconcentration and *ascites.

ovariectomy *n. see* OOPHORECTOMY.

ovariotomy *n.* literally, incision of an ovary. However, the term commonly refers to surgical removal of an ovary (*oophorectomy).

ovaritis *n. see* OOPHORITIS.

ovary *n.* the main female reproductive organ, which produces ova (egg cells) and steroid hormones in a regular cycle (*see* MENSTRUAL CYCLE) in response to hormones (*gonadotrophins) from the anterior pituitary gland. There are two ovaries, situated in the lower abdomen, one on each side of the uterus (*see* REPRODUCTIVE SYSTEM). Each ovary contains numerous **follicles**, within which the ova develop (see illustration), but only a small proportion of them reach maturity (*see* GRAAFIAN FOLLICLE, OOGENESIS). The follicles secrete *oestrogen and small amounts of androgen. After ovulation a *corpus luteum forms at the site of the ruptured follicle and secretes progesterone. Oestrogen and progesterone regulate the changes in the uterus throughout the menstrual cycle and pregnancy. —**ovarian** *adj.*

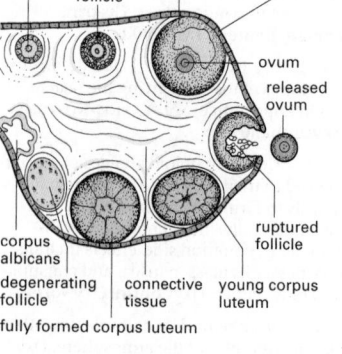

Ovary. A section of the ovary showing ova in various stages of maturation.

overbite *n.* the vertical overlap of the upper incisor teeth over the lower ones.

overcompensation *n.* (in psychology) the situation in which a person tries to overcome a disability by making greater efforts than are required. This may result in the person becoming extremely efficient in what he (or she) is trying to achieve; alternatively, excessive overcompensation may be harmful to the person.

overjet *n.* the horizontal overlap of the upper incisor teeth in front of the lower ones.

overt *adj.* plainly to be seen or detected: applied to diseases with observable signs and symptoms, as opposed to those whose presence may not be suspected for years despite the fact that they cause insidious damage. An infectious disease becomes overt only at the end of an incubation period.

over-the-counter drug (OTC drug) a drug that may be purchased directly from a pharmacist without a doctor's prescription. Current government policy is to extend the range of OTC drugs: a number have already been derestricted (e.g. ibuprofen, ranitidine) and this trend is increasing, which will place an additional advisory responsibility on pharmacists.

overtube *n.* a flexible plastic tube (25–45 cm long) designed to fit over the shaft of an *endoscope. It is used in cases where multiple introductions of the endoscope are required and also as a stiffening device for the endoscope. It can be used with a *gastroscope, *cholangioscope, *enteroscope, or colonoscope (*see* COLONOSCOPY). An overtube is usually placed over the shaft of an endoscope prior to its insertion; once the endoscope is in the desired place, the overtube is lubricated and slid in position over the shaft. This then makes removal and reinsertion of the endoscope relatively easy and without significant discomfort to the patient. It is commonly used in combination with a gastroscope for removal of ingested foreign bodies from the oesophagus or stomach.

ovi- (**ovo-**) *combining form denoting* an egg; ovum.

oviduct *n. see* FALLOPIAN TUBE.

ovulation *n.* the process by which an ovum is released from a mature *Graafian follicle. The fluid-filled follicle distends the surface of the ovary until a thin spot breaks down and the ovum floats out surrounded by a cluster of follicle cells (the cumulus oophoricus) and starts to travel down the Fallopian tube to the uterus. Ovulation is stimulated by the secretion of *luteinizing hormone by the anterior pituitary gland.

ovum (egg cell) *n.* the mature female sex cell (*see* GAMETE). The term is often applied to the secondary *oocyte although this is technically incorrect. The final stage of meiosis occurs only when the oocyte has been activated by fertilization.

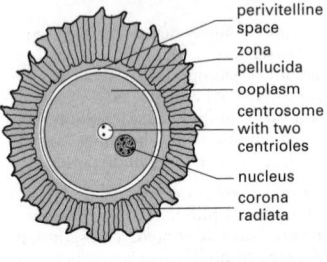

perivitelline space
zona pellucida
ooplasm
centrosome with two centrioles
nucleus
corona radiata

A mature ovum (magnification about ×600).

oxalic acid an extremely poisonous acid, $C_2H_2O_4$. It is a component of some bleaching powders and is found in many plants, including sorrel and the leaves of rhubarb. Oxalic acid is a powerful local irritant; when swallowed it produces burning sensations in the mouth and throat, vomiting of blood, breathing difficulties, and circulatory collapse. Treatment is with calcium lactate or other calcium salts, lime water, or milk.

oxaliplatin *n.* a third-generation analogue of *cisplatin that is useful in the treatment of gastrointestinal malignancies, particularly colorectal cancer. Administered by intravenous infusion in combination with fluorouracil and folinic acid, it has less toxic side-effects than cisplatin, although it can cause a typical *peripheral neuropathy exacerbated by cold temperatures. Trade name: **Eloxatin**.

oxalosis *n.* an inborn defect of metabolism causing deposition of oxalate in the kidneys and elsewhere and eventually leading to renal failure.

oxaluria *n.* the presence in the urine of oxalic acid or oxalates, especially calcium oxalate. Excessive amounts of oxalates are excreted in *oxalosis.

oxazepam *n.* a *benzodiazepine drug used to relieve severe anxiety and tension. It is administered by mouth and commonly causes drowsiness. *See also* ANXIOLYTIC.

oxidant *n.* (in biological systems) a molecule that serves as an electron acceptor. In human disease oxidants are derived from normal intracellular processes and released by inflammatory cells. They are counteracted by *antioxidants, such as beta-carotene.

oxidase *n. see* OXIDOREDUCTASE.

oxidoreductase *n.* one of a group of enzymes that catalyse oxidation-reduction reactions. This class includes the enzymes formerly known either as **dehydrogenases** or as **oxidases**.

oximeter *n.* an instrument for measuring the proportion of oxygenated haemoglobin (oxyhaemoglobin) in the blood.

oxprenolol *n.* a drug that controls the activity of the heart (*see* BETA BLOCKER), used mainly to treat angina, high blood pressure, and abnormal heart rhythm. It is administered by mouth; side-effects may include dizziness, drowsiness, headache, and digestive upsets. Trade names: **Slow-Trasicor**, **Trasicor**.

oxybutynin *n.* an *antimuscarinic drug administered orally or in transdermal (skin) patches to reduce frequency and urgency of passing urine associated with an unstable bladder or overactivity of the *detrusor muscle of the bladder wall. It acts by relaxing the bladder muscle. Side-effects include a dry mouth, loss of appetite, constipation, and blurred vision. Trade names: **Cystrin**, **Ditropan**, **Kentera**, **Lyrinel XL**.

oxycephaly (turricephaly) *n.* a deformity of the bones of the skull giving the head a pointed appearance. *See* CRANIOSYNOSTOSIS. —**oxycephalic** *adj.*

oxycodone *n.* an opioid analgesic (*see* OPIATE) used to treat moderate or severe pain, primarily in terminally ill patients. It is administered orally, intravenously, or subcutaneously; common side-effects include drowsiness, dizziness, nausea, and constipation. Trade names: **OxyContin**, **OxyNorm**.

oxygen *n.* an odourless colourless gas that makes up one-fifth of the atmosphere. Oxygen is essential to most forms of life in that it combines chemically with glucose (or some other fuel) to provide energy for metabolic processes. It is absorbed into the blood from air breathed into the lungs. Oxygen is administered therapeutically in various conditions in which the tissues are unable to obtain an adequate supply through the lungs (*see* OXYGENATOR, (OXYGEN) TENT). Symbol: O.

oxygenator *n.* a machine that oxygenates blood outside the body. It is used together with pumps to maintain the patient's circulation while he or she is undergoing open heart surgery (*see* HEART-LUNG MACHINE) or to improve the circulation of a patient with heart or lung disorders that lower the amount of blood oxygen.

oxygen deficit a physiological condition that exists in cells during periods of temporary oxygen shortage. During periods of violent exertion the body requires extra energy, which is obtained by the breakdown of glucose in the absence of oxygen, after the available oxygen has been used up. The breakdown products are acidic and cause muscle pain. The oxygen required to get rid of the breakdown products (called the oxygen deficit) must be made available after the exertion stops.

oxygen tent *see* TENT.

oxyhaemoglobin *n.* the bright-red substance formed when the pigment *haemoglobin in red blood cells combines reversibly with oxygen. Oxyhaemoglobin is the form in which oxygen is transported from the lungs to the tissues, where the oxygen is released. *Compare* METHAEMOGLOBIN.

oxyntic cells (parietal cells) cells of the *gastric glands that secrete hydrochloric acid in the fundic region of the stomach.

oxytetracycline *n.* an antibiotic used to treat infections caused by a wide variety of bacteria, including *Chlamydia* and mycoplasmas, and acne. It is administered by mouth; side-effects are those of the other *tetracyclines.

oxytocic *n.* any agent that induces or accelerates labour by stimulating the muscles of the uterus to contract. *See also* OXYTOCIN.

oxytocin *n.* a hormone, released by the pituitary gland, that causes contraction of the uterus during labour and stimulates milk flow from the breasts by causing contraction of muscle fibres in the milk ducts. Intravenous infusions or injections of oxytocin (**Syntocinon**) are used to induce labour and to control or prevent postpartum haemorrhage. Combined with *ergometrine (in **Syntometrine**), oxytocin is used for active management of the third stage of labour.

oxyuriasis *n. see* ENTEROBIASIS.

Oxyuris *n. see* THREADWORM.

ozaena *n.* a disorder of the nose in which the mucous membranes inside the nose become atrophied, with the production of an offensive discharge and crusts.

ozone *n.* a poisonous gas containing three oxygen atoms per molecule. Ozone is a very powerful oxidizing agent and is formed when oxygen or air is subjected to electric discharge. Ozone in the troposphere (the atmospheric layer closest to the earth's surface), as found in photochemical smog, can cause health problems. Ozone at very high altitudes (the **ozone layer**) is responsible for absorbing a large proportion of the sun's ultraviolet radiation. Without this absorption by ozone the earth would be subjected to a lethal amount of ultraviolet radiation.

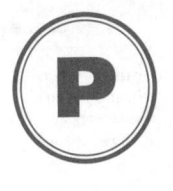

p53 *n.* a tumour-suppressor gene located on chromosome 17. p53 protein binds DNA, which stimulates genes involved in suppressing division and inducing *apoptosis. Mutations of *p53* result in uncontrolled division of cells and formation of tumours; they occur in breast, skin, and various other cancers.

PA *see* POSTEROANTERIOR.

Pacchionian body *see* ARACHNOID VILLUS. [A. Pacchioni (1665–1726), Italian anatomist]

pacemaker *n.* **1.** a device used to produce and maintain a normal heart rate in patients who have *bradycardia. The unit consists of a battery that stimulates the heart through one or more insulated electrode wires (*leads) attached to the surface of the ventricle (**epicardial pacemaker**) or lying in contact with the lining of the heart (**endocardial pacemaker**). The pacemaker senses when the natural heart rate falls below a predetermined value and then stimulates the heart (**demand pacemaker**). A pacemaker may be used as a temporary measure with an external battery or it may be permanent, when the whole apparatus is surgically implanted under the skin. In most cases the right atrium and right ventricle are paced (**dual-chamber pacing**), but in a proportion of patients only right ventricular (**single-chamber**) **pacing** is required. **2.** the part of the heart that regulates the rate at which it beats: the *sinoatrial node.

pachy- *combining form denoting* **1.** thickening of a part or parts. **2.** the dura mater.

pachydactyly *n.* abnormal enlargement of the fingers and toes, occurring either as a congenital abnormality or as part of an acquired disease (such as *acromegaly).

pachyglossia *n.* abnormal thickness of the tongue.

pachymeningitis *n.* inflammation of the dura mater, one of the membranes (meninges) covering the brain and spinal cord (*see* MENINGITIS).

pachymeninx *n.* the *dura mater, outermost of the three meninges.

pachymeter *n.* an instrument used to measure the thickness of the cornea. **—pachymetry** *n.*

pachyonychia congenita a rare genetically determined skin disorder (*see* GENODERMATOSIS) characterized by thickening of the nails together with other ectodermal abnormalities.

pachysomia *n.* thickening of parts of the body, which occurs in certain diseases.

pachytene *n.* the third stage of the first prophase of *meiosis, in which *crossing over begins.

Pacinian corpuscles sensory receptors for touch in the skin, consisting of sensory nerve endings surrounded by capsules of membrane in 'onion-skin' layers. They are especially sensitive to changes in pressure and so detect vibration particularly well. [F. Pacini (1812–83), Italian anatomist]

pack *n.* a pad of folded moistened material, such as cotton-wool, applied to the body or inserted into a cavity.

packed cell volume (haematocrit) the volume of the red cells (erythrocytes) in blood, expressed as a fraction of the total volume of the blood. The packed cell volume is determined by centrifuging blood in a tube and measuring the height of the red-cell column as a fraction of the total. Automated instruments calculate packed cell volume as the product of the erythrocyte count and the measured mean red cell volume (**mean corpuscular volume; MCV**).

paclitaxel *n.* a *cytotoxic anticancer drug (*see* TAXANE). Administered by intravenous infusion, it is used mainly to treat ovarian cancer, breast cancer, and *non-small-cell lung cancer. Typical side-effects include damage to bone marrow (*see* MYELOSUPPRESSION), loss of hair, and peripheral neuropathy. Trade names: **Abraxane, Taxol**.

PACS (picture archiving and communication system) a computer network enabling the storage and transfer of digital images for display on high-resolution monitors. Images can be viewed at multiple sites simultaneously. The system also allows the manipulation of images on screen. *See* DIGITAL RADIOGRAPHY, COMPUTERIZED RADIOGRAPHY, COMPUTERIZED TOMOGRAPHY, DIGITIZATION.

pad *n.* cotton-wool, foam rubber, or other material used to protect a part of the body from friction, bruising, or other unwanted contact.

paed- (paedo-) *combining form denoting* children.

paediatric dentistry the branch of dentistry concerned with the oral health care of children and adolescents.

paediatrics *n.* the general medicine of childhood. Handling the sick child requires a special approach at every age from birth (or preterm birth) to adolescence and also a proper understanding of parents. It also requires detailed knowledge of genetics, obstetrics, psychological development, management of handicaps at home and in school, and effects of social conditions on child health. The preventive measures associated with all these aspects of paediatrics are the concern of *public health consultants and *community paediatricians. *See also* CHILD HEALTH CLINIC. —**paediatrician** *n.*

(((●))) SEE WEB LINKS
• Website of Action for Sick Children: includes information for health-care professionals

paedophilia *n.* sexual attraction to children (of either sex) that may cause deviant behaviour. Sexual activity with any children under the age of 16 is illegal in the UK for adults. Paedophiles who have been arrested may be forced to undergo treatment: *behaviour therapy can be used, or the sexual drive can be reduced by drug treatment. —**paedophile** *n.* —**paedophilic** *adj.*

Paget's disease **1.** a chronic disease of bones, occurring in the elderly and most frequently affecting the skull, backbone, pelvis, and long bones. Affected bones become thickened and their structure disorganized: X-rays reveal patchy *sclerosis. There are often no symptoms, but pain, deformity, and fracture can occur; when the skull is affected, blindness and deafness can occur due to nerve compression. There is a very small (1%) risk of malignant change (*osteosarcoma). Treatment is with *bisphosphonates

or calcitonin. Medical name: **osteitis deformans**. **2.** a malignant condition of the nipple, resembling eczema in appearance, associated with underlying infiltrating cancer of the breast. *See also* BREAST CANCER. **3.** an uncommon condition of the vulva characterized by an epithelial lesion that histologically resembles the lesion of Paget's disease of the nipple. It may be associated with locally invasive *adenocarcinomas of the surrounding skin, as well as tumours at other sites. [Sir J. Paget (1814–99), British surgeon]

pain *n.* an unpleasant sensation ranging from mild discomfort to agonized distress, associated with real or potential tissue damage. Pain is a response to impulses from the peripheral nerves in damaged tissue, which pass to nerves in the spinal cord, where they are subjected to a gate control. This gate modifies the subsequent passage of the impulses in accordance with descending controls from the brain. Because attention is a crucial component of pain, distraction can act as a basis for pain therapy. On the other hand, anxiety and depression focus the attention and exaggerate the pain. If the nerve pathways are damaged, the brain can increase the amplification in the pathway, maintaining the sensation as a protective mechanism.

pain clinic a clinic that specializes in the management and relief of pain. Pain clinics are usually directed by anaesthetists.

paint *n.* (in pharmacy) a liquid preparation that is applied to the skin or mucous membranes. Paints usually contain antiseptics, astringents, caustics, or analgesics.

palaeo- *combining form denoting* **1.** ancient. **2.** primitive.

palaeocerebellum *n.* the anterior lobe of the cerebellum. In evolutionary terms it is one of the earliest parts of the hindbrain to develop in mammals.

palaeopathology *n.* the study of the diseases of humans and other animals in prehistoric times, from examination of their bones or other remains. By examining the bones of specimens of Neanderthal man it has been discovered that spinal arthritis was a disease that existed at least 50,000 years ago.

palaeostriatum *n. see* PALLIDUM.

palaeothalamus *n.* the anterior and central part of the *thalamus, older in evolutionary terms than the lateral part, the neothalamus, which is well developed in apes and humans.

palate *n.* the roof of the mouth, which separates the mouth from the nasal cavity and consists of two portions. The **hard palate**, at the front of the mouth, is formed by processes of the maxillae and palatine bones and is covered by mucous membrane. The **soft palate**, further back, is a movable fold of mucous membrane that tapers at the back of the mouth to form a fleshy hanging flap of tissue – the **uvula**.

palatine bone either of a pair of approximately L-shaped bones of the face that contribute to the hard *palate, the nasal cavity, and the orbits. *See* SKULL.

palato- *combining form denoting* 1. the palate. 2. the palatine bone.

palatoplasty *n.* surgery to alter the shape or physical characteristics of the palate. This can be plastic surgery of the roof of the mouth, usually to correct cleft palate or other defects present at birth. Other palatoplasty operations are carried out under local or general anaesthesia to shorten and/or stiffen the palate in the treatment of snoring or obstructive sleep apnoea. They may use conventional surgical techniques (*uvulopalatopharyngoplasty), laser (*laser-assisted uvulopalatoplasty), or injection of sclerosants. It is also possible to use radiofrequency energy in a process called **radiofrequency palatal myoplasty** (RPM), also known as **somnoplasty**.

palatorrhaphy *n. see* STAPHYLORRHAPHY.

pali- (palin-) *combining form denoting* repetition or recurrence.

palilalia *n.* a disorder of speech in which a word spoken by the individual is rapidly and involuntarily repeated. It is seen, with other tics, in *Tourette's syndrome. It is also encountered when encephalitis or other processes damage the *extrapyramidal system of the brain.

palindromic *adj.* relapsing: describing diseases or symptoms that recur or get worse.

paliphrasia *n.* repetition of phrases while speaking: a form of *stammering or a kind of *tic.

palliative 1. *adj.* providing relief from the symptoms of a disease but without effecting a cure. Palliative care is often used in the treatment of terminal illness. 2. *n.* a palliative medicine.

pallidotomy (pallidectomy) *n.* a neurosurgical operation to destroy or modify the effects of the globus pallidus (*see* BASAL GANGLIA), formerly used for the relief of *parkinsonism and other conditions in which involuntary movements were prominent before the advent of modern drug therapies. The development of more accurate techniques to localize the globus pallidus has led to a revival in its use: in the modern form of pallidotomy, a lesion is made in the globus pallidus by stereotactic surgery (*see* STEREOTAXY). New techniques achieving better results involve the implantation of stimulators (pallidal stimulation).

pallidum (palaeostriatum) *n.* one of the dense collections of grey matter, deep in each cerebral hemisphere, that go to make up the *basal ganglia.

pallium *n.* the outer wall of the cerebral hemisphere as it appears in the early stages of evolution of the mammalian brain. In the modern brain it corresponds to the *cerebral cortex.

pallor *n.* abnormal paleness of the skin, due to reduced blood flow or lack of normal pigments. Pallor may be associated with an indoor mode of life; it may also indicate shock, anaemia, cancer, or other diseases.

palmitic acid *see* FATTY ACID.

palpation *n.* the process of examining part of the body by careful feeling with the hands and fingertips. Using palpation it is possible, in many cases, to distinguish between swellings that are solid and those that are cystic (*see* FLUCTUATION). Palpation is also used to discover the presence of a fetus in the uterus (*see* BALLOTTEMENT).

palpebral *adj.* relating to the eyelid (palpebra).

palpitation *n.* an awareness of the heartbeat. This is normal with fear, emotion, or exertion. It may also be a symptom of neurosis, arrhythmias, heart disease, and overactivity of the circulation (as in thyrotoxicosis).

PALS *see* PATIENT ADVICE AND LIAISON SERVICE.

palsy *n.* paralysis. This archaic word is retained in compound terms, such as *Bell's palsy, *cerebral palsy, and *Todd's paralysis (or palsy).

paludism *n. see* MALARIA.

pamidronate (disodium pamidronate) *n.* a *bisphosphonate drug used to treat malignant *hypercalcaemia, breast cancer that has spread to the bones, and Paget's disease. It is administered by intravenous infusion; side-effects include flulike symptoms, nausea, and vomiting. Trade name: **Aredia Dry Powder**.

pan- (pant(o)-) *combining form denoting* all; every: hence (in medicine) affecting all parts of an organ or the body; generalized.

panacea *n.* a medicine said to be a cure for all diseases and disorders, no matter what their nature. Unfortunately panaceas do not exist, despite the claims of many patent medicine manufacturers.

Panadol *n. see* PARACETAMOL.

pancarditis *n. see* ENDOMYOCARDITIS.

Pancoast syndrome pain and paralysis involving the lower branches of the brachial plexus due to infiltration by a malignant tumour of the apical region of the lung. *Horner's syndrome may also be present. [H. K. Pancoast (1875–1939), US radiologist]

pancreas *n.* a compound gland, about 15 cm long, that lies behind the stomach. One end lies in the curve of the duodenum; the other end touches the spleen. It is composed of clusters (**acini**) of cells that secrete *pancreatic juice. This contains a number of enzymes concerned in digestion. The juice drains into small ducts that open into the **pancreatic duct**. This unites with the common *bile duct and the secretions pass into the duodenum. Interspersed among the acini are the *islets of Langerhans – isolated groups of cells that secrete the hormones *insulin and *glucagon into the bloodstream.

pancreas divisum a congenital abnormality in which the pancreas develops in two parts draining separately into the duodenum, the small ventral pancreas through the main ampulla and the larger dorsal pancreas through an accessory papilla. In rare instances this is associated with recurrent abdominal pain, probably due to inadequate drainage of the dorsal pancreas. Diagnosis is usually made by CT scanning, magnetic resonance cholangiopancreatography (MRCP), or *ERCP.

pancreatectomy *n.* surgical removal of the pancreas. **Total pancreatectomy (Whipple's operation)** involves the entire gland and part of the duodenum. In **subtotal pancreatectomy** most of the gland is removed, usually leaving a small part close to the duodenum. In **partial pancreatectomy** only a portion of the gland is removed. The operations are performed for tumours in the gland or because of chronic or relapsing *pancreatitis. After total or subtotal pancreatectomy it is necessary to administer pancreatic enzymes with food to aid its digestion and insulin injections to replace that normally secreted by the gland.

pancreatic juice the digestive juice secreted by the *pancreas. Its production is stimulated by hormones secreted by the duodenum, which in turn is stimulated by contact with food from the stomach. If the duodenum produces the hormone *secretin the pancreatic juice contains a large amount of sodium bicarbonate, which neutralizes the acidity of the stomach contents. Another hormone (*see* CHOLECYSTOKININ) stimulates the production of a juice rich in digestive enzymes, including trypsinogen and chymotrypsinogen (which are converted to *trypsin and *chymotrypsin in the duodenum), *amylase, *lipase, and *maltase.

pancreatic polypeptide a hormone released from the D cells of the *islets of Langerhans of the pancreas in response to protein in the small intestine. Its actions are to inhibit pancreatic bicarbonate and protein enzyme secretion and to relax the gall bladder. It belongs to a family of similar hormones that have actions on appetite and food metabolism.

pancreatin *n.* an extract obtained from the *pancreas, containing the pancreatic enzymes. Pancreatin is administered to treat conditions in which pancreatic secretion is deficient; for example, in pancreatitis.

pancreatitis *n.* inflammation of the pancreas. **Acute pancreatitis** is a sudden illness in which the patient experiences severe pain in the upper abdomen and back, with shock; its cause is not always discovered, but it may be associated with gallstones or alcoholism. It may be mistaken for a perforated peptic ulcer but differs from this condition in that the level of the enzyme *amylase in the blood is raised. The main complication is the formation of a *pseudocyst. Treatment consists of intravenous feeding (no food or drink should be given by mouth), antibiotics, and *antimuscarinic drugs. **Relapsing pancreatitis**, in which the above symptoms are recurrent and less severe, may be associated with gallstones or alcoholism; prevention is by removal of gallstones and avoidance of alcohol and fat. Operations may be done to improve drainage of the pancreatic duct. **Chronic pancreatitis** may produce symptoms similar to relapsing pancreatitis or may be painless; it can lead to pancreatic failure causing *malabsorption and *diabetes mellitus. The pancreas often becomes calcified, producing visible shadowing on X-rays. The malabsorption is treated by a low-fat diet with pancreatic enzyme supplements, and the diabetes with insulin. **Autoimmune pancreatitis** is a recently described condition in which an autoimmune process leads to inflammation and swelling of the pancreas. Although abdominal pain is minimal or absent, jaundice is usually present. Radiologically it is characterized by diffuse 'sausage-shaped' enlargement of the pancreas and narrowing of the main pancreatic duct. The presence of raised serum IgG4 is a serological marker. Treatment involves immunosuppressant agents (e.g. corticosteroids or azathioprine). There is an association with other autoimmune disorders.

pancreatogram *n.* a radiographic image of the pancreatic ducts obtained by injecting a contrast medium into them by direct puncture under ultrasound guidance, at the time of laparotomy or by *ERCP. It has largely been replaced by noninvasive techniques involving MRCP (*see* CHOLANGIOGRAPHY).

pancreatotomy *n.* surgical opening of the duct of the pancreas in order to inspect the duct, to join the duct to the intestine, or to inject contrast material in order to obtain X-ray pictures of the duct system.

pancreozymin *n.* the name originally given to the fraction of the hormone *cholecystokinin that acts on the pancreas.

pancuronium *n. see* MUSCLE RELAXANT.

pancytopenia *n.* a simultaneous decrease in the numbers of red cells (*anaemia), white cells (*neutropenia), and platelets (*thrombocytopenia) in the blood. It occurs in a variety of disorders, including aplastic *anaemias, *hypersplenism, and tumours of the bone marrow. It may also occur after chemotherapy or total body irradiation.

panda sign a sign of bilateral periorbital *haematoma associated with injury to the anterior cranial fossa, the front of the skull cavity that supports the frontal lobes of the brain. The name derives from its similarity in appearance to the black eye patches of a panda.

pandemic *n.* an *epidemic so widely spread that vast numbers of people in different countries are affected. The Black Death, the epidemic plague that ravaged Europe in the fourteenth century and killed over one third of the population, was a classical pandemic. AIDS is currently considered to be pandemic. —**pandemic** *adj.*

panic disorder a condition featuring recurrent episodes of acute distress, mental confusion, and fear of impending death or disaster. The heart beats rapidly, breathing is deep and fast, and sweating occurs. Overbreathing (hyperventilation) often makes the attack worse. These **panic attacks** last 10 minutes or less and usually occur about twice a week (but may be more frequent); they are especially common in people with *agoraphobia. Treatment is with *antidepressant drugs and *behaviour therapy.

panmixis *n.* random mating within a population, i.e. when there is no selection of partners on religious, racial, social, or other grounds.

panniculitis *n.* inflammation of the layer of fat beneath the skin, leading to multiple tender nodules in the legs and trunk. There are many clinical patterns (including *erythema nodosum) and many causes.

panniculus *n.* a membranous sheet of tissue. For example, the **panniculus adiposus** is the fatty layer of tissue underlying the skin.

pannus *n.* vascularized *granulation tissue in the superficial layers of the cornea, growing in from the conjunctiva. It is seen as a result of inflammation of the cornea or conjunctiva, particularly in *trachoma.

panophthalmitis *n.* inflammation involving the whole of the interior of the eye.

Panstrongylus *n.* a genus of large bloodsucking bugs (*see* REDUVIID). *P. megistus* is important in transmitting *Chagas' disease to humans in Brazil.

pant- (panto-) *combining form. see* PAN-.

pantaloon hernia a double sac comprising the sac of an indirect (external) and a direct (internal) inguinal *hernia on the same side.

pantoprazole *n. see* PROTON-PUMP IN-HIBITOR.

pantothenic acid a B vitamin that is a constituent of *coenzyme A. It plays an important role in the transfer of acetyl groups in the body. Pantothenic acid is widely distributed in food and a deficiency is therefore unlikely to occur.

pantropic *adj.* describing a virus that can invade and affect many different tissues of the body, for example the nerves, skin, or liver, without showing a special affinity for any one of them.

papain *n.* a preparation that contains one or more protein-digesting enzymes. It is obtained from the pawpaw fruit and is used as a digestant.

Papanicolaou test (Pap test) *see* CERVICAL SCREENING. [G. N. Papanicolaou (1883–1962), Greek physician, anatomist, and cytologist]

papaverine *n.* an alkaloid, derived from opium, that relaxes smooth muscle. In combination with *morphine and *codeine (a mixture called **papaveretum**), it is administered by injection as a preanaesthetic medication and for relief of postoperative pain, but is now rarely used. It may cause abnormal heart rate. Papaverine may also be given by injection into the corpora cavernosa of the penis to treat erectile dysfunction.

papilla *n.* (*pl.* **papillae**) any small nipple-shaped protuberance. Several different kinds of papillae occur on the *tongue, in association with the taste buds. The **optic papilla** is an alternative name for the *optic disc.

papillary *adj.* nipple-like. Papillary epithelial neoplasms are composed of slender fronds of epithelial cells supported by fine fibrovascular cores. *See* PAPILLOMA.

papillitis *n.* inflammation of the first part of the optic nerve (the optic disc or optic papilla), i.e. where the nerve leaves the eyeball.

papilloedema *n.* swelling of the first part of the optic nerve (the optic disc or optic papilla) when viewed through an ophthalmoscope. It can be a sign of raised intracranial pressure or inflammation of the optic nerve (papillitis).

papilloma *n.* a benign tumour of nonglandular and nonsecretory epithelium forming a nipple-like growth on the surface of the skin or a mucous membrane. Examples include **bladder papillomas**. —**papillomatous** *adj.*

papillomatosis *n.* a condition in which many *papillomas grow on an area of skin or mucous membrane.

papillotomy *n.* the operation of cutting the *ampulla of Vater to widen its outlet in order to improve bile drainage and allow the passage of stones from the common bile duct. It is usually performed using a diathermy wire through a *duodenoscope following *ERCP.

papovavirus *n.* one of a group of small DNA-containing viruses producing tumours in animals (subgroup **polyomaviruses**) and in animals and humans (subgroup **papillomaviruses**). *See also* HUMAN PAPILLOMAVIRUS.

PAPP-A pregnancy-associated plasma protein A: a plasma protein in the serum of pregnant women that is used as a marker for Down's syndrome (levels are decreased in comparison to normal pregnancies). Measurement of PAPP-A and *human chorionic gonadotrophin (hCG) can be combined in a *prenatal screening test during the first 12 weeks of pregnancy.

Pappataci fever *see* SANDFLY FEVER.

papule *n.* a small raised spot on the skin, often dome-shaped, less than 5 mm in diameter.

papulo- *combining form denoting* a papule or pimple.

papulosquamous *adj.* describing a rash that is both papular and scaly.

para- *combining form denoting* **1.** beside or close to. Example: **paranasal** (near the nasal cavity). **2.** resembling. Example: **paradysentery** (a mild form of dysentery). **3.** abnormal. Example: **paralalia** (abnormal speech).

paracentesis *n.* tapping: the process of drawing off fluid from a part of the body through a hollow needle or *cannula. In ophthalmology, it involves an incision into the anterior chamber of the eye.

paracetamol (acetaminophen) *n.* an *analgesic drug that also reduces fever. It is widely used to treat mild or moderate pain, such as headache, toothache, and dysmenorrhoea, and as an antipyretic in colds, influenza, etc. It is administered by mouth, intravenous infusion, or as suppositories; side-effects are rare, but overdosage causes liver damage. Trade names: **Calpol**, **Disprol**, **Panadol**, etc.

Paracoccidioides *n.* a genus of yeast-like fungi causing infection of the skin and mucous membranes. The species *P. brasiliensis* causes a chronic skin disease, South American *blastomycosis.

paracrine *adj.* describing a hormone that is secreted by an endocrine gland and affects the function of nearby cells, rather than being transported distally by the blood or lymph.

paracusis *n.* any distortion of hearing.

paradidymis *n.* the vestigial remains of part of the embryonic *mesonephros that are found near the testis of the adult. Some of the mesonephric collecting tubules persist as the functional *vasa efferentia but the rest degenerate almost completely. A similar vestigial structure (the **paroophoron**) is found in females.

paradox *n.* (in *family therapy) a surprising interpretation or suggestion made in the course of therapy in order to demonstrate the relationship between a psychological symptom and a system of family relationships.

paradoxical breathing breathing movements in which the chest wall moves in on inspiration and out on expiration, in reverse of the normal movements. It may be seen in children with respiratory distress of any cause, which leads to indrawing of the intercostal spaces during inspiration. Patients with chronic airways obstruction also show indrawing of the lower ribs during inspiration, due to the distorted action of a depressed and flattened diaphragm. Crush injuries of the chest, with fractured ribs and sternum, can lead to a severe degree of paradoxical breathing.

paraesthesia *n.* a spontaneously occurring tingling sensation, sometimes described as **pins and needles**. It may be due to partial and temporary damage to a peripheral nerve, such as that caused by external pressure on the affected part, but can also result from damage to sensory fibres in the spinal cord or from peripheral vascular disease. *Compare* DYSAESTHESIA.

paraffin *n.* one of a series of hydrocarbons derived from petroleum. **Paraffin wax (hard paraffin)**, a whitish mixture of solid hydrocarbons melting at 45–60°C, is used in medicine mainly as a base for ointments and in microscopy for *embedding specimens. **Liquid paraffin** is a mineral oil formerly used as a laxative; combined with **soft paraffin** (white or yellow), it is used as an emollient (**Cetraben**, **E45**, etc.), as a lubricating ointment for treating dry eyes (**Lacri-Lube**, **Lubi-Tears**), and to impregnate gauze dressings to prevent the fibres from sticking.

paraganglioma *n.* a tumour, related to *phaeochromocytoma arising from *paraganglion cells. Such tumours can occur around the aorta, the carotid artery (carotid body tumour), and the cervical portion of the vagus nerve (*glomus tumour), as well as in the abdomen and the eye. They are usually benign and treated by surgery, but occasionally can be malignant, requiring systemic treatment.

paraganglion *n.* one of the small oval masses of cells found in the walls of the ganglia of the sympathetic nervous system, near the spinal cord. They are *chromaffin cells, like those of the adrenal gland, and may secrete adrenaline.

parageusia (parageusis) *n.* abnormality of the sense of taste.

paragonimiasis (endemic haemoptysis) *n.* a tropical disease that occurs principally in Asia, caused by the presence of the fluke *Paragonimus westermani* in the lungs or other organs. The infection is acquired by eating inadequately cooked shellfish. Early symptoms include fever, cough, chest pain, fatigue, and sweating. Later symptoms vary depending on which organs are affected: in the case of the lungs, symptoms resemble those of tuberculosis. Paragonimiasis is treated with praziquantel.

Paragonimus *n.* a genus of large tropical parasitic *flukes that are particularly prevalent in the Far East. The adults of *P. westermani* live in the human lungs, where they cause destruction and bleeding of the tissues (*see* PARAGONIMIASIS). However, they may also be found in other organs of the body. Eggs are passed out in the sputum and the larvae undergo their development in two other hosts, a snail and a crab.

paragranuloma *n.* a former name for one of the types of *Hodgkin's disease. It is now known as **lymphocyte-predominant Hodgkin's disease** and has the best prognosis of all the types.

parainfluenza viruses a group of large RNA-containing viruses that cause infections of the respiratory tract producing mild influenza-like symptoms. They are included in the paramyxovirus group (*see* MYXOVIRUS).

paraldehyde *n.* an *anticonvulsant drug used to control seizures in *status epilepticus. It is administered by enema; side-effects include rashes.

paralysis *n.* muscle weakness that varies in its extent, its severity, and the degree of spasticity or flaccidity according to the nature of the underlying disease and its distribution in the brain, spinal cord, peripheral nerves, or muscles. *See* FLACCID (PARALYSIS), SPASTIC PARALYSIS. *See also* DIPLEGIA, HEMIPLEGIA, PARAPLEGIA, POLIOMYELITIS. —**paralytic** *adj.*

paramedian *adj.* situated close to or beside the *median plane.

paramedical *adj.* describing or relating to the professions closely linked to the medical profession and working in conjunction with them. *See* ALLIED HEALTH PROFESSIONAL.

paramesonephric duct *see* MÜLLERIAN DUCT.

parameter *n.* (in medicine) a measurement of some factor, such as blood pressure, pulse rate, or haemoglobin level, that may have a bearing on the condition being investigated.

parametric test *see* SIGNIFICANCE.

parametritis (pelvic cellulitis) *n.* inflammation of the loose connective tissue and smooth muscle around the uterus (the parametrium). The condition may be associated with *puerperal infection.

parametrium *n.* the layer of connective tissue surrounding the uterus.

paramnesia *n.* a distorted memory, such as *confabulation or *déjà vu.

paramyotonia congenita a rare disorder in which prolonged contraction of muscle fibres (*see* MYOTONIA) is precipitated by cold and exercise. It is due to a mutation in the sodium-channel gene.

paramyxovirus *n. see* MYXOVIRUS.

paranasal sinuses the air-filled spaces, lined with mucous membrane, within some of the bones of the skull. They open into the nasal cavity, via the meatuses, and are named according to the bone in which they are situated. They comprise the **frontal sinuses** and the **maxillary sinuses** (one pair of each), the **ethmoid sinuses** (consisting of many spaces inside the ethmoid bone), and the two **sphenoid sinuses**. See illustration.

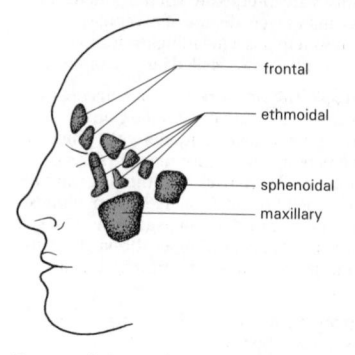

Paranasal sinuses (projected to the surface).

paraneoplastic syndrome signs or symptoms occurring in a patient with cancer that result from antibodies produced by the cancer and are not due directly to local effects of the cancer cells. Examples are *myasthenia gravis secondary to a tumour of the thymus, a cerebellar syndrome in patients with lung cancer (due to anti-*Purkinje cell antibody), and a peripheral neuropathy in patients with breast cancer. Removal of the cancer usually leads to resolution of the problem.

paranoia *n.* **1.** a mental illness or a symptom of a mental illness characterized by *delusions, sometimes organized into a system. *Antipsychotic medication is often beneficial. **2.** a state of mind in which the individual has a strong belief that he or she is persecuted by others and therefore displays behaviour marked by suspiciousness. Severe paranoia can lead to the diagnosis of *personality disorder.

paranoid *adj.* **1.** describing a mental state characterized by fixed and logically elaborated *delusions. There are many causes, including paranoid *schizophrenia, bipolar affective disorder, organic psychoses, *alcoholism, and severe emotional stress. **2.** describing a personality disorder distinguished by such traits as excessive sensitivity to rejection by others, suspiciousness, hostility, and self-importance.

paraparesis *n.* weakness of both legs, resulting from disease of the nervous system.

paraphasia *n.* a disorder of language in which unintended syllables, words, or phrases are interpolated in the patient's speech. A severe degree of paraphasia results in speech that is a meaningless jumble of words and sounds, called **jargon aphasia**.

paraphimosis *n.* retraction and constriction of the foreskin behind the glans penis. This occurs in some patients with *phimosis on erection of the penis: the tight foreskin cannot be drawn back over the glans and becomes painful and swollen. Manual replacement of the foreskin can usually be achieved under local or general anaesthesia, but *circumcision is required to prevent a recurrence.

paraphrenia *n.* a former name for *late-onset schizophrenia.

paraplegia *n.* *paralysis of both legs, usually due to disease or injury of the spinal cord. It is often accompanied by loss of sensation below the level of the injury and disturbed bladder function. —**paraplegic** *adj.*, *n.*

paraprotein *n.* an abnormal protein of the *immunoglobulin series. Paraproteins appear in malignant disease of the spleen, bone marrow, liver, etc. Examples of paraproteins are *myeloma globulins, *Bence-Jones protein, and *macroglobulin.

parapsoriasis *n.* an obsolete name for the earliest phase of *mycosis fungoides.

parapsychology *n.* the study of extrasensory perception, psychokinesis, and other mental abilities that appear to defy natural law.

Paraquat *n. Trademark.* the chemical compound dimethyl dipyridilium, widely used as a weed-killer. When swallowed it exerts its most serious effects upon the lungs, the tissues of which it destroys after a few days. Paraquat poisoning is almost invariably fatal.

parasite *n.* any living thing that lives in (*see* ENDOPARASITE) or on (*see* ECTOPARASITE)

another living organism (*see* HOST). The parasite, which may spend all or only part of its existence with the host, obtains food and/or shelter from the host and contributes nothing to its welfare. Some parasites cause irritation and interfere with bodily functions; others destroy host tissues and release toxins into the body, thus injuring health and causing disease. Human parasites include fungi, bacteria, viruses, protozoa, and worms. *See also* COMMENSAL, SYMBIOSIS. —**parasitic** *adj.*

parasiticide *n.* an agent that destroys parasites (excluding bacteria and fungi). *See also* ACARICIDE, ANTHELMINTIC, TRYPANOCIDE.

parasitology *n.* the study and science of parasites.

parasternal *adj.* situated close to the sternum. The **parasternal line** is an imaginary vertical line parallel to and midway between the lateral margin of the sternum and the vertical line through the nipple.

parasuicide *n. see* DELIBERATE SELF-HARM.

parasympathetic nervous system one of the two divisions of the *autonomic nervous system, having fibres that leave the central nervous system from the brain and the lower portion of the spinal cord and are distributed to blood vessels, glands, and the majority of internal organs. The system works in balance with the *sympathetic nervous system, the actions of which it frequently opposes.

parasympatholytic *adj.* opposing the effects of the *parasympathetic nervous system. *Antimuscarinic drugs have this effect by preventing acetylcholine from acting as a neurotransmitter.

parasympathomimetic *n.* a drug that has the effect of stimulating the *parasympathetic nervous system. The actions of parasympathomimetic drugs are **cholinergic** (resembling those of *acetylcholine) and include stimulation of skeletal muscle, *vasodilatation, depression of heart rate, increasing the tension of smooth muscle, increasing secretions (such as saliva), and constricting the pupil of the eye. They are used in the treatment of *myasthenia gravis (*see* ANTICHOLINESTERASE), glaucoma (*see* MIOTIC), and urinary retention (e.g. *distigmine).

paratenon *n.* the tissue of a tendon sheath that fills up spaces round the tendon.

parathion *n.* an organic phosphorus compound, used as a pesticide, that causes poisoning when inhaled, ingested, or absorbed through the skin. Like several other organic phosphorus compounds, it attacks the enzyme *cholinesterase and causes excessive stimulation of the parasympathetic nervous system. The symptoms are headache, sweating, salivation, lacrimation, vomiting, diarrhoea, and muscular spasms. Treatment is by administration of *atropine.

parathormone *n. see* PARATHYROID HORMONE.

parathyroidectomy *n.* surgical removal of the parathyroid glands, usually as part of the treatment of *hyperparathyroidism.

parathyroid glands two pairs of yellowish-brown *endocrine glands that are situated behind, or sometimes embedded within, the *thyroid gland. They are stimulated to produce *parathyroid hormone by a decrease in the amount of calcium in the blood.

parathyroid hormone (parathormone) a hormone, synthesized and released by the parathyroid glands, that controls the distribution of calcium and phosphate in the body. A high level of the hormone causes transfer of calcium from the bones to the blood; a deficiency lowers blood calcium levels, causing *tetany. This condition may be treated by injections of calcium gluconate. *Compare* CALCITONIN.

parathyroid hormone-related protein (PTH-RP) a protein that is secreted by certain malignant tumours and is the main cause of malignant *hypercalcaemia. PTH-RP, which has effects similar to *parathyroid hormone, stimulates generalized bone resorption and excessive calcium reabsorption in the kidney tubules. It is most commonly produced by lung tumours, squamous cell carcinomas of other organs, melanomas, and tumours of the breast, liver, pancreas, bladder, and prostate.

paratyphoid fever an infectious disease caused by the bacterium *Salmonella paratyphi A, B,* or *C.* Bacteria are spread in the faeces of patients or carriers, and outbreaks occur as a result of poor sanitation or unhygienic food-handling. After an incubation period of 1–10 days, symptoms, including diarrhoea, mild fever, and a pink rash on the chest, appear and last for about a week. Treatment with chloramphenicol is effective.

The *TAB vaccine provides temporary immunity against paratyphoid A and B.

pareidolia *n.* misperception of random stimuli as real things or people, as when faces are vividly seen in the flames of a fire.

parenchyma *n.* the functional part of an organ, as opposed to the supporting tissue (**stroma**).

parental order *see* SECTION 30 ORDER.

parental responsibility the legal status that, by virtue of the Children Act 1989, requires adults to act in the interests of a child's welfare. A birth mother will always have parental responsibility unless it is removed by an adoption order. Originally, parental responsibility was automatically shared only when the couple was married; in the case of unmarried couples, the male partner had to apply for a parental responsibility order. However, following a change in the law and since 1 December 2003, unmarried men who are named in the birth registration automatically acquire parental responsibility. In medical ethics, a person with parental responsibility can consent to, or refuse, treatment on behalf of a child who is too young to have capacity to make his or her own decisions about health care. However, the entitlement to act on behalf of a child is limited to the extent to which a person with parental responsibility is acting in the child's best interests. *See also* GILLICK COMPETENCE.

parenteral *adj.* administered by any way other than through the mouth: applied, for example, to the introduction of drugs or other agents into the body by injection.

paresis *n.* muscular weakness caused by disease of the nervous system. It implies a lesser degree of weakness than *paralysis, although the two words are often used interchangeably.

paries *n.* (*pl.* **parietes**) 1. the enveloping or surrounding part of an organ or other structure. 2. the wall of a cavity.

parietal *adj.* 1. of or relating to the inner walls of a body cavity, as opposed to the contents: applied particularly to the membranes lining a cavity (*see* PERITONEUM, PLEURA). 2. of or relating to the parietal bone.

parietal bone either of a pair of bones forming the top and sides of the cranium. *See* SKULL.

parietal cells *see* OXYNTIC CELLS.

parietal lobe one of the major divisions of each cerebral hemisphere (*see* CEREBRUM), lying behind the frontal lobe, above the temporal lobe, and in front of the occipital lobe. It is thus beneath the crown of the skull. It contains the *sensory cortex and *association areas.

parity *n.* a term used to indicate the number of pregnancies a woman has had that have each resulted in the birth of an infant capable of survival, as distinct from gravidity (*see* GRAVID). *See also* GRAND MULTIPARITY.

parkinsonism (akinetic rigid syndrome) *n.* a clinical picture characterized by tremor, rigidity, slowness of movement, and postural instability. The commonest symptom is tremor, which often affects one hand, spreading first to the leg on the same side and then to the other limbs. It is most pronounced in resting limbs, interfering with such actions as holding a cup. The patient has an expressionless face, an unmodulated voice, an increasing tendency to stoop, and a shuffling walk. Parkinsonism is a disease process affecting the basal ganglia of the brain and associated with a deficiency of the neurotransmitter *dopamine. Sometimes a distinction is made between **Parkinson's disease**, a degenerative disorder, and parkinsonism due to other causes. For example, it may be induced by the long-term use of *antipsychotic drugs and uncommonly it can be attributed to the late effects of *encephalitis or coal-gas poisoning, or to *Wilson's disease, or to multiple strokes (vascular parkinsonism). Other syndromes of which parkinsonism is a feature are *multiple system atrophy and *progressive supranuclear palsy. Relief of the symptoms may be obtained with *antimuscarinic drugs, dopamine-receptor agonists (*see* DOPAMINE), *levodopa, and subcutaneous *apomorphine injections and infusions. New surgical treatments include stereotactic *pallidotomy and pallidal stimulation. The latter procedure involves placing an electronic stimulator in the globus pallidus that can be controlled by an external switch or control panel. [J. Parkinson (1755–1824), British physician]

(⊕) **SEE WEB LINKS**

• Website of the Parkinson's Disease Society

paronychia (whitlow) *n.* an inflamed swelling of the *nail folds. **Acute paronychia** is usually caused by infection with *Staphylococcus aureus*. **Chronic paronychia** occurs mainly in those who habitually engage in wet work; it is associated with secondary infection with *Candida albicans*. It is vital to keep the hands dry in order to control chronic paronychia.

paroophoron *n.* the vestigial remains of part of the Wolffian duct (*see* MESONEPHROS) in the female, situated next to each ovary. It is associated with a similar structure, the **epoophoron**. Both are without known function.

parosmia *n.* any disorder of the sense of smell.

parotid gland one of a pair of *salivary glands situated in front of each ear. The openings of the parotid ducts (**Stensen's ducts**) are on the inner sides of the cheeks, opposite the second upper molar teeth.

parotitis *n.* inflammation of the parotid salivary glands. *See* MUMPS (INFECTIOUS PAROTITIS).

parous *adj.* having given birth to one or more children.

paroxetine *n.* an antidepressant drug that acts by prolonging the action of the neurotransmitter serotonin (5-hydroxytryptamine) in the brain (*see* SSRI). It is taken by mouth for the treatment of depression, obsessive–compulsive disorder, panic disorder, posttraumatic stress disorder, and some other anxiety disorders; side-effects may include nausea, indigestion, abdominal pain, diarrhoea, and rash. Trade name: **Seroxat**.

paroxysm *n.* **1.** a sudden violent attack, especially a spasm or convulsion. **2.** the abrupt worsening of symptoms or recurrence of disease. —**paroxysmal** *adj.*

paroxysmal nocturnal haemoglobinuria (PNH) a type of acquired haemolytic *anaemia that results from an abnormality of the red blood cell membrane. It is due to a defect in the formation of glycosylphosphatidylinositol (GPI), whose role is to anchor proteins to the lipid framework of the membrane. This leads to increased *complement-mediated destruction of red blood cells, which results in the release of haemoglobin in the circulation and then in the urine, giving the latter a reddish colour. Some patients may develop blood clots.

PARP inhibitor a drug that blocks the action of the PARP enzyme, which is required for *DNA repair in cancer cells with faulty *BRCA1* and *BRCA2* genes. Such drugs, including **olaparib**, are undergoing therapeutic trials for the treatment of cancer in patients with *BRCA1* or *BRCA2* mutations.

parrot disease *see* PSITTACOSIS.

pars *n.* a specific part of an organ or other structure, such as any of parts of the pituitary gland.

Part III accommodation residential accommodation provided by local authorities, under the terms of Part III of the National Assistance Act 1948, for adults who, because of age, disability, illness, or any other reason, are in need of care and support.

parthenogenesis *n.* reproduction in which an organism develops from an unfertilized ovum. It is common in plants and occurs in some lower animals (e.g. aphids).

partial volume artifact an apparent decrease in the visibility of a structure in a *cross-sectional imaging technique, such as CT or MRI, when either the thickness of the object is much less than that of the slice being used to make the image, or when the object is only partially within the slice. *See* ARTIFACT.

particularism *n.* a school of moral thought proposing that attention to the specifics and details of a situation is required to determine the preferred course of action. Such an approach is contrary to theories that depend on universal norms or principles, such as *Kantian ethics.

partogram *n.* a graphic record of the course of labour, designed to monitor its progress and enable early recognition of any problems. It includes information on the mother's blood pressure, heart rate, and temperature; length, frequency, and strength of contractions; and heart rate and amniotic fluid in the baby.

parturition *n.* childbirth. *See* LABOUR.

parvi- (parvo-) *combining form denoting* small size.

parvovirus *n.* any member of a genus of small DNA-containing viruses. **Human parvovirus B19** is the only member to cause disease in humans. It destroys red blood cells and is responsible for severe anaemia in patients with sickle-cell disease. Infection during pregnancy may adversely affect the fetus, resulting in *hydrops fetalis. The

virus is also the causative agent of the childhood infection *erythema infectiosum.

pascal *n.* the *SI unit of pressure, equal to 1 newton per square metre. Symbol: Pa.

Paschen bodies particles that occur in the cells of skin rashes in patients with *cowpox or *smallpox; they are thought to be the virus particles. [E. Paschen (1860–1936), German pathologist]

passive movement movement not brought about by a patient's own efforts. Passive movements are induced by manipulation of the joints by a physiotherapist. They are useful in maintaining function when a patient has nerve or muscle disorders that prevent voluntary movement.

passivity *n.* (in psychiatry) a *Schneiderian first-rank symptom in which a patient has the impression that his or her feelings or actions are those of another or others, usually an unknown outside power.

paste *n.* (in pharmacy) a medicinal preparation of a soft sticky consistency, which is applied externally.

Pasteurella a genus of small rodlike Gram-negative bacteria that are parasites of animals and humans. The species *P. multocida* usually infects animals but may be transmitted to humans through bites or scratches.

pasteurization *n.* the treatment of milk by heating it to 65°C for 30 minutes, or to 72°C for 15 minutes, followed by rapid cooling, to kill such bacteria as those of tuberculosis and typhoid.

pastille *n.* a medicinal preparation containing gelatine and glycerine, usually coated with sugar, that is dissolved in the mouth so that the medication is applied to the mouth or throat.

Patau syndrome a chromosome disorder in which there are three no. 13 chromosomes (instead of the usual two), causing abnormal brain development, severe mental retardation, and defects in the heart, kidney, and scalp. Affected individuals rarely survive. [K. Patau (20th century), US geneticist]

patch test a specialist test to discover which allergen is responsible for contact *dermatitis in a patient. Very low (validated) concentrations of potentially relevant allergens are applied under patches on the back.

These are removed after two days and the underlying skin is examined then, and again after a further two days. International criteria exist for interpreting results. A positive test will show an eczematous reaction, although differentiating allergic from irritant reactions is sometimes difficult. The commonest allergens are nickel (e.g. from costume jewellery), fragrances (from toiletries), and hair dye chemicals. Establishing the relevance of the reactions is critical.

patella *n.* the lens-shaped bone that forms the kneecap. It is situated in front of the knee in the tendon of the quadriceps muscle of the thigh. *See also* SESAMOID BONE.

patellar reflex (knee jerk) reflex contraction of the quadriceps (thigh) muscle so that the leg kicks, elicited in a patient sitting with one knee crossed over the other by sharply tapping the tendon of the muscle below the kneecap. The reflex is mediated through nerves emanating from the third and fourth lumbar spinal levels (*see* SPINAL NERVES). This is a test of the connection between the sensory nerves attached to stretch receptors in the muscle, the spinal cord, and the motor neurons running from the cord to the thigh muscle, all of which are involved in the reflex. The patellar reflex is reduced or absent when there is disease or damage of the spinal cord at or below the level of the reflex and exaggerated in disorders above the level of the reflex.

patent ductus arteriosus *see* DUCTUS ARTERIOSUS.

paternalism *n.* an attitude or policy that overrides a person's own wishes (*autonomy) in pursuit of his or her *best interests. Such an approach is contrary to the Kantian *imperative to treat people as ends in themselves and never as a means to an end. The question of when, if ever, a measure of paternalism may be justified remains one of the most contested in ethics. The philosopher John Stuart Mill argued that intervention was justified only when trying to prevent a person from causing harm to others, not to himself. In practice, however, we accept certain paternalistic constraints in our everyday lives in the interests of welfare, such as the legal requirement to wear seat belts when driving. In general, Western medical ethics takes the view that the autonomy of the individual is paramount and his or her wishes are sacrosanct. However, a form of paternalism may be justified when a person

lacks the capacity to make decisions for him- or herself, assuming there is no valid *advance statement, decision, or directive or a proxy with *lasting power of attorney to represent the patient's wishes. *See also* THERAPEUTIC PRIVILEGE. —**paternalistic** *adj.*

path- (patho-) *combining form denoting* disease. Example: **pathophobia** (morbid fear of).

pathogen *n.* a microorganism, such as a bacterium, that parasitizes an animal (or plant) or a human and produces a disease.

pathogenic *adj.* capable of causing disease. The term is applied to a parasitic microorganism (especially a bacterium) in relation to its host. —**pathogenicity** *n.*

pathognomonic *adj.* describing a symptom or sign that is characteristic of or unique to a particular disease. The presence of such a sign or symptom allows positive diagnosis of the disease.

pathological *adj.* relating to or arising from disease.

pathological fracture a fracture through diseased or abnormal bone, usually resulting from a force insufficient to fracture a normal bone. Tumour, infection, congenital bone defects, and osteoporosis are among the causes.

pathology *n.* the study of disease processes with the aim of understanding their nature and causes. This is achieved by observing samples of blood, urine, faeces, and diseased tissue obtained from the living patient or at autopsy, by the use of X-rays, and by many other techniques. (*See* BIOPSY.) **Clinical pathology** is the application of the knowledge gained to the treatment of patients. —**pathologist** *n.*

-pathy *combining form denoting* **1.** disease. Example: **nephropathy** (of the kidney). **2.** therapy. Example: **osteopathy** (by manipulation).

Patient Advice and Liaison Service (PALS) (in England) a confidential service provided by each NHS trust to support patients, their families, and carers by giving advice and information in response to questions and concerns about local NHS services. *See also* ADVOCACY.

patient and public involvement *see* LOCAL INVOLVEMENT NETWORKS.

547

pauciarthritis *n. see* ARTHRITIS.

pavementation (pavementing) *n.* the sticking of white blood cells to the linings of the finest blood vessels (capillaries) when inflammation occurs.

PBC *see* PRACTICE-BASED COMMISSIONING.

PCA3 a gene that is expressed (i.e. manifests its effects) to a significantly greater degree in cancerous prostate tissue than in benign prostate tissue. A test for *PCA3* can be performed on urine passed just after a digital rectal examination of the prostate; **uPM3** – the first such test to be developed – is a far more specific and sensitive indicator of the presence of prostate cancer than tests for *prostate specific antigen (PSA), increased amounts of which are produced in both malignant and nonmalignant prostate tissue.

PCI *see* PERCUTANEOUS CORONARY INTERVENTION.

PCNL *see* PERCUTANEOUS NEPHROLITHOTOMY.

PCO *see* POLYCYSTIC OVARY.

PCOS *see* POLYCYSTIC OVARY SYNDROME.

PCP *Pneumocystis jiroveci* (formerly *carinii*) pneumonia. Although the causative organism has been reclassified and renamed, the original abbreviation continues to be used for this type of pneumonia. *See* PNEUMOCYSTIS.

PCR *see* POLYMERASE CHAIN REACTION.

PCT *see* PRIMARY CARE TRUST.

PDGF platelet-derived growth factor (*see* GROWTH FACTOR).

peak expiratory flow rate (PEFR) the maximum rate at which a person can forcibly expel air from the lungs at any time, expressed usually in litres per minute (occasionally in litres per second). A low value can help diagnose asthma in the correct clinical context, and differences between the morning and evening values can also be a feature of poor control of asthma. There is a place for PEFR in the monitoring of acute exacerbations of chronic pulmonary obstructive disease (COPD) but not in the diagnosis of COPD.

peau d'orange a dimpled appearance of the skin over a breast tumour, resembling the surface of an orange. The skin is thick-

ened and the openings of hair follicles and sweat glands are enlarged.

PECT positron emission computed tomography (*see* POSITRON EMISSION TOMOGRAPHY).

pecten *n.* **1.** the middle section of the anal canal, below the anal valves (*see* ANUS). **2.** a sharp ridge on the upper branch of the pubis (part of the hip bone). —**pectineal** *adj.*

pectoral *adj.* relating to the chest.

pectoral girdle *see* SHOULDER GIRDLE.

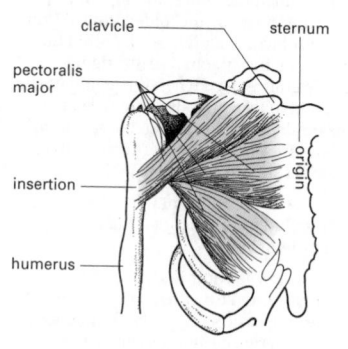

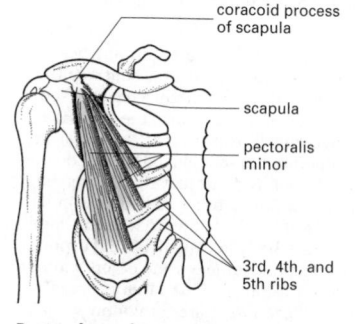

Pectoral muscles.

pectoral muscles the chest muscles (see illustration). The **pectoralis major** is a large fan-shaped muscle that works over the shoulder joint, drawing the arm forward across the chest and rotating it medially. Beneath it, the **pectoralis minor** depresses the shoulder and draws the scapula down towards the chest.

pectoriloquy *n.* abnormal transmission of

the patient's voice sounds through the chest wall so that they can be clearly heard through a stethoscope. Whispered sounds (**whispering pectoriloquy**) can be heard over the lung of a patient with pneumonia.

pectus *n.* the chest or breast.

pectus carinatum *see* PIGEON CHEST.

pectus excavatum *see* FUNNEL CHEST.

pedicle *n.* **1.** the narrow neck of tissue connecting some tumours to the normal tissue from which they have developed. **2.** (in plastic surgery) a narrow folded tube of skin by means of which a piece of skin used for grafting remains attached to its original site. A pedicle graft is used when the recipient site is unsuited to take an independent skin graft (for example, because of poor blood supply). *See also* FLAP, SKIN GRAFT. **3.** (in anatomy) any slender stemlike process.

pediculicide *n.* an agent that kills lice; examples include *dimeticone, *malathion, and *permethrin.

Pediculoides (Pyemotes) *n.* a genus of widely distributed tiny predaceous mites. *P. ventricosus* occasionally attacks humans and causes an allergic dermatitis called **grain itch**. This complaint most usually affects those people coming into contact with stored cereal products, such as hay and grain.

pediculosis *n.* an infestation with lice, which causes intense itching; continued scratching by the patient may result in secondary bacterial infection of the skin. **Head lice** (**pediculosis capitis**; *see* PEDICULUS) are quite common in schoolchildren and do not indicate poor hygiene; they may be treated with *malathion or other pediculicide lotions and/or by the use of a fine-toothed nit comb. By contrast, **body lice** (**pediculosis corporis**) often affect the homeless and others without access to washing facilities. **Pubic** (or **crab**) **lice** (*Phthirus pubis*) are commonly sexually transmitted and respond to the same treatment as head lice.

Pediculus *n.* a widely distributed genus of lice. There are two varieties of the species affecting humans: *P. humanus capitis*, the head louse; and *P. humanus corporis*, the body louse. The presence of these parasites can irritate the skin (*see* PEDICULOSIS), and in some parts of the world body lice are involved in transmitting *relapsing fever and *typhus.

pedometer *n.* a small portable device that records the number of paces walked, and thus the approximate distance covered. A pedometer is usually attached to the leg or hung at the belt.

peduncle *n.* a narrow process or stalklike structure, serving as a support or a connection. For example, the **middle cerebellar peduncle** connects the pons and cerebellum.

pedunculated *adj.* having a stalk or stemlike attachment to an epithelial surface. Pedunculated tumours are commonly, but not invariably, benign.

PEFR *see* PEAK EXPIRATORY FLOW RATE.

PEG percutaneous endoscopic *gastrostomy.

pegaptanib *n. see* RANIBIZUMAB.

peginterferon alfa *n. see* INTERFERON.

pegvisomant *n. see* GROWTH HORMONE.

pellagra *n.* a nutritional disease due to a deficiency of *nicotinic acid (a B vitamin). Pellagra results from the consumption of a diet that is poor in either nicotinic acid or the amino acid tryptophan, from which nicotinic acid can be synthesized in the body. It is common in maize-eating communities. The symptoms of pellagra are scaly dermatitis on exposed surfaces, diarrhoea, and depression.

pellicle *n.* a thin layer of skin, membrane, or any other substance.

pelvic-floor exercises *see* KEGEL EXERCISES.

pelvic girdle (hip girdle) the bony structure to which the bones of the lower limbs are attached. It consists of the right and left *hip bones.

pelvic inflammatory disease (PID) an acute or chronic condition in which the uterus, Fallopian tubes, and ovaries are infected. It is usually the result of infection ascending from the vagina; *Chlamydia trachomatis* and *Neisseria gonorrhoeae* have been identified as causative agents. PID may be associated with lower abdominal pain, irregular vaginal bleeding, and vaginal discharge. An acute infection may respond to treatment with antibiotics, but in the chronic state, when pelvic *adhesions have developed, surgical removal of the diseased tissue may be necessary. Blocking of the Fallopian tubes is a common result of pelvic inflammatory disease; this can lead to *ectopic pregnancy or infertility.

pelvimetry *n.* measurement of the four internal diameters of the pelvis (transverse, anteroposterior, left oblique, and right oblique) on an X-ray image or by means of CT or MR scanning. Pelvimetry may be used to determine if a vaginal delivery will be possible, but it is an unreliable predictor of obstetric outcome and its use is controversial.

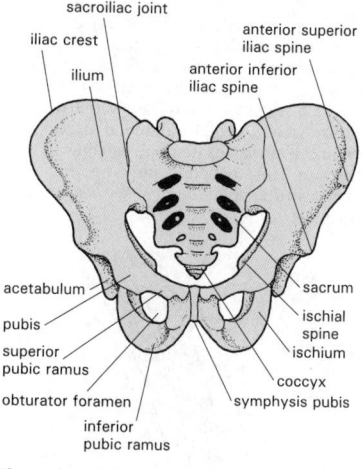

The male pelvis (ventral view).

Labels: sacroiliac joint; iliac crest; ilium; anterior superior iliac spine; anterior inferior iliac spine; acetabulum; pubis; superior pubic ramus; obturator foramen; inferior pubic ramus; sacrum; ischial spine; ischium; coccyx; symphysis pubis

pelvis *n.* (*pl.* **pelves**) **1.** the bony structure formed by the *hip bones, *sacrum, and *coccyx: the bony pelvis (see illustration). The hip bones are fused at the back to the sacrum to form a rigid structure that protects the organs of the lower abdomen and provides attachment for the bones and muscles of the lower limbs. The female pelvis may be one of four shapes (see illustration). In the **android** pelvis the cavity is funnel-shaped with a contracted outlet; the **anthropoid** pelvis is long, narrow, and oval. The classical shape, **gynaecoid**, has a transversely oval outlet and a roomy pelvic cavity; the **platypelloid** pelvis is wide and flattened at the brim, with the promontory of the sacrum pushed forward. **2.** the lower part of the abdomen. **3.** the cavity within the bony pelvis. **4.** any structure shaped like a basin, e.g. the expanded part of the ureter in the kidney (**renal pelvis**). —**pelvic** *adj.*

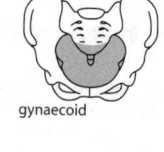
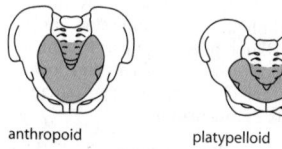

android   gynaecoid

anthropoid   platypelloid

The female pelvis.

pemetrexed *n.* an *antimetabolite used for treating pleural *mesothelioma and advanced *non-small-cell lung cancer. It is administered by intravenous infusion; side-effects include *myelosuppression, gastrointestinal symptoms, and skin disorders. Trade name: **Alimta**.

pemphigoid (bullous pemphigoid) *n.* a chronic itchy blistering disorder most common in the elderly. The blisters most commonly occur on the limbs and may persist for several days, unlike those of *pemphigus. Pemphigoid is an *autoimmune disease and responds to treatment with corticosteroids or immunosuppressant drugs. **Ocular pemphigoid** is a potentially blinding disease in which there is dryness, blistering, and scarring of the conjunctiva, leading to shortening of the *fornices due to adhesions (*symblepharon).

pemphigoid gestationalis (pemphigoid gestationis) a rare autoimmune condition (1 in 10,000–1 in 60,000 pregnancies) that usually starts in the second trimester with itching preceding a widespread *polymorphic eruption with vesicles and blisters. It is associated with *intrauterine growth restriction and preterm delivery.

pemphigus (pemphigus vulgaris) *n.* a rare but serious *autoimmune disease marked by successive outbreaks of blisters. The blisters are superficial and do not remain intact for long; the mouth and other mucous membranes, as well as the skin, are usually affected. A number of milder variants of the disease exist. Systemic immunosuppressant treatment is required.

Pena operation a recommended surgical

treatment of congenital anal maldevelopment.

Pendred's syndrome goitre associated with congenital deafness due to deficiency of *peroxidase, an enzyme that is essential for the utilization of iodine. [V. Pendred (1869–1946), British physician]

penetrance *n.* the frequency with which the characteristic controlled by a gene is seen in the individuals possessing it. Complete penetrance occurs when the characteristic is seen in all individuals known to possess the gene. If a percentage of individuals with the gene do not show its effects, penetrance is incomplete. In this way a characteristic in a family may appear to 'skip' a generation.

-penia *combining form denoting* lack or deficiency. Example: **neutropenia** (of neutrophils).

penicillamine *n.* a drug that binds metals and therefore aids their excretion (*see* CHELATING AGENT). It is used to treat *Wilson's disease, lead poisoning, and severe rheumatoid arthritis (*see* DISEASE-MODIFYING ANTIRHEUMATIC DRUG). It is administered by mouth and may cause blood disorders (blood counts should be carried out during treatment); other side-effects include nausea, loss of taste, and rashes. Trade name: **Distamine**.

penicillin *n.* an *antibiotic that was derived from the mould *Penicillium rubrum* and first became available for treating bacterial infections in 1941. Since then, a number of naturally occurring penicillins have been developed to treat a wide variety of infections, notably **benzylpenicillin** (**penicillin G**), administered by injection, and **phenoxymethylpenicillin** (**penicillin V**), which is administered orally. There are few serious side-effects, but some patients are allergic to penicillin and develop such reactions as skin rashes and potentially fatal *anaphylaxis. Many antibiotics are derived from the penicillins, including *amoxicillin, *ampicillin, and *ticarcillin; these are known as **semisynthetic penicillins**. All penicillins except *flucloxacillin are *beta-lactam antibiotics and are sensitive to penicillinase.

penicillinase *n.* an enzyme, produced by some bacteria, that is capable of antagonizing the antibacterial action of penicillin and other *beta-lactam antibiotics. Purified penicillinase may be used to treat reactions to penicillin. It is also used in diagnostic tests to isolate microorganisms from the blood of patients receiving penicillin.

Penicillium *n.* a genus of mouldlike fungi that commonly grow on decaying fruit, bread, or cheese. The species *P. rubrum* is the major natural source of the antibiotic *penicillin. Some species of *Penicillium* are pathogenic to humans, causing diseases of the skin and respiratory tract.

penile prosthesis *see* PROSTHESIS.

penis *n.* the male organ that carries the *urethra, through which urine and semen are discharged (see illustration). Most of the organ is composed of erectile tissue (*see* CORPUS CAVERNOSUM, CORPUS SPONGIOSUM), which becomes filled with blood under conditions of sexual excitement, causing an erection. The erect penis can enter the vagina and ejaculate semen. *See also* GLANS, PREPUCE.

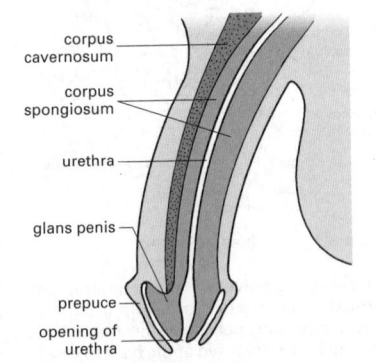

corpus cavernosum

corpus spongiosum

urethra

glans penis

prepuce

opening of urethra

The penis (median section).

pent- (penta-) *combining form denoting* five.

pentamidine *n.* a drug effective against protozoans and used in the treatment of *Pneumocystis pneumonia in AIDS patients and *leishmaniasis. It is administered by deep intramuscular injection, intravenous infusion, or inhalation. Possible side-effects include low blood pressure, heart irregularity, low blood sugar (hypoglycaemia), low white blood cell count, and kidney damage. Trade name: **Pentacarinat**.

pentose *n.* a simple sugar with five carbon atoms: for example, ribose and xylose.

pentostatin *n.* a *cytotoxic drug that is used in treating *hairy cell leukaemia; it works by interfering with the action of the enzyme adenosine deaminase. Pentostatin is administered by intravenous injection; side-effects, which may be severe, include *myelosuppression. Trade name: **Nipent**.

pentosuria *n.* an inborn defect of sugar metabolism causing abnormal excretion of pentose in the urine. There are no serious ill-effects.

pepsin *n.* an enzyme in the stomach that begins the digestion of proteins by splitting them into peptones (*see* PEPTIDASE). It is produced by the action of hydrochloric acid on **pepsinogen**, which is secreted by the gastric glands. Once made, pepsin itself can act on pepsinogen to produce more pepsin.

pepsinogen *n. see* PEPSIN.

peptic *adj.* **1.** relating to pepsin. **2.** relating to digestion.

peptic ulcer a breach in the protective lining (mucosa) of the digestive tract caused by digestion of the mucosa by pepsin and acid. This may occur when pepsin and acid are present in abnormally high concentrations or when some other mechanism reduces the normal protective mechanisms of the mucosa. These include *Helicobacter pylori* infection and the use of aspirin and other NSAIDs. A peptic ulcer may be found in the oesophagus (**oesophageal ulcer**, associated with reflux *oesophagitis); the stomach (*see* GASTRIC ULCER); duodenum (*see* DUODENAL ULCER); jejunum (**jejunal ulcer**, usually in the *Zollinger-Ellison syndrome); in a Meckel's *diverticulum; and close to a *gastroenterostomy (**stomal ulcer, anastomotic ulcer, marginal ulcer**).

peptidase *n.* one of a group of digestive enzymes that split proteins in the stomach and intestine into their constituent amino acids. The group is divided into the *endopeptidases and *exopeptidases.

peptide *n.* a molecule consisting of two or more *amino acids linked by bonds between the amino group (–NH) and the carboxyl group (–CO). This bond is known as a **peptide bond**. *See also* POLYPEPTIDE.

peptone *n.* a large protein fragment produced by the action of enzymes on proteins in the first stages of protein digestion.

peptonuria *n.* the presence in the urine of *peptones, intermediate compounds formed during the digestion of proteins.

perception *n.* (in psychology) the process by which information about the world, as received by the senses, is analysed and made meaningful. Abnormalities of perception include *hallucinations, *illusions, and *agnosia.

percussion *n.* the technique of examining part of the body by tapping it with the fingers or an instrument (**plessor**) and sensing the resultant vibrations. With experience it is possible to detect the presence of abnormal solidification or enlargement in different organs and the presence of fluid, for example in the lungs.

percutaneous *adj.* through the skin: often applied to the route of administration of drugs in ointments, etc., which are absorbed through the skin.

percutaneous coronary intervention (PCI) treatment of coronary artery disease delivered by cardiac *catheterization. This usually means *coronary angioplasty followed by insertion of a coronary *stent, but also includes more specialized procedures, such as rotational *atherectomy (rotablation). **Primary PCI** is the initial *reperfusion treatment: the use of coronary stents rather than *thrombolysis as the first-line treatment for myocardial infarction to relieve coronary obstruction caused by thrombosis. **Rescue PCI** is used in the event of unsuccessful thrombolysis.

percutaneous epididymal sperm aspiration *see* PESA.

percutaneous nephrolithotomy (PCNL) a technique of removing stones from the kidney via a *nephroscope passed into the kidney through a track from the skin surface previously established by the presence of a catheter.

percutaneous transhepatic cholangiopancreatography a method for outlining the bile ducts and pancreatic ducts with radiopaque dyes, which are introduced by a catheter inserted into the ducts from the surface of the skin (*see also* CHOLANGIOGRAPHY). The procedure is often performed prior to insertion of a biliary drain or stent when this is not possible via *ERCP in cases of obstructive *jaundice.

percutaneous transluminal coronary angioplasty (PTCA) dilatation of a nar-

p

rowed coronary artery using a balloon catheter advanced to the heart through a peripheral artery. It is now more commonly referred to as *percutaneous coronary intervention to take into account the fact that a coronary *stent is nearly always also deployed. *See* ANGIOPLASTY.

perforation *n.* the creation of a hole in an organ, tissue, or tube. This may occur in the course of a disease (e.g. a *duodenal ulcer, colonic *diverticulitis, or stomach cancer), allowing the contents of the intestine to enter the peritoneal cavity, which causes acute inflammation (*peritonitis) with sudden severe abdominal pain and shock. Treatment is usually by surgical repair of the perforation, but conservative treatment with antibiotics may result in spontaneous healing. Perforation may also be caused accidentally by instruments – for example a gastroscope may perforate the stomach, a curette may perforate the uterus – or by injury, for example to the eardrum.

perforin *n.* a protein produced by *cytotoxic T cells and *natural killer cells that are in contact with virus-infected target cells. It creates pores in the target-cell membrane, which facilitates the delivery of *granzymes to the cell to induce cell death (*apoptosis).

perfusion *n.* **1.** the passage of fluid through a tissue, especially the passage of blood through the lung tissue to pick up oxygen from the air in the alveoli, which is brought there by *ventilation, and release carbon dioxide. If ventilation is impaired deoxygenated venous blood is returned to the general circulation. If perfusion is impaired insufficient gas exchange takes place. **2.** the deliberate introduction of fluid into a tissue, usually by injection into the blood vessels supplying the tissue.

perfusion scan a technique for demonstrating an abnormal blood supply to an organ by injecting a radioactive *tracer or *contrast medium. One of the most common uses, often in conjunction with ventilation scanning (*see* VENTILATION-PERFUSION SCANNING), is to detect obstruction of pulmonary arteries due to embolism by thrombus (*see* PULMONARY EMBOLISM). Particles labelled with radioactive tracer are injected intravenously and become temporarily lodged in the capillaries in the lungs. Areas not being perfused show up as holes on the gamma-camera images. In *magnetic resonance imaging or *computerized tomography, con-

trast medium is injected and a series of images is obtained. The rate of change of enhancement is an index of the blood supply to the area of interest. This technique can be used to study blood supply to the brain, heart, or kidneys (in particular), to help diagnose arterial strictures or blockages, or tumours in which blood supply may be increased by abnormal vessels.

pergolide *n.* a drug that stimulates *dopamine receptors in the brain and is used in the treatment of Parkinson's disease. It is administered by mouth. Possible side-effects include confusion, hallucinations, sleepiness, heart irregularity, nausea, breathing difficulties, and double vision. Trade name: **Celance**.

peri- *prefix denoting* near, around, or enclosing. Examples: **perianal** (around the anus); **pericardial** (around the heart); **peritonsillar** (around a tonsil).

periadenitis *n.* inflammation of tissues surrounding a gland.

perianal haematoma (external haemorrhoid) a small painful swelling beside the anus, occurring after a bout of straining to pass faeces or coughing. Perianal haematomas are caused by the rupture of a small vein in the anus. They often heal spontaneously but occasionally rupture. Rarely this is followed by abscess formation. If severe pain continues, surgical removal can be undertaken. *See also* HAEMORRHOIDS.

periapical *adj.* around an apex, particularly the apex of a tooth. The term is applied to bone surrounding the apex and to X-ray views of this area.

peri-arrest period the recognized period, either just before or just after a full *cardiac arrest, when the patient's condition is very unstable and care must be taken to prevent progression or regression into a full cardiac arrest.

periarteritis nodosa *see* POLYARTERITIS NODOSA.

periarthritis *n.* inflammation of tissues around a joint capsule, including tendons and *bursae. **Chronic periarthritis**, which may be spontaneous or follow injury, is a common cause of pain and stiffness of the shoulder; it usually responds to local steroid injections or physiotherapy.

periarticular *adj.* around a joint, including the joint margins and surrounding area immediately adjacent to the joint capsule. The term is commonly used to specify fractures, tumours, and types of internal fixation devices. *See also* EXTRA-ARTICULAR, INTRA-ARTICULAR.

peribulbar *adj.* (in ophthalmology) denoting the area around the eyeball.

pericard- (pericardio-) *combining form* denoting the pericardium.

pericardiectomy (pericardectomy) *n.* surgical removal of the membranous sac surrounding the heart (pericardium). It is used in the treatment of chronic constrictive pericarditis and chronic pericardial effusion (*see* PERICARDITIS).

pericardiocentesis *n.* removal of excess fluid from within the sac (pericardium) surrounding the heart by means of needle *aspiration. *See* PERICARDITIS, HYDROPERICARDIUM.

pericardiolysis *n.* the surgical separation of *adhesions between the heart and surrounding structures within the ribcage (**adherent pericardium**). The operation has now fallen into disuse.

pericardiorrhaphy *n.* the repair of wounds in the membrane surrounding the heart (pericardium), such as those due to injury or surgery.

pericardiostomy *n.* an operation in which the membranous sac around the heart is opened and the fluid within drained via a tube. It is sometimes used in the treatment of septic pericarditis.

pericardiotomy (pericardotomy) *n.* surgical opening or puncture of the membranous sac (pericardium) around the heart. It is required to gain access to the heart in heart surgery and to remove excess fluid from within the pericardium.

pericarditis *n.* acute or chronic inflammation of the membranous sac (pericardium) surrounding the heart. Pericarditis may be seen alone or as part of pancarditis (*see* ENDOMYOCARDITIS). It has numerous causes, including virus infections, uraemia, and cancer. **Acute pericarditis** is characterized by fever, chest pain, and a pericardial friction rub. Fluid may accumulate within the pericardial sac (**pericardial effusion**). Rarely, chronic thickening of the pericardium (**chronic constrictive pericarditis**) develops.

This interferes with activity of the heart and has many features in common with *heart failure, including oedema, pleural effusions, ascites, and engorgement of the veins. Constrictive pericarditis most often results from tubercular infection.

The treatment of pericarditis is directed to the cause. Pericardial effusions may be aspirated by a needle inserted through the chest wall. Chronic constrictive pericarditis is treated by surgical removal of the pericardium (**pericardiectomy**).

pericardium *n.* the membrane surrounding the heart, consisting of two portions. The outer **fibrous pericardium** completely encloses the heart and is attached to the large blood vessels emerging from the heart. The internal **serous pericardium** is a closed sac of *serous membrane: the inner visceral portion (**epicardium**) is closely attached to the muscular heart wall and the outer parietal portion lines the fibrous pericardium. Within the sac is a very small amount of fluid, which prevents friction as the two surfaces slide over one another as the heart beats. —**pericardial** *adj.*

pericardotomy *n. see* PERICARDIOTOMY.

perichondritis *n.* inflammation of cartilage and surrounding soft tissues, usually due to chronic infection. A common site is the external ear.

perichondrium *n.* the dense layer of fibrous connective tissue that covers the surface of *cartilage.

pericoronitis *n.* inflammation around the crown of a tooth, particularly a partially erupted third molar.

pericranium *n.* the *periosteum of the skull.

pericystitis *n.* inflammation in the tissues around the bladder, causing pain in the pelvis, fever, and symptoms of *cystitis. It usually results from infection in the Fallopian tubes or uterus, but can occasionally arise from severe infection in a *diverticulum of the bladder itself. Treatment of pericystitis is directed to the underlying cause and usually involves antibiotic therapy. Pericystitis associated with a pelvic abscess clears when the abscess is surgically drained.

periderm *n. see* EPITRICHIUM.

perihepatitis *n.* inflammation of the membrane covering the liver (capsule). It is usually associated with abnormalities of the liver (including liver abscess, cirrhosis, tuberculosis) or chronic peritonitis.

perikaryon *n. see* CELL BODY.

perilymph *n.* the fluid between the bony and membranous *labyrinths of the ear.

perimenopause *n.* the period of time around the *menopause in which marked changes in the menstrual cycle occur, usually accompanied by hot flushes, and in which no 12 consecutive months of *amenorrhoea have yet occurred.

perimeter *n.* an instrument for mapping the extent of the *visual field. The patient fixes his or her gaze on a target in the centre of the inner surface of the hemisphere. Objects are presented on this surface and the patient says if they can be seen. The area of the visual field can be defined and any gaps in the field can be detected. There are several types of perimeter. In the **static perimeter** the movable object is replaced by a system of tiny lights that can be flashed briefly. A patient with a field defect will fail to see the lights that flash in the area of the defect. Modern visual field testing uses computer-assisted **automated perimeters** to map out and analyse visual fields and thus detect very subtle field defects (**computerized perimetry**). Automated perimeters are commonly used in the diagnosis and follow-up of glaucoma. —**perimetry** *n.*

perimetritis *n.* inflammation of the membrane on the outer surface of the uterus. The condition may be associated with *parametritis.

perimetrium *n.* the *peritoneum of the uterus.

perimysium *n.* the fibrous sheath that surrounds each bundle of *muscle fibres.

perinatal *adj.* relating to the period starting a few weeks before birth and including the birth and a few weeks after birth.

perinatal mortality rate (PNM) the total number of babies born dead after 24 weeks' gestation (*stillbirths) and of live-born babies that die in the first week of life, regardless of gestational age at birth (**early neonatal deaths**), per 1000 live births and stillbirths. *See* INFANT MORTALITY RATE. *See also* CONFIDENTIAL ENQUIRIES.

perindopril *n. see* ACE INHIBITOR.

perineal descent abnormal bulging down of the *perineum as a result of weakness of the pelvic floor muscles. It often accompanies problems with defecation and micturition.

perineal repair *see* COLPORRHAPHY.

perineal tear (perineal trauma) an injury to the perineum, which may be sustained during childbirth. Perineal tears can be classified by degree. Second-degree tears involve the perineal muscles but not the anal sphincter. Third-degree tears involve the anal sphincter complex: the external anal sphincter (EAS) and internal anal sphincter (IAS). These are subclassified as 3a (less than 50% of EAS thickness torn), 3b (more than 50% of EAS thickness torn), and 3c (IAS torn). Fourth-degree tears involve the anal sphincter complex (EAS and IAS) and the rectal mucosa. It is vitally important that these injuries are recognized and repaired by competent personnel. *See also* OBSTETRIC ANAL SPHINCTER INJURY.

perineoplasty *n.* an operation designed to enlarge the vaginal opening by incising the hymen and part of the perineum (**Fenton's operation**).

perineorrhaphy *n.* the surgical repair of a damaged perineum. The damage is usually the result of a tear in the perineum sustained during childbirth.

perinephric abscess a collection of pus around the kidney, usually secondary to *pyonephrosis.

perinephritis *n.* inflammation of the tissues around the kidney. This is usually due to spread of infection from the kidney itself (*see* PYELONEPHRITIS, PYONEPHROSIS). The patient has pain in the loins, fever, and fits of shivering. Prompt treatment of the underlying renal infection is required to prevent progression to an abscess.

perineum *n.* the region of the body between the anus and the urethral opening, including both skin and underlying muscle. In females it is perforated by the vaginal opening. —**perineal** *adj.*

perineurium *n.* the sheath of connective tissue that surrounds individual bundles (fascicles) of nerve fibres within a large *nerve.

periocular *adj.* adjacent to the eyeball.

periodic acid–Schiff reaction (PAS reac-

tion) a test for the presence of glycoproteins, polysaccharides, certain mucopolysaccharides, glycolipids, and certain fatty acids in tissue sections. The tissue is treated with periodic acid, followed by *Schiff's reagent. A positive reaction is the development of a red or magenta coloration.

periodic fever *see* MALARIA.

periodontal *adj.* denoting or relating to the tissues surrounding the teeth.

periodontal abscess an abscess that arises in the periodontal tissues and is usually an acute manifestation of periodontal disease.

periodontal disease disease of the tissues that support and attach the teeth – the gums, periodontal membrane, and alveolar bone. It is caused by the metabolism of bacterial *plaque on the surfaces of the teeth adjacent to these tissues. Periodontal disease includes *gingivitis and the more advanced stage of **periodontitis**, which results in the formation of spaces between the gums and the teeth (**periodontal pockets**), the loss of some fibres that attach the tooth to the jaw, and the loss of bone. The disease is widespread and is the most common cause of tooth loss in older people. Poor oral hygiene is a major contributory factor, but the resistance of the patient also has some influence; for example, the reduced resistance of patients with AIDS may predispose to periodontal disease.

periodontal membrane (periodontal ligament) the ligament around a *tooth, by which it is attached to the bone.

periodontal pocket a space between the gingival tissues and tooth occurring in periodontitis. *See* PERIODONTAL DISEASE.

periodontium *n.* the tissues that support and attach the teeth to the jaw: the gums (*see* GINGIVA), *periodontal membrane, alveolar bone, and *cementum.

periodontology *n.* the branch of dentistry concerned with the tissues that support and attach the teeth and the prevention and treatment of *periodontal disease.

perioperative *adj.* denoting the period that extends from the day before to the first few days after surgery, during which drugs (e.g. analgesics, antibiotics, anticoagulants) may need to be administered and *vital signs are monitored.

periorbital *adj.* **1.** around the eye socket (*orbit). **2.** relating to the periosteum within the orbit.

periosteum *n.* a layer of dense connective tissue that covers the surface of a bone except at the articular surfaces. The outer layer of the periosteum is extremely dense and contains a large number of blood vessels. The inner layer is more cellular in appearance and contains osteoblasts and fewer blood vessels. The periosteum provides attachment for muscles, tendons, and ligaments.

periostitis *n.* inflammation of the membrane surrounding a bone (*see* PERIOSTEUM). **Acute periostitis** results from direct injury to the bone and is associated with a *haematoma, which may later become infected. The uncomplicated condition subsides quickly with rest and anti-inflammatory analgesics. **Chronic periostitis** sometimes follows but is more often due to an inflammatory disease, such as tuberculosis or syphilis, or to a chronic ulcer overlying the bone involved. Chronic periostitis causes thickening of the underlying bone, which is evident on X-ray.

peripheral nervous system all parts of the nervous system lying outside the central nervous system (brain and spinal cord). It includes the *cranial nerves and *spinal nerves and their branches, which link the receptors and effector organs with the brain and spinal cord. *See also* AUTONOMIC NERVOUS SYSTEM.

peripheral neuropathy (polyneuropathy, peripheral neuritis) any of a group of disorders affecting the sensory and/or motor nerves in the peripheral nervous system. They tend to start distally, in the fingers and toes, and progress proximally. Symptoms include pins and needles, stabbing pains and a numbness on the sensory side, and weakness of the muscles. The most common causes of peripheral neuropathy are diabetes, alcohol, certain drugs, and such infections as HIV; genetic causes of peripheral neuropathy include amyloidosis and *Charcot-Marie-Tooth disease. The diagnosis may be established by neurophysiological tests, blood tests, and occasionally a nerve biopsy.

periphlebitis *n.* inflammation of the tissues around a vein: seen as an extension of *phlebitis.

perisalpingitis *n.* inflammation of the peritoneal membrane on the outer surface of a Fallopian tube.

perisplenitis *n.* inflammation of the external coverings of the spleen.

peristalsis *n.* a wavelike movement that progresses along some of the hollow tubes of the body. It occurs involuntarily and is characteristic of tubes that possess circular and longitudinal muscles, such as the *intestines. It is induced by distension of the walls of the tube. Immediately behind the distension the circular muscle contracts. In front of the distension the circular muscle relaxes and the longitudinal muscle contracts, which pushes the contents of the tube forward. —**peristaltic** *adj.*

peritendineum *n.* the fibrous covering of a tendon.

peritendinitis *n. see* TENOSYNOVITIS.

peritomy *n.* an eye operation in which an incision of the conjunctiva is made in a complete circle around the cornea.

peritoneal dialysis (PD) a form of renal replacement therapy (*see* DIALYSIS) that utilizes the peritoneum as the semipermeable membrane separating blood and *dialysate. Peritoneal dialysis can be given as a temporary and emergency treatment using a rigid percutaneous cannula to deliver fluid into the peritoneal cavity; this cannula usually needs removal and/or replacement within a few days. Alternatively, PD can be used as a chronic treatment, either in the form of chronic ambulatory peritoneal dialysis (*see* CAPD) or **automated peritoneal dialysis (APD)**, in which case fluid delivery is through a soft silastic catheter that is tunnelled subcutaneously out of the peritoneal cavity and is designed to stay in place for years. In all cases, the dialysis fluid is left within the peritoneal cavity for a period of time during which substances in the bloodstream diffuse into the fluid according to their concentration gradient and the permeability of the peritoneal membrane.

peritoneoscope *n. see* LAPAROSCOPE.

peritoneum *n.* the *serous membrane of the abdominal cavity (see illustration). The **parietal peritoneum** lines the walls of the abdomen, and the **visceral peritoneum** covers the abdominal organs. *See also* MESENTERY, OMENTUM. —**peritoneal** *adj.*

peritonitis *n.* inflammation of the *peritoneum. **Primary peritonitis** is caused by bacteria spread via the bloodstream: examples are **pneumococcal peritonitis** and

tuberculous peritonitis. Symptoms are diffuse abdominal pain and swelling, with fever and weight loss. Fluid may accumulate in the peritoneal cavity (*see* ASCITES) or the infection may complicate existing ascites (**spontaneous bacterial peritonitis**). **Secondary peritonitis** is due to perforation or rupture of an abdominal organ (for example, a duodenal ulcer or the vermiform appendix), allowing access of bacteria and irritant digestive juices to the peritoneum. This produces sudden severe abdominal pain, first at the site of rupture but becoming generalized. Shock develops, and the abdominal wall becomes rigid; X-ray examination may reveal gas within the peritoneal cavity. Treatment is usually by surgical repair of the perforation, but in some cases conservative treatment using antibiotics and intravenous fluid may be used. *Subphrenic abscess is a possible complication. **Meconium peritonitis** occurs in newborn infants as a result of a perforated intestine; it is initially a sterile contamination of the peritoneum.

peritonsillar abscess *see* QUINSY.

peritrichous *adj.* describing bacteria in which the flagella cover the entire cell surface.

perityphlitis *n. Archaic.* inflammation of the tissues around the caecum.

periureteritis *n.* inflammation of the tissues around a ureter. This is usually associated with inflammation of the ureter itself (*ureteritis) often behind an obstruction caused by a stone or stricture. Treatment is directed to relieving any obstruction of the

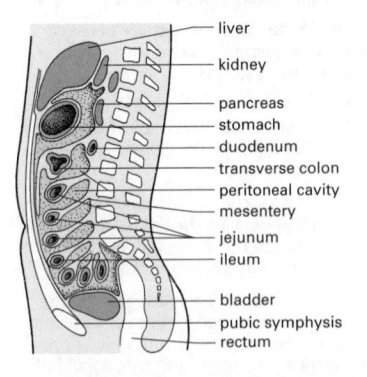

— liver
— kidney
— pancreas
— stomach
— duodenum
— transverse colon
— peritoneal cavity
— mesentery
— jejunum
— ileum
— bladder
— pubic symphysis
— rectum

Peritoneum. Sagittal section of the abdomen to show arrangement of the peritoneum.

ureter and controlling the infection with antibiotics.

periurethral injection   the injection of a bulking agent (e.g. collagen) into the tissues around the urethra, used for the treatment of urodynamic stress *incontinence. Such injections have a low morbidity and are easy to administer, and results are better in women with good bladder-neck support but poor urethral function. The short-term success rates of these procedures are reasonable, but long-term success rates are poor.

periventricular haemorrhage (PVH) a significant cause of morbidity and mortality in infants who are born prematurely in which bleeding occurs from fragile blood vessels around the *ventricles in the brain. Bleeding extending into the lateral ventricles is termed **intraventricular haemorrhage** (IVH) and in severe cases can extend into the brain tissue (cerebral parenchyma). Surviving infants may have long-term neurological deficits, such as cerebral palsy, developmental delay, or seizures.

periventricular leucomalacia (PVL) softening of white matter around the ventricles of the brain in preterm infants due to a decreased blood supply to the brain, usually associated with *hypoxic-ischaemic encephalopathy. Diagnosis is by ultrasound, which shows increased density and, later, cysts in the periventricular area. The brain damage can cause visual impairment and cerebral palsy.

PERLA pupils equal, react to light and accommodation: used in hospital notes.

perle   *n.* a soft capsule containing medicine.

perleche   *n.* dryness and cracking of the corners of the mouth, sometimes with infection. Perleche may be caused by persistent lip licking or by a vitamin-deficient diet.

permethrin   *n.* a synthetic derivative of the naturally occurring insecticide pyrethrin that is applied externally as a cream to treat pubic lice and scabies. Trade name: **Lyclear**.

pernicious   *adj.* describing diseases that are highly dangerous or likely to result in death if untreated. *See also* PERNICIOUS ANAEMIA.

pernicious anaemia a form of *anaemia

resulting from deficiency of *vitamin B$_{12}$. This in turn results either from failure to produce the substance (*intrinsic factor) that facilitates absorption of B$_{12}$ from the bowel or from dietary deficiency of the vitamin. Pernicious anaemia is characterized by defective production of red blood cells and the presence of *megaloblasts in the bone marrow. In severe forms the nervous system is affected (*see* SUBACUTE COMBINED DEGENERATION OF THE CORD). The condition is treated by injections of vitamin B$_{12}$.

pernio   *n.* the medical name for a chilblain (*see* CHILBLAINS).

perniosis   *n. see* CHILBLAINS.

pero-   *combining form denoting* deformity; defect. Example: **peromelia** (of the limbs).

peroneal   *adj.* relating to or supplying the outer (fibular) side of the leg.

peroneus   *n.* one of the muscles of the leg that arises from the fibula. The **peroneus longus** and **peroneus brevis** are situated at the side of the leg and inserted into the metatarsal bones of the foot. They help to turn the foot outwards.

peroxidase   *n.* an enzyme, found mainly in plants but also present in leucocytes and milk, that catalyses the dehydrogenation (oxidation) of various substances in the presence of hydrogen peroxide (which acts as a hydrogen acceptor, being converted to water in the process).

peroxisome   *n.* a small structure within a cell that is similar to a *lysosome but contains different enzymes, some of which may take part in reactions involving hydrogen peroxide.

perphenazine   *n.* a phenothiazine *antipsychotic drug used to treat schizophrenia, mania, anxiety, and severe agitation and to prevent and treat severe nausea and vomiting. It is administered by mouth; side-effects are similar to those of *fluphenazine. Trade name: **Fentazin**.

perseveration   *n.* **1.** excessive persistence at a task that prevents the individual from turning his or her attention to new situations. It is a symptom of organic disease of the brain and sometimes of obsessional neurosis. **2.** the phenomenon in which an image continues to be perceived briefly in the absence of the object. This is a potentially serious neurological disorder.

persistent idiopathic facial pain (atypical facial pain, chronic idiopathic facial pain) a neuralgia that has no known cause and is typified by pain in the face that does not fit the distribution of nerves. It may be stress-related, and in some cases appears to be associated with defective metabolism of *tyramine. Treatment may involve the use of antidepressants.

persistent vegetative state (PVS) the condition that is diagnosed after a patient has been in the *vegetative state for more than 12 months after a head injury or more than 6 months after other causes of brain damage. Following the high-profile case of Tony Bland, who was in PVS following injuries sustained in the Hillsborough Football Stadium disaster, the law currently allows medical treatment, such as *artificial nutrition and hydration, to be withdrawn from patients in PVS but permission must first be granted by the courts.

personality *n.* (in psychology) an enduring disposition to act and feel in particular ways that differentiate one individual from another. These patterns of behaviour are sometimes conceptualized as different categories (*see* PERSONALITY DISORDER) and sometimes as different dimensions (*see* EXTROVERSION, NEUROTICISM).

personality disorder a deeply ingrained and maladaptive pattern of behaviour, persisting over many years. It is usually manifest by the time the individual is adolescent. The abnormality of behaviour must be sufficiently severe that it causes suffering, either to the patient or to other people (or to both). Some individuals with such personalities mature into people who are less debilitated by their personality development. Certain types of psychotherapy are of some therapeutic value, but treatment is mostly aimed at mitigating the worst consequences of the personality disorder rather than cure. *See* ANANKASTIC, ANTISOCIAL PERSONALITY DISORDER, AVOIDANT, EMOTIONALLY UNSTABLE PERSONALITY DISORDER, HYSTERICAL, PARANOID, SCHIZOID PERSONALITY, SCHIZOTYPAL PERSONALITY DISORDER.

personhood *n.* in ethics, a concept that is often debated as part of efforts to establish the unique moral status of human beings (*see* HUMANITY) and to consider specific moral problems (e.g. the status of the embryo in assisted reproduction, abortion, and euthanasia). The distinguishing or defining characteristics of being a person have been said to include consciousness and the ability to reason, to reflect on oneself and one's actions, to form relationships, to inspire love and protection, to have an interest in one's future, and to have the potential to become human. The Australian philosopher Peter Singer has famously argued that the approach of most ethicists to moral status is 'speciesist' in that it discriminates against nonhuman animals, which may have more cognitive ability than some humans (e.g. comparing a high-functioning sheep dog or ape with newborn babies or patients in a persistent vegetative state).

perspiration *n.* *sweat or the process of sweating. **Insensible perspiration** is sweat that evaporates immediately from the skin and is therefore not visible; **sensible perspiration** is visible on the skin in the form of drops.

Perthes' disease *see* LEGG-CALVÉ-PERTHES DISEASE.

pertussis *n. see* WHOOPING COUGH.

pes *n.* (in anatomy) the foot or a part resembling a foot.

PESA (percutaneous epididymal sperm aspiration) a method of assisted conception in which spermatozoa are removed directly from the *epididymis under local anaesthetic. The sperm are then used to fertilize egg cells in vitro (*see* ICSI).

pes cavus *see* CLAW-FOOT.

pes planus *see* FLAT-FOOT.

pessary *n.* **1.** a plastic device, often ring-shaped, that fits into the vagina and keeps the uterus in position: used to treat *prolapse. The usual type is a **ring pessary** but occasionally a **Hodge pessary** is used. **2. (vaginal suppository)** a plug or cylinder of cocoa butter or some other soft material containing a drug that is fitted into the vagina for the treatment of gynaecological disorders (e.g. vaginitis) or for the induction of labour (a Prostin pessary containing prostaglandin).

pesticide *n.* a chemical agent used to kill insects or other organisms harmful to crops and other cultivated plants. Some pesticides, such as *parathion and *dieldrin, have caused poisoning in human beings and livestock after accidental exposure.

PET *see* POSITRON EMISSION TOMOGRAPHY.

PET/CT scanning an imaging system that allows a PET scan (*see* POSITRON EMISSION TOMOGRAPHY) and a CT scan (*see* COMPUTERIZED TOMOGRAPHY) to be performed very close together, with minimal movement of the patient between scans. This means that the images produced can be co-registered (*see* CO-REGISTRATION), giving very accurate anatomical localization (from the CT scan) of areas of increased activity (identified on the PET scan). This is very important for determining the site of disease in order to plan treatment.

petechiae *pl. n.* small round flat dark-red spots caused by bleeding into the skin or beneath the mucous membrane. Petechiae occur, for example, in the *purpuras.

pethidine *n.* a potent opioid analgesic (*see* OPIATE) with mild sedative action, used to relieve moderate or severe pain of short duration (including that associated with childbirth). It is administered by mouth or injection; side-effects may include nausea, dizziness, and dry mouth. Trade name: **Pamergan P100**.

petit mal *see* EPILEPSY.

Petri dish a flat shallow circular glass or plastic dish with a pillbox-like lid, used to hold solid agar or gelatin media for culturing bacteria. [J. R. Petri (1852–1921), German bacteriologist]

petrissage *n.* kneading: a form of *massage in which the skin is lifted up, pressed down and squeezed, and pinched and rolled. Alternate squeezing and relaxation of the tissues stimulates the local circulation and may have a pain-relieving effect in muscular disorders.

petrositis *n.* inflammation of the petrous part of the *temporal bone (which encloses the inner ear), usually due to an extension of *mastoiditis.

petrous bone *see* TEMPORAL BONE.

Peutz-Jeghers syndrome a hereditary disorder in which the presence of multiple *polyps in the lining of the small intestine (intestinal *polyposis) is associated with pigmented areas (similar to freckles) around the lips, on the inside of the mouth, and on the palms and soles. The polyps can also occur in the colon and stomach. They may bleed, resulting in anaemia, or may cause obstruction of the bowel. Half of the patients develop malignant tumours (not necessarily of

the bowel). [J. L. A. Peutz (1886–1957), Dutch physician; H. J. Jeghers (1904–90), US physician]

-pexy *combining form denoting* surgical fixation. Example: **omentopexy** (of the omentum).

Peyer's patches oval masses of *lymphoid tissue on the mucous membrane lining the small intestine. [J. C. Peyer (1653–1712), Swiss anatomist]

Peyronie's disease a dense fibrous plaque in the penis, which can be felt in the erectile tissue as an irregular hard lump. The penis curves or angulates at this point on erection and pain often results. The cause is unknown. The penis can be straightened surgically by means of *Nesbit's operation. [F. de la Peyronie (1678–1747), French surgeon]

PGD *see* PREIMPLANTATION GENETIC DIAGNOSIS.

pH a measure of the concentration of hydrogen ions in a solution, and therefore of its acidity or alkalinity. A pH of 7 indicates a neutral solution, a pH below 7 indicates acidity, and a pH in excess of 7 indicates alkalinity.

PHA *n. see* PHYTOHAEMAGGLUTININ.

phaco- (phako-) *combining form denoting* the lens of the eye.

phacoemulsification (phakoemulsification) *n.* the use of a high-frequency *ultrasound probe to break up a cataract so that it can be removed through a very small incision. This is now the most popular method of performing cataract surgery in the developed world.

phaeochromocytoma *n.* a small vascular tumour of the inner region (medulla) of the adrenal gland. Many tumours function by their uncontrolled and irregular secretion of the hormones *adrenaline and *noradrenaline. They cause attacks of raised blood pressure, increased heart rate, palpitations, and headache.

phag- (phago-) *combining form denoting* **1.** eating. **2.** phagocytes.

phage *n. see* BACTERIOPHAGE.

-phagia *combining form denoting* a condition involving eating.

phagocyte *n.* a cell that is able to engulf

and digest bacteria, protozoa, cells and cell debris, and other small particles. Phagocytes include many white blood cells (*see* LEUCO-CYTE) and *macrophages, which play a major role in the body's defence mechanism. —**phagocytic** *adj.*

phagocytosis *n.* the engulfment and digestion of bacteria and other foreign particles by a cell (*see* PHAGOCYTE). *Compare* PINOCYTOSIS.

phakic *adj.* denoting an eye with the natural crystalline lens still in place, as contrasted with aphakic (*see* APHAKIA) or pseudophakic (*see* PSEUDOPHAKIA).

phako- *combining form. see* PHACO-.

phalangeal cells rows of supporting cells between the sensory hair cells of the organ of Corti (*see* COCHLEA).

phalangectomy *n.* surgical removal of one or more of the small bones (phalanges) in the fingers or toes.

phalanges *n.* (*sing.* **phalanx**) the bones of the fingers and toes (digits). The first digit (thumb/big toe) has two phalanges. Each of the remaining digits has three phalanges. —**phalangeal** *adj.*

phalangitis *n.* inflammation of a finger or toe, causing swelling and pain. The condition may be caused by infection of the soft tissues, tendon sheaths, bone, or joints or by some rheumatic diseases, such as *psoriatic arthritis. *See also* DACTYLITIS.

phalanx *n. see* PHALANGES.

Phalen's sign a diagnostic sign for *carpal tunnel syndrome. The patient is asked to hold his or her wrists in full flexion with the dorsal surfaces of both hands pushing against each other with fingers pointing downwards for 30–60 seconds. This manoeuvre increases pressure on the median nerve: tingling and numbness or pain in the thumb, index, middle, and ring fingers suggests carpal tunnel syndrome. *See also* TINEL'S SIGN. [G. S. Phalen (1911–98), US orthopaedist]

phalloplasty *n.* surgical reconstruction or repair of the penis. It is required for congenital deformity of the penis, as in *hypospadias or *epispadias, and sometimes also following injury to the penis with loss of skin.

phallus *n.* the embryonic penis, before the urethral duct has reached its final state of development.

phanero- *combining form denoting* visible; apparent.

phantom limb the sensation that an arm or leg, or part of an arm or leg, is still attached to the body after it has been amputated. Pain may seem to come from the amputated part. This may arise because of stimulation of the amputation stump, which contains severed nerves that formerly carried messages from the removed portion, but more usually occurs because the neural representation of the limb is still present in the brain and may become activated.

phantom pregnancy *see* PSEUDOCYESIS.

phantom tumour 1. an accumulation of fluid (pleural effusion) in the lung in patients with heart failure, which resembles a lung tumour on radiological examination. 2. a swelling in the abdomen or elsewhere, caused by local muscular contraction or the accumulation of gases, that mimics a swelling caused by a tumour.

pharmaceutical *adj.* relating to pharmacy.

pharmacist *n.* a person who is qualified by examination and registered and authorized to dispense medicines or to keep open a shop for the sale and dispensing of medicines.

pharmaco- *combining form denoting* drugs. Example: **pharmacophobia** (morbid fear of).

pharmacodynamics *n.* the interaction of drugs with cells. It includes such factors as the binding of drugs to cells, their uptake, and intracellular metabolism.

pharmacogenomics *n.* the study of how genes affect the actions of drugs. The enormous growth of knowledge about the human genome, arising from the *Human Genome Project, has revolutionized drug treatment, enabling the precise targeting of drugs against the products of specific mutations causing disease (*see* TARGETED AGENT). In addition, it will be possible to identify those genetic variations that affect how drugs are metabolized in the body and their potential for causing adverse effects. Thus analysis of genetic data from individuals will enable safer and more effective treatment.

pharmacognosy n. the knowledge or study of pharmacologically active principles derived from plants.

pharmacokinetics n. the study of how drugs are handled within the body, including their absorption, distribution, metabolism, and excretion. It is concerned with such matters as how drug concentration in the body changes with time, how drugs pass across cell membranes, how often they should be given, what the effect of long-term administration may be, how drugs interact with each other, and how individual variations affect all these things.

pharmacology n. the science of the properties of drugs and their effects on the body. —**pharmacological** adj.

pharmacopoeia n. a book containing a list of the drugs used in medicine, with details of their formulae, methods of preparation, dosages, standards of purity, etc.

pharmacy n. 1. the preparation and dispensing of drugs. 2. premises registered to dispense medicines and sell poisons.

pharyng- (pharyngo-) combining form denoting the pharynx. Example: **pharyngopathy** (disease of).

pharyngeal arch (branchial arch, visceral arch) any of the paired segmented ridges of tissue in each side of the throat of the early embryo that correspond to the gill arches of fish. Each arch contains a cartilage, a cranial nerve, and a blood vessel. Between each arch there is a *pharyngeal pouch.

pharyngeal cleft (branchial cleft, visceral cleft) any of the paired segmented clefts in each side of the throat of the early embryo that correspond to the gills of fish. Soon after they have formed they close to form the *pharyngeal pouches, except for the first cleft, which persists as the external auditory meatus.

pharyngeal pouch (branchial pouch, visceral pouch) any of the paired segmented pouches in the side of the throat of the early embryo. They give rise to the tympanic cavity, the parathyroid glands, the thymus, and probably the thyroid gland.

pharyngeal reflex see GAG REFLEX.

pharyngectomy n. surgical removal of part of the pharynx.

pharyngitis n. inflammation of the part of the throat behind the soft palate (pharynx). It produces *sore throat and may be associated with *tonsillitis.

pharyngocele n. a pouch or cyst opening off the pharynx (see BRANCHIAL CYST).

pharyngoscope n. an *endoscope for the examination of the pharynx.

pharynx n. a muscular tube, lined with mucous membrane, that extends from the beginning of the oesophagus (gullet) up to the base of the skull. It is divided into the *nasopharynx, *oropharynx, and *hypopharynx (see illustration) and it communicates with the posterior *nares, *Eustachian tube, the mouth, larynx, and oesophagus. The pharynx acts as a passageway for food from the mouth to the oesophagus, and as an air passage from the nasal cavity and mouth to the larynx. It also acts as a resonating chamber for the sounds produced in the larynx. —**pharyngeal** adj.

The pharynx (longitudinal section).

phenelzine n. a drug used to relieve depression (see MAO INHIBITOR). It is administered by mouth; side-effects include dizziness and a fall in blood pressure on standing up. Trade name: **Nardil**.

phenindione n. an *anticoagulant drug administered by mouth to prevent or treat thrombosis in the blood vessels of the heart and limbs. The main adverse effect is bleeding (*see* WARFARIN); other side-effects may include rashes and other allergic reactions.

phenobarbital (phenobarbitone) *n.* a *barbiturate drug that has been used as an anticonvulsant in the treatment of epilepsy, but is no longer commonly prescribed. It is administered by mouth or injection; side-effects may include drowsiness and skin sensitivity reactions, and dependence may result from continued use.

phenol (carbolic acid) *n.* a strong *disinfectant. Derivatives of phenol (**phenolics**) may be used for disinfecting the skin before surgery. **Oily phenol** is administered by injection for *sclerotherapy of haemorrhoids.

phenothiazines *pl. n.* a group of chemically related compounds with various pharmacological actions. Some (e.g. *chlorpromazine and *trifluoperazine) are *antipsychotic drugs; others (e.g. *piperazine) are anthelmintics.

phenotype *n.* **1.** the observable characteristics of an individual, which result from interaction between the genes he possesses (*genotype) and the environment. **2.** the expression in a person or on a cell of characteristics determined by genes that are not fully defined.

phenoxybenzamine *n.* a drug that dilates blood vessels (*see* ALPHA BLOCKER). It is used to reduce high blood pressure in patients with *phaeochromocytoma. It is administered by mouth or injection and may cause dizziness and fast heartbeat. Trade name: **Dibenyline**.

phenoxymethylpenicillin (penicillin V) *n. see* PENICILLIN.

phentolamine *n.* a drug that dilates blood vessels (*see* ALPHA BLOCKER) and is used to reduce high blood pressure in patients with *phaeochromocytoma. It is administered by intravenous injection; side-effects include fast heartbeat and digestive upsets. Trade name: **Rogitine**.

phenylalanine *n.* an *essential amino acid that is readily converted to tyrosine. Blockade of this metabolic pathway gives rise to *phenylketonuria, which is associated with abnormally large amounts of phenylalanine and phenylpyruvic acid in the blood and retarded mental development.

phenylephrine *n.* a drug that constricts

blood vessels (*see* SYMPATHOMIMETIC) and may be given by injection to increase blood pressure in the emergency treatment of hypotension. It is also administered in eye drops (with atropine) in the treatment of anterior *uveitis; irritation may occur when applied. Trade name: **Minims Phenylephrine Hydrochloride**.

phenylketonuria *n.* an inherited defect of protein metabolism (*see* INBORN ERROR OF METABOLISM) causing an excess of the amino acid phenylalanine in the blood, which damages the nervous system and leads to severe mental retardation. Screening of newborn infants by testing a blood sample for phenylalanine (*see* GUTHRIE TEST) enables the condition to be detected soon enough for dietary treatment to prevent any brain damage: the baby's diet contains proteins from which phenylalanine has been removed. The gene responsible for phenylketonuria is recessive, so that a child is affected only if both parents are carriers of the defective gene.

phenylthiocarbamide (PTC) *n.* a substance that tastes bitter to some individuals but is tasteless to others. Response to PTC appears to be controlled by a single pair of genes (*alleles): ability to taste PTC is *dominant to the inability to taste it.

phenytoin *n.* an *anticonvulsant drug used to control tonic–clonic and partial epileptic seizures and status epilepticus. It is administered by mouth or intravenous injection; side-effects include nausea and vomiting, confusion, dizziness, headache, tremor, insomnia, and (more rarely) gum hypertrophy, hirsutism, and skin rashes. Overdosage causes unsteadiness and slurred speech. Trade name: **Epanutin**.

phial *n.* a small glass bottle for storing medicines or poisons.

Philadelphia chromosome an abnormal form of chromosome 22 that has a foreshortened long arm due to a reciprocal *translocation with chromosome 9. It is most commonly seen in the marrow cells of patients with chronic *myeloid leukaemia.

-philia *combining form denoting* morbid craving or attraction. Example: **nyctophilia** (for darkness).

phimosis *n.* narrowing of the opening of the foreskin, which cannot therefore be drawn back over the underlying glans penis. This predisposes to inflammation (*see* BAL-

ANITIS, BALANOPOSTHITIS), which results in further narrowing. Treatment is by surgical removal of the foreskin (*circumcision).

phleb- (phlebo-) *combining form denoting* a vein or veins. Example: **phlebectopia** (abnormal position of).

phlebectomy *n.* the surgical removal of a vein (or part of a vein), sometimes performed for the treatment of varicose veins in the legs (**varicectomy**).

phlebitis *n.* inflammation of the wall of a vein, which is most commonly seen in the legs as a complication of *varicose veins. A segment of vein becomes painful and tender and the surrounding skin feels hot and appears red. Thrombosis commonly develops (see THROMBOPHLEBITIS). Treatment consists of elastic support together with drugs, such as NSAIDs, to relieve the inflammation and pain. Anticoagulants are not used (*compare* PHLEBOTHROMBOSIS). Phlebitis may also complicate sepsis (see PYLEPHLEBITIS) or cancer, especially of the stomach, bronchus, or pancreas. In pancreatic cancer the phlebitis may affect a variety of veins (**thrombophlebitis migrans**).

phlebography *n. see* VENOGRAPHY.

phlebolith *n.* a stone-like structure, usually found incidentally on abdominal X-ray, that results from deposition of calcium in a venous blood clot. It appears as a small round white opacity in the pelvic region. It does not produce symptoms and requires no treatment.

phlebosclerosis (venosclerosis) *n.* a rare degenerative condition, of unknown cause, that affects the leg veins of young men. The vein walls become thickened and feel like cords under the skin. It is not related to arteriosclerosis and needs no treatment.

phlebothrombosis *n.* obstruction of a vein by a blood clot, without preceding inflammation of its wall. It is most common within the deep veins of the calf of the leg – **deep vein thrombosis** (**DVT**) – in contrast to *thrombophlebitis, which affects superficial leg veins. Prolonged immobility, heart failure, pregnancy, injury, and surgery predispose to thrombosis by encouraging sluggish blood flow. Many of these conditions are associated with changes in the clotting factors in the blood that increase the tendency to thrombosis; these changes also occur in some women taking oral contraceptives.

The affected leg may become swollen and tender. The main danger is that the clot may become detached and give rise to *pulmonary embolism. Regular leg exercises help to prevent deep vein thrombosis, and anticoagulant drugs (such as heparin and warfarin) are used in prevention and treatment. Large clots may be removed surgically in the operation of **thrombectomy** to relieve leg swelling.

Phlebotomus *n. see* SANDFLY.

phlebotomy (venesection) *n.* the surgical opening or puncture of a vein in order to remove blood (e.g. in the treatment of *polycythaemia) or to infuse fluids, blood, or drugs in the treatment of many conditions. It may also be required for cardiac *catheterization. A **phlebotomist** is a clinical support worker or assistant health-care scientist who collects blood from patients for diagnostic laboratory testing.

phlegm *n.* a nonmedical term for *sputum.

phlegmon *n. Archaic.* inflammation of connective tissue, leading to ulceration.

phlycten *n.* a small pinkish-yellow nodule surrounded by a zone of dilated blood vessels that occurs in the conjunctiva or in the cornea. It develops into a small ulcer that heals without trace in the conjunctiva but produces some residual scarring in the cornea. Phlyctens, which are prone to recur, are thought to be due to a type of allergy to certain bacteria.

phobia *n.* a pathologically strong *fear of a particular event or thing. Avoiding the feared situation may severely restrict one's life and cause much suffering. The main kinds of phobia are **specific phobias** (isolated fears of particular things, such as sharp knives), *agoraphobia, *claustrophobia, **social phobias** of encountering people, and **animal phobias**, as of spiders, rats, or dogs (see also PREPAREDNESS). Treatment is with behaviour therapy, especially *desensitization, *graded self-exposure, or *flooding. *Cognitive behavioural therapy and drug therapies are also useful.

-phobia *combining form denoting* morbid fear or dread.

phocomelia *n.* congenital absence of the upper arm and/or upper leg, the hands or feet or both being attached to the trunk by a short stump. The condition is extremely rare except as a side-effect of the drug *thalidomide taken during early pregnancy.

pholcodine *n.* a drug that suppresses coughs and reduces irritation in the respiratory system (*see* ANTITUSSIVE). It is administered by mouth as a linctus for the relief of dry or painful coughs and sometimes causes nausea and drowsiness. Trade names: **Galenphol, Pavacol-D**.

phon *n.* a unit of loudness of sound. The intensity of a sound to be measured is compared by the human ear to a reference tone of 2×10^{-5} pascal sound pressure and 1000 hertz frequency. The intensity of the reference tone is increased until it appears to be equal in loudness to the sound being measured; the loudness of this sound in phons is then equal to the number of decibels by which the reference tone has had to be increased.

phon- (phono-) *combining form denoting* sound or voice.

phonasthenia *n.* weakness of the voice, especially when due to fatigue.

phonation *n.* the production of vocal sounds, particularly speech.

phoniatrics *n.* the study of the voice and its disorders.

phonocardiogram *n. see* ELECTROCARDIO- PHONOGRAPHY. —**phonocardiography** *n.*

phonophobia *n.* excessive sensitivity to certain specific sounds. *See* HYPERACUSIS, MISOPHONIA.

phonosurgery *n.* surgery performed on the larynx externally or endoscopically to improve or modify the quality of the voice.

-phoria *combining form denoting* (in ophthalmology) an abnormal deviation of the eyes or turning of the visual axis. Example: **heterophoria** (tendency to squint).

Phormia *n.* a genus of non-bloodsucking flies, commonly known as blowflies. The maggot of *P. regina* normally breeds in decaying meat but it has occasionally been found in suppurating wounds, giving rise to a type of *myiasis.

phosgene *n.* a poisonous gas developed during World War I. It is a choking agent, acting on the lungs to produce *oedema, with consequent respiratory and cardiac failure.

phosphagen *n.* creatine phosphate (*see* CREATINE).

phosphataemia *n.* the presence of phosphates in the blood. Sodium, calcium, potassium, and magnesium phosphates are normal constituents.

phosphatase *n.* one of a group of enzymes capable of catalysing the hydrolysis of phosphoric acid esters. An example is glucose-6-phosphatase, which catalyses the hydrolysis of glucose-6-phosphate to glucose and phosphate. Phosphatases are important in the absorption and metabolism of carbohydrates, nucleotides, and phospholipids and are essential in the calcification of bone. **Acid phosphatase** is present in kidney, semen, serum, and the prostate gland. **Alkaline phosphatase** occurs in teeth, developing bone, plasma, kidney, and intestine.

phosphatidylcholine *n. see* LECITHIN.

phosphatidylserine *n.* a cephalin-like phospholipid containing the amino acid serine. It is found in brain tissue. *See also* CEPHALIN.

phosphaturia (phosphuria) *n.* the presence of an abnormally high concentration of phosphates in the urine, making it cloudy. The condition may be associated with the formation of stones (calculi) in the kidneys or bladder.

phosphocreatine *n.* creatine phosphate (*see* CREATINE).

phosphofructokinase *n.* an enzyme that catalyses the conversion of fructose-6-phosphate to fructose-1,6-diphosphate. This is an important reaction occurring during the process of *glycolysis.

phospholipid *n.* a *lipid containing a phosphate group as part of the molecule. Phospholipids are constituents of all tissues and organs, especially the brain. They are synthesized in the liver and small intestine and are involved in many of the body's metabolic processes. Examples of phospholipids are *cephalins, *lecithins, sphingolipids, plasmalogens, and phosphatidylserine.

phosphonecrosis *n.* the destruction of tissues caused by excessive amounts of phosphorus in the system. The tissues likely to suffer in phosphorus poisoning are the liver, kidneys, muscles, bones, and the cardiovascular system.

565

phosphorus *n.* a nonmetallic element. Phosphorus compounds are major constituents in the tissues of both plants and animals. In humans, phosphorus is mostly concentrated in *bone. However, certain phosphorus-containing compounds – for example adenosine triphosphate (*ATP) and *creatine phosphate – play an important part in energy conversions and storage in the body. In a pure state, phosphorus is toxic. Symbol: P.

phosphorylase *n.* any enzyme that catalyses the combination of an organic molecule (usually glucose) with a phosphate group (phosphorylation). Phosphorylase is found in the liver and kidney, where it is involved in the breakdown of glycogen to glucose-1-phosphate.

phot- (photo-) *combining form denoting* light.

photalgia *n.* pain in the eye caused by very bright light.

photoablation *n.* the use of light or lasers to destroy tissue.

photochemotherapy *n. see* PHOTODYNAMIC THERAPY, PUVA.

photocoagulation *n.* the destruction of tissue by heat released from the absorption of light shone on it. In eye disorders the technique is used to destroy diseased retinal tissue, occurring, for example, as a complication of diabetes (diabetic *retinopathy) and *macular degeneration; and to produce scarring between the retina and choroid, thus binding them together, in cases of *retinal detachment. Photocoagulation of the retina is usually done with an *argon or *diode laser.

Photocoagulation is also a method of arresting bleeding by causing coagulation, usually using an infrared light source.

photodermatosis *n.* any of various skin diseases caused by exposure to light of varying wavelength (*see* PHOTOSENSITIVITY). The facial prominences and the 'V' of the neck are most commonly affected, the shadow areas behind the ears and below the chin being protected. A common photodermatosis is **polymorphous light eruption**, which affects 10% of the population. It appears with the first sunshine of spring and abates by late summer. The photodermatoses include certain *porphyrias, notably porphyria cutanea tarda.

photodynamic diagnosis a technique for improving the sensitivity and specificity of bladder cancer diagnosis at cystoscopy using a light-sensitive agent. This agent is instilled into the bladder, taken up by the epithelial cells, and converted into a porphyrin that accumulates only in malignant and premalignant cells. It fluoresces under light of a specific wavelength and is thus highlighted against normal bladder mucosa.

photodynamic therapy (PDT, photoradiation therapy, phototherapy, photochemotherapy) **1.** a treatment for some types of superficial cancers. A light-sensitive agent (**porfimer sodium** [Photofrin] or **temoporfin** [Foscan]) is injected into the bloodstream and remains in cancer cells for a longer time than in normal cells. Exposure to laser radiation produces an active form of oxygen that destroys the treated cancer cells. The laser radiation can be directed through a fibreoptic bronchoscope into the airways, through a gastroscope into the oesophagus, or through a cystoscope into the bladder. PDT causes minimal damage to healthy tissue, but as it cannot pass through more than about 3 cm of tissue, it is restricted to treating tumours on or just under the skin or on the lining of internal organs. Photodynamic therapy makes the skin and eyes sensitive to light for six weeks or more after treatment. **2.** a treatment for wet age-related *macular degeneration that involves the intravenous injection of a light-sensitive agent (**verteporfin**, Visudyne) which passes to the abnormal leaking blood vessels in the retina. The agent is activated when a cold laser light is directed at the macula, sealing the abnormal vessels and thus preventing further leakage and macular damage. The effect is to limit visual loss and stabilize vision.

photomicrograph *n.* an enlarged photographic record of an object taken through an optical or electron microscope. *Compare* MICROPHOTOGRAPH.

photomultiplier tube an electronic device that magnifies the light emitted from a *scintillator by accelerating electrons in a high-voltage field. The resulting signal can be used to display the scintillations on a TV screen. Such devices are commonly used in *gamma cameras.

photophobia *n.* discomfort caused by exposure to light. In most cases the light simply aggravates already existing discomfort from eye disease; contraction of the eyelids and other reactions aimed at avoiding the light follow. Photophobia may be associated with dilation of the pupils as a result of eye drops or with migraine, measles, German measles, meningitis, iritis, or disruption of the sensitive corneal epithelium.

photophthalmia *n.* inflammation of the eye due to exposure to light. It is usually caused by the damaging effect of ultraviolet light on the cornea, for example in snow blindness or when lying under a sunbed.

photopic *adj.* relating to or describing conditions of bright illumination. For example, **photopic vision** is vision in bright light, in which the *cones of the retina are responsible for visual sensation. —**photopia** *n.*

photopsia *n.* the sensation of flashes of light caused by mechanical stimulation of the retina of the eye, usually due to traction by the attached vitreous humour when the eye is moved.

photoradiation *n. see* PHOTODYNAMIC THERAPY.

photorefractive keratectomy (PRK) *see* KERATECTOMY.

photoretinitis *n.* damage to the retina of the eye caused by looking at the sun without adequate protection for the eyes. The retina may be burnt by the intense light focused on it; this affects the central part of the visual field, which may be permanently lost (**sun blindness**).

photoselective vaporization of the prostate (PVP) a technique to vaporize the prostate by means of a laser, used to relieve *lower urinary tract symptoms due to benign prostatic hyperplasia (*see* PROSTATE GLAND). It is associated with fewer problems than a traditional TURP (*see* RESECTION), but cannot be easily used on very large prostates.

photosensitivity *n.* abnormal reaction of the skin to sunlight. This characterizes certain skin diseases (*see* PHOTODERMATOSIS). Photosensitivity reactions may also occur in those taking such drugs as thiazide diuretics, furosemide, amiodarone, and NSAIDs. In these cases the effect may resemble severe sunburn. —**photosensitive** *adj.*

photosynthesis *n.* the process whereby green plants and some bacteria manufacture carbohydrates from carbon dioxide and water, using energy absorbed from sunlight by the green pigment chlorophyll. In green plants this complex process may be summarized thus:

$$6CO_2 + 6H_2O \rightarrow C_6H_{12}O_6 + 6O_2$$

phototaxis *n.* movement of a cell or organism in response to a stimulus of light.

phototherapeutic keratectomy *see* KERATECTOMY.

phototherapy *n.* **1.** treatment that involves exposure to ultraviolet or infrared radiation. For example, ultraviolet B radiation is used for treating severe psoriasis. *See also* PUVA. **2.** *see* PHOTODYNAMIC THERAPY.

phototoxicity *n.* damage caused by prolonged exposure to light; for example, **retinal phototoxicity** is damage to the retina of the eye as a result of prolonged exposure to light.

photuria *n.* the excretion of phosphorescent urine, which glows in the dark, due to the presence of certain phosphorus-containing compounds derived from phosphates.

phren- (phreno-) *combining form denoting* **1.** the mind or brain. **2.** the diaphragm. **3.** the phrenic nerve.

-phrenia *combining form denoting* a condition of the mind. Example: **hebephrenia** (schizophrenia affecting young adults).

phrenic crush 1. damage to the phrenic nerve as a result of trauma. **2.** formerly, surgical crushing of a portion of the *phrenic nerve. This paralyses the diaphragm on the side operated upon, which is then pushed upwards by the abdominal contents, thus pressing on the lung and partially collapsing it. This operation was formerly often combined with *pneumoperitoneum in the treatment of pulmonary tuberculosis but is now obsolete.

phrenic nerve the nerve that supplies the muscles of the diaphragm. On each side it arises in the neck from the third, fourth, and fifth cervical spinal roots and passes downwards between the lungs and the heart to reach the diaphragm. Impulses through the nerves from the brain bring about the regular contractions of the diaphragm during breathing.

phrenology *n.* the study of the bumps on the outside of the skull in order to determine a person's character. It is based on the mistaken theory that the skull becomes modified over the different functional areas of the cortex of the brain.

Phrygian cap the normal radiological appearance of the tip of the gall bladder, seen in a minority of cholecystograms (*see* CHOLE-CYSTOGRAPHY). Its name is derived from its resemblance to the characteristic Balkan headgear.

Phthirus *n.* a widely distributed genus of lice. The crab (or pubic) louse, *P. pubis*, is a common parasite of humans that lives permanently attached to the body hair, particularly that of the pubic or perianal regions but also on the eyelashes and the hairs in the armpits. Crab lice are not known to transmit disease but their bites can irritate the skin (*see* PEDICULOSIS). An infestation may be acquired during sexual intercourse or from hairs left on clothing, towels, and lavatory seats.

phthisis *n.* **1.** any disease resulting in wasting of tissues. **Phthisis bulbi** is a shrunken eyeball that has lost its function due to disease or damage. **2.** a former name for pulmonary *tuberculosis.

phycomycosis *n.* a disease caused by parasitic fungi of the genera *Rhizopus*, *Absidia*, and *Mucor*. The disease affects the sinuses, the central nervous system, the lungs, and the skin tissues. The fungi are able to grow within the blood vessels of the lungs and nervous tissue, thus causing blood clots which cut off the blood supply (*see* INFARCTION). Treatment with the antibiotic *amphotericin has proved effective.

phylogenesis *n.* the evolutionary history of a species or individual.

physi- (physio-) *combining form denoting* **1.** physiology. **2.** physical.

physical *adj.* (in medicine) relating to the body rather than to the mind. For example, a **physical sign** is one that a doctor can detect when examining a patient, such as abnormal dilation of the pupils or the absence of a knee-jerk reflex (*see also* FUNCTIONAL DISORDER, ORGANIC DISORDER).

physical medicine a medical specialty established by the Royal Society of Medicine in 1931. Initially the members pioneered clinics devoted to the diagnosis and management of rheumatic diseases, but later extended their interests to the *rehabilitation of patients with physical disabilities ranging from asthma and hand injuries to back trou-

ble and poliomyelitis. The term has caused confusion in recent years, with many doctors preferring the description **rheumatology and rehabilitation** for this specialist activity. Since 1972, however, when the Royal College of Physicians approved it, physical medicine has become the generally accepted term. *See also* RHEUMATOLOGY.

physician *n.* a registered medical practitioner who specializes in the diagnosis and treatment of disease by other than surgical means. In the USA the term is applied to any authorized medical practitioner. *See also* DOCTOR.

physiological saline *see* SALINE.

physiological solution one of a group of solutions used to maintain tissues in a viable state. These solutions contain specific concentrations of substances that are vital for normal tissue function (e.g. sodium, potassium, calcium, chloride, magnesium, bicarbonate, and phosphate ions, glucose, and oxygen). An example of such a solution is *Ringer's solution.

physiology *n.* the science of the functioning of living organisms and of their component parts. —**physiological** *adj.* —**physiologist** *n.*

physiotherapy *n.* the branch of treatment that employs physical methods to promote healing, including the use of light, infrared and ultraviolet rays, heat, electric current, ultrasound, massage, manipulation, hydrotherapy, and remedial exercise.

physis (growth plate) a horizontal band of tissue located between the ends (*epiphyses) of a long bone and the growing zone (*metaphysis) of the shaft. It is composed of cartilaginous, bony, and fibrous components that combine to allow for longitudinal and latitudinal growth and remodelling of the developing bone (endochondral *ossification). See illustration overleaf. *See also* SALTER-HARRIS CLASSIFICATION.

physo- *combining form denoting* air or gas.

phyt- (phyto-) *combining form denoting* plants; of plant origin.

phytohaemagglutinin (PHA) *n.* a plant-derived alkaloid that stimulates T lymphocytes to divide in the test tube.

phytomenadione *n.* a form of *vitamin K occurring naturally in green plants and synthesized for use as an antidote to overdosage

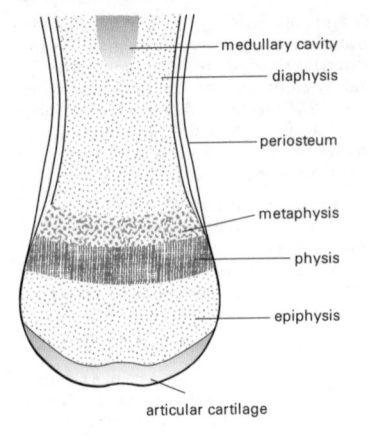

medullary cavity

diaphysis

periosteum

metaphysis

physis

epiphysis

articular cartilage

Physis. Growth areas of a long bone.

with anticoagulant drugs and to prevent *haemorrhagic disease of the newborn. Administered by mouth or injection, it promotes the production of prothrombin, essential for the normal coagulation of blood. Trade name: **Konakion.**

phytophotodermatitis *n.* an eruption of linear blisters occurring after exposure to light in people who have been in contact with certain plants, such as wild parsnip or cow parsley, to which they are sensitive. A particularly dramatic reaction occurs with giant hogweed (*Heracleum mantegazzianum*).

phytotherapy *n.* medical treatment based exclusively on plant extracts and products. Plants have provided a wide range of important drugs (*taxanes among others) and current research into drugs from plants continues to be fruitful. However, it is essential that any drugs derived directly from plants should be extracted, purified, assayed, and tested before being used as medication. The use of crude plant extracts as medicines can be dangerous because seemingly identical samples of the same plant may contain widely differing amounts of the active ingredient.

phytotoxin *n.* any poisonous substance (toxin) produced by a plant, such as any of the toxins produced by fungi of the genus *Amanita*.

pia (pia mater) *n.* the innermost of the three *meninges surrounding the brain and spinal cord. The membrane is closely at-

tached to the surface of the brain and spinal cord, faithfully following each fissure and sulcus. It contains numerous finely branching blood vessels that supply the nerve tissue within. The subarachnoid space separates it from the arachnoid.

pian *n. see* YAWS.

pica *n.* the indiscriminate eating of non-nutritious or harmful substances, such as grass, stones, or clothing. It is common in early childhood but may also be found in patients with learning disabilities or psychosis. Although previously thought to be completely nonadaptive, some evidence suggests that in rare cases patients showing pica may have particular mineral deficiencies.

Pick's disease a cause of *dementia. The damage is mainly in the frontal and temporal lobes of the brain, in contrast with the more diffuse degeneration of *Alzheimer's disease. [A. Pick (1851–1924), Czech psychiatrist]

pico- *prefix denoting* one million-millionth (10^{-12}).

picornavirus *n.* one of a group of small RNA-containing viruses (pico = small; hence pico-RNA-virus). The group includes *Coxsackie viruses, *polioviruses, and *rhinoviruses.

picric acid (trinitrophenol) a yellow crystalline solid used as a dye and as a tissue *fixative.

picture archiving and communication system *see* PACS.

PICU (psychiatric intensive care unit) a unit especially designed for nursing the most acutely and severely mentally ill. PICUs are often locked wards with increased staffing levels. Usually patients stay on a PICU ward for the shortest possible period before being transferred to an open psychiatric ward.

PID 1. *see* PELVIC INFLAMMATORY DISEASE. 2. *see* PROLAPSED INTERVERTEBRAL DISC.

Pierre Robin syndrome a congenital disease in which affected infants have a very small lower jawbone (mandible) and a cleft palate. They are susceptible to feeding and respiratory problems. [Pierre Robin (1867–1950), French dentist]

piezoelectric *adj.* denoting or relating to an electrically generated pulse or polarity that is caused by pressure.

pigeon chest forward protrusion of the breastbone resulting in deformity of the chest. The condition is painless and harmless. Medical name: **pectus carinatum**.

pigeon toes an abnormal posture in which the toes are turned inwards. It is often associated with *knock-knee.

pigment *n.* a substance giving colour. Physiologically important pigments include the blood pigments (especially *haemoglobin), *bile pigments, and retinal pigment (*see* RHODOPSIN). The pigment *melanin occurs in the skin and in the iris of the eye. Important plant pigments include *chlorophyll and the *carotenoids.

pigmentation *n.* coloration produced in the body by the deposition of one pigment, especially in excessive amounts. Pigmentation may be produced by natural pigments, such as bile pigments (as in jaundice) or melanin, or by foreign material, such as lead or arsenic in chronic poisoning.

pigment epitheliopathy an inflammatory disease of the retinal pigment epithelium (RPE; *see* RETINA). Acute posterior multifocal placoid pigment epitheliopathy (APMPPE) is characterized by the presence of multiple cream-coloured irregular lesions scattered in the posterior segment of the eye. The disease occurs in young adults and usually affects both eyes. Visual acuity usually recovers with time.

pig-tail stents *see* STENT.

piles *n.* *see* HAEMORRHOIDS.

pili (fimbriae) *pl. n.* (*sing.* **pilus**, **fimbria**) hairlike processes present on the surface of certain bacteria. They are thought to be involved in adhesion of bacteria to other cells and in transfer of DNA during *conjugation.

pill *n.* **1.** a small ball of variable size, shape, and colour, sometimes coated with sugar, that contains one or more medicinal substances in solid form. It is taken by mouth. **2.** *see* ORAL CONTRACEPTIVE.

pillar *n.* (in anatomy) an elongated apparently supportive structure. For example, the **pillars of the fauces** are folds of mucous membrane on either side of the opening from the mouth to the pharynx.

pilo- *combining form denoting* hair. Example: **pilosis** (excessive development of).

pilocarpine *n.* a *parasympathomimetic drug administered as eye drops or gel to reduce the pressure inside the eye in glaucoma (*see* MIOTIC). It is also administered orally to treat *dry mouth; side-effects may include headache, frequent urination, and sweating. Trade names: **Minims Pilocarpine Nitrate**, **Pilogel**, **Salagen**.

pilomotor nerves sympathetic nerves that supply muscle fibres in the skin, around the roots of hairs. Activity of the sympathetic nervous system causes the muscles to contract, raising the hairs and giving the *gooseflesh effect of fear or cold.

pilonidal sinus a short tract leading from an opening in the skin in or near the cleft at the top of the buttocks and containing hairs. The sinus may be recurrently infected, leading to pain and the discharge of pus. Treatment is by surgical opening and cleaning of the sinus.

pilosebaceous *adj.* relating to the hair follicles and their associated sebaceous glands.

pilus *n.* a hair. *See also* PILI.

pimecrolimus *n.* *see* CALCINEURIN INHIBITORS.

pimel- (pimelo-) *combining form denoting* fat; fatty.

pimozide *n.* an *antipsychotic drug used to treat schizophrenia and some delusional disorders. It is administered by mouth and may cause serious disturbances of heart rhythm. Trade name: **Orap**.

pimple *n.* a small inflamed swelling on the skin that contains pus. It may be the result of bacterial infection of a skin pore that has become obstructed with fatty secretions from the sebaceous glands. Pimples occurring in large numbers on the chest, back, and face are usually described as *acne, a common condition of adolescence.

PIN *see* PROSTATIC INTRAEPITHELIAL NEOPLASIA.

pinard *n.* an instrument used by midwives to auscultate the fetal heart. *See* INTERMITTENT AUSCULTATION.

pincement *n.* one of the techniques used in massage, in which pinches of the patient's flesh are taken between finger and thumb and twisted or rolled before release. This is said to improve the tone of the skin, improve circulation, and alleviate underlying pain.

pineal gland (pineal body) a pea-sized

mass of nerve tissue attached by a stalk to the posterior wall of the third ventricle of the brain, deep between the cerebral hemispheres at the back of the skull. It secretes the hormone *melatonin. The gland becomes calcified as age progresses, providing a useful landmark in X-rays of the skull. Anatomical name: **epiphysis**.

pinguecula *n.* a degenerative change in the conjunctiva of the eye, seen most commonly in the elderly and in those who live in hot dry climates. Thickened yellow triangles develop on the conjunctiva at the inner and outer margins of the cornea.

pink disease a severe illness of children of the teething age, marked by pink cold clammy hands and feet, heavy sweating, raised blood pressure, rapid pulse, photophobia, loss of appetite, and insomnia. Affected infants are very prone to secondary infection, which may be fatal. It has been suggested that the condition is an allergic reaction to mercury, since it used to occur when teething powders, lotions, and ointments containing mercury were used. Although there is no definite proof of this, the disease has virtually disappeared since all mercury-containing paediatric preparations have been banned. Medical names: **acrodynia**, **erythroedema**, **erythromelalgia**.

pink eye *see* CONJUNCTIVITIS.

pink puffer the typical appearance of a patient with chronic obstructive pulmonary disease, who is breathless and flushed. *See also* BLUE BLOATER.

pinna (auricle) *n.* the flap of skin and cartilage that projects from the head at the exterior opening of the external auditory meatus of the *ear (see illustration). In humans the pinna is largely vestigial but it may be partly

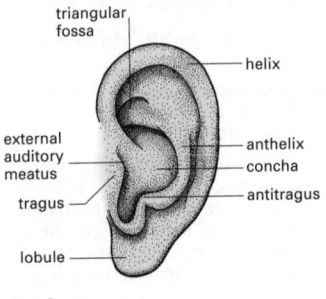

The pinna.

concerned with detecting the direction of sound sources.

pinnaplasty *n. see* OTOPLASTY.

pinocytosis *n.* the intake of small droplets of fluid by a cell by cytoplasmic engulfment. It occurs in many white blood cells and in certain kidney and liver cells. *Compare* PHAGOCYTOSIS.

pins and needles *see* PARAESTHESIA.

pinta *n.* a skin disease, prevalent in tropical America, that is caused by the spirochaete *Treponema carateum*. The disease is thought to be transmitted either by direct contact between individuals or by flies that carry the infective spirochaetes on their bodies. Symptoms include thickening and eventual loss of pigment of the skin, particularly on the hands, wrists, feet, and ankles. Pinta is treated with penicillin G.

pinworm *n. see* THREADWORM.

pioglitazone *n. see* THIAZOLIDINEDIONES.

pipelle *n.* a disposable flexible plastic endometrial sampling device consisting of an inner plunger and a 3-mm outer sheath, which is inserted through the cervix into the endometrial cavity to obtain a blind endometrial biopsy by gentle suction.

piperazine *n.* a drug used to treat infestations by roundworms and threadworms. It is administered by mouth; side-effects do not usually occur, but continued treatment at high doses may cause nausea, vomiting, headache, tingling sensations, and rashes. Trade name: **Pripsen**.

piriform fossae two pear-shaped depressions that lie on either side of the opening to the larynx.

piroxicam *n.* a nonsteroidal anti-inflammatory drug (*see* NSAID) used to relieve pain and stiffness in osteoarthritis, rheumatoid arthritis, gout, and ankylosing spondylitis. It is administered by mouth or topically; side-effects, which can be severe, include skin rash and gastrointestinal symptoms. Trade names: **Brexidol**, **Feldene**.

pisiform bone the smallest bone of the wrist (*carpus): a pea-shaped bone that articulates with the triquetral bone and, indirectly by cartilage, with the ulna.

pit *n.* (in anatomy) a hollow or depression, such as any of the depressions on the surface of an embryo marking the site of future organs.

pithing *n.* the laboratory procedure in which a part or the whole of the central nervous system of an experimental animal (such as a frog) is destroyed, usually by inserting a probe through the foramen magnum, in preparation for physiological or pharmacological experiments.

pitting *n.* the formation of depressed scars, as occurs on the skin following acne or (formerly) smallpox. **Pitting oedema** is swelling of the tissues due to excess fluid in which fingertip pressure leaves temporary indentations in the skin.

pituicyte *n.* a type of cell found in the posterior lobe of the pituitary gland, similar in appearance to an *astrocyte, with numerous fine branches that end in contact with the lining membrane of the blood channels in the gland.

pituitary apoplexy acute intrapituitary haemorrhage, usually into an existing tumour, presenting as severe headache and collapse. It is a medical emergency. Due to the sudden expansion in size of the gland with the haemorrhage, it is accompanied by lesions of the cranial nerves running close to the pituitary gland, causing paralysis of the muscles of the orbit and occasionally the face. Anterior pituitary insufficiency usually results, but posterior pituitary function survives. Surprisingly, pituitary function usually recovers.

pituitary gland (hypophysis) the master endocrine gland: a pea-sized body attached beneath the *hypothalamus in a bony cavity at the base of the skull. It has an anterior lobe (**adenohypophysis**), which secretes *thyroid-stimulating hormone, *ACTH (adrenocorticotrophic hormone), the *gonadotrophins, *growth hormone, *prolactin, *lipotrophin, and *melanocyte-stimulating hormone. The secretion of all these hormones is regulated by specific **releasing hormones**, which are produced in the hypothalamus (*see also* CORTICOTROPHIN-RELEASING HORMONE, GONADOTROPHIN-RELEASING HORMONE, THYROTROPHIN-RELEASING HORMONE). The posterior lobe (**neurohypophysis**) secretes *vasopressin and *oxytocin, which are synthesized in the hypothalamus and transported to the pituitary, where they are stored before release.

pityriasis *n.* (originally) any of a group of skin diseases typified by the development of fine branlike scales. The term is now used only with a modifying adjective. **Pityriasis alba** is a common condition in children in which pale scaly patches occur on the face; it is related to atopic *eczema. **Pityriasis rosea** is a common skin rash, believed to be viral in origin, starting with a single patch (a **herald patch**) on the trunk and followed by an eruption of oval pink scaly *macules. The spots are often aligned along the ribs. The rash usually clears completely in about eight weeks. **Pityriasis versicolor** is a common chronic infection of the skin caused by the yeast *Malassezia furfur*, which produces a persistent pale or brown scaly rash on the trunk. Treatment with *selenium sulphide shampoo or with oral itraconazole readily kills the organism but the skin may take months to regain its normal colour. *See also* DANDRUFF (PITYRIASIS CAPITIS).

Pityrosporum *n. see* MALASSEZIA.

pivmecillinam *n.* a *penicillin-type antibiotic used mainly to treat urinary-tract infections caused by many Gram-negative bacteria. It is administered by mouth: possible side-effects include allergic reactions, nausea, and vomiting. Trade name: **Selexid**.

pivot joint *see* TROCHOID JOINT.

pixel *n.* short for 'picture element', the smallest individual component of an electronically produced image. Numerical values are ascribed to each pixel, which describe its position and relative intensity and/or colour. A two-dimensional *matrix of pixels produces the final image.

pizotifen *n.* an antihistamine drug used to prevent severe migraine and cluster headaches. Administered by mouth, it acts by inhibiting the effects of *serotonin. Possible side-effects include dizziness, drowsiness, and weight gain. Trade name: **Sanomigran**.

placebo *n.* a medicine that is ineffective but may help to relieve a condition because the patient has faith in its powers. New drugs are tested against placebos in clinical trials: the drug's effect is compared with the **placebo response**, which occurs even in the absence of any pharmacologically active substance in the placebo. Use of placebos in treatment is controversial, with some believing that such treatment compromises the patient's *autonomy and compromises the virtue of honesty, thereby potentially undermining the doctor–patient relationship.

placenta *n.* an organ within the uterus by means of which the embryo is attached to the wall of the uterus. Its primary function is to provide the embryo with nourishment, eliminate its wastes, and exchange respiratory gases. This is accomplished by the close proximity of the maternal and fetal blood systems within the placenta. It also functions as a gland, secreting *human chorionic gonadotrophin, *progesterone, and oestrogens, which regulate the maintenance of pregnancy. *See also* AFTERBIRTH. —**placental** *adj.*

placenta accreta a condition in which the placenta is abnormally strongly attached to the wall of the uterus with superficial penetration of chorionic *villi into the underlying *myometrium. Women with *placenta praevia and at least one previous Caesarean delivery are considered to be at high risk for placenta accreta. When placenta accreta is thought to be likely, consultant obstetric and anaesthetic input are vital in planning and conducting the delivery. Radiological input with temporary uterine balloon tamponade may be considered, and methotrexate has been used. The risk of haemorrhage, blood transfusion, and hysterectomy should be discussed. In **placenta increta** the chorionic villi extend into the myometrium; a **placenta percreta** occurs where the chorionic villi penetrate through the myometrial wall. An emergency hysterectomy is usually necessary in these rare cases.

placental abruption *see* ABRUPTIO PLACENTAE.

placenta praevia a condition in which the placenta is situated wholly or partially in the lower and noncontractile part of the uterus. When this becomes elongated and stretched during the last few weeks of pregnancy, and the cervix becomes stretched either before or during labour, placental separation and haemorrhage will occur. The cause is not known. In the more severe degrees of placenta praevia, where the placenta is situated entirely before the presenting part of the fetus, delivery must be by Caesarean section. In lesser degrees of placenta praevia, vaginal delivery may be considered.

placentography (sonoplacentography) *n.* imaging of the pregnant uterus by ultrasonography in order to determine the position of the placenta.

placode *n.* any of the thickened areas of ectoderm in the embryo that will develop into nerve ganglia or the special sensory structures of the eye, ear, or nose.

plagiocephaly *n.* any distortion or lack of symmetry in the shape of the head, usually due to irregularity in the closure of the sutures between the bones of the skull.

plague *n.* **1.** any epidemic disease with a high death rate. **2.** an acute epidemic disease of rats and other wild rodents caused by the bacterium *Yersinia pestis*, which is transmitted to humans by rat fleas. **Bubonic plague**, the most common form of the disease, has an incubation period of 2–6 days. Headache, fever, weakness, aching limbs, and delirium develop and are followed by acute painful swellings of the lymph nodes (*see* BUBO). In favourable cases the buboes burst after about a week, releasing pus, and then heal. In other cases bleeding under the skin, producing black patches, can lead to ulcers, which may prove fatal (hence the former name **Black Death**). In the most serious cases bacteria enter the bloodstream (**septicaemic plague**) or lungs (**pneumonic plague**); if untreated, these are nearly always fatal. Treatment with tetracycline, streptomycin, and chloramphenicol is effective; vaccination against the disease provides only partial protection.

plane *n.* a level or smooth surface, especially any of the imaginary flat surfaces – oriented in various directions – used to divide the body; for example, the *coronal and *sagittal planes.

planoconcave *adj.* describing a structure, such as a lens, that is flat on one side and concave on the other.

planoconvex *adj.* describing a structure, such as a lens, that is flat on one side and convex on the other.

plantar *adj.* relating to the sole of the foot (**planta**). *See also* FLEXION.

plantar arch the arch in the sole of the foot formed by anastomosing branches of the plantar arteries.

plantar fasciitis (policeman's heel) inflammation of the point of attachment of the *fascia in the sole of the foot to the calcaneus (heel bone), causing pain and localized tenderness of the heel. Treatment is a pad under the heel, anti-inflammatory medication, or steroid injections. The inflammation takes 6–12 months to subside.

plantar reflex a reflex obtained by drawing a bluntly pointed object (such as a key) along the outer border of the sole of the foot from the heel to the little toe. The normal **flexor response** is a bunching and downward movement of the toes. An upward movement of the big toe is called an **extensor response** (or **Babinski reflex** or **response**). In all persons over the age of 18 months this is a sensitive indication of damage to the *pyramidal system in either the brain or spinal cord.

plantar wart a *wart occurring on the sole of the foot.

plantigrade *adj.* walking on the entire sole of the foot: a habit of humans, bears, and some other animals.

plaque *n.* **1.** a layer that forms on the surface of a tooth, principally at its neck, composed of bacteria in an organic matrix (*biofilm). Under certain conditions the plaque may cause *gingivitis, *periodontal disease, or *dental caries. The purpose of oral hygiene is to remove plaque. **2.** a raised patch on the skin, formed by *papules enlarging or coalescing to form an area 2 cm or more across. **3.** a deposit, consisting of a fatty core covered with a fibrous cap, that develops on the inner wall of an artery in atherosclerosis (*see* ATHEROMA). **4.** any flat and often raised patch, for example on mucous membrane, resulting from local damage.

-plasia *combining form denoting* formation; development. Example: **hyperplasia** (excessive tissue formation).

plasm- (plasmo-) *combining form denoting* **1.** blood plasma. **2.** protoplasm or cytoplasm.

plasma (blood plasma) *n.* the straw-coloured fluid in which the blood cells are suspended. It consists of a solution of various inorganic salts of sodium, potassium, calcium, etc., with a high concentration of protein (approximately 70 g/l) and a variety of trace substances.

plasma cells antibody-producing cells found in blood-forming tissue and also in the epithelium of the lungs and gut. They develop in the bone marrow, lymph nodes, and spleen when antigens stimulate B *lymphocytes to produce the precursor cells that give

rise to them. Malignant proliferation of plasma cells results in either a *plasmacytoma or multiple *myeloma.

plasma coagulation a type of *electrocoagulation used to arrest haemorrhage or destroy abnormal tissue. A stream of inert gas, such as argon or helium, is ionized, thereby carrying electrical energy to adjacent tissue; there is no physical contact between the plasma coagulation apparatus and the tissue.

plasmacytoma *n.* a malignant tumour of plasma cells, often known as a 'solitary myeloma'. Although usually occurring as a single tumour in bone marrow or more rarely soft tissue (**extramedullary plasmacytoma**), it may be multiple, in which case it is classified as a multiple myeloma. All of these tumours may produce the abnormal gammaglobulins that are characteristic of myeloma, and they may progress to widespread myeloma. The soft-tissue tumours often respond to radiotherapy and to such drugs as melphalan and cyclophosphamide; the bone tumours are less responsive. Tumours originating in soft tissue (usually the airways) may spread to bone, producing an appearance on X-ray identical to myeloma deposits; these secondary growths often resolve completely after treatment.

plasmalogen *n.* a phospholipid, found in brain and muscle, similar in structure to *lecithin and *cephalin.

plasmapheresis *n.* a procedure for removing a quantity of plasma from the blood. Blood is withdrawn through a vein from the patient and passed through a machine (a cell separator). Plasma is removed and the rest of the blood is returned to the patient through another vein.

plasmin (fibrinolysin) *n.* an enzyme that digests the protein fibrin. Its function is the dissolution of blood clots (*see* FIBRINOLYSIS). Plasmin is not normally present in the blood but exists as an inactive precursor, **plasminogen**.

plasminogen *n.* a substance normally present in the blood plasma that may be activated to form *plasmin. *See* FIBRINOLYSIS, PLASMINOGEN ACTIVATORS.

plasminogen activators enzymes that convert the inactive substance *plasminogen to the active enzyme *plasmin, which digests blood clots (*see* FIBRINOLYSIS). There are two types of plasminogen activators, *tissue-type plasminogen activator (tPA) and urokinase-like plasminogen activator (uPA). *See* BLOOD COAGULATION.

plasmoditrophoblast *n. see* TROPHO-BLAST.

Plasmodium *n.* a genus of protozoans (*see* SPOROZOA) that live as parasites within human red blood cells and liver cells. The parasite undergoes its asexual development (*see* SCHIZOGONY) in humans and completes the sexual phase of its development (*see* SPOROGONY) in the stomach and digestive glands of a bloodsucking *Anopheles* mosquito. Four species cause *malaria: *P. vivax*, *P. ovale*, *P. falciparum*, and *P. malariae*.

plasmolysis *n.* a process occurring in bacteria and plants in which the protoplasm shrinks away from the rigid cell wall when the cell is placed in a *hypertonic solution. Plasmolysis is due to withdrawal of water from the cell by *osmosis.

plaster *n.* adhesive tape used in shaped pieces or as a bandage to keep a dressing in place.

plaster model (in dentistry) an accurate cast of the teeth and jaws made from modified plaster of Paris. A pair of models are used to study the dentition, particularly before treatment. Models are also used to construct dentures, orthodontic appliances, and such restorations as crowns.

plaster of Paris a preparation of gypsum (calcium sulphate) that sets hard when water is added. It is used in various modified forms in dentistry to make *plaster models. It is also used in orthopaedics for preparing plaster *casts.

Plastibell device a plastic device that facilitates *circumcision while protecting the glans penis. It is widely used for circumcisions in newborn boys.

plastic lymph a transparent yellowish liquid produced in a wound or other site of inflammation, in which connective tissue cells and blood vessels develop during healing.

plastic surgery a branch of surgery dealing with the reconstruction of deformed or damaged parts of the body. It also includes the replacement of parts of the body that have been lost. If performed simply to improve appearances plastic surgery

is called **cosmetic surgery** (or **aesthetic plastic surgery**), but most plastic surgery involves the treatment and repair of disfigurement and disability caused by burns, major accidents, and cancer and the correction of congenital defects, such as cleft lip and cleft palate.

plastron *n.* the breastbone (*sternum) together with the costal cartilages attached to it.

-plasty *combining form denoting* plastic surgery. Example: **labioplasty** (of the lips).

platelet (**thrombocyte**) *n.* a disc-shaped cell structure, 1–2 μm in diameter, that is present in the blood. With *Romanowsky stains platelets appear as fragments of pale-blue cytoplasm with a few red granules. They have several functions, all relating to the arrest of bleeding (*see* BLOOD COAGULATION, PLATELET ACTIVATION). There are normally $150–400 \times 10^9$ platelets per litre of blood. *See also* THROMBOPOIESIS.

platelet activation the process whereby platelets adhere to collagen released from endothelial cells in damaged blood vessels

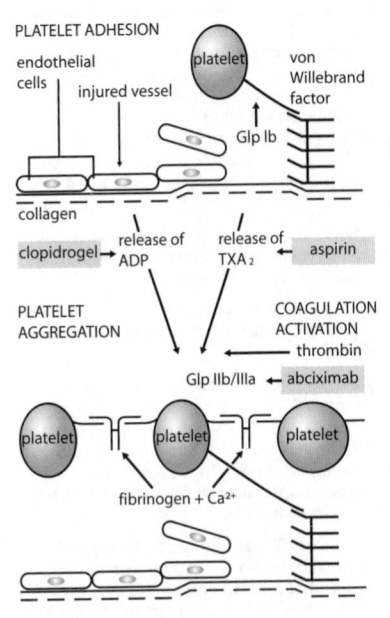

Platelet activation. The stages of the process and sites of action of antiplatelet drugs.

and aggregate to form a plug. An important metabolic pathway in platelets converts membrane phospholipids to *thromboxane A_2 (TXA_2), which can activate platelets. ADP, released from platelet granules, and *thrombin are other activators. The adhesive and aggregation reactions of platelets are mediated through surface membrane glycoproteins (Glp): Glp Ib and Glp IIb/IIIa. Aspirin acts as an *antiplatelet drug by irreversibly inhibiting one of the enzymes of this pathway, cyclo-oxygenase. *Clopidrogel inhibits the ADP receptor on platelet membranes, and *abciximab blocks platelet aggregation by inhibiting Glp IIb/IIIa (see illustration).

platelet-derived growth factor (PDGF) *see* GROWTH FACTOR.

platy- *combining form denoting* broad or flat.

platyhelminth *n. see* FLATWORM.

platysma *n.* a broad thin sheet of muscle that extends from below the collar bone to the angle of the jaw. It depresses the jaw.

pledget *n.* a small wad of dressing material, such as lint, used either to cover a wound or sore or as a plug. It is also used during operations, mounted on an instrument, to wipe away blood or other fluids.

-plegia *combining form denoting* paralysis. Example: **hemiplegia** (of one side of the body).

pleio- (pleo-) *combining form denoting* 1. multiple. 2. excessive.

pleiotropy *n.* a situation in which a single gene is responsible for more than one effect in the *phenotype. The mutation of such a gene will therefore have multiple effects. —**pleiotropic** *adj.*

pleocytosis *n.* the presence of an abnormally large number of lymphocytes in the cerebrospinal fluid, which bathes the brain and spinal cord.

pleomastia (polymastia) *n.* multiple breasts or nipples. These are usually symmetrically arranged along a line between the mid point of the collar bone and the pelvis (the nipple line).

pleomorphism *n.* 1. the condition in which an individual assumes a number of different forms during its life cycle. The malarial parasite (*Plasmodium*) displays pleomorphism. 2. a feature of malignant neoplastic cells, which show a marked variation in the shapes of individual cells and cell nuclei.

pleoptics *n.* special techniques practised by orthoptists (*see* ORTHOPTICS) for developing normal function of the macula (the most sensitive part of the retina), in people whose macular function has previously been disturbed because of strabismus (squint).

plerocercoid *n.* a larval stage of certain tapeworms, such as *Diphyllobothrium latum*. It differs from the *cysticercus (another larval form) in being solid and in lacking a cyst or bladder.

plessimeter (pleximeter) *n.* a small plate of bone, ivory, or other material pressed against the surface of the body and struck with a *plessor in the technique of *percussion.

plessor (plexor) *n.* a small hammer used to investigate nervous reflexes and in the technique of *percussion.

plethora *n.* any excess of any bodily fluid, especially blood (*see* HYPERAEMIA). —**plethoric** *adj.*

plethysmography *n.* the process of recording the changes in the volume of a limb caused by alterations in blood pressure. The limb is inserted into a fluid-filled watertight casing (**oncometer**) and the pressure variations in the fluid are recorded.

pleur- (pleuro-) *combining form denoting* 1. the pleura. 2. the side of the body.

pleura *n.* the covering of the lungs (**visceral pleura**) and of the inner surface of the chest wall (**parietal pleura**). (See illustration.) The covering consists of a closed sac of *serous membrane, which has a smooth shiny moist surface due to the secretion of small amounts of fluid. This fluid lubricates

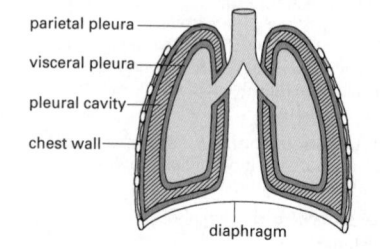

parietal pleura

visceral pleura

pleural cavity

chest wall

diaphragm

The pleura.

the opposing visceral and parietal surfaces so that they can slide painlessly over each other during breathing. —**pleural** *adj.*

pleural cavity the space between the visceral and parietal *pleura, which is normally very small as the pleural membranes are in close contact. The introduction of fluid (**pleural effusion**) or gas separates the pleural surfaces and increases the volume of the pleural space.

pleurectomy *n.* surgical removal of part of the *pleura, which is sometimes done to prevent further recurrences of spontaneous *pneumothorax or to remove diseased areas of pleura.

pleurisy *n.* inflammation of the *pleura, often due to pneumonia in the underlying lung. The normally shiny and slippery pleural surfaces lose their sheen and become slightly sticky, so that there is pain on deep breathing and a characteristic 'rub' can be heard through a stethoscope. Pleurisy is always associated with some other disease in the lung, chest wall, diaphragm, or abdomen.

pleurocele *n.* herniation of the pleura. *See* HERNIA.

pleurocentesis (thoracentesis, thoracocentesis) *n.* the insertion of a hollow needle into the *pleural cavity through the chest wall in order to withdraw fluid, blood, pus, or air.

pleurodesis *n.* the artificial production of pleurisy by chemical or mechanical means to obliterate the *pleural cavity, in order to prevent recurrent, usually malignant, pleural effusions.

pleurodynia *n.* severe paroxysmal pain arising from the muscles between the ribs. It is usually thought to be of rheumatic origin.

pleurolysis (pneumolysis) *n.* surgical stripping of the parietal *pleura from the chest wall to allow the lung to collapse. The procedure was used to help tuberculosis to heal, before the advent of effective antituberculous drugs.

pleuropneumonia *n.* inflammation involving both the lung and pleura. *See* PLEURISY, PNEUMONIA.

pleurotyphoid *n.* *typhoid fever involving the lungs.

pleximeter *n. see* PLESSIMETER.

plexor *n. see* PLESSOR.

plexus *n.* a network of nerves or blood vessels. *See* BRACHIAL PLEXUS.

plica *n.* a fold of tissue; for example, the **plica sublingualis**, the mucous fold in the floor of the mouth. —**plicate** *adj.*

plication *n.* a surgical technique in which the size of a hollow organ is reduced by taking tucks or folds in the walls.

ploidy *n.* the condition of having multiple the normal number of chromosomes for the species. An increase in ploidy in the cells of a malignant tumour usually indicates greater aggressiveness and ability to invade.

plombage *n.* **1.** a technique used in surgery for the correction of retinal detachment. A small piece of silicone plastic is sewn on the outside of the eyeball to produce an indentation over the retinal hole or tear to allow the retina to reattach. **2.** the insertion of plastic balls into the pleural cavity to cause collapse of the lung. This was done in the days before effective antituberculous drugs to help tuberculosis to heal.

plumbism *n.* lead poisoning. *See* LEAD[1].

Plummer's disease a hyperfunctioning, usually benign, *adenoma of the thyroid gland, which can be palpated and appears as a 'hot nodule' on radioactive thyroid scanning. Treatment is to control the nodule with antithyroid drugs and then remove it surgically or destroy it permanently with radioactive iodine. [H. S. Plummer (1874–1937), US physician]

pluri- *combining form denoting* more than one; several.

pluripotent *adj. see* STEM CELL.

PMS *see* PREMENSTRUAL SYNDROME.

pneo- *combining form denoting* breathing; respiration.

pneum- *combining form. see* PNEUMO-.

pneumat- (pneumato-) *combining form denoting* **1.** the presence of air or gas. **2.** respiration.

pneumatization *n.* the presence of air-filled cavities in bone, such as the sinuses of the skull.

pneumatocele *n.* herniation of lung tissue. *See* HERNIA.

pneumatosis *n.* the occurrence of gas

cysts in abnormal sites in the body. **Pneumatosis cystoides intestinalis** is the occurrence of multiple gas cysts in the wall of the lower intestines. Its cause is unknown; it can be treated by *hyperbaric oxygenation.

pneumaturia *n.* the presence in the urine of bubbles of air or other gas, due to the formation of gas by bacteria infecting the urinary tract or to an abnormal connection (fistula) between the urinary tract and bowel.

pneumo- (pneum-) *combining form denoting* **1.** the presence of air or gas. Example: **pneumocolon** (within the colon). **2.** the lung(s). Example: **pneumogastric** (relating to the lungs and stomach). **3.** respiration.

pneumocephalus (pneumocele) *n.* the presence of air within the skull, usually resulting from a fracture passing through one of the air sinuses. There may be a leak of cerebrospinal fluid at the site of the fracture, manifested as a watery discharge from the nose. Pneumocephalus can be detected by plain X-rays of the skull, which show air and a fluid level inside a cavity, or by CT and MRI scanning.

pneumococcal vaccine a vaccine that protects against infection by the bacterium *Streptococcus pneumoniae*, which can cause serious diseases, including pneumonia, septicaemia, and *meningitis. Children under 2 years of age and adults over 65 years are at particular risk. Since September 2006, the pneumococcal vaccine has become part of the childhood *immunization programme.

pneumococcus *n.* (*pl.* **pneumococci**) the bacterium *Streptococcus pneumoniae*, which is associated with pneumonia and pneumococcal meningitis. —**pneumococcal** *adj.*

pneumoconiosis *n.* a group of lung diseases caused by inhaling dust. The dust particles must be less than 0.5 μm in diameter to reach the depths of the lung and there is usually a long period after initial exposure before shadows appear on the chest X-ray and breathlessness develops. In practice industrial exposure to coal dust (*see* COALWORKER'S PNEUMOCONIOSIS), silica (*see* SILICOSIS), and asbestos (*see* ASBESTOSIS) produces most of the cases of pneumoconiosis. In Britain such cases are examined by the Medical Boarding Centres (Respiratory Diseases), on whose advice statutory compensation for industrial injury may be awarded.

Pneumocystis *n.* a genus of protozoans. The species *P. jiroveci* (formerly *carinii*) causes pneumonia in immunosuppressed patients, usually following intensive chemotherapy. *Pneumocystis jiroveci* (*carinii*) pneumonia (PCP) is fatal in 10–30% of cases if untreated, but it can be overcome with high doses of *co-trimoxazole or *pentamidine.

pneumocyte *n.* a type of cell that lines the walls separating the air sacs (*see* ALVEOLUS) in the lungs. Type I pneumocytes are flat and inconspicuous. Type II pneumocytes are cuboidal and secrete *surfactant.

pneumoencephalography *n.* a technique used in the X-ray diagnosis of disease within the skull. Air is introduced into the cavities (ventricles) of the brain to displace the cerebrospinal fluid, thus acting as a *contrast medium. X-ray photographs show the size and disposition of the ventricles and the subarachnoid spaces. The technique has largely been superseded by CT and MRI scanning.

pneumograph *n.* an instrument used to record the movements made during respiration.

pneumolysis *n. see* PLEUROLYSIS.

pneumomediastinum *n.* air in the mediastinum visible on chest X-ray. It can be a complication of surgical *emphysema due to pneumothorax, but the air can originate from the upper airways or the upper gastrointestinal tract. A rare cause is gas-forming organisms. *See* HAMMAN'S SIGN.

pneumon- (pneumono-) *combining form denoting* the lung(s). Example: **pneumonopexy** (surgical fixation to the chest wall).

pneumonectomy *n.* surgical removal of a lung, usually for cancer.

pneumonia *n.* inflammation of the lung caused by bacteria, in which the air sacs (*alveoli) become filled with inflammatory cells and the lung becomes solid (*see* CONSOLIDATION). The symptoms include those of any infection (fever, malaise, headaches, etc.), together with cough and chest pain. Pneumonias may be classified in different ways.

(1) According to the X-ray appearance. **Lobar pneumonia** affects whole lobes and is usually caused by *Streptococcus pneumoniae*, while **lobular pneumonia** refers to

multiple patchy shadows in a localized or segmental area. When these multiple shadows are widespread, the term **bronchopneumonia** is used. In bronchopneumonia, the infection starts in a number of small bronchi and spreads in a patchy manner into the alveoli. **Interstitial pneumonia** is the result of an inflammatory process centred within the alveolar walls rather than the alveolar airspaces. It may be due to a variety of factors, including certain infections, drugs, inhalation of fumes, and exposure to high concentrations of oxygen.

(2) According to the infecting organism. The most common organism is *Streptococcus pneumoniae*, but *Haemophilus influenzae*, *Staphylococcus aureus*, *Legionella pneumophila*, and *Mycoplasma pneumoniae* (among others) may all be responsible for the infection. *See also* ATYPICAL PNEUMONIA, VIRAL PNEUMONIA.

(3) According to the clinical and environmental circumstances under which the pneumonia is acquired. These infections are divided into **community-acquired pneumonia**, **hospital-acquired (nosocomial) pneumonia**, and pneumonias occurring in immunocompromised subjects (including those with AIDS). The organisms responsible for community-acquired pneumonia are totally different from those in the other groups.

Appropriate antibiotic therapy, based on the clinical situation and on microbiological studies, will result in complete recovery in the majority of patients.

pneumonitis *n.* inflammation of the lung that is confined to the walls of the air sacs (alveoli) and often caused by viruses or unknown agents. It may be acute and transient or chronic, leading to increasing respiratory disability. It does not respond to antibiotics but corticosteroids may be helpful. *Compare* PNEUMONIA.

pneumopericardium *n.* the presence of air within the membranous sac surrounding the heart. *See* HYDROPNEUMOPERICARDIUM.

pneumoperitoneum *n.* air or gas in the peritoneal or abdominal cavity, usually due to a perforation of the stomach or bowel. Pneumoperitoneum may be induced for diagnostic purposes (e.g. *laparoscopy). A former treatment of tuberculosis was the deliberate injection of air into the peritoneal cavity to allow the tuberculous lung to be rested (**artificial pneumoperitoneum**); this

was frequently combined with *phrenic crush.

pneumoradiography *n.* X-ray examination of part of the body using a gas, such as air or carbon dioxide, as a contrast medium. The technique was used to examine the ventricles of the brain (pneumoencephalography). It is now largely obsolete, apart from *double contrast examinations of the bowel and in CT *colography.

pneumoretinopexy *n.* a surgical technique in which an inert gas bubble is injected into the eye to press and seal breaks in the retina. When the retina is flat, a laser beam or *cryoretinopexy is applied to cause scarring and permanently seal the tear.

pneumothorax *n.* air in the *pleural cavity. Any breach of the lung surface or chest wall allows air to enter the pleural cavity, causing the lung to collapse. The leak can occur without apparent cause, in otherwise healthy people (**spontaneous pneumothorax**), or result from injuries to the chest (**traumatic pneumothorax**). In **tension pneumothorax** a breach in the lung surface acts as a valve, admitting air into the pleural cavity when the patient breathes in but preventing its escape when he breathes out. This air must be let out by surgical incision.

A former treatment for pulmonary tuberculosis – **artificial pneumothorax** – was the deliberate injection of air into the pleural cavity to collapse the lung and allow the tuberculous areas to heal.

pneumotonometer *n.* an instrument that blows a puff of air at the cornea to cause flattening and hence measure intraocular pressure. It is commonly used by optometrists in tests for glaucoma.

PNH *see* PAROXYSMAL NOCTURNAL HAEMOGLOBINURIA.

PNM *see* PERINATAL MORTALITY RATE.

-pnoea *combining form denoting* a condition of breathing. Example: **dyspnoea** (breathlessness).

pock *n.* a small pus-filled eruption on the skin characteristic of *chickenpox and *smallpox rashes. *See also* PUSTULE.

pocket *n.* (in dentistry) *see* PERIODONTAL POCKET.

pocket resuscitation mask a compressible and easily carried mask, which can be expanded and fitted over the mouth and nose of a nonbreathing patient in order to perform mouth-to-mouth resuscitation through a small valve without contact between the mouth of the rescuer and that of the patient.

pod- *combining form denoting* the foot.

podagra *n.* gout of the foot, especially the big toe.

podalic version (internal podalic version) a procedure in which the position of a fetus in the uterus is altered so that its feet will emerge first at birth. It is used mainly to deliver a second twin that is presenting transversely or obliquely. *See also* CEPHALIC VERSION.

podiatry (chiropody) *n.* the study and care of the foot, including its normal structure, its diseases, and their treatment. The main role of a **podiatrist** (**chiropodist**) is to assess, diagnose, and treat abnormalities and diseases of the foot and to give advice on proper foot care and the prevention of foot problems.

podocyte *n.* an epithelial cell in the glomerulus that spreads over the capillary basement membrane and has branching tentacle-like processes that interdigitate with adjacent cells. The podocytes leave gaps or thin filtration slits. The slits are covered by slit diaphragms, which are composed of a number of cell-surface proteins including *nephrin, podocalyxin, and P-cadherin, which ensure that large molecules, such as albumin and gammaglobulin, are not filtered. Podocytes are damaged in *minimal change nephropathy and a major target of injury in *HIVAN.

podopompholyx *n. see* POMPHOLYX.

POEMS syndrome a syndrome, mostly reported in Japanese males, consisting of *polyneuropathy, organomegaly, endocrine failure, M protein (immunoglobulins) in the plasma, and skin changes, such as thickening, hirsutism, or excess sweating. Each of the components occurs with varying consistency. The cause is not known but it is not thought to be autoimmune in nature.

-poiesis *combining form denoting* formation; production. Example: **haemopoiesis** (of blood cells).

poikilo- *combining form denoting* variation; irregularity.

poikilocyte *n.* an abnormally shaped red

blood cell (*erythrocyte). Poikilocytes may be classified into a variety of types on the basis of their shape; for example elliptocytes (ellipsoid) and schistocytes (semilunar). *See also* POIKILOCYTOSIS.

poikilocytosis *n.* the presence of abnormally shaped red cells (*poikilocytes) in the blood. Poikilocytosis is particularly marked in *myelofibrosis but can occur to some extent in almost any blood disease.

poikiloderma *n.* a combination of pale and darkened skin with telangiectasia (*see* TELANGIECTASIS) and atrophy (wrinkled thin skin). This may be a sign of *cutaneous T-cell lymphoma.

poikilothermic *adj.* cold-blooded: being unable to regulate the body temperature, which fluctuates according to that of the surroundings. Reptiles and amphibians are cold-blooded. *Compare* HOMOIOTHERMIC. —**poikilothermy** *n.*

pointillage *n.* a procedure in massage in which the therapist's fingers are pressed, fingertip first, deep into the patient's skin. This is done to manipulate underlying structures and break up adhesions that may have formed following injury.

poison *n.* any substance that irritates, damages, or impairs the activity of the body's tissues. In large enough doses almost any substance acts as a poison, but the term is usually reserved for substances, such as arsenic, cyanide, and strychnine, that are harmful in relatively small amounts.

polar body one of the small cells produced during the formation of an ovum from an *oocyte that does not develop into a functional egg cell.

pole *n.* (in anatomy) the extremity of the axis of the body, an organ, or a cell.

poli- (polio-) *combining form denoting* the grey matter of the nervous system.

policeman's heel *see* PLANTAR FASCIITIS.

polioencephalitis *n.* a virus infection of the brain causing particular damage to the *grey matter of the cerebral hemispheres and the brainstem. The term is now usually restricted to infections of the brain by the poliomyelitis virus.

polioencephalomyelitis *n.* any virus infection of the central nervous system affecting the grey matter of the brain and spinal cord. *Rabies is the outstanding example.

poliomyelitis (infantile paralysis, polio) *n.* an infectious virus disease affecting the central nervous system. The virus is excreted in the faeces of an infected person and the disease is therefore most common where sanitation is poor. However, epidemics may occur in more hygienic conditions, where individuals have not acquired immunity to the disease during infancy. Symptoms commence 7–12 days after infection. In most cases paralysis does not occur: in **abortive poliomyelitis** only the throat and intestines are infected and the symptoms are those of a stomach upset or influenza; in **nonparalytic poliomyelitis** these symptoms are accompanied by muscle stiffness, particularly in the neck and back. **Paralytic poliomyelitis** is much less common. The symptoms of the milder forms of the disease are followed by weakness and eventual paralysis of the muscles: in **bulbar poliomyelitis** the muscles of the respiratory system are involved and breathing is affected. *See also* POST-POLIO SYNDROME.

There is no specific treatment, apart from measures to relieve the symptoms: cases of bulbar polio may require the use of a *ventilator. Immunization, using the *Sabin vaccine (taken orally) or the *Salk vaccine (injected), is highly effective.

poliovirus *n.* one of a small group of RNA-containing viruses causing *poliomyelitis. They are included within the *picornavirus group.

pollex *n.* (*pl.* **pollices**) the thumb.

pollinosis *n.* a more precise term than *hay fever for an allergy due to the pollen of grasses, trees, or shrubs.

poly- *combining form denoting* 1. many; multiple. 2. excessive. 3. generalized; affecting many parts.

polyarteritis nodosa (periarteritis nodosa) a disease of unknown cause in which there is patchy inflammation of the walls of the arteries. It is one of the *connective-tissue diseases. Common manifestations are arthritis, neuritis, asthma, skin rashes, hypertension, kidney failure, and fever. The inflammation is suppressed by corticosteroid drugs (such as prednisolone).

polyarthritis *n.* disease involving several to many joints, either together or in se-

quence, causing pain, stiffness, swelling, tenderness, and loss of function. *Rheumatoid arthritis is the most common cause.

polychromasia (polychromatophilia) *n.* the presence of certain blue red blood cells (*erythrocytes) seen in blood films stained with *Romanowsky stains, as well as the normal pink cells. The cells that appear blue are juvenile erythrocytes (*see* RETICULOCYTE).

polyclinic *n. see* HEALTH CENTRE.

polycoria *n.* a rare congenital abnormality of the eye in which there are one or more holes in the iris in addition to the pupil.

polycystic disease of the kidneys either of two inherited disorders in which renal cysts are a common feature. **Autosomal recessive polycystic kidney disease** (**ARPKD**) occurs in about 1 in 20,000 live births. It is due to a single mutation on chromosome 6 for the gene encoding the protein fibrocystin. The majority of cases are diagnosed before or at birth. The most severely affected fetuses have enlarged kidneys and *oligohydramnios due to poor fetal renal output. These fetuses develop the 'Potter' phenotype with characteristic facies, pulmonary hypoplasia, and deformities of the spine and limbs. Those surviving the neonatal period (50–70%) develop varying degrees of renal impairment but this may not proceed to end-stage until early adulthood. **Autosomal dominant polycystic kidney disease** (**ADPKD**) affects between 1 in 400 and 1 in 1000 individuals and is one of the most common hereditary diseases. Two types have been defined. ADPKD 1 is the commonest and responsible for about 85% of cases. It is due to a mutation in the *PKD1* gene on chromosome 16, which encodes **polycystin 1**, an *ion-channel-regulating protein. ADPKD2 is due to a mutation in the *PKD2* gene on chromosome 4, which encodes the protein **polycystin 2**, a calcium-release channel. ADPKD2 tends to be a milder disease with later presentation.

ADPKD is a multisystem disorder that is also associated with cyst formation in other organs (particularly the liver), cardiovascular disorders, and colonic diverticular disease. Renal disease presents in early adult life with haematuria, loin pain, urinary tract infection, hypertension, renal stone disease, or the finding of a mass in the abdomen. Other cases are identified by family contact tracing; the findings of a few cysts on renal ultrasonography in a young adult with a family history of ADPKD is highly suggestive of the disease. Renal disease is progressive and about 50% of patients will have reached end-stage by the time they enter their seventh decade. The progress of the renal failure can be slowed by good blood pressure control. In the UK, patients with ADPKD are responsible for 5–10% of the total on renal replacement therapy.

There are a number of separate rare autosomal dominant conditions other than ADPKD1 and ADPKD 2 that can present with polycystic kidneys. These include *von Hippel-Lindau disease and *tuberous sclerosis.

polycystic ovary (PCO) the presence of more than 12 follicles in each ovary (2–9 mm in diameter), or increased ovarian volume (>10 ml), or both. The presence of enlarged ovaries with multiple small cysts and a hypervascularized androgen-secreting stroma (connective tissue) is associated with signs of androgen excess (*see* POLYCYSTIC OVARY SYNDROME).

polycystic ovary syndrome (PCOS, Stein-Leventhal syndrome) a heterogeneous disorder characterized by *hyperandrogenism (clinical hirsutism, biochemical hyperandrogenism, or both) and ovarian dysfunction (with *polycystic ovaries), which results in amenorrhoea or oligomenorrhoea (absent or infrequent menstrual periods) and is associated with subfertility (from lack of ovulatory menstrual cycles). The condition is associated with obesity and *insulin resistance, which increase the risk of type 2 *diabetes mellitus, endometrial cancer, and cardiovascular disease. Treatment is based on dietary and exercise advice, *metformin, hormones to regulate the menstrual cycle, and in cases of subfertility, *clomifene to induce ovulation; the hyperandrogenism usually responds to *anti-androgens.

polycystin *n. see* POLYCYSTIC DISEASE OF THE KIDNEYS.

polycythaemia *n.* an increase in the *packed cell volume (haematocrit) in the blood. This may be due either to a decrease in the total volume of the plasma (**relative polycythaemia**) or to an increase in the total volume of the red cells (**absolute polycythaemia**). The latter may occur as a primary disease (*see* POLYCYTHAEMIA VERA) or as a secondary condition in association with various respiratory or circulatory disorders that cause deficiency of oxygen in the tissues and with certain tumours, such as carcinoma of the kidney.

polycythaemia vera (polycythaemia rubra vera, Vaquez-Osler disease) a disease in which the number of red cells in the blood is greatly increased (*see also* POLYCYTHAEMIA). There is often also an increase in the numbers of white blood cells and platelets. Symptoms include headache, thromboses, *cyanosis, *plethora, and itching. Polycythaemia vera may be treated by blood-letting, but more severe cases may need to be treated with cytotoxic drugs. The cause of the disease is not known.

polydactylism *n. see* HYPERDACTYLISM.

polydipsia *n.* abnormally intense thirst, leading to the drinking of large quantities of fluid. This is a symptom typical of *diabetes mellitus and *diabetes insipidus but it can occur in the absence of any metabolic abnormality (**psychogenic polydipsia**). *See also* WATER-DEPRIVATION TEST.

polygene *n.* one of a number of genes that together control a single characteristic in an individual. Each polygene has only a slight effect and the expression of a set of polygenes is the result of their combined interaction. Characteristics controlled by polygenes are usually of a quantitative nature, e.g. height. *See also* MULTIFACTORIAL. —**polygenic** *adj.*

polyhydramnios (hydramnios) *n.* an increase in the amount of *amniotic fluid surrounding the fetus, which occurs usually in the third *trimester and may be associated with maternal diabetes, multiple pregnancy, any fetal anomaly causing impaired swallowing, or placental abnormality.

polymastia *n. see* PLEOMASTIA.

polymer *n.* a substance formed by the linkage of a large number of smaller molecules known as **monomers**. An example of a monomer is glucose, whose molecules link together to form glycogen, a polymer. Polymers may have molecular weights from a few thousands to many millions. Polymers made up of a single type of monomer are known as **homopolymers**; those of two or more monomers as **heteropolymers**.

polymerase chain reaction (PCR) a

technique of molecular genetics in which a particular sequence of DNA can be isolated and amplified sufficiently to enable genetic analysis. The technique may be utilized, for example, in the identification of viruses in tissue samples, e.g. human papillomavirus in cervical smears.

polymorph (polymorphonuclear leuco-cyte) *n.* a type of white blood cell with a lobed nucleus. *See* BASOPHIL, EOSINOPHIL, NEUTROPHIL.

polymorphic eruption of pregnancy (PEP) intensely itchy papules and weals on the abdomen (except the umbilicus), upper limbs, and buttocks, usually within the *striae gravidarum; it is also known as **PUPPP** (pruritic urticarial papules and plaques of pregnancy). It occurs in 1 in 250 first pregnancies late in the third trimester. This condition is harmless to mother and baby, but can be very annoying. It lasts an average of 6 weeks and resolves spontaneously 1–2 weeks after delivery. The most severe itching normally lasts for no more than a week.

polymorphous light eruption *see* PHO-TODERMATOSIS.

polymorphism *n.* (in genetics) the occurrence of a chromosome or a genetic character in more than one form, resulting in the coexistence of more than one morphological type in the same population.

polymyalgia rheumatica a rheumatic disease causing aching and progressive stiffness of the muscles of the shoulders and hips after inactivity. These symptoms are typically associated with loss of appetite, fatigue, night sweats, and a raised *ESR. The condition is most common in the elderly, rarely occurring before the age of 50. The symptoms respond rapidly and effectively to corticosteroid treatment, which must usually be continued for several years. It is sometimes associated with temporal *arteritis.

polymyositis *n.* a generalized disease of the muscles that may be acute or chronic. It particularly affects the muscles of the shoulder and hip girdles, which are weak and tender to the touch. Microscopic examination of the affected muscles shows diffuse inflammatory changes; treatment is with *corticosteroids and other immunosuppressant drugs. The skin may be reddened and atrophic. *See also* DERMATOMYOSITIS.

polymyxin B an *antibiotic used to treat severe infections caused by Gram-negative bacteria. Formulated with other drugs, it is administered as a solution or ointment for ear, eye, and skin infections.

polyneuritis *n. see* PERIPHERAL NEUROPA-THY.

polyneuropathy *n. see* PERIPHERAL NEU-ROPATHY.

polynucleotide *n.* a long chain of linked *nucleotides, of which molecules of DNA and RNA are made.

polyopia *n.* the sensation of multiple images of one object. It is sometimes experienced by people with early cataract. *See also* DIPLOPIA.

polyorchidism *n.* a congenital abnormality resulting in more than two testes.

polyp (polypus) *n.* a growth, usually benign, protruding from a mucous membrane. Polyps are commonly found in the nose and sinuses, giving rise to obstruction, chronic infection, and discharge. They are often present in patients with allergic rhinitis, in whom they may develop in response to long-term antigenic stimulation. Other sites of occurrence include the ear, the stomach, and the colon. Colonic polyps in the adult population are common above the age of 50 and approximately 25% are multiple. Adenomatous colonic polyps have malignant potential, which often is associated with large size (>1 cm). Colonoscopy helps to detect and remove colonic polyps. **Juvenile polyps** occur in the intestine (usually colon or rectum) of infants or young people; sometimes they are multiple (**juvenile polyposis**). In the latter form there is a risk of malignant change (25% of cases) but most juvenile polyps are benign (*see also* POLYPOSIS, PEUTZ-JEGHERS SYN-DROME). Polyps are usually removed endoscopically (*see* POLYPECTOMY); polyps that are large, difficult to remove, or malignant need bowel surgery.

polypectomy *n.* the endoscopic or surgical removal of a *polyp. The technique used depends upon the site and size of the polyp. Endoscopically, polyps can be removed by various methods. A **hot biopsy** involves coagulation of a small polyp with a *diathermy current and obtaining a specimen at the same time. **Snare polypectomy** is done by cutting across the base using a wire loop (snare) through which a coagulating *diathermy current is passed to reduce the risk of bleeding while cutting the polyp tissue. **Cold biopsy** involves removal of a very small polyp using forceps without diathermy, decreasing the perforation risk. **Endoscopic mucosal resection** (EMR) involves lifting a flat polyp in the mucosa by injecting a hypertonic solution under the polyp followed by snare polypectomy with diathermy.

polypeptide *n.* a molecule consisting of three or more amino acids linked together by *peptide bonds. *Protein molecules are polypeptides.

polyphagia *n.* gluttonous excessive eating.

polypharmacy *n.* treatment of a patient with more than one type of medicine.

polyphyletic *adj.* describing a number of individuals, species, etc., that have evolved from more than one ancestral group. *Compare* MONOPHYLETIC.

polyploid *adj.* describing cells, tissues, or individuals in which there are three or more complete sets of chromosomes. *Compare* DIPLOID, HAPLOID. —**polyploidy** *n.*

polypoid *adj.* having the appearance of a *polyp.

polyposis *n.* a condition in which numerous *polyps form in an organ or tissue. **Familial adenomatous polyposis** (**FAP**) is a hereditary disease (caused by a defective dominant gene) in which multiple *adenomas develop in the intestine, usually the large bowel or rectum, at an early age. As these polyps almost invariably become malignant, patients are usually advised to undergo total removal of the affected bowel. *See also* PEUTZ-JEGHERS SYNDROME. *Compare* HEREDITARY NONPOLYPOSIS COLORECTAL CANCER, PSEUDOPOLYPOSIS.

polypus *n. see* POLYP.

polyradiculitis (polyradiculopathy) *n.* any disorder of the peripheral nerves (*see* NEUROPATHY) in which the brunt of the disease falls on the nerve roots where they emerge from the spinal cord. An abnormal allergic response in the nerve fibres is thought to be one cause of this condition; the *Guillain-Barré syndrome is an example. Other causes include infections (such as syphilis), herpesviruses, and tumours (such as lymphoma or other forms of cancer).

polyribosome *n. see* POLYSOME.

polysaccharide *n.* a *carbohydrate formed from many monosaccharides joined together in long linear or branched chains. Polysaccharides have two important functions: (1) as storage forms of energy; for example *glycogen in animals and *starch in plants, and (2) as structural elements; for example *mucopolysaccharides in animals and *cellulose in plants.

polyserositis *n.* inflammation of the membranes that line the chest, abdomen, and joints, with accumulation of fluid in the cavities. Commonly the condition is inherited and intermittent and is termed **familial Mediterranean fever**. If complicated by infiltration of major organs by a glycoprotein (*see* AMYLOIDOSIS) the disease usually proves fatal. Regular administration of colchicine will prevent the attacks in 95% of patients.

polysome (polyribosome) *n.* a structure that occurs in the cytoplasm of cells and consists of a group of *ribosomes linked together by *messenger RNA molecules: formed during protein synthesis.

polysomnograph *n.* a record of measurements of various bodily parameters during sleep. It is used in the diagnosis of sleep disorders, such as *obstructive sleep apnoea.

polyspermia *n.* 1. excessive formation of semen. 2. *see* POLYSPERMY.

polyspermy (polyspermia) *n.* fertilization of a single ovum by more than one spermatozoon: the development is abnormal and the embryo dies.

polythelia *n.* a congenital excess of nipples (*see* PLEOMASTIA).

polyuria *n.* the production of large volumes of urine, which is dilute and of a pale colour. The phenomenon may be due simply to excessive liquid intake or to disease, particularly diabetes mellitus, diabetes insipidus, and kidney disorders.

pompholyx *n.* *eczema of the hands (*see also* CHEIROPOMPHOLYX) and feet (**podopompholyx**). Because the horny layer of the skin in these parts is so thick, the vesicles typical of eczema cannot rupture; they therefore persist in the skin, looking like sago grains. There is intense itching until the skin eventually peels. There may be secondary infection due to scratching. Pompholyx is commonest in early adulthood and attacks occur suddenly, lasting some weeks. The disease may be recurrent or persist as a chronic condition.

pons *n.* 1. (pons Varolii) the part of the *brainstem that links the medulla oblongata and the thalamus, bulging forwards in front of the cerebellum, from which it is separated by the fourth ventricle. It contains numerous nerve tracts between the cerebral cortex and the spinal cord and several nuclei of grey matter. From its front surface the *trigeminal nerves emerge. 2. any portion of tissue that joins two parts of an organ.

pontic *n.* (in dentistry) *see* BRIDGE.

popliteus *n.* a flat triangular muscle at the back of the knee joint, between the femur and tibia, that helps to flex the knee. —**popliteal** *adj.*

porcelain *n.* (in dentistry) a ceramic material that is used to construct tooth-coloured crowns, inlays, or veneers.

pore *n.* a small opening; for example, **sweat pores** are the openings of the sweat glands on the surface of the skin.

porencephaly *n.* an abnormal communication between the lateral *ventricle and the surface of the brain. This is usually a consequence of brain injury or cerebrovascular disease; uncommonly it may be a developmental defect, when it would most likely affect both lateral ventricles.

porfimer sodium *see* PHOTODYNAMIC THERAPY.

porocephaliasis *n.* a rare infestation of the nasal cavities, windpipe, lungs, liver, or spleen by the nymphs of the parasitic arthropod *Porocephalus*. Humans become infected on consumption of water or uncooked vegetables contaminated with the parasite's eggs. There may be some abdominal pain while the parasite is in the gut but in many cases there are no symptoms.

Porocephalus *n.* a genus of wormlike arthropods occurring mainly in tropical Africa and India. The legless adults are parasites in the lungs of snakes. The eggs, which are ejected with the snake's bronchial secretions, may be accidentally swallowed by humans. The larva bores through the gut wall and usually migrates to the liver, where it develops into a nymph (*see* POROCEPHALIASIS).

porphin *n.* a complex nitrogen-containing ring structure and parent compound of the *porphyrins.

porphobilinogen *n.* a pigment that appears in the urine of individuals with acute *porphyria, causing it to darken if left standing.

porphyria *n.* one of a group of rare disorders due to *inborn errors of metabolism in which there are deficiencies in the enzymes involved in the biosynthesis of haem. The accumulation of the enzyme's substrate gives rise to symptoms of the disorder. The defect may be primarily in the liver (**hepatic porphyria**) or in the bone marrow (**erythropoietic porphyria**) or both. The prominent features include the excretion of *porphyrins and their derivatives in the urine, which may change colour on standing (*see* PORPHOBILINOGEN); sensitivity of the skin to sunlight causing chronic inflammation or blistering; inflammation of the nerves (neuritis); mental disturbances; and attacks of abdominal pain. The commonest porphyria is **porphyria cutanea tarda**, which affects up to 1 in 5000 people in some countries. It is a hereditary or acquired hepatic porphyria in which light-exposed areas of the skin become blistered and fragile. **Acute intermittent porphyria** is a hereditary hepatic porphyria characterized by recurrent attacks of acute abdominal pain, severe constipation, and psychotic behaviour. Factors triggering attacks include alcohol and many drugs.

porphyrin *n.* one of a number of pigments derived from *porphin, which are widely distributed in living things. All porphyrins form chelates with iron, magnesium, zinc, nickel, copper, and cobalt. These chelates are constituents of *haemoglobin, *myoglobin, the *cytochromes, and chlorophyll, and are thus important in many oxidation/reduction reactions in all living organisms. *See also* PROTOPORPHYRIN IX.

porphyrinuria *n.* the presence in the urine of breakdown products of the red blood pigment haemoglobin (porphyrins), sometimes causing discoloration. *See* PORPHYRIA, PORPHOBILINOGEN.

porta *n.* the aperture in an organ through which its associated vessels pass. Such an opening occurs in the liver (**porta hepatis**).

portable *adj.* (in radiography) referring to images obtained using light-weight equipment, away from the main department. The quality of portable radiographs is usually limited due to compromises in the equipment design to keep it light and movable, which is necessary when patients cannot easily be moved (for example, on intensive therapy units).

portacaval anastomosis (portacaval shunt) **1.** a surgical technique in which the hepatic portal vein is joined to the inferior vena cava. Blood draining from the abdominal viscera is thus diverted past the liver. It is used in the treatment of *portal hypertension, since – by lowering the pressure within the veins of the stomach and oesophagus – it prevents serious bleeding into the gastrointestinal tract. **2.** any of the natural communications between the branches of the hepatic portal vein in the liver and the inferior vena cava.

portal *adj.* **1.** relating to the portal vein or system. **2.** relating to a porta.

portal hypertension a state in which the pressure within the hepatic *portal vein is increased, causing enlargement of the spleen, enlargement of veins in the oesophagus (gullet) (which may rupture to cause severe bleeding), and accumulation of fluid in the peritoneal cavity (ascites). The commonest cause is *cirrhosis, but other diseases of the liver or thrombosis of the portal vein will also produce it. Treatment is by *diuretic drugs, by surgery to join the portal vein to the inferior vena cava (bypassing the liver; *see* PORTACAVAL ANASTOMOSIS), or by implanting a *stent within the liver to join portal tract veins to a hepatic vein tributary (**TIPSS – transjugular intrahepatic porto-systemic shunt**).

portal image an electronic image taken during radiotherapy treatment to verify the position of radiation beams.

portal system a vein or group of veins that terminates at both ends in a capillary bed. The best known is the **hepatic portal system**, which consists of the *portal vein and its tributaries (see illustration). Blood is drained from the spleen, stomach, pancreas, and small and large intestines into veins that merge to form the portal vein leading to the liver. Here the portal vein branches, ending in many small capillaries called *sinusoids. These permit the passage into the liver cells of nutrients absorbed by blood from the intestines.

portal vein a short vein, about 8 cm long,

forming part of the hepatic *portal system. It receives many tributaries, including the splenic vein from the spleen and pancreas, the gastric vein from the stomach, the mesenteric vein from the small and large intestines, and the rectal vein from the rectum and anus.

port-wine stain *see* NAEVUS.

positive-pressure ventilation *see* NON-INVASIVE VENTILATION.

positive symptoms (in psychiatry) symptoms of schizophrenia characterized by a distortion of some aspect of functioning, such as delusions, hallucinations, or disordered speech. *Compare* NEGATIVE SYMPTOMS.

positron *n.* an electrically charged particle released in some radioactive decays, notably fluorine-18 or nitrogen-13, that has the same mass as an electron but opposite charge. It has a very short lifetime as it quickly reacts with an electron to produce a pair of *gamma rays, which are emitted in diametrically opposite directions. The energy of each gamma ray is always 511 keV.

positron emission tomography (PET, positron emission computed tomography, PECT) a technique in nuclear medicine for *cross-sectional imaging that enables a noninvasive assessment and localization of metabolic activity to be made. Originally used to study activity in the brain, PET is now also used for investigating the chest and abdomen. Emission of a *positron by a radioisotope results in annihilation of

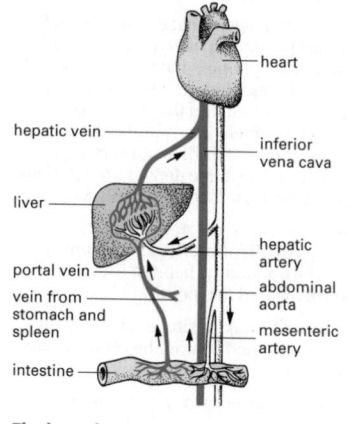

The hepatic portal system.

the positron on collision with an electron, and the creation of two gamma rays of known energy travelling in exactly opposite directions. The PET scanner has detectors on each side of the patient to detect the simultaneous arrival of the gamma rays. Images are created using reconstruction *algorithms similar to CT scanning. *Fluorodeoxyglucose, labelled with fluorine-18, is used to examine glucose metabolism, and ammonia, labelled with nitrogen-13, gives information on perfusion. Carbon-11 and oxygen-15 can also be used as radioisotopes for PET scanning. Some diseases result in decreased uptake of the radio-labelled material due to decreased function; others show increased glucose metabolism and concentrate the isotope avidly. In this way functional activity of the tissues can be compared with anatomical images obtained by CT or MRI scanning (*see* PET/CT SCANNING). Localized areas of increased glucose uptake revealed by PET scans can sometimes signify functional activity of malignant cells, which use more glucose than normal cells, although other processes, such as infection, can produce similar scans. PET scans can help to localize metastatic disease (*see* METASTASIS) that is not identified by other scanning techniques. *See also* TOMOGRAPHY. *Compare* COMPUTERIZED TOMOGRAPHY.

posology *n.* the science of the dosage of medicines.

posset *n.* a small amount of milk that is regurgitated, usually with some wind, by many babies after feeding.

Possum *n.* a device that enables severely paralysed patients to use typewriters, adding machines, telephones, and a wide variety of other machines. Modern Possums are operated by micro-switches that require only the slightest movement in any limb. The original device worked by blowing and sucking a mouthpiece. The name derives from **Patient-Operated Selector Mechanism** (**POSM**).

post- *prefix denoting* 1. following; after. Example: **postepileptic** (after an epileptic attack). 2. (in anatomy) behind. Example: **postoral** (behind the mouth).

postcentral *adj.* 1. situated behind any centre. 2. situated behind the central fissure of the brain.

postcibal *adj.* occurring after eating.

postcoital bleeding genital-tract bleeding in females occurring after sexual intercourse. This is an important symptom and may be caused by sexually transmitted infections, vaginal candidiasis, atrophic *vaginitis, cervical *ectropion, cervical polyp, or cervical cancer.

postcoital contraception (emergency contraception) prevention of pregnancy after intercourse has taken place. This can be achieved by two methods, which aim to prevent implantation of the fertilized ovum in the uterus: (1) two spaced oral doses of *levonorgestrel (**Levonelle**) taken within 72 hours of unprotected intercourse; and (2) insertion of an *IUCD within five days of unprotected intercourse.

postcoital test a test used in the investigation of infertility. A specimen of cervical mucus, taken 6–24 hours after coitus, is examined under a microscope. The appearance of 10 or more progressively motile spermatozoa per high-power field in the specimen indicates that there is no abnormal reaction between spermatozoa and mucus. The test should be undertaken in the postovulatory phase of the menstrual cycle.

posterior *adj.* situated at or near the back of the body or an organ. The **posterior chamber** of the eye is the rear section, behind the lens, which is filled with vitreous humour.

postero- *combining form denoting* posterior. Example: **posterolateral** (behind and at the side of).

posteroanterior (PA) *adj.* from the back to the front. In radiography it refers to the direction of the X-ray beam (i.e. from the back to the front of the patient); thus a PA radiograph is taken with the X-ray film in front of the patient. Normally, a chest radiograph will be PA: since the heart is in the front of the chest, its size can be most accurately assessed if the X-ray film is in front of the chest. *Compare* DECUBITUS, ANTEROPOSTERIOR.

postganglionic *adj.* describing a neuron in a nerve pathway that starts at a ganglion and ends at the muscle or gland that it supplies. In the sympathetic nervous system, postganglionic fibres are *adrenergic, unlike those in the parasympathetic system, which are *cholinergic. *Compare* PREGANGLIONIC.

postgastrectomy syndrome *see* DUMPING SYNDROME.

posthitis *n.* inflammation of the foreskin. This usually occurs in association with inflammation of the glans penis (**balanitis**; *see* BALANOPOSTHITIS). Pain, redness, and swelling of the foreskin occurs due to bacterial infection. Treatment is by antibiotic administration, and subsequent *circumcision prevents further attacks.

posthumous birth 1. delivery of a child by *Caesarean section after the mother's death. 2. birth of a child after the father's death.

postmature *adj.* describing a baby born after 42 weeks of gestation (calculated from the first day of the last menstrual period). Such a birth can be associated with maternal diabetes or with *anencephaly in the fetus. —**postmaturity** *n.*

postmenopausal bleeding (PMB) bleeding from the female genital tract occurring more than 12 months after the last menstrual period. Endometrial cancer is present in 10% cases, and atrophic *vaginitis is also a common cause.

postmenopause *n.* the period of a woman's life after the *menopause. The term 'menopause' is often used in reference to the postmenopausal period.

postmicturition dribble a *lower urinary tract symptom in which a dribble occurs after voiding has been completed, often after leaving the toilet. It is quite common in men but is not caused by benign prostatic hyperplasia.

post mortem Latin: after death. *See* AUTOPSY.

postnasal space *see* NASOPHARYNX.

postnatal depression *depression that starts after childbirth. *Bonding between the mother and child can be impaired (particularly in the case of male children), leading to *attachment disorders if the illness is not diagnosed and treated. Postnatal depression occurs in about 10% of women (in the UK women are routinely screened for it after childbirth) and responds to the treatment strategies used for other forms of depression, such as *antidepressant medication and *cognitive behavioural therapy; in rare cases hospital admission is needed. *Compare* BABY BLUES, PUERPERAL PSYCHOSIS.

postoperative *adj.* following surgery: referring to the condition of a patient or to the treatment given at this time.

postpartum *adj.* relating to the period of a few days immediately after birth.

postpartum blues *see* BABY BLUES.

postpartum haemorrhage (PPH) excessive bleeding (>500 ml) from the genital tract after delivery. Primary PPH occurs within 24 hours of delivery; secondary PPH occurs after 24 hours. Atonic PPH is due to failure of the uterus to contract after delivery; it may be caused by retained products of conception or may occur after a long labour. *See also* B-LYNCH BRACE SUTURE, RUSCH CATHETER.

post-polio syndrome insidious numbness in muscles that develops 15–20 years after an attack of *poliomyelitis; the muscles may or may not have been previously affected. It may be caused by loss of nerve cells that have been under greater strain than normal as a result of the polio; there is no evidence of reactivation of the poliovirus. The syndrome also includes other symptoms, such as fatigue and pain, which may be due to secondary mechanical causes.

postprandial *adj.* occurring after eating.

post-processing *n.* (in radiology) the electronic manipulation of digitally acquired images (*see* DIGITIZATION) following an examination in order to improve diagnostic accuracy.

postresuscitation care medical care given to an individual who has survived a *cardiac arrest. This will usually consist of a 12-lead electrocardiogram (*see* LEAD[2]), a chest X-ray, a number of venous and arterial blood tests, and transfer to a high-dependency or coronary care unit for further intensive monitoring and drug administration.

post-term pregnancy a pregnancy that has gone beyond 42 weeks gestation or 294 days from the first date of the last menstrual period.

post-traumatic stress disorder (PTSD) an anxiety disorder caused by a major physical or emotional trauma, such as an injury, assault, rape, or exposure to warfare or a disaster involving many casualties. The onset is at least one month after the traumatic event. The patient experiences the persistent recurrence of images or memories of the event, together with nightmares, insomnia, a sense of isolation, guilt, irritability, and loss of concentration. Emotions may be deadened and depression may develop. The condition usually settles with time, but support and skilled counselling may be needed. More severe cases may be treated by *eye movement desensitization and reprocessing therapy (EMDR), *cognitive behavioural therapy, and/or *SSRIs.

postural hypotension *see* HYPOTENSION.

postural muscles (antigravity muscles) muscles (principally extensors) that serve to maintain the upright posture of the body against the force of gravity.

postviral fatigue syndrome *see* CFS/ME/PVF.

potassium *n.* a mineral element and an important constituent of the human body. It is the main base ion of intracellular fluid. Together with *sodium, it helps to maintain the electrical potential of the nervous system and is thus essential for the functioning of nerve and muscle. Normal blood levels are between 3.5 and 5 mmols/litre. High concentrations occur particularly in kidney failure and may lead to *arrhythmia and finally to cardiac arrest. Low values result from fluid loss, e.g. due to vomiting or diarrhoea, and this may lead to general muscle paralysis. Symbol: K.

potassium-channel activator any one of a class of drugs that enhance the movement of potassium ions through the *ion channels in cell membranes. In the case of smooth muscle cells, such as those in the walls of arteries, their sensitivity to the normal stimuli to contract is reduced. The result is relaxation of the muscle fibres and widening of the arteries. Potassium-channel activators are used for improving the blood supply to the heart muscle in angina pectoris. Possible side-effects include headache, flushing, vomiting, dizziness, and weakness. A currently available member of the class is **nicorandil** (Ikorel), administered orally.

potassium chloride a salt of potassium used to prevent and treat potassium deficiency, especially during treatment with digoxin or anti-arrhythmic drugs. It is administered by mouth; some irritation in the digestive system may occur. Severe potassium deficiency may be treated by intravenous infusion. Trade names: **Kay-Cee-L**, **Sando-K**, **Slow-K**.

potassium permanganate a salt of potassium having antiseptic and astringent properties. Potassium permanganate solution is applied to the skin to treat weeping eczema. It irritates mucous membranes and is poisonous if taken into the body. Trade name: **Permitabs**.

Potter syndrome a congenital condition characterized by absence of kidneys, resulting in decreased amniotic fluid (*see* OLIGOHYDRAMNIOS) and compression of the fetus. Babies have poorly developed lungs, a characteristic wrinkled and flattened facial appearance, and leg deformities and do not usually survive. [E. L. Potter (20th century), US pathologist]

Pott's disease *tuberculosis of the backbone. Untreated, it can lead to a hunchback deformity. Treatment is antituberculous chemotherapy and occasionally surgery. [P. Pott (1714–88), British surgeon]

pouch *n.* **1.** (in anatomy) a small sac-like structure, especially occurring as an outgrowth of a larger structure. The **pouch of Douglas** is a pouch of peritoneum occupying the space between the rectum and uterus. **2.** (in surgery) a sac created from a loop of intestine and used to replace a section of rectum that has been surgically removed, for example for ulcerative colitis (*see* ILEAL POUCH), or to replace the bladder after *cystectomy.

poultice (fomentation) *n.* a preparation of hot moist material applied to any part of the body to increase local circulation, alleviate pain, or soften the skin to allow matter to be expressed from a boil. Poultices containing kaolin retain heat for a considerable period during use.

Poupart's ligament *see* INGUINAL LIGAMENT. [F. Poupart (1661–1708), French anatomist]

poverty of speech brief hesitant speech using few words (often monosyllables) and lacking spontaneity. It occurs in patients with schizophrenia and depression.

powder *n.* (in pharmacy) a medicinal preparation consisting of a mixture of two or more drugs in the form of fine particles.

power of attorney *see* LASTING POWER OF ATTORNEY.

pox *n.* **1.** an infectious disease causing a

skin rash. **2.** a rash of pimples that become pus-filled, as in *chickenpox and *smallpox.

poxvirus *n.* one of a group of large DNA-containing viruses including those that cause *smallpox (variola) and *cowpox (vaccinia) in humans, and pox and tumours in animals.

PPH *see* POSTPARTUM HAEMORRHAGE.

PPI forum (in England) patient and public involvement forum: *see* LOCAL INVOLVEMENT NETWORKS.

PPROM preterm prelabour (or premature) rupture of membranes: spontaneous rupture of fetal membranes prior to 37 weeks gestation in the absence of regular painful contractions.

practice-based commissioning (PBC) a new initiative across England that will result in a change in financial flows. Since April 2005 all practices or groups of practices have been eligible to receive their own budget from the primary care trust (PCT) to commission services to suit the needs of the local community. Unlike the old fundholding system, PBC is intended to be less bureaucratic, more equitable, and focused on improving the quality of patient care. It is being implemented in a variety of ways under the direction of individual PCTs.

practice manager the person responsible for running a doctor's surgery, whose role involves managing staff, accounts, and medical records as well as developing the practice's business strategy. Practice managers also liaise with external bodies, such as local NHS trusts and social service departments, to ensure efficient communication between the various organizations.

practice nurse a trained nurse caring for the patients of one or more general practitioners in the consulting room and on domiciliary consultations. In Britain, practice nurses are usually employed directly by GPs. However, they may also be employed by *primary care trusts as practice nurses or *district nurses.

Prader orchidometer *see* ORCHIDOMETER.

Prader-Willi syndrome (Prader-Willi-Labhart syndrome) a congenital condition that is inherited as an autosomal *dominant trait and is due to an abnormality of chromosome 15 (*see* IMPRINTING). It is marked by pathological overeating and resulting obesity (affected children often subsequently develop type 2 diabetes), lethargy, short stature, a characteristic facial expression, learning disabilities, and underactivity of the testes or ovaries (*hypogonadism) due to lack of pituitary gonadotrophins. It is a cause of delayed puberty. [A. Prader, H. Willi, and A. Labhart (20th century), Swiss paediatricians]

pravastatin *n.* a drug used to reduce abnormally high levels of cholesterol and other lipids in the blood (*see* STATIN). Its actions and side-effects are similar to those of *atorvastatin. Trade name: **Lipostat**.

praziquantel *n.* an *anthelmintic drug used to eliminate tapeworms and schistosomes. It is administered by mouth. Possible side-effects include nausea, abdominal discomfort, fever, sweating, and drowsiness. Trade name: **Cysticide**.

prazosin *n.* a drug used in the treatment of high blood pressure (hypertension) and also to relieve urinary retention due to benign enlargement of the *prostate gland (*see* ALPHA BLOCKER). It is administered by mouth; common side-effects include dizziness, headache, palpitations, and nausea. Trade name: **Hypovase**.

pre- *prefix denoting* **1.** before; preceding. Example: **premenstrual** (before menstruation); **prenatal** (before birth). **2.** (in anatomy) in front of; anterior to. Example: **precardiac** (in front of the heart); prepatellar (in front of the patella).

pre-agonal *adj.* relating to the phenomena that precede the moment of death. *See also* AGONAL.

precancerous *adj.* describing a nonmalignant condition that is known to become malignant if left untreated. *Leukoplakia of the vulva is known to be a precancerous condition. *See also* METAPLASIA.

precipitin *n.* any antibody that combines with its antigen to form a complex that comes out of solution and is seen as a precipitate. The antibody-antigen reaction is specific; the precipitin reaction is therefore a useful means of confirming the identity of an unknown antigen or establishing that a serum contains antibodies to a known disease. This test may be performed in watery solution or in a semisolid medium such as agar gel. *See also* AGGLUTINATION.

precipitinogen *n.* any antigen that is precipitated from solution by a *precipitin.

precision attachment (in dentistry) a special machined joint that holds certain types of partial *dentures in place. The attachment is in two parts, one fixed to the denture and the other fixed to a crown on one of the teeth abutting the denture.

precocious puberty the development at an early age of the physical and physiological changes associated with *puberty. In girls this is usually taken as development of breasts or pubic hair before the age of six or menstruation before the age of eight. In boys development of pubic hair or other adult sexual features below the age of nine is considered to be precocious. In girls 90% of cases have no underlying abnormalities, but in boys approximately half have a serious underlying cause, of which malignant testicular tumours and malignant adrenal tumours are the most common.

precocity *n.* an acceleration of normal development. The intellectually precocious child has a high IQ and may become isolated from his or her contemporaries or frustrated at school. —**precocious** *adj.*

precordial thump a thump delivered directly to the chest wall over the heart as the first stage in treatment of a *cardiac arrest if the arrest has been witnessed (i.e. just happened) and monitored (i.e. diagnosis is immediately confirmed). The shock in that early stage can depolarize enough of the heart muscle to allow the normal *pacemaker systems within the heart to take over and restore normal cardiac output.

precordium *n.* the region of the thorax immediately over the heart. —**precordial** *adj.*

precuneus *n.* an area of the inner surface of the cerebral hemisphere on each side, above and in front of the *corpus callosum. *See* CEREBRUM.

predisposition *n.* a tendency to be affected by a particular disease or kind of disease. Such a tendency may be hereditary or may arise because of such factors as lack of vitamins, food, or sleep. *See also* DIATHESIS.

prednisolone *n.* a synthetic *corticosteroid used to treat rheumatic diseases, inflammatory and allergic conditions (e.g. inflammatory bowel disease and asthma), and some cancers (e.g. leukaemia, lymphoma). It is administered by mouth or rectally, injected into joints or muscles, or applied in drops (to treat eye or ear conditions). Side-effects are those of *cortisone. Trade names: **Deltacortril Enteric, Deltastab, Minims Prednisolone Sodium Phosphate, Predenema, Predfoam, Predsol**.

pre-eclampsia *n.* the combination of *pregnancy-induced hypertension and *proteinuria (>0.3 g in 24 hours) with or without oedema. *See also* ECLAMPSIA, HELLP SYNDROME.

prefrontal lobe the region of the brain at the very front of each cerebral hemisphere (*see* FRONTAL LOBE). The functions of the lobe are concerned with emotions, memory, learning, and social behaviour. Nerve tracts in the lobe are cut during the operation of prefrontal *leucotomy.

pregabalin *n. see* GABAPENTIN.

preganglionic *adj.* describing fibres in a nerve pathway that end in a ganglion, where they form synapses with *postganglionic fibres that continue the pathway to the effector organ, muscle or gland.

pre-gangrene *n.* the penultimate stage of vascular insufficiency before *gangrene sets in; the term is usually applied to *ischaemia of the lower limb.

pregestational diabetes pre-existing diabetes mellitus in a woman who becomes pregnant. Pregnancy has profound effects on diabetic control and insulin requirements, which are almost doubled, and hypoglycaemia is more common. There is an increased risk of many complications, including fetal *macrosomia and *shoulder dystocia, and pre-eclampsia is twice as common in diabetic pregnancies. *Polyhydramnios and preterm labour are also more common. Even in well-controlled cases, delivery is normally indicated approximately two weeks before the estimated date due to the size of the baby and falling insulin requirements with late gestation, which can affect the uteroplacental flow.

pregnancy *n.* the period during which a woman carries a developing fetus, normally in the uterus (*compare* ECTOPIC PREGNANCY). Pregnancy lasts for approximately 266 days, from *conception until the baby is born, or 280 days from the first day of the last menstrual period (*see* NAEGELE RULE). During pregnancy menstruation is absent, there may be a great increase in appetite, and the breasts increase in size; the woman may also experience *morning sickness. These and other changes are brought about by a hormone (*progesterone) produced at first by the ovary and later by the *placenta. Definite evidence of pregnancy is provided by various *pregnancy tests, by the detection of the heartbeat of the fetus, and by ultrasound. Medical name: **cyesis**. See also PSEUDOCYESIS (PHANTOM PREGNANCY). —**pregnant** adj.

pregnancy-induced hypertension (PIH) raised blood pressure (>140/90 mmHg) developing in a woman during the second half of pregnancy. It usually resolves within six weeks of delivery and is associated with a better prognosis than *pre-eclampsia.

pregnancy test any of several methods used to demonstrate whether or not a woman is pregnant. Most pregnancy tests are based on the detection of a hormone, *human chorionic gonadotrophin (hCG), in the urine. The sample of urine is mixed with serum containing antibodies to hCG and marker particles (sheep red cells or latex particles) coated with hCG. In the absence of pregnancy, the antibodies will cause *agglutination of the marker particles. If the urine is from a pregnant woman, the antibodies will be absorbed and no agglutination will occur. These tests may be positive for pregnancy as early as 30 days after the date of the last normal period and are 98% accurate. Newer tests using *monoclonal antibodies (**beta hCG**) are more easily interpreted. When carried out on serum rather than urine, these tests give even earlier positive results.

pregnanediol n. a steroid that is formed during the metabolism of the female sex hormone *progesterone. It occurs in the urine during pregnancy and certain phases of the menstrual cycle.

pregnenolone n. a steroid synthesized in the adrenal glands, ovaries, and testes. Pregnenolone is an important intermediate product in steroid hormone synthesis and can – depending on the pathways followed – be converted to corticosteroids (glucocorticoids or mineralocorticoids), androgens, or oestrogens.

preimplantation genetic diagnosis (PGD) a diagnostic procedure carried out on embryos at the earliest stage of development, before implantation in the uterus. Access to these early embryos requires the *in vitro fertilization of egg cells: three days after fertilization one or two cells are aspirated from the six-cell embryo; alternatively, tissue is removed from an embryo at five or six days, when it has reached the *blastocyst stage. Isolated cells can then be genetically analysed, allowing the transfer of selected embryos to the mother. One of the major applications of PGD is for the detection (using the *FISH technique) of chromosomal abnormalities, especially *aneuploidies (e.g. Down's syndrome), and the procedure is used mainly in women who have had repeated miscarriages or have failed to achieve pregnancy after several IVF treatment cycles, which could be due to the presence of such abnormalities in the embryo. PGD can also be used to detect defective genes responsible for hereditary disorders (e.g. the commonest form of cystic fibrosis, Huntington's disease) and genes associated with susceptibility to certain cancers. When a defect is detected, *genetic counselling is offered.

premature beat see ECTOPIC BEAT.

premature birth see PRETERM BIRTH.

premature ejaculation emission of semen (and consequent loss of erection) before insertion of the penis into the vagina or immediately afterwards.

premature ovarian failure menopause occurring before the age of 40. It may be caused by autoimmunity, chemotherapy, radiotherapy, or genetic factors, for example a mutation in the FSH receptor gene causing excess secretion of gonadotrophins and small underdeveloped ovaries. Treatment is by hormone replacement, either with the contraceptive pill or HRT. *Oocyte donation should be discussed if the patient wishes it.

premature rupture of membranes see PROM, PPROM.

premedication n. drugs administered to a patient before an operation (usually one in which an anaesthetic is used). Premedication usually comprises injection of a sedative (such as a *benzodiazepine, to calm the patient down, together with a drug, such as *hyoscine, to dry up the secretions of the lungs (which might otherwise be inhaled during anaesthesia).

premenstrual syndrome (PMS) a group of symptoms experienced in varying degrees by women of reproductive age in the week before menstruation. These include altered mental stability, fatigue, bloating, breast tenderness, and headaches. Since social and work functioning and family life can be severely affected, medical help is often sought. Treatments include stress management, salt restriction and low-dose diuretics to relieve fluid retention, and analgesia for aches and pains; hormone therapy with progestogens, combined oral contraceptives, and *gonadorelin analogues may be required.

premolar *n.* either of the two teeth on each side of each jaw behind the canines and in front of the molars in the adult *dentition.

premyelocyte *n. see* PROMYELOCYTE.

prenatal diagnosis (antenatal diagnosis) diagnostic procedures carried out on pregnant women in order to detect the presence of genetic or other abnormalities in the developing fetus. Ultrasound scanning (*see* ULTRASONOGRAPHY) remains the cornerstone of prenatal diagnosis. Other procedures include chromosome and enzyme analysis of fetal cells obtained by *amniocentesis or, at an earlier stage of pregnancy, by *chorionic villus sampling (CVS). *Compare* PRENATAL SCREENING.

prenatal screening *screening tests carried out to estimate the risk of chromosomal or other abnormalities being present in a developing fetus. They include blood tests to measure levels of *human chorionic gonadotrophin (hCG), *PAPP-A, *alpha-fetoprotein (AFP), and *unconjugated oestriol (uE$_3$) (*see also* TRIPLE TEST) and also ultrasound scanning for the presence of soft markers (*see* ULTRASOUND MARKER, NUCHAL TRANSLUCENCY SCANNING). If the results indicate a high risk of abnormalities being present, a diagnosis may be confirmed by more invasive procedures (*see* PRENATAL DIAGNOSIS).

preneoplastic *adj.* preceding the formation of a benign or malignant tumour (neoplasm). Preneoplastic lesions have the potential to give rise to tumours at that site. For example, mammary ductal epithelial *hyperplasia can give rise to *ductal carcinoma in situ. Preneoplastic conditions may result in tumours at that site or elsewhere. For example, ulcerative colitis predisposes to the development of colorectal *adenocarcinoma and *cholangiocarcinoma.

preoperative *adj.* before operation: referring to the condition of a patient or to treatment, such as sedation, given at this time.

preparedness *n.* (in psychology) a quality of some stimuli that makes them much more likely to trigger a pathological fear. For example, animals or high places are much more likely to become the subject of a *phobia than are plants or clothes. One theory is that individuals are genetically predisposed to *conditioning of fear to objects that have been a biological threat during human evolution.

prepatellar bursitis *see* HOUSEMAID'S KNEE.

prepubertal *adj.* relating to or occurring in the period before puberty.

prepuce (foreskin) *n.* the fold of skin that grows over the end (glans) of the penis. On its inner surface modified sebaceous glands (**preputial glands**) secrete a lubricating fluid over the glans. The accumulation of this secretion is known as *smegma. The foreskin is often surgically removed in infancy (*see* CIRCUMCISION). The fold of skin that surrounds the clitoris is also called the prepuce. —**preputial** *adj.*

preputial glands modified sebaceous glands on the inner surface of the *prepuce.

prepyramidal *adj.* 1. situated in the middle lobe of the cerebellum, in front of the *pyramid. 2. describing nerve fibres in tracts that descend from the cerebral cortex to the spinal cord, before the crossing over that occurs at the pyramid of the medulla oblongata.

presby- (presbyo-) *combining form denoting* old age.

presbyacusis *n.* the progressive sensorineural *deafness that occurs with age.

presbyopia *n.* difficulty in reading at the usual distance (about one foot from the eyes) and in performing other close work, due to the decline with age in the ability of the eye to alter its focus to see close objects clearly. This is caused by gradual loss of elasticity of the lens of the eye which thus becomes progressively less able to increase its curvature in order to focus on near objects.

prescribed disease one of a number of *occupational diseases for which benefits are payable. These diseases arise as a result of employment requiring close contact with a hazardous substance or circumstance. Prescribed diseases are categorized by cause: physical, biological, chemical, or other. Examples include poisoning by such chemicals as mercury or benzene, decompression sickness in divers, and infections such as *anthrax in those handling wool. Some diseases that occur widely in the population may be prescribed in relation to a specific occupation (e.g. deafness in those working with pneumatic drills or tuberculosis in mortuary attendants). *See also* COSHH.

prescription *n.* a written direction from a registered medical practitioner to a pharmacist for preparing and dispensing a drug.

presenility *n.* premature ageing of the mind and body, so that a person shows the reduction in mental and physical abilities normally found only in old age. *See also* DEMENTIA, PROGERIA. —**presenile** *adj.*

present *vb.* **1.** of a patient) to come forward for examination and treatment because of experiencing specific symptoms (**presenting symptoms**). **2.** (in obstetrics) *see* PRESENTATION.

presentation *n.* the part of the fetus that is closest to the birth canal and can be felt on inserting a finger into the vagina. Normally the back of the head (vertex) presents, the most favourable position for delivery being occipital anterior (*see* OCCIPUT). However, the buttocks may present (*see* BREECH PRESENTATION) or, if the fetus lies transversely across the uterus, the shoulder or arm may present (*see* MALPRESENTATION). These abnormal presentations may cause complications during childbirth, and attempts may be made to correct them. *See also* DENOMINATOR.

pressor *n.* an agent that raises blood pressure. *See* VASOCONSTRICTOR.

pressure index (PI) the ratio of the pressure in the posterior tibial artery to that in the brachial artery, which reflects the degree of arterial obstruction in the artery of the lower limb.

pressure point a point at which an artery lies over a bone on which it may be compressed by finger pressure, to arrest haemorrhage beyond. For example, the femoral artery may be compressed against the pelvic bone in the groin.

pressure sore (bedsore, decubitus ulcer) an ulcerated area of skin caused by continuous pressure on part of the body: a hazard to be guarded against in all bedridden (especially unconscious) patients. Healing is hin-dered by the reduced blood supply to the area, and careful nursing is necessary to prevent local gangrene. The patient's position should be changed frequently (pressure-relieving mattresses are extremely helpful), and the buttocks, heels, elbows, and other regions at risk kept dry and clean.

presymptomatic *adj.* describing or relating to a symptom that occurs before the typical symptoms of a disease. *See also* PRODROMAL.

presystole *n.* the period in the cardiac cycle just preceding systole.

preterm birth (premature birth) birth of a baby before 37 weeks (259 days) of gestation (calculated from the first day of the mother's last menstrual period); a birth at less than 23 weeks is at present incompatible with life. Such factors as *pre-eclampsia, multiple pregnancies (e.g. twins), maternal infection, and *cervical incompetence may all result in preterm births, but in the majority of cases the cause is unknown. Conditions affecting preterm babies may include *respiratory distress syndrome, feeding difficulties, inability to maintain normal body temperature, *apnoea, infection, *necrotizing enterocolitis, and brain haemorrhages. Supportive treatment is provided in an incubator in a neonatal unit; many infants survive with no residual handicap but the shorter the gestation period, the more serious are the problems to be overcome.

prevalence *n.* a measure of morbidity based on current levels of disease in a population, estimated either at a particular time (**point prevalence**) or over a stated period (**period prevalence**). It can be expressed either in terms of affected people (persons) or episodes of sickness per 1000 individuals at risk. *Compare* INCIDENCE RATE.

preventive dentistry the branch of dentistry concerned with the prevention of dental disease. It includes dietary counselling, advice on oral hygiene, and the application of *fluoride and *fissure sealants to the teeth.

preventive medicine the branch of medicine whose main aim is the prevention of disease. This is a wide field, in which workers tackle problems ranging from the immunization of persons against infectious diseases, such as diphtheria or whooping cough, to finding methods of eliminating *vectors, such as malaria-carrying mosquitoes. *See* PRIMARY PREVENTION, SECONDARY PREVEN-

TION, TERTIARY PREVENTION. *See also* WORLD HEALTH ORGANIZATION.

preventive resin restoration a hybrid between a *fissure sealant and a conventional *filling that is used to treat early dental caries involving dentine.

priapism *n.* a persistent and usually painful erection of the penis that requires urgent decompression; occasionally, however, it can be painless, in which case its treatment is less urgent. A prolonged erection (i.e. of greater than six hours duration), resulting from administration of *papaverine, intracorporeal *alprostadil, or a similar drug, can be successfully treated by draining the blood from the corpora cavernosa of the penis with a 19 SWG butterfly needle and instilling a *vasoconstrictor (e.g. phenylephrine). Priapism may also occur in patients with sickle-cell disease and those undergoing *haemodialysis. An unrelieved priapism results in eventual fibrosis of the spongy tissue of the corpora and no further erections are possible.

prickle cells cells with cytoplasmic processes that form intercellular bridges. The germinative layer of the *epidermis is sometimes called the prickle cell layer.

prickly heat an itchy rash of small raised red spots. It occurs usually on the face, neck, back, chest, and thighs. Infants and obese people are susceptible to prickly heat, which is most common in hot moist weather. It is caused by blockage of the sweat ducts and the only treatment is removal of the patient to a cool (air-conditioned) place. Medical name: **miliaria rubra**.

prilocaine *n.* a local *anaesthetic used particularly in dentistry. It is administered by injection; high doses of the drug may cause methaemoglobinaemia and cyanosis. Prilocaine is also a constituent of *EMLA cream. Trade name: **Citanest**.

prima facie an obligation or essential principle that, on first sight, is a valid way to address an ethical question and must be explicitly rebutted if an alternative approach is to be followed. The *four principles are said to be prima facie in medical ethics by those who subscribe to a principalist approach to medical ethics. *See also* KANTIAN ETHICS.

primaquine *n.* a drug used in the treatment of benign *malarias. It is administered by mouth after treatment with *chloroquine.

High doses may cause blood disorders (such as methaemoglobinaemia or haemolytic anaemia) and digestive upsets.

primary care health care provided by *general practitioners or other health professionals to whom patients seeking medical treatment have direct access and to whom they can usually self-refer. As well as via the GP service, primary care is also provided through *primary care trust medical services, which allow the PCT to deliver primary care services directly, and alternative provider medical services, where services are provided by outside contractors, such as private health companies. Other primary care services provided by the NHS include the general dental and ophthalmic services, together with *NHS walk-in centres and other community services outside the hospital service. *See also* COMMUNITY HEALTH, DOMICILIARY SERVICES, GENERAL DENTAL SERVICES, HEALTH CENTRE, NHS DIRECT. *Compare* SECONDARY CARE, TERTIARY CARE.

primary care trust (PCT) one of a group of free-standing statutory bodies within the *National Health Service, accountable to their local *strategic health authority. The 152 PCTs have responsibility for the healthcare needs of their local community; their aim is to improve the health of and address *health inequalities in their communities. They control the bulk of the NHS budget and receive allocations from the Department of Health to commission and provide primary care and community services across the local area and to commission hospital services for patients. *Compare* CARE TRUST, SPECIALIZED COMMISSIONING GROUP.

primary prevention avoidance of the onset of disease by behaviour modification or treatment. For example, limiting alcohol intake reduces the risk of developing cirrhosis, and routine childhood *immunization prevents the development of infections of childhood. *See also* PREVENTIVE MEDICINE, SECONDARY PREVENTION, TERTIARY PREVENTION.

primary teeth the first set of teeth, which develop in infancy. These teeth are normally shed just before the eruption of their permanent successors. In the absence of permanent successors they can remain functional for many years. *See* DENTITION.

prime *vb.* (in chemotherapy) to administer small doses of a *cytotoxic drug prior to high-dose chemotherapy and/or radio-therapy. This causes proliferation of the primitive bone marrow cells and aids subsequent regeneration of the bone marrow.

prime mover *see* AGONIST.

primidone *n.* an *anticonvulsant drug used to treat major and partial epilepsy and essential tremor. It is administered by mouth; common side-effects, which are usually transient, include drowsiness, muscle incoordination, nausea, and sight disturbances. Trade name: **Mysoline.**

primigravida *n.* a woman experiencing her first pregnancy.

primipara *n.* a woman who has given birth to one infant capable of survival.

primitive streak the region of the embryo that proliferates rapidly, producing mesoderm cells that spread outwards between the layers of ectoderm and endoderm.

primordial *adj.* (in embryology) describing cells or tissues that are formed in the early stages of embryonic development.

primum non nocere an ancient dictum of medical ethics, usually translated from the Latin as "first do no harm". This statement of the principle of *nonmaleficence is often mistakenly believed to form part of the *Hippocratic oath: its source is not known. Commonly in medical treatment, harm in the form of risks or discomfort precede benefits, e.g. the pain of inserting an intravenous line comes before the effects of the medication delivered via the line. As such, it has been suggested that the correct interpretation is to weigh, avoid, and minimize risks and maximize the benefits rather than to strictly (but unrealistically) ensure benefit occurs in advance of harm. *See also* RISK–BENEFIT ANALYSIS.

P–R interval the interval on an *electrocardiogram between the onset of atrial activity and ventricular activity. It represents the time required for the impulse from the *sinoatrial node to reach the ventricles.

prion *n.* an abnormal form of a constituent protein (PrP) of brain cells. The abnormal proteins are very stable: they are not removed by the normal cellular processes of degradation and are resistant to radiation and sterilization (therefore surgical instruments need first to undergo *decontamination). They are believed to interact with

normal PrP in such a way as to convert it to the abnormal form, which accumulates in the brain. Prions are now widely accepted as being the causal agents of a range of serious diseases including *Creutzfeldt-Jakob disease, *Gerstmann-Straussler-Scheinker syndrome, and *kuru, all of which are *spongiform encephalopathies. Different mutations in the *PrP* gene are believed to be responsible for the different forms of these so-called **prion disorders**.

privacy *n.* the condition of being withdrawn from public view. The law now recognizes privacy as a *human right by virtue of the Human Rights Act 1998, although there are occasions when this right may be overridden (for example, in legal proceedings). In medical ethics, the concept is associated with a doctor's duty of *confidentiality, which helps to maintain a patient's privacy and builds trust.

PRK photorefractive keratectomy (*see* KERATECTOMY).

pro- *prefix denoting* 1. before; preceding. 2. a precursor. 3. in front of.

probability *n. see* SIGNIFICANCE.

proband *n. see* PROPOSITUS.

probang *n.* a long flexible rod with a small sponge, ball, or tuft at the end, used to remove obstructions from the larynx or oesophagus (gullet). A probang is also used to apply medication to these structures.

probe *n.* 1. a thin rod of pliable metal, such as silver, with a blunt swollen end. The instrument is used for exploring cavities, wounds, fistulae, and sinus channels. 2. (**dental probe**) a hand instrument designed for specific exploratory examination procedures (e.g. for dental caries, endodontics, or periodontics). 3. (**ultrasound probe**) *see* ULTRASOUND, TRANSDUCER. 4. (**gene probe**) a radioactively labelled cloned section of DNA that is used to detect identical sections of nucleic acid by means of pairing between complementary bases. *See* NORTHERN BLOT ANALYSIS, SOUTHERN BLOT ANALYSIS.

probenecid *n.* a drug that reduces the level of uric acid in the blood (*see* URICOSURIC DRUG). It is administered by mouth to prevent the toxic effects on the kidney of the antiviral drug cidofovir (Vistide), used in treating severe cytomegalovirus eye infection in AIDS patients. Mild side-effects, such as digestive upsets, dizziness, and frequent urination, may occur.

probing depth a measurement of the depth of a periodontal pocket (*see* PERIODONTAL DISEASE).

probiotics *pl. n.* **1.** bacteria (e.g. **Lactobacillus*) or other microorganisms that are said to be beneficial to the human body and occur in or are added to certain foods (e.g. yoghurt) and supplements. **2.** the foods or supplements containing these microorganisms. —**probiotic** *adj.*

procarbazine *n.* a drug that inhibits growth of cancer cells by preventing cell division and is used to treat such cancers as Hodgkin's disease. It is administered by mouth; side-effects may include loss of appetite, nausea, *myelosuppression, and rash.

procarcinogen *n.* a chemical substance that does not itself cause cancer but which can be converted by enzymatic action to another substance that can cause cancer (the ultimate *carcinogen).

process *n.* (in anatomy) a thin prominence or protuberance; for example, any of the processes of a vertebra.

prochlorperazine *n.* a phenothiazine *antipsychotic drug used to treat schizophrenia and other psychoses and severe vertigo, nausea, and vomiting. It is administered by mouth or deep intramuscular injection; possible side-effects include drowsiness and dry mouth, and high doses may cause tremors and abnormal muscle movements. Trade names: **Buccastem**, **Stemetil**.

procidentia *n.* the complete downward displacement (*prolapse) of an organ, especially the uterus (**uterine procidentia**), which protrudes from the vaginal opening. Uterine procidentia may result from injury to the floor of the pelvic cavity, invariably the result of childbirth.

proct- (procto-) *combining form denoting* the anus and/or rectum.

proctalgia (proctodynia) *n.* pain in the rectum or anus. In **proctalgia fugax** severe pain suddenly affects the rectum and may last for minutes or hours; attacks may be days or months apart. There is no structural disease and the pain is probably due to muscle spasm (*see* IRRITABLE BOWEL SYNDROME). Relief is sometimes obtained from a bowel

action, inserting a finger into the rectum, or from a hot bath, but it may be prevented by measures used in treating the irritable bowel syndrome.

proctatresia *n. see* IMPERFORATE ANUS.

proctectasia *n.* enlargement or widening of the rectum, usually due to long-standing constipation (*see* DYSCHEZIA).

proctectomy *n.* surgical removal of the rectum. It is usually performed for cancer of the rectum and may require the construction of a permanent opening in the colon (*see* COLOSTOMY). If the anus is left, an *ileal pouch can be constructed to replace the rectum.

proctitis *n.* inflammation of the rectum. Symptoms are ineffectual straining to empty the bowels (*tenesmus), diarrhoea, urgency, and often bleeding. Proctitis is invariably present in ulcerative *colitis and sometimes in *Crohn's disease. Rarer causes include damage by irradiation (for example in radiation therapy for cervical or prostate cancer), by *lymphogranuloma venereum, or after a colostomy has rendered the rectum nonfunctional (**diversion proctitis**).

proctocele *n. see* RECTOCELE.

proctocolectomy *n.* a surgical operation in which the rectum and colon are removed. In **panproctocolectomy** the whole rectum and colon are removed, necessitating either a permanent opening of the ileum (*see* ILEOSTOMY) or the construction of an *ileal pouch. This is usually performed for ulcerative *colitis.

proctocolitis *n.* inflammation of the rectum and colon, usually due to ulcerative *colitis. *See also* PROCTITIS.

proctodeum *n.* the site of the embryonic anus, marked by a depression lined with ectoderm. The membrane separating it from the hindgut breaks down in the third month of gestation. *Compare* STOMODEUM.

proctodynia *n. see* PROCTALGIA.

proctogram *n.* an X-ray photograph of the rectum taken after the introduction into it of a contrast medium. A **defecating proctogram** demonstrates problems of abnormal defecation.

proctology *n.* the study of disorders of the rectum and anus.

proctorrhaphy *n.* a surgical operation to stitch tears of the rectum or anus.

proctoscope *n.* an illuminated instrument through which the lower part of the rectum and the anus may be inspected and minor procedures (such as injection or banding therapy for haemorrhoids) carried out. —**proctoscopy** *n.*

proctosigmoiditis *n.* inflammation of the rectum and the sigmoid (lower) colon. *See also* PROCTOCOLITIS.

proctotomy *n.* incision into the rectum or anus to relieve *stricture (narrowing) of these canals or to open an imperforate (closed) anus.

procyclidine *n.* an *antimuscarinic drug used to reduce muscle tremor and rigidity in parkinsonism. It is administered by mouth or injection; common side-effects include dry mouth, blurred vision, and giddiness. Trade names: **Arpicolin**, **Kemadrin**.

prodromal *adj.* relating to the period of time between the appearance of the first symptoms of an infectious disease and the development of a rash or fever. A **prodromal rash** is one preceding the full rash of an infectious disease.

prodrome *n.* a symptom indicating the onset of a disease.

prodrug *n.* a drug that requires metabolism in the liver before becoming biologically active. Examples are *carbimazole, which is metabolized to the pharmacologically active compound methimazole; and *capecitabine, which is metabolized to *fluorouracil.

proenzyme (zymogen) *n.* the inactive form in which certain enzymes (e.g. digestive enzymes) are originally produced and secreted. The existence of this inactive form prevents the enzyme from breaking down the cells in which it was made. Once the proenzyme has been secreted it is converted to the active form.

proerythroblast *n.* the earliest recognizable precursor of the red blood cell (erythrocyte). It is found in the bone marrow and has a large nucleus and a cytoplasm that stains deep blue with *Romanowsky stains. *See also* ERYTHROBLAST, ERYTHROPOIESIS.

profunda *adj.* describing blood vessels that are deeply embedded in the tissues they supply.

profundaplasty *n.* surgical enlargement of the junction of the femoral artery and its deep branch, a common operation to relieve narrowing by atherosclerosis at this point.

progeria *n.* a very rare condition in which all the signs of old age appear and progress in a child, so that 'senility' is reached before puberty.

progesterone *n.* a steroid hormone secreted by the *corpus luteum of the ovary, the placenta, and also (in small amounts) by the adrenal cortex and testes. It is responsible for preparing the inner lining (endometrium) of the uterus for pregnancy. If fertilization occurs it maintains the uterus throughout pregnancy and prevents the further release of eggs from the ovary. *See also* MENSTRUAL CYCLE, PROGESTOGEN.

progestogen *n.* one of a group of naturally occurring or synthetic steroid hormones, including *progesterone, that maintain the normal course of pregnancy. Progestogens are used to treat premenstrual tension, *amenorrhoea, and abnormal bleeding from the uterus. Because they prevent ovulation, progestogens are a major constituent of *oral contraceptives and other forms of hormonal *contraception. Synthetic progestogens may be taken by mouth but the naturally occurring hormone must be given by intramuscular injection or subcutaneous implant, as it is rapidly broken down in the liver.

proglottis *n.* (*pl.* **proglottids** or **proglottides**) one of the segments of a *tapeworm. Mature segments, situated at the posterior end of the worm, each consist mainly of a branched uterus packed with eggs.

prognathism *n.* abnormal protrusion of one or both jaws. —**prognathic** *adj.*

prognosis *n.* an assessment of the future course and outcome of a patient's disease, based on knowledge of the course of the disease in other patients together with the general health, age, and sex of the patient.

progressive lenses *see* VARIFOCAL LENSES.

progressive supranuclear palsy (Steele-Richardson-Olszewski syndrome) a progressive neurological disorder resulting from degeneration of the motor neurons, basal ganglia, and brainstem. Starting in late middle age, it is characterized by a staring facial expression due to impaired ability to move the eyes up and down, progressing to difficulties in swallowing, speech, balance, and movement and general spasticity. The condition enters the differential diagnosis of *parkinsonism, with which it is often confused in its early stages.

proguanil *n.* a drug that kills malaria parasites and is used in combination with atovaquone (as **Malarone**) for the prevention and treatment of malignant (falciparum) *malaria. Alone or (more usually) in combination with *chloroquine (as **Paludrine/Avloclor**), it may be used for the prevention of malaria. It is administered by mouth and rarely causes side-effects. Trade name: **Paludrine**.

proinsulin *n.* a substance produced in the pancreas from which the hormone *insulin is derived.

projection *n.* (in psychology) the attribution of one's own qualities to other people. This is one of the *defence mechanisms; people who cannot tolerate their own feelings (e.g. anger) may cope by imagining that other people have those feelings (e.g. are angry).

projective test (in psychology) a way of measuring aspects of personality, in which the subject is asked to talk freely about ambiguous objects. His responses are then analysed. Examples are the *Rorschach test and the Thematic Apperception Test (in which the subject invents stories about a set of pictures).

prokinetic agent an agent that induces peristaltic movement, especially intestinal activity.

prolactin (lactogenic hormone, luteotrophic hormone, luteotrophin) *n.* a hormone, synthesized and stored in the anterior pituitary gland, that stimulates milk production after childbirth and also stimulates production of *progesterone by the *corpus luteum in the ovary. Excessive secretion of prolactin, resulting in raised serum levels of the hormone (**hyperprolactinaemia**), is usually due to the presence of a pituitary adenoma (*see* PROLACTINOMA); other causes include *dopamine receptor antagonists (e.g. antipsychotic drugs) and chronic renal failure.

prolactinoma *n.* a benign tumour (an *adenoma) of the pituitary gland that secretes excessive amounts of prolactin. Symptoms include loss of sexual drive,

amenorrhoea or impotence, and sometimes production of breast milk in men and women. If the tumour is large enough it may compress and damage adjacent structures. Treatment is with dopamine receptor agonist drugs, such as *bromocriptine, as dopamine inhibits prolactin production and may also shrink and harden the tumour, facilitating later surgical removal.

prolapse *n.* downward displacement of an organ or tissue from its normal position, usually the result of weakening of the supporting tissues. Prolapse of the uterus and/or vagina is, in most cases, caused by stretching and/or tearing of the supporting tissues during childbirth. The cervix may be visible at the vaginal opening or the uterus and vagina may be completely outside the opening (procidentia). Treatment is by surgical shortening of the supporting ligaments and narrowing of the vagina and vaginal orifice (*see* COLPORRHAPHY, COLPOPERINEOR-RHAPHY). In prolapse of the rectum, the rectum descends to lie outside the anus.

prolapsed intervertebral disc (PID) a 'slipped disc': protrusion of the pulpy inner material of an *intervertebral disc through a tear in the fibrous outer coat, causing pressure on adjoining nerve roots, ligaments, etc. The condition often results from sudden twisting or bending of the backbone or lifting. Pressure on the sciatic nerve root causes *sciatica, and if severe may damage the nerve's function, leading to abnormalities or loss of sensation, muscle weakness, or loss of tendon reflexes. 70–80% of patients improve with conservative treatment of rest and analgesics, and traction may help. If these fail, the protruding portion of the disc is surgically removed (*see* DISCECTOMY, LAMINECTOMY, MICRODISCECTOMY).

proline *n.* an *amino acid found in many proteins.

PROM prelabour (or premature) rupture of membranes: spontaneous rupture of membranes prior to the onset of labour. The majority of women who demonstrate this phenomenon will go into active labour spontaneously within the following 48 hours.

promazine *n.* a phenothiazine *antipsychotic drug used to relieve agitation, confusion, and restlessness. It is administered by mouth; common side-effects are drowsiness and dizziness.

promegakaryocyte *n.* an immature cell,

found in the bone marrow, that develops into a *megakaryocyte.

promethazine *n.* a powerful *antihistamine drug used to treat allergic conditions and – because of its sedative action – insomnia; it is also used as a premedication and an *antiemetic. Promethazine is administered by mouth or injection; side-effects include drowsiness, dizziness, and confusion. Trade names: **Avomine, Phenergan**.

prominence *n.* (in anatomy) a projection, such as a projection on a bone.

promontory *n.* (in anatomy) a projecting part of an organ or other structure.

promoter (in oncogenesis) *n.* a substance that, in conjunction with an *initiator, leads to the production of a cancer.

prompting *n.* a technique used in *behaviour modification to elicit a response not previously present. The subject is made to engage passively in the required behaviour by instructions or by being physically put through the movements. The behaviour can then be rewarded (*see* REINFORCEMENT). This is followed by **fading**, in which the prompting is gradually withdrawn and the reinforcement maintained.

promyelocyte (premyelocyte) *n.* the developmental stage of a *granulocyte (a type of white blood cell) between the *myeloblast and the *myelocyte. It has abundant cytoplasm that, with *Romanowsky stains, appears blue with reddish granules. Promyelocytes are normally found in the blood-forming tissue of the bone marrow but may appear in the blood in a variety of diseases. *See also* GRANULOPOIESIS.

pronation *n.* the act of turning the hand so that the palm faces downwards. In this position the bones of the forearm (radius and ulna) are crossed. *Compare* SUPINATION.

pronator *n.* any muscle that causes pronation of the forearm and hand; for example, the **pronator teres**, a two-headed muscle arising from the humerus and ulna, close to the elbow, and inserted into the radius.

prone *adj.* **1.** lying with the face downwards. **2.** (of the forearm) in the position in which the palm of the hand faces downwards (*see* PRONATION). *Compare* SUPINE.

pronephros *n.* the first kidney tissue that develops in the embryo. It is not functional

and soon disappears. *Compare* MESONEPHROS, METANEPHROS.

pronucleus *n.* (*pl.* **pronuclei**) the nucleus of either the ovum or spermatozoon after fertilization but before the fusion of nuclear material. The pronuclei are larger than the normal nucleus and have a diffuse appearance.

propantheline *n.* an *antimuscarinic drug that decreases activity of smooth muscle (*see* ANTISPASMODIC) and is used to treat disorders of the digestive system and (in adults) *enuresis. It is administered by mouth; side-effects include dry mouth and blurred vision. Trade name: **Pro-Banthine**.

properdin *n.* a group of substances in blood plasma that, in combination with *complement and magnesium ions, is capable of destroying certain bacteria and viruses. The properdin complex occurs naturally, rather than as the result of previous exposure to microorganisms, and its activity is not directed against any particular species. *Compare* ANTIBODY.

proper officer *see* PUBLIC HEALTH CONSULTANT.

prophase *n.* the first stage of *mitosis and of each division of *meiosis, in which the chromosomes become visible under the microscope. The first prophase of meiosis ocurs in five stages (*see* LEPTOTENE, ZYGOTENE, PACHYTENE, DIPLOTENE, DIAKINESIS).

prophylactic *n.* an agent that prevents the development of a condition or disease. An example is *glyceryl trinitrate, which is used to prevent attacks of angina.

prophylaxis *n.* any means taken to prevent disease, such as immunization against diphtheria or whooping cough, or *fluoridation to prevent dental decay in children. —**prophylactic** *adj.*

propofol *n. see* ANAESTHETIC.

propositus (proband) *n.* the first individual studied in an investigation of several related patients with an inherited or familial disorder.

propranolol *n.* a drug (*see* BETA BLOCKER) used to treat abnormal heart rhythm, angina, and high blood pressure; it is also taken to relieve the symptoms of thyrotoxicosis and anxiety associated with palpitation or tremor and to prevent migraine headaches. It is administered by mouth or injection; common side-effects include digestive upsets, sleep disturbances, lassitude, and coldness of extremities. Trade names: **Half-Inderal LA**, **Inderal**, **Inderal-LA**.

proprietary name (in pharmacy) the trade name of a drug: the name assigned to it by the firm that manufactured it. For example, Taxotere is the proprietary name of docetaxel.

proprioceptor *n.* a specialized sensory nerve ending (*see* RECEPTOR) that monitors internal changes in the body brought about by movement and muscular activity. Proprioceptors located in muscles and tendons transmit information that is used to co-ordinate muscular activity (*see* STRETCH RECEPTOR, TENDON ORGAN). *See also* MECHANORECEPTOR.

proptometer *n. see* EXOPHTHALMOMETER.

proptosis *n.* forward displacement of an organ, especially the eye (*see* EXOPHTHALMOS).

propylthiouracil *n.* a *thionamide antithyroid drug that is used to treat *thyrotoxicosis and to prepare patients for surgical removal of the thyroid gland. It is administered by mouth; side-effects may include rashes and digestive upsets.

prorennin *n. see* RENNIN.

Proscar *n. see* FINASTERIDE.

prosect *vb.* to dissect a cadaver (or part of one) for anatomical demonstration. —**prosection** *n.* —**prosector** *n.*

prosencephalon *n.* the forebrain.

prosop- (**prosopo-**) *combining form denoting* the face. Example: **prosopodynia** (pain in).

prosopagnosia *n.* inability to recognize faces, either in person or in photographs, due to damage in the right occipito-temporal area of the brain. Causes include stroke and brain tumours.

prospective study 1. a forward-looking review of a group of individuals in relation to morbidity. 2. *see* COHORT STUDY.

prostacyclin *n.* a derivative of *prostaglandin H produced by the endothelium lining blood vessel walls. It inhibits blood clotting by preventing platelet aggregation and causes vasodilatation (*compare*

THROMBOXANE A₂). *Epoprostenol is a pharmaceutical preparation of prostacyclin.

prostaglandin *n.* one of a group of hormone-like substances present in a wide variety of tissues and body fluids (including the uterus, brain, lungs, kidney, and semen). Prostaglandins have many actions; for example, they cause contraction of smooth muscle (including that of the uterus), dilation of blood vessels, and are mediators in the process of inflammation (aspirin and other *NSAIDs act by blocking their production). They are also involved in the production of mucus in the stomach, which provides protection against acid gastric juice; use of NSAIDs reduces this effect and predisposes to peptic ulceration, the principal side-effect of these drugs. There are nine classes of prostaglandins (PGA–I), within which individual prostaglandins are denoted by numerals (e.g. PGE$_1$). Synthetic prostaglandins are used to induce labour or produce abortion (*see* DINOPROSTONE, GEMEPROST) and to treat peptic ulcers (*see* MISOPROSTOL), congenital heart disease in newborn babies (*see* ALPROSTADIL), and glaucoma (*see* LATANOPROST).

prostate cancer a malignant tumour (*carcinoma) of the prostate gland, a common form of cancer in elderly men. In most men it progresses slowly over many years and gives symptoms similar to those of benign enlargement of the prostate (*see* PROSTATE GLAND). Before it was possible to test for *prostate specific antigen (PSA), the tumour had often invaded locally, spread to regional lymph nodes, and metastasized to bone before clinical presentation. By checking elevated levels of PSA or *PCA3, prostate cancer can be detected 5–10 years before the tumour would present symptomatically. If the disease is confined to the prostate, the patient may have a radical *prostatectomy, radical radiotherapy, or *brachytherapy; in elderly patients, it may be enough to monitor the tumour growth. If the disease is outside the prostate, androgen deprivation therapy may be used; this may be achieved by *gonadorelin analogues, *anti-androgens, surgical castration, or oestrogen therapy.

prostatectomy *n.* surgical removal of the prostate gland. The operation is necessary to relieve retention of urine due to enlargement of the prostate or to reduce *lower urinary tract symptoms thought to be due to benign prostatic hyperplasia (*see* PROSTATE GLAND).

The operation can be performed through the bladder (**transvesical prostatectomy**) or through the surrounding capsule of the prostate (**retropubic prostatectomy**). In the operation of **transurethral prostatectomy** (or **transurethral resection**) some or all the obstructing prostate can be removed through the urethra using a resectoscope (*see* RESECTION).

Radical (or **total**) **prostatectomy** is undertaken for the treatment of prostate cancer that is confined to the gland. It entails removal of the prostate together with its capsule and the seminal vesicles. Continuity of the urinary tract is achieved by anastomosing the bladder to the divided urethra. Radical prostatectomy may be performed by laparoscopy, sometimes with the aid of a robot (**robotic prostatectomy**): the three-armed da Vinci robot can be operated by the surgeon via a console and provides three-dimensional displays of the operation site and surrounding structures.

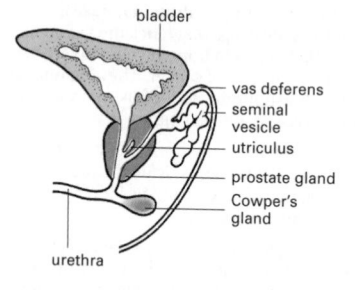

The prostate gland and associated structures (median view).

prostate gland a male accessory sex gland that opens into the urethra just below the bladder and vas deferens (see illustration). During ejaculation it secretes an alkaline fluid that forms part of the *semen. The prostate may become enlarged in elderly men (**benign prostatic hyperplasia; BPH**). This may result in obstruction of the neck of the bladder, impairing urination. The bladder dilates and the increased pressure is transmitted through the ureters to the kidney nephrons, leading to damage and impaired function of the kidneys. Treatment is by transurethral *resection of the prostate (*see also* PROSTATECTOMY) or by means of drugs (e.g. *finasteride, alpha blockers).

prostate specific antigen (PSA) an enzyme produced by the glandular epithelium of the prostate. Increased quantities are secreted when the gland becomes enlarged or inflamed, and levels of PSA in the blood are significantly elevated in cancer of the prostate. Although there is no clear 'cut-off' level for normality, over 4 ng/ml in the blood is associated with a 20% risk of prostate cancer, even in patients with normal-feeling prostates on rectal examination. Newer PSA assays can measure free PSA and compare it to the total PSA in the blood. Low free:total PSA ratios indicate a greater risk of prostate cancer and improve the discrimination between cancer and benign disease in men with a PSA in the range 4–10 ng/ml. PSA levels tend to be much higher in advanced prostate cancer and the rate of fall on treatment (e.g. after radical prostatectomy or radiotherapy) is a good prognostic indicator of response.

prostatic intraepithelial neoplasia (PIN) abnormal cells in the prostate that are not cancer, but are associated with cancer within the prostate. Typically, PIN will be found in prostate biopsies taken because levels of *prostate specific antigen are elevated, and its presence normally leads to another set of prostate biopsies being taken in the future.

prostatism *n. see* LOWER URINARY TRACT SYMPTOMS.

prostatitis *n.* inflammation of the prostate gland. This may be due to bacterial infection and can be either acute or chronic. In acute prostatitis the patient has all the symptoms of a urinary infection, including pain in the perineal area, temperature, and shivering. Treatment is by antibiotic administration. In chronic prostatitis, patients commonly complain of pain in the area between the scrotum and the anus, accompanied by *lower urinary tract symptoms. Some of these cases are due to bacterial infection, in which case antibiotics are required. In others, no bacterial infection is demonstrated, although there may be evidence of inflammation. Treatment in these cases involves alpha blockers, anti-inflammatory agents, and occasionally antibiotics. In some men, vigorous prostate massage performed under a general anaesthetic can significantly alleviate symptoms.

prostatorrhoea *n.* an abnormal discharge of fluid from the prostate gland. This occurs in some patients with acute *prostatitis, who complain of a profuse discharge from the urethra. The discharge is usually thin and watery and is often sterile on culture. The discharge usually subsides when the underlying prostatitis is controlled.

prosthesis *n.* (*pl.* **prostheses**) any artificial device that is attached to the body as an aid. Prostheses include bridges, dentures, artificial parts of the face, artificial limbs, hearing aids and cochlear implants, implanted pacemakers, and many other substitutes for parts of the body that are missing or nonfunctional. **Penile prostheses** are malleable, semirigid, or inflatable rods inserted into the corpora cavernosa of the penis to produce rigidity sufficient for vaginal penetration in men with erectile dysfunction. —**prosthetic** *adj.*

prosthodontics (prosthetic dentistry) *n.* the branch of dentistry concerned with the provision of *dentures, *bridges, and *implant-retained prostheses.

protamine *n.* one of a group of simple proteins that can be conjugated with nucleic acids to form nucleoproteins. **Protamine sulphate** (Prosulf) is injected as an antidote to heparin overdosage in oral anticoagulant therapy.

protanopia *n.* a defect in colour vision in which affected individuals are insensitive to red light and confuse reds, yellows, and greens. *Compare* DEUTERANOPIA, TRITANOPIA.

protease *n.* any enzyme that catalyses the splitting of a protein. *See also* PROTEOLYTIC ENZYME.

protease inhibitor any one of a class of drugs used in the treatment of HIV infection and *AIDS. Used in combination with other *antiretroviral drugs, they act by inhibiting the action of protease, an enzyme produced by HIV that cleaves two precursor proteins into smaller fragments. These fragments are required for viral growth, infectivity, and replication. Protease inhibitors include **atazanavir** (Reyataz), **indinavir** (Crixivan), **lopinavir** and **ritonavir** (combined in Kaletra), **nelfinavir** (Viracept), **saquinavir** (Invirase), and **tipranavir** (Aptivus). They are administered by mouth; side-effects include nausea, vomiting, diarrhoea, and rashes; these drugs are also associated with hyperglycaemia and *lipodystrophy.

proteasome *n.* a multi-enzyme complex in cells that breaks down proteins into short peptides.

protein *n.* one of a group of organic compounds of carbon, hydrogen, oxygen, and nitrogen (sulphur and phosphorus may also be present). The protein molecule is a complex structure made up of one or more chains of *amino acids, which are linked by peptide bonds. Proteins are essential constituents of the body; they form the structural material of muscles, tissues, organs, etc., and are equally important as regulators of function, as enzymes and hormones. Proteins are synthesized in the body from their constituent amino acids, which are obtained from the digestion of protein in the diet. Excess protein, not required by the body, can be converted into glucose and used as an energy source.

protein kinase an enzyme that catalyses the transfer of a phosphate group from ATP to a specific amino acid residue of an intracellular protein (usually serine, threonine, or tyrosine), thereby affecting the biological activity of the protein. **Protein kinase inhibitors** are drugs that block the action of protein kinases in tumour cells and are used in the treatment of cancer. They include *sorafenib, *sunitinib, and *temsirolimus. *See also* TYROSINE KINASE INHIBITOR.

proteinuria *n.* the presence of protein in the urine. This may indicate the presence of damage to, or disease of, the kidneys. *See also* ALBUMINURIA.

proteolysis *n.* the process whereby complex protein molecules, obtained from the diet, are broken down by digestive enzymes in the stomach and small intestine into their constituent amino acids, which are then absorbed into the bloodstream. *See* ENDOPEPTIDASE, EXOPEPTIDASE. —**proteolytic** *adj.*

proteolytic enzyme a digestive enzyme that causes the breakdown of protein. *See* ENDOPEPTIDASE, EXOPEPTIDASE.

proteose *n.* a product of the hydrolytic decomposition of protein.

Proteus *n.* a genus of rodlike Gram-negative flagellate highly motile bacteria common in the intestines and in decaying organic material. All species can decompose urea. Some species may cause disease in humans: *P. vulgaris* can cause urinary tract infections.

prothrombin *n.* a substance, present in blood plasma, that is the inactive precursor from which the enzyme *thrombin is derived during the process of *blood coagulation. *See also* COAGULATION FACTORS.

prothrombin time (PT) the time taken for blood clotting to occur in a sample of blood to which calcium and thromboplastin have been added. A prolonged PT (compared with a control sample) indicates a deficiency of *coagulation factors, which – with calcium and thromboplastin – are required for the conversion of prothrombin to thrombin to occur in the final stages of blood coagulation. Measurement of PT is used to control anticoagulant therapy (e.g. with warfarin). *See* INR.

proto- *combining form denoting* **1.** first. **2.** primitive; early. **3.** a precursor.

protodiastole *n.* the short period in the cardiac cycle between the end of systole and the closure of the *aortic valve marking the start of diastole.

proton pump the enzyme in the *oxyntic (parietal) cells of the stomach that causes acid secretion by producing hydrogen ions in exchange for potassium ions.

proton-pump inhibitor a drug that reduces gastric acid secretion by blocking the *proton pump within the *oxyntic (parietal) cells. Proton-pump inhibitors include **esomeprazole** (Nexium), **lansoprazole** (Zoton), *omeprazole, **pantoprazole** (Protium), and **rabeprazole** (Pariet); they are used for treating gastric and duodenal ulcers, reflux oesophagitis, and the hypersecretion caused by *gastrinoma.

proton therapy a type of radiotherapy that uses a beam of protons. These charged particles are produced by a *cyclotron and penetrate only a predictable distance into the body depending on the energy. This is the radiotherapy treatment of choice for many childhood cancers, particularly brain and spinal tumours, as it can avoid more normal tissue and reduce the risk of long-term complications compared to photon (X-ray) beams.

proto-oncogene *n.* a gene in a normal cell that is of identical structure to certain viral genes. Some are important regulators of cell division and damage may change them into *oncogenes.

protopathic *adj.* describing the ability to perceive only strong stimuli of pain, heat, etc. *Compare* EPICRITIC.

protoplasm *n.* the material of which living cells are made, which includes the cytoplasm and nucleus. —**protoplasmic** *adj.*

protoplast *n.* a bacterial or plant cell without its cell wall.

protoporphyrin IX the most common type of *porphyrin found in nature. It is a constituent of haemoglobin, myoglobin, most of the cytochromes, and the commoner chlorophylls.

protozoa *pl. n.* a group of microscopic single-celled organisms. Most protozoa are free-living but some are important disease-causing parasites of humans; for example, *Plasmodium, *Leishmania, and *Trypanosoma* cause *malaria, *kala-azar, and *sleeping sickness respectively. *See also* AMOEBA.

protozoan *n.* a microorganism of the group *protozoa.

protozoology *n.* the study of *protozoa.

protrusion *n.* (in dentistry) **1.** forward movement of the lower jaw. **2.** a *malocclusion in which some of the teeth are further forward than usual. *Compare* RETRUSION.

protuberance *n.* (in anatomy) a rounded projecting part, e.g. the projecting part of the chin (**mental protuberance**).

provitamin *n.* a substance that is not itself a vitamin but can be converted to a vitamin in the body. An example is β-carotene, which can be converted into vitamin A.

proximal *adj.* (in anatomy) situated close to the origin or point of attachment or close to the median line of the body. *Compare* DISTAL.

proxy decision a decision made with or on behalf of a person who lacks full legal capacity to *consent to or refuse medical treatment. In the case of children under the age of 16 years who are not Gillick-competent (*see* GILLICK COMPETENCE) because they are deemed insufficiently mature or understanding of their situation, people with parental responsibility will usually be asked to take a proxy decision about their care. However, parents can only consent to, or refuse, treatment on behalf of their children in so far as they are considered to be acting in the child's *best interests. For adults, a person previously nominated by the patient while he or she had capacity can be granted a *lasting power of attorney and may make health-care decisions on the patient's behalf. The decision itself may be based on either a judgment of the patient's best interests or a judgment as to what he or she would wish in the circumstances (a *substituted judgment). *See also* ADVANCE STATEMENT, DECISION, OR DIRECTIVE; ADVOCACY.

Prozac *n. see* FLUOXETINE.

prune belly syndrome (Eagle-Barrett syndrome) a hereditary condition, occurring exclusively in males, characterized by a deficiency of abdominal muscles, complex malformation of the urinary tract, and bilateral undescended testes. The lungs may be underdeveloped. The name derives from the typically wrinkled appearance of the skin over the abdomen.

prurigo *n.* an intensely itchy eruption of small papules. **Besnier's prurigo** is a type of chronic atopic *eczema that is lichenified (*see* LICHENIFICATION). **Nodular prurigo** is a condition of unknown cause, although it is usually found in atopic individuals (*see* ATOPY). Very severe itching characterizes these nodules, which mostly occur on the distal limbs. **Prurigo of pregnancy** occurs in 1 in 300 women in the middle trimester of pregnancy, affecting mainly the abdomen and the extensor surfaces of the limbs. It may recur in later pregnancies. It is linked to abnormal blood hormone levels, particularly elevated levels of gonadotrophins and lower levels of cortisol and oestrogen. **Pruritic folliculitis of pregnancy** is a similar pruritic eruption, predominantly on the trunk and thighs, consisting of follicular papules and pustules. It usually presents in the latter half of pregnancy and resolves early after delivery.

pruritus *n.* itching. Mediated by histamine and other vasoactive chemicals, it is the predominant symptom of atopic *eczema, *lichen planus, and many other skin diseases. It also occurs in the elderly and may be a manifestation of psychological illness. Perineal itching is common: itching of the vulva in women (**pruritus vulvae**) may be accompanied by itching of the anal region (**pruritus ani**), although the latter is more common in men. Causes of perineal itching include poor hygiene, *candidiasis, *threadworms, and itchy skin diseases (such as eczema). Pruritus also occurs as a symptom of dry skin and of certain systemic disorders, such as chronic renal failure, *cholestasis, and iron deficiency. **Pruritus gravidarum** is

generalized itching during pregnancy that starts in the first trimester. It is associated with *obstetric cholestasis and requires monitoring of liver function and bile acids, high levels of which endanger the fetus. Other conditions marked by pregnancy-related itch include *polymorphic eruption of pregnancy, *prurigo of pregnancy, pruritic folliculitis of pregnancy, and *pemphigoid gestationalis; all of these are associated with a rash. Treatment of pruritus is determined by the cause.

prussic acid *see* HYDROCYANIC ACID.

PSA *see* PROSTATE SPECIFIC ANTIGEN.

psammoma *n.* a tumour containing gritty sandlike particles (**psammoma bodies**). It is typical of cancer of the ovary but may also be found in the meninges (the membranes surrounding the brain).

pseud- (**pseudo-**) *combining form denoting* superficial resemblance to; false.

pseudarthrosis (nearthrosis) *n.* a 'false' joint. Congenital pseudarthrosis occurs in childhood, when an apparent fracture in the tibia or clavicle is followed by non-*union. A pseudarthrosis can form in adulthood when a fracture fails to unite and the bone ends are separated by fibrous tissue, which allows some movement across the fracture site.

pseudoagglutination *n.* the misleading appearance of clumping that occurs during an antiserum-antigen test as a result of incorrect temperature or acidity of the solutions used.

pseudoaneurysm *n. see* ANEURYSM.

pseudocholinesterase *n.* an enzyme found in the blood and other tissues that – like *cholinesterase – breaks down acetylcholine, but much more slowly. Not being localized at nerve endings, it plays little part in the normal breakdown of acetylcholine in synapses and at neuromuscular junctions.

pseudocoxalgia *n. see* LEGG-CALVÉ-PERTHES DISEASE.

pseudocrisis *n.* a false *crisis: a sudden but temporary change in a condition, such as a fall of temperature in a patient with fever.

pseudocryptorchidism *n.* apparent absence of the testes. This is quite common in young boys, who retract their testes into the groin due to involuntary or reflex contraction of the cremasteric muscle of the suspensory cord. The condition is only important in that it needs to be distinguished from true failure of descent of the testes into the scrotum, which requires early surgical treatment (*see* CRYPTORCHIDISM).

pseudocyesis (phantom pregnancy, false pregnancy) *n.* a condition in which a nonpregnant woman exhibits symptoms of pregnancy, e.g. enlarged abdomen, increased weight, morning sickness, and absence of menstruation. The condition usually has an emotional basis.

pseudocyst *n.* a fluid-filled space without a proper wall or lining, within an organ. A **pancreatic pseudocyst** may develop in cases of chronic pancreatitis or as a complication of acute pancreatitis. As the pseudocyst, which is filled with enzyme-rich pancreatic juice, slowly expands it may cause episodes of abdominal pain accompanied by a rise in the level of enzymes in the blood. It may be felt by abdominal examination or seen by radiology or ultrasound examination. Treatment is by drainage, usually by the technique of joining the pseudocyst to the stomach performed endoscopically under ultrasonic guidance or surgically (*marsupialization).

pseudodementia *n.* a condition in which symptoms of *dementia, including memory disorders, are caused by depression rather than organic brain disease. It is most commonly seen in elderly depressed individuals.

pseudoexfoliation syndrome the appearance of white dandruff-like deposits on structures in the anterior chamber of the eye, which are especially prominent around the pupil margin and on the anterior lens capsule. It is a sign of zonular weakness and indicates an increased risk of secondary glaucoma.

pseudogout *n.* joint pain and swelling, resembling gout, caused by crystals of calcium pyrophosphate in the synovial membrane and fluid (*see* SYNOVITIS). It usually affects large joints (e.g. the knee) in middle-aged women. X-rays may show signs of *chondrocalcinosis.

pseudohallucination *n.* **1.** an especially vivid mental image that cannot substantially be changed by an effort of will, in contrast to ordinary *imagery. **2.** (in modern psychiatry) an experience described by the patient as a genuine hallucination, but in the psychi-

atrist's judgment is not perceived by the patient to be arising from an external stimulus. It may sometimes be seen as an attempt by patients to pretend that they suffer from genuine hallucinations. The term is generally unhelpful because it implies a value judgment. Moreover, it does not make sense because it is impossible to have a 'pretend' form of something that does not exist in the first place.

pseudohermaphroditism *n.* the condition in which an individual is genetically male (XY) or female (XX) and has normal internal sex organs but whose external genitalia resemble those of the opposite sex. For example, a woman would have enlarged labia and clitoris, resembling a scrotum and penis respectively.

pseudohypertrophy *n.* increase in the size of an organ or structure caused by excessive growth of cells that have a packing or supporting role but do not contribute directly to its functioning. The result is usually a decline in the efficiency of the organ although it becomes larger. —**pseudohypertrophic** *adj.*

pseudohypoparathyroidism *n.* a syndrome of mental retardation, restricted growth, and bony abnormalities due to a genetic defect that causes lack of response to the hormone secreted by the *parathyroid glands. Treatment with calcium and vitamin D can reverse most of the features. *See also* ALBRIGHT'S HEREDITARY OSTEODYSTROPHY.

pseudomembrane *n.* a false membrane, consisting of a layer of exudate on the surface of the skin or a mucous membrane. In diphtheria a pseudomembrane forms in the throat. In **pseudomembranous colitis**, a disease caused by *Clostridium difficile* that usually follows antibiotic therapy, pseudomembranes develop in the colon, resulting in profuse diarrhoea.

pseudomembranous colitis *see* CLOSTRIDIUM, PSEUDOMEMBRANE.

Pseudomonas *n.* a genus of rodlike motile pigmented Gram-negative bacteria. Most live in soil and decomposing organic matter; they are involved in recycling nitrogen, converting nitrates to ammonia or free nitrogen. The species *P. aeruginosa* is pathogenic to humans, occurring in pus from wounds; it is associated with urinary tract infections. *P. pseudomallei* is the causative agent of *melioidosis.

pseudomyxoma *n.* a mucoid tumour of the peritoneum, often seen in association with *myxomas of the ovary. In **pseudomyxoma peritonei** there are recurrent deposits of mucin-producing cells in the abdomen, which can be difficult to clear by surgery and may prove fatal.

pseudoneuritis *n.* a condition that resembles *retrobulbar neuritis but is not due to inflammation. The most usual cause is blockage of blood vessels in the optic nerve (**ischaemic optic neuropathy**).

pseudo-obstruction (Ogilvie's syndrome) *n.* apparent obstruction of the colon without evidence of mechanical narrowing (**acute colonic pseudo-obstruction**). It commonly occurs in hospitalized patients with serious illness, probably caused by abnormality in colonic autonomic regulation and often associated with trauma (nonoperative), sepsis (pneumonia), postoperative state (after abdominal, pelvic, or orthopaedic surgery), or cardiac dysfunction (heart failure, infarction). Nausea, vomiting, and abdominal pain with associated abdominal distension are usually present. Management is usually conservative and involves treatment of the underlying condition, the 'drip and suck' approach (*see* ILEUS), decompression of the colon, and neostigmine therapy. Surgery is required when the conservative approach fails or in cases of perforation.

pseudophakia *n.* the state of the eye after the natural lens has been replaced by a synthetic lens implanted inside the eye, approximately in the position previously occupied by the natural lens. This is the current form of surgery for *cataract. —**pseudophakic** *adj.*

pseudopodium *n.* (*pl.* **pseudopodia**) a temporary and constantly changing extension of the body of an amoeba or an amoeboid cell (*see* PHAGOCYTE). Pseudopodia engulf bacteria and other particles as food and are responsible for the movements of the cell.

pseudopolyposis *n.* a condition in which the bowel lining (mucosa) is covered by elevated or protuberant plaques (**pseudopolyps**) that are not true *polyps but abnormal growths of inflamed mucosa. It is usually found in patients with chronic ulcerative *colitis. The pseudopolyps may be seen with the sigmoidoscope or the colonoscope

(through which they may be sampled for microscopic examination) or by barium enema examination.

pseudopseudohypoparathyroidism *n.* a condition in which all the symptoms of *pseudohypoparathyroidism are present but the patient's response to parathyroid hormone is normal. It is often found in families affected with pseudohypoparathyroidism.

pseudotumour cerebri *see* BENIGN INTRACRANIAL HYPERTENSION.

pseudoxanthoma elasticum a hereditary disease in which elastic fibres (*see* ELASTIC TISSUE) become calcified. The skin becomes lax and yellowish papules develop in affected areas; this is accompanied by degenerative changes in the blood vessels and *angioid streaks in the retina.

psilosis *n. see* SPRUE.

psittacosis (parrot disease, ornithosis) *n.* an endemic infection of birds, especially parrots, budgerigars, canaries, finches, pigeons, and poultry, caused by a small intracellular bacterium, *Chlamydia psittaci*. The birds are often asymptomatic carriers. The infection is transmitted to humans by inhalation from handling the birds or by contact with feathers, faeces, or cage dust, but person-to-person transmission also occurs. The symptoms include fever, dry cough, severe muscle pain, and headache; occasionally a severe generalized systemic illness results. The condition responds to tetracycline or erythromycin.

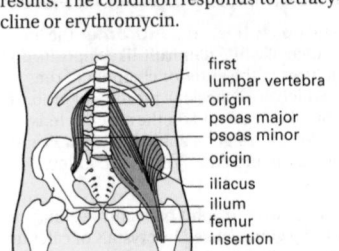

first
lumbar vertebra
origin
psoas major
psoas minor
origin
iliacus
ilium
femur
insertion

Psoas and iliacus muscles.

psoas (psoas major) *n.* a muscle in the groin that acts jointly with the iliacus muscle to flex the hip joint (see illustration). A smaller muscle, **psoas minor**, has the same action but is often absent.

psoralen *n. see* PUVA.

psoriasis *n.* a chronic disease in which scaly pink patches form on the elbows, knees, scalp, and other parts of the body. Psoriasis is one of the commonest skin diseases in Britain, affecting about 2% of the population, although many mild cases are undiagnosed. The most common time of onset is in adolescence. It may occur in association with arthritis (*see* PSORIATIC ARTHRITIS), and severe psoriasis is associated with a higher risk of diabetes mellitus and cardiovascular disease. The disease may be very severe, affecting much of the skin and causing considerable disability and psychological stress. Psoriasis is partly of genetic origin with polygenic influences. Exacerbations of psoriasis may be associated with streptococcal infection and drugs such as lithium and beta blockers.

There is no cure, but first-line treatments include *coal tar, *dithranol, and topical corticosteroids and vitamin D analogues (e.g. *calcipotriol). Narrow-band UVB or *PUVA can also be effective as can systemic therapies, such as *methotrexate, *retinoids, and *ciclosporin. Biological treatments, such as *infliximab, adalimumab, and *etanercept, are potent but expensive.

(⊕) SEE WEB LINKS

• Website of the Psoriasis Association: information on psoriasis, psoriatic arthritis, and treatment options

psoriatic arthritis arthritis associated with *psoriasis. It occurs in only a small minority of patients with psoriasis but may be painful and disabling. It often affects small joints, such as the terminal joints of the fingers and toes, or the spine (*spondylitis) and the sacroiliac joints (*sacroiliitis).

psych- (psycho-) *combining form denoting* 1. the mind; psyche. 2. psychology.

psyche *n.* the mind or the soul; the mental (as opposed to the physical) functioning of the individual.

psychedelic *adj.* describing drugs that induce changes in the level of consciousness of the mind. Psychedelic drugs, which include *lysergic acid diethylamide (LSD) and *cannabis, are *hallucinogens and are used legally only for experimental purposes.

psychiatric intensive care unit *see* PICU.

psychiatrist *n.* a medically qualified physician who specializes in the study and treatment of mental disorders. In the UK psychiatrists classically qualify by specialist training for at least six years after medical school and *Foundation Programme years.

psychiatry *n.* the study of mental disorders and their diagnosis, management, and prevention. —**psychiatric** *adj.*

psychic *adj.* 1. of or relating to the *psyche. 2. relating to parapsychological phenomena. 3. describing a person who is allegedly endowed with extrasensory or psychokinetic powers.

psychoanalysis *n.* a school of psychology and a method of treating mental disorders based upon the teachings of Sigmund Freud (1856–1939). Psychoanalysis employs the technique of *free association in the course of intensive *psychotherapy in order to bring repressed fears and conflicts to the conscious mind, where they can be dealt with (*see* REPRESSION). It stresses the dynamic interplay of unconscious forces and the importance of sexual development in childhood for the development of personality. —**psychoanalyst** *n.* —**psychoanalytic** *adj.*

psychodrama *n.* a form of group psychotherapy in which individuals acquire insight into themselves by acting out situations from their past with other group members. *See* GROUP THERAPY.

psychogenic *adj.* having an origin in the mind rather than in the body. The term is applied particularly to symptoms and illnesses.

psychogenic polydipsia *see* POLYDIPSIA.

psychogeriatrics *n.* the branch of psychiatry that deals with the mental disorders of old people. —**psychogeriatric** *adj.*

psychologist *n.* a person who is engaged in the scientific study of the mind. A psychologist studies psychology for at least three years and then may work in a university, in industry, in schools, or in a hospital. A **clinical psychologist** has been trained in aspects of the assessment and treatment of the ill and handicapped. He or she usually works in a hospital, often as one of a multidisciplinary team. An **educational psychologist** has been trained in aspects of the cognitive and emotional development of children. He or she usually works in close association with schools and advises on the management of children.

psychology *n.* the scientific study of behaviour and its related mental processes. Psychology is concerned with such matters as memory, rational and irrational thought, intelligence, learning, personality, perceptions, and emotions and their relationship to behaviour. Schools of psychology differ in their philosophy and methods. They include the introspectionist Freudian, Jungian, and Adlerian schools and the gestaltist, behaviourist, and cognitive schools; contemporary psychology tends strongly towards the latter (*see* COGNITIVE PSYCHOLOGY). Many practical psychologists profess not to belong to any school; some take an eclectic position. The branches of psychology, on the other hand, are functional or professional subspecialities based on practical considerations. They include abnormal, analytic, applied, clinical, comparative, developmental, educational, experimental, geriatric, industrial, infant, physiological, and social psychology. —**psychological** *adj.*

psychometrics *n.* the measurement of individual differences in psychological functions (such as intelligence and personality) by means of standardized tests. —**psychometric** *adj.*

psychomotor *adj.* relating to muscular and mental activity. The term is applied to disorders in which muscular activities are affected by cerebral disturbance.

psychomotor epilepsy *see* EPILEPSY.

psychoneuroimmunology *n.* the study of the effects of the mind on the functioning of the immune system, especially in relation to the influence of the mind on susceptibility to disease and the progression of a disease.

psychopath *n.* a person who behaves in an antisocial way and shows little or no guilt for antisocial acts and little capacity for forming emotional relationships with others. Psychopaths tend to respond poorly to treatment and do not learn from punishment, but many mature as they age. *See also* ANTISOCIAL PERSONALITY DISORDER. —**psychopathic** *adj.* —**psychopathy** *n.*

psychopathology *n.* **1.** the study of mental disorders, with the aim of explaining and describing aberrant behaviour. *Compare* PSYCHIATRY. **2.** the symptoms, collectively, of a mental disorder. —**psychopathological** *adj.*

psychopharmacology *n.* the study of the effects of drugs on mental processes and behaviour, particularly *psychotropic drugs.

psychophysiology *n.* the branch of psychology that records physiological measurements, such as the electrical resistance of the skin, the heart rate, the size of the pupil, and the electroencephalogram, and relates them to psychological events. —**psychophysiological** *adj.*

psychosexual development the process by which an individual becomes more mature in his sexual feelings and behaviour. Gender identity, sex-role behaviour, and choice of sexual partner are the three major areas of development. In Freudian psychoanalysis the phrase is sometimes used specifically for a sequence of stages, supposed by psychoanalytic psychologists to be universal, in which oral, anal, phallic, latency, and genital stages successively occur. These stages reflect the parts of the body on which sexual interest is concentrated during childhood development.

psychosis *n.* one of a group of *mental illnesses that feature loss of contact with reality. The psychoses include *schizophrenia, major disorders of affect (*see* BIPOLAR AFFECTIVE DISORDER), major *paranoid states, drug intoxication, and organic mental disorders. They can be chronic or transient. Psychotic disorders manifest some of the following: *delusions, *hallucinations, severe thought disturbances, abnormal alteration of mood, poverty of thought, ego disturbances, and inappropriate *affect. Many cases of psychotic illness respond well to *antipsychotic drugs. —**psychotic** *adj.*

psychosocial assessment an interviewing technique that combines psychiatric history taking with elements of problem solving in *psychotherapy: after a psychiatric history has been elicited, the interviewer summarizes the patient's difficulties and offers potential solutions. It is often used in patients who have presented with *deliberate self-harm, and research suggests that it offers the possibility of reducing repetition rates in such patients.

psychosomatic *adj.* relating to or involving both the mind and body: usually applied to illnesses that are caused by the interaction of mental and physical factors. Certain physical illnesses, including asthma, eczema, and peptic ulcer, are thought to be in part a response to psychological and social stresses.

Psychological treatments sometimes have a marked effect, but are usually much less effective than physical treatments for such illnesses.

psychosurgery *n.* surgery on the brain to relieve psychological symptoms. The procedure is irreversible and is therefore reserved for the most severe and intractable of symptoms, particularly severe chronic anxiety, obsessive–compulsive disorder, depression, and untreatable pain. Side-effects can be severe but are less common with modern selective operations. In the UK psychosurgery cannot be performed without the patient's specific informed *consent and a second opinion by another psychiatrist. —**psychosurgical** *adj.*

psychotherapy *n.* psychological (as opposed to physical) methods for the treatment of mental disorders and psychological problems. There are many different approaches to psychotherapy, including *psychoanalysis, *client-centred therapy, *group therapy, and *family therapy. These approaches share the views that the relationship between therapist and client is of prime importance, that the goal is to help personal development and self-understanding generally rather than only to remove symptoms, and that the therapist does not direct the client's decisions. They have all been very widely applied to differing clinical conditions; in the treatment of *mental illness, various psychotherapeutic approaches are used with success, for example *cognitive behavioural therapy in depression and anxiety and psychosocial interventions in schizophrenia. *See also* BEHAVIOUR THERAPY, COUNSELLING. —**psychotherapeutic** *adj.* —**psychotherapist** *n.*

psychoticism *n.* a dimension of personality derived from psychometric tests, characterized by aggression, emotional coldness, and manipulativeness, indicating a susceptibility to psychosis.

psychotropic *adj.* describing drugs that affect mood. *Antidepressants, *sedatives, CNS *stimulants, and *antipsychotics are psychotropic.

psychro- *combining form denoting* cold.

psychrophilic *adj.* describing organisms, especially bacteria, that grow best at temperatures of 0–25°C. *Compare* MESOPHILIC, THERMOPHILIC.

PTA pure tone *audiogram.

PTC 1. percutaneous transhepatic cholangiography (*see* CHOLANGIOGRAPHY). 2. *see* PHENYLTHIOCARBAMIDE.

pterion *n.* the point on the side of the skull at which the sutures between the *parietal, *temporal, and *sphenoid bones meet.

pteroylglutamic acid *see* FOLATE.

pterygium *n.* a triangular overgrowth of the cornea, usually the inner side, by thickened and degenerative conjunctiva. It is most commonly seen in people from dry hot climates, is caused by prolonged exposure to sunlight, and only rarely interferes with vision.

pterygo- *combining form denoting* the pterygoid process of the sphenoid bone. Example: **pterygomaxillary** (of the pterygoid process and the maxilla).

pterygoid process either of two large processes of the *sphenoid bone.

PTH-RP *see* PARATHYROID HORMONE-RELATED PROTEIN.

ptomaine *n.* any of various substances produced in decaying foodstuffs and responsible for the unpleasant taste and smell of such foods. These compounds – which include putrescine, cadaverine, and neurine – were formerly thought to be responsible for food poisoning, but although they are often associated with toxic bacteria they themselves are harmless.

ptosis (blepharoptosis) *n.* drooping of the upper eyelid, for which there are several causes. It may be due to a disorder of the third cranial nerve (*oculomotor nerve), in which case it is likely to be accompanied by paralysis of eye movements causing double vision and an enlarged pupil. When part of *Horner's syndrome, ptosis is accompanied by a small pupil and an absence of sweating on that side of the face. It may be due to *myasthenia gravis, in which the ptosis increases with fatigue and is part of a more widespread fatiguable weakness. Ptosis is associated with the severe pain and other symptoms of a *cluster headache. It may also occur as an isolated congenital feature or as part of a disease of the eye muscles, when it is associated with weak or absent eye movements.

-ptosis *combining form denoting* a lowered

position of an organ or part; prolapse. Example: **colpoptosis** (of the vagina).

PTSD *see* POST-TRAUMATIC STRESS DISORDER.

PTTK partial thromboplastin time with kaolin, also known as activated partial thromboplastin time (**APTT**): a method for estimating the degree of anticoagulation induced by heparin therapy for venous thrombosis.

ptyal- (ptyalo-) *combining form denoting* saliva. Example: **ptyalorrhoea** (excessive flow of).

ptyalin *n.* an enzyme (an *amylase) found in saliva.

ptyalism (sialorrhoea) *n.* the excessive production of saliva: a symptom of certain nervous disorders, poisoning (by mercury, mushrooms, or organophosphates), or infection (rabies). *Compare* DRY MOUTH.

ptyalith *n.* a stone (*calculus) in a salivary gland or duct.

ptyalography *n. see* SIALOGRAPHY.

puberty *n.* the time at which the onset of sexual maturity occurs and the reproductive organs become functional (*see* GONADARCHE). This is manifested in both sexes by the appearance of *secondary sexual characteristics (e.g. deepening of the voice in boys; growth of breasts in girls) and in girls by the start of *menstruation. These changes are brought about by an increase in sex hormone activity due to stimulation of the ovaries and testes by pituitary hormones. *See also* ADRENARCHE, ANDROGEN, OESTROGEN, PRECOCIOUS PUBERTY. —**pubertal** *adj.*

pubes *n.* **1.** the body surface that overlies the pubis, at the front of the pelvis. It is covered with **pubic hair**. **2.** *see* PUBIS. —**pubic** *adj.*

pubiotomy *n.* an operation to divide the pubic bone near the symphysis, the front midline where the left and right pubic bones meet. Pubiotomy is now only rarely performed during childbirth if it is necessary to increase the size of an abnormally small pelvis to allow passage of the child and a Caesarean section is contraindicated. It is occasionally also done to facilitate access to the base of the bladder and the urethra during complex urological procedures (e.g. *urethroplasty).

pubis *n.* (*pl.* **pubes**) a bone forming the lower and anterior part of each side of the *hip bone (*see also* PELVIS). The two pubes meet at the front of the pelvis at the **pubic symphysis**. *See also* PUBES.

public access defibrillation programmes programmes of lay education in the UK that aim to provide training in cardiac resuscitation up to and including *defibrillation. Together with programmes to increase the availability of *automated external defibrillators in public places (e.g. shops and railway stations), they recognize that the best outcomes from cardiac resuscitation are obtained with early defibrillation and good bystander basic life support.

publication ethics the standards expected from those who write, publish, and disseminate research. In response to a number of high-profile research fraud cases, the Committee on Publication Ethics (COPE) was established in 1997. It is a registered UK charity but has an international membership with most of the major academic biomedical journals represented. Specific issues that fall within the broad remit of COPE and the subject of publication ethics include research misconduct, plagiarism, so-called gift authorship, determination of contribution to research, and peer review processes.

public health consultant (in Britain) a medical consultant with postgraduate training in public health. Formerly known as **community physicians**, such consultants undertake public health functions in the *National Health Service, either as *Directors of Public Health or as consultants in public health. Usually Directors of Public Health or *Consultants in Communicable Disease Control will act as **proper officers** to the appropriate local authority, giving epidemiological and other medical advice to the *Environmental Health Officer.

public health ethics the moral dimensions of health relating to populations, epidemiology, disease prevention, health promotion, *justice, and *equality. Public health ethics is commonly concerned with the tensions between individual *autonomy and *communitarianism and/or *utilitarianism.

Public Health Inspector (in Britain) the former title of an Environmental Health Officer.

public health medicine the specialty concerned with preventing disease and improving health in populations as distinct from individuals. Formerly known as **community medicine** or **social medicine**, it includes *epidemiology, *health promotion, *health service planning, *health protection, and evaluation. *See also* PUBLIC HEALTH CONSULTANT.

public health nurse *see* HEALTH VISITOR.

public health specialist a public health practitioner with postgraduate training in public health or with demonstrated competence in key areas of public health practice. These consultants undertake public health functions in the National Health Service either as *Directors of Public Health or as public health specialists.

public interest disclosure 1. the expression of concern about performance or competence that is privileged at law by virtue of the Public Interest Disclosure Act 1998. The statute provides that where an employee acts in good faith in questioning the behaviour or performance of another member of staff or an organization, he or she should be protected from such penalties as disciplinary procedures, suspension, or dismissal. *See also* WHISTLE-BLOWING. 2. circumstances in which *confidentiality can be breached because there is a serious risk of physical harm to an identifiable individual or individuals. The basis on which confidentiality can be breached in the public interest were defined in the case of *W v Egdell*, in which the court held that the risk had to be of physical harm to identifiable person(s) and must not be merely 'fanciful'. Where there is a serious risk of physical harm to a specific person, there is an entitlement but not a duty to breach confidentiality, and the *General Medical Council requires that doctors must be prepared to justify their decision either way.

pubovaginal sling a band of material inserted directly under the bladder neck as a treatment for women with stress *incontinence. The sling can be constructed from fascia (connective tissue) obtained from the patient or it can be synthetic. *Compare* TENSION-FREE VAGINAL TAPE.

pudendal nerve the nerve that supplies the lowest muscles of the pelvic floor and the anal sphincter. It is often damaged in childbirth, causing incontinence.

pudendum *n.* (*pl.* **pudenda**) the external genital organs, especially those of the female (*see* VULVA). —**pudendal** *adj.*

puerperal *adj.* relating to childbirth or the period that immediately follows it.

puerperal cardiomyopathy a rare complication of pregnancy, occurring from the sixth month of pregnancy until six months postnatally (usually within six weeks of delivery). It is characterized by palpitations, dyspnoea, oedema (peripheral and central), and impaired exercise tolerance. The diagnosis is confirmed on echocardiography. It has a high mortality and morbidity. Treatment of heart failure, anticoagulation, and in some cases immunosuppressant therapy is required; in some cases heart transplantation may be considered.

puerperal infection infection of the female genital tract arising as a complication of childbirth.

puerperal psychosis a *psychosis that is triggered by childbirth and usually arises in the first two weeks after giving birth. It affects 1 in 200 women; those suffering from bipolar affective disorder or schizophrenia or those who have a history of puerperal psychosis are at particularly high risk. The symptoms develop very rapidly and the patient needs to be hospitalized, ideally in a mother and baby psychiatric unit to avoid separation; most patients respond well to *antipsychotic medication.

puerperal pyrexia a temperature of 38°C occurring on any two days within 14 days of childbirth or miscarriage.

puerperium *n.* the period of up to about six weeks after childbirth, during which the mother's body returns to its prepregnant state and her uterus returns to its normal size (i.e. involution takes place).

Pulex *n.* a genus of widely distributed *fleas. *P. irritans*, the human flea, is a common parasite whose bite may give rise to intense irritation and bacterial infection. It is an intermediate host for larvae of the tapeworms *Hymenolepis and *Dipylidium*, which it can transmit to humans, and it may also be involved in the transmission of plague.

pulmo- (pulmon(o)-) *combining form denoting* the lung(s).

pulmonary *adj.* relating to, associated with, or affecting the lungs.

pulmonary artery the artery that conveys blood from the heart to the lungs for oxygenation: the only artery in the body containing deoxygenated blood. It leaves the right ventricle and passes upwards for 5 cm before dividing into two, one branch going to each lung. Within the lungs each pulmonary artery divides into many fine branches, which end in capillaries in the alveolar walls. *See also* PULMONARY CIRCULATION.

pulmonary capillary wedge pressure (PCWP) an indirect measurement of the pressure of blood in the left atrium of the heart, which indicates the adequacy of left heart function. It is measured using a catheter wedged in the most distal segment of the pulmonary artery. *See also* SWAN-GANZ CATHETER.

pulmonary circulation a system of blood vessels effecting transport of blood between the heart and lungs. Deoxygenated blood leaves the right ventricle by the pulmonary artery and is carried to the alveolar capillaries of the lungs. Gaseous exchange occurs, with carbon dioxide leaving the circulation and oxygen entering. The oxygenated blood then passes into small veins leading to the pulmonary veins, which leave the lungs and return blood to the left atrium of the heart. The oxygenated blood can then be pumped around the body via the *systemic circulation.

pulmonary embolism obstruction of the *pulmonary artery or one of its branches by an *embolus, usually a blood clot derived from *phlebothrombosis of the leg veins (deep vein thrombosis). Large pulmonary emboli result in acute heart failure or sudden death. Smaller emboli cause death of sections of lung tissue, pleurisy, and haemoptysis (coughing of blood). Minor pulmonary emboli respond to the *anticoagulant drugs heparin and warfarin. Major pulmonary embolism is treated by *embolectomy or by dissolution of the blood clot with an infusion of *streptokinase. Recurrent pulmonary embolism may result in *pulmonary hypertension.

pulmonary hypertension a condition in which there is raised blood pressure within the blood vessels supplying the lungs (the pulmonary artery blood pressure is normally much lower than the pressure within the aorta and its branches). Pulmonary hypertension may complicate pulmonary em-

bolism, *septal defects, heart failure, diseases of the mitral valve, and chronic lung diseases. It may also develop without any known cause (**primary pulmonary hypertension**). The right ventricle enlarges and heart failure, fainting, and chest pain occur. The treatment is that of the cause; drugs used to control *hypertension are ineffective.

pulmonary regurgitation leakage of the pulmonary valve in the heart. Mild regurgitation is a common normal finding, but severe congenital pulmonary regurgitation may require surgical correction.

pulmonary stenosis congenital narrowing of the outlet of the right ventricle of the heart to the pulmonary artery. The defect may be in the pulmonary valve (**valvular stenosis**) or in the outflow tract of the right ventricle below the valve (**infundibular stenosis**). It may be isolated or combined with other heart defects (e.g. *tetralogy of Fallot). Severe pulmonary stenosis may produce angina pectoris, faintness, and heart failure. The defect is corrected by surgery.

pulmonary tuberculosis *see* TUBERCULOSIS.

pulmonary valve a valve in the heart lying between the right ventricle and the pulmonary artery. It is a *semilunar valve that prevents blood returning to the ventricle from the pulmonary artery.

pulmonary vein a vein carrying oxygenated blood from the lung to the left atrium. *See* PULMONARY CIRCULATION.

pulp *n.* **1.** a soft mass of tissue (for example, of the *spleen, in which there is both **red pulp** and **white pulp**). **2.** the mass of connective tissue in the **pulp cavity**, at the centre of a *tooth. It is surrounded by dentine except where it communicates with the rest of the body at the apex. The pulp within the crown portion of the pulp cavity is described as **coronal pulp**; that within the root canal is the **radicular pulp**. **3.** the fleshy cushion on the flexor surface of the fingertip.

pulp capping the procedure of covering an exposed tooth pulp following trauma with a medicament (usually based on calcium hydroxide), which is then covered with a temporary or permanent *restoration.

pulpitis *n.* inflammation of the pulp of a tooth: a frequent cause of toothache.

pulpotomy *n.* a procedure in which part

of the pulp of a tooth damaged by trauma or caries is cut back and then covered with a medicament and *restoration.

pulsatile *adj.* characterized by regular rhythmical beating.

pulse *n.* a series of pressure waves within an artery caused by contractions of the left ventricle and corresponding with the **heart rate** (the number of times the heart beats per minute). It is easily detected on such superficial arteries as the radial artery near the wrist and the carotid artery in the neck (see illustration). The average adult pulse rate at rest is 60–80 per minute, but exercise, injury, illness, and emotion may produce much faster rates.

carotid
brachial
radial
femoral
popliteal
posterior tibial
dorsalis pedis

Peripheral pulses.

pulseless disease *see* TAKAYASU'S DISEASE.

pulseless electrical activity (**electromechanical dissociation**) the appearance of normal-looking complexes on the electrocardiogram that are, however, associated with a state of *cardiac arrest. It is usually caused by large pulmonary emboli (*see* PULMONARY EMBOLISM), *cardiac tamponade, tension *pneumothorax, severe disturbance of body salt levels, severe haemorrhage, or hypothermia causing severe lack of oxygen to the heart muscle.

pulsus alternans alternate variation of the force of the pulse due to variation in force of heart muscle contraction. It is a sign of cardiomyopathy and heart failure.

pulsus paradoxus an exaggerated fall in systolic blood pressure and pulse volume when the patient breathes in. It is seen in constrictive *pericarditis, pericardial effusion, and asthma.

pulvinar *n.* the expanded posterior end of the *thalamus.

punch-drunk syndrome a group of symptoms consisting of progressive *dementia, tremor of the hands, epilepsy, and parkinsonism. It is a consequence of repeated blows to the head that have been severe enough to cause *concussion.

punctum *n.* (*pl.* **puncta**) (in anatomy) a point or small area, especially the **puncta lacrimalia** – the two openings of the tear ducts in the inner corners of the upper and lower eyelids (*see* LACRIMAL APPARATUS).

puncture 1. *n.* a wound made accidentally or deliberately by a sharp object or instrument. Puncture wounds need careful treatment as a small entry hole in the skin can disguise serious injury in an underlying organ or tissue. Punctures are also performed for diagnostic purposes using a hollow needle, in order to withdraw a sample of tissue or fluid for examination; needle punctures are used especially for obtaining tissue samples for the liver, bone marrow, or breast. *See also* LUMBAR PUNCTURE. 2. *vb.* to pierce a tissue with a sharp instrument or needle.

pupil *n.* the circular opening in the centre of the *iris, through which light passes into the lens of the eye. —**pupillary** *adj.*

pupillary reflex (**light reflex**) the reflex change in the size of the pupil according to the amount of light entering the eye. Bright light reaching the retina stimulates nerves of the *parasympathetic nervous system, which cause the pupil to contract. In dim light the pupil opens, due to stimulation of the *sympathetic nervous system. *See also* IRIS.

pupilloplasty *n.* a surgical procedure to alter the shape or function of the pupil. It is usually performed to repair a pupil damaged after trauma.

PUPPP *see* POLYMORPHIC ERUPTION OF PREGNANCY.

pure tone audiogram (PTA) *see* AUDIO-GRAM.

purgation *n.* the use of drugs to stimulate intestinal activity and clear the bowels. *See* LAXATIVE.

purgative *n. see* LAXATIVE.

purine *n.* a nitrogen-containing compound with a two-ring molecular structure. Examples of purines are adenine and guanine, which form the *nucleotides of nucleic acids, and uric acid, which is the end-product of purine metabolism.

Purkinje cells nerve cells found in great numbers in the cortex of the cerebellum. The cell body is flask-shaped, with numerous dendrites branching from the neck and extending fanwise among other cells towards the surface and a long axon that runs from the base deep into the cerebellum. [J. E. Purkinje (1787–1869), Bohemian physiologist]

Purkinje fibres *see* ATRIOVENTRICULAR BUNDLE.

purpura *n.* a skin rash resulting from bleeding into the skin from small blood vessels (capillaries); the individual purple spots of the rash are called **petechiae**. Purpura may be due either to defects in the capillaries (**nonthrombocytopenic purpura**) or to a deficiency of blood platelets (**thrombocytopenic purpura**). *See* HENOCH-SCHÖNLEIN PURPURA, IDIOPATHIC THROMBOCYTOPENIC PURPURA, THROMBOCYTOPENIA, THROMBOTIC THROMBOCYTOPENIC PURPURA.

purulent *adj.* forming, consisting of, or containing pus.

pus *n.* a thick yellowish or greenish liquid formed at the site of an established infection. Pus contains dead white blood cells, both living and dead bacteria, and fragments of dead tissue. *See also* MUCOPUS, SEROPUS.

push-bang technique a technique for removing a stone from the ureter. It consists of 'pushing' the stone back into the renal pelvis, where it can be destroyed by *lithotripsy ('bang').

pustule *n.* a small pus-containing blister on the skin.

putamen *n.* a part of the lenticular nucleus (*see* BASAL GANGLIA).

putrefaction *n.* the process whereby proteins are decomposed by bacteria. This is ac-companied by the formation of amines (such as **putrescine** and **cadaverine**) having a strong and very unpleasant smell.

putrescine *n.* an amine formed during *putrefaction.

PUVA (photochemotherapy) *p*soralen + *u*ltra*v*iolet A: the combination of a **psoralen** (a light-sensitive drug) and exposure to long-wave (315–400 nm) ultraviolet light (UVA). It was used in the East in ancient times, with natural sunlight as the light source, for the treatment of *vitiligo. It is now principally used for treating *psoriasis; a number of other conditions also respond. The psoralen is usually taken as tablets but may be administered in a bath. The UVA is administered in light cabinets, but the increased risk of skin cancer limits its use.

P value *see* SIGNIFICANCE.

PVP *see* PHOTOSELECTIVE VAPORIZATION OF THE PROSTATE.

PVS *see* PERSISTENT VEGETATIVE STATE.

py- (pyo-) *combining form denoting* pus; a purulent condition. Example: **pyoureter** (pus in a ureter).

pyaemia *n.* blood poisoning by pus-forming bacteria released from an abscess. The widespread formation of abscesses may develop, with fatal results. *Compare* SAPRAE-MIA, SEPTICAEMIA, TOXAEMIA.

pyarthrosis *n.* an infected joint filled with pus (*see* SEPTIC ARTHRITIS).

pyel- (pyelo-) *combining form denoting* the pelvis of the kidney. Example: **pyelecta-sis** (dilation of).

pyelitis *n.* inflammation of the pelvis of the kidney (the part of the kidney from which urine drains into the ureter). This is usually caused by a bacterial infection, which may develop in any condition causing obstruction to the flow of urine. The patient experiences pain in the loins, shivering, and a high temperature. Treatment is by the administration of a suitable antibiotic, together with analgesics and a high fluid intake. Any underlying abnormality of the urinary system must be relieved to prevent further attacks.

pyelocystitis *n.* inflammation of the renal pelvis and urinary bladder (*see* PYELITIS, CYSTITIS).

pyelogram *n. see* PYELOGRAPHY.

pyelography *n.* X-ray examination of the pelvis of the kidney using *radiopaque contrast material. **Anterograde pyelography** is performed by puncturing the renal pelvis directly with a needle through the skin and injecting contrast material. **Intravenous pyelography** is usually part of an examination of the whole urinary tract (*see* INTRAVENOUS UROGRAPHY). **Retrograde pyelography** is performed after a tube has been inserted through the bladder and up the ureter at cystoscopy. Contrast material is injected up this tube as it is withdrawn and X-ray images taken. All techniques are used to show the anatomy of the renal pelvis and its drainage, as well as to demonstrate the presence of tumours and stones.

pyelolithotomy *n.* surgical removal of a stone from the kidney through an incision made in the pelvis of the kidney. The incision is usually made into the posterior surface of the pelvis (**posterior pyelotomy**) to gain access to the stone, which can then be lifted clear.

pyelonephritis *n.* bacterial infection of the kidney substance. In **acute pyelonephritis**, the patient has pain in the loins, a high temperature, and shivering fits. Treatment is by the administration of an appropriate antibiotic, and a full urological investigation is conducted to determine any underlying abnormality and prevent recurrence. In **chronic pyelonephritis**, the kidneys become small and scarred and kidney failure ensues. *Vesicoureteric reflux in childhood is one of the causes.

pyeloplasty *n.* an operation to relieve obstruction at the junction of the pelvis of the kidney and the ureter. *See* HYDRONEPHROSIS, DIETL'S CRISIS.

pyelotomy *n.* surgical incision into the pelvis of the kidney. This operation is usually undertaken to remove a stone (*see* PYELO-LITHOTOMY) but is also necessary when surgical drainage of the kidney is required by a catheter or tube.

Pyemotes *n. see* PEDICULOIDES.

pyg- (pygo-) *combining form denoting* the buttocks.

pykno- *combining form denoting* thickness or density.

pyknosis *n.* the process in which the cell nucleus is thickened into a dense mass, which occurs when cells die. —**pyknotic** *adj.*

pyl- (pyle-) *combining form denoting* the portal vein.

pylephlebitis (portal pyaemia) *n.* septic inflammation and thrombosis of the hepatic portal vein. This is a rare result of the spread of infection within the abdomen (as from appendicitis). The condition causes severe illness, with fever, liver abscesses, and *ascites. Treatment is by antibiotic drugs and surgical drainage of abscesses.

pylethrombosis *n.* obstruction of the portal vein by a blood clot (*see* THROMBOSIS). It can result from infection of the umbilicus in infants, pylephlebitis, cirrhosis of the liver, and liver tumours. *Portal hypertension is a frequent result.

pylor- (pyloro-) *combining form denoting* the pylorus. Example: **pyloroduodenal** (of the pylorus and duodenum).

pylorectomy *n.* a surgical operation in which the muscular outlet of the stomach (*pylorus) is removed. *See* ANTRECTOMY, PYLOROPLASTY.

pyloric stenosis narrowing of the muscular outlet of the stomach (*pylorus). This causes delay in passage of the stomach contents to the duodenum, which leads to repeated vomiting (sometimes of food eaten more than 24 hours earlier), and sometimes visible distension and movement of the stomach. If the condition persists the patient loses weight, becomes dehydrated, and develops *alkalosis. **Congenital hypertrophic pyloric stenosis** occurs in babies about 3–5 weeks old (particularly boys) in which the thickened pyloric muscle can be felt as a nodule. Treatment is by the surgical operation of *pyloromyotomy (Ramstedt's operation). Recovery is usually complete and the condition does not recur. Pyloric stenosis in adults is caused either by a *peptic ulcer close to the pylorus or by a cancerous growth invading the pylorus. Stenosis from peptic ulceration may be treated by healing the ulcer with an *antisecretory drug and dilating the pylorus with a *balloon, or by surgical removal or bypass (*see* GASTRO-ENTEROSTOMY). Surgery is usually required for cancerous obstruction, although in unfit patients a stent can be placed to relieve the obstruction.

pyloromyotomy (Ramstedt's operation) *n.* a surgical operation in which the muscle around the outlet of the stomach (pylorus) is

p

divided down to the lining (mucosa) in order to relieve congenital *pyloric stenosis.

pyloroplasty *n.* a surgical operation in which the outlet of the stomach (pylorus) is widened by a form of reconstruction. It is done to allow the contents of the stomach to pass more easily into the duodenum, particularly combined with a *vagotomy to treat peptic ulcers (which would otherwise cause delay in gastric emptying).

pylorospasm *n.* closure of the outlet of the stomach (pylorus) due to muscle spasm, leading to delay in the passage of stomach contents to the duodenum and vomiting. It is usually associated with duodenal or pyloric ulcers.

pylorus *n.* the lower end of the *stomach, which leads to the duodenum. It terminates at a ring of muscle – the **pyloric sphincter** – which contracts to close the opening by which the stomach communicates with the duodenum. —**pyloric** *adj.*

pyo- *combining form. see* PY-.

pyocele *n.* a swelling caused by an accumulation of pus in a part of the body.

pyocolpos *n.* the presence of pus in the vagina.

pyocyanin *n.* an antibiotic substance produced by the bacterium *Pseudomonas aeruginosa* and active principally against Gram-positive bacteria.

pyoderma gangrenosum an acute destructive ulcerating process of the skin, especially the legs. It may be associated with ulcerative *colitis or *Crohn's disease or with *rheumatoid arthritis or other forms of arthritis affecting many joints. Treatment is with ciclosporin, high doses of corticosteroids, or other immunosuppressants.

pyogenic *adj.* causing the formation of pus. Pyogenic bacteria include *Staphylococcus aureus, Streptococcus hemolyticus*, and *Neisseria gonorrhoeae.*

pyogenic arthritis *see* SEPTIC ARTHRITIS.

pyogenic granuloma a common rapidly growing nodule on the surface of the skin. Resembling a redcurrant or, if large, a raspberry, it is composed of small blood vessels and therefore bleeds readily after the slightest injury. The nodule never becomes malignant and is treated by *curettage and cautery; it may recur and require excision.

pyometra *n.* the presence of pus in the uterus.

pyometritis *n.* inflammation of the uterus, with the formation of pus.

pyomyositis *n.* bacterial or fungal infection of a muscle resulting in painful inflammation.

pyonephrosis *n.* obstruction and infection of the kidney resulting in pus formation. A kidney stone is the usual cause of the obstruction, and the kidney becomes distended by pus and destroyed by the inflammation, which extends into the kidney substance itself and sometimes into the surrounding tissues (*see* PERINEPHRITIS). Treatment is urgent *nephrectomy under antibiotic cover.

pyopneumothorax *n.* pus and gas or air in the *pleural cavity. The condition can arise if gas is produced by gas-forming bacteria as part of an *empyema or if air is introduced during attempts to drain the pus from an empyema. Alternatively a *hydropneumothorax may become infected.

pyorrhoea *n.* a former name for *periodontal disease.

pyosalpingitis *n.* inflammation of a Fallopian tube, with the formation of pus.

pyosalpingo-oophoritis *n.* inflammation of an ovary and Fallopian tube, with the formation of pus.

pyosalpinx *n.* the accumulation of pus in a Fallopian tube.

pyosis *n.* the formation and discharge of pus.

pyothorax *n. see* EMPYEMA.

pyr- (pyro-) *combining form denoting* **1.** fire. **2.** a burning sensation. **3.** fever.

pyramid *n.* **1.** one of the conical masses that make up the medulla of the *kidney, extending inwards from a base inside the cortex towards the pelvis of the kidney. **2.** one of the elongated bulging areas on the anterior surface of the *medulla oblongata in the brain, extending downwards to the spinal cord. **3.** one of the divisions of the vermis of the *cerebellum in the middle lobe. **4.** a protrusion of the medial wall of the vestibule of the middle ear.

pyramidal cell a type of neuron found in the *cerebral cortex, with a pyramid-shaped cell body, a branched dendrite extending from the apex towards the brain surface, several dendrites extending horizontally from the base, and an axon running in the white matter of the hemisphere.

pyramidal system a collection of nerve fibres in the central nervous system that extend from the *motor cortex in the brain to the spinal cord and are responsible for initiating movement. In the medulla oblongata the fibres form a *pyramid (hence the name), within which they cross from one side of the brain to the opposite side of the spinal cord; this is called the **decussation of the pyramids**. Damage to the pyramidal system manifests in a specific pattern of weakness in the face, arms, and legs, abnormally brisk reflexes, and an extensor *plantar reflex (Babinski response).

pyrazinamide *n.* a drug administered by mouth, in combination with other drugs, to treat tuberculosis. Side-effects may include digestive upsets, loss of appetite, joint pains, gout, fever, and rashes, and high doses may cause liver damage.

pyret- (pyreto-) *combining form denoting* fever.

pyrexia *n. see* FEVER.

pyridostigmine *n.* an *anticholinesterase drug used in the treatment of *myasthenia gravis. It is administered by mouth; side-effects may include nausea, vomiting, abdominal pain, diarrhoea, sweating, and increased salivation. Trade name: **Mestinon**.

pyridoxal phosphate a derivative of vitamin B_6 that is an important *coenzyme in certain reactions of amino-acid metabolism. *See* TRANSAMINATION.

pyridoxine *n. see* VITAMIN B_6.

pyrimethamine *n.* a drug administered by mouth in combination with the *sulphonamide sulfadoxine (as **Fansidar**) for the treatment of malignant (falciparum) *malaria. It is also used, in combination with *sulfadiazine, in the treatment of toxoplasmosis. Possible side-effects include loss of appetite and vomiting, and prolonged use may interfere with red blood cell production (pyrimethamine is a *dihydrofolate reductase inhibitor). Trade name: **Daraprim**.

pyrimidine *n.* a nitrogen-containing compound with a ring molecular structure. The commonest pyrimidines are cytosine, thymine, and uracil, which form the *nucleotides of nucleic acids.

pyrogen *n.* any substance or agent producing fever. —**pyrogenic** *adj.*

pyrosis *n.* another name (chiefly US) for *heartburn.

pyruvic acid (pyruvate) a compound, derived from carbohydrates, that may be oxidized via a complex series of reactions in the *Krebs cycle to yield carbon dioxide and energy in the form of ATP.

pyuria *n.* the presence of pus in the urine, making it cloudy. This is a sign of bacterial infection in the urinary tract.

p

QALYs quality-adjusted life years. *See* QUALITY OF LIFE.

qat *n. see* KHAT.

Q fever an acute infectious disease of many animals, including cattle, sheep, goats, deer, and dogs, that is caused by a *rickettsia, *Coxiella burnetii*; it can be transmitted to humans primarily through inhalation of infected particles or consumption of contaminated unpasteurized milk but also via ticks, which can act as vectors. After an incubation period of up to three weeks a severe influenza-like illness develops, sometimes with pneumonia. The disease lasts about two weeks; treatment with tetracyclines or chloramphenicol is effective. *See also* TYPHUS.

qinghaosu *n. see* ARTEMISININ.

QOF *see* QUALITY AND OUTCOMES FRAMEWORK.

QRS complex the element of an *electrocardiogram that precedes the *S–T segment and indicates electrical activation of the ventricles.

Q–T interval the interval on an *electrocardiogram between the beginning of ventricular depolarization (*Q wave) and the beginning of *repolarization (the T wave). *See also* LONG QT SYNDROME.

quadrantanopia *n.* absence or loss of one quarter of the *visual field (i.e. upper nasal (inner), upper temporal (outer), lower nasal (inner), or lower temporal (outer)).

quadrate lobe one of the lobes of the *liver.

quadratus *n.* any of various four-sided muscles. The **quadratus femoris** is a flat muscle at the head of the femur, responsible for lateral rotation of the thigh.

quadri- *combining form denoting* four. Example: **quadrilateral** (having four sides).

quadriceps *n.* one of the great extensor muscles of the legs. It is situated in the thigh and is subdivided into four distinct portions: the **rectus femoris** (which also flexes the

thigh), **vastus lateralis**, **vastus medialis**, and **vastus intermedius** (see illustration).

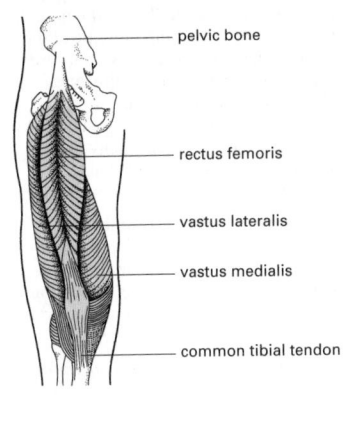

- pelvic bone
- rectus femoris
- vastus lateralis
- vastus medialis
- common tibial tendon

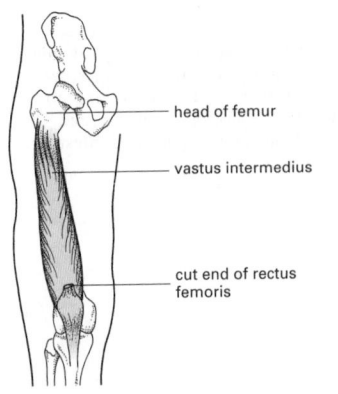

- head of femur
- vastus intermedius
- cut end of rectus femoris

Components of the quadriceps femoris.

quadriplegia (tetraplegia) *n.* paralysis affecting all four limbs, which may or may not be total. —**quadriplegic** *adj., n.*

Quality and Outcomes Framework (QOF) a system, introduced as part of the new general medical services (nGMS) contract (*see* GENERAL PRACTITIONER), whereby practices are rewarded for implementing good medical practice. There are four main domains: clinical, organizational, patient experience, and additional services. Each domain has various criteria based on best practice, which have a number of points allocated for achievement. The points are collated at the end of the financial year and converted into payment for the practice. The system is overseen and audited by the relevant *primary care trust.

quality assurance setting, monitoring, and maintaining standards for the quality of a service. *See* CLINICAL GOVERNANCE.

quality of life a measure of a person's wellbeing that is relevant in two ways in medical ethics. (1) The experience, burden, and effects of disease as opposed to its duration are often invoked in debates about *abortion, *assisted suicide, *euthanasia, and the withholding or withdrawal of medical treatment. The criteria for determining another person's wellbeing are complex and contested. Some commentators have sought to distinguish quality of life judgments. (2) The formal evaluation of losses and gains is employed to determine who will benefit most from a treatment and, on this basis, who should receive priority where resources are scarce. In such cases a calculation of **quality-adjusted life years** (**QALYs**) is made, rather than a simpler estimate of how long a successfully treated patient can expect to live. Each expected year of full health is scored 1, each expected year with various degrees of illness or disability less than 1, and death 0. Research priorities are often made on the basis of a related metric, **disability-adjusted life years** (**DALYs**), which seeks to minimize the burden of disease. Both metrics have been criticized for discriminating against those with prior medical conditions, which lower their baseline score, and the elderly, whose longevity is short. *See also* NEED.

quantitative digital radiography a method of detecting *osteoporosis. A narrow X-ray beam is directed at the area of interest (usually the spine and hip), which enables a measurement to be made of its calcium content (density). In this way the likelihood of fracture can be assessed and preventive measures considered.

quarantine *n.* the period for which a person (or animal) is kept in isolation in order to prevent the spread of a contagious disease. The original quarantine was a period of 40 days, but different diseases now have different quarantine periods.

quartan fever *see* MALARIA.

Queckenstedt test a part of the routine *lumbar puncture procedure. It is used to determine whether or not the flow of cerebrospinal fluid is blocked in the spinal canal. [H. H. G. Queckenstedt (1876–1918), German physician]

quellung reaction a reaction in which antibodies against the bacterium *Streptococcus pneumoniae* combine with the bacterial capsule, which becomes swollen and visible to light microscopy.

quetiapine *n. see* ANTIPSYCHOTIC.

quickening *n.* the first movement of a fetus in the uterus felt by the mother. Quickening is usually experienced after about 16 weeks of pregnancy, although it may occur earlier.

quiescent *adj.* describing a disease that is in an inactive or undetectable phase.

quinine *n.* a drug used in the treament of *malaria due to *Plasmodium falciparum*. It is administered by mouth or injection; large doses can cause severe poisoning, symptoms of which include headache, fever, vomiting, confusion and damage to sight and hearing (*see* CINCHONISM). Small doses of quinine are used to treat nocturnal leg cramps.

quinism *n.* the symptoms of overdosage or prolonged treatment with quinine. *See* CINCHONISM.

quinolone *n.* one of a group of chemically related synthetic antibiotics that includes *ciprofloxacin, *nalidixic acid, and *ofloxacin. These drugs act by inactivating an enzyme, DNA gyrase, that is necessary for replication of the microorganisms and are often useful for treating infections with organisms that have become resistant to other antibiotics. Possible side-effects of quinolones include nausea, vomiting, diarrhoea, abdominal pain, headache, dizziness, and itching. Confusion, joint pains, skin troubles, and tendinitis occasionally occur.

quinsy *n.* pus in the space between the tonsil and the wall of the pharynx. The patient has severe pain with difficulty opening the mouth (*trismus) and swallowing. Treatment is with antibiotics. Surgical incision of the abscess may be necessary to release the

q

collection of pus. Medical name: **peritonsillar abscess**.

quotidian fever *see* MALARIA.

Q wave the downward deflection on an *electrocardiogram that indicates the beginning of ventricular depolarization. An abnormally deep and wide Q wave is an indication of prior heart muscle damage due to heart attack.

q

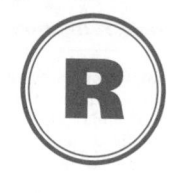

rabbit fever *see* TULARAEMIA.

rabies (hydrophobia) *n.* an acute virus disease of the central nervous system that affects all warm-blooded animals and is usually transmitted to humans by a bite from an infected dog. Symptoms appear after an incubation period ranging from 10 days to over a year and include malaise, fever, difficulty in breathing, salivation, periods of intense excitement, hallucinations, and painful muscle spasms of the throat induced by swallowing. In the later stages of the disease the mere sight of water induces convulsions and paralysis; death occurs within 4–5 days. Daily injections of rabies vaccine, together with an injection of rabies antiserum, may prevent the disease from developing in a person bitten by an infected animal. —**rabid** *adj.*

racemose *adj.* resembling a bunch of grapes. The term is applied particularly to a compound gland the secretory part of which consists of a number of small sacs.

rachi- (rachio-) *combining form denoting* the spine.

rachis *n. see* BACKBONE.

rachischisis *n. see* SPINA BIFIDA.

rachitic *adj.* afflicted with rickets.

rad *n.* a former unit of absorbed dose of ionizing radiation. It has been replaced by the *gray.

radial *adj.* relating to or associated with the radius (a bone in the forearm).

radial artery a branch of the brachial artery, beginning at the elbow and passing superficially down the forearm to the styloid process of the radius at the wrist. It then winds around the wrist and enters the palm of the hand, sending out branches to the fingers.

radial keratotomy an operation for short-sightedness (myopia). Deep cuts into the tissue of the cornea are placed radially around the outer two-thirds of the cornea; this flattens the curvature of the central part of the cornea and reduces the myopia. This procedure is now rarely performed, having been superseded by *excimer laser treatment.

radial nerve an important mixed sensory and motor nerve of the arm, forming the largest branch of the *brachial plexus. It extends downwards behind the humerus, supplying muscles of the upper arm, to the elbow, which it supplies with branches, and then runs parallel with the radius. It supplies sensory branches to the base of the thumb and a small area of the back of the hand.

radial reflex flexion of the forearm (and sometimes also of the fingers) that occurs when the lower end of the radius is tapped. It is due to contraction of the brachioradialis muscle, which is stimulated by tapping its point of insertion in the radius.

radiation *n.* energy in the form of waves or particles, especially **electromagnetic radiation**, which includes (in order of increasing energy) radio waves, microwaves, *infrared rays (radiant heat), visible light, *ultraviolet rays, *X-rays, and *gamma rays. The latter two are described as ionizing radiation due to their effect on other atoms and are potentially harmful. Particle radiation is described as alpha (a helium nucleus), beta (an electron), or *positron emission. Only the latter is commonly used for diagnostic imaging (*see* POSITRON EMISSION TOMOGRAPHY).

radiation protection measures designed to limit the dose of harmful radiation to patients and workers. Medical exposure to radiation is governed in the UK by the Ionising Radiation (Medical Exposures) Regulations 2000 (**IRMER**). A guiding theme of protection is the **ALARA principle** ("as low as reasonably achievable").

radiation sickness an acute illness caused by extreme exposure to rays emitted by radioactive substances, e.g. X-rays or gamma rays. Very high doses cause death within hours from destructive lesions of the central nervous system. Lower doses, which may eventually prove fatal, cause nausea, vomiting, and diarrhoea followed after a week or more by bleeding and other symptoms of damage to the bone marrow, loss of hair, and bloody diarrhoea. Some of the milder symptoms can occur after *radiotherapy during treatment of cancer.

radical treatment vigorous treatment that aims at the complete cure of a disease rather than the mere relief of symptoms. *Compare* CONSERVATIVE TREATMENT.

radicle *n.* (in anatomy) **1.** a small *root. **2.** the initial fibre of a nerve or the origin of a vein. —**radicular** *adj.*

radiculitis *n.* inflammation of the root of a nerve. *See* POLYRADICULITIS.

radio- *combining form denoting* **1.** radiation. **2.** radioactive substances.

radioactive iodine therapy the administration of an estimated amount of the radioactive isotope iodine-131 as a drink in order to treat an overactive thyroid gland (*see* THYROTOXICOSIS). The iodine concentrates in the thyroid and thus delivers its beta radiation locally, with little effect on other tissues. The gland will shrink and become euthyroid over the succeeding 8–12 weeks but there is a high incidence of subsequent hypothyroidism (up to 80%), which requires lifetime treatment with thyroxine. The treatment cannot be used if there is any suspicion of pregnancy, and the patient must stay away from young children and pregnant women for around ten days after administration. Despite these drawbacks, radioactive iodine remains a popular form of treatment for any cause of hyperthyroidism.

radioactivity *n.* disintegration of the nuclei of certain elements, with the emission of energy in the form of alpha, beta, or gamma rays. As particles are emitted the elements 'decay' into other elements. Naturally occurring radioactive elements include radium and uranium. There are many artificially produced isotopes, including iodine-131 and cobalt-60 used in *radiotherapy; technetium-99m is used in *nuclear medicine. *See* RADIOISOTOPE. —**radioactive** *adj.*

radioautography *n. see* AUTORADIOGRAPHY.

radiobiology *n.* the study of the effects of radiation on living cells and organisms. Studies of the behaviour of cancer cells exposed to radiation have important applications in *radiotherapy, revealing why some tumours fail to respond to the treatment;

this has led to the development of new radiotherapy techniques that make tumours more susceptible to attack by radiation.

radiodermatitis *n.* inflammation of the skin after exposure to ionizing radiation. This may occur after a short dose of heavy radiation (radiotherapy or atomic explosions) or prolonged exposure to small doses, as may happen accidentally to X-ray workers. The skin becomes dry, hairless, and atrophied, losing its colouring.

radiofrequency ablation the selective destruction of abnormal conducting tissue in the heart by the targeted delivery of radiofrequency energy via a catheter (*see* CATHETERIZATION) under X-ray and electrocardiographic guidance. It is usually curative in patients with supraventricular *re-entry tachycardia and is the treatment of choice for this condition (*see* SUPRAVENTRICULAR TACHYCARDIA, WOLFF-PARKINSON-WHITE SYNDROME). It can be used for a variety of other arrhythmias with varying degrees of success.

radiofrequency palatal myoplasty (RPM) *see* PALATOPLASTY.

radiographer *n.* **1.** (diagnostic radiographer) a person who is trained in the technique of taking X-ray pictures of parts of the body. In modern practice a radiographer may also perform other imaging techniques, including *magnetic resonance imaging, *ultrasound, and *nuclear medicine. **2.** (therapeutic radiographer) a person who is trained in the technique of treatment by *radiotherapy.

radiography *n.* diagnostic radiology: traditionally, the technique of examining the body by directing *X-rays through it to produce images (**radiographs**) on photographic film or a fluoroscope. Increasingly radiography includes the production of images by *computerized tomography and *nuclear medicine. It is used to produce images of disease in all parts of the body, to be interpreted by radiologists for physicians and surgeons. It is also widely used in dentistry for detecting dental caries, periodontal disease, periapical disease, the presence and position of unerupted teeth, and disease of the jaws. *See also* RADIOGRAPHER, RADIOLOGY.

radioimmunoassay *n.* a technique using radioactive antibodies as *tracers to estimate the levels of natural substances in a blood sample. The antibodies bind to antigens, and the amount of radioactivity trapped is a measure of the amount of the target antigen present. The technique is widely used in the estimation of hormone levels.

radioimmunolocalization *n.* a method of identifying the site of a tumour (e.g. colorectal cancer) that relies on its uptake of radioactive isotopes attached to an appropriate anticancer immune cell. As yet this technique is little used in clinical practice.

radioimmunotherapy *n.* treatment in which a radioactive substance is linked to an antibody that attaches to a specific type of tumour cell, thus delivering the radiation to the tumour and limiting damage to healthy cells. *See* MONOCLONAL ANTIBODY.

radioisotope *n.* an *isotope of an element that emits alpha, beta, or gamma radiation during its decay into another element. Artificial radioisotopes, produced by bombarding elements with beams of neutrons, are widely used in medicine as *tracers and as sources of radiation for the different techniques of *radiotherapy.

radiologist *n.* a doctor specialized in the interpretation of X-rays and other imaging techniques for the diagnosis of disease. An **interventional radiologist** specializes in the use of imaging to guide *interventional radiology techniques.

radiology *n.* the branch of medicine involving the study of radiographs or other imaging technologies (such as *ultrasound and *magnetic resonance imaging) to diagnose or treat disease. A physician specializing in this field is known as a *radiologist. *See also* INTERVENTIONAL RADIOLOGY, RADIOGRAPHY.

radiology information system (RIS) a computer system responsible for keeping details of all the patients coming to a clinical radiology department, including the time and place of their examination. This is vital to the functioning of a picture archiving and communications system (*see* PACS).

radiolucent *adj.* having the property of being transparent to X-rays. Radiopacity decreases with atomic number of the element. Radiolucent materials, such as beryllium, are used to construct windows in X-ray tubes to allow the X-rays to escape from the tube. Gases are relatively radiolucent to X-rays and can be used as a negative *contrast medium in X-ray examinations, e.g. in *double-

contrast barium examinations of the bowel or carbon dioxide *arteriography.

radionecrosis *n.* death (*necrosis) of tissue, commonly bone or skin, caused by exposure to ionizing radiation, as in *radiotherapy. It can be induced by subsequent injury or surgery. *See* IONIZATION.

radionuclide *n.* a substance containing a radioactive atomic nucleus. Radionuclides can be used as *tracers for diagnosis in *nuclear medicine.

radiopaque *adj.* having the property of absorbing, and therefore being opaque to, X-rays. Radiopacity increases with atomic weight. Radiopaque materials, such as those containing iodine or barium, are used as *contrast media in radiography. Metallic foreign bodies in tissues are also radiopaque and can be detected by radiography. Such heavy elements as lead and barium can be used in shielding to protect people from unnecessary exposure to ionizing radiation. —**radiopacity** *n.*

radio pill a capsule containing a miniature radio transmitter that can be swallowed by a patient. During its passage through the digestive tract it transmits information about internal conditions (acidity, etc.) that can be monitored by means of a radio receiver near the patient. Such capsules can contain video cameras and light sources to examine the bowel.

radiosensitive *adj.* describing certain forms of cancer cell that are particularly susceptible to radiation and are likely to be dealt with successfully by radiotherapy.

radiosensitizer *n.* a substance that increases the sensitivity of cells to radiation. The presence of oxygen and other compounds with a high affinity for electrons will increase radiosensitivity. Chemotherapy drugs such as fluorouracil can be used concurrently with radiotherapy as radiosensitizers.

radiotherapist *n.* a doctor who specializes in treatment with radiotherapy.

radiotherapy *n.* therapeutic radiology: the treatment of disease with penetrating radiation, such as X-rays, beta rays, or gamma rays, which may be produced by machines or given off by radioactive isotopes. Beams of radiation may be directed at a diseased part from a distance (*see* TELETHERAPY), or radioactive material, in the form of needles, wires, or pellets, may be implanted in the body (*see* BRACHYTHERAPY). Many forms of cancer are destroyed by radiotherapy.

radium *n.* a radioactive metallic element that emits alpha and gamma rays during its decay into other elements. The gamma radiation was formerly employed in *radiotherapy for the treatment of cancer. Because *radon, a radioactive gas, is released from radium, the metal was enclosed in gas-tight containers during use. Radium is stored in lead-lined containers, which give protection from the radiation. Symbol: Ra.

radius *n.* the outer and shorter bone of the forearm (*compare* ULNA). It partially revolves about the ulna, permitting *pronation and *supination of the hand. The head of the radius articulates with the *humerus. The lower end articulates both with the scaphoid and lunate bones of the *carpus (wrist) and with the ulna (via the **ulnar notch** on the side of the bone). —**radial** *adj.*

radix *n. see* ROOT.

radon *n.* a radioactive gaseous element that is produced during the decay of *radium. Sealed in small capsules called **radon seeds**, it is used in *radiotherapy for the treatment of cancer, but has largely been replaced by newer agents and techniques. It emits alpha and gamma radiation. Symbol: Rn.

rale *n. see* CREPITATION.

raloxifene *n.* a drug used to prevent and treat osteoporosis that develops after the menopause. Raloxifene is a *selective (o)estrogen receptor modulator (SERM): it mimics the protective action of oestrogen in the bones without the risk of the adverse effects (e.g. on the breast and uterus) associated with *hormone replacement therapy. However, it does not relieve menopausal symptoms. It is administered by mouth; side-effects include hot flushes, and there is a risk of *thromboembolism and *thrombophlebitis. Trade name: **Evista**.

raltegravir *n.* an *antiretroviral (ARV) drug used, in combination with other ARVs, for treating refractory HIV infection. It acts by inhibiting integrase, an enzyme required by the virus to replicate and infect other cells. It is administered by mouth; side-effects include abdominal pain, constipation, and *lipodystrophy. Trade name: **Isentress**.

ramipril *n. see* ACE INHIBITOR.

Ramsay Hunt syndrome a form of *herpes zoster affecting the facial nerve, associated with facial paralysis and loss of taste. It also produces pain in the ear and other parts supplied by the nerve. [J. R. Hunt (1872–1937), US neurologist]

Ramstedt's operation *see* PYLOROMY-OTOMY. [W. C. Ramstedt (1867–1963), German surgeon]

ramus *n.* (*pl.* **rami**) **1.** a branch, especially of a nerve fibre or blood vessel. **2.** a thin process projecting from a bone, e.g. the rami of the *mandible.

Randall's plaque the initial deposit of calcium-loaded material on a renal *pyramid that develops into a kidney stone. [A. Randall (1883–1951), US urologist]

randomized controlled trial *see* INTERVENTION STUDY.

random sample a subgroup of a total population selected by a random process ensuring that each member of the population has an equal chance of being included in the sample. It is sometimes **stratified** so that separate samples are drawn from each of several layers of the population, usually on the basis of age, sex, and socio-economic group. Selection is sometimes facilitated by identifying, in advance, groups of individuals (e.g. towns or neighbourhoods) who will together represent the whole (a so-called **sampling frame**).

ranibizumab *n.* a recombinant *monoclonal antibody fragment used for the treatment of wet age-related *macular degeneration. It inhibits *vascular endothelial growth factor and therefore choroidal *neovascularization. Ranibizumab is injected into the eye; the most common side-effects are conjunctival hemorrhage, eye pain, *floaters, increased intraocular pressure, and intraocular inflammation. **Pegaptanib** (Macugen) has similar uses and effects. Trade name: **Lucentis**.

ranitidine *n.* an H_2-receptor antagonist (*see* ANTIHISTAMINE) that is used in the treatment of gastric and duodenal ulcers and gastro-oesophageal reflux disease. It can be administered by mouth, intravenously, or rarely intramuscularly; side-effects include headache, diarrhoea, rash, and drowsiness. Trade name: **Zantac**.

ranula *n.* a cyst found under the tongue, formed when the duct leading from a salivary or mucous gland is obstructed and distended.

rapamycin *n. see* SIROLIMUS.

raphe *n.* a line, ridge, seam, or crease in a tissue or organ, especially the line that marks the junction of two embryologically distinct parts that have fused to form a single structure in the adult. For example, the **raphe of the tongue** is the furrow that passes down the centre of the dorsal surface of the tongue.

rarefaction *n.* thinning of bony tissue sufficient to cause decreased density of bone to X-rays, as in osteoporosis.

rash *n.* a temporary eruption on the skin, usually typified by discrete red spots or generalized reddening, that may be accompanied by itching. A rash may be a local skin reaction or the outward sign of a disorder affecting the body. Rashes commonly occur with infectious diseases, such as chickenpox and measles.

Rasmussen's encephalitis a focal encephalitis, found most commonly in children, that results in continual focal seizures (*see* EPILEPSY). The underlying cause is unknown but it may be due to a viral infection or an autoimmune process. Patients who are unresponsive to medical (antiepileptic) therapy may undergo surgery of the abnormal brain to try and control the seizures. [G. L. Rasmussen (20th century), US anatomist]

raspatory *n.* a filelike surgical instrument used for scraping the surface of bone (see illustration).

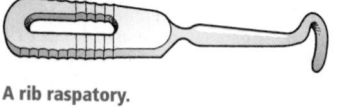

A rib raspatory.

raspberry tumour an *adenoma of the umbilicus.

rat-bite fever (**sodokosis**) a disease, contracted from the bite of a rat, due to infection by either the bacterium *Spirillum minus*, which causes ulceration of the skin and recurrent fever, or by the fungus *Streptobacillus moniliformis*, which causes inflammation of the skin, muscular pains, and vomiting. Both infections respond well to penicillin.

Rathke's pouch *see* CRANIOPHARYNGIOMA.

rationalization *n.* (in psychology) the explanation of events or behaviour in terms that avoid giving the true reasons. For example, someone may claim to have been too tired to go to a party whereas in fact he or she was afraid of meeting new people.

rationing *n.* the process of allocating health-care resources among a population when demand outstrips supply. Where "first come first served" is not considered an appropriate policy, access to treatment may be rationed on a basis of *need, effectiveness, or *quality of life. *See* EQUALITY, JUSTICE, NATIONAL INSTITUTE FOR HEALTH AND CLINICAL EXCELLENCE.

rauwolfia *n.* the dried root of the shrub *Rauwolfia serpentina*, which contains several alkaloids, including **reserpine**. Rauwolfia and its alkaloids lower blood pressure and depress activity of the central nervous system. They were formerly used as tranquillizers and to treat hypertension, but have been replaced by more effective and reliable drugs.

Raynaud's disease a condition of unknown cause in which the arteries of the fingers are unduly reactive and enter spasm (**angiospasm** or **vasospasm**) when the hands are cold. This produces attacks of pallor, numbness, and discomfort in the fingers. A similar condition (**Raynaud's phenomenon**) may result from atherosclerosis, connective-tissue diseases, ingestion of ergot derivatives, or the frequent use of vibrating tools. Gangrene or ulceration of the fingertips may result from lack of blood to the affected part. Warm gloves and peripheral *vasodilators may relieve the condition. In unresponsive cases *sympathectomy is of value. [M. Raynaud (1834–81), French physician]

reaction formation (in psychoanalysis) a *defence mechanism by which unacceptable unconscious ideas are replaced in consciousness by their opposites. For instance, a man might make an ostentatious show of affection to someone for whom he has an unconscious hatred.

reactive *adj.* (in psychiatry) describing mental illnesses thought to be precipitated by events in the psychological environment. *See also* ENDOGENOUS.

reactive arthritis *see* REITER'S SYNDROME.

reactive hypoglycaemia a condition of

postprandial *hypoglycaemia, of varying severity, induced by excessive levels of insulin release from the pancreas. It can be divided into early and late forms, depending on whether the insulin release occurs less than or more than three hours after the meal. The early form is due to the rapid discharge of ingested carbohydrate from the stomach into the small bowel, immediately triggering hyperinsulinaemia. It can occur without obvious cause but is most commonly associated with upper-bowel surgery. The late form is due to a loss of the early-phase insulin response causing excessive postprandial *hyperglycaemia, which then itself triggers an exaggerated insulin response with subsequent hypoglycaemia.

reagin *n*. a type of *antibody, formed against an allergen, that has special affinity for cell membranes and remains fixed in various tissues. Subsequent contact with the allergen causes damage to the tissues when the antigen-antibody reaction occurs. The damaged cells, particularly *mast cells, release histamine and serotonin, which are responsible for the local inflammation of an allergy or the very severe effects of anaphylactic shock (*see* ANAPHYLAXIS). Reagins belong to the IgE class of *immunoglobulins.

reality orientation therapy that aims to improve cognitive functioning and behaviour in elderly people with dementia by using repetition and a range of resources to help the memory. It involves regularly reminding the person of such information as the time, the date, where he or she is, and planned events for that day. The information is given verbally by a carer or written on boards placed in prominent positions in the person's home.

real-time imaging the rapid acquisition and manipulation of ultrasound information from a scanning probe by electronic circuits to enable images to be produced on TV screens almost instantaneously. The operator can place the scanning probe accurately on the region of interest in order to observe its structure and appreciate moving structures within it (*see* DOPPLER ULTRASOUND). Using similar techniques, the instantaneous display of other imaging modalities, such as *computerized tomography scanning and *magnetic resonance imaging, can now be achieved. Real-time imaging is useful in guiding *interventional radiology procedures, for example, allowing a needle to

be guided accurately as it is passed into the body.

reamer *n*. an instrument used in *endodontics to prepare the walls of a root canal for *root canal treatment.

rebound *n*. the return or increase of a condition after cessation of treatment or other stimulus. **Rebound headache**, which may be worse than the initial headache, may occur after stopping medication, particularly if too much was taken. Similarly, **rebound insomnia** may occur after the cessation of sleeping pills, particularly after long-term treatment.

reboxetine *n*. an *antidepressant drug that acts by inhibiting reabsorption of the neurotransmitter *noradrenaline, thus prolonging its action in the brain. It is administered by mouth to treat major depression; side-effects include dry mouth, constipation, insomnia, and dizziness. Trade name: **Edronax**.

receptaculum *n*. the dilated portion of a tubular anatomical part. The **receptaculum** (or **cisterna**) **chyli** is the dilated end of the *thoracic duct, into which lymph vessels from the lower limbs and intestines drain.

receptor *n*. **1.** a cell or group of cells specialized to detect changes in the environment and trigger impulses in the sensory nervous system. All sensory nerve endings act as receptors, whether they simply detect touch, as in the skin, or chemical substances, as in the nose and tongue, or sound or light, as in the ear and eye. *See* EXTEROCEPTOR, INTEROCEPTOR, MECHANORECEPTOR, PROPRIOCEPTOR. **2.** a specialized area of a cell membrane, consisting of a specially adapted protein, that can bind with a specific hormone (e.g. *oestrogen receptors), neurotransmitter (e.g. *adrenoceptors), drug, or other chemical, thereby initiating a change within the cell.

recess *n*. (in anatomy) a hollow chamber or a depression in an organ or other part.

recessive *adj*. describing a gene (or its corresponding characteristic) whose effect is shown in the individual only when its *allele is the same, i.e. when two such alleles are present (the **double recessive** condition). Many hereditary diseases (including cystic fibrosis) are due to the presence of a defective gene as a double recessive. They are said to show **autosomal recessive** inheritance, since the gene is carried on an autosome (any chromosome other than a sex chromosome). *Compare* DOMINANT. —**recessive** *n.*

recipient *n.* a person who receives something from a *donor, such as a blood transfusion or a kidney transplant.

recombinant DNA DNA that contains genes from different sources that have been combined by the techniques of *genetic engineering rather than by breeding experiments. Genetic engineering is therefore also known as **recombinant DNA technology**.

record linkage the means by which information about health events from several different sources (e.g. hospital attendance, vaccination, and consultation with general practitioners) are all related to a specific individual in a common file or more usually a computerized record. This contrasts with data in which events only are recorded (*see* HOSPITAL EPISODE STATISTICS) and two individuals treated for the same disease cannot be distinguished from one individual treated on two separate occasions.

recovery position a first-aid position into which an unconscious but breathing patient can be laid to afford maximum protection to the airway. It involves laying the patient on his or her side, with the uppermost leg bent at the knee and hip and the lower arm behind the back to prevent rolling onto the front or back into a position in which the patient could smother or choke.

recrudescence *n.* a fresh outbreak of a disorder in a patient after a period during which its signs and symptoms had died down and recovery seemed to be taking place.

recruitment *n.* **1.** (in physiology) the phenomenon whereby an increase in the strength of a stimulus or repetition of the stimulus will stimulate increasing numbers of nerve cells to respond. **2.** (in audiology) the phenomenon in which a person with sensorineural deafness cannot hear quiet sounds but can perceive loud sounds just as loudly as, or even more loudly than, a person with normal hearing.

rect- (recto-) *combining form denoting* the rectum. Examples: **rectouterine** (relating to the rectum and uterus); **rectovesical** (relating to the rectum and bladder).

rectal bleeding *see* HAEMATOCHESIA.

rectocele (proctocele) *n.* bulging or pouching of the rectum, usually a forward protrusion of the rectum into the posterior wall of the vagina often in association with prolapse of the uterus. It is repaired by posterior *colporrhaphy.

rectosigmoid *n.* the region of the large intestine around the junction of the sigmoid colon and the rectum.

rectum *n.* the terminal part of the large *intestine, about 12 cm long, which runs from the sigmoid colon to the anal canal. Faeces are stored in the rectum before defecation. —**rectal** *adj.*

rectus *n.* any of several straight muscles. The **rectus muscles of the orbit** are some of the extrinsic *eye muscles. **Rectus abdominis** is a long flat muscle that extends bilaterally along the entire length of the front of the abdomen. The rectus muscles acting together serve to bend the trunk forwards; acting separately they bend the body sideways. The **rectus femoris** forms part of the *quadriceps.

recurrent *adj.* (in anatomy) describing a structure, such as a nerve or blood vessel, that turns back on its course, forming a loop.

recurrent miscarriage *see* MISCARRIAGE.

red blood cell *see* ERYTHROCYTE.

redia *n.* (*pl.* **rediae**) the third-stage larva of a parasitic *fluke. Rediae develop within the body of a freshwater snail and undergo a process of asexual reproduction, giving rise to many fourth-stage larvae called *cercariae. *See also* MIRACIDIUM, SPOROCYST.

red reflex the red area seen through the pupil as a result of the reflection of light from the retina. It is usually seen on *fundoscopy and sometimes in photographs taken using a flashlight.

Reductil *n. see* SIBUTRAMINE.

reduction *n.* (in surgery) the restoration of a displaced part of the body to its normal position by manipulation or operation. The fragments of a broken bone are reduced before a splint is applied; a dislocated joint is reduced to its normal seating; or a hernia is reduced when the displaced organ or tissue is returned to its usual anatomical site.

reduction division the first division of *meiosis, in which the chromosome number is halved. The term is sometimes used as a synonym for the whole of meiosis.

reduplication *n.* doubling of the heart sounds, which may be heard in healthly individuals and shows variation with respiration due to the slightly asynchronous closure of the heart valves.

reduviid *n.* any one of a group of winged insects (Reduviidae) whose mouthparts – adapted for piercing and sucking – take the form of a long proboscis that is tucked beneath the head when not in use. Some South American genera, notably *Panstrongylus*, *Rhodnius*, and *Triatoma* – the kissing bugs, are nocturnal bloodsucking insects that transmit the parasite causing *Chagas' disease.

Reduvius *n.* a genus of predatory bloodsucking reduviid bugs. *R. personatus*, widely distributed in Europe, normally preys upon insects but occasionally attacks humans. Its bite causes various allergic symptoms, including rash, nausea, and palpitations.

Reed-Sternberg cell a large binucleate cell that is characteristic of *Hodgkin's disease. [D. Reed Mendenhall (1874–1964), US pathologist; C. Sternberg (1872–1935), Austrian pathologist]

re-entry tachycardia a rapid heart rate due to a self-sustaining circulation of electrical impulses from the atria to the ventricles and back again. This **re-entry circuit** requires the presence of an abnormal *accessory pathway of electrical conduction in addition to the *atrioventricular node.

refeeding syndrome a potentially fatal condition that may affect severely malnourished patients in response to the reintroduction of a protein- and calorie-rich diet. It is thought to be due to severe fluid and *electrolyte shifts (especially low phosphate, magnesium, and potassium levels in the blood) and related metabolic complications (e.g. raised levels of insulin in the blood). Its manifestations include shortness of breath, *paraesthesia, muscle weakness, palpitations (due to cardiac *arrhythmia), fitting, and death in serious cases. An assessment to identify patients at risk before the introduction of feed, and regular monitoring and prompt correction of serum electrolyte concentration, helps to prevent the condition.

referred pain (synalgia) pain felt in a part of the body other than where it might be expected. An abscess beneath the diaphragm, for example, may cause a referred pain in the shoulder area, while heart disorders may cause pain in the left arm and fingers. The confusion arises because sensory nerves from different parts of the body share common pathways when they reach the spinal cord.

reflective practice the process of considering one's own professional practice during or after events in order to review one's values and to understand the emotions and reasons behind one's actions and decisions and the effect of those actions and decisions on others. Reflection is seen as essential to developing and maintaining ethical medical practice. *See* AUTONOMY.

reflex *n.* an automatic or involuntary activity brought about by relatively simple nervous circuits, without consciousness being necessarily involved. Thus a painful stimulus such as a pinprick will bring about the reflex of withdrawing the finger before the brain has had time to send a message to the muscles involved. *See* CONDITIONED REFLEX, PATELLAR REFLEX, PLANTAR REFLEX, PUPILLARY REFLEX, ROOTING REFLEX..

reflex arc the nervous circuit involved in a *reflex, being at its simplest a sensory nerve with a receptor, linked at a synapse in the brain or spinal cord with a motor nerve, which supplies a muscle or gland (see illustration). In a simple reflex (such as the *patellar reflex) only two neurons may be involved, but in other reflexes there may be several *interneurons in the arc.

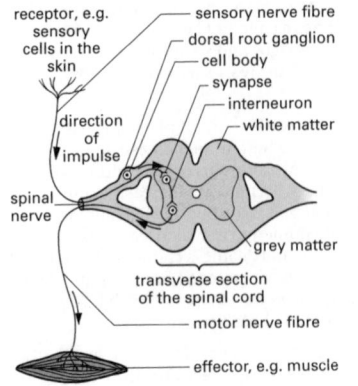

The reflex arc.

reflexology *n.* a complementary therapy based on the theory that reflex points on the feet correspond with all body parts. Firm pressure is applied to the relevant reflex points using the thumb or fingers. Reflexology is said to be able to help with specific illnesses and may also restore the body's natural balance and harmony. It can be used for people of any age and there are very few contraindications.

reflex sympathetic dystrophy (RSD, complex regional pain syndrome, Sudek's atrophy) neurological dysfunction in a limb following trauma, surgery, or disease, characterized by intense burning pain, swelling, stiffness, and sweaty shiny mottled skin. It is caused by overactivity of the sympathetic nervous system. The *ESR is often elevated, X-rays may reveal some patchy osteoporosis, and a bone scan usually demonstrates increased blood flow. Early treatment with splinting and physiotherapy are essential, in combination with *sympatholytic drugs, corticosteroids, and regional sympathetic blocks; *sympathectomy may be required in chronic cases.

reflux *n.* a backflow of liquid, against its normal direction of movement. *See also* (REFLUX) OESOPHAGITIS, VESICOURETERIC REFLUX.

reformatting *n.* the process of changing the way that information already obtained is presented to the viewer. Typical examples are three-dimensional reconstructions and *multiplanar reconstructions.

refraction *n.* **1.** the change in direction of light rays when they pass obliquely from one transparent medium to another, of a different density. Refraction occurs as light enters the eye, when it passes from air to the media of the eye, i.e. cornea, aqueous humour, lens, and vitreous humour, to come to a focus on the retina. Errors of refraction, in which light rays do not come to a focus on the retina due to defects in the refracting media or shape of the eyeball, include astigmatism and long- and short-sightedness. **2.** determination of the power of refraction of the eye. This gives the degree to which the eye differs from normal, which will determine whether or not the patient needs glasses and, if so, how strong they should be.

refractive error an abnormality of the eye resulting in a blurred image on the retina as a result of abnormal focusing, which can be corrected by glasses, contact lenses, or *refractive surgery. Refractive errors include *myopia, *hypermetropia, and *astigmatism.

refractive surgery any surgical procedure that has as its primary objective the correction of any refractive error. It includes such procedures as clear lens extraction, *LASIK, *LASEK, and photorefractive *keratectomy.

refractometer *n. see* OPTOMETER.

refractory *adj.* unresponsive: applied to a condition that fails to respond satisfactorily to a given treatment.

refractory period (in neurology) the time of recovery needed for a nerve cell that has just transmitted a nerve impulse or for a muscle fibre that has just contracted. During the refractory period a normal stimulus will not bring about excitation of the cell, which is undergoing *repolarization.

refrigeration *n.* lowering the temperature of a part of the body to reduce the metabolic activity of its tissues or to provide a local anaesthetic effect.

Refsum's disease an inherited disorder of lipid metabolism resulting in abnormal accumulation of phytanic acid (a fatty acid) in body tissues. This results in a *peripheral neuropathy affecting the sensory and motor nerves, diminishing vision due to *retinitis pigmentosa, and unsteadiness (*ataxia) caused by damage to the cerebellum. [S. Refsum (20th century), Norwegian physician]

regimen *n.* (in therapeutics) a prescribed systematic form of treatment, such as a diet, course of drugs, or special exercises, for curing disease or improving health.

regional ileitis *see* CROHN'S DISEASE.

regional specialty *see* CATCHMENT AREA.

registrar *n. see* CONSULTANT.

regression *n.* (in psychiatry) reversion to a more immature level of functioning. The term may be applied to the state of a patient in hospital who becomes incontinent and demanding. It may also be applied to a single psychological function; for example, psychoanalysts speak of the *libido regressing to an early stage of development.

regulations *pl. n.* explicit rules to govern behaviour that are enforced by specified institutions or agencies. Where regulations are breached, the relevant regulatory authority can impose sanctions. Regulations may derive from statute, for example the Medical Act 1983 (as amended), from professional bodies (e.g. the General Medical Council), or from a designated individual with appropriate authority (e.g. a chief executive of a NHS trust).

regulatory T cell (Treg cell) a type of T *lymphocyte that suppresses immune responses.

regurgitation n. 1. the bringing up of undigested material from the stomach to the mouth (*see* VOMITING). 2. the flowing back of a liquid in a direction opposite to the normal one, as when blood surges back through a defective valve in the heart after the heart has contracted (*see* AORTIC REGURGITATION, MITRAL REGURGITATION).

rehabilitation 1. (in *physical medicine) the treatment of an ill, injured, or disabled patient with the aim of restoring normal health and function or to prevent the disability from getting worse. 2. any means for restoring the independence of a patient after diseases or injury, including employment retraining.

Reifenstein's syndrome (partial androgen insensitivity syndrome) a congenital resistance to androgen hormones (*see* ANDROGEN INSENSITIVITY SYNDROME) resulting in poor development of the male sexual characteristics, which often becomes more obvious at puberty. Some features of feminization may occur (e.g. breast development). [E. C. Reifenstein (1908–75), US endocrinologist]

reiki n. a complementary therapy based on an ancient healing system rediscovered in the 20th century by a Buddhist monk. It involves a therapist putting his or her hands on or very close to a patient to boost the patient's natural invisible energy fields (reiki means 'universal life force'). It is often used as an adjunct to other therapies and is said to be helpful for many conditions.

reimplantation n. *see* REPLANTATION.

reinforcement n. (in psychology) the strengthening of a conditioned reflex (*see* CONDITIONING). In classical conditioning this takes place when a conditioned stimulus is presented at the same time as – or just before – the unconditioned stimulus. In operant conditioning it takes place when a pleasurable event (or **reinforcer**), such as a reward, follows immediately after some behaviour. The **reinforcement schedule** governs how often and when such behaviour is rewarded. Different schedules produce different effects on behaviour.

Reissner's membrane the membrane that separates the scala vestibuli and the scala media of the *cochlea of the ear. [E. Reissner (1824–78), German anatomist]

Reiter's syndrome (reactive arthritis) a condition characterized by nongonococcal inflammation of the urethra (*see* URETHRITIS), conjunctivitis, and polyarthritis, usually developing after a gastrointestinal or genitourinary (especially chlamydial) infection. Horny areas may develop on the skin. [H. Reiter (1881–1969), German physician]

rejection n. (in transplantation) the destruction by immune mechanisms of a tissue grafted from another individual. Antibodies, complement, clotting factors, and platelets are involved in the failure of the graft to survive. *Allograft rejection is a vigorous response that can be modified by drugs (such as ciclosporin and corticosteroids) and antibodies against T cells; *xenograft rejection is an acute response that is at present beyond therapeutic control.

relapse n. a return of disease symptoms after recovery had apparently been achieved or the worsening of an apparently recovering patient's condition during the course of an illness.

relapsing fever an infectious disease caused by bacteria of the genus *Borrelia*, which is transmitted by ticks or lice and results in recurrent fever. The first episode of fever occurs about a week after infection: it is accompanied by severe headache and aching muscles and joints and lasts 2–8 days. Subsequent attacks are milder and occur at intervals of 3–10 days; untreated, the attacks may continue for up to 12 weeks. Treatment with antibiotics, such as tetracycline or erythromycin, is effective.

relative analgesia a sedation technique, used particularly in dentistry, in which a mixture of *nitrous oxide and oxygen is given. The patient remains conscious throughout; the technique is used to supplement local anaesthesia for nervous patients.

relative density *see* SPECIFIC GRAVITY.

relativism n. a theoretical approach proposing that morality is not absolute but is instead subjectively located in the specific social context in which it occurs. As such, moral judgments depend not on universal norms but on an assessment of the individual and the situation. In medical ethics, the concept is often applied to cultural relativism, whereby the assumption is that because health-care traditions and practices vary, so too must definitions of what constitutes ethical practice. *Compare* KANTIAN ETHICS. *See also* PARTICULARISM.

relaxant *n.* an agent that reduces tension and strain, particularly in muscles (*see* MUSCLE RELAXANT).

relaxation *n.* (in physiology) the diminution of tension in a muscle, which occurs when it ceases to contract: the state of a resting muscle.

relaxation therapy treatment by teaching patients to decrease their anxiety by reducing the tone in their muscles. This can be used by itself to help people cope with stressful situations or as a part of *desensitization to specific fears.

relaxin *n.* a hormone, secreted by the placenta in the terminal stages of pregnancy, that causes the cervix (neck) of the uterus to dilate and prepares the uterus for the action of *oxytocin during labour.

Relenza *n. see* ZANAMIVIR.

reline *n.* the procedure by which the fitting surface of a denture is rebased to make it fit a jaw that has undergone resorption since the denture was originally made. The procedure is often necessary for dentures that were fitted immediately after extraction of the teeth.

rem *n.* roentgen equivalent man: a former unit dose of ionizing radiation equal to the dose that gives the same biological effect as that due to one roentgen of X-rays. The rem has been replaced by the *sievert.

REM rapid eye movement: describing a stage of *sleep during which the muscles of the eyeballs are in constant motion behind the eyelids. People woken up during this stage of sleep generally report that they were dreaming at the time.

Remicade *n. see* INFLIXIMAB.

remission *n.* **1.** a lessening in the severity of symptoms or their temporary disappearance during the course of an illness. **2.** a reduction in the size of a cancer and the symptoms it is causing.

remittent fever *see* FEVER.

renal *adj.* relating to or affecting the kidneys.

renal artery either of two large arteries arising from the abdominal aorta and supplying the kidneys. Each renal artery divides into an anterior and a posterior branch before entering the kidney.

renal cell carcinoma (Grawitz tumour, hypernephroma) a malignant tumour of kidney cells, so called because it is said to resemble part of the adrenal gland and at one time was thought to originate from this site. It may be present for some years before giving rise to symptoms, which include fever, loin pain and swelling, and blood in the urine. Treatment is by surgery, but tumours are apt to recur locally or spread via the bloodstream and can often be seen growing along the renal vein. Secondary growths from a renal cell carcinoma in the lung have a characteristic 'cannon-ball' appearance. These tumours are relatively insensitive to radiotherapy and cytotoxic drugs but some respond to such hormones as progestogens. Targeted therapy (*see* TARGETED AGENT) is with sorafenib and sunitinib.

renal function tests tests for assessing the function of the kidneys. These include measurements of the specific gravity of urine, creatinine *clearance time, and blood urea levels; intravenous urography; and renal angiography.

renal osteodystrophy *see* OSTEODYSTROPHY.

renal transplantation *see* TRANSPLANTATION.

renal tubular acidosis (RTA) metabolic acidosis due to failure of the kidney to excrete acid into the urine. Three types of RTA are recognized. **Type I** (**distal RTA**) results from a reduction in net acid secretion in the distal convoluted tubule (*see* NEPHRON) and an inability to acidify the urine. Hypokalaemia is often present and may be severe. The condition can be either genetically determined or, more commonly, the result of systemic disease (e.g. autoimmune disorders) or drugs (e.g. amphotericin). **Type II** (**proximal RTA**) is due to a lowered threshold for bicarbonate reabsorption; eventually a steady state is established with a low serum bicarbonate but capacity to acidify the urine. Hypokalaemia is present due to *aldosteronism caused by the increased delivery of sodium to the distal tubule. Proximal RTA usually occurs as part of more widespread proximal tubule dysfunction with the *Fanconi syndrome. **Type IV RTA** results from impaired excretion of both acid and potassium and results in acidosis with hyperkalaemia. It is most commonly seen with aldosterone deficiency. This may be isolated, especially in diabetics, or it may be induced by drugs (angiotensin II antagonists or ACE inhibitors).

renal tubule (uriniferous tubule) the fine tubular part of a *nephron, through which water and certain dissolved substances are reabsorbed back into the blood.

reni- (reno-) *combining form denoting* the kidney.

renin *n.* an enzyme released into the blood by the kidney in response to stress. It reacts with a substrate from the liver to produce *angiotensin, which causes constriction of blood vessels and thus an increase in blood pressure. Excessive production of renin results in the syndrome of *renovascular hypertension.

rennin *n.* an enzyme produced in the stomach that coagulates milk. It is secreted by the gastric glands in an inactive form, **prorennin**, which is activated by hydrochloric acid. Rennin converts caseinogen (milk protein) into insoluble casein in the presence of calcium ions. This ensures that the milk remains in the stomach, exposed to protein-digesting enzymes, for as long as possible. The largest amounts of rennin are present in the stomachs of young mammals.

renography (isotope renography) *n.* the radiological study of the kidneys by a *gamma camera following the intravenous injection of a radioactive *tracer, which is concentrated and excreted by the kidneys. The radioactive isotope (usually *technetium-99m) emits gamma rays, which are recorded by the camera positioned over the kidneys. A graph of the radioactivity in each kidney over time provides information on its function and rate of drainage. *See* DMSA, DTPA, MAG3.

renovascular hypertension disease affecting the arterial supply to the kidneys, leading to ischaemia and resultant stimulation of the renin-*angiotensin-aldosterone axis. In the major vessels, the most common cause is atheromatous plaque disease. Other causes are fibromuscular dysplasia and *Takayasu's disease.

reovirus *n.* one of a group of small RNA-containing viruses that infect both respiratory and intestinal tracts without producing specific or serious diseases (and were therefore termed *r*espiratory *e*nteric *o*rphan viruses). *Compare* ECHOVIRUS.

repaglinide *n. see* MEGLITINIDES.

reperfusion *n.* restoration of blood flow to a tissue that follows relief of an arterial occlusion, most commonly following the correction of acute coronary artery occlusion by coronary *stenting or *thrombolysis in the context of heart attack.

repetitive strain injury (RSI) pain in an upper limb associated with frequent repetition of a particular movement, usually related to keyboard usage. Symptoms often occur in the absence of clear signs, such as *tenosynovitis or *tendovaginitis, which presents difficulties both in treatment and in claiming compensation from an employer (if an industrial cause can be identified).

repetitive transcranial magnetic stimulation (rTMS) *see* TRANSCRANIAL MAGNETIC STIMULATION.

replacement bone a bone that is formed by replacing cartilage with bony material.

replantation *n.* **1.** the reattachment of severed limbs (or parts of limbs) and other body parts (e.g. the nose) using *microsurgery to rejoin nerves and vessels. **2. (reimplantation)** (in dentistry) the reinsertion of a tooth into its socket after its accidental or deliberate removal. The prognosis for the tooth is improved if the tooth is not allowed to dry out prior to replantation. —**replant** *vb.*

replication *n.* the process by which *DNA makes copies of itself when the cell divides. The two strands of the DNA molecule unwind and each strand directs the synthesis of a new strand complementary to itself (see illustration).

repolarization *n.* the process in which the membrane of a nerve cell returns to its normal electrically charged state after a nerve impulse has passed. During the passage of a nerve impulse a temporary change in the molecular structure of the membrane allows a surge of ions across the membrane (*see* ACTION POTENTIAL). During repolarization ions diffuse back to restore the charge and the nerve becomes ready to transmit further impulses. *See* REFRACTORY PERIOD.

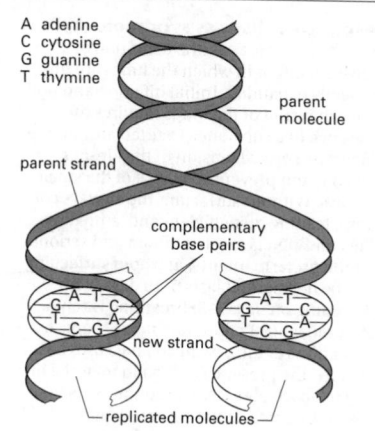

A adenine
C cytosine
G guanine
T thymine

parent molecule

parent strand

complementary base pairs

new strand

replicated molecules

Replication of a DNA molecule.

repositor *n.* an instrument used to return a displaced part of the body – for instance, a prolapsed uterus – to its normal position.

repression *n.* (in *psychoanalysis) the process of excluding an unacceptable wish or an idea from conscious mental life. The repressed material may give rise to symptoms. One goal of psychoanalysis is to return repressed material to conscious awareness so that it may be dealt with rationally.

reproduction rate *see* FERTILITY RATE.

reproductive system the combination of organs and tissues associated with the process of reproduction. In males it includes the testes, vasa deferentia, prostate gland, seminal vesicles, urethra, and penis; in females it includes the ovaries, Fallopian tubes, uterus, vagina, and vulva. (See illustration.)

research ethics committee *see* ETHICS COMMITTEE.

resection *n.* surgical removal of a portion of any part of the body. For example, a section of diseased intestine may be removed and the healthy ends sewn together. A **submucous resection** is removal of part of the cartilage septum (central division) of the nose that has become deviated, usually by injury. **Transurethral resection of the prostate (TURP)** – an operation performed when the prostate gland becomes enlarged – involves removal of portions of the gland through the urethra using an instrument called a **resectoscope**.

resectoscope *n.* a type of surgical instrument (an *endoscope) used in resection of the prostate or in the removal of bladder tumours.

reserpine *n. see* RAUWOLFIA.

reserve volume the extra volume of air that an individual could inhale or exhale when breathing to the limit of his or her capacity.

residual volume the volume of air that remains in the lungs after the individual has breathed out as much as he can. This volume is increased in *emphysema.

resistance *n.* **1.** the degree of *immunity

r

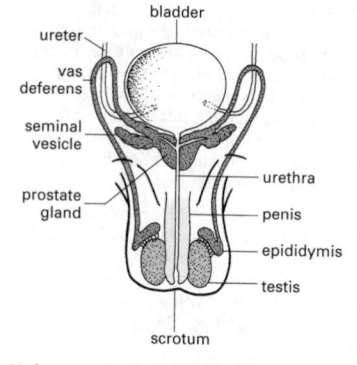

bladder

ureter

vas deferens

seminal vesicle

prostate gland

urethra

penis

epididymis

testis

scrotum

Male reproductive system.

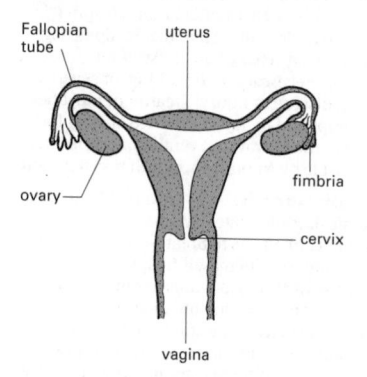

Fallopian tube

uterus

ovary

fimbria

cervix

vagina

Female reproductive system.

that the body possesses: a measure of its ability to withstand disease. **2.** the degree to which a disease or disease-causing organism remains unaffected by antibiotics or other drugs.

resolution *n.* **1.** the stage during which inflammation gradually disappears. **2.** the degree to which individual details can be distinguished by the eye, as through a *microscope.

resorption *n.* loss of substance through physiological or pathological means.

respiration *n.* the process of gaseous exchange between an organism and its environment. This includes both **external respiration**, which involves *breathing, in which oxygen is taken up by the capillaries of the lung *alveoli and carbon dioxide is released from the blood, and **internal respiration**, during which oxygen is released to the tissues and carbon dioxide absorbed by the blood. Blood provides the transport medium for the gases between the lungs and tissue cells. In addition, it contains a pigment, *haemoglobin, with special affinity for oxygen. Once inside the cell oxygen is utilized in metabolic processes resulting in the production of energy (*see* ATP), water, and waste materials (including carbon dioxide). *See also* LUNG. —**respiratory** *adj.*

respirator *n.* **1.** a face mask for administering oxygen or other gas or for filtering harmful fumes, dust, etc. **2.** *see* VENTILATOR.

respiratory arrest cessation of breathing, which – without treatment – will very quickly be followed by *cardiac arrest. It may result from airway obstruction, brain or spinal injury, overdose of certain medications (e.g. opioids), disease of the muscles and/or nerves necessary for breathing, or severe lung disease or injury. Treatment must be prompt and include clearance of any blockage in the airway and ventilatory support, for example by *mouth-to-mouth resuscitation.

respiratory distress severe difficulty in achieving adequate oxygenation in spite of significant efforts to breathe: it is usually associated with increased *respiratory rate and the use of *accessory muscles in the chest wall. It can occur in both obstructive and nonobstructive lung conditions. *See* ADULT RESPIRATORY DISTRESS SYNDROME, AIRWAY OBSTRUCTION, DYSPNOEA, RESPIRATORY DISTRESS SYNDROME, STRIDOR.

respiratory distress syndrome (hyaline membrane disease) the condition of a newborn infant in which the lungs are imperfectly expanded. Initial inflation and normal expansion of the lungs requires the presence of a substance (*surfactant) that reduces the surface tension of the air sacs (alveoli) and prevents collapse of the small airways. Without surfactant the airways collapse, leading to inefficient and 'stiff' lungs. The condition is most common and serious among preterm infants, in whom surfactant may be deficient. It lasts 5–10 days, with worsening on days 2–3. Breathing is rapid, laboured, and shallow, and microscopic examinations of lung tissue in fatal cases has revealed the presence of *hyalin material in the collapsed air sacs. The condition is treated by careful nursing, intravenous fluids, and oxygen, with or without positive-pressure ventilation (*see* NONINVASIVE VENTILATION). Recently, surfactant administered at birth has produced encouraging results. *See also* ADULT RESPIRATORY DISTRESS SYNDROME.

respiratory quotient (RQ) the ratio of the volume of carbon dioxide transferred from the blood into the alveoli to the volume of oxygen absorbed into the alveoli. The RQ is usually about 0.8 because more oxygen is taken up than carbon dioxide excreted.

respiratory rate (RR) breathing rate: the number of breaths per minute. Normally between 6 and 12, it increases after exercise and in cases of *respiratory distress and decreases after head injury and opioid overdosage.

respiratory syncytial virus (RSV) a paramyxovirus (*see* MYXOVIRUS) that causes infections of the nose and throat. It is a major cause of bronchiolitis and pneumonia in young children. In tissue cultures infected with the virus, cells merge together to form a conglomerate (**syncytium**). RSV is thought to have a role in *sudden infant death syndrome. Vulnerable children can be treated with *ribavirin, but most children just require supportive measures.

respiratory system the combination of organs and tissues associated with *breathing. It includes the nasal cavity, pharynx, larynx, trachea, bronchi, bronchioles, and lungs and also the diaphragm and other muscles associated with breathing movements.

response *n.* the way in which the body or

part of the body reacts to a *stimulus. For example, a nerve impulse may produce the response of a contraction in a muscle that the nerve supplies.

response prevention a form of *behaviour therapy given for severe *obsessions. Patients are encouraged to abstain from rituals and repetitive acts while they are in situations that arouse anxiety. For example, a hand-washing ritual might be treated by stopping washing while being progressively exposed to dirt. The anxiety then declines, and with it the obsessions.

restenosis n. recurrent *stenosis, usually in a blood vessel after such procedures as angioplasty or insertion of a stent. Restenosis can complicate 20–50% of such procedures.

restiform body a thick bundle of nerve fibres that conveys impulses from tracts in the spinal cord to the cortex of the anterior and posterior lobes of the cerebellum.

resting cell a cell that is not undergoing division. See INTERPHASE.

restless legs syndrome (Ekbom's syndrome) a condition in which a sense of uneasiness, restlessness, and itching, often accompanied by twitching and pain, is felt in the calves of the legs when sitting or lying down, especially in bed at night. The only relief is walking or moving the legs, which often leads to insomnia. The cause is unknown: it may be inadequate circulation, nerve damage (see PERIPHERAL NEUROPATHY), deficiency of iron, vitamin B_{12}, or folate, or a reaction to antipsychotic or antidepressant drugs. In severe cases treatment with a *dopamine receptor agonist (e.g. pramipexole) may be helpful.

restoration n. (in dentistry) any type of dental *filling or *crown, which is aimed at restoring a tooth to its normal form, function, and appearance. A **sealant restoration** (or **preventive resin restoration**) is a combination of a *fissure sealant and a small filling.

rest pain pain without prior exertion, usually experienced in the feet or chest (*angina pectoris), that indicates an extreme degree of *ischaemia.

restriction enzyme (restriction endonuclease) an enzyme, obtained from bacteria, that cuts DNA into specific short segments.

Restriction enzymes are widely used in *genetic engineering.

resuscitation n. the restoration of a person who appears to be dead by the revival of cardiac and respiratory function. See CARDIOPULMONARY RESUSCITATION, MOUTH-TO-MOUTH RESUSCITATION. See also ADVANCE STATEMENT, DECISION, OR DIRECTIVE; DNAR ORDER.

resuscitation mannikin a life-size model of a person for practising all aspects of basic and advanced life support, including endotracheal *intubation and *defibrillation.

retainer n. (in dentistry) **1.** a component of a partial *denture that keeps it in place. **2.** an *orthodontic appliance that holds the teeth in position at the end of active treatment. **3.** a component of a *bridge that is fixed to a natural tooth.

retardation n. the slowing up of a process. **Psychomotor retardation** is a marked slowing down of activity and speech, which can reach a degree where a patient can no longer care for him- or herself. It is a symptom of severe *depression. The term *mental retardation implies a delay in intellectual development rather than a qualitative defect.

retching n. repeated unavailing attempts to vomit.

rete n. a network of blood vessels, nerve fibres, or other strands of interlacing tissue in the structure of an organ. The **rete testis** is a network of tubules conducting sperm from the seminiferous tubules of the *testis to the vasa efferentia.

retention n. inability to pass urine, which is retained in the bladder. The condition may be acute and painful or chronic and painless. **Acute urinary retention** (**AUR**) can be precipitated by surgery, urinary infection, constipation, and drugs; spontaneous AUR is usually caused by enlargement of the prostate gland in men, although many other conditions may result in obstruction of bladder outflow. Retention is relieved by catheter drainage of the bladder, after which the underlying problem is dealt with. See also INTERMITTENT SELF-CATHETERIZATION.

retention defect (in psychology) a memory defect in which items that have been registered in the memory are lost from storage. It is a feature of *dementia.

reteplase *n. see* FIBRINOLYTIC, TISSUE-TYPE PLASMINOGEN ACTIVATOR.

reticular activating system the system of nerve pathways in the brain concerned with the level of consciousness – from the states of sleep, drowsiness, and relaxation to full alertness and attention. The system integrates information from all of the senses and from the cerebrum and cerebellum and determines the overall activity of the brain and the autonomic nervous system and patterns of behaviour during waking and sleeping.

reticular fibres microscopic, almost nonelastic, branching fibres of *connective tissue that join together to form a delicate supportive meshwork around blood vessels, muscle fibres, glands, nerves, etc. They are composed of a collagen-like protein (**reticulin**) and are particularly common in lymph nodes, the spleen, liver, kidneys, and muscles.

reticular formation a network of nerve pathways and nuclei throughout the *brainstem, connecting motor and sensory nerves to and from the spinal cord, the cerebellum and the cerebrum, and the cranial nerves. It is estimated that a single neuron in this network may have synapses with as many as 25,000 other neurons.

reticulin *n.* a protein that is the major constituent of *reticular fibres.

reticulocyte *n.* an immature red blood cell (erythrocyte). Reticulocytes may be detected and counted by staining living red cells with certain basic dyes that result in the formation of a blue precipitate (**reticulum**) within the reticulocytes. They normally comprise about 1% of the total red cells and are increased (**reticulocytosis**) whenever the rate of red cell production increases.

reticulocytosis *n.* an increase in the proportion of immature red blood cells (reticulocytes) in the bloodstream. It is a sign of increased output of new red cells from the bone marrow.

reticuloendothelial system (RES) a community of cells – *phagocytes – spread throughout the body. It includes *macrophages and *monocytes. The RES is concerned with defence against microbial infection and with the removal of worn-out blood cells from the bloodstream. *See also* SPLEEN.

reticulosis *n.* abnormal overgrowth, usu-

ally malignant, of any of the cells of the lymphatic glands or the immune system. *See* LYMPHOMA, HODGKIN'S DISEASE, BURKITT'S LYMPHOMA, MYCOSIS FUNGOIDES.

reticulum *n.* a network of tubules or blood vessels. *See* ENDOPLASMIC RETICULUM, SARCOPLASMIC RETICULUM.

retin- (retino-) *combining form denoting* the retina. Example: **retinopexy** (fixation of a detached retina).

retina *n.* the light-sensitive layer that lines the interior of the eye. The outer part of the retina (**retinal pigment epithelium; RPE**), next to the *choroid, is pigmented to prevent the passage of light. The inner part, next to the cavity of the eyeball, contains *rods and *cones (light-sensitive cells) and their associated nerve fibres (see illustration). A large number of cones is concentrated in a depression in the retina at the back of the eyeball called the *fovea. —**retinal** *adj.*

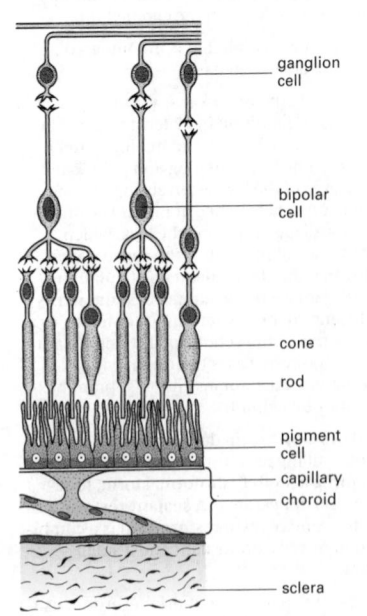

ganglion cell

bipolar cell

cone

rod

pigment cell

capillary

choroid

sclera

The structure of the retina.

retinaculum *n.* (*pl.* **retinacula**) a thickened band of tissue that serves to hold various tissues in place. For example, **flexor**

retinacula are found over the flexor tendons in the wrist and ankle.

retinal 1. (retinene) *n.* the aldehyde of retinol (*vitamin A). *See also* RHODOPSIN. 2. *adj. see* RETINA.

retinal artery occlusion blockage of arterial blood supply to the retina, usually as a result of *thrombosis or *embolism. The central retinal artery enters the eye at the optic disc and then divides into branches to supply different parts of the retina. Blockage of the central retinal artery (**central retinal artery occlusion**) usually results in sudden painless loss of vision. Blockage of one of the branches of the central retinal artery (**branch retinal artery occlusion**) results in *ischaemia of the retina supplied by the occluded vessel and related visual field loss.

retinal detachment (detached retina) separation of the inner nervous layer of the *retina from the outer pigmented layer (retinal pigment epithelium, RPE). It commonly occurs when a break (hole or tear) allows fluid from the vitreous cavity of the eyeball to accumulate under the retina (rhegmatogenous) but can also occur when fluid accumulates by leakage from the RPE (nonrhegmatogenous). Vision is lost in the affected part of the retina. The retina can be reattached by surgical means, such as external *plombage or internal *vitrectomy, or by creating patches of scar tissue between the retina and the choroid by application of extreme cold (*see* CRYOSURGERY) or heat (*see* PHOTOCOAGULATION).

retinal dialysis separation of the retina from its insertion at the ora serrata (the anterior margin of the retina, lying just posterior to the ciliary body). This acts as a retinal tear and causes a *retinal detachment.

retinal vein occlusion blockage of a vein carrying blood from the retina. Small branch veins carry blood from different parts of the retina and drain into the central retinal vein, which leaves the eye at the optic disc. Blockage of the central retinal vein (**central retinal vein occlusion**) usually results in sudden painless reduction of vision. Distended veins, haemorrhages, and *cotton-wool spots are seen in the retina and the optic disc may become swollen. Blockage of a branch of the central retinal vein (**branch retinal vein occlusion**) results in painless reduction of vision in the affected area, where engorged veins, haemorrhages, and cotton-wool spots may be seen.

retinene *n. see* RETINAL.

retinitis *n.* inflammation of the retina caused mainly by viral infection; for example, *cytomegalovirus (CMV) retinitis, HIV retinitis. In practice, the term is often used for noninflammatory conditions; for example, *retinitis pigmentosa. For such conditions the term *retinopathy is becoming more widely used.

retinitis pigmentosa a hereditary condition characterized by progressive degeneration of the *retina due to malfunctioning of the retinal pigment epithelium. It starts in childhood with *night blindness and limited peripheral vision and may progress to complete loss of vision. Progression and visual function are both extremely variable, depending on the type of retinitis pigmentosa.

retinoblastoma *n.* a rare malignant tumour of the retina, occurring mainly in developing retinal cells in children under the age of two years.

retinoid *n.* any one of a group of drugs derived from vitamin A. They bind to one or more of six specific receptors that are found on many cells. On the skin they act to cause drying and peeling and a reduction in oil (sebum) production. These effects can be useful in the treatment of severe *acne, *psoriasis, *ichthyosis, and other skin disorders. Retinoids include *isotretinoin, *tretinoin, **acitretin** (Neotigason), and **tazarotene** (Zorac); they are administered by mouth or applied as a cream, gel, or lotion. **Alitretinoin** (Toctino) is an oral treatment for severe chronic hand eczema. Possible side-effects, which may be serious, include severe fetal abnormalities (if taken by pregnant women), toxic effects on babies (if taken by breastfeeding mothers), liver and kidney damage, excessive drying, redness and itching of the skin, and muscle pain and stiffness.

retinol *n. see* VITAMIN A.

retinopathy *n.* any of various disorders of the retina resulting in impairment or loss of vision. It is usually due to damage to the blood vessels of the retina, occurring (for example) as a complication of longstanding diabetes (**diabetic retinopathy**), high blood pressure, or AIDS (**AIDS retinopathy**). In diabetic retinopathy, haemorrhaging or exudation may occur, either from damaged vessels into the retina or from new abnormal vessels (*see* NEOVASCULARIZATION) into the vitreous humour. Treatment of the later stages requires laser surgery (*see* PHOTOCOAGULATION). Diabetic retinopathy can be detected by careful eye examination before it causes a deterioration in vision. **Retinopathy of prematurity** (**ROP**), formerly known as **retrolental fibroplasia**, is the abnormal growth of developing retinal blood vessels seen in premature infants. It may be mild and resolve spontaneously or severe enough to lead to blindness if untreated.

retinopexy *n.* any surgical procedure used to repair a *retinal detachment. *See* PNEUMORETINOPEXY, CRYORETINOPEXY.

retinoschisis *n.* splitting of the layers of the neurosensory retina with accumulation of fluid between the layers. This is usually static or it may progress very slowly compared to other types of *retinal detachment.

retinoscope *n.* an instrument used to determine the power of spectacle lens required to correct *refractive errors of the eye. It is held in the hand and casts a beam of light into the subject's eye. The examiner looks along the beam and sees the reflection in the subject's pupil. By interpreting the way the reflection moves as the instrument is moved, and by altering this by lenses held in the other hand near the subject's eye, the examiner is able to determine the degree of refractive error. —**retinoscopy** *n.*

retinotomy *n.* a surgical incision into the retina.

retraction *n.* **1.** (in obstetrics) the state of uterine muscle fibres remaining shortened after contracting during labour. This results in a gradual progression of the fetus downwards through the pelvis. The basal portion of the uterus becomes thicker and pulls up the dilating cervix over the presenting part. **2.** (in dentistry) the drawing back of one or more teeth into a better position by an *orthodontic appliance.

retraction ring a depression in the uterine wall marking the junction between the actively contracting muscle fibres of the upper segment of the uterus and the muscle fibres of the lower segment. This depression is not always visible and is normal. In obstructed labour (e.g. contracted pelvis or malposition of the fetus resulting in shoulder presentation), the muscle fibres of the upper segment become shorter and thicker; the muscle fibres of the lower segment, on the other hand, become elongated and thinner. The junction between the two becomes more distinct as it rises into the abdomen from the pelvis. This abnormal ring is known as **Bandl's ring** and is a sign of impending rupture of the lower segment of the uterus, which becomes progressively thinner as Bandl's ring rises upwards. Immediate action to relieve the obstruction is then necessary, usually in the form of Caesarean section.

retractor *n.* a surgical instrument used to expose the operation site by drawing aside the cut edges of skin, muscle, or other tissues. There are several types of retractors for different operations (see illustration).

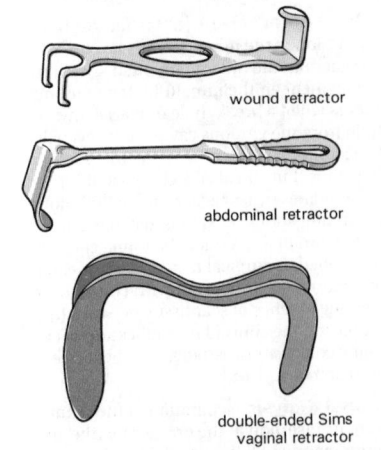

wound retractor

abdominal retractor

double-ended Sims vaginal retractor

Retractors.

retro- *prefix denoting* at the back or behind. Examples: **retrobulbar** (at the back of the eyeball); **retroperitoneal** (behind the peritoneum).

retrobulbar neuritis (**optic neuritis**) inflammation of the optic nerve behind the eye, causing increasingly blurred vision. When the inflammation involves the first part of the nerve and can be seen at the optic disc, it is called **optic papillitis**. Retrobulbar neuritis is one of the symptoms of multiple sclerosis but it can also occur as an isolated lesion, in the absence of any other involvement of the nervous system, with the patient recovering vision completely.

retroflexion *n*. the bending backward of an organ or part of an organ, especially the abnormal bending backward of the upper part of the uterus (i.e. the part furthest from the cervix).

retrograde *adj*. going backwards, or moving in the opposite direction to the normal. (*See* (RETROGRADE) PYELOGRAPHY.) **Retrograde amnesia** is a failure to remember events immediately preceding an illness or injury.

retrolental fibroplasia *see* RETINOPATHY (OF PREMATURITY).

retroperitoneal fibrosis (RPF) a condition in which a dense plaque of fibrous tissue develops behind the peritoneum adjacent to the abdominal aorta. The ureters become encased and hence obstructed, causing acute *anuria and renal failure. The obstruction can be relieved by *nephrostomy or the insertion of double J *stents. In the acute phase steroid administration may help, but in established RPF *ureterolysis is required.

retroperitoneal space the region between the posterior parietal *peritoneum and the front of the *lumbar vertebrae. It contains important structures, including the kidneys, adrenal glands, pancreas, lumbar spinal nerve roots, sympathetic ganglia and nerves, and the abdominal *aorta and its major branches.

retropulsion *n*. a compulsive tendency to walk backwards. It is a symptom of *parkinsonism.

retrospective study 1. a review of the characteristics of a group of individuals, some of whom have a specific disease or condition, to investigate possible causes by comparing affected and unaffected individuals in terms of past experience. *See also* CASE CONTROL STUDY. 2. *see* COHORT STUDY.

retroversion *n*. an abnormal position of the uterus in which it is tilted backwards, with the base lying in the *pouch of Douglas, against the rectum, instead of on the bladder. It occurs in about 20% of women.

retrovirus *n*. an RNA-containing virus that can convert its genetic material into DNA by means of the enzyme *reverse transcriptase, which enables it to become integrated into

the DNA of its host's cells. Retroviruses have been implicated in the development of some cancers and are associated with conditions characterized by an impaired immune system (*HIV is a retrovirus). They are also used as *vectors in gene therapy.

retrusion *n*. (in dentistry) 1. backward movement of the lower jaw. 2. a malocclusion in which some of the teeth are further back than usual. *Compare* PROTRUSION.

Rett's syndrome a disorder affecting young girls, in which stereotyped movements (*see* STEREOTYPY) and social withdrawal appear during early childhood. Intellectual development is often impaired and special educational help is needed. [A. Rett (1924–1997), Austrian paediatrician]

revalidation *n*. the process, not yet introduced, in which doctors, in order to retain their medical licence, will be required to demonstrate to the *General Medical Council, at regular intervals, that they remain fit to practise medicine. The procedure will make doctors more accountable to the public. *See* LICENSING. *See also* CLINICAL GOVERNANCE.

revascularization *n*. 1. the regrowth of blood vessels following disease or injury so that normal blood supply to an organ, tissue, or part is restored. 2. the restoration of blood flow to an organ by *angioplasty/ *stenting or surgical *bypass grafting. *See* CORONARY REVASCULARIZATION.

reverse transcriptase an enzyme, found mainly in *retroviruses, that catalyses the synthesis of DNA from RNA. It enables the viral RNA to be integrated into the host DNA. **Reverse transcriptase inhibitors** are antiviral drugs that inhibit this process; they include *zidovudine and *didanosine, used in the treatment of HIV infection; and **lamivudine** (Epivir, Zeffix) and **tenofovir disoproxil** (Viread), for treating HIV infection and chronic hepatitis B.

Revlimid *n*. *see* LENALIDOMIDE.

Reye's syndrome a rare disorder occurring in childhood. It is characterized by the symptoms of *encephalitis combined with evidence of liver failure. Often, the symptoms develop in the apparent recovery phase of a viral infection. Treatment is aimed at controlling cerebral *oedema and correcting metabolic abnormalities in order to allow spontaneous recovery, but there is still a significant mortality and there may be resid-

r

ual brain damage. The cause is not known, but *aspirin has been implicated and this drug should not be used in children below the age of 16 unless specifically indicated. [R. D. K. Reye (1912–77), Australian histopathologist]

rhabdomyolysis *n.* the rapid breakdown of skeletal muscle cells, with the release of myoglobin and other potentially toxic cell components. Blood levels of *creatine kinase are raised. It can result in *hyperkalaemia, *hypovolaemia, *myoglobinuric acute renal failure, and *disseminated intravascular coagulation. Causes include muscle trauma and crush injury, alcohol abuse, seizures, and medications (notably statins).

rhabdomyoma *n.* a rare benign tumour of skeletal muscle or heart muscle.

rhabdomyosarcoma *n.* a rare malignant tumour, usually of childhood, originating in, or showing the characteristics of, striated muscle. **Pleomorphic rhabdomyosarcoma** occurs in late middle age, in the muscles of the limbs. **Embryonal rhabdomyosarcomas**, affecting infants, children, and young adults, are classified as **botryoid** (in the vagina (*see* SARCOMA BOTRYOIDES), bladder, ear, etc.), **embryonal** (most common in the head and neck, particularly the orbit); and **alveolar** (at the base of the thumb). The pleomorphic and alveolar types respond poorly to treatment; botryoid tumours are treated with a combination of radiotherapy, surgery, and drugs. The embryonal type, if treated at an early stage, can often be cured with a combination of radiotherapy and drugs (including vincristine, dactinomycin, and cyclophosphamide).

rhagades *pl. n.* cracks or long thin scars in the skin, particularly around the mouth or other areas of the body subjected to constant movement. The fissures around the mouth and nose of babies with congenital syphilis eventually heal to form rhagades.

rhegmatogenous *adj.* resulting from a break or tear in the retina. For example, **rhegmatogenous retinal detachment** results as a consequence of a tear in the retina.

rheo- *combining form denoting* 1. a flow of liquid. 2. an electric current.

rhesus factor (Rh factor) a group of *antigens that may or may not be present on the surface of the red blood cells; it forms the basis of the rhesus blood group system. Most

people have the rhesus factor, i.e. they are **Rh-positive**. People who lack the factor are termed **Rh-negative**. Incompatibility between Rh-positive and Rh-negative blood is an important cause of blood transfusion reactions and *haemolytic disease of the newborn. *See also* BLOOD GROUP.

rhesus prophylaxis *see* ANTI-D IMMUNOGLOBULIN.

rheumatic fever (acute rheumatism) a disease affecting mainly children and young adults that arises as a delayed complication of infection of the upper respiratory tract with haemolytic streptococci (*see* STREPTOCOCCUS). The main features are fever, arthritis progressing from joint to joint, reddish circular patches on the skin, small painless nodules formed on bony prominences such as the elbow, abnormal involuntary movements of the limbs and head (Sydenham's *chorea), and inflammation of the heart muscle, its valves, and the membrane surrounding the heart. The condition may progress to **chronic rheumatic heart disease**, with scarring and chronic inflammation of the heart and its valves leading to heart failure, murmurs, and damage to the valves. The initial infection is treated with antibiotics (e.g. penicillin) and bed rest, with aspirin to relieve the joint pain. Following an acute attack, long-term prophylaxis with penicillin is often recommended to prevent a relapse. Rheumatic fever is now rare in developed countries.

rheumatism *n.* any disorder in which aches and pains affect the muscles and joints. *See* RHEUMATOID ARTHRITIS, RHEUMATIC FEVER, OSTEOARTHRITIS, GOUT.

rheumatoid arthritis the second most common form of *arthritis (after *osteoarthritis). It typically involves the joints of the fingers, wrists, feet, and ankles, with later involvement of the hips, knees, shoulders, and neck. It is a disease of the synovial lining of joints; the joints are initially painful, swollen, and stiff and are usually affected symmetrically. As the disease progresses the ligaments supporting the joints are damaged and there is erosion of the bone, leading to deformity of the joints. Tendon sheaths can be affected, leading to tendon rupture. Onset can be at any age, and there is a considerable range of severity. Women are at greater risk. Rheumatoid arthritis is an *autoimmune disease, and most patients show the presence of **rheumatoid factor** in their serum. There are characteristic changes on X-ray. In the early stages there is soft tissue swelling and periarticular osteoporosis; late stages are characterized by marginal bony erosions, narrowing of the articular space, articular destruction, and joint deformity.

Treatment is with a variety of drugs, including anti-inflammatory analgesics (*see* NSAID), steroids, and *disease-modifying antirheumatic drugs. Surgical treatment is by excision of the synovium in early cases or by *fusion or joint replacement once bony changes have occurred. (*See also* HIP REPLACEMENT.) The condition may resolve spontaneously, but is usually relapsing and remitting with steady progression. It may finally burn itself out, leaving severely deformed joints.

rheumatology *n.* the medical specialty concerned with the diagnosis and management of disease involving joints, tendons, muscles, ligaments, and associated structures. *See also* PHYSICAL MEDICINE. —**rheumatologist** *n.*

rhexis *n.* the breaking apart of a blood vessel, organ, tissue, or cellular component.

Rh factor *see* RHESUS FACTOR.

rhin- (rhino-) *combining form denoting* the nose.

rhinencephalon *n.* the parts of the brain, collectively, that in early stages of evolution were concerned mainly with the sense of smell. The rhinencephalon includes the olfactory nerve, olfactory tract, and the regions now usually classified as belonging to the *limbic system.

rhinitis *n.* inflammation of the mucous membrane of the nose. It may be caused by virus infection (**acute rhinitis**; *see* (COMMON) COLD) or an allergic reaction (**allergic rhinitis**; *see* HAY FEVER). In **atrophic rhinitis** the mucous membrane becomes thinned and fragile. In **perennial** (or **vasomotor**) **rhinitis** there is overgrowth of, and increased secretion by, the membrane.

rhinolith *n.* a stone (calculus) in the nose, usually formed around a foreign body.

rhinology *n.* the branch of medicine concerned with disorders of the nose and nasal passages.

rhinomycosis *n.* fungal infection of the lining of the nose.

rhinophyma *n.* a bulbous craggy swelling of the nose, usually in men. It is a complication of *rosacea and in no way related to alcohol intake. Paring by plastic surgery may be necessary for cosmetic purposes.

rhinoplasty *n.* surgery to alter the shape of the nose, sometimes using tissue (skin, cartilage, or bone) from elsewhere in the body or artificial implants.

rhinorrhoea *n.* a persistent watery mucous discharge from the nose, as in the common cold.

rhinoscleroma *n.* the formation of nodules in the interior of the nose and *nasopharynx, which become thickened. It is caused by bacterial infection (with *Klebsiella rhinoscleromatis*).

rhinoscopy *n.* examination of the interior of the nose using a speculum or endoscope.

rhinosinusitis *n.* inflammation of the lining of the nose and paranasal sinuses. Rhinosinusitis is a common condition caused by allergies, infection, immune deficiencies, *mucociliary transport abnormalities, trauma, drugs, or tumours. *See* RHINITIS, SINUSITIS.

rhinosporidiosis *n.* an infection of the mucous membranes of the nose, larynx, eyes, and genitals that is caused by the fungus *Rhinosporidium seeberi* and is characterized by the formation of tiny *polyps. It occurs most commonly in Asia.

rhinovirus *n.* any one of a group of RNA-containing viruses that cause respiratory infections resembling the common cold. They are included in the *picornavirus group.

Rhipicephalus *n.* a genus of hard *ticks widely distributed in the tropics. The dog tick (*R. sanguineus*) can suck human blood and is commonly involved in the transmission of diseases caused by rickettsiae (*see* TYPHUS).

rhiz- (rhizo-) *combining form denoting* a root. Example: **rhizonychia** (the root of a nail).

rhizotomy *n.* a surgical procedure in which selected nerve roots are cut at the point where they emerge from the spinal cord. In **posterior rhizotomy** the posterior (sensory) nerve roots are cut for the relief of intractable pain in the organs served by these nerves. An **anterior rhizotomy** – the cutting of the anterior (motor) nerve roots –

is sometimes done for the relief of severe muscle spasm or *dystonia.

Rhodnius *n.* a genus of large bloodsucking bugs (*see* REDUVIID). *R. prolixus* is important in the transmission of *Chagas' disease in Central America and the northern part of South America.

rhodopsin (visual purple) *n.* a pigment in the retina of the eye, within the *rods, consisting of **retinal** – an aldehyde of retinol (*vitamin A) – and a protein. The presence of rhodopsin is essential for vision in dim light. It is bleached in the presence of light and this stimulates nervous activity in the rods.

rhombencephalon *n. see* HINDBRAIN.

rhomboid *n.* either of two muscles (**rhomboid major** and **rhomboid minor**) situated in the upper part of the back, between the backbone and shoulder blade. They help to move the shoulder blade backwards and upwards.

rhonchus *n.* (*pl.* **rhonchi**) an abnormal musical noise produced by air passing through narrowed bronchi. It is heard through a stethoscope, usually when the patient breathes out.

rhythm method a contraceptive method in which sexual intercourse is restricted to the **safe period** at the beginning and end of the *menstrual cycle. The safe period is calculated either on the basis of the length of the menstrual cycle or by reliance on the change of body temperature that occurs at ovulation. A third possible indicator (*see* BILLINGS METHOD) is the change that occurs with ovulation in the stickiness of the mucus at the neck (cervix) of the uterus. The method depends for its reliability on the woman having uniform regular periods and its failure rate is higher than with mechanical methods, approaching 25 pregnancies per 100 woman-years.

rib *n.* a curved, slightly twisted, strip of bone forming part of the skeleton of the thorax, which protects the heart and lungs. There are 12 pairs of ribs. The head of each rib articulates with one of the 12 thoracic vertebrae of the backbone; the other end is attached to a section of cartilage (*see* COSTAL CARTILAGE). The first seven pairs – the **true ribs** – are connected directly to the sternum by their costal cartilages. The next three pairs – the **false ribs** – are attached indirectly: each is connected by its cartilage to the rib above it. The last two pairs of ribs – the **floating ribs** – end freely in the muscles of the body wall. Anatomical name: **costa**.

ribavirin *n.* an antiviral drug effective against a range of DNA and RNA viruses, including the herpes group, *respiratory syncytial virus, and *hepatitis C. It is administered by a small-particle aerosol inhaler or by mouth. Possible side-effects include breathing difficulty, bacterial pneumonia, and *pneumothorax (when inhaled) and haemolytic anaemia (with oral treatment); it also antagonizes the action of *zidovudine against HIV. Trade names: **Copegus**, **Rebetol**, **Virazole**.

riboflavin *n. see* VITAMIN B$_2$.

ribonuclease *n.* an enzyme, located in the *lysosomes of cells, that splits RNA at specific places in the molecule.

ribonucleic acid *see* RNA.

ribose *n.* a pentose sugar (i.e. one with free carbon atoms) that is a component of *RNA and several coenzymes. Ribose is also involved in intracellular metabolism.

ribosome *n.* a particle, consisting of RNA and protein, that occurs in cells and is the site of protein synthesis in the cell (*see* TRANSLATION). Ribosomes are either attached to the *endoplasmic reticulum or free in the cytoplasm as *polysomes. —**ribosomal** *adj.*

ribozyme *n.* an RNA molecule that can act as an enzyme, catalysing changes to its own molecular structure (before its discovery it was assumed that all enzymes were proteins). Research into the ability of genetically engineered ribozymes to destroy the RNA of HIV (the AIDS virus) is ongoing.

ricin *n.* a highly toxic albumin obtained from castor-oil seeds (*Ricinus communis*) that inhibits protein synthesis and becomes attached to the surface of cells, resulting in gastroenteritis, hepatic congestion and jaundice, and cardiovascular collapse. It is lethal to most species, even in minute amounts (1 μg/kg body weight); it is most toxic if injected intravenously or inhaled as fine particles. Ricin is being investigated as a treatment for certain lymphomas, which depends on its delivery to the exact site of the tumour in order to avoid destruction of healthy cells (*see* IMMUNOTOXIN).

rickets *n.* a disease of childhood in which the bones do not harden due to a deficiency of *vitamin D. Without vitamin D, not enough calcium salts are deposited in the bones to make them rigid: consequently they become soft and malformed. This is particularly noticeable in the long bones, which become bowed, and in the front of the ribcage, where a characteristic rickety 'rosary' may become apparent. The deficiency of vitamin D may be dietary or due to lack of exposure to sunlight, which is important in the conversion of vitamin D to its active form. In the UK rickets is more common in Asian immigrant families.

Renal rickets is due to impaired kidney function causing bone-forming minerals to be excreted in the urine, which results in softening of the bones.

rickettsiae *pl. n.* (*sing.* **rickettsia**) a group of very small nonmotile spherical or rodlike parasitic bacteria that cannot reproduce outside the bodies of their hosts. Rickettsiae infect arthropods (ticks, mites, etc.), through which they can be transmitted to mammals (including humans), in which they can cause severe illness. The species *Rickettsia akari* causes *rickettsial pox, *R. conorii, R. prowazekii, R. tsutsugamushi,* and *R. typhi* cause different forms of *typhus, *R. rickettsii* causes *Rocky Mountain spotted fever, and *Coxiella burnetii* causes *Q fever. —**rickettsial** *adj.*

rickettsial pox a disease of mice caused by the bacterium *Rickettsia akari* and transmitted to humans by mites: it produces chills, fever, muscular pain, and a rash similar to that of *chickenpox. The disease is mild and runs its course in 2–3 weeks. *See also* TYPHUS.

ridge *n.* 1. (in anatomy) a crest or a long narrow protuberance, e.g. on a bone. 2. (in dental anatomy) the crest of the jawbone following tooth loss. *See* ALVEOLUS.

Riedel's struma a rare fibrosing destructive disorder of the thyroid gland that may spread to adjacent tissues and obstruct the airway. It is sometimes associated with fibrosis in other parts of the body, such as the bile duct or *retroperitoneal fibrosis. The treatment is surgical removal. [B. M. C. L. Riedel (1846–1916), German surgeon]

rifampicin *n.* an antibiotic used to treat various infections, particularly tuberculosis and leprosy. It is administered by mouth or intravenous infusion; digestive upsets and

sensitivity reactions sometimes occur. Trade names: **Rifadin, Rimactane.**

Rift Valley fever a virus disease of East Africa transmitted from animals to humans by mosquitoes and causing symptoms resembling those of *influenza.

right 1. *adj.* in accordance with ethical principles or accepted professional standards. There may be more than one right action in any given circumstance. The tradition of *Kantian ethics maintains that an action may be right irrespective of any *good that flows from it; *consequentialism denies this. 2. *n.* any moral or legal entitlement. *See* HUMAN RIGHTS.

rigidity *n.* (in neurology) resistance to the passive movement of a limb that persists throughout its range. It is a symptom of *parkinsonism. The smooth resistance through the whole range of movement is also known as **lead-pipe rigidity**; with superimposed tremor, as in parkinsonism, it is called **cogwheel rigidity**. *Compare* SPASTICITY.

rigor *n.* 1. an abrupt attack of shivering and a sensation of coldness, accompanied by a rapid rise in body temperature. This often marks the onset of a fever and may be followed by a feeling of heat, with copious sweating. 2. *see* RIGOR MORTIS.

rigor mortis the stiffening of a body that occurs within some eight hours of death in temperate climates, due to chemical changes in muscle tissue. It usually starts to disappear after about 24 hours.

riluzole *n.* a drug used to prolong the lives of patients with amyotrophic lateral *sclerosis (*see* MOTOR NEURON DISEASE). It is administered by mouth; side-effects include nausea, vomiting, and dizziness. Trade name: **Rilutek.**

rima *n.* (in anatomy) a cleft. The **rima glottidis** (or glottis) is the space between the vocal folds.

ring *n.* (in anatomy) *see* ANNULUS.

ring block a circumferential ring of local anaesthetic solution used to block the nerves of a digit for purposes of minor surgery (*see* NERVE BLOCK). Precautions are necessary to avoid vascular damage leading to gangrene.

Ringer's solution (Ringer's mixture) a clear colourless *physiological solution of sodium chloride (common salt), potassium

r

chloride, and calcium chloride prepared with recently boiled pure water. The osmotic pressure of the solution is the same as that of blood serum. Ringer's solution is used for maintaining organs or tissues alive outside the animal or human body for limited periods. Sterile Ringer's solution may be injected intravenously to treat dehydration. [S. Ringer (1835–1910), British physiologist]

ringworm (tinea) *n.* a fungal infection of the skin, the scalp, or the nails. Ringworm is caused by the dermatophyte fungi – species of *Microsporum*, *Trichophyton*, and *Epidermophyton* – and also affects animals, a source of infection for humans. It can be spread by direct contact or via infected materials. The lesions of ringworm may form partial or complete rings and may cause intense itching. The commonest form of ringworm is **athlete's foot (tinea pedis)**, which affects the skin between the toes. Another common type is ringworm of the scalp (**tinea capitis**). There is currently an epidemic of scalp ringworm in industrialized nations spread by human-to-human contact. It targets people of African or Afro-Caribbean extraction and is caused by *Trichophyton tonsurans*. Ringworm also affects the groin and thighs (**tinea cruris**) and the skin under a beard (**tinea barbae**). The disease is treated with antifungal agents taken by mouth (such as itraconazole or terbinafine, especially necessary with tinea capitis or nail involvement) or applied locally (for tinea on the body).

Rinne's test a test to determine whether *deafness is conductive or sensorineural. A vibrating tuning fork is held first in the air, close to the ear, and then with its base placed on the bone (mastoid process) behind the ear. If the sound conducted by air is heard louder than the sound conducted by bone the test is positive and the deafness sensorineural; a negative result, when the sound conducted by bone is heard louder, indicates conductive deafness. [H. A. Rinne (1819–68), German otologist]

RIS *see* RADIOLOGY INFORMATION SYSTEM.

risk assessment (in psychiatry) an assessment of the risk that a patient may pose at a given time, which is part of every *mental state examination. Risk assessments are based primarily on past behaviour and certain aspects of current behaviour. They are usually divided into risk to the patient himself or herself, risk to others, and risk of neglect.

Such assessments are more reliable for predicting short-term risk than long-term risk.

risk–benefit analysis an analytical process used to weigh up the probability of forseeable risks and benefits of an action or policy. In medical ethics, it provides a means of reconciling the principles of *beneficence and *nonmaleficence where a particular intervention has dangers as well as benefits. *Compare* COST–BENEFIT ANALYSIS. *See also* CONSEQUENTIALISM.

risk factor an attribute, such as a habit (e.g. cigarette smoking) or exposure to some environmental hazard, that leads the individual concerned to have a greater likelihood of developing an illness. The relationship is one of probability and as such can be distinguished from a *causal agent.

risk management a feature of *clinical governance. Risk management principles are applied to clinical and nonclinical aspects of health care to increase patient safety by identifying potential hazards, assessing the degree of risk, and reducing the risk or determining an acceptable balance between risk and benefit. Risk management should include systems for learning from untoward, significant, or critical incidents and near misses.

risk of malignancy index (RMI) a scoring system that combines ultrasound findings, menopausal status and age, and serum *CA125 levels to give an estimate of the risk of malignancy in a woman with a mass in the Fallopian tubes or ovaries. If the total RMI score is <200 the risk of malignancy is considered to be low. If the total RMI score is >200 the chances of malignancy are raised and management should be planned with a gynaecological oncologist.

risk register 1. a list of infants who have experienced some event in their obstetric and/or perinatal history known to be correlated with a higher than average likelihood of serious abnormality. Problems associated with risk registers include limiting the designation of predisposing conditions, so to contain the number on the register within reasonable proportions, and ensuring that children not on the register receive adequate surveillance. 2. (**at-risk register**) *see* CHILD PROTECTION REGISTER.

risperidone *n.* an atypical *antipsychotic drug used in the treatment of schizophrenia, mania, and other psychoses. Side-effects, which are fewer and less severe than those of the older antipsychotics, include nausea, *akathisia, headache, and fatigue. Trade name: **Risperdal**.

risus sardonicus an abnormal grinning expression resulting from involuntary prolonged contraction of facial muscles, as seen in *tetanus.

ritodrine *n. see* SYMPATHOMIMETIC.

ritonavir *n. see* PROTEASE INHIBITOR.

Ritter's disease *see* STAPHYLOCOCCAL SCALDED SKIN SYNDROME. [G. Ritter von Rittershain (1820–83), German physician]

rituximab *n.* a *monoclonal antibody that acts against the protein CD20, located mainly on the surface of B lymphocytes; it is used in the treatment of many lymphomas and leukaemias. It is also licensed for the treatment of severe rheumatoid arthritis. It is administered by intravenous infusion; side-effects include hypersensitivity reactions and immunosuppression. Trade name: **MabThera**.

rivastigmine *n. see* ACETYLCHOLINESTERASE INHIBITOR.

river blindness *see* ONCHOCERCIASIS.

RMI *see* RISK OF MALIGNANCY INDEX.

RNA (ribonucleic acid) a *nucleic acid, occurring in the nucleus and cytoplasm of cells, that is concerned with synthesis of proteins (*see* MESSENGER RNA, RIBOSOME, TRANSFER RNA, TRANSLATION). In some viruses RNA is the genetic material. The RNA molecule is a single strand made up of units called *nucleotides.

RNA interference (RNAi) a mechanism, either natural or the result of biotechnological manipulation, by which *RNA suppresses or interferes with the expression of a gene or genes. Its possible role in gene-specific therapy is under investigation.

robotic prostatectomy *see* PROSTATECTOMY.

Rocky Mountain spotted fever (spotted fever, tick fever) a disease of rodents and other small mammals in the USA caused by the bacterium *Rickettsia rickettsii* and transmitted to humans by ticks. Symptoms include fever, muscle pains, and a profuse reddish rash like that of measles. If untreated the disease may be fatal, but treatment with

tetracycline or chloramphenicol is effective. *See also* TYPHUS.

rocuronium *n. see* MUSCLE RELAXANT.

rod *n.* one of the two types of light-sensitive cells in the *retina of the eye (*compare* CONE). The human eye contains about 125 million rods, which are necessary for seeing in dim light. They contain a pigment, *rhodopsin (or visual purple), which is broken down (bleached) in the light and regenerated in the dark. Breakdown of visual purple gives rise to nerve impulses; when all the pigment is bleached (i.e. in bright light) the rods no longer function. *See also* DARK ADAPTATION, LIGHT ADAPTATION.

rodent ulcer *see* BASAL CELL CARCINOMA.

roentgen *n.* a unit of exposure dose of X- or gamma-radiation equal to the dose that will produce 2.58×10^{-4} coulomb on all the ions of one sign, when all the electrons released in a volume of air of mass 1 kilogram are completely stopped.

Rokitansky-Küster-Hauser syndrome *see* MAYER-ROKITANSKY-KÜSTER-HAUSER SYNDROME.

role playing acting out another person's expected behaviour, usually in a contrived situation, in order to understand that person better. It is used in family psychotherapy, in teaching social skills to patients, and also in the training of psychiatric (and other) staff.

Romaña's sign an early clinical sign of *Chagas' disease, appearing some three weeks after infection. There is considerable swelling of the eyelids of one or both eyes. This may be due to the presence of the parasites causing the disease but it may also be an allergic reaction to the repeated bites of their insect carriers. [C. Romaña (20th century), Brazilian physician]

Romanowsky stains a group of stains used for microscopical examination of blood cells, consisting of variable mixtures of thiazine dyes, such as azure B, with eosin. Romanowsky stains give characteristic staining patterns, on the basis of which blood cells are classified. The group includes the stains of Leishmann, Wright, May-Grünwald, Giemsa, etc. [D. L. Romanowsky (1861–1921), Russian physician]

Romberg's sign a finding on examination suggesting a sensory disorder affecting those nerves that transmit information to the brain about the position of the limbs and joints and the tension in the muscles. The patient is asked to stand upright. Romberg's sign is positive if he maintains his posture when his eyes are open but sways and falls when his eyes are closed. [M. Romberg (1795–1873), German neurologist]

rongeur *n.* powerful biting forceps for cutting tissue, particularly bone.

root *n.* **1.** (in neurology) a bundle of nerve fibres at its emergence from the spinal cord. The 31 pairs of *spinal nerves have two roots on each side, an anterior root containing motor nerve fibres and a posterior root containing sensory fibres. The roots merge outside the cord to form mixed nerves. **2.** (in dentistry) the part of a *tooth that is not covered by enamel and is normally attached to the alveolar bone by periodontal fibres. **3.** the origin of any structure, i.e. the point at which it diverges from another structure. Anatomical name: **radix**.

root canal treatment (in *endodontics) the procedure of removing the remnants of the pulp of a tooth, cleaning and shaping the canal inside the tooth, and filling the root canal (*see* ROOT FILLING). The entire treatment usually extends over several visits. It is used to treat toothache and apical abscesses.

root end resection *see* APICECTOMY.

root filling **1.** the final stage of *root canal treatment, in which the prepared canal inside a tooth root is filled with a suitable material. **2.** the material used to fill the canal in the root, usually a core of *gutta-percha with a thin coating of sealing cement.

root induction (in *endodontics) a procedure to allow continued root formation in an immature tooth with a damaged pulp. *See* APEXOGENESIS.

rooting reflex a primitive reflex present in newborn babies: if the cheek is stroked near the mouth, the infant will turn its head to the same side to suckle.

ropinirole *n.* a dopamine receptor agonist (*see* DOPAMINE) used to treat Parkinson's disease (either alone or in conjunction with levodopa) and restless legs syndrome. It is administered by mouth; side-effects include nausea, drowsiness, and swelling (oedema) of the legs. Trade names: **Adartrel**, **Requip**.

Rorschach test a test to measure aspects of personality, consisting of ten inkblots, half of which are in various colours and the other half in black and white. The responses to the different inkblots are used to derive hypotheses about the subject. The use of the test for the diagnosis of brain damage or schizophrenia is no longer generally supported. *See also* PROJECTIVE TEST. [H. Rorschach (1884–1922), Swiss psychiatrist]

rosacea *n.* a chronic inflammatory disease of the face in which the skin becomes abnormally flushed. At times it becomes pustular and there may be an associated *keratitis. The disease occurs in both sexes and at all ages but is most common in women in their thirties; the cause is unknown. Treatment is with topical metronidazole; oral tetracyclines, erythromycin, or isotretinoin; or pulsed dye laser.

roseola (roseola infantum, exanthem subitum) *n.* a condition of young children in which a fever lasting for three or four days is followed by a rose-coloured maculopapular rash that fades after two days. The commonest exanthematous fever in young children, it is caused by human herpesvirus 6.

rosiglitazone *n. see* THIAZOLIDINEDIONES.

Ross River fever a viral disease caused by an *alphavirus transmitted by mosquitoes. Various vertebrates can be infected, and wild rodents may be reservoirs of the infection. The virus can cause epidemics of *polyarthritis and skin rashes (macules and papules). It occurs in Australia and the western Pacific region.

rostellum *n.* (*pl.* **rostella**) a mobile and retractable knob bearing hooks, present on the head (scolex) of certain *tapeworms, e.g. *Taenia* and *Echinococcus*.

rostrum *n.* (*pl.* **rostra**) (in anatomy) a beaklike projection, such as that on the sphenoid bone. —**rostral** *adj.*

rotablation *n. see* ATHERECTOMY.

rotator *n.* a muscle that brings about rotation of a part. The **rotatores** are small muscles situated deep in the back between adjacent vertebrae. They help to extend and rotate the vertebrae.

rotavirus *n.* any member of a genus of viruses that occur in birds and mammals and cause diarrhoea (often severe) in children. The viruses are excreted in the faeces of infected individuals and are usually transmitted in food prepared with unwashed hands. Rotavirus infection is endemic worldwide.

Rothera's test a method of testing urine for the presence of acetone or acetoacetic acid: a sign of *diabetes mellitus. Strong ammonia is added to a sample of urine saturated with ammonium sulphate crystals and containing a small quantity of sodium nitroprusside. A purple colour confirms the presence of acetone or acetoacetic acid. [A. C. H. Rothera (1880–1915), Australian biochemist]

Roth spot a pale area surrounded by haemorrhage sometimes seen in the retina, with the aid of an *ophthalmoscope, in those who have bacterial endocarditis, septicaemia, or leukaemia. [M. Roth (1839–1915), Swiss physician]

roughage *n. see* DIETARY FIBRE.

rouleau *n.* (*pl.* **rouleaux**) a cylindrical structure in the blood formed from several red blood cells piled one upon the other and adhering by their rims.

round window *see* FENESTRA (ROTUNDA).

roundworm *n. see* NEMATODE.

RPE retinal pigment epithelium. *See* RETINA.

RPM radiofrequency palatal myoplasty. *See* PALATOPLASTY.

-rrhagia (-rrhage) *combining form denoting* excessive or abnormal flow or discharge from an organ or part. Examples: **haemorrhage** (excessive bleeding); **menorrhagia** (excessive menstrual flow).

-rrhaphy *combining form denoting* surgical sewing; suturing. Example: **herniorrhaphy** (of a hernia).

-rrhexis *combining form denoting* splitting or rupture of a part.

-rrhoea *combining form denoting* a flow or discharge from an organ or part. Example: **rhinorrhoea** (from the nose).

RSI *see* REPETITIVE STRAIN INJURY.

RSV *see* RESPIRATORY SYNCYTIAL VIRUS.

rTMS repetitive *transcranial magnetic stimulation.

rubber dam (in dentistry) a sheet of rubber used to isolate one or more teeth during treatment.

rubefacient *n.* an agent that causes reddening and warming of the skin. Rubefa-

cients are often used as *counterirritants for the relief of muscular pain.

rubella *n. see* GERMAN MEASLES.

rubeola *n. see* MEASLES.

rubeosis iridis (rubeosis) growth of blood vessels onto the iris, usually as a result of ischaemia of the eye. This occurs, for example, in diabetic *retinopathy and central *retinal vein occlusion.

rubidium-81 *n.* an artificial radioactive isotope that has a half-life of about four hours and decays into the radioactive gas *krypton-81m, emitting radiations as it does so. It provides a useful source of krypton-81m for use in *ventilation-perfusion scanning. Symbol: Rb-81.

rubor *n.* redness: one of the classical signs of inflammation in a tissue, the other three being *calor (heat), *dolor (pain) and *tumor (swelling). The redness of inflamed tissue is due to the increase in size of the small blood vessels in the area, which therefore contain more blood.

rubrospinal tract a tract of *motor neurons that extends from the midbrain down to different levels in the spinal cord, carrying impulses that have travelled from the cerebral and cerebellar cortex via the nucleus ruber (red nucleus). The tract plays an important part in the control of skilled and dextrous movements.

ruga *n.* (*pl.* **rugae**) a fold or crease, especially one of the folds of mucous membrane that line the stomach.

rule of nines a method for quickly assessing the area of the body covered by burns in order to assist calculation of the amount of intravenous fluid to be given. The body is divided into areas of skin comprising approximately 9% each of the total body surface. These are as follows: each arm = 9%, the head = 9%, each leg = 18%, the back of the torso (including the buttocks) = 18%, the front of the torso = 18%, with the external genitalia making up the final 1%. The rule is not applicable to children, whose body proportions change with age (in younger children the head represents a greater proportion of the total body surface area).

rumination *n.* (in psychiatry) an obsessional type of thinking in which the same thoughts or themes are experienced repetitively, to the exclusion of other forms of mental activity. Rumination is a feature of obsessive–compulsive disorder.

rupture 1. *n. see* HERNIA. 2. *n.* the bursting apart or open of an organ or tissue; for example, the splitting of the membranes enclosing an infant during childbirth. 3. *vb.* (of tissues, etc.) to burst apart or open.

Rusch catheter a catheter traditionally used for prostate surgery but now successful in the management of *postpartum haemorrhage as an alternative to hysterectomy. The catheter is inserted into the uterine cavity and the balloon filled passively with up to 500 ml warm saline to achieve a *tamponade effect.

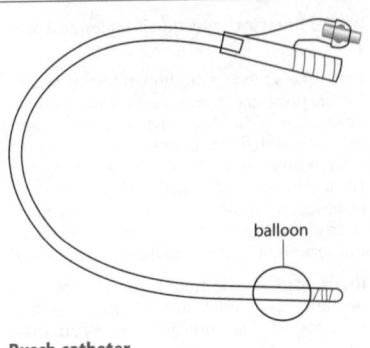

balloon

Rusch catheter.

Russell-Silver syndrome (Silver-Russell syndrome) a congenital condition characterized by short stature, a triangular face with a small mandible (lower jaw), and asymmetry of the body. [A. Russell (20th century), British paediatrician; H. K. Silver (1918–), US paediatrician]

Russian spring-summer encephalitis an influenza-like viral disease that affects the brain and nervous system and occurs in Russia and central Europe. It is transmitted to humans either through the bite of forest-dwelling ticks of the species *Ixodes persulcatus* or by drinking the milk of infected goats. Infection of the meninges results in paralysis of the limbs and of the muscles of the neck and back. The disease, which is often fatal, can be prevented by vaccination.

Ryle's tube a thin flexible tube of rubber or plastic, inserted through the nose of a patient and used for withdrawing fluid from the stomach or giving a test meal. [J. A. Ryle (1889–1950), British physician]

r

Sabin vaccine an oral vaccine against poliomyelitis, prepared by culture of the virus under special conditions so that it loses its virulence (i.e. it becomes attenuated) but retains its ability to stimulate antibody production. [A. B. Sabin (1906–93), US bacteriologist]

sac *n.* a pouch or baglike structure. Sacs can enclose natural cavities in the body, e.g. in the lungs (*see* ALVEOLUS) or in the *lacrimal apparatus of the eye, or they can be pathological, as in a hernia.

saccade *n.* (*pl.* **saccades**) a rapid movement of the eye used to shift gaze from one object to another. It can be done voluntarily or occurs as a reflex triggered by a visual stimulus in the peripheral visual field.

sacchar- (saccharo-) *combining form denoting* sugar.

saccharide *n.* a carbohydrate. *See also* DISACCHARIDE, MONOSACCHARIDE, POLYSACCHARIDE.

saccharine *n.* a sweetening agent. Saccharine is 300 times as sweet as sugar and has no energy content. It is very useful as a sweetener in diabetic and low-calorie foods. Saccharine is stable at high temperatures and therefore can be used in cooking.

Saccharomyces *n. see* YEAST.

saccule (sacculus) *n.* the smaller of the two membranous sacs within the vestibule of the ear: it forms part of the membranous *labyrinth. It is filled with fluid (endolymph) and contains a *macula. This responds to gravity and relays information to the brain about the position of the head.

saccus *n.* a sac or pouch. The **saccus endolymphaticus** is the small sac connected to the saccule and utricle of the inner ear by the *endolymphatic duct.

sacral agenesis (caudal regression syndrome) a severe neural tube defect specific to diabetic pregnancies. The risk may be correlated with the *glycated haemoglobin (HbA_{1c}) level.

sacralization *n.* abnormal fusion of the fifth lumbar vertebra with the sacrum.

sacral nerves the five pairs of *spinal nerves that emerge from the spinal column in the sacrum. The nerves carry sensory and motor fibres from the upper and lower leg and from the anal and genital regions.

sacral vertebrae the five vertebrae that are fused together to form the *sacrum.

sacro- *combining form denoting* the sacrum. Examples: **sacrococcygeal** (relating to the sacrum and coccyx); **sacrodynia** (pain in); **sacroiliac** (relating to the sacrum and ilium).

sacrocolpopexy *n.* surgical treatment of *vault prolapse, which can be an abdominal or laparoscopic procedure. It involves suspending the prolapsed vaginal vault to the sacral promontory using a synthetic mesh or biological material; however, it is associated with a significant risk of haemorrhage and mesh erosion. **Posterior intravaginal slingplasty** (or **infracoccygeal sacropexy**) is a new technique in which an artificial uterosacral ligament (which supports the vagina) is formed. This helps to relocate the vaginal apex and restore the normal vaginal axis. The procedure appears to have similar efficacy to those currently in use but with minimal surgical morbidity.

sacroiliitis *n.* inflammation of the sacroiliac joint. Involvement of both joints is a common feature of ankylosing *spondylitis and associated rheumatic diseases, including *Reiter's syndrome and *psoriatic arthritis. The resultant low back pain and stiffness may be alleviated by rest and anti-inflammatory analgesics.

sacrospinous ligament fixation a surgical technique to correct vaginal *vault prolapse after hysterectomy. A stitch is made from the apex of the vagina to the sacrospinous ligament (which supports the vagina) approximately 2 cm medial to the ischial spine. The main complication is bleeding and formation of a haematoma.

sacrum *n.* (*pl.* **sacra**) a curved triangular

element of the *backbone consisting of five fused vertebrae (**sacral vertebrae**). It articulates with the last lumbar vertebra above, the coccyx below, and the hip bones laterally. *See also* VERTEBRA. —**sacral** *adj.*

SAD (seasonal affective disorder) a disorder marked by changes of mood at particular times of the year. Typically, with the onset of winter, there is depression, general slowing of mind and body, excessive sleeping, and overeating. These symptoms resolve with the coming of spring. The phenomenon may partly account for the known seasonal variation in suicide rates. Prevalence increases with latitude and younger people (especially women) are most likely to be affected. There is evidence that mood is related to light, which suppresses the release of the hormone *melatonin from the pineal gland. Exposure to additional light during the day may relieve symptoms.

saddle joint a form of *diarthrosis (freely movable joint) in which the articulating surfaces of the bones are reciprocally saddle-shaped. It occurs at the carpometacarpal joint of the thumb.

safe period the days in each *menstrual cycle when conception is least likely. Ovulation generally occurs at the midpoint of each cycle, and in women with regular periods it is possible to calculate the days at the beginning and end of the cycle when coitus is unlikely to result in pregnancy. *See* RHYTHM METHOD.

safranin (safranine) *n.* a group of water- and alcohol-soluble basic dyes used to stain cell nuclei and as counterstains for Gram-negative bacteria.

sagittal *adj.* describing a dorsoventral plane that extends down the long axis of the body, parallel to the median plane, dividing it into right and left parts (see illustration).

sagittal suture *see* SUTURE.

Saint's triad the coexistence of *gallstones, colonic diverticula (*see* DIVERTICULUM), and hiatus *hernia in a patient. It is important to identify which of these conditions, if any, is causing the symptoms of dyspepsia. [C. F. M. Saint (1886–1973), South African surgeon]

salaam attacks *see* INFANTILE SPASMS.

salbutamol *n.* a drug that stimulates β_2 adrenoceptors (*see* SYMPATHOMIMETIC): a short-acting beta agonist used as a *bronchodilator to relieve asthma and other reversible obstructive airways diseases. It is administered by inhalation, mouth, or injection; side-effects may include dizziness, tremor, and fast heart rate, particularly after large doses. Trade names: **Airomir**, **Asmasal Clickhaler**, **Ventolin**, etc.

salcatonin *n. see* CALCITONIN.

salicylic acid a drug that causes the skin to peel and destroys bacteria and fungi. It is applied to the skin, alone or in combination with other agents, to treat warts, corns, calluses, acne, dandruff, psoriasis, and fungal nail infections. Skin sensitivity reactions may occur after continued use. Trade names: **Cuplex**, **Duofilm**, **Salactol**, **Verrugon**, etc.

salicylism *n.* poisoning due to an overdose of aspirin or other salicylate-containing compounds. The main symptoms are headache, dizziness, ringing in the ears (tinnitus), disturbances of vision, vomiting, and – in severe cases – delirium and collapse. There is often severe *acidosis.

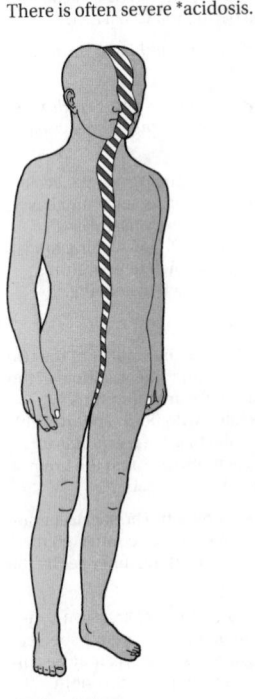

Sagittal plane.

saline (normal saline, physiological saline) *n.* a solution containing 0.9% *sodium chloride. Saline may be used clinically for irrigating wounds, treating sodium depletion (by intravenous infusion), as a diluent for drugs, and as an ingredient of plasma substitutes.

saline infusion sonohysterography (SIS) *see* SONOHYSTEROGRAPHY.

saliva *n.* the alkaline liquid secreted by the *salivary glands and the mucous membrane of the mouth. Its principal constituents are water, mucus, buffers, and enzymes (e.g. amylase). The functions of saliva are to keep the mouth moist, to aid swallowing of food, to minimize changes of acidity in the mouth, and to digest starch. *See also* DRY MOUTH. —**salivary** *adj.*

salivary gland a gland that produces *saliva. There are three pairs of salivary glands: the *parotid glands, *sublingual glands, and *submandibular glands (see illustration). They are stimulated by reflex action, which can be initiated by the taste, smell, sight, or thought of food.

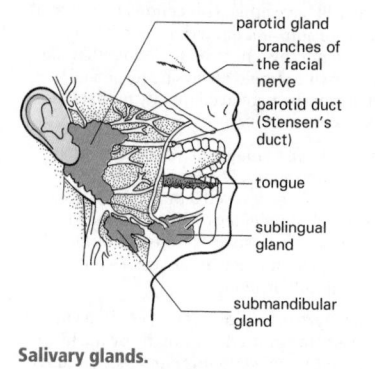

parotid gland
branches of the facial nerve
parotid duct (Stensen's duct)
tongue
sublingual gland
submandibular gland

Salivary glands.

salivary stone *see* SIALOLITH.

salivation *n.* the secretion of saliva by the salivary glands of the mouth, increased in response to the chewing action of the jaws or to the thought, taste, smell, or sight of food. A small but regular flow of saliva is maintained to promote cleanliness in the mouth even when food is not being eaten. *See also* PTYALISM.

Salk vaccine a vaccine against poliomyelitis, formed by treating the virus with formalin, which prevents it from causing disease but does not impair its ability to stimulate antibody production. It is administered by injection. [J. E. Salk (1914–95), US bacteriologist]

salmeterol *n.* a *sympathomimetic drug: a long-acting beta agonist used, with inhaled corticosteroids, as a *bronchodilator to control chronic asthma and chronic obstructive pulmonary disease. It is administered by inhaler. Possible side-effects include palpitations, a paradoxical worsening of the condition, and a lowering of the blood potassium level. Trade name: **Serevent**.

Salmonella *n.* a genus of motile rodlike Gram-negative bacteria that inhabit the intestines of animals and humans and cause disease. They ferment glucose, usually with the formation of gas. The species *S. paratyphi* causes *paratyphoid fever, and *S. typhi* causes *typhoid fever. Other species of *Salmonella* cause *food poisoning, gastroenteritis, and septicaemia.

salmonellosis *n.* an infestation of the digestive system by bacteria of the genus *Salmonella. See also* FOOD POISONING.

salping- (**salpingo-**) *combining form denoting* 1. the Fallopian tube. 2. the auditory tube (meatus).

salpingectomy *n.* the surgical removal of a Fallopian tube. The operation involving both tubes is a permanent and completely effective method of contraception (*see* STERILIZATION) since it prevents the egg cells passing from the ovaries to the uterus.

salpingitis *n.* inflammation of a tube, most commonly applied to inflammation of one or both of the Fallopian tubes caused by bacterial infection spreading from the vagina or uterus or carried in the blood. In **acute salpingitis** there is a sharp pain in the lower abdomen, which may be mistaken for appendicitis, and the infection may spread to the membrane lining the abdominal cavity (*see* PERITONITIS). In severe cases the tubes may become blocked with scar tissue and the patient will be unable to conceive. The condition is treated with antibiotics and later, if necessary, by the surgical removal of the diseased tube(s).

salpingography *n.* *radiography of one or both Fallopian tubes after a *radiopaque substance has been introduced into them via an injection into the uterus. **Standardized selective salpingography** enables occluded

S

tubes, visualized by salpingography, to be restored to patency by means of tubal *catheterization.

salpingolysis *n.* a surgical operation carried out to restore patency to blocked Fallopian tubes; it involves the *division and removal of adhesions around the ovarian ends of the tubes.

salpingo-oophorectomy *n.* surgical removal of the Fallopian tube and ovary.

salpingo-oophoritis *n.* inflammation of a Fallopian tube and an ovary.

salpingostomy *n.* the operation performed to restore free passage through a blocked Fallopian tube. The blocked portion of the tube is removed surgically and the continuity is then restored. It is performed in women who have been sterilized previously by tubal occlusion (*see* STERILIZATION) and in others whose Fallopian tubes have become blocked as a result of pelvic infection.

salt depletion excessive loss of sodium chloride (common salt) from the body. This may result from sweating, persistent vomiting or diarrhoea, or loss of fluid in wounds. The main symptoms are muscular weakness and cramps. Miners and workers in hot climates are particularly at risk, and salt tablets are often taken as a preventive measure.

Salter-Harris classification (S-H classification) a classification of fractures involving the growth plate of bones (*see* PHYSIS), which is useful for their prognosis and treatment. There are five S-H categories of fracture. [R. Salter and R. I. Harris (20th century), Canadian orthopaedic surgeons]

salvage procedure surgical measures to palliate the worst effects of a tumour but with no aim to effect a cure.

Salvarsan *n. see* ARSENIC.

Salzmann's degeneration a noninflammatory condition of the cornea resulting in yellow-white nodules under the epithelium in the central area. These may cause symptoms if the epithelium over them breaks down or if they are located along the visual axis. [M. Salzmann (1862–1954), German ophthalmologist]

Samaritans *n.* a British voluntary organization providing a telephone service for the suicidal and despairing. Started in 1953 by the Rev. Chad Varah in the cellars of a London church (St Stephen, Walbrook) with one telephone, it now has over 200 branches throughout the country manned by some 22,000 volunteers. It offers a free, nonprofessional, confidential, and (if required) anonymous service at all hours. Samaritans offer little advice, believing that their clients will be helped to make their own decisions by talking to someone who cares.

sampling frame *see* RANDOM SAMPLE.

Samter's triad a syndrome characterized by the presence of asthma, nasal *polyps, and hypersensitivity to aspirin. [M. Samter (1908–99) German-born US physician]

sanatorium *n.* **1.** a hospital or institution for the rehabilitation and convalescence of patients of any kind. **2.** an institution for patients who have suffered from pulmonary tuberculosis.

sanctity of life the belief that all human life is intrinsically valuable. The concept often, but not always, derives from a faith-based belief that life is a gift from God and, as such, should never be deliberately harmed or destroyed. Those who hold such a view will have ethical objections to euthanasia, abortion, and embryo research. The phrase may also be used to denote that the value of life should always be respected, whatever the perceived quality of that life. *See also* HUMANITY, PERSONHOOD.

sandfly *n.* a small hairy fly of the widely distributed genus *Phlebotomus*. Adult sandflies rarely exceed 3 mm in length and have long slender legs. The blood-sucking females of certain species transmit various diseases, including *leishmaniasis, *sandfly fever, and *bartonellosis.

sandfly fever (Pappataci fever) a viral disease transmitted to humans by the bite of the sandfly *Phlebotomus papatasii*. Sandfly fever occurs principally in countries surrounding the Persian Gulf and the tropical Mediterranean; it occurs during the warmer months, does not last long, and is never fatal. Symptoms resemble those of influenza. There is no specific treatment apart from aspirin and codeine to relieve the symptoms.

sandwich therapy a combination of treatments in which one type of therapy is 'sandwiched' between exposures to another therapy. For example, surgical removal of a tumour may be 'sandwiched' between pre- and postoperative courses of radiotherapy.

See also CHEMORADIOTHERAPY, COMBINED THERAPY.

SANE a British charity whose role is to raise the awareness of mental health issues. It also initiates research into serious mental illness and offers telephone support for those with mental health problems and for those caring for them.

sangui- (sanguino-) *combining form denoting* blood.

sanguineous *adj.* 1. stained, containing, or covered with blood. 2. of tissues) containing more than the normal quantity of blood.

sanies *n.* a foul-smelling watery discharge from a wound or ulcer, containing serum, blood, and pus.

sanitarian *n. see* MEDICAL ASSISTANT.

saphena *n. see* SAPHENOUS VEIN.

saphena varix an abnormal dilatation of the terminal section of the long *saphenous vein in the groin.

saphenous nerve a large branch of the *femoral nerve that arises in the upper thigh, travels down on the inside of the leg, and supplies the skin from the knee to below the ankle with sensory nerves.

saphenous vein (saphena) either of two superficial veins of the leg, draining blood from the foot. The **long saphenous vein** – the longest vein in the body – runs from the foot, up the medial side of the leg, to the groin, where it joins the femoral vein. The **short saphenous vein** runs up the back of the calf to join the popliteal vein at the back of the knee.

sapr- (sapro-) *combining form denoting* 1. putrefaction. 2. decaying matter.

sapraemia *n.* blood poisoning by toxins of saprophytic bacteria (bacteria living on dead or decaying matter). *Compare* PYAEMIA, SEPTICAEMIA, TOXAEMIA.

saprophyte *n.* any free-living organism that lives and feeds on the dead and putrefying tissues of animals or plants. *Compare* PARASITE. —**saprophytic** *adj.*

saquinavir *n. see* PROTEASE INHIBITOR.

sarc- (sarco-) *combining form denoting* 1. flesh or fleshy tissue. 2. muscle.

Sarcocystis *n.* a genus of parasitic protozoans (*see* SPOROZOA) that infect birds, reptiles, and herbivorous mammals. *S. lindemanni*, which occasionally infects humans, forms cylindrical cysts (**sarcocysts**) in the muscle fibres. In heavy infections these cysts can cause tissue degeneration and therefore provoke muscular pain and weakness. Sarcocysts have, in the few positively diagnosed cases, been located in the heart muscles, arm muscles, and larynx.

sarcoid 1. *adj.* fleshy. 2. *n.* a fleshy tumour.

sarcoidosis (Boeck's disease) *n.* a chronic disorder of unknown cause in which the lymph nodes in many parts of the body are enlarged and small fleshy nodules (*see* GRANULOMA) develop in the lungs, liver, and spleen. The skin, nervous system, eyes, and salivary glands are also commonly affected (*see* UVEOPAROTITIS), and the condition has features similar to *tuberculosis. Recovery is complete with minimal after-effects in two-thirds of all cases.

sarcolemma *n.* the cell membrane that encloses a muscle cell (muscle fibre).

sarcoma *n.* any *cancer of connective tissue. These tumours may occur in any part of the body, as they arise in the tissues that make up an organ rather than being restricted to a particular organ. They can arise in fibrous tissue, muscle, fat, bone, cartilage, synovium, blood and lymphatic vessels, and various other tissues. *See also* CHONDROSARCOMA, FIBROSARCOMA, LEIOMYOSARCOMA, LIPOSARCOMA, LYMPHANGIOSARCOMA, OSTEOSARCOMA, RHABDOMYOSARCOMA. —**sarcomatous** *adj.*

sarcoma botryoides the most common tumour of the cervix and vagina in children and adolescents under the age of 16; 90% occur in children under five years. Symptoms are vaginal bleeding and a bloody discharge; in young girls the tumour may protrude from the cervix. It is a highly malignant *rhabdomyosarcoma with the appearance of a bunch of grapes. Treatment is with triple chemotherapy with or without radiotherapy prior to hysterectomy and vaginectomy.

sarcomatosis *n.* *sarcoma that has spread widely throughout the body, most commonly through the bloodstream. It is treated with drugs, typically one or a combination of the following: cyclophosphamide, ifosfamide, vincristine, dactinomycin, methotrexate, or doxorubicin. The prognosis is very poor.

sarcomere *n.* one of the basic contractile units of which *striated muscle fibres are composed.

Sarcophaga *n.* a genus of widely distributed non-bloodsucking flies, the flesh flies. Maggots are normally found in carrion or excrement but occasionally females will deposit their eggs in wounds or ulcers giving off a foul-smelling discharge; the presence of the maggots causes a serious *myiasis. Rarely, maggots may be ingested with food and give rise to an intestinal myiasis.

sarcoplasm (myoplasm) *n.* the cytoplasm of muscle cells.

sarcoplasmic reticulum an arrangement of membranous vesicles and tubules found in the cytoplasm of striated muscle fibres. The sarcoplasmic reticulum plays an important role in the transmission of nervous excitation to the contractile parts of the fibres.

Sarcoptes *n.* a genus of small oval mites. The female of *S. scabiei*, the scabies mite, tunnels into the skin, where it lays its eggs. The presence of the mites causes severe irritation, which eventually leads to *scabies.

sarcostyle *n.* a bundle of muscle fibrils.

SARS (severe acute respiratory syndrome) an *atypical pneumonia caused by a virus, SARS coronavirus (SARS CoV), and spread by close contact with an infected person, that first appeared in November 2002 in Guangdong province, China. Over the next few months it spread to many countries in Asia, Europe, and North and South America before being contained (the last case in this outbreak occurred in June 2003). According to the World Health Organization (WHO), a total of 8098 people worldwide contracted SARS during the 2003 outbreak; 774 of these died. Over the next two years the number of cases declined until the disease itself was declared eradicated by the WHO (in May 2005).

sartorius *n.* a narrow ribbon-like muscle at the front of the thigh, arising from the anterior superior spine of the ilium and extending to the tibia, just below the knee. The longest muscle in the body, the sartorius flexes the leg on the thigh and the thigh on the abdomen.

SAS sleep apnoea syndrome (*see* OBSTRUCTIVE SLEEP APNOEA).

saturated fatty acid a *fatty acid in which all the carbon atoms are linked by single bonds and the molecule is unable to accept additional atoms (i.e. it cannot undergo addition reactions with other molecules). These fats occur mainly in animal and dairy products, and a diet high in these foods may contribute to a high serum cholesterol level, which may increase the risk of *coronary artery disease. *Compare* UNSATURATED FATTY ACID.

saucerization *n.* **1.** an operation in which tissue is cut away from a wound to form a saucer-like depression. It is carried out to facilitate healing and is commonly used to treat injuries or disorders in which bone is infected. **2.** the concave appearance of the upper surface of a vertebra that has been fractured by compression.

Sayre's jacket a plaster of Paris cast shaped to fit around and support the backbone. It is used in cases where the vertebrae have been severely damaged by disease, such as tuberculosis. [L. A. Sayre (1820–1900), US surgeon]

scab *n.* a hard crust of dried blood, serum, or pus that develops during the body's wound-healing process over a sore, cut, or scratch.

scabicide *n.* a drug that kills the mites causing *scabies.

scabies *n.* a skin infection caused by the mite *Sarcoptes scabiei*. Scabies is typified by severe itching (particularly at night), red papules, and often secondary infection. The female mite invades the skin to lay her eggs and the newly hatched mites pass from person to person by close prolonged contact. The intense itching represents a true allergic reaction to the mite, its eggs, and its faeces. Commonly infected areas are the penis, nipples, and the finger webs. Treatment is by application of a scabicide, usually *permethrin or *malathion, to all areas of the body from the neck down; benzyl benzoate may be used but is more irritant. All members of a family need treatment, but clothing and bedding need not be disinfested.

scala *n.* one of the spiral canals of the *cochlea. The **scala media** (**cochlear duct**) is the central membranous canal, containing the sensory apparatus of the cochlea; the **scala vestibuli** and **scala tympani** are the two bony canals of the cochlea.

scald *n.* a *burn produced by a hot liquid or vapour, such as boiling water or steam.

scale 1. *n.* any of the flakes of dead epidermal cells shed from the skin. 2. *vb.* to scrape deposits of calculus (tartar) from the teeth (*see* SCALER).

scalenus *n.* one of four paired muscles of the neck (**scalenus anterior**, **medius**, **minimus**, and **posterior**), extending from the cervical (neck) vertebrae to the first and second ribs. They are responsible for raising the first and second ribs in inspiration and for bending the neck forward and to either side.

scalenus syndrome (thoracic outlet syndrome) the group of symptoms caused by compression of the subclavian artery and the lower roots of the brachial plexus against the fibrous and bony structures of the outlet of the upper thoracic vertebrae. Loss of sensation, wasting, and vascular symptoms may be found in the affected arm, which may also be painful.

scaler *n.* an instrument for removing calculus from the teeth. It may be a hand instrument (usually sickle or curette) or one energized by rapid ultrasonic vibrations.

scalpel *n.* a small pointed surgical knife used by surgeons for cutting tissues. It has a straight handle and usually detachable disposable blades of different shapes.

scan 1. *n.* examination of the body or a part of the body using *ultrasonography, *computerized tomography (CT), *magnetic resonance imaging (MRI), or scintigraphy (*see* SCINTIGRAM). 2. *n.* the image obtained from such an examination. 3. *vb.* to examine the body using any of these techniques.

scanning laser ophthalmoscope *see* OPHTHALMOSCOPE.

scanning speech a disorder of articulation in which the syllables are inappropriately separated and equally stressed. It is caused by disease of the cerebellum or its connecting fibres in the brainstem.

scaphocephaly *n.* an abnormally long and narrow skull due to premature closure of the suture between the two parietal bones, along the top of the skull. —**scaphocephalic** *adj.*

scaphoid bone a boat-shaped bone of the wrist (*see* CARPUS). It articulates with the trapezium and trapezoid bones in front, with the radius behind, and with the capitate and lunate medially. It is commonly injured by falls on the wrist.

scaphoid fracture a fracture of the scaphoid bone in the wrist, usually caused by a fall onto the outstretched hand. There is pain and swelling in the *anatomical snuffbox and movements of the wrist and thumb are painful. If the fracture is suspected but not initially visible on X-ray, advanced imaging (a bone scan, CT scan, or MRI) is now increasingly used to confirm the diagnosis without delay. Treatment is with a cast for an undisplaced fracture and by internal fixation for a displaced fracture. Due to the anatomy of its blood supply, healing can take a long time, and a *bone graft and internal fixation may be required for non-*union.

scapul- (scapulo-) *combining form denoting* the scapula.

scapula *n.* (*pl.* **scapulas** or **scapulae**) the shoulder blade: a triangular bone, a pair of which form the back part of the shoulder girdle (see illustration). The **spine** on its dorsal (back) surface ends at the **acromion process** at the top of the shoulder. This process turns forward and articulates with the collar bone (*clavicle) at the **acromioclavicular joint**; it overhangs the **glenoid fossa**, into which the humerus fits to form the socket of the shoulder joint. The **coracoid process** curves upwards and forwards from the neck of the scapula and provides attachment for ligaments and muscles. —**scapular** *adj.*

Right scapula (dorsal surface).

scar *n.* a permanent mark left after wound healing. A **hypertrophic scar** is an abnormal raised scar that tends to settle after a year or so, as distinct from a *keloid, which is not only permanent but tends to extend beyond the original wound.

scarification *n.* the process of making a series of shallow cuts or scratches in the skin to allow a substance to penetrate the body. This was commonly performed during vaccination against smallpox; the vaccine was administered as a droplet left in contact with the scarified area.

scarlatina *n. see* SCARLET FEVER.

scarlet fever a highly infectious disease caused by a strain of *Streptococcus* bacteria that produces toxins. Symptoms begin 2–4 days after exposure and include fever, tonsillitis, and a characteristic widespread scarlet rash. The tongue is also affected; initially covered by a thick white material, it then becomes bright red (the 'strawberry tongue'). Treatment with antibiotics shortens the course of the disease and reduces the risk of secondary complications, which include kidney and ear inflammation. Medical name: **scarlatina**. *Compare* GERMAN MEASLES.

Scarpa's triangle *see* FEMORAL TRIANGLE. [A. Scarpa (1747–1832), Italian anatomist and surgeon]

scat- (scato-) *combining form denoting* faeces.

scatter diagram (in statistics) *see* CORRELATION.

SCC *see* SQUAMOUS CELL CARCINOMA.

SCDS *see* SUPERIOR CANAL DEHISCENCE SYNDROME.

Scheuermann's disease (adolescent kyphosis) a disorder of spinal growth in which a sequence of three or more vertebrae become slightly wedge-shaped. It arises in adolescence and usually occurs in the thoracic spine, causing poor posture, backache, fatigue, and exaggerated *kyphosis. X-ray findings include *Schmorl's nodes. [H. W. Scheuermann (1877–1960), Danish surgeon]

Schick test a test to determine whether a person is susceptible to diphtheria. A small quantity of diphtheria toxin is injected under the skin; a patch of reddening and swelling shows that the person has no immunity and – if at particular risk – should be immunized. With safer *toxoids, this test is no longer necessary. [B. Schick (1877–1967), US paediatrician]

Schiff's reagent aqueous *fuchsin solution decolourized with sulphur dioxide. A blue coloration develops in the presence of aldehydes. [H. Schiff (1834–1915), German chemist]

Schilling test a test used to assess a patient's capacity to absorb vitamin B_{12} from the bowel. Radioactive vitamin B_{12} is given by mouth and urine collected for 24 hours. A normal individual will excrete at least 10% of the original dose over this period; a patient with *pernicious anaemia will excrete less than 5%. [R. F. Schilling (1919–   ), US physician]

schindylesis *n.* a form of *synarthrosis (immovable joint) in which a crest of one bone fits into a groove of another.

-schisis *combining form denoting* a cleft or split.

schisto- *combining form denoting* a fissure; split.

schistoglossia *n.* fissuring of the tongue. Congenital fissures are transverse, whereas those due to disease (such as syphilis) are usually longitudinal.

Schistosoma (Bilharzia) *n.* a genus of blood *flukes, three species of which are important parasites of humans causing one of the most serious of tropical diseases (*see* SCHISTOSOMIASIS). *S. japonicum* is common in the Far East; *S. mansoni* is widespread in Africa, the West Indies, and South and Central America; and *S. haematobium* occurs in Africa and the Middle East.

schistosomiasis (bilharziasis) *n.* a tropical disease caused by blood flukes of the genus *Schistosoma*. Eggs present in the stools or urine of infected people undergo part of their larval development within freshwater snails living in water contaminated with human sewage. The disease is contracted when *cercaria larvae, released from the snails, penetrate the skin of anyone bathing in infected water. Adult flukes eventually settle in the blood vessels of the intestine (*S. mansoni* and *S. japonicum*) or the bladder (*S. haematobium*); the release of their spiked eggs causes anaemia, inflammation, and the formation of scar tissue. Additional intestinal symptoms are diarrhoea, dysentery, enlargement of the spleen and liver, and cirrhosis of the liver. If the bladder is affected, blood is passed in the urine and cystitis and cancer of the bladder may develop. The disease is treated with praziquantel.

schiz- (schizo-) *combining form denoting* a split or division.

schizogony *n.* a phase of asexual reproduction in the life cycle of a sporozoan (protozoan parasite) that occurs in the liver or red blood cells. The parasite grows and divides many times to form a **schizont**, which contains many *merozoites. The eventual release of merozoites of *Plasmodium*, the malaria parasite, from the blood cells produces fever in the patient.

schizoid personality a personality characterized by solitariness, emotional coldness to others, inability to experience pleasure, lack of response to praise and criticism, withdrawal into a fantasy world, excessive introspection, and eccentricity of behaviour. Some schizophrenics have this personality before their illness, but most schizoid personalities do not become schizophrenic. *See* PERSONALITY DISORDER.

schizont *n.* one of the stages that occurs during the asexual phase of the life cycle of a sporozoan. *See* SCHIZOGONY.

schizonticide *n.* any agent used for killing *schizonts.

schizophrenia *n.* a severe *mental illness characterized by a disintegration of the process of thinking, of contact with reality, and of emotional responsiveness. *Positive symptoms, such as *delusions and *hallucinations (especially of voices), are common, and any *Schneiderian first-rank symptoms are particularly indicative of the illness. *Negative symptoms include social withdrawal, impairment of ego boundaries, and loss of energy and initiative. Schizophrenia is diagnosed only if symptoms persist for at least one month. The illness can spontaneously remit, run a course with infrequent or frequent relapses, or become chronic. The prognosis has improved with *antipsychotic drugs and with vigorous psychological and social management and rehabilitation. The many causes include genetic factors, environmental stress, and various triggering factors. —**schizophrenic** *adj.*

(⊕) SEE WEB LINKS

• Website of Rethink (formerly National Schizophrenia Fellowship): includes information on the causes, symptoms, and treatment of schizophrenia

schizotypal personality disorder a personality disorder characterized by cold aloof feelings, eccentricities of behaviour, odd ways of thinking and talking, and occasional short periods of intense illusions, hallucinations, or delusion-like ideas. The condition is more common in people who are genetically related to schizophrenics.

Schlemm's canal a channel in the eye, at the junction of the cornea and the sclera, through which the aqueous humour drains. [F. Schlemm (1795–1858), German anatomist]

Schmidt's syndrome the autoimmune destruction of a combination of the thyroid, the adrenals, and the beta cells of the islets of Langerhans, causing type 1 *diabetes mellitus. It is often associated with failure of the ovaries (causing an early menopause), the parathyroids, and the parietal cells of the *gastric glands (causing pernicious anaemia). [M. B. Schmidt (1863–1949), German physician]

Schmorl's node (Schmorl's nodule) a lucent area seen on X-ray of the backbone that denotes extrusion of some nucleus pulposus from an *intervertebral disc into the body of a vertebra. [C. G. Schmorl (1861–1932), German pathologist]

Schneiderian first- and second-rank symptoms symptoms of *schizophrenia first classified by German psychiatrist Kurt Schneider (1887–1967) in 1938. First-rank symptoms were considered by Schneider to be particularly indicative of schizophrenia; they include all forms of *thought alienation, *delusional perception, *passivity, and third-person auditory *hallucinations in the form of either a running commentary or voices talking about the patient among themselves. Some schizophrenic patients never exhibit first-rank symptoms or only experience them in some psychotic episodes. They may also occur in *mania. Second-rank symptoms are common symptoms of schizophrenia but also often occur in other forms of mental illness. They include *delusions of reference, paranoid and persecutory *delusions, and second-person auditory hallucinations.

Schönlein-Henoch purpura *see* HENOCH-SCHÖNLEIN PURPURA.

school health service (in Britain) a service concerned with promotion of health and wellbeing in schoolchildren, including the early detection of health and social problems and their subsequent treatment and surveillance. The service is now the responsibility of the local *primary care trust.

school nurse a member of the *school health service who undertakes health improvement activities, including health education and promotion, developmental screening, and vaccinations. *Health visitors sometimes work in this capacity.

Schwann cells the cells that lay down the *myelin sheath around the axon of a medullated nerve fibre. Each cell is responsible for one length of axon, around which it twists as it grows, so that concentric layers of membrane envelop the axon. The gap between adjacent Schwann cells forms a *node of Ranvier. [T. Schwann (1810–82), German anatomist and physiologist]

schwannoma *n. see* NEUROFIBROMA, VESTIBULAR SCHWANNOMA.

sciatica pain radiating from the buttock into the thigh, calf, and occasionally the foot. Although it is in the distribution of the sciatic nerve, sciatica is rarely due to disease of this nerve. Pain felt down the back and lateral aspect of the thigh, leg, and foot is often caused by degeneration or displacement of an intervertebral disc (*see* PROLAPSED INTERVERTEBRAL DISC), which encroaches upon and irritates a lower lumbar or an upper sacral spinal nerve root. The onset may be sudden, brought on by an awkward lifting or twisting movement that causes a tear in the fibrous coat of the disc, or more gradual, from progressive narrowing secondary to degenerative changes in the disc. The back is often stiff and painful and there may be numbness and weakness in the leg. Bed rest will often relieve the pain but surgical treatment is occasionally necessary (*see* LAMINECTOMY, DISCECTOMY, MICRODISCECTOMY).

sciatic nerve the major nerve of the leg and the nerve with the largest diameter. It runs down behind the thigh from the lower end of the spine; above the knee joint it divides into two main branches, the **tibial** and **common peroneal nerves**, which are distributed to the muscles and skin of the lower leg.

SCID *see* SEVERE COMBINED IMMUNE DEFICIENCY.

scintigram *n.* a diagram showing the distribution of radioactive *tracer in a part of

the body, produced by recording the flashes of light given off by a *scintillator as it is struck by radiation of different intensities. This technique is called **scintigraphy**. By scanning the body, section by section, a 'map' of the radioactivity in various regions is built up, aiding the diagnosis of cancer or other disorders. Such a record is known as a **scintiscan**. These images are now usually obtained using a *gamma camera.

scintillation counter a device to measure and record the fluorescent flashes in a *scintillator exposed to high-energy radiation.

scintillator *n.* a substance that produces a fluorescent flash when struck by high-energy radiation, such as beta or gamma rays. In medicine the most commonly used scintillator is a crystal of thallium-activated sodium iodide, which forms the basis of a *gamma camera. *See also* SCINTIGRAM.

scintiscan *n. see* SCINTIGRAM.

scirrhous *adj.* describing carcinomas that are stony hard to the touch. Such a carcinoma (for example of the breast) is known as a **scirrhus**.

scissor leg a disability in which one leg becomes permanently crossed over the other as a result of spasticity of its *adductor muscles or deformity of the hips. The condition occurs in children with brain damage and in adults after strokes. A *tenotomy or injections with *botulinum toxin may reduce the degree of disability.

scissura (scissure) *n.* a cleft or splitting, such as the splitting of the tip of a hair or the splitting open of tissues when a hernia forms.

scler- (sclero-) *combining form denoting* 1. hardening or thickening. 2. the sclera. 3. sclerosis.

sclera (sclerotic coat) *n.* the white fibrous outer layer of the eyeball. At the front of the eye it becomes the cornea. *See* EYE. —**scleral** *adj.*

sclerectomy *n.* an operation in which a portion of the sclera (the thick white layer of the eyeball) is removed.

scleritis *n.* inflammation of the sclera (the white of the eye).

scleroderma *n.* thickening of the skin, either localized (*see* MORPHOEA) or generalized, resulting in waxy ivory-coloured areas. Treatment is unsatisfactory, but spontaneous resolution may occur. Scleroderma is thought to be an *autoimmune disease. *Systemic sclerosis is a related multisystem disorder.

scleromalacia *n.* thinning of the sclera (white of the eye) as a result of inflammation. Sometimes the sclera fades away completely in an area, and the underlying dark-bluish tissue (usually the ciliary body) bulges beneath the conjunctiva. This state is known as **scleromalacia perforans**.

sclerosis *n.* hardening of tissue, usually due to scarring (fibrosis) after inflammation or to ageing. It can affect the lateral columns of the spinal cord and the medulla of the brain (**amyotrophic lateral sclerosis** or **Lou Gehrig's disease**), causing progressive muscular paralysis (*see* MOTOR NEURON DISEASE). It can also occur in scattered patches throughout the brain and spinal cord (*see* MULTIPLE SCLEROSIS) or in the walls of the arteries (*see* ARTERIOSCLEROSIS, ATHEROSCLEROSIS). *See also* TUBEROUS SCLEROSIS.

sclerotherapy *n.* treatment of varicose veins by the injection of an irritant solution. This causes thrombophlebitis, which encourages obliteration of the varicose vein by thrombosis and subsequent scarring. Sclerotherapy is also used for treating haemorrhoids and oesophageal varices.

sclerotic 1. (**sclerotic coat**) *n. see* SCLERA. 2. *adj.* affected with *sclerosis.

sclerotome *n.* 1. a surgical knife used in the operation of *sclerotomy. 2. (in embryology) the part of the segmented mesoderm (*see* SOMITE) in the early embryo that gives rise to all the skeletal tissue of the body. The vertebrae and ribs retain the segmented structure, which is lost in the skull and limbs.

sclerotomy *n.* an operation in which an incision is made in the sclera (white of the eye).

scolex *n.* (*pl.* **scolices**) the head of a *tapeworm. The presence of suckers and/or hooks on the scolex enables the worm to attach itself to the wall of its host's gut.

scoliosis *n.* lateral (sideways) deviation of the backbone, caused by congenital or acquired abnormalities of the vertebrae, muscles, and nerves. Treatment may require spinal braces and, in cases of severe deformity, surgical correction by fusion or *osteotomy. *See also* KYPHOSIS, KYPHOSCOLIOSIS.

-scope *combining form denoting* an instrument for observing or examining. Example: **gastroscope** (instrument for examining the stomach).

ScopeGuide *n. Trademark. see* 3-D MAGNETIC IMAGER.

scopolamine *n. see* HYOSCINE.

scorbutic *adj.* affected with scurvy.

scoring system any of various methods in which the application of an agreed numerical scale is used as a means of estimating the degree of a clinical situation, e.g. the severity of an injury, the degree of patient recovery, or the extent of malignancy. Examples include the *Glasgow Coma Scale (or scoring system) and the *injury scoring system.

scoto- *combining form denoting* darkness.

scotoma *n.* (*pl.* **scotomata**) a small area of abnormally less sensitive or absent vision in the visual field, surrounded by normal sight. There is a *blind spot in the visual field of each eye due to the optic disc, which is not sensitive to light. Similar islands of total visual loss in other parts of the field are referred to as **absolute scotomata**. A **relative scotoma** is a spot where the vision is decreased but still present.

scotometer *n.* an instrument used for mapping defects in the visual field. *See also* PERIMETER.

scotopic *adj.* relating to or describing conditions of poor illumination. For example, **scotopic vision** is vision in dim light in which the *rods of the retina are involved (*see* DARK ADAPTATION).

screening test a test carried out on a large number of apparently healthy people to separate those who may have a specified disease and could benefit from further testing from those who probably do not. Examples include newborn blood spot screening, cervical screening, and breast screening. The appropriateness of screening depends on the severity and *epidemiology of the disease and the efficacy and availability of treatment. Other factors to be taken into account are the safety, acceptability, cost, *sensitivity, and specificity of the test. No screening test is perfect, and all screening is associated with *false positives and *false negatives. *See also* GENETIC SCREENING.

scrofula *n.* *tuberculosis of lymph nodes, usually those in the neck, causing the formation of abscesses. Untreated, these burst through the skin and form running sores, which leave scars when they heal. Treatment with antituberculous drugs is effective. The disease, which is now rare in the developed world, most commonly affects young children. —**scrofulous** *adj.*

scrofuloderma *n.* tuberculosis of the skin in which the skin breaks down over suppurating tuberculous glands, with the formation of irregular-shaped ulcers with blue-tinged edges. Treatment is with antituberculous drugs, to which scrofuloderma responds better than *lupus vulgaris, another type of skin tuberculosis.

scrototomy *n.* an operation in which the scrotum is surgically explored, usually undertaken to investigate patients with probable obstructive *azoospermia.

scrotum *n.* the paired sac that holds the testes and epididymides outside the abdominal cavity. Its function is to allow the production and storage of spermatozoa to occur at a lower temperature than that of the abdomen. Further temperature control is achieved by contraction or relaxation of muscles in the scrotum. —**scrotal** *adj.*

scrub typhus (tsutsugamushi disease) a disease, widely distributed in SE Asia, caused by the parasitic bacterium *Rickettsia tsutsugamushi* and transmitted to humans through the bite of mites. Only larval mites of the genus *Trombicula* are involved as vectors. Symptoms include headache, chills, high temperature (104°F), a red rash over most of the body, a cough, and delirium. A small ulcer forms at the site of the bite. Scrub typhus is treated with tetracycline and other broad-spectrum antibiotics. *See also* RICKETTSIAE, TYPHUS.

scrum-pox *n.* a form of *herpes simplex found in rugby players and wrestlers. It is caused by abrasive contact.

scruple *n.* a unit of weight used in pharmacy. 1 scruple = 1.295 g (20 grains). 3 scruples = 1 drachm.

scurvy *n.* a disease that is caused by a deficiency of *vitamin C (ascorbic acid). It results from a lack of fresh fruit and vegetables in the diet (unlike most animals, humans

cannot synthesize ascorbic acid and must obtain it from food). The first sign of scurvy is swollen bleeding gums, and a rash of tiny bleeding spots around the hair follicles is characteristic. This may be followed by subcutaneous bleeding and the opening of previously healed wounds. Vitamin C is used in treatment and for prevention of scurvy in those at risk (mainly the elderly).

seasickness *n. see* MOTION SICKNESS.

seasonal affective disorder *see* SAD.

seat-belt syndrome thoracic injuries that arise from violent contact with a restraining seat belt in motor vehicle accidents occurring at high speeds.

sebaceous cyst 1. a pale or flesh-coloured dome-shaped cyst that commonly occurs in adults, especially on the face, neck, or trunk. It is firm, with a central dot, and contains keratin, not sebum; such cysts are therefore more correctly referred to as **epidermoid cysts**. They are usually removed surgically. 2. a cyst of the sebaceous glands occurring in multiple form in a rare inherited condition, **steatocystoma multiplex**.

sebaceous gland any of the simple or branched glands in the *skin that secrete an oily substance, *sebum. They open into hair follicles and their secretion is produced by the disintegration of their cells. Some parts of the skin have many sebaceous glands, others few. Activity varies with age: the glands are most active at puberty.

seborrhoea *n.* excessive secretion of sebum by the *sebaceous glands. The glands are enlarged, especially on the nose and central face. The condition predisposes to acne and is common at puberty, usually lasting for a few years. Seborrhoea may be associated with a kind of *eczema (seborrhoeic eczema). —**seborrhoeic** *adj.*

sebum *n.* the oily substance secreted by the *sebaceous glands and reaching the skin surface through small ducts that lead into the hair follicles. Sebum provides a thin film of fat over the skin, which slows the evaporation of water; it also has an antibacterial effect.

second *n.* the *SI unit of time, equal to the duration of 9,192,631,770 periods of the radiation corresponding to the transition between two hyperfine levels of the ground state of the caesium-133 atom. This unit is now the basis of all time measurements. Symbol: s.

secondary care health care provided by hospital clinicians for patients whose *primary care was provided by the *general practitioner or other health professional who first assessed, diagnosed, or treated the patient. Secondary care cannot be accessed directly by patients. For example, a general practitioner who assesses a patient with an unusual skin condition may refer the patient to a dermatologist, who then becomes the source of secondary care. *Compare* TERTIARY CARE.

secondary prevention the avoidance or alleviation of disease by early detection and appropriate management. Secondary prevention approaches include population *screening tests that identify disease in asymptomatic people, enabling timely treatment; and *thrombolysis in people who have had a heart attack (*myocardial infarction) or ischaemic *stroke. *See also* PREVENTIVE MEDICINE, PRIMARY PREVENTION, TERTIARY PREVENTION.

secondary sexual characteristics the physical characteristics that develop after puberty as a result of sexual maturation. In boys they include the growth of facial and pubic hair and the breaking of the voice. In girls they include the growth of pubic hair and the development of the breasts.

second messenger an organic molecule that acts within a cell to initiate the response to a signal carried by a chemical messenger (e.g. a hormone) that does not itself enter the cell. Examples of second messengers are *inositol triphosphate and cyclic *AMP.

second-rank symptom *see* SCHNEIDER-IAN FIRST- AND SECOND-RANK SYMPTOMS.

secretin *n.* a hormone secreted from the small intestine (duodenum) when acidified food leaves the stomach. It stimulates the secretion of relatively enzyme-free alkaline juice by the pancreas (*see* PANCREATIC JUICE) and of bile by the liver.

secretion *n.* 1. the process by which a gland isolates constituents of the blood or tissue fluid and chemically alters them to produce a substance that it discharges for use by the body or excretes. The principal methods of secretion – *apocrine, *holocrine, and *merocrine – are illustrated in the

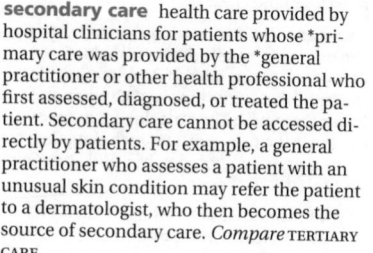

Methods of secretion.

diagram. 2. the substance that is produced by a gland.

secretor *n.* a person in whose saliva and other body fluids are found traces of the water-soluble A, B, or O agglutinogens that determine *blood group.

section 1. *n.* (in surgery) the act of cutting (the cut or division made is also called a section). For example, an **abdominal section** is performed for surgical exploration of the abdomen (*see* LAPAROTOMY). A **transverse section** is a cut made at right angles to a structure's long axis. *See also* CAESAREAN SECTION. 2. *n.* (in imaging) a three-dimensional reconstruction of body scans obtained by computerized tomography or magnetic resonance imaging. These are reconstituted as transverse and sagittal plane sections, less commonly as coronal plane sections. 3. *n.* (in microscopy) a thin slice of the specimen to be examined under a microscope. 4. *vb.* (in psychiatry) to issue an order for the compulsory admission of a patient to a psychiatric hospital for assessment and/or treatment under the appropriate provision or section of the *Mental Health Act 1983 as amended by the Mental Health Act 2007. There are formal procedures, such as review and right to appeal, to ensure this legislation is not abused. A patient who otherwise has capacity may still consent to or refuse treatment for conditions unrelated to the mental disorder for which he or she is detained.

section 30 order (parental order) a court order made under the Human Fertilization and Embryology Act 1990 that enables a married couple to be regarded as the legal parents of a child born to a *surrogate mother commissioned by that couple. Application must be made within six months of the child's birth and the child's home must be with the husband and wife at the time of the application.

section 47 removal a section of the National Assistance Act 1948 that enables a local authority to arrange for the compulsory removal to a place of care of a person who is unwilling to go voluntarily from his or her own home. Individuals who are suffering from a grave chronic disease, or are physically incapacitated, or are living in insanitary conditions because of old age or infirmity can be removed if they are unable to care for themselves and do not receive care and attention from others. A proper officer (*see* PUBLIC HEALTH CONSULTANT) and another registered medical practitioner (usually the patient's general practitioner) must certify that removal is in the interests of the patient or that it would prevent injury to the health of, or serious nuisance to, other people.

security object a particular item that brings comfort and a sense of security to a young child, often for a number of years. Security objects are usually associated in some way with bed and are often made of soft material. A scrap of an old blanket or of a former night garment, a teddy bear, even an old nappy may be chosen as a comforter and these are often pressed to the face as the child settles down to sleep. There is no reason to suppose that security objects are in any way undesirable, at any age.

sedation *n*. the production of a restful state of mind, particularly by the use of drugs (*see* SEDATIVE).

sedative *n*. a drug that has a calming effect, relieving anxiety and tension. Sedatives are *hypnotic drugs administered in lower doses than those needed for sleep (drowsiness is a common side-effect). See also* ANXIOLYTIC.

sedimentation rate the rate at which solid particles sink in a liquid under the influence of gravity. *See also* ESR (ERYTHROCYTE SEDIMENTATION RATE).

see-saw breathing a pattern of breathing seen in complete (or almost complete) airway obstruction. As the patient attempts to breathe, the diaphragm descends, causing the abdomen to lift and the chest to sink. The reverse happens as the diaphragm relaxes. It is almost always associated with use of the *accessory muscles of respiration and drawing in (recession) of the *intercostal muscles of the chest wall.

segment *n*. (in anatomy) a portion of a tissue or organ, usually distinguishable from other portions by lines of demarcation. For example, the uterus consists of **upper** and **lower segments**. The **anterior segment** of the eye is the front portion, including the cornea, anterior chamber, iris, and lens. *See also* SOMITE.

Seidel sign 1. a sickle-shaped *scotoma appearing as an upward or downward extension of the blind spot. 2. a test to confirm leakage of the aqueous humour. *Fluorescein sodium dye is instilled and viewed with cobalt blue light; a bright green flow of liquid is seen at the site of the leakage. [E. Seidel (1882–1948), German ophthalmologist]

Seip-Beradinelli syndrome *see* LIPODYSTROPHY. [M. Seip (20th century), Scandinavian physician; W. Beradinelli (1903–56), Argentinian physician]

Seldinger technique a technique for introducing a catheter into a blood vessel or cavity. A needle is used to puncture the structure, then a *guidewire is passed through the needle. The needle is removed, and the catheter is introduced over the wire. The technique is used in angiography, cardiac catheterization, cannulation of large veins, and drainage of abscesses and other body cavities. [S. I. Seldinger (1921–98), Swedish radiologist]

selective (o)estrogen receptor modulator (SERM) a drug that has oestrogen-like activity in some tissues and an anti-oestrogenic effect in others, depending on the manner of its binding with the oestrogen receptors. *Tamoxifen was the first SERM to be introduced. Because of its activity as an *anti-oestrogen it is used in the treatment of breast cancer, but its oestrogenic activity may cause side-effects. *Raloxifene is used in the treatment of osteoporosis for its oestrogenic effects on bone density.

selective laser trabeculoplasty (SLT) *see* TRABECULOPLASTY.

selective serotonin and noradrenaline reuptake inhibitor *see* SNRI.

selegiline *n*. an *MAO inhibitor that inhibits *monoamine oxidase B and is used in the treatment of Parkinson's disease. Administered by mouth, selegiline is thought to retard the breakdown of *dopamine. Possible side-effects include faintness on standing up, nausea, involuntary movements, and confusion. Trade names: **Eldepryl**, **Zelapar**.

selenium *n.* a *trace element that is an essential component of the enzyme glutathione peroxidase, which catalyses the oxidation of *glutathione by hydrogen peroxide. It thus has important *antioxidant properties. Dietary deficiency of selenium results in *cardiomyopathy. Symbol: Se.

selenium sulphide a selenium compound with antifungal properties, used to treat *dandruff and scalp infections. It is administered in a shampoo. Trade name: **Selsun**.

self-inflating bag a device for delivering emergency artificial ventilation by means of a tight-fitting face mask, a *laryngeal mask, or an endotracheal tube (*see* INTUBATION). It consists of a stiff plastic bag, which is squeezed to deliver its gas contents into the patient's airway; when the pressure is released, it is reinflated from the atmosphere or an attached oxygen supply. Flow into and out of the bag is controlled by a system of simple valves. With an attached oxygen supply, high concentrations of oxygen can be given.

self-limiting *adj.* describing a condition that runs a predicted course and is unaffected by any treatment.

sella turcica a depression in the body of the sphenoid bone that encloses the pituitary gland.

semeiology *n. see* SYMPTOMATOLOGY.

semen (seminal fluid) *n.* the fluid ejaculated from the penis at sexual climax. Each ejaculate may contain 300–500 million spermatozoa suspended in a fluid secreted by the *prostate gland and *seminal vesicles with a small contribution from *Cowper's glands. It contains fructose, which provides the spermatozoa with energy, and *prostaglandins, which affect the muscles of the uterus and may therefore assist transport of the spermatozoa. —**seminal** *adj.*

semi- *prefix denoting* half.

semicircular canals three tubes that form part of the membranous *labyrinth of the ear. They are concerned with balance and each canal registers movement in a different plane. At the base of each canal is a

small swelling (an **ampulla**), which contains a *crista. When the head moves the fluid (endolymph) in the canals presses on the cristae, which register the movement and send nerve impulses to the brain.

semilunar cartilage one of a pair of crescent-shaped cartilages in the knee joint situated between the femur and tibia.

semilunar valve either of the two valves in the heart situated at the origin of the aorta (*see* AORTIC VALVE) and the pulmonary artery (*see* PULMONARY VALVE). Each consists of three flaps (cusps), which maintain the flow of blood in one direction.

seminal analysis analysis of a specimen of semen, which should be obtained after five days of abstinence from coitus, in order to assess male fertility. Normal values are as follows: volume of ejaculate: 2–6.5 ml; liquefaction complete in 30 minutes; sperm concentration: 20–200 million spermatozoa per ml (**sperm count** refers to the total number of spermatozoa in the ejaculate); motility: 60% moving progressively at 30 minutes to 3 hours; abnormal forms: less than 20%. Analysis of three separate specimens is necessary before confirming the presence of an abnormal result.

seminal vesicle either of a pair of male accessory sex glands that open into the vas deferens before it joins the urethra. The seminal vesicles secrete most of the liquid component of *semen.

seminiferous tubule any of the long convoluted tubules that make up the bulk of the *testis.

seminoma *n.* a malignant tumour of the testis, appearing as a swelling, often painless, in the scrotum. It tends to occur in an older age group than the *teratomas. The treatment for localized disease is surgery involving removal of the testis (*see* ORCHIDECTOMY). Secondary tumours in the lungs can be treated with chemotherapy and radiotherapy to the draining lymph nodes. A similar tumour occurs in the ovary (*see* DYSGERMINOMA).

semipermeable membrane a membrane that allows the passage of some molecules but not others. Cell membranes (*see* CELL) are semipermeable. Semipermeable membranes are used clinically in *haemodialysis for patients with kidney failure.

semiprone *adj.* describing the position of

a patient lying face downwards, but with one or both knees flexed to one side so that the body is not lying completely flat. *Compare* PRONE, SUPINE.

Semont liberatory manoeuvre a series of head and body movements used to move microscopic debris from the posterior *semicircular canal in the inner ear. It is used in the treatment of *benign paroxysmal positional vertigo.

SEN *see* SPECIAL EDUCATIONAL NEEDS.

senescence *n.* the process of ageing, which is often marked by a decrease in physical and mental abilities. —**senescent** *adj.*

senile dementia a *dementia of old age.

senior house officer *see* CONSULTANT.

senna *n.* any of various preparations of the dried fruits of certain shrubs of the genus *Cassia*, used as a stimulant *laxative to relieve constipation. It is administered by mouth; side-effects do not usually occur, but severe diarrhoea may follow large doses. Trade name: **Manevac**.

sensation *n.* a feeling: the result of messages from the body's sensory receptors registering in the brain as information about the environment. Messages from *exteroceptors are interpreted as specific sensations – smell, taste, temperature, pain, etc. – in the conscious mind. Messages from *interoceptors, however, rarely reach the consciousness to produce sensation.

sense *n.* one of the faculties by which the qualities of the external environment are appreciated – sight, hearing, smell, taste, or touch.

sense organ a collection of specialized cells (*receptors), connected to the nervous system, that is capable of responding to a particular stimulus from either outside or inside the body. Sense organs can detect light (the eyes), heat, pain, and touch (the skin), smell (the nose), and taste (the taste buds).

sensibility *n.* the ability to be affected by, and respond to, changes in the surroundings (*see* STIMULUS). Sensibility is a characteristic of cells of the nervous system.

sensitive *adj.* possessing the ability to respond to a *stimulus. The cells of the retina, for example, are sensitive to the stimulus of light and respond by sending nerve impulses to the brain. Other *receptors are sensitive to

different specific stimuli, such as pressure or the presence of chemical substances.

sensitivity *n.* 1. (in microbiology) the degree to which a disease-causing organism responds to treatment by *antibiotics or other drugs. 2. (in preventive medicine) a measure of the reliability of a *screening test based on the proportion of people with a specific disease who react positively to the test (the higher the sensitivity the fewer *false negatives). This contrasts with **specificity**, which is the proportion of people free from disease who react negatively to the test (i.e. the higher the specificity the fewer the *false positives). Most screening tests operate such that if the sensitivity is increased the specificity is reduced and the proportion of false positives may rise to unacceptable proportions.

sensitization *n.* 1. alteration of the responsiveness of the body to the presence of foreign substances. In the development of an *allergy, an individual becomes sensitized to a particular allergen and reaches a state of hypersensitivity. The phenomena of sensitization are due to the production of antibodies. 2. (in behaviour therapy) a form of *aversion therapy in which anxiety-producing stimuli are associated with the unwanted behaviour. In **covert sensitization** the behaviour and an unpleasant feeling (such as disgust) are evoked simultaneously by verbal cues.

sensory *adj.* relating to the input division of the nervous system, which carries information from *receptors throughout the body towards the brain and spinal cord.

sensory cortex the region of the *cerebral cortex responsible for receiving incoming information relayed by sensory nerve pathways from all parts of the body. Different areas of cortex correspond to different parts of the body and to the various senses. *Compare* MOTOR CORTEX.

sensory deprivation a major reduction in incoming sensory information. The main input sensory channels are the eyes, ears, skin, and nose. If input from all of these is blocked, there is loss of the sense of reality, distortion of time and imagined space, hallucinations, bizarre thought patterns, and other indications of neurological dysfunction. Even minimal sensory deprivation in early childhood can have a serious effect on the personality.

sensory nerve a nerve that carries information inwards, from an outlying part of the body towards the central nervous system. Different sensory nerves convey information about temperature, pain, touch, taste, etc., to the brain. Compare MOTOR NERVE.

sentinel lymph node the first lymph node to show evidence of metastasis (spread) of a malignant tumour (e.g. breast cancer) via the lymphatic system. Absence of cancer cells in the sentinel node indicates that more distal lymph nodes will also be free of metastasis. In breast cancer, the change in practice to perform axillary lymph node dissection only if the sentinel node contains metastatic tumour has reduced the risk of arm lymphoedema.

separation anxiety a state of distress and fear at the prospect of leaving familiar people (e.g. parents) and secure surroundings, such as is experienced by some children when they first go to school. It may be caused by insecure *attachment.

sepsis *n.* the putrefactive destruction of tissues by disease-causing bacteria or their toxins.

sept- (septi-) *combining form denoting* 1. seven. 2. (septo-) a septum, especially the nasal septum. 3. sepsis.

septal defect a hole in the partition (septum) between the left and right halves of the heart. This abnormal communication is usually congenital due to an abnormality of heart development in the fetus, but can occasionally occur as a complication of *myocardial infarction. It may be found between the two atria (see ATRIAL SEPTAL DEFECT) or between the ventricles (see VENTRICULAR SEPTAL DEFECT). A septal defect permits abnormal circulation of blood from the left side of the heart, where pressures are higher, to the right. This abnormal circulation is called a **shunt** and results in excessive blood flow through the lungs. *Pulmonary hypertension develops and *heart failure may occur with large shunts. A heart *murmur is normally present. Large defects are closed surgically or by using percutaneous catheter techniques (see ATRIAL SEPTAL DEFECT) but small defects do not require treatment.

septic *adj.* relating to or affected with *sepsis.

septicaemia *n.* widespread destruction of tissues due to absorption of disease-causing bacteria or their toxins from the bloodstream. The term is also used loosely for any form of *blood poisoning. Compare PYAEMIA, SAPRAEMIA, TOXAEMIA.

septic arthritis (pyogenic arthritis) infection in a joint. The joint is swollen, hot, and tender, and movement causes severe pain. The infecting organism (usually *Staphylococcus aureus*) can enter the joint via the bloodstream, from an injection or penetrating injury, or by direct spread from an adjacent area of osteomyelitis. The condition is a surgical emergency as it can lead to rapid destruction of articular cartilage, loss of joint function, and septicaemia. Treatment is by *arthrotomy or irrigation of the joint by arthroscopy, with appropriate antibiotic therapy.

septic shock *see* SHOCK.

Septrin *n. see* CO-TRIMOXAZOLE.

septum *n.* (*pl.* **septa**) a partition or dividing wall within an anatomical structure. For example, the **atrioventricular septum** divides the atria of the heart from the ventricles. —**septal** *adj.* —**septate** *adj.*

sequela *n.* (*pl.* **sequelae**) any disorder or pathological condition that results from a preceding disease or accident.

sequestration *n.* 1. the formation of a fragment of dead bone (see SEQUESTRUM) and its separation from the surrounding tissue. 2. (in development) a separated part of an organ; a developmental anomaly.

sequestrectomy *n.* surgical removal of a *sequestrum.

sequestrum *n.* (*pl.* **sequestra**) a portion of dead bone formed in an infected bone in chronic *osteomyelitis. It is surrounded by an envelope (**involucrum**) of sclerotic bone and fibrous tissue and can be seen as a dense area within the bone on X-ray. It can cause irritation and the formation of pus, which may discharge through a *sinus, and is usually surgically removed (**sequestrectomy**).

ser- (sero-) *combining form denoting* 1. serum. 2. serous membrane.

serine *n. see* AMINO ACID.

SERM *see* SELECTIVE (O)ESTROGEN RECEPTOR MODULATOR.

seroconvert *vb.* to produce specific antibodies in response to the presence of an antigen (e.g. a vaccine or a virus). In HIV-positive patients **seroconversion** occurs within about two weeks of the initial infection. It is marked by a sore throat, swollen lymph nodes, fever, aches and pains, and fatigue. *See* AIDS.

serofibrinous *adj.* describing an exudate of serum that contains a high proportion of the protein fibrin.

serology *n.* the study of blood serum and its constituents, particularly their contribution to the protection of the body against disease. *See* AGGLUTINATION, COMPLEMENT FIXATION, PRECIPITIN. —**serological** *adj.*

sero-negative arthritis an arthritis in which rheumatoid factor is not present in the serum. *See also* SPONDYLOARTHROPATHY.

seropus *n.* a mixture of serum and pus, which forms, for example, in infected blisters.

serosa *n. see* SEROUS MEMBRANE.

serositis *n.* inflammation of a *serous membrane, such as the lining of the thoracic cavity (pleura). *See* POLYSEROSITIS.

serotherapy *n.* the use of serum containing known antibodies (*see* ANTISERUM) to treat a patient with an infection or to confer temporary passive *immunity upon a person at special risk. The use of antisera prepared in animals carries its own risks (for example, a patient may become hypersensitive to horse protein); the risk is reduced if the serum is taken from an immune human being.

serotonin (5-hydroxytryptamine) *n.* a compound widely distributed in the tissues, particularly in the blood platelets, intestinal wall, and central nervous system. Serotonin is thought to play a role in inflammation similar to that of *histamine and it is involved in the genesis of a migrainous headache. Drugs that act like serotonin are used in the treatment of migraine (*see* $5HT_1$ AGONIST). It also acts as a *neurotransmitter, and its levels in the brain are believed to have an important influence on mood. Drugs that prolong its effects are used as antidepressants (*see* SNRI, SSRI).

serotype *n.* a category into which material is placed based on its serological activity, particularly in terms of the antigens it contains or the antibodies that may be produced against it. Thus bacteria of the same species may be subdivided into serotypes that pro-

duce slightly different antigens. The serotype of an infective organism is important when treatment or prophylaxis with a vaccine is being considered.

serous *adj.* **1.** relating to or containing serum. **2.** resembling serum or producing a fluid resembling serum.

serous membrane (serosa) a smooth transparent membrane, consisting of *mesothelium and underlying elastic fibrous connective tissue, lining certain large cavities of the body. The *peritoneum of the abdomen, *pleura of the chest, and *pericardium of the heart are all serous membranes. Each consists of two portions: the **parietal** portion lines the walls of the cavity, and the **visceral** portion covers the organs concerned. The two are continuous, forming a closed sac with the organs essentially outside the sac. The inner surface of the sac is moistened by a thin fluid derived from blood serum, which allows frictionless movement of organs within their cavities. *Compare* MUCOUS MEMBRANE.

serpiginous *adj.* describing a creeping or extending skin lesion, especially one with a wavy edge.

serratus *n.* any of several muscles arising from or inserted by a series of processes that resemble the teeth of a saw. An example is the **serratus anterior**, a muscle situated between the ribs and shoulder blade in the upper and lateral parts of the thorax. It is the chief muscle responsible for pushing and punching movements.

Sertoli cells cells found in the walls of the seminiferous tubules of the *testis. Compared with the germ cells they appear large and pale. They anchor and probably nourish the developing germ cells, especially the *spermatids, which become partly embedded within them. A **Sertoli-cell tumour** is a rare testicular tumour causing *feminization. [E. Sertoli (1842–1910), Italian histologist]

sertraline *n.* an antidepressant drug that acts by prolonging the action of the neurotransmitter serotonin (5-hydroxytryptamine) in the brain (*see* SSRI). It is taken by mouth for the treatment of depression and obsessive–compulsive disorder; side-effects may include dizziness, agitation, tremor, nausea, diarrhoea, and drowsiness. Trade name: **Lustral**.

serum (blood serum) *n.* the fluid that separates from clotted blood or blood plasma that is allowed to stand. Serum is essentially similar in composition to *plasma but lacks fibrinogen and other substances that are used in the coagulation process.

serum hepatitis *see* HEPATITIS.

serum sickness a reaction that sometimes occurs 7–12 days after injection of a quantity of foreign antigen and is characterized by the deposition of large immune complexes. Since the complexes are deposited in the arteries, kidneys, and joints, the symptoms are those of vasculitis, nephritis, and arthritis.

sesamoid bone an oval nodule of bone that lies within a tendon and slides over another bony surface. The patella (kneecap) and certain bones in the hand and foot are sesamoid bones.

sessile *adj.* (of a tumour) attached directly by its base without a peduncle (stalk).

seton *n.* a form of treatment in which a thread is passed through a *fistula and tied in a loop. The seton acts as a wick to drain off pus and can be tightened to open the track. This method can be used to treat high anal fistulas because it has a reduced risk of causing incontinence.

severe combined immune deficiency (SCID) a rare disorder that usually manifests itself within the first three months of life by severe bacterial, fungal, and viral infection and *failure to thrive. It is due to reduced numbers of T and B *lymphocytes – white blood cells necessary for fighting infection. Some cases are caused by *adenosine deaminase (ADA) deficiency. The only treatment currently available is a bone-marrow transplant, but *gene therapy offers hope for the future.

Sever's disease *apophysitis caused by pulling at the point of insertion of the Achilles tendon into the calcaneus (heel bone), causing heel pain. [J. W. Sever (20th century), US orthopaedic surgeon]

sevoflurane *n.* a rapid-acting general *anaesthetic administered by inhalation, used for inducing and maintaining anaesthesia during surgery.

sexarche *n.* the age when a person first engages in sexual intercourse.

sex chromatin *chromatin found only in female cells and believed to represent a single X chromosome in a nondividing cell. It can be used to discover the sex of a baby before birth by examination of cells obtained by *amniocentesis or *chorionic villus sampling. There are two main kinds: (1) the **Barr body**, a small object that stains with basic dyes, found on the edge of the nucleus just inside the nuclear membrane; (2) a drumstick-like appendage to the nucleus in neutrophils (a type of white blood cell).

sex chromosome a chromosome that is involved in the determination of the sex of the individual. Women have two *X chromosomes; men have one X chromosome and one *Y chromosome. *Compare* AUTOSOME.

sex hormone any steroid hormone, produced mainly by the ovaries or testes, that is responsible for controlling sexual development and reproductive function. *Oestrogens and *progesterone are the female sex hormones; *androgens are the male sex hormones.

sex-limited *adj.* describing characteristics that are expressed differently in the two sexes but are controlled by genes not on the sex chromosomes, e.g. baldness in men.

sex-linked *adj.* describing genes (or the characteristics controlled by them) that are carried on the sex chromosomes, usually the *X chromosome. The genes for certain disorders, such as *haemophilia, are carried on the X chromosome; these genes and disorders are described as **X-linked**. Since these sex-linked genes are *recessive, men are more likely to have the diseases since they have only one X chromosome; women can carry the genes but their harmful effects are usually masked by the dominant (normal) alleles on their second X chromosome.

sexology *n.* the study of sexual matters, including anatomy, physiology, behaviour, and techniques.

sex ratio the proportion of males to females in a population, usually expressed as the number of males per 100 females. The **primary sex ratio**, at the time of fertilization, is in theory 50% male. The **secondary sex ratio**, found at birth, usually indicates slightly fewer girls than boys.

sex reversal on Y (SRY) *see* Y CHROMOSOME.

sexual abuse *see* CHILD ABUSE, PAEDOPHILIA.

sexual deviation any sexual behaviour regarded as abnormal by society. The deviation may relate to the sexual object (as in *fetishism) or the activity engaged in (for example, sadism and exhibitionism). The activity is sexually pleasurable.

The definition of what is normal varies with different cultures, and treatment is appropriate only when the deviation causes suffering. Some people may find that *counselling helps them to adjust to their deviation. Others may wish for treatment to change the deviation: *aversion therapy may be used, also *conditioning normal sexual fantasies to pleasurable behaviour. The only helpful effect of drugs is to reduce sexual drive generally.

sexually transmitted disease (STD) any disease transmitted by sexual intercourse, formerly known as **venereal disease**. STDs include *AIDS, *syphilis, *gonorrhoea, some *Chlamydia* infections, genital *herpes, and *soft sore. The medical specialty concerned with STDs is **genitourinary medicine**.

SGA *see* SMALL FOR GESTATIONAL AGE.

SGOT (serum glutamic oxaloacetic transaminase) *see* ASPARTATE AMINOTRANSFERASE.

SGPT (serum glutamic pyruvic transaminase) *see* ALANINE AMINOTRANSFERASE.

SHA *see* STRATEGIC HEALTH AUTHORITY.

shaking palsy an archaic name for Parkinson's disease (*see* PARKINSONISM).

shaping *n.* a technique of *behaviour modification used in the teaching of complex skills or in encouraging rare forms of behaviour. At first the therapist rewards actions that are similar to the desired behaviour; thereafter the therapist rewards successively closer approximations, until eventually only the desired behaviour is rewarded and thereby learned.

S-H classification *see* SALTER-HARRIS CLASSIFICATION.

sheath *n.* **1.** (in anatomy) the layer of connective tissue that envelops structures such as nerves, arteries, tendons, and muscles. **2.** a *condom.

Sheehan's syndrome a condition in which *amenorrhoea and infertility follow a major haemorrhage in pregnancy. It is caused by necrosis (death) of the anterior lobe of the pituitary gland as a direct result of the haemorrhage reducing the blood supply to the gland. *Compare* ASHERMAN SYNDROME. [H. L. Sheehan (20th century), British pathologist]

sheltered housing specially converted (or adapted) accommodation, designed to meet the special needs of people who are capable of a degree of self-care. A warden is generally in attendance. The extent to which meals and other services are provided on a continuous basis varies; so too in Britain does the per capita payment from the appropriate social service department.

Sheridan-Gardiner test a test for detecting visual handicap in children who are too young to be able to read the *Snellen chart. A series of cards, each marked with a single letter of a specific size, are held up at a distance of 6 metres from the child being tested. The child is provided with an identification card containing a selection of letters and is asked to point to the letter that is the same as the one on the card in the distance. The test is suitable for children between the ages of two and seven.

Shigella *n.* a genus of nonmotile rodlike Gram-negative bacteria normally present in the intestinal tract of warm-blooded animals. They ferment carbohydrates without the formation of gas. Some *Shigella* species are pathogenic. *S. dysenteriae* is associated with bacillary *dysentery.

shigellosis *n.* an infestation of the digestive system by bacteria of the genus *Shigella*, causing bacillary *dysentery.

shingles *n.* herpes zoster (*see* HERPES).

shock *n.* the condition associated with circulatory collapse, when the arterial blood pressure is too low to maintain an adequate supply of blood to the tissues. The patient has a cold sweaty pallid skin, a weak rapid pulse, irregular breathing, dry mouth, dilated pupils, a decreased level of consciousness, and a reduced flow of urine.

Shock may be due to a decrease in the volume of blood (**hypovolaemic shock**), as occurs after internal or external *haemorrhage, burns, dehydration, or severe vomiting or diarrhoea. It may be caused by reduced activity of the heart (**cardiogenic shock**), as in coronary thrombosis, myocardial infarction, or pulmonary embolism. It may also be due to widespread dilation of the blood vessels so that there is insufficient blood to fill them.

This may be caused by severe sepsis (**septic**, **bacteraemic**, or **toxic shock**), with a resultant systemic inflammatory response associated with *disseminated intravascular coagulation and multiple organ failure. It may also be caused by a severe allergic reaction (**anaphylactic shock**: *see* ANAPHYLAXIS), overdosage with such drugs as opioids or barbiturates, or the emotional shock due to a personal tragedy or disaster (**neurogenic shock**). Sometimes shock may result from a combination of any of these causes, as in *peritonitis. The treatment of shock is determined by the cause.

short-sightedness *n. see* MYOPIA.

short Synacthen test a test used to assess the ability of the adrenal cortex to produce cortisol. Serum cortisol is measured before and then 30 minutes after an intramuscular injection of 250 µg tetracosactide (Synacthen), an analogue of *ACTH. The adrenal glands are considered to be inadequate if there is a low baseline concentration of cortisol or the rise is less than a certain predefined amount.

shoulder *n.* the ball-and-socket joint (*see* ENARTHROSIS) between the glenoid cavity of the *scapula and the upper end (head) of the humerus. It is a common site of dislocation. The joint is surrounded by a capsule closely associated with many tendons: it is the site of many strains and inflammations ('cuff injuries').

shoulder dystocia a difficult birth (*see* DYSTOCIA) in which the anterior or, less commonly, the posterior fetal shoulder impacts on the maternal symphysis or sacral promontory. It is an obstetric emergency and is diagnosed when the shoulders fail to deliver after the fetal head when gentle downward traction has failed. Additional obstetric manoeuvres (e.g. *McRobert's manoeuvre) are required to release the shoulders from below the pubic symphysis. It occurs in approximately 1% of vaginal births. There are well-recognized risk factors, such as diabetes, fetal *macrosomia, and maternal obesity, but it is often difficult to predict. There can be a high *perinatal mortality rate and morbidity associated with the condition, even when it is managed appropriately. The most common fetal injuries are to the brachial plexus, causing an *Erb's palsy or *Klumpke's paralysis, and *hypoxic-ischaemic encephalopathy. Maternal morbidity is also increased, particularly

postpartum haemorrhage and fourth-degree *perineal tears (OASIS).

shoulder girdle (pectoral girdle) the bony structure to which the bones of the upper limbs are attached. It consists of the right and left *scapulas (**shoulder blades**) and clavicles (collar bones).

shunt *n.* a passage connecting two anatomical channels and diverting blood or other fluid (e.g. cerebrospinal fluid) from one to the other. It may occur as a congenital abnormality (as in *septal defects of the heart) or be surgically created. *See also* ANASTOMOSIS.

shunt nephritis nephritis associated with infected indwelling shunts. The infection is usually with staphylococci (*S. epidermidis*) and patients present with anorexia, malaise, arthralgia, and low-grade fever. Purpura, anaemia, and hepatosplenomegaly may be found and urine analysis shows heavy proteinuria, often with a *nephrotic syndrome and haematuria. Treatment usually involves removal of the infected shunt as well as antibiotics.

SIADH *see* SYNDROME OF INAPPROPRIATE SECRETION OF ANTIDIURETIC HORMONE.

sial- (sialo-) *combining form denoting* 1. saliva. 2. a salivary gland.

sialadenitis *n.* inflammation of a salivary gland.

sialagogue *n.* a drug that promotes the secretion of saliva. *Parasympathomimetic drugs have this action.

sialic acid an amino sugar. Sialic acid is a component of some *glycoproteins, *gangliosides, and bacterial cell walls.

sialography *n.* a technique for X-ray examination of the salivary glands. A series of X-ray images is taken after introducing a quantity of radiopaque contrast medium through a cannula into the ducts of the *parotid or *submandibular glands in the mouth. It enables the presence of degenerative disease or stones blocking the ducts to be detected.

sialolith *n.* a stone (calculus) in a salivary gland or duct, most often the duct of the submandibular gland. The flow of saliva is obstructed, causing swelling and intense pain. Treatment is primarily by surgery to remove the stone or the whole gland but in a few cases *lithotripsy is used.

S

sialorrhoea *n. see* PTYALISM.

Siamese twins *see* CONJOINED TWINS.

sib *n. see* SIBLING.

sibilant *adj.* whistling or hissing. The term is applied to certain high-pitched abnormal sounds heard through a stethoscope.

sibling (**sib**) *n.* one of a number of children of the same parents, i.e. a brother or sister.

sibutramine *n.* a drug that acts on the central nervous system to suppress the appetite: it inhibits the reuptake of noradrenaline and serotonin. Sibutramine is used in the treatment of obesity; it is prescribed mainly for those with a *body mass index of 30 or over who have failed to respond to standard weight-reduction measures. It is administered by mouth; side-effects include dry mouth, constipation, and insomnia. Trade name: **Reductil**.

sickle-cell disease (**drepanocytosis**) a hereditary blood disease that mainly affects people of African ancestry but also occurs in the Mediterranean region and reaches high frequencies in parts of Saudi Arabia and India. It occurs when the sickle-cell gene has been inherited from both parents and is characterized by the production of an abnormal type of *haemoglobin – **sickle-cell haemoglobin** (**Hbs**) – which precipitates in the red cells when the blood is deprived of oxygen, forming crystals that distort the cells into the characteristic sickle shape: this process is known as **sickling**. An excess of sickle cells in the circulation results in blockage of small blood vessels, producing episodes of severe pain (a **sickle-cell crisis**). Sickle cells are rapidly removed from the circulation, leading to anaemia and jaundice. There is no satisfactory treatment; the highest mortality is in childhood but some patients may live to an age of 60–70 years.

The carrier condition (**sickle-cell trait**) occurs when the defective gene is inherited from only one parent. It generally causes no symptoms but confers some protection from malaria, which accounts for the high frequency of the gene in malarious areas. If a general anaesthetic is to be given to a patient with this condition, the anaesthetist should be alerted.

sickle-cell nephropathy progressive renal disease developing in 5–8% of patients with *sickle-cell disease. Infarcts in the cortex can occur with sickle-cell crises and present with pain and haematuria. Acute or more insidious damage to the medulla will lead to a urinary concentrating defect and later to papillary necrosis and/or fibrosis. Occlusion of vessels within the glomerular capillary tuft leads to a secondary form of *focal segmental glomerulosclerosis and can present with the *nephrotic syndrome.

side-effect *n.* an effect produced by a drug in addition to its desired therapeutic effects. **Adverse effects** are often undesirable and may be harmful.

sidero- *combining form denoting* iron.

sideroblast *n.* a red blood cell precursor (*see* ERYTHROBLAST) in which iron-containing granules can be demonstrated by suitable staining techniques. Sideroblasts may be seen in normal individuals and are absent in iron deficiency. A certain type of anaemia (**sideroblastic anaemia**) is characterized by the presence of abnormal **ringed sideroblasts**. —**sideroblastic** *adj.*

siderocyte *n.* a red blood cell in which granules of iron-containing protein (**Pappenheimer bodies**) can be demonstrated by suitable staining techniques. These granules are normally removed by the spleen and siderocytes are characteristically seen when the spleen is absent.

sideropenia *n.* iron deficiency. This may result from dietary inadequacy; increased requirement of iron by the body, as in pregnancy or childhood; or increased loss of iron from the body, usually due to chronic bleeding. The most important manifestation of iron deficiency is *anaemia, which is readily corrected by iron therapy.

siderosis *n.* the deposition of iron oxide dust in the lungs, occurring in silver finishers, arc welders, and haematite miners. Iron oxide itself is inert, but pulmonary *fibrosis may develop if fibrogenic dusts such as silica are also inhaled.

SIDS *see* SUDDEN INFANT DEATH SYNDROME.

siemens *n.* the *SI unit of electrical conductance, equal to the conductance between two points on a conductor when a potential difference of 1 volt between these points causes a current of 1 ampere to flow between them. Symbol: S.

sievert *n.* the *SI unit of dose equivalent, being the dose equivalent when the absorbed dose of ionizing radiation multiplied by the stipulated dimensionless factors is 1 J kg^{-1}. As different types of radiation cause different effects in biological tissue a weighted absorbed dose, called the dose equivalent, is used in which the absorbed dose is modified by multiplying it by dimensionless factors stipulated by the International Commission on Radiological Protection. The sievert has replaced the *rem. Symbol: Sv.

sigmoid- *combining form denoting* the sigmoid colon. Example: **sigmoidotomy** (incision into).

sigmoid colon (sigmoid flexure) the S-shaped terminal part of the descending *colon, which leads to the rectum.

sigmoid colectomy (sigmoidectomy) removal of the sigmoid colon by surgery. It is performed for tumours, severe *diverticular disease, or for an abnormally long sigmoid colon that has become twisted (*see* VOLVULUS).

sigmoidoscope *n. see* SIGMOIDOSCOPY.

sigmoidoscopy *n.* an examination of the rectum and sigmoid colon with a device (**sigmoidoscope**) inserted through the anus. There are two main types of sigmoidoscopy. **Rigid sigmoidoscopy** utilizes a rigid sigmoidoscope, approximately 30 cm in length, to assess anorectal disease. The second type is **flexible sigmoidoscopy**, which is more commonly used and utilizes a flexible endoscope to assess the rectum, sigmoid, and the left side of the colon. It can be used to identify the causes of diarrhoea and rectal bleeding, such as colitis or cancer.

sign *n.* an indication of a particular disorder that is detected by a physician while examining a patient but is not apparent to the patient. *Compare* SYMPTOM.

significance *n.* (in statistics) a relationship between two groups of observations indicating that the difference between them is unlikely to have occurred by chance alone. An assumption is made that there is no difference between the two populations from which the two groups come (**null hypothesis**). This is tested, and a calculation indicating that there is a **probability** of less than 5% (**P value** <0.05) that the difference observed occurred by chance is categorized as **statistically significant** and the null hypothesis is rejected. Some tests are **parametric**, based on the assumption that the range of

observations are distributed by chance in a **normal** or **Gaussian distribution**, where 95% of observations lie within two *standard deviations of the *mean (**Student's t test** to compare means). Nonparametric tests (**Mann-Whitney U tests**) make no assumptions about distribution patterns. *See also* FREQUENCY DISTRIBUTION, STANDARD ERROR.

sign language (signed language) a form of communication that uses movements of the hands and other parts of the body together with facial expressions instead of sound. There are many different forms of sign language throughout the world. British Sign Language (BSL) is the form most commonly used in Great Britain. In Northern Ireland, Northern Irish Sign Language (NISL), BSL, and Irish Sign Language (ISL; the most common form in Ireland) are all used.

sign of Dance (Dance's sign, signe de Dance) a feeling of emptiness on palpation of the right lower quadrant of the abdomen, which is thought to be characteristic of *intussusception. [J. B. H. Dance (1797–1832), French physician]

sildenafil *n.* a drug administered orally for the treatment of erectile dysfunction. By inhibiting the action of the enzyme phosphodiesterase type 5, it elevates local *nitric oxide levels, causing smooth muscle relaxation and increased blood flow to the corpus cavernosum of the penis, which results in erection during sexual stimulation. Sildenafil is also licensed for the treatment of pulmonary hypertension. Side-effects include headache, facial flushing, dyspepsia, nasal congestion, and dizziness. Because of severe adverse reactions, the drug is contraindicated in patients taking nitrate-based drugs, such as *glyceryl trinitrate. **Tadalafil** (Cialis) and **vardenafil** (Levitra) are drugs with similar actions and effects. Trade names: **Revatio, Viagra**.

silicosis *n.* a lung disease – a form of *pneumoconiosis – produced by inhaling silica dust particles. It affects workers in hard-rock mining and tunnelling, quarrying, stone dressing, sand blasting, and boiler scaling. Silica stimulates *fibrosis of lung tissue, which produces progressive breathlessness and considerably increased susceptibility to tuberculosis.

silver nitrate a salt of silver with *astringent, *caustic, and *disinfectant properties. Available as a stick, it is used to destroy

S

warts. Application discolours the skin bluish-black. Trade name: **AVOCA.**

Silver-Russell syndrome *see* RUSSELL-SILVER SYNDROME.

simeticone (activated dimeticone) *n.* a silicone-based material with antifoaming properties, used in the treatment of infantile colic and also incorporated into antacid remedies. Trade names: **Dentinox, Infacol**.

Simmonds disease loss of sexual function, loss of weight, and other features of failure of the pituitary gland (*hypopituitarism) caused by trauma or tumours or occurring in women after childbirth complicated by bleeding (postpartum haemorrhage). [M. Simmonds (1885–1925), German physician]

Sims's position the left-sided knees-up position commonly assumed by patients undergoing examinations of the anus and rectum or vagina. [J. M. Sims (1813–83), US gynaecologist]

simulator *n.* an X-ray device used in radiotherapy to localize accurately the exact position of the radiation fields before treatment begins.

Simulium *n. see* BLACK FLY.

simvastatin *n.* a drug used to reduce abnormally high levels of cholesterol in the blood (*see* STATIN). Its actions and side-effects are similar to those of *atorvastatin. Trade name: **Zocor.**

Sinemet *n. see* LEVODOPA.

sinew *n.* a tendon.

singer's nodule a pearly white nodule that may develop on the vocal folds of people who use their voice excessively or in those with poor vocal technique.

single photon emission computed tomography *see* SPECT SCANNING.

singular nerve a small subdivision of the *vestibular nerve that carries information from the posterior *semicircular canal to the brain. **Singular neurectomy** is a surgical procedure to divide the singular nerve, occasionally used in the treatment of *benign paroxysmal positional vertigo.

singultus *n. see* HICCUP.

sinistr- (sinistro-) *combining form denoting* left or the left side.

sino- (sinu-) *combining form denoting* **1.** a sinus. **2.** the sinus venosus.

sinoatrial node (SA node) the pacemaker of the heart: a microscopic area of specialized cardiac muscle located in the upper wall of the right atrium near the entry of the vena cava. Fibres of the SA node are self-excitatory, contracting rhythmically at around 70 times per minute. Following each contraction, the impulse spreads throughout the atrial muscle and into fibres connecting the SA node with the *atrioventricular node. The SA node is supplied by fibres of the autonomic nervous system; impulses arriving at the node accelerate or decrease the heart rate.

sinus *n.* **1.** an air cavity within a bone, especially any of the cavities within the bones of the face or skull (*see* PARANASAL SINUSES). **2.** any wide channel containing blood, usually venous blood. **Venous sinuses** occur, for example, in the dura mater and drain blood from the brain. **3.** a pocket or bulge in a tubular organ, especially a blood vessel; for example, the *carotid sinus. **4. (sinus tract)** an infected blind-ending epithelium-lined tract leading from a focus of infection to the surface of the skin or a hollow organ. *See* PILONIDAL SINUS.

sinus arrhythmia a normal variation in the heart rate, which accelerates slightly on inspiration and slows on expiration. It is common in young fit individuals.

sinusitis *n.* inflammation of one or more of the mucous-membrane-lined air spaces in the facial bones that communicate with the nose (the paranasal sinuses). It is often associated with inflammation of the nasal lining (*rhinitis) and may be acute or chronic (*see* RHINOSINUSITIS). Symptoms may include pain, purulent discharge from the nose, nasal obstruction, and disturbances of the sense of smell. Many cases are self-limiting. Others require treatment with antibiotics, decongestants, or steroid nose drops. A few cases need surgery, such as sinus washouts, *antrostomy, or functional *endoscopic sinus surgery (FESS).

sinusoid *n.* a small blood vessel found in certain organs, such as the adrenal gland and liver. Large numbers of sinusoids occur in the liver. They receive oxygen-rich blood from the hepatic artery and nutrients from the intestines via the portal vein. Oxygen and nutrients diffuse through the capillary walls into the liver cells. The sinusoids are drained by the hepatic veins. *See also* PORTAL SYSTEM.

sinus rhythm a normal heart rhythm, usually as recorded on an electrocardiogram. The *sinoatrial node, located in the right atrium, normally functions as the natural pacemaker for the heart.

sinus venosus a chamber of the embryonic heart that receives blood from several veins. In the adult heart it becomes part of the right atrium.

siphonage *n.* the transfer of liquid from one container to another by means of a bent tube. The procedure is used in gastric *lavage, when the stomach is filled with water through a funnel and rubber tube, and the tube is then bent downwards to act as a siphon and empty the stomach of its contents.

Siphunculina *n.* a genus of flies. *S. funicola*, the eye fly of India, feeds on the secretions of the tear glands and in landing on or near the eyes contributes to the spread of *conjunctivitis.

Sipple's syndrome *see* MENS. [J. H. Sipple (1930–), US physician]

sirenomelia (mermaid syndrome, symmelia, sympodia) *n.* a rare and fatal developmental abnormality in which the legs are fused, the kidneys fail to develop, and the sacrum, bladder, and rectum are absent.

sirolimus (rapamycin) *n.* an immunosuppressant drug used to prevent rejection in kidney transplantation. Sirolimus was first discovered as a product of the bacterium *Streptomyces hygroscopicus* in a soil sample from Rapa Nui (the Polynesian name for Easter Island), hence the alternative name. Administered by mouth, it blocks the activation of B and T lymphocytes by *interleukin 2 (IL-2). Trade name: **Rapamune**.

Sister Mary Joseph nodule a metastatic tumour nodule in the umbilicus that originates from a tumour in the pelvis or abdomen, particularly ovarian and stomach cancer. [Sister Mary Joseph Dempsey (1856–1939), US nurse]

sito- *combining form denoting* food.

sitz bath a hip bath in which the person is seated so that water or saline solution soaks only the hips and buttocks. Sitz baths are used to treat haemorrhoids and anal fissures (among other conditions).

SI units (Système International d'Unités) the internationally agreed system of units now in use for all scientific purposes. Based on the metre-kilogram-second system, SI units have seven base units and two supplementary units. Measurements of all other physical quantities are expressed in derived units, consisting of two or more base units. Tables 1.1 and 1.2 (Appendix) list the base units and the derived units having special names; all these units are defined in the dictionary.

Decimal multiples of SI units are expressed using specified prefixes; where possible a prefix representing 10 raised to a power that is a multiple of three should be used. Prefixes are listed in Table 1.3 (Appendix).

Sjögren's syndrome an autoimmune condition affecting the salivary and lacrimal glands, resulting in a *dry mouth and dryness of the eyes. In the systemic form of the disease other glands may be affected, causing dryness of the airways, vagina, or skin, as well as the joints (producing a relatively mild form of arthritis) and muscles (which ache), and there may be tiredness and lethargy. Sjögren's syndrome may also occur secondarily to other conditions (e.g. rheumatoid arthritis). Symptomatic treatment, including saliva and tear substitutes, is available. Patients are susceptible to dental caries, and preventive measures are important. [H. S. C. Sjögren (1899–1986), Swedish ophthalmologist]

skatole (methyl indole) *n.* a derivative of the amino acid tryptophan, excreted in the urine and faeces.

skeletal muscle *see* STRIATED MUSCLE.

skeleton *n.* the rigid framework of connected *bones that gives form to the body, protects and supports its soft organs and tissues, and provides attachments for muscles and a system of levers essential for locomotion. The 206 named bones of the body are organized into the **axial skeleton** (of the head and trunk) and the **appendicular skeleton** (of the limbs). See illustration overleaf. —**skeletal** *adj.*

skew deviation a neurological condition of the eyes in which one eye turns down while the other turns up. It is seen in disorders of the *cerebellum or *brainstem.

skia- *combining form denoting* shadow.

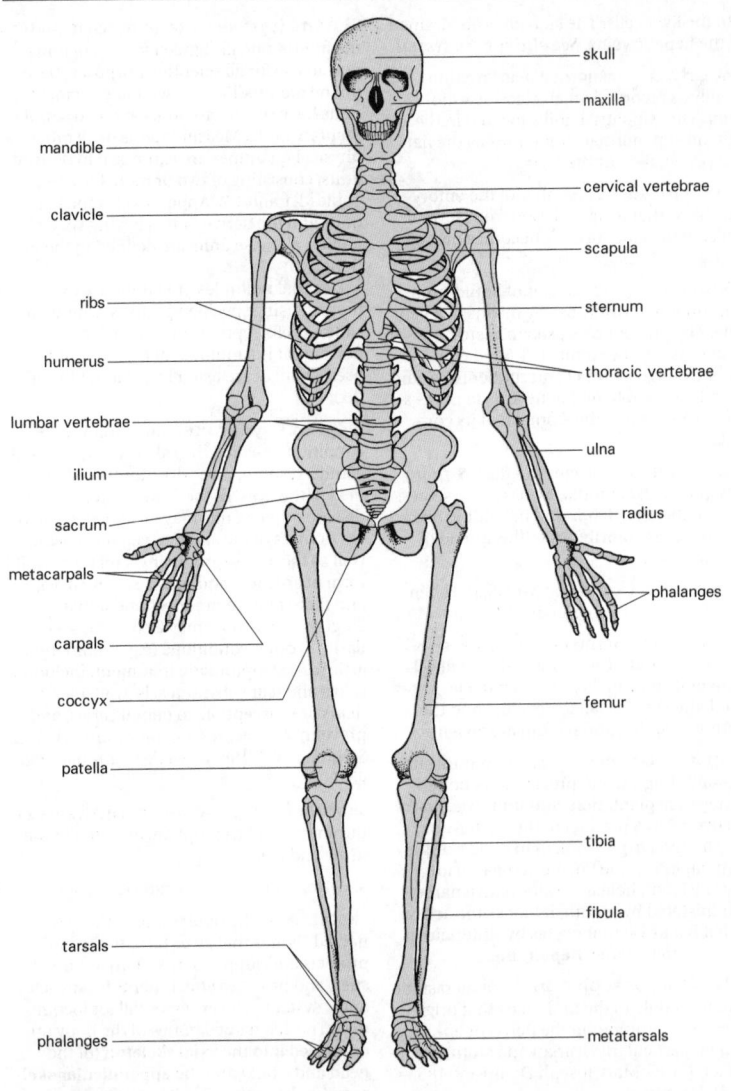

The skeleton.

skier's thumb (gamekeeper's thumb) an injury to the ulnar collateral ligament of the thumb, caused by forced abduction across the metacarpophalangeal joint, at the base of the thumb. Treatment is by splintage or, in the case of severe injuries, by surgical repair of the torn ligament ends.

skin *n.* the outer covering of the body, consisting of an outer layer, the *epidermis, and an inner layer, the *dermis (see illustration).

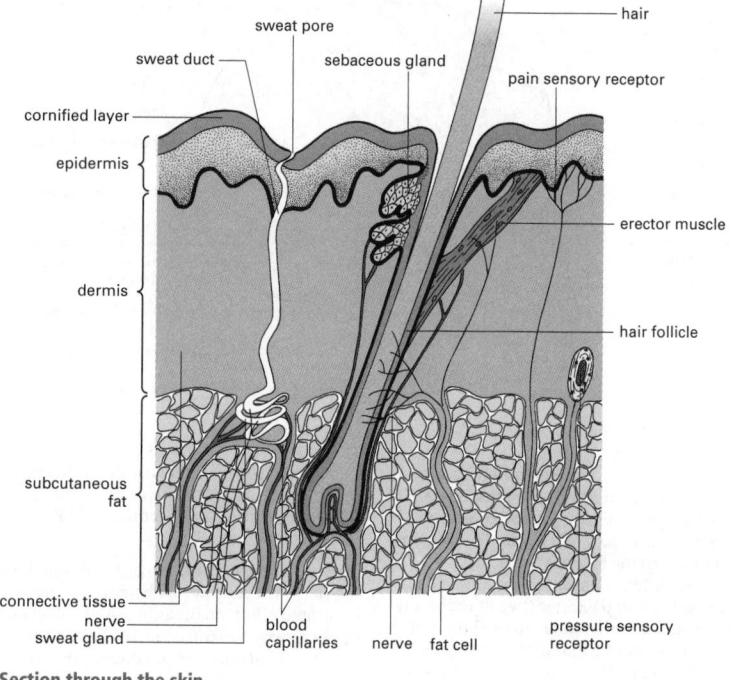

cornified layer
epidermis
dermis
subcutaneous fat
connective tissue
nerve
sweat gland

sweat pore
sweat duct
sebaceous gland
hair
pain sensory receptor
erector muscle
hair follicle
blood capillaries
nerve
fat cell
pressure sensory receptor

Section through the skin.

Beneath the dermis is a layer of fatty tissue. The skin has several functions. The epidermis protects the body from injury and also from invasion by parasites. It also helps to prevent the body from becoming dehydrated. The combination of erectile hairs, *sweat glands, and blood capillaries in the skin form part of the temperature-regulating mechanism of the body. When the body is too hot, loss of heat is increased by sweating and by the dilation of the capillaries. When the body is too cold the sweat glands are inactive, the capillaries contract, and a layer of air is trapped over the epidermis by the erected hairs. The skin also acts as an organ of excretion (by the secretion of *sweat) and as a sense organ (it contains receptors that are sensitive to heat, cold, touch, and pain). The layer of fat that lies underneath the dermis can act as a reservoir of food and water. Anatomical name: **cutis**.

skin graft a portion of healthy skin cut from one area of the body and used to cover a part that has lost its skin, usually as a result of injury, burns, or operation. A skin graft is normally taken from another part of the body of the same patient (an *autograft), but occasionally skin may be grafted from one person to another as a temporary healing measure (an *allograft). The full thickness of skin may be taken for a graft (see FLAP) or the surgeon may use three-quarters thickness, thin sheets of skin (see SPLIT-SKIN GRAFT), or a pinch skin graft. The type used depends on the condition and size of the damaged area to be treated. The skin graft may be free or attached by a *pedicle.

ski-stick injury a penetrating injury by a ski stick.

skull *n.* the skeleton of the head and face, which is made up of 22 bones. It can be divided into the cranium, which encloses the brain, and the face (including the lower jaw (mandible)). The **cranium** consists of eight bones. The frontal, parietals (two), occipital, and temporals (two) form the vault of the skull (**calvaria**) and are made up of two thin

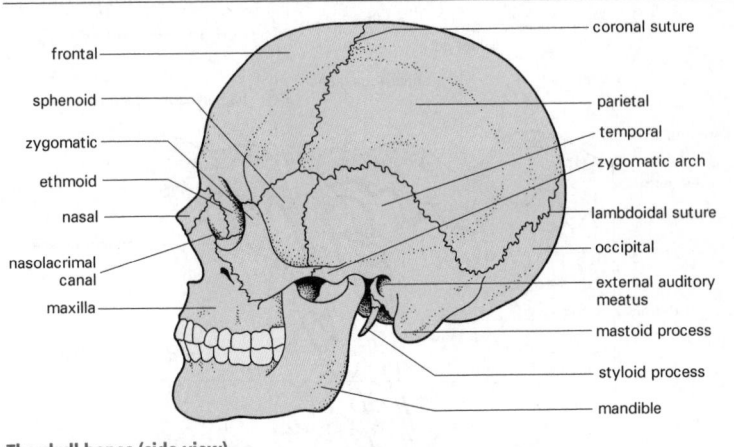

The skull bones (side view).

layers of compact bone separated by a layer of spongy bone (**diploë**). The remaining bones of the cranium – the sphenoid and ethmoid – form part of its base. The 14 bones that make up the face are the nasals, lacrimals, inferior nasal conchae, maxillae, zygomatics, and palatines (two of each), the vomer, and the mandible. All the bones of the skull except the mandible are connected to each other by immovable joints (*see* SUTURE). The skull contains cavities for the eyes (*see* ORBIT) and nose (*see* NASAL CAVITY) and a large opening at its base (**foramen magnum**) through which the spinal cord passes. See illustration.

slapped cheek syndrome *see* ERYTHEMA (INFECTIOSUM).

SLE systemic lupus erythematosus. *See* LUPUS ERYTHEMATOSUS.

sleep *n.* a state of natural unconsciousness, during which the brain's activity is not apparent (apart from the continued maintenance of basic bodily functions, such as breathing) but can be detected by means of an electroencephalogram (EEG). Different stages of sleep are recognized by different EEG wave patterns. Drowsiness is marked by short irregular waves; as sleep deepens the waves become slower, larger, and more irregular. This slow-wave sleep is periodically interrupted by episodes of paradoxical, or *REM (rapid-eye-movement), sleep, when the EEG pattern is similar to that of an awake and alert person. Dreaming occurs during

REM sleep. The two states of sleep alternate in cycles of from 30 to 90 minutes, REM sleep constituting about a quarter of the total sleeping time.

sleep apnoea cessation of breathing during sleep, which may be **obstructive**, due to frustrated efforts to breathe against blocked upper airways (*see* OBSTRUCTIVE SLEEP APNOEA), or **central**, in which there is no evidence of any voluntary effort.

sleep apnoea syndrome (SAS) *see* OBSTRUCTIVE SLEEP APNOEA.

sleeping sickness (African trypanosomiasis) a disease of tropical Africa caused by the presence in the blood of the parasitic protozoans *Trypanosoma gambiense* or *T. rhodesiense*. The parasites are transmitted through the bite of *tsetse flies. Initial symptoms include fever, headache, and chills, followed later by enlargement of the lymph nodes, anaemia, and pains in the limbs and joints. After a period of several months or even years, the parasites invade the minute blood vessels supplying the central nervous system. This causes drowsiness and lethargy, and ultimately – if untreated – the patient dies. Rhodesian sleeping sickness is the more virulent form of the disease. Drugs used to treat the acute stage of the disease include eflornithine, pentamidine, and suramin; melarsoprol (a drug containing arsenic) is used after the brain is affected. Eradication of tsetse flies helps prevent spread of the infection.

sleep paralysis a terrifying inability to move or speak while remaining fully alert. It occurs in up to 60% of patients with *narcolepsy and may occur in other conditions, such as severe anxiety.

sleep-walking *n. see* SOMNAMBULISM.

sling *n.* a bandage arranged to support and rest an injured limb so that healing is not hindered by activity. The most common sling is a *triangular bandage tied behind the neck to support the weight of a broken arm. The arm is bent at the elbow and held across the body.

sling procedure any of a group of surgical procedures for treating stress incontinence in women. *See* COLPOSUSPENSION, PUBOVAGINAL SLING, TENSION-FREE VAGINAL TAPE.

slipped disc a colloquial term for a herniated intervertebral disc (*see* PROLAPSED INTERVERTEBRAL DISC).

slippery slope argument a position assuming that a relatively innocuous or small first step will result in significant consequences (often considered to be negative in effect) that will be difficult, if not impossible, to prevent. Such an approach may assume or overestimate causation between one act and its likely consequences. In medical ethics, a negative chain of consequences is often cited in debates about *euthanasia. *See also* CONSEQUENTIALISM.

slit lamp a device for providing a narrow beam of light, used in conjunction with a special microscope. It can be used to examine minutely the structures within the eye, one layer at a time.

slough *n.* dead tissue, such as skin, that separates from healthy tissue after inflammation or infection.

slow virus one of a group of infective disease agents that resemble *viruses in some of their biological properties but whose physical properties (e.g. sensitivity to radiation) suggest that they may not contain nucleic acid. They are now more commonly known as *prions.

SLT selective laser *trabeculoplasty.

SMA *see* SPINAL MUSCULAR ATROPHY.

small-bowel enema (enteroclysis) a technique for examining the jejunum and ileum by passing a tube through the nose, oesophagus, and stomach into the small bowel and directly injecting barium. It gives excellent detail of the lining of the small bowel but is more uncomfortable than a *small-bowel meal. It is particularly useful for showing small-intestinal diseases, such as coeliac disease and Crohn's disease, as well as strictures, tumours, and obstructions.

small-bowel meal (barium follow-through) a technique for examining the small bowel, often used when small-bowel enema is not tolerated. The patient swallows dilute *barium sulphate suspension and then a series of abdominal radiographs are taken. It is important that barium reaches the caecum for a complete examination. The technique is particularly useful for showing inflammatory bowel disease, particularly *Crohn's disease.

small-cell lung cancer (SCLC) a type of bronchial carcinoma characterized by **small cells** (or **oat cells**), small round or oval cells with darkly staining nuclei and scanty indistinct cytoplasm. Small-cell carcinoma is usually related to smoking and accounts for about one-quarter of bronchial carcinomas; it carries a poor prognosis but can be cured in the early stages by chemotherapy and radiotherapy. *Compare* NON-SMALL-CELL LUNG CANCER.

small for gestational age (SGA) describing a fetus or baby that has failed to reach the size or birth weight expected for its gestational age. This may be because the fetus or baby is constitutionally small or it may be due to *intrauterine growth restriction in the fetus. In the latter case, the perinatal outcome is less favourable.

smallpox *n.* an acute infectious virus disease causing high fever and a rash that scars the skin. It is transmitted chiefly by direct contact with a patient. Symptoms commence 8–18 days after exposure and include headache, backache, high fever, and vomiting. On the third day, as the fever subsides, red spots appear on the face and spread to the trunk and extremities. Over the next 8–9 days all the spots (macules) change to pimples (papules), then to pea-sized blisters that are at first watery (vesicles) but soon become pus-filled (pustules). The fever returns, often causing delirium. On the eleventh or twelfth day the rash and fever abate. Scabs formed by drying out of pustules fall off 7–20 days later, leaving permanent scars. The patient remains infectious until all scabs have been shed. Most patients recover but serious complications, such as nephritis or pneumonia, may develop. Treatment with thiosemicarbazone is effective. An attack usually confers immunity; immunization against smallpox has now totally eradicated the disease. Medical name: **variola**. *See also* ALASTRIM, COWPOX.

smear *n.* a specimen of tissue or other material taken from part of the body and smeared on a microscope slide for examination. *See* CERVICAL SMEAR.

smegma *n.* the secretion of the glands of the foreskin (*prepuce), which accumulates under the foreskin and has a white cheesy appearance. It becomes readily infested by a harmless bacterium that resembles the tubercle bacillus.

Smith's fracture a fracture just above the wrist, across the distal (far) end of the radius, resulting in volar (forward) displacement of the hand and wrist below the fracture. It is the reverse of *Colles' fracture. [R. W. Smith (1807–73), Irish surgeon]

smooth muscle (involuntary muscle) muscle that produces slow long-term contractions of which the individual is unaware. Smooth muscle occurs in hollow organs, such as the stomach, intestine, blood vessels, and bladder. It consists of spindle-shaped cells within a network of connective tissue (see illustration) and is under the control of the autonomic nervous system. *Compare* STRIATED MUSCLE.

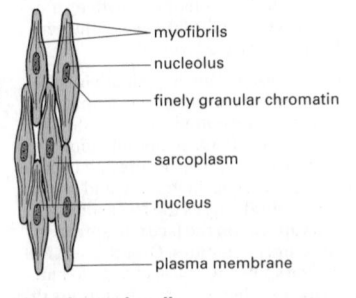

Smooth muscle cells.

snare *n.* an instrument consisting of a wire loop designed to remove polyps, tumours, and other projections of tissue, particularly those occurring in body cavities (see illustration). The loop is used to encircle the base of

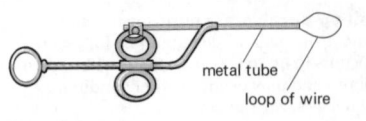

A nasal snare.

the tumour and is then pulled tight. *See also* DIATHERMY.

sneeze 1. *n.* an involuntary violent reflex expulsion of air through the nose and mouth provoked by irritation of the mucous membrane lining the nasal cavity. 2. *vb.* to produce a sneeze.

Snellen chart the commonest chart used for testing sharpness of distant vision (*see* VISUAL ACUITY). It consists of rows of capital letters, called **test types**, the letters of each row becoming smaller down the chart. The large letter at the top is of such a size that it can be read by a person with normal sight from a distance of 60 metres. A normally sighted person can read successive lines of letters from 36, 24, 18, 12, 9, 6, and 5 metres respectively. There is sometimes a line for 4 metres. The subject sits 6 metres from the chart and one eye is tested at a time. If he can only read down as far as the 12-metre line the visual acuity is expressed as 6/12. Normally sighted people can read the 6-metre line, i.e. normal acuity is 6/6, and many people read the 5-metre line with ease. A smaller chart on the same principle is available for testing near vision. In North America the test is done at a distance of 20 feet: 20/20 vision is the same as 6/6. [H. Snellen (1834–1908), Dutch ophthalmologist]

snoring *n.* noisy breathing while asleep due to vibration of the soft palate, uvula, pharyngeal walls, or epiglottis. In children it is often associated with enlargement of the tonsils and adenoids. Treatments of snoring include weight loss, tobacco and alcohol avoidance, adenoidectomy, tonsillectomy, nasal airway surgery, *uvulopalatopharyngoplasty, or other forms of *palatoplasty.

snow blindness a painful disorder of the cornea of the eye due to excessive exposure to ultraviolet light reflected from the snow. Recovery usually follows within 24 hours of covering the eyes.

SNRI (selective serotonin and noradrenaline reuptake inhibitor) any one of a class of *antidepressant drugs that increase the availability of *serotonin and *noradrenaline by blocking the reabsorption of these neurotransmitters by nerve endings in the brain. Side-effects include gastrointestinal disturbances, giddiness, nausea, and sweating. The group includes **venlafaxine** (which is also licensed for the treatment of *generalized anxiety disorder), **duloxetine** (also licensed for treating stress *incontinence in women), and **milnacipran** (also used for treating chronic pain syndromes).

snuffles *n.* 1. partial obstruction of breathing in infants, caused by the common cold. 2. (formerly) discharge through the nostrils associated with necrosis of the nasal bones: seen in infants with congenital syphilis.

social anxiety disorder an extreme fear of humiliating or embarrassing oneself in social situations (e.g. dating, parties, eating with other people, asking questions, etc.). Symptoms include shaking, blushing, gastrointestinal disturbances, sweating, and other signs of anxiety; people with social anxiety disorder may avoid social situations. Treatment includes behavioural therapy and medication (e.g. antidepressants, anxiolytics, or beta blockers).

social class *see* NATIONAL STATISTICS SOCIO-ECONOMIC CLASSIFICATION.

social marketing the application of marketing techniques to achieve behaviour change for a social benefit, for example reduction in *health inequalities.

social medicine *see* PUBLIC HEALTH MEDICINE.

social services advice and practical help with problems associated with social circumstances. Every local authority is responsible for establishing and staffing a social service department. Basic training for social work involves completing an approved degree in social work; there are also social workers with medical and psychiatric training who are seconded for work in hospitals (*see* HOSPITAL SOCIAL WORKER) and specialist social workers in areas such as criminal justice. Social workers assess the eligibility of clients for such social services as care assistants and meals on wheels or refer them to the appropriate statutory or voluntary services; difficulties may sometimes arise when the hospital *catchment area is not coterminous with the local authority. In relation to mental health, social workers may obtain

court orders for *compulsory admission where necessary and provide surveillance and support for those being treated at home or in designated hostel accommodation, including those discharged from hospital. (*See also* AFTERCARE.) **Case work** involves identifying the causes of the client's problem and, where appropriate, advising how best to correct them and/or adapt to the circumstances.

social worker *see* SOCIAL SERVICES.

socio-economic group *see* NATIONAL STATISTICS SOCIO-ECONOMIC CLASSIFICATION.

socket *n.* (in anatomy) a hollow or depression into which another part fits, such as the cavity in the alveolar bone of the jaws into which the root of a tooth fits. *See also* DRY SOCKET.

sodium *n.* a mineral element and an important constituent of the human body (average sodium content of the adult body is 4000 mmol). Sodium controls the volume of extracellular fluid in the body and maintains the acid-base balance. It also helps maintain electrical potentials in the nervous system and is thus necessary for the functioning of nerves and muscles. Sodium is contained in most foods and is well absorbed, the average daily intake in the UK being 200 mmol. The amount of sodium in the body is controlled by the kidneys. An excess of sodium leads to the condition of **hypernatraemia**, which often results in *oedema. This may develop in infants fed on bottled milk, which has a much higher sodium content than human milk. Since babies are less able to remove sodium from the body than adults the feeding of a high-sodium diet to babies is dangerous and may lead to dehydration. Sodium is also implicated in hypertension: a high-sodium diet is thought to increase the risk of hypertension in later life. Symbol: Na.

sodium bicarbonate a salt of sodium that neutralizes acid and is used to treat metabolic acidosis (particularly *renal tubular acidosis) and to reduce the acidity of the urine in mild urinary-tract infections; it is usually administered by mouth. Sodium bicarbonate is also an ingredient of many *antacid preparations and is used in the form of drops to soften earwax.

sodium channel *see* ION CHANNEL.

sodium chloride common salt: a salt of *sodium that is present in all tissues and is important in maintaining the *electrolyte balance of the body. Sodium chloride infusions are the basis of fluid replacement therapy after operations and for conditions associated with salt depletion, including shock and dehydration (*see* SALINE). Sodium chloride is also a basic constituent of *oral rehydration therapy and is used to irrigate the eye (e.g. for intraocular surgery).

sodium cromoglicate *see* CROMOGLICATE.

sodium fluoride a salt of sodium used to prevent tooth decay. It is administered by mouth or applied to the teeth as a paste, mouthwash, or gel. Taken in excess by mouth, it may cause digestive upsets and large doses may cause fluorine poisoning. *See also* FLUORIDATION. Trade names: **Duraphat**, **En-De-Kay**, **Fluor-a-day**, **FluoriGard**.

sodium fusidate an antibiotic used to treat penicillin-resistant infections caused by *Staphylococcus*, including osteomyelitis. It is administered by mouth or intravenous infusion; common side-effects are nausea and vomiting. Trade name: **Fucidin**. *See also* FUSIDIC ACID.

sodium hydroxide (caustic soda) a powerful alkali in widespread use as a cleaning agent. It attacks the skin, causing severe chemical burns that are best treated by washing the area with large quantities of water. When swallowed it causes burning of the mouth and throat, which should be treated by giving water, milk, or other fluid to dilute the stomach contents and by gastric lavage.

sodium hypochlorite a salt of sodium used in solution as a disinfectant. In dentistry a 0.5–5.0% solution is used for washing out, cleaning, and disinfecting infected root canals.

sodium nitrite a sodium salt used, with **sodium thiosulphate**, to treat cyanide poisoning. Both drugs are administered by intravenous injection and may cause headache and flushing.

sodium valproate an *anticonvulsant drug used to treat all types of epilepsy. It is administered by mouth or intravenously; side-effects may include digestive upsets, weight gain, and (rarely) impaired liver function. It should be used with caution in pregnant women because of a risk of abnormalities developing in the fetus. Trade name: **Epilim**.

sodokosis *n. see* RAT-BITE FEVER.

soft sore (chancroid) a sexually transmitted disease caused by the bacterium *Haemophilus ducreyi*, resulting in enlargement and ulceration of lymph nodes in the groin. Treatment with sulphonamides is effective.

solarium *n.* a room in which patients are exposed to either sunlight or artificial sunlight (a blend of visible light and infrared and ultraviolet radiation directed from special lamps).

solar plexus (coeliac plexus) a network of sympathetic nerves and ganglia high in the back of the abdomen.

soleus *n.* a broad flat muscle in the calf of the leg, beneath the *gastrocnemius muscle. The soleus flexes the foot, so that the toes point downwards.

solifenacin *n.* an *antimuscarinic drug administered by mouth to relieve urinary frequency, urgency, and incontinence due to overactivity of the *detrusor muscle of the bladder. It has few side-effects. Trade name: **Vesicare**.

soma *n.* 1. the entire body excluding the germ cells. 2. the body as distinct from the mind.

somat- *combining form denoting* 1. the body. 2. somatic.

somatic *adj.* 1. relating to the nonreproductive parts of the body. A somatic mutation cannot be inherited. 2. relating to the body wall (i.e. excluding the viscera), e.g. somatic *mesoderm. *Compare* SPLANCHNIC. 3. relating to the body rather than the mind.

somatization disorder a psychiatric disorder characterized by multiple physical symptoms in the absence of physical disorders that could explain them. The disorder is chronic and is often accompanied by depression and anxiety. It can disrupt personal and family relationships and lead to unnecessary medical and surgical treatment. It is sometimes treated with *cognitive behavioural therapy, *psychotherapy, and/or *antidepressants.

somatoform disorders a group of disorders in which there is a history of repeated physical complaints with no physical basis. They include *somatization disorder and hypochondriasis (*see* HYPOCHONDRIA). Also included (in DSM-IV but not in ICD-10) is *conversion disorder.

somatomedin *n.* a protein hormone, produced by the liver in response to stimulation by growth hormone, that stimulates protein synthesis and promotes growth. It is biochemically similar to *insulin and has some actions similar to insulin; it is therefore sometimes said to have **insulin-like activity** (**ILA**) or is referred to as **insulin-like growth factor** (**IGF**).

somatopleure *n.* the body wall of the early embryo, which consists of a simple layer of ectoderm lined with mesoderm. The amnion is a continuation of this structure outside the embryo. *Compare* SPLANCHNO-PLEURE.

somatostatin (growth-hormone-release inhibiting hormone) a hormone produced by the hypothalamus and some extraneural tissues, including the gastrointestinal tract and pancreas (*see* ISLETS OF LANGERHANS), that acts to inhibit the secretion of many hormones. For example, in the pituitary gland it inhibits the release of *growth hormone (somatotrophin) and in the pancreas it suppresses secretion of insulin and glucagon. **Somatostatin analogues** are used to treat *acromegaly (caused by overproduction of growth hormone) and to relieve the symptoms caused by hormone-secreting neuroendocrine tumours, including *carcinoid tumours. They include **lanreotide** (Somatuline, also licensed for the treatment of thyroid tumours) and **octreotide** (Sandostatin, also used to reduce vomiting in palliative care and to treat *oesophageal varices), which are administered by injection; gastrointestinal upsets (e.g. nausea, loss of appetite, abdominal pain, diarrhoea) are the most common side-effects.

somatostatinoma *n.* a rare tumour of the *islets of Langerhans that produces excessive amounts of somatostatin. It is an example of an *apudoma. In severe cases it can cause the **somatostatinoma syndrome**, consisting of diabetes, gall-bladder disease, and *steatorrhoea due to malabsorption.

somatotrophin *n. see* GROWTH HORMONE.

somatotype *n. see* BODY TYPE.

somite *n.* any of the paired segmented divisions of *mesoderm that develop along the length of the early embryo. The somites differentiate into voluntary muscle, bones, con-

nective tissue, and the deeper layers of the skin (*see* DERMATOME, MYOTOME, SCLEROTOME).

somnambulism *n.* sleep-walking: walking about and performing other actions in a semiautomatic way during sleep without later memory of doing so. It is common during childhood and may persist into adult life. It can arise spontaneously or as the result of stress or hypnosis; it may also be a side-effect of a hypnotic drug. —**somnambulistic** *adj.*

somnolism *n.* a hypnotic trance. *See* HYP-NOSIS.

somnoplasty *n. see* PALATOPLASTY.

Somogyi effect *see* DAWN PHENOMENON. [M. Somogyi (1883–1971), US biochemist]

sonography *n. see* ULTRASONOGRAPHY.

sonohysterography (saline infusion sonohysterography, SIS) *n.* an ultrasound technique for examining the uterus in which evaluation of the endometrial cavity is augmented by the use of saline, which distends the uterine cavity separating the two layers of endometrium and creating a contrast. This can help identify intracavitary lesions (e.g. submucous *fibroids) and determine the amount of cavity distortion.

sonoplacentography *n. see* PLACENTOG-RAPHY.

soporific *n. see* HYPNOTIC.

sorafenib *n.* a drug used in the management of advanced renal cell carcinoma and liver cancer. It is an inhibitor of multiple kinases (*see* PROTEIN KINASE, TYROSINE KINASE INHIBITOR), preventing the mediation of cell growth and proliferation, and blocks *vascular endothelial growth factor receptors on tumour cells, preventing new vessel formation. It is administered by mouth; side-effects include rash, diarrhoea, and hypertension. Trade name: **Nexavar**.

sorbitol *n.* a carbohydrate with a sweet taste, used as a substitute for cane sugar in foods suitable for diabetics since it is absorbed slowly from the intestine.

sordes *pl. n.* the brownish encrustations that form around the mouth and teeth of patients suffering from fevers.

sore *n.* a lay term for any ulcer or other open wound of the skin or mucous membranes, which may be caused by injury or infection. *See also* PRESSURE SORE, SOFT SORE.

sore throat pain at the back of the mouth, commonly due to bacterial or viral infection of the tonsils (*tonsillitis) or the pharynx (*pharyngitis). If infection persists the lymph nodes in the neck may become tender and enlarged (cervical adenitis).

sotalol *n.* a drug (*see* BETA BLOCKER) used to treat and prevent abnormal heart rhythm (*see* ARRHYTHMIA). It is administered by mouth or injection; side-effects may include digestive upsets, tiredness, and dizziness. Trade names: **Beta-Cardone**, **Sotacor**.

Sotos syndrome (cerebral gigantism) a rare inherited disorder resulting in excessive physical growth during the first 2–3 years of life. It presents in childhood with a characteristic facial appearance, a disproportionately large head, large hands and feet, abnormally widely spaced eyes (ocular *hypertelorism), developmental delay, and tall stature for age. Children with Sotos syndrome tend to be large at birth and taller and heavier, stabilizing after about five years to achieve normal adult height. Most cases occur sporadically, although familial cases have been reported. [J. F. Sotos (1927–), U.S. paediatrician]

souffle *n.* a soft blowing sound heard through the stethoscope, usually produced by blood flowing in vessels.

sound (in surgery) **1.** *n.* a long rodlike instrument, often with a curved end, used to explore body cavities (such as the bladder) or to dilate *strictures in the urethra or other canals. **2.** *vb.* to explore a cavity using a sound.

Soundbridge *n. see* IMPLANTABLE HEARING AID.

Southern blot analysis a technique for identifying a specific form of DNA in cells. The DNA is extracted from the cells and restriction enzymes used to cut it into small fragments. The fragments are separated and a gene *probe known to match the DNA fragment being sought is used. *Compare* NORTHERN BLOT ANALYSIS, WESTERN BLOT ANALYSIS. [E. M. Southern (1938–), US biologist]

Southey's tubes fine-calibre tubes for insertion into subcutaneous tissue to drain excess fluid. They are rarely used in practice today. [R. Southey (1835–99), British physician]

space maintainer an orthodontic appliance that maintains an existing space in the dentition.

Spanish fly the blister beetle, *Lytta vesicatoria*: source of the irritant and toxic chemical compound *cantharidin.

sparganosis *n.* a disease caused by the migration of certain tapeworm larvae (*see* SPARGANUM) in the tissues beneath the skin, between the muscles, and occasionally in the viscera and brain. The larvae, which normally develop in frogs and reptiles, are transferred to humans who eat the uncooked flesh of these animals or drink water contaminated with minute crustaceans infected with the tapeworm larvae. The larvae cause inflammation, swelling, and fibrosis of the tissues. Treatment of the condition, common in the Far East, involves surgical removal of the larvae.

sparganum *n.* the larvae of certain tapeworms, including species of *Diphyllobothrium* and *Spirometra*, which may infect humans (*see* SPARGANOSIS). They are actually *plerocercoids, but the generic name *Sparganum* is sometimes given to them since they fail to develop into adults and definite classification of the species is not possible from the larvae alone.

spasm *n.* a sustained involuntary muscular contraction, which may occur either as part of a generalized disorder, such as a *spastic paralysis, or as a local response to an otherwise unconnected painful condition. **Carpopedal spasm** affects the muscles of the hands and feet and is caused by a reduction in the blood calcium level (often transitory, as in hyperventilation). *See also* MAIN D'ACCOUCHEUR.

spasmo- *combining form denoting* spasm.

spasmodic *adj.* occurring in spasms or resembling a spasm.

spasmolytic *n.* a drug that relieves spasm of smooth muscle. *See also* ANTISPASMODIC.

spasmus nutans a combination of symptoms including a slow nodding movement of the head, *nystagmus (involuntary movements of the eyes), and spasm of the neck muscles. It affects infants and it normally disappears within a year or two.

spasticity *n.* resistance to the passive movement of a limb that is maximal at the beginning of the movement and gives way as more pressure is applied. Also known as **clasp-knife rigidity**, it is a symptom of damage to the *pyramidal system in the brain or spinal cord. It is usually accompanied by weakness in the affected limb (*see* SPASTIC PARALYSIS). *Compare* RIGIDITY.

spastic paralysis weakness of a limb or limbs associated with increased reflex activity. This results in resistance to passive movement of the limb (*see* SPASTICITY). It is caused by disease affecting the nerve fibres of the *pyramidal system, which in health not only initiate movement but also inhibit the stretch reflexes to allow the movements to take place. *See also* CEREBRAL PALSY.

spatula *n.* an instrument with a blunt blade used to spread ointments or plasters and, particularly in dentistry, to mix materials. A flat spatula is used to depress the tongue during examination of the oropharynx.

spatulation *n.* the technique of widening the orifice of an anatomical tube prior to joining it up, which makes the join more secure and less prone to narrowing.

special educational needs (SEN) the requirements of children who have difficulties in learning or in accessing education. Children with SEN can be supported via mainstream schools or may attend a *special school. Children identified as having SEN that cannot be met by a mainstream school should be assessed by their local authority, which may issue a **statement of special educational needs**. This statement describes the child and the additional help needed.

special hospitals hospitals for the care of mentally ill patients who are also dangerous and must therefore be kept securely. There are four in the UK: Broadmoor, Rampton, Ashworth, and Carstairs. Most (but not all) patients are there compulsorily under a hospital order made by a court according to the *Mental Health Act 1983.

specialist registrar (in a hospital) *see* CONSULTANT.

specialized commissioning group (in England) a group working on behalf of a consortium of *primary care trusts to undertake collaborative commissioning of specialized services and *tertiary care. The specialized commissioning groups were established in response to the 2006 Carter review of specialized services. The 35 specialized services are those that are not provided in all local areas, including haemophilia services and specialized mental health services. There are 10 specialized commissioning groups, each covering a population of about five million people and conterminous with the strategic health authorities. A National Specialized Commissioning Group oversees the specialized commissioning groups and undertakes collaborative decision-making and commissioning on behalf of these groups.

special school (in Britain) an education establishment for children with *special educational needs. The identification and assessment of those needing to attend a special school may occur long before school age. Special schools exist for children with different types of need, including physical disability and hearing impairment. Special education for children with severe disabilities may start as early as 2 years.

species *n.* the smallest unit used in the classification of living organisms. Members of the same species are able to interbreed and produce fertile offspring. Similar species are grouped together within one *genus.

specific 1. *n.* a medicine that has properties especially useful for the treatment of a particular disease. **2.** *adj.* (of a disease) caused by a particular microorganism that causes no other disease. **3.** *adj.* of or relating to a species.

specific gravity the ratio, more correctly known as **relative density**, of the density of a substance at 20°C to the density of water at its temperature of maximum density (4°C). Measurement of the specific gravity of urine is one of the tests of renal function.

specificity *n.* (in screening tests) *see* SENSITIVITY.

spectrograph *n.* an instrument (a *spectrometer or *spectroscope) that produces a photographic record (**spectrogram**) of the intensity and wavelength of electromagnetic radiations.

spectrometer *n.* any instrument for measuring the intensity and wavelengths of visible or invisible electromagnetic radiations. *See also* SPECTROSCOPE.

spectrophotometer *n.* an instrument (a spectrometer) for measuring the intensity of the wavelengths of the components of light (visible or ultraviolet).

spectroscope *n.* an instrument used to split up light or other radiation into components of different wavelengths. The simplest spectroscope uses a prism, which splits white light into the rainbow colours of the visible spectrum.

SPECT scanning (single photon emission computing tomography) (in nuclear medicine) a *cross-sectional imaging technique for observing an organ or part of the body using a *gamma camera; images are produced after injecting a radioactive *tracer. The camera is rotated around the patient being scanned. Using a computer reconstruction *algorithm similar to that of a *computerized tomography scanner, multiple 'slices' are made through the area of interest. SPECT scanning is used particularly in cardiac nuclear medicine imaging (*see* MUGA SCAN). It differs from PET scanning in that radioactive decay gives off only a single gamma ray.

specular reflection (in *ultrasonics) the reflection of sound waves from the surface of an internal structure, which can be used to produce a picture of the surface as a sonogram (*see* ULTRASONOGRAPHY). A specular reflection contrasts with vaguer diffuse echoes produced by minor differences in tissue density.

speculum *n.* (*pl.* **specula**) a metal instrument for inserting into and holding open a cavity of the body, such as the vagina, rectum, or nasal orifice, in order that the interior may be examined (see illustration).

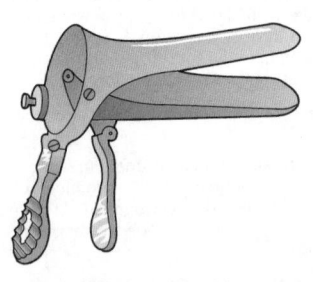

Vaginal speculum (Cusco's).

speech and language therapy the treatment of patients who have problems with communication or eating or drinking because of congenital causes, accidents, or illness (e.g. stroke). Speech and language

therapists are *allied health professionals who have special training in this field.

sperm *n. see* SPERMATOZOON.

sperm- (spermi(o)-, spermo-) *combining form denoting* sperm or semen.

spermat- (spermato-) *combining form denoting* 1. sperm. 2. organs or ducts associated with sperm.

spermatic artery either of two arteries that originate from the abdominal aorta and travel downwards to supply the testes.

spermatic cord the cord, consisting of the *vas deferens, nerves, and blood vessels, that runs from the abdominal cavity to the testicle in the scrotum. The *inguinal canal, through which the spermatic cord passes, becomes closed after the testes have descended.

spermatid *n.* a small cell produced as an intermediate stage in the formation of spermatozoa. Spermatids become embedded in *Sertoli cells in the testis. They are transformed into spermatozoa by the process of spermiogenesis (*see* SPERMATOGENESIS).

spermatocele *n.* a cystic swelling in the scrotum containing sperm. The cyst arises from the epididymis (the duct conveying sperm from the testis) and can be felt as a lump above the testis. Needle *aspiration of the cyst reveals a milky opalescent fluid that contains sperm. Treatment is by surgical removal.

spermatocyte *n.* a cell produced as an intermediate stage in the formation of spermatozoa (*see* SPERMATOGENESIS). Spermatocytes develop from spermatogonia in the walls of the seminiferous tubules of the testis; they are known as either **primary** or **secondary spermatocytes** according to whether they are undergoing the first or second division of meiosis.

spermatogenesis *n.* the process by which mature spermatozoa are produced in the testis (see illustration). *Spermatogonia, in the outermost layer of the seminiferous tubules, multiply throughout reproductive life. Some of them divide by meiosis into *spermatocytes, which produce haploid *spermatids. These are transformed into mature spermatozoa by the process of **spermiogenesis**. The whole process takes 70–80 days.

spermatogonium *n.* (*pl.* **spermatogonia**) a cell produced at an early stage in

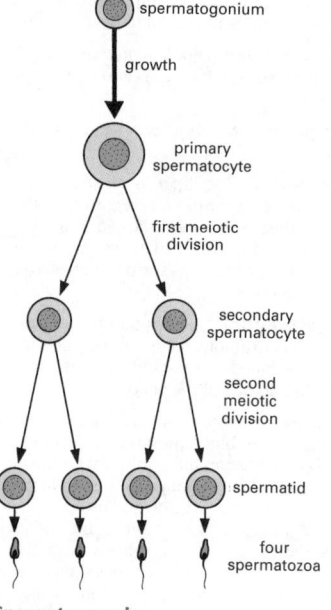

Spermatogenesis.

the formation of spermatozoa (*see* SPERMATO-
GENESIS). Spermatogonia first appear in the
testis of the fetus but do not multiply significantly until after puberty. They act as stem
cells in the walls of the seminiferous tubules,
dividing continuously by mitosis and giving
rise to *spermatocytes.

spermatorrhoea *n.* the involuntary discharge of semen without orgasm. Semen is
usually produced by ejaculation at orgasm
and does not normally discharge at other
times. If, however, the mechanism of ejaculation is lost, spermatorrhoea may occur.

spermatozoon (sperm) *n.* (*pl.* **spermatozoa**) a mature male sex cell (*see* GAMETE).
The tail of a sperm enables it to swim, which
is important as a means for reaching and fer-
tilizing the ovum (although muscular movements of the uterus may assist its journey
from the vagina). *See also* ACROSOME, FERTIL-
IZATION.

spermaturia *n.* the presence of spermatozoa in the urine. Spermatozoa are occasionally seen on microscopic examination of the
urine and their presence is not abnormal. If
present in large numbers, the urine becomes

cloudy, usually towards the end of micturition. Abnormal ejaculation into the bladder
on orgasm (retrograde ejaculation) may
occur after *prostatectomy or other surgical
procedures or in neurological conditions
that destroy the ability of the bladder neck to
close on ejaculation.

sperm bank a facility that collects,
freezes, and stores human sperm for future
use in *artificial insemination (*see* CRYO-
PRESERVATION). Sperm is donated by men
who relinquish legal rights to any future
child, but in the UK donors do not have the
right to remain anonymous. In some cases,
men store their sperm for their own future
use if they are to undergo a medical treatment that might leave them sterile.

sperm count *see* SEMINAL ANALYSIS.

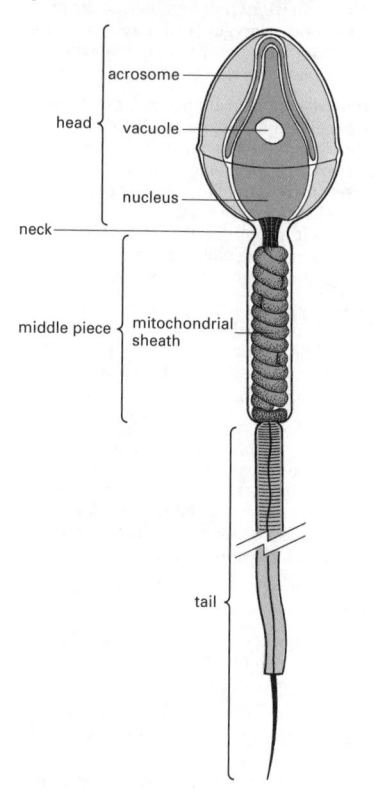

A spermatozoon.

spermicide *n.* an agent that kills spermatozoa. Creams and jellies containing chemical spermicides are used – in conjunction with a *diaphragm – as contraceptives. —**spermicidal** *adj.*

spermiogenesis *n.* the process by which spermatids become mature spermatozoa within the seminiferous tubules of the testis. *See* SPERMATOGENESIS.

spheno- *combining form denoting* the sphenoid bone. Examples: **sphenomaxillary** (relating to the sphenoid and maxillary bones); **sphenopalatine** (relating to the sphenoid bone and palate).

sphenoid bone a bone forming the base of the cranium behind the eyes. It consists of a **body**, containing air spaces continuous with the nasal cavity (*see* PARANASAL SINUSES); two **wings** that form part of the orbits; and two **pterygoid processes** projecting down from the point where the two wings join the body. *See* SKULL.

spherocyte *n.* an abnormal form of red blood cell (*erythrocyte) that is spherical rather than disc-shaped. In blood films spherocytes appear smaller and stain more densely than normal red cells. They are characteristically seen in some forms of haemolytic anaemia. Spherocytes tend to be removed from the blood as they pass through the spleen. *See also* SPHEROCYTOSIS.

spherocytosis *n.* the presence in the blood of abnormally shaped red cells (*spherocytes). Spherocytosis may occur as a hereditary disorder (**hereditary spherocytosis**) or in certain haemolytic *anaemias.

sphincter *n.* a specialized ring of muscle that surrounds an orifice. Contractions of the sphincter partly or completely close the orifice. Sphincters are found, for example, around the anus (**anal sphincter**) and at the opening between the stomach and duodenum (**pyloric sphincter**).

sphincter- *combining form denoting* a sphincter.

sphincterectomy *n.* **1.** the surgical removal of any sphincter muscle. **2.** the complete division of a sphincter.

sphincterotomy *n.* **1.** surgical division, usually partial, of any sphincter muscle. *See also* ANAL FISSURE. **2.** surgical incision of part of the iris in the eye at the border of the pupil.

sphingolipid *n.* a *phospholipid that con-

tains sphingosine. Sphingolipids are found in large amounts in brain and nerve tissue.

sphingosine *n.* a lipid alcohol that is a constituent of sphingolipids and cerebrosides.

sphygmo- *combining form denoting* the pulse.

sphygmocardiograph *n.* an apparatus for producing a continuous record of both the heartbeat and the subsequent pulse in one of the blood vessels. The recording can be shown on a moving tape or on an electronic screen.

sphygmograph *n.* an apparatus for producing a continuous record of the pulse in one of the blood vessels, showing the strength and rate of the beats.

sphygmomanometer *n.* an instrument for measuring *blood pressure in the arteries. It consists of an inflatable cuff connected to a graduated scale gauge calibrated in millimetres of mercury (mmHg). The cuff is applied to a limb (usually the arm) and inflated to exert pressure on a large artery until the blood flow stops. The pressure is then slowly released and, with the aid of a stethoscope to listen to the pulse, it is possible to determine both the systolic and diastolic pressures (which can be read on the scale). Automated electronic devices are increasingly used.

sphygmophone *n.* a device to record the heartbeat or pulse in the form of amplified sound waves played through a loudspeaker or earphones.

sphygmoscope *n.* a device for showing the heartbeat or pulse as a visible signal, especially a continuous wave signal on a cathode-ray tube.

spica *n.* a bandage wound spirally around an injured limb. At each turn it is given a twist so that the slack material is taken up at the overlap.

spicule *n.* a small splinter of bone.

spider naevus a dilated arteriole forming a red papule from which radiate prominent capillaries, so that it resembles a spider. Excessive numbers of spider naevi are a sign of liver cirrhosis, hepatitis, thyrotoxicosis, and rheumatoid arthritis; they are also a feature of normal pregnancy. *See also* TELANGIECTASIS.

spina bifida (**rachischisis**) a developmental defect in which the newborn baby has part of the spinal cord and its coverings exposed through a gap in the backbone. The symptoms may include paralysis of the legs, incontinence, and learning disabilities from the commonly associated brain defect, *hydrocephalus. Spina bifida is associated with an abnormally high level of *alpha-fetoprotein in the amniotic fluid surrounding the embryo. The condition can be diagnosed at about the 16th week of pregnancy by a maternal blood test and confirmed by amniocentesis and ultrasound. The risk of spina bifida is reduced if supplements of *folic acid are taken by women while trying to conceive and during the first three months of pregnancy. *See also* NEURAL TUBE DEFECTS.

(🌐) SEE WEB LINKS

• Website of the Association for Spina Bifida and Hydrocephalus

spina bifida occulta a defect in the bony arch of the spine that (unlike spina bifida) has a normal skin covering; there may be an overlying hairy patch. The condition is usually an incidental finding on X-ray and it is not associated with neurological involvement.

spinal accessory nerve *see* ACCESSORY NERVE.

spinal anaesthesia 1. suppression of sensation, usually in the lower part of the body, by the injection of a local anaesthetic into the *subarachnoid space. A very fine needle is used to reduce the amount of cerebrospinal fluid that escapes as the needle penetrates the dura. The technique has complications (headache, sepsis, paraplegia). The injection site for spinal anaesthetics is most often in the lumbar region of the vertebral column, the needle being inserted between the vertebrae (anywhere between the second and fifth). The extent of the area anaesthetized depends upon the amount and strength of local anaesthetic injected. Dilute local anaesthetic solutions are used when the sensory nerves are targeted rather than the motor nerves. Spinal anaesthesia is useful in patients whose condition makes them unsuitable for a general anaesthetic, perhaps because of chest infection; to reduce the requirements for general anaesthetic drugs; or in circumstances where a skilled anaesthetist is not readily available to administer a general anaesthetic. 2. loss of sensation in part of the body as a result of injury or disease to the spinal cord. The area of the body affected depends upon the site of the lesion: the lower it is in the cord the less the sensory disability.

spinal column *see* BACKBONE.

The spinal cord (transverse section).

spinal cord the portion of the central nervous system enclosed in the vertebral column, consisting of nerve cells and bundles of nerves connecting all parts of the body with the brain. It contains a core of grey matter surrounded by white matter (see illustration p. 687). It is enveloped in three layers of membrane, the *meninges, and extends from the medulla oblongata in the skull to the level of the second lumbar vertebra. From it arise 31 pairs of *spinal nerves.

spinal muscular atrophy (SMA) a hereditary condition in which cells of the spinal cord die and the muscles in the arms and legs become progressively weaker. Eventually the respiratory muscles are affected and death usually results from respiratory infection. Most affected individuals are wheelchair-bound by the age of 20 and few survive beyond the age of 30. The gene responsible has been located: in affected children it is inherited as a double *recessive. There are three forms of the disease, based on severity of the symptoms and the age at which they appear. Type 1 (infantile spinal muscular atrophy) is the most acute and aggressive form of the condition (*see* WERDNIG-HOFFMANN DISEASE). Type 2 develops between the ages of 6 months and 2 years and type 3 (**Kugelberg-Welander disease**), the least severe form, appears between 2 and 17 years of age.

spinal nerves the 31 pairs of nerves that leave the spinal cord and are distributed to the body, passing out from the vertebral canal through the spaces between the arches of the vertebrae (see illustration). Each nerve has two *roots, an anterior, carrying motor nerve fibres, and a posterior, carrying sensory fibres. Immediately after the roots leave the spinal cord they merge to form a mixed spinal nerve on each side.

spinal shock a state of *shock accompanied by temporary paralysis of the lower extremities that results from injury to the spine and is often associated with *ileus. If the spinal cord is transected, permanent motor paralysis persists below the level of spinal-cord division.

spindle *n.* a collection of fibres seen in a cell when it is dividing. The fibres radiate from the two ends (**poles**) and meet at the centre (the **equator**) giving a structure shaped like two cones placed base to base. It plays an important part in chromosome

movement in *mitosis and *meiosis and is also involved in division of the cytoplasm.

spine *n.* 1. a sharp process of a bone. 2. the vertebral column (*see* BACKBONE). —**spinal** *adj.*

spino- *combining form denoting* 1. the spine. 2. the spinal cord.

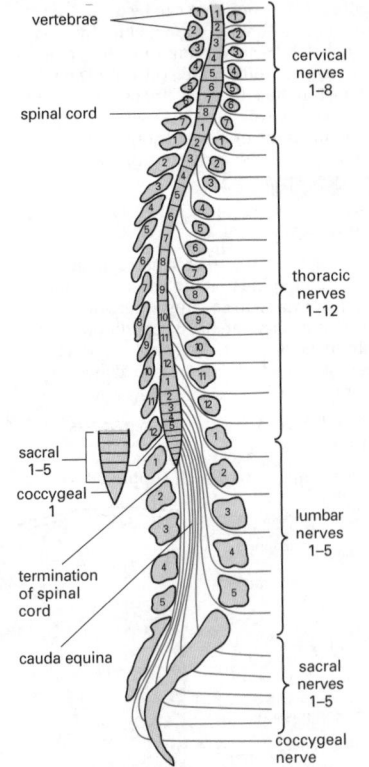

vertebrae

spinal cord

cervical nerves 1–8

thoracic nerves 1–12

sacral 1–5
coccygeal 1

termination of spinal cord

cauda equina

lumbar nerves 1–5

sacral nerves 1–5

coccygeal nerve

The spinal nerves (one side only).

spinocerebellar degeneration any of a group of inherited disorders of the cerebellum and corticospinal tracts in the brain. They are characterized by *spasticity of the limbs and cerebellar *ataxia.

spiral bandage a bandage wound round a part of the body, overlapping the previous section at each turn.

spiral CT scanning (helical CT scanning)

a development of conventional *computerized tomography (CT) scanning in which the X-ray tube rotates continuously around the patient as he or she passes through the scanner. This allows the acquisition of images throughout a specified volume of tissue much more quickly. Since these images are digitally acquired (*see* DIGITIZATION), *postprocessing can produce images in numerous planes, without further exposure of the patient to ionizing radiation. *See also* MULTI-DETECTOR COMPUTERIZED TOMOGRAPHY.

spiral organ *see* ORGAN OF CORTI.

Spirillum *n.* a genus of highly motile rigid spiral-shaped bacteria usually found in fresh and salt water containing organic matter. They bear tufts of flagella at one or both ends of the cell. Most species are saprophytes, but *S. minus* causes *rat-bite fever.

spiro- *combining form denoting* **1.** spiral. **2.** respiration.

spirochaete *n.* any one of a group of spiral-shaped bacteria that lack a rigid cell wall and move by means of muscular flexions of the cell. The group includes the genera *Borrelia*, *Leptospira*, and *Treponema*.

spirograph *n.* an instrument for recording breathing movements. The record (a tracing) obtained is called a **spirogram**. —**spirography** *n.*

spirometer *n.* an instrument for measuring the volume of air inhaled and exhaled. It is used in tests of *ventilation. —**spirometry** *n.*

spironolactone *n.* a synthetic corticosteroid that inhibits the activity of the hormone *aldosterone and is used as a potassium-sparing *diuretic to treat fluid retention (oedema) in cirrhosis, *ascites, and severe heart failure. It is also used in treating aldosteronism. Spironolactone is administered by mouth; side-effects may include headache, stomach upsets, breast enlargement and impotence (in men), and menstrual disturbances (in women). Trade name: **Aldactone**.

Spitz-Holter valve a one-way valve used to drain cerebrospinal fluid in order to control *hydrocephalus. The device is inserted into the ventricles of the brain and passes via a subcutaneous tunnel to drain into either the right atrium or the peritoneum.

splanch- (splanchno-) *combining form denoting* the viscera.

splanchnic *adj.* relating to the viscera, e.g. splanchnic *mesoderm. *Compare* SOMATIC.

splanchnic nerves the series of nerves in the sympathetic system that are distributed to the blood vessels and viscera, passing forwards and downwards from the chain of sympathetic ganglia near the spinal cord to enter the abdomen and branch profusely.

splanchnocranium *n.* the part of the skull that is derived from the *pharyngeal arches, i.e. the mandible (lower jaw).

splanchnopleure *n.* the wall of the embryonic gut, which consists of a layer of endoderm with a layer of mesoderm outside it. The yolk sac is a continuation of this structure. *Compare* SOMATOPLEURE.

spleen *n.* a large dark-red ovoid organ situated on the left side of the body below and behind the stomach. It is enclosed within a fibrous capsule that extends into the spongy interior – the **splenic pulp** – to form a supportive framework. The pulp consists of aggregates of *lymphoid tissue (**white pulp**) within a meshwork of *reticular fibres packed with red blood cells (**red pulp**). The spleen is a major component of the *reticuloendothelial system, producing lymphocytes in the newborn and containing *phagocytes, which remove worn-out red blood cells and other foreign bodies from the bloodstream. It also acts as a reservoir for blood and, in the fetus, as a source of red blood cells. Anatomical name: **lien**. —**splenic** *adj.*

splen- (spleno-) *combining form denoting* the spleen. Example: **splenorenal** (relating to the spleen and kidney).

splenectomy *n.* surgical removal of the spleen. This is sometimes necessary in the emergency treatment of bleeding from a ruptured spleen and in the treatment of some blood diseases. Splenectomy in children may diminish the immune response to infections.

splenitis *n.* inflammation of the spleen. *See also* PERISPLENITIS.

splenium *n.* the thickest part of the *corpus callosum, rounded and protruding backwards over the thalami, the pineal gland, and the midbrain.

splenomegaly *n.* enlargement of the

spleen. It most commonly occurs in *malaria, *schistosomiasis, and other disorders caused by parasites; in infections; in blood disorders, including some forms of anaemia and lack of platelets (*thrombocytopenia); in *leukaemia; and in *Hodgkin's disease. *See also* HYPERSPLENISM.

splenorenal anastomosis a method of treating *portal hypertension by joining the splenic vein to the left renal vein. *Compare* PORTACAVAL ANASTOMOSIS.

splenunculus *n.* a small sphere of splenic tissue occurring at a site other than the spleen. Splenunculi are present in many people.

splint *n.* a rigid appliance (*orthosis) used to support or hold a limb or digit in position until healing has occurred. Splints can be used to treat fractures and dislocations and to assist in the healing of soft-tissue injuries.

splinter haemorrhage a linear haemorrhage below the nails, usually the result of trauma but also occurring in such conditions as subacute bacterial *endocarditis or severe rheumatoid arthritis.

split-skin graft (SSG, Thiersch's graft) a type of skin graft in which thin partial thicknesses of skin are cut in narrow strips or sheets and placed onto the wound area to be healed.

splitting *n.* a *defence mechanism by which people deal with an emotional conflict by viewing some people as all good and others as all bad: they fail to integrate themselves or other people into complex but coherent images. It is common in people with an *emotionally unstable personality disorder.

spondyl- (spondylo-) *combining form denoting* a vertebra or the spine.

spondylitis *n.* inflammation of the synovial joints of the backbone. **Ankylosing spondylitis** is a *sero-negative arthritis; 90% of cases carry the tissue-type antigen HLA-B27 (*see* HLA SYSTEM). Ankylosing spondylitis predominantly affects young adult Caucasian males and the inflammation affects the joint capsules and their attached ligaments and tendons, principally the intervertebral joints and sacroiliac joints (*see* SACROILIITIS). The resultant pain and stiffness are treated by analgesics (including *NSAIDs) and physiotherapy. The disorder can lead to severe deformities of the spine

(*see* KYPHOSIS, ANKYLOSIS) and the hip joint, in which case surgical correction or *arthroplasty may be required.

spondyloarthropathy any *sero-negative arthritis that is characterized by the presence of the tissue-type antigen HLA-B27 (*see* HLA SYSTEM) and the absence of rheumatoid factor. Spondyloarthropathies include ankylosing *spondylitis, *Reiter's syndrome, and *psoriatic arthritis.

spondylolisthesis *n.* a forward shift (slippage) of one vertebra upon another, due to a defect in the bone or in the joints that normally bind them together. This may be congenital or develop after injury. The vertebral displacement is most likely to occur in the lumbar (lower back) or cervical (neck) regions of the backbone. The majority of cases in which pain is present are treated with rest, analgesics, and NSAIDs. In a small minority, showing severe disability, pressure on nerve roots, or slippage of more than 50%, surgical fusion may be required.

spondylolysis *n.* a bony defect in a vertebra between the *lamina and the *transverse process, thought to be due to a *stress fracture and common in gymnasts.

spondylosis *n.* a spinal condition resulting from degeneration and flattening of the intervertebral discs in the cervical, thoracic, or lumbar regions. Symptoms include pain and restriction of movement, and in advanced cases tingling, numbness, and weakness may develop due to pressure on nerve roots. Spondylosis produces a characteristic appearance on X-ray, including narrowing of the space occupied by the disc and the presence of *osteophytes; these features of the disease (**radiological spondylosis**) may not be accompanied by any signs and symptoms. Pain is relieved by analgesics, NSAIDs, and physiotherapy; painful movements are prevented by wearing a neck orthosis (when the neck region is affected) or a lumbosacral corset (for the lower spine). Very severe cases sometimes require surgical fusion.

spondylosyndesis *n.* surgical fusion of the intervertebral joints of the backbone.

spongiform encephalopathy any one of a group of rapidly progressive degenerative neurological diseases that include scrapie in sheep, bovine spongiform encephalopathy (BSE) in cattle, and *kuru, *Creutzfeldt-Jakob disease, and *Gerstmann-Straussler-Scheinker syndrome in humans. In humans the spongiform encephalopathies are characterized by rapidly progressive dementia associated with myoclonic jerks (*see* MYOCLONUS); on pathological examination the brains of affected individuals show a characteristic cystic degeneration. The diseases are thought to be caused by unconventional transmissible agents (*see* PRION).

spongioblast *n.* a type of cell that forms in the early stages of development of the nervous system, giving rise to *astrocytes and *oligodendrocytes.

spontaneous *adj.* arising without apparent cause or outside aid. The term is applied in medicine to certain conditions, such as pathological fractures, that arise in the absence of outside injury; also to recovery from a disease without the aid of specific treatment.

spontaneous intracranial hypotension *see* INTRACRANIAL HYPOTENSION HEADACHE.

sporadic *adj.* describing a disease that occurs only occasionally or in a few isolated places. *Compare* ENDEMIC, EPIDEMIC.

spore *n.* a small reproductive body produced by plants and microorganisms. Some kinds of spores function as dormant stages of the life cycle, enabling the organism to survive adverse conditions. Other spores are the means by which the organism can spread vegetatively. *See also* ENDOSPORE.

sporicide *n.* an agent that kills spores (e.g. bacterial spores). Some disinfectants that liberate chlorine are sporicides, but most other germicides are ineffective since spores are very resistant to chemical action. —**sporicidal** *adj.*

sporocyst *n.* the second-stage larva of a parasitic *fluke, found within the tissues of a freshwater snail. A sporocyst develops from a first stage larva (*see* MIRACIDIUM) and gives rise either to the next larval stage (*see* REDIA) or daughter sporocysts. The latter develop directly into the final larval stage (*see* CERCARIA) without the intermediate redia stage.

sporogony *n.* the formation of *sporozoites during the life cycle of a sporozoan. The contents of the zygote, formed by the fusion of sex cells, divide repeatedly and eventually release a number of sporozoites. *Compare* SCHIZOGONY.

sporotrichosis *n.* a chronic infection of the skin and superficial lymph nodes that is caused by the fungus *Sporothrix schenckii* and results in the formation of abscesses and ulcers. It occurs mainly in the tropics.

Sporozoa *n.* a group of parasitic protozoans that includes *Plasmodium*, the malaria parasite. Most sporozoans do not have cilia or flagella. Sporozoan life cycles are complex and usually involve both sexual and asexual stages. Some sporozoans are parasites of invertebrates, and the parasites are passed to new hosts by means of spores. Sporozoans that parasitize vertebrates are transmitted from host to host by invertebrates, which act as intermediate hosts. For example, the mosquito *Anopheles* is the intermediate host of *Plasmodium*.

sporozoite *n.* one of the many cells formed as a result of *sporogony during the life cyle of a sporozoan. In *Plasmodium* sporozoites are formed by repeated divisions of the contents of the *oocyst inside the body of the mosquito. The released sporozoites ultimately pass into the insect's salivary glands and await transmission to a human host at the next blood meal.

sports injury any injury related to the practice of a sport, often resulting from the overuse and stretching of muscles, tendons, and ligaments.

sports medicine a specialty concerned with the treatment of *sports injuries and measures designed to prevent or minimize them (e.g. in the design of sports equipment).

spotted fever *see* MENINGITIS, ROCKY MOUNTAIN SPOTTED FEVER, TYPHUS.

sprain *n.* injury to a ligament, caused by sudden overstretching. As the ligament is not severed it gradually heals, but this may take several months. Sprains should be treated by cold compresses (ice-packs) at the time of injury, and later by restriction of activity.

Sprengel's deformity a congenital abnormality of the scapula (shoulder blade), which is small and positioned high in the shoulder. It is caused by failure of the normal development and descent of this bone. [O. G. K. Sprengel (1852–1915), German surgeon]

sprue (psilosis) *n.* deficient absorption of food due to disease of the small intestine.

Tropical sprue is seen in people from temperate regions who stay in tropical climates for weeks or months. It is characterized by diarrhoea (usually *steatorrhoea), an inflamed tongue (glossitis), anaemia, and weight loss; the lining of the small intestine is inflamed and atrophied, probably because of infection, but the cause of this condition is not clearly known. Treatment with antibiotics and *folic acid is usually effective, but the condition often improves spontaneously on return to a temperate climate. *See also* COELIAC DISEASE (NONTROPICAL SPRUE), MALABSORPTION.

spud *n.* a blunt needle used for removing foreign bodies embedded in the cornea of the eye.

spur *n.* a sharp projection, especially one of bone.

sputum *n.* material coughed up from the respiratory tract. Its characteristics, including colour, consistency, volume, smell, and the appearance of any solid material within it, often provide important information affecting the diagnosis and management of respiratory disease. Pathological examination of sputum for microorganisms and for abnormal cells may add further information.

squalene *n.* an unsaturated hydrocarbon (a terpene), synthesized in the body, from which *cholesterol is derived.

squama *n.* (*pl.* **squamae**) 1. a thin plate of bone. 2. a scale, such as any of the scales from the cornified layer of the *epidermis.

squamo- *combining form denoting* 1. the squamous portion of the temporal bone. 2. squamous epithelium.

squamous bone *see* TEMPORAL BONE.

squamous cell carcinoma (SCC) any cancer of squamous epithelium, arising from such tissues as the skin and the lining of the upper airways and digestive tract (especially in the head and neck). SCC is the second commonest form of skin cancer (after *basal cell carcinoma), occurring usually in late-middle and old age. Cumulative sun exposure is the commonest cause but other environmental carcinogens may be responsible. SCC is mainly found on areas exposed to light and is three times more common in men than in women. Renal transplant patients are at particularly high risk of this tumour. SCC grows faster than basal cell carcinoma; it spreads locally at first but later

may spread to sites distant from its origin (*see* METASTASIS). Treatment is usually by surgical excision or radiotherapy.

squamous epithelium *see* EPITHELIUM.

squint *n. see* STRABISMUS.

SRY sex reversal on Y. *See* Y CHROMOSOME.

SSG *see* SPLIT-SKIN GRAFT.

SSPE *see* SUBACUTE SCLEROSING PANENCEPHALITIS.

SSRI (selective serotonin reuptake inhibitor) any one of a group of *antidepressant drugs that exert their action by blocking the reabsorption of the neurotransmitter *serotonin by the nerve endings in the brain. Their effect is to prolong the action of serotonin in the brain. As well as depression, SSRIs are used to treat anxiety, generalized anxiety disorder, panic disorder, obsessive–compulsive disorder, post-traumatic stress disorder, and phobias. The group includes *citalopram, **escitalopram** (Cipralex), *fluoxetine, *fluvoxamine, *paroxetine, and *sertraline. Nausea, indigestion, abdominal pain, and other gastrointestinal disturbances are the most common side-effects.

stadium *n.* (*pl.* **stadia**) a stage in the course of a disease; for example, the **stadium invasionis** is the period between exposure to infection and the onset of symptoms.

stage *vb.* (in oncology) to classify a primary tumour by its size and the presence or absence of metastases. In addition to clinical examination, a variety of imaging and surgical techniques may be employed to provide a more accurate assessment. Staging tumours is of importance in prognosis and defining appropriate treatment. *See also* TNM CLASSIFICATION.

staghorn calculus a branched stone forming a cast of the collecting system of the kidney and therefore filling the calyces and pelvis. The stone is usually associated with infected urine, the commonest organism being *Proteus vulgaris*. The combination of obstruction and infection can cause *pyonephrosis and, if neglected, a *perinephric abscess.

stagnant loop syndrome *see* BLIND LOOP SYNDROME.

stain 1. *n.* a dye used to colour tissues and other specimens for microscopical examination. In an **acid stain** the colour is carried by an acid radical and the stain is taken up by parts of the specimen having a basic (alkaline) reaction. In a **basic stain** the colour, carried by a basic radical, is attracted to parts of the specimen having an acidic reaction. **Neutral stains** have neither acidic nor basic affinities. A **contrast stain** is used to give colour to parts of a tissue not affected by a previously applied stain. A **differential stain** allows different elements in a specimen to be distinguished by staining them in different colours. **2.** *vb.* to treat a specimen for microscopical study with a stain.

Stamey procedure an outdated operation devised to cure stress incontinence of urine in women in which specially designed needles are employed to sling or hitch up the neck of the bladder to the anterior abdominal wall with unabsorbable suture material. *See also* COLPOSUSPENSION. [T. A. Stamey, US surgeon]

stammering (stuttering) *n.* halting articulation with interruptions to the normal flow of speech and repetition of the initial consonants of words or syllables. It usually first appears in childhood and the symptoms are most severe when the stammerer is under any psychological stress. It is not a symptom of organic disease and it will usually respond to the re-education of speech by a trained therapist. —**stammerer** *n.*

standard deviation (in statistics) a measure of the scatter of observations about their arithmetic *mean, which is calculated from the square root of the **variance** of the readings in the series. The arithmetic sum of the amounts by which each observation varies from the mean must be zero, but if these variations are squared before being summated, a positive value is obtained: the mean of this value is the variance. In practice a more reliable estimate of variance is obtained by dividing the sum of the squared deviations by one *less* than the total number of observations. *See also* SIGNIFICANCE.

standard error (of a *mean) the extent to which the means of several different samples would vary if they were taken repeatedly from the same population.

standardized mortality ratio (SMR) the ratio of observed mortality rate to expected mortality rate (calculated using indirect standardization), expressed as an integer where 100 represents agreement between observed and expected rates. *See* STANDARDIZED RATES.

standardized rates rates used to summarize the *morbidity or *mortality experience of a population. Age-specific rates and population structures from a study population and a reference or *standard population are used to produce a weighted average. Standardized rates can be used to compare the health experience of populations with different structures. **Direct standardization** requires application of age-specific rates from a study population to a reference population structure (e.g. the European standard population) to produce a (**directly**) **standardized rate**. **Indirect standardization** requires application of age-specific rates from a standard population (e.g. England and Wales) to a study population structure to produce an expected morbidity or mortality rate. *Compare* CRUDE RATE.

standard population a notional population used in standardization (*see* STANDARDIZED RATES). The **European standard population** is a population of two million, with a defined age structure. It is younger than the England population, and has similar age structures for males and females.

St Anthony's fire an old colloquial name for the inflammation of the skin associated with ergot poisoning. *See* ERGOTISM.

stapedectomy *n.* surgical removal of the third ear ossicle (stapes), enabling it to be replaced with a prosthetic bone in the treatment of *otosclerosis. A modification of this procedure involves creating a small hole in the base (footplate) of the stapes using a microdrill or laser, rather than completely removing the stapes. This allows insertion of the prosthesis through the hole and is referred to as **stapedotomy**. Many surgeons consider this procedure to be safer than stapedectomy.

stapes *n.* a stirrup-shaped bone in the middle *ear that articulates with the incus and is attached to the membrane of the fenestra ovalis. *See* OSSICLE.

staphylectomy *n. see* UVULECTOMY.

staphylococcal scalded skin syndrome (Ritter's disease) a potentially serious condition of young infants (and occasionally seen in adults) in which the skin becomes reddened and tender and then peels off, giving the appearance of a scald.

The area of skin loss may be quite extensive and is usually centred on the armpits and groin. The underlying cause is an infection by certain bacteria of the genus *Staphylococcus*. It is contagious and may occur in clusters. Treatment is by antibiotics (usually intravenous), but careful nursing is essential to prevent skin damage.

Staphylococcus *n.* a genus of Gram-positive nonmotile spherical bacteria occurring in grapelike clusters. Some species are saprophytes; others parasites. Many species produce *exotoxins. The species *S. aureus* is commonly present on skin and mucous membranes; it causes boils and internal abscesses. More serious infections caused by staphylococci include pneumonia, bacteraemia, osteomyelitis, and enterocolitis. *See also* MRSA. —**staphylococcal** *adj.*

staphyloma *n.* abnormal bulging of the cornea or sclera (white) of the eye. **Anterior staphyloma** is a bulging scar in the cornea to which a part of the iris is attached. It is usually the site of a healed corneal ulcer that has penetrated right through the cornea; the iris blocks the hole and prevents the further leakage of fluid from the front chamber of the eye. In **ciliary staphyloma** the sclera bulges over the ciliary body as a result of high pressure inside the eyeball. A bulging of the sclera at the back of the eye (**posterior staphyloma**) occurs in some severe cases of short-sightedness.

staphylorrhaphy (palatorrhaphy, uraniscorrhaphy) *n.* surgical suture of a cleft palate.

staple *n.* (in surgery) a piece of metal used to join up pieces of tissue. Staples can be used as an alternative to *sutures for an *anastomosis or to bring together the skin edges of an incision; stapling machines have been produced for this purpose. *See also* ENDOSTAPLER.

starch *n.* the form in which *carbohydrates are stored in many plants and a major constituent of the diet. Starch consists of linked glucose units and occurs in two forms, **α-amylose** and **amylopectin**. In α-amylose the units are in the form of a long unbranched chain; in amylopectin they form a branched chain. The presence of starch can be detected using iodine: α-amylose gives a blue colour with iodine; amylopectin a red colour. Starch is digested by means of the enzyme *amylase. *See also* DEXTRIN.

Starling's law a law stating that, within certain limits, a muscle (including the heart muscle) responds to increased stretching at rest by an increased force of contraction when stimulated. [E. H. Starling (1866–1927), British physiologist]

startle reflex *see* MORO REFLEX.

starvation *n. see* MALNUTRITION.

stasis *n.* stagnation or cessation of flow; for example, of blood or lymph whose flow is obstructed or of the intestinal contents when onward movement (peristalsis) is hindered.

-stasis *combining form denoting* stoppage of a flow of liquid; stagnation. Example: **haemostasis** (of blood).

statementing *n.* the provision by a local authority of a statement of *special educational needs for children attending school who have mental or physical disabilities severe enough to require extra help at school.

static reflex the reflex maintenance of muscular tone for posture.

statin *n.* any one of a class of drugs that inhibit the action of an enzyme involved in the liver's production of cholesterol (*see* HMG CoA REDUCTASE). Statins can lower the levels of *low-density lipoproteins (LDLs) by 25–45% and are used mainly to treat hypercholesterolaemia but also to reduce the risk of coronary heart disease in susceptible patients. Muscle inflammation and breakdown (*see* RHABDOMYOLYSIS) is a rare but serious side-effect of statins. The class includes *atorvastatin, **fluvastatin** (Lescol), *pravastatin, **rosuvastatin** (Crestor), and *simvastatin.

status asthmaticus a severe attack of asthma, which often follows a period of poorly controlled asthma. Patients are distressed and very breathless and may die from respiratory failure if not vigorously treated with inhaled oxygen, nebulized or intravenous bronchodilators, and corticosteroid therapy; sedatives are absolutely contraindicated. These patients need hospital care in an intensive care unit.

status epilepticus the occurrence of repeated epileptic seizures without any recovery of consciousness between them. Its control is a medical emergency, since prolonged status epilepticus may lead to the patient's death or long-term disability.

status lymphaticus enlargement of the

thymus gland and other parts of the lymphatic system, formerly believed to be a predisposing cause to sudden death in infancy and childhood associated with hypersensitivity to drugs or vaccines.

Statutory Sick Pay benefit payable to employees who are unable to work because of illness.

STD *see* SEXUALLY TRANSMITTED DISEASE.

steapsin *n. see* LIPASE.

stearic acid *see* FATTY ACID.

steat- (steato-) *combining form denoting* fat; fatty tissue.

steatoma *n.* any cyst or tumour of a sebaceous gland.

steatopygia *n.* the accumulation of large quantities of fat in the buttocks.

steatorrhoea *n.* the passage of abnormally increased amounts of fat in the faeces (more than 5 g/day) due to reduced absorption of fat by the intestine (*see* MALABSORPTION). The faeces are pale, smell offensive, may look greasy, and are difficult to flush away.

steatosis *n.* infiltration of *hepatocytes with fat. This may occur in pregnancy, alcoholism, malnutrition, obesity, hepatitis C infection, or with some drugs.

Steele-Richardson-Olszewski syndrome *see* PROGRESSIVE SUPRANUCLEAR PALSY. [J. C. Steele and J. C. Richardson (20th century), Canadian neurologists; J. Olszewski (1913–64), Polish-born Canadian neuropathologist]

Stein-Leventhal syndrome *see* POLYCYSTIC OVARY SYNDROME. [I. F. Stein and M. L. Leventhal (20th century), U.S. gynaecologists]

stellate fracture a star-shaped fracture of the kneecap caused by a direct blow. The bone may be either split or severely shattered; if the fragments are displaced, the bone may need to be surgically repaired or rarely removed (**patellectomy**).

stellate ganglion a star-shaped collection of sympathetic nerve cell bodies in the root of the neck, from which sympathetic nerve fibres are distributed to the face and neck and to the blood vessels and organs of the thorax.

Stellwag's sign apparent widening of the

distance between the upper and lower eyelids (the palpebral fissure) due to retraction of the upper lid and protrusion of the eyeball. It is a sign of exophthalmic *goitre. [C. Stellwag von Carion (1823–1904), Austrian ophthalmologist]

stem cell an undifferentiated cell that is able to renew itself and produce specialized cells. **Embryonic stem cells** at the *blastocyst stage of development can differentiate into almost any cell type (except placental cells); they are described as **pluripotent**. Embryonic cells preceeding the blastocyst, produced by the first 3–4 divisions of the fertilized egg, are capable of producing all the different cell types required by the developing embryo (i.e. they are **totipotent**). **Adult stem cells** (also known as **somatic stem cells**) occur in many tissues and organs, including bone marrow (*see* HAEMOPOIETIC STEM CELL), muscle, liver, pancreas, etc., and can produce the specialized cells needed in the particular tissue or organ in which they arise (i.e. they are **multipotent**). *See also* UMBILICAL CORD BLOOD BANKED STEM CELLS.

STEMI S–T elevation *myocardial infarction.

steno- *combining form denoting* **1.** narrow. Example: **stenocephaly** (narrowness of the head). **2.** constricted.

stenopaeic *adj.* (in ophthalmology) describing an optical device consisting of an opaque disc punctured with a fine slit or hole (or holes), which is placed in front of the eye in the same position as glasses and enables sharper vision in cases of gross long- or short-sightedness or astigmatism. It sharpens the image formed on the retina because it confines the light reaching the eye to one or more fine beams, which pass through the centre of the lens undeviated by refractive error. The same principle is used in the pin-hole camera.

stenosis *n.* the abnormal narrowing of a passage or opening, such as a blood vessel or heart valve. *See* AORTIC STENOSIS, CAROTID ARTERY STENOSIS, MITRAL STENOSIS, PULMONARY STENOSIS, PYLORIC STENOSIS.

stenostomia (stenostomy) *n.* the abnormal narrowing of an opening, such as the opening of the bile duct.

Stensen's duct the long secretory duct of the *parotid salivary gland. [N. Stensen (1838–86), Danish physician]

stent *n.* a tube placed inside a duct or canal to reopen it or keep it open. It may be a simple tube, usually plastic, or an expandable, usually sprung mesh metal, tube (**self-expanding metal stent**, **SEMS**). The former is more easily removable, while the latter gives a larger lumen for a given outer diameter. Stents may be used at operation to aid healing of an anastomosis, for example of a ureter. Alternatively they can be placed across an obstruction to maintain an open lumen, for example in obstruction due to tumour in the oesophagus, stomach, bile ducts, colon, or ureter. In an artery after *angioplasty, stents help to prevent *restenosis (narrowing) and are increasingly used in coronary artery disease in place of coronary artery bypass grafting (*see* PERCUTANEOUS CORONARY INTERVENTION). **Drug-eluting stents** are coronary stents coated with a drug that inhibits growth of the scar tissue responsible for recurrent stenosis.

Double J (or **pig-tail**) **stents** are slender catheters with side holes that are passed over a guide wire either through an endoscope or at open operation to drain urine from the kidney pelvis to the bladder, via the ureter. On removal of the guide wire both the upper and lower extremities of the stent assume a J-shape, hence preventing both upward and downward migration. They are commonly used to splint a damaged ureter and to relieve obstruction.

stepping reflex a primitive reflex in newborn babies that should disappear by the age of two months. If the baby is held in a 'walking' position with the feet touching the ground, the feet move in a 'stepping' manner. Persistence of this reflex beyond two months is suggestive of *cerebral palsy.

sterco- *combining form denoting* faeces.

stercobilin *n.* a brownish-red pigment formed during the metabolism of the *bile pigments biliverdin and bilirubin, which are derived from haemoglobin. Stercobilin is subsequently excreted in the urine or faeces.

stercolith *n.* a stone formed of dried compressed faeces.

stereognosis *n.* the ability to recognize the three-dimensional shape of an object by touch alone. This is a function of the *association areas of the parietal lobe of the brain. *See also* AGNOSIA.

stereoisomers *pl. n.* compounds having the same molecular formula but different three-dimensional arrangements of their atoms. The atomic structures of stereoisomers are mirror images of each other.

stereopsis *n. see* STEREOSCOPIC VISION.

stereoscopic vision (stereopsis) perception of the shape, depth, and distance of an object as a result of having *binocular vision. The brain receives two distinct images from the eyes, which it interprets as a single three-dimensional image.

stereotactic localization the accurate localization of structures within the body by using three-dimensional measurements. It enables the accurate positioning within the body of radiotherapy beams or sources for the treatment of tumours and of localizing wires for the biopsy of small tumours. *See also* STEREOTAXY (STEREOTACTIC SURGERY), CYBERKNIFE, GAMMA KNIFE.

stereotaxy (stereotactic surgery) *n.* a surgical procedure in which a deep-seated area in the brain is operated upon after its position has been established very accurately by three-dimensional measurements using CT or MRI. The operation may be performed using an electrical current or by heat, cold, or mechanical techniques. *See also* LEUCOTOMY.

stereotypy *n.* the constant repetition of a complex action, which is carried out in the same way each time. It is seen in *catatonia and infantile *autism; sometimes it is an isolated symptom in mental retardation. It is more common in patients who live in institutions where they are bored and unstimulated. It can prevent a patient from carrying on normal life, and sometimes causes physical injury to the patient.

sterile *adj.* **1.** (of a living organism) barren; unable to reproduce its kind (*see* STERILITY). **2.** (of inanimate objects) completely free from bacteria, fungi, viruses, or other microorganisms that could cause infection.

sterility *n.* inability to have children, either due to *infertility or (in someone who has been fertile) deliberately induced by surgical procedures as a means of contraception (*see* STERILIZATION). Sterility may also be an incidental result of an operation or drug treatment undertaken for other reasons, such as removal of the uterus (*hysterectomy) because of cancer.

sterilization *n.* **1.** a surgical operation or any other process that induces *sterility in men or women. In women, hysterectomy and bilateral oophorectomy (surgical removal of both ovaries) are 100% effective and permanent. Alternatively, the Fallopian tubes may be removed (*see* SALPINGECTOMY) or divided and/or ligated. These operations can be performed through the abdomen or the vagina. The modern technique (**tubal occlusion**) is to occlude (close) permanently the inner (lower) half of the Fallopian tube through a *laparoscope. The occluding device is usually a clip (the **Hulka-Clemens** or **Filshie clips**) or a small plastic ring (**Falope ring**); *diathermy coagulation carries greater dangers (e.g. bowel burns) and is now little used. A more recent method is the use of a rapid-setting plastic introduced into the tubes through a hysteroscope (*see* HYSTEROSCOPY). Men are usually sterilized by *vasectomy. *See also* CASTRATION. **2.** the process by which all types of microorganisms (including spores) are destroyed. This is achieved by the use of heat, radiation, chemicals, or filtration. *See also* AUTOCLAVE.

stern- (sterno-) *combining form denoting* the sternum. Example: **sternocostal** (relating to the sternum and ribs).

Sternberg-Reed cell *see* REED-STERNBERG CELL.

sternebra *n.* (*pl.* **sternebrae**) one of the four parts that fuse during development to form the body of the sternum.

sternocleidomastoid muscle *see* STERNOMASTOID MUSCLE.

sternohyoid *n.* a muscle in the neck, arising from the sternum and inserted into the hyoid bone. It depresses the hyoid bone.

sternomastoid muscle (sternocleidomastoid muscle) a long muscle in the neck, extending from the mastoid process to the sternum and clavicle. It serves to rotate the neck and flex the head.

sternomastoid tumour a small painless nonmalignant swelling in the lower half of the *sternomastoid muscle, appearing a few days after birth. It occurs when the neck of the fetus is in an abnormal position in the uterus, which interferes with the blood supply to the affected muscle, and it is most common after breech births. The tumour may cause a slight tilt of the head towards the tumour and turning of the face to the other side. This can be corrected by physio-

therapy aimed at increasing all movements of the body, but without stretching the neck.

sternotomy *n.* surgical division of the breastbone (sternum), performed to allow access to the heart and its major vessels.

sternum *n.* (*pl.* **sterna**) the breastbone: a flat bone, 15–20 cm long, extending from the base of the neck to just below the diaphragm and forming the front part of the skeleton of the thorax. The sternum articulates with the collar bones (*see* CLAVICLE) and the costal cartilages of the first seven pairs of ribs. It consists of three sections: the middle and longest section – the **body** or **gladiolus** – is attached to the *manubrium at the top and the *xiphoid (or ensiform) process at the bottom. The manubrium slopes back from the body so that the junction between the two parts forms an angle (**angle of Louis** or **sternal angle**). —**sternal** *adj.*

steroid *n.* one of a group of compounds having a common structure based on the **steroid nucleus**, which consists of three six-membered carbon rings and one five-membered carbon ring. The naturally occurring steroids include the male and female sex hormones (*androgens and *oestrogens), the hormones of the adrenal cortex (*see* CORTICOSTEROID), *progesterone, *bile salts, and *sterols. Synthetic steroids have been produced for therapeutic purposes.

steroid card a card that must be carried by patients taking long-term corticosteroid medication, particularly if high doses are used. The card states that in an emergency treatment with steroids must not be suddenly stopped since this may precipitate an *Addisonian crisis.

sterol *n.* one of a group of *steroid alcohols. The most important sterols are *cholesterol and *ergosterol.

stertor *n.* a snoring type of noisy breathing heard in deeply unconscious patients.

steth- (stetho-) *combining form denoting* the chest.

stethoscope *n.* an instrument used for listening to sounds within the body, such as those in the heart and lungs (*see* AUSCULTATION). A simple stethoscope usually consists of a diaphragm or an open bell-shaped structure (which is applied to the body) connected by rubber or plastic tubes to earpieces for the examiner. More complicated devices may contain electronic amplification systems to aid diagnosis.

sthenia *n.* a state of normal or greater than normal strength. *Compare* ASTHENIA. —**sthenic** *adj.*

stigma *n.* (*pl.* **stigmata**) **1.** a mark that characterizes a particular disease, such as the *café au lait spots characteristic of neurofibromatosis. **2.** any spot or lesion on the skin.

stilet (**stylet, stylus**) *n.* **1.** a slender probe. **2.** a wire placed in the lumen of a catheter to give it rigidity while the instrument is passed along a body canal (such as the urethra).

stillbirth *n.* birth of a fetus that shows no evidence of life (heartbeat, respiration, or independent movement) at any time later than 24 weeks after conception. Under the Stillbirth (Definition) Act 1992, there is a legal obligation to notify all stillbirths to the appropriate authority. The number of such births expressed per 1000 births (live and still) is known as the **stillbirth rate**. In legal terms, viability is deemed to start at the 24th week of pregnancy and a fetus born dead before this time is known as a *miscarriage or *abortion. However, some fetuses born alive before the 24th week may now survive as a result of improved perinatal care. *See also* CONFIDENTIAL ENQUIRIES.

(((●))) **SEE WEB LINKS**

• Website of Sands (Stillbirth and Neonatal Death Society)

Still's disease *see* JUVENILE CHRONIC ARTHRITIS. [Sir G. F. Still (1868–1941), British physician]

stimulant *n.* an agent that promotes the activity of a body system or function. *Amphetamines, *methylphenidate, and *caffeine are stimulants of the central nervous system; *doxapram is a respiratory stimulant (*see* ANALEPTIC).

stimulator *n.* any apparatus designed to stimulate nerves and muscles for a variety of purposes. It can be used to stimulate particular areas of the brain or to block pain (as in *transcutaneous electrical nerve stimulation).

stimulus *n.* (*pl.* **stimuli**) any agent that provokes a response, or particular form of activity, in a cell, tissue, or other structure, which is said to be sensitive to that stimulus.

stippling *n.* a spotted or speckled appearance, such as is seen in the retina in certain eye diseases or in abnormal red blood cells stained with basic dyes.

stirrup *n.* (in anatomy) *see* STAPES.

stitch *n.* **1.** a sharp localized pain, commonly in the abdomen, associated with strenuous physical activity (such as running), especially shortly after eating. It is a form of cramp. **2.** *see* SUTURE.

stock culture *see* CULTURE.

Stokes-Adams syndrome (Adams-Stokes syndrome) attacks of temporary loss of consciousness (*syncope) that occur when blood flow ceases due to severe *bradycardia. This syndrome may complicate *heart block. [W. Stokes (1804–78) and R. Adams (1791–1875), Irish physicians]

stoma *n.* (*pl.* **stomata**) **1.** (in anatomy) the mouth or any mouthlike part. **2.** (in surgery) the artificial opening of a tube (e.g. the colon or ileum) that has been brought to the abdominal surface (*see* COLOSTOMY, ILEOSTOMY). **Stoma therapists** are nurses specially trained in the care of these artificial openings and the appliances used with them. —**stomal** *adj.*

stomach *n.* a distensible saclike organ that forms part of the alimentary canal between the oesophagus (gullet) and the duodenum (see illustration). It communicates with the former by means of the **lower oesophageal sphincter** (**LOS**), or **cardiac sphincter**, and with the latter by the **pyloric sphincter**. The stomach lies just below the diaphragm, to the right of the spleen and partly under the liver. Its function is to continue the process of digestion that begins in the mouth. *Gastric juice, secreted by gastric glands in the mucosa, contains hydrochloric acid and the enzyme *pepsin, which contribute to chemical digestion. This – together with the churning action of the muscular layers of the stomach – reduces the food to a semiliquid partly digested mass that passes on to the duodenum.

stomach stapling (gastric stapling, vertical banded gastroplasty) restrictive *bariatric surgery in which staples are inserted into the wall of the stomach to form a small pouch, which restricts the amount of food that can be eaten. At the same time a gastric band is applied to limit the size of the opening between the pouch and the rest of the stomach.

stomat- (stomato-) *combining form denoting* the mouth.

stomatitis *n.* inflammation of the mucous lining of the mouth.

stomatology *n.* the branch of medicine concerned with diseases of the mouth.

stomodeum *n.* the site of the embryonic mouth, marked by a depression lined with ectoderm from which the teeth develop. The membrane separating it from the foregut

breaks down by the end of the first month of pregnancy. *Compare* PROCTODEUM.

-stomy (-ostomy) *combining form denoting* a surgical opening into an organ or part. Example: **colostomy** (into the colon).

stone *n. see* CALCULUS.

stool *n.* *faeces discharged from the anus.

stop needle a surgical needle with a shank that has a protruding collar to stop it when the needle has been pushed a pre-

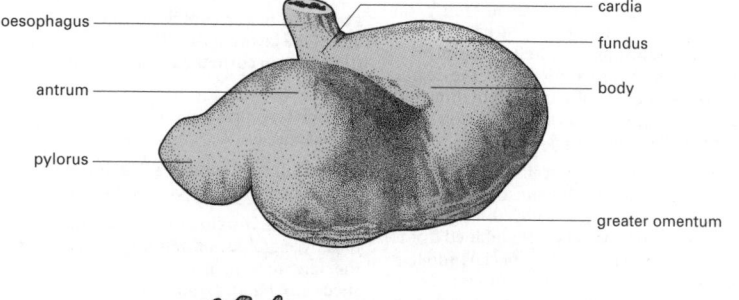

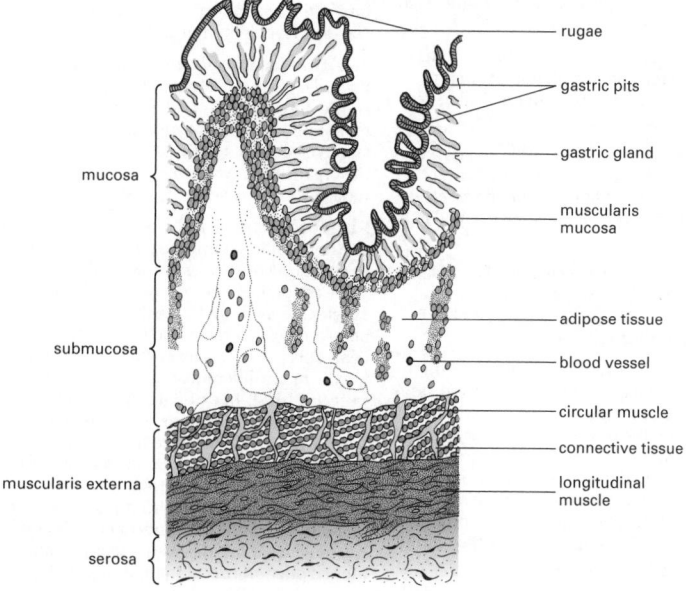

Stomach. Regions of the stomach seen from the front (above); layers of the stomach wall (below).

scribed distance into the tissue. A stop needle has the eye at the tip.

strabismus (heterotropia) *n.* squint: abnormal alignment of the two eyes. The strabismus is most commonly horizontal – **convergent strabismus** (or **esotropia**) or **divergent strabismus** (**exotropia**) – but it may be vertical (**hypertropia**, in which the eye looks upwards, or **hypotropia**, in which it looks downwards). In rare cases both eyes look towards the same point but one is twisted clockwise or anticlockwise in relation to the other (**cyclotropia**). Usually strabismus is **concomitant**, i.e. the abnormal alignment of the two eyes remains fairly constant, in whatever direction the person is looking. Strabismus acquired by injury or disease is usually **incomitant**, i.e. the degree of misalignment varies in different directions of gaze. *See also* COVER TEST, DEVIATION, DIVERGENCE, HETEROPHORIA.

strain 1. *n.* excessive stretching or working of a muscle, resulting in pain and swelling of the muscle. *Compare* SPRAIN. 2. *n.* a group of organisms, such as bacteria, obtained from a particular source or having special properties distinguishing them from other members of the same species. 3. *vb.* to damage a muscle by overstretching.

strain gauge a sensitive instrument for measuring tension and alterations in pressure. It is extensively used in medical instruments.

strangulated *adj.* describing a part of the body whose blood supply has been interrupted by compression of a blood vessel, as may occur in a loop of intestine trapped in a *hernia.

strangulation *n.* the closure of a passage, such as the main airway to the lungs (resulting in the cessation of breathing), a blood vessel, or the gastrointestinal tract.

strangury *n.* severe pain in the urethra referred from the base of the bladder and associated with an intense desire to pass urine. It occurs when the base of the bladder is irritated by a stone or an indwelling catheter. It is also noted in patients with an invasive cancer of the base of the bladder or severe *cystitis or *prostatitis, when the strong desire to urinate is accompanied by the painful passage of a few drops of urine.

Strassman procedure an operation to correct a double uterus (*see* UTERUS DIDEL-

PHYS). It has now largely been replaced by hysteroscopic techniques. [P. F. Strassman (1866–1938), German obstetrician and gynaecologist]

strategic health authority (SHA) a statutory organization in England responsible for strategic leadership, building capacity, organizational development, and performance management in the local *National Health Service. SHAs (28 of them) were established in 2002 by merging the existing health authorities, and each SHA area contains various NHS *trusts. In July 2006 the number of SHAs was reduced to 10.

stratum *n.* a layer of tissue or cells, such as any of the layers of the *epidermis of the skin (the **stratum corneum** is the outermost layer).

strawberry mark (strawberry naevus) *see* NAEVUS.

streak *n.* (in anatomy) a line, furrow, or narrow band. *See also* PRIMITIVE STREAK.

Streptobacillus *n.* a genus of Gram-negative aerobic nonmotile rodlike bacteria that tend to form filaments. The single species, *S. moniliformis*, is a normal inhabitant of the respiratory tract of rats but causes *rat-bite fever in humans.

streptococcal toxic shock syndrome a bacterial disease characterized by fever, shock, and multiple organ failure. It is similar to the *toxic shock syndrome caused by staphylococci, but in these cases the infecting organisms are *Streptococcus Type A bacteria. *See also* NECROTIZING FASCIITIS.

Streptococcus *n.* a genus of Gram-positive nonmotile spherical bacteria occurring in chains. Most species are saprophytes; some are pathogenic. Many pathogenic species are **haemolytic**, i.e. they have the ability to destroy red blood cells in blood agar. This provides a useful basis for classifying the many different strains. Strains of *S. pyogenes* (the β-haemolytic streptococci) are associated with many infections, including *scarlet fever, and produce many *exotoxins. Strains of the α-haemolytic streptococci are associated with bacterial *endocarditis. The species *S. pneumoniae* (formerly *Diplococcus pneumoniae*) – the **pneumococcus** – is associated with serious diseases, including pneumonia, pneumococcal *meningitis, and septicaemia; it is also a common bacterial cause of ear infections (*see also* PNEUMOCOC-

CAL VACCINE). It occurs in pairs, surrounded by a capsule (*see* QUELLUNG REACTION). *S. mutans* has been shown to cause dental caries. *See also* LANCEFIELD CLASSIFICATION, STREPTOKINASE. —**streptococcal** *adj.*

streptodornase *n.* an enzyme produced by some haemolytic bacteria of the genus *Streptococcus* that is capable of liquefying pus. *See also* STREPTOKINASE.

streptokinase *n.* an enzyme produced by some haemolytic bacteria of the genus *Streptococcus* that is capable of liquefying blood clots (*see also* FIBRINOLYTIC). It is injected to treat blockage of blood vessels, including deep vein thrombosis, myocardial infarction, and pulmonary embolism. Side-effects may include digestive upsets, haemorrhage, and fever. Trade name: **Streptase**.

streptolysin *n.* an *exotoxin that is produced by strains of *Streptococcus* bacteria and destroys red blood cells.

Streptomyces *n.* a genus of aerobic mouldlike bacteria. Most species live in the soil, but some are parasites of animals, humans, and plants; in humans they cause *Madura foot. They are important medically as a source of such antibiotics as *streptomycin, *neomycin, *dactinomycin, and *chloramphenicol.

streptomycin *n.* an *aminoglycoside antibiotic, derived from the bacterium *Streptomyces griseus*, that is used in combination with other drugs for treating tuberculosis and brucellosis. It is administered by intramuscular injection; side-effects causing ear and kidney damage may develop in some patients.

stress *n.* any factor that threatens the health of the body or has an adverse effect on its functioning, such as injury, disease, overwork, or worry. The existence of one form of stress tends to diminish resistance to other forms. Constant stress brings about changes in the balance of hormones in the body.

stress fracture a fracture occurring in normal bone that has been subjected to excessive and repetitive trauma resulting in cumulative microscopic fractures. Over time, these microfractures exceed the capacity of the normal healing process, resulting in the development of a macroscopic fracture (also known as a **fatigue fracture**). Patients are usually long-distance runners, ballet

dancers, footballers, and others who undergo regular intensive training. Pain, localized tenderness, and swelling gradually develop; initially, X-rays are normal, but a bone scan or MRI will usually allow diagnosis to be made. Treatment includes protected weight bearing, rest, cross-training, and (less commonly) surgery.

stress incontinence *see* INCONTINENCE.

stress ulcers gastric or duodenal ulcers that can be associated with stress from severe head injury (**Cushing's ulcers**) or major burns (**Curling's ulcers**).

stretch receptor a cell or group of cells found between muscle fibres that responds to stretching of the muscle by transmitting impulses to the central nervous system through the sensory nerves. Stretch receptors are part of the *proprioceptor system necessary for the performance of coordinated muscular activity.

stretch reflex (**myotatic reflex**) the reflex contraction of a muscle in response to its being stretched.

stria *n.* (*pl.* **striae**) (in anatomy) a streak, line, or thin band. The **striae gravidarum** (stretch marks) are the lines that appear on the the skin of the abdomen of pregnant women, due to excessive stretching of the elastic fibres. Red or purple during pregnancy, they become white after delivery. The **stria terminalis** is a white band that separates the thalamus from the ventricular surface of the caudate nucleus in the brain.

striated muscle a tissue comprising the bulk of the body's musculature. It is also known as **skeletal muscle**, because it is attached to the skeleton and is responsible for the movement of bones, and **voluntary muscle**, because it is under voluntary control. Striated muscle is composed of parallel bundles of multinucleate fibres (each containing many **myofibrils**), which reveal cross-banding when viewed under the microscope. This effect is caused by the alternation of **actin** and **myosin** protein filaments within each myofibril (see illustration). According to the 'sliding filament' theory, when muscle contraction takes place, the two sets of filaments slide past each other, so reducing the length of each unit (**sarcomere**) of the myofibril. The sliding is caused by a series of cyclic reactions, requiring ATP, resulting in a change in orientation of projections on the myosin filaments; each projection is first attached to muscle fibre

Structure of striated muscle.

an actin filament but contracts and releases it to become reattached at a different site.

stricture *n.* a narrowing of any tubular structure in the body, such as the oesophagus (gullet), biliary tract, bowel, ureter, or urethra. A stricture may result from inflammation, muscular spasm, growth of a tumour within the affected part, or from pressure on it by neighbouring organs. For example, a **urethral stricture** is a fibrous narrowing of the urethra, usually resulting from injury or inflammation. The patient has increasing difficulty in passing urine and may develop *retention. The site and length of the stricture is assessed by *urethrography and urethroscopy, and treatment is by periodic dilatation of the urethra using *sounds, *urethrotomy, or *urethroplasty. Strictures in the alimentary canal are dilated by *balloon or treated surgically (*stricturoplasty). Symptomatic malignant strictures can be managed by insertion of a *stent, especially in cases of oesophageal, colonic, or biliary strictures.

stricturoplasty *n.* an operation in which a stricture (usually in the small intestine) is widened by cutting it longitudinally and suturing transversely.

stridor *n.* the noise heard on breathing in when the trachea or larynx is obstructed. It tends to be louder and harsher than *wheeze.

strobila *n.* (*pl.* **strobilae**) the entire chain of segments that make up the body of an adult *tapeworm.

stroke (apoplexy) *n.* a sudden attack of weakness usually affecting one side of the body. It is the consequence of an interruption to the flow of blood to the brain. An **ischaemic stroke** occurs when the flow of blood is prevented by clotting (*see* THROMBOSIS) or by a detached clot, either from the heart or a large vessel (such as the carotid artery), that lodges in an artery (*see* EMBOLISM). A **haemorrhagic stroke** results from rupture of an artery wall (*see* CEREBRAL HAEMORRHAGE). Prolonged reduction of blood pressure may result in more diffuse brain damage, as after a cardiorespiratory arrest. A stroke can vary in severity from a passing weakness or tingling in a limb (*see* TRANSIENT ISCHAEMIC ATTACK) to a profound paralysis, coma, and death.

(((⊕))) SEE WEB LINKS

• Website of the Stroke Association: includes resources for professionals

stroma *n.* the connective tissue basis of an organ, as opposed to the functional tissue (**parenchyma**). For example, the stroma of the erythrocytes is the spongy framework of protein strands within a red blood cell in which the blood pigment haemoglobin is packed; the stroma of the cornea is the transparent fibrous tissue making up the main body of the cornea.

Strongyloides *n.* a genus of small slender nematode worms that live as parasites inside the small intestines of mammals. *S. stercoralis* infects the human small intestine (*see* STRONGYLOIDIASIS); its larvae, which are passed out in the stools, develop quickly into infective forms.

strongyloidiasis (strongyloidosis) *n.* an infestation of the small intestine with the parasitic nematode worm *Strongyloides stercoralis*, common in humid tropical regions. Larvae, present in soil contaminated with human faeces, penetrate the skin of a human host and may produce an itching rash. They migrate to the lungs, where they cause tissue destruction and bleeding, and then via the windpipe and gullet to the intestine. Adult worms burrow into the intestinal wall and may cause ulceration, diarrhoea, abdominal pain, nausea, anaemia, and weakness. Treatment involves use of ivermectin or albendazole.

strontium *n.* a yellow metallic element, absorption of which causes bone damage when its atoms displace calcium in bone. The radioactive isotope **strontium-90**, which emits beta rays, is used in radiotherapy for the *contact therapy of skin and eye tumours and in *radioimmunotherapy in combination with *monoclonal antibodies. Another isotope, **strontium-89** (Metastron), has an established role in the treatment of metastatic carcinoma: it is given by intravenous injection for the relief of pain due to bone metastases. Symbol: Sr.

struma *n.* (*pl.* **strumae**) a swelling of the thyroid gland (*see* GOITRE). *See also* RIEDEL'S STRUMA.

struma ovarii a *teratoma of the ovary containing thyroid tissue that becomes overactive and causes thyrotoxicosis. It is diagnosed by radioiodine scanning showing a high uptake in the pelvis; the treatment is surgical removal of the affected ovary.

strychnine *n.* a poisonous alkaloid produced in the seeds of the East Indian tree *Strychnos nux-vomica*. In small doses it was formerly widely used in 'tonics'. Poisoning causes painful muscular spasms similar to those of tetanus; the back becomes arched (the posture known as **opisthotonos**) and death is likely to occur from spasm in the respiratory muscles.

S–T segment the segment on an *electrocardiogram that represents the interval between the end of ventricular *depolarization (QRS complex) and the beginning of ventricular *repolarization (T wave). The S–T segment is usually depressed by *ischaemia of the heart muscle but raised in the initial phase of myocardial infarction. It is therefore very useful for diagnosis in patients presenting with chest pain.

Student's t test *see* SIGNIFICANCE. [Pseudonym of W. S. Gosset (1876–1937), British statistician]

Studer pouch *see* CYSTECTOMY.

stupe *n.* any piece of material, such as a wad of cottonwool, soaked in hot water (with or without medication) and used to apply a poultice.

stupor *n.* a condition of near unconsciousness, with apparent mental inactivity and reduced ability to respond to stimulation.

Sturge-Weber syndrome *see* ANGIOMA. [W. A. Sturge (1850–1919) and F. P. Weber (1863–1962), British physicians]

stuttering *n. see* STAMMERING.

St Vitus' dance an archaic name for *Sydenham's chorea.

Stycar tests Standard Tests for Young Children and Retardates: tests to detect visual problems in children between the ages of six months and five years. They consist of a series of standardized balls, toys, or letters. The tests were developed by the paediatrician Mary Sheridan.

stye *n.* acute inflammation of a gland at the base of an eyelash, caused by bacterial infection. The gland becomes hard and tender and a pus-filled cyst develops at its centre. Styes are treated by bathing in warm water or removal of the eyelash involved. Medical name: **hordeolum**.

stylet *n. see* STILET.

stylo- *combining form denoting* the styloid process of the temporal bone. Example: **stylomastoid** (relating to the styloid and mastoid processes).

styloglossus *n.* a muscle that extends from the tongue to the styloid process of the temporal bone. It serves to draw the tongue upwards and backwards.

stylohyoid *n.* a muscle that extends from the styloid process of the temporal bone to the hyoid bone. It serves to draw the hyoid bone backwards and upwards.

styloid process 1. a long slender downward-pointing spine projecting from the lower surface of the *temporal bone of the skull. It provides attachment for muscles and ligaments of the tongue and hyoid bone. 2. any of various other spiny projections; occurring, for example, at the lower ends of the ulna and radius.

stylus *n.* 1. a pencil-shaped instrument, commonly used for applying external medication; for example, to apply silver nitrate to warts. 2. *see* STILET.

styptic *n. see* HAEMOSTATIC.

sub- *prefix denoting* 1. below; underlying. Examples: **subcostal** (below the ribs); **sub-**

lingual (below the tongue); **submandibular** (below the mandible). **2.** partial or slight.

subacute *adj.* describing a disease that progresses more rapidly than a *chronic condition but does not become *acute.

subacute combined degeneration of the cord the neurological disorder complicating a deficiency of *vitamin B$_{12}$ or folate and often combined with *pernicious anaemia, which causes malabsorption of the vitamin B$_{12}$ by the production of intrinsic factor antibodies. There is selective damage to the motor and sensory nerve fibres in the spinal cord, resulting in *spasticity of the limbs and a sensory *ataxia. It may also be accompanied by damage to the peripheral nerves and the optic nerve and by dementia. It is treated by giving vitamin B$_{12}$ injections.

subacute sclerosing panencephalitis (SSPE) a rare and late complication of *measles characterized by a slow progressive neurological deterioration that is usually fatal. It can occur four to ten years after the initial infection.

subaponeurotic haemorrhage bleeding under the *aponeurosis of the scalp resulting from trauma to blood vessels crossing the space from the skull to the overlying scalp. It results from delivery by forceps or vacuum extraction. It is very uncommon but can be fatal. *See also* CEPHAL-HAEMATOMA, CHIGNON.

subarachnoid haemorrhage sudden bleeding into the subarachnoid space surrounding the brain, which causes severe headache with stiffness of the neck. The usual source of such a haemorrhage is a cerebral *aneurysm that has burst. The diagnosis is confirmed by CT scan or by finding blood-stained cerebrospinal fluid at *lumbar puncture. Identification of the site of the aneurysm, upon which decisions about treatment will be based, is achieved by cerebral *angiography.

subarachnoid space the space between the arachnoid and pia *meninges of the brain and spinal cord, containing circulating cerebrospinal fluid and large blood vessels. Several large spaces within it are known as **cisternae**.

subclavian artery either of two arteries supplying blood to the neck and arms. The right subclavian artery branches from the in-

nominate artery; the left subclavian arises directly from the aortic arch.

subclavian steal syndrome a syndrome produced by proximal narrowing of the subclavian artery. There are no symptoms at rest, but when the affected arm is exercised blood is diverted to the arm down the main subclavian artery, away from smaller branches that arise just beyond the narrowing (i.e. 'stolen' from these branches). If branches to the brain are affected, *syncope may result. The syndrome may result in chest pain in people in whom an internal mammary artery branch of the subclavian artery has been used to bypass a coronary narrowing (*see* CORONARY ARTERY BYPASS GRAFT).

subclinical *adj.* describing a disease that is suspected but is not sufficiently developed to produce definite signs and symptoms in the patient.

subconscious *adj.* **1.** describing mental processes of which a person is not aware. **2.** (in psychoanalysis) denoting the part of the mind that includes memories, motives, and intentions that are momentarily not present in consciousness but can more or less readily be recalled to awareness. *Compare* UNCONSCIOUS.

subcutaneous *adj.* beneath the skin. A **subcutaneous injection** is given beneath the skin. **Subcutaneous tissue** is loose connective tissue, often fatty, situated under the dermis.

subdural *adj.* below the dura mater (the outermost of the meninges); relating to the space between the dura mater and arachnoid. *See also* HAEMATOMA.

subglottis *n.* that part of the *larynx that lies below the vocal folds.

subinvolution *n.* failure of the uterus to revert to its normal size during the six weeks following childbirth.

sublimation *n.* the replacement of socially undesirable means of gratifying motives or desires by means that are socially acceptable. *See also* DEFENCE MECHANISM, REPRESSION.

subliminal *adj.* subconscious: beneath the threshold of conscious perception.

sublingual *adj.* below the tongue. Tablets and capsules of some drugs are administered by being placed beneath the tongue, where they dissolve.

sublingual gland one of a pair of *salivary glands situated in the lower part of the mouth, one on either side of the tongue. The sublingual glands are the smallest salivary glands; each gland has about 20 ducts, most of which open into the mouth directly above the gland.

subluxation *n.* partial *dislocation of a joint, so that the bone ends are misaligned but still in contact.

submandibular gland (submaxillary gland) one of a pair of *salivary glands situated below the parotid glands. Their ducts (**Wharton's ducts**) open in two papillae under the tongue, on either side of the frenulum.

submaxillary gland *see* SUBMANDIBULAR GLAND.

submentovertical (SMV) *adj.* denoting an X-ray view of the base of the skull.

submucosa *n.* the layer of loose connective (*areolar) tissue underlying a mucous membrane; for example, in the wall of the intestine. —**submucosal** *adj.*

subphrenic abscess a collection of pus in the space below the diaphragm, usually on the right side, between the liver and diaphragm. Causes include postoperative infection (particularly after stomach or bowel surgery) and perforation of an organ (e.g. perforated peptic ulcer). Prompt treatment with antibiotics together with radiological or surgical drainage of the abscess is usually required.

substance abuse the nonclinical, or recreational, use of pharmacologically active substances such that continued use results in adverse physiological or psychological effects (*see* DEPENDENCE). Substances commonly abused include alcohol (*see* ALCOHOLISM), *amphetamines, *cannabis, *cocaine, *Ecstasy, *heroin, *lysergic acid diethylamide (LSD), and organic solvents (by inhalation).

substituted judgment a decision made by someone on behalf of a patient lacking capacity that is judged to reflect what the patient would have wanted had he or she had the mental capacity to decide for him- or herself. This judgment is best made by someone close to the patient who has a good

knowledge of the patient's beliefs, opinions, and character. Nevertheless, there may still be potentially conflicting and partial interests at play. *See also* LASTING POWER OF ATTORNEY, PROXY DECISION.

substitution *n.* **1.** (in psychoanalysis) the replacement of one idea by another: a form of *defence mechanism. **2. (symptom substitution)** the supposed process whereby removing one psychological symptom leads to another symptom appearing if the basic psychological cause has not been removed. It is controversial whether this happens.

substitution therapy provision of a less harmful alternative to a drug or remedy that a patient has been receiving. It is used when the patient has become addicted to a drug or is placing too much reliance upon a particular remedy. An example is the replacement of heroin in an opioid-dependent patient with methadone.

substrate *n.* the specific substance or substances on which a given *enzyme acts. For example, starch is the substrate for salivary amylase; RNA is the substrate for ribonuclease.

subsultus *n.* abnormal twitching or tremor of muscles, such as may occur in feverish conditions.

subtertian fever a form of *malaria resulting from repeated infection by *Plasmodium falciparum* and characterized by continuous fever.

subthalamic nucleus a collection of grey matter, shaped like a biconvex lens, lying beneath the *thalamus and close to the *corpus striatum, to which it is connected by nerve tracts. It has connections with the cerebral cortex and several other nuclei nearby. Stimulation of this nucleus is now being used in the treatment of Parkinson's disease.

subtotal *adj.* almost complete or partial: applied, for example, to surgical procedures (e.g. subtotal *thyroidectomy) or to occlusion (usually of an artery).

subzonal insemination (Suzi) a method of assisting conception in cases of infertility caused by the inability of the spermatozoa to penetrate the barriers surrounding the ovum. Using *in vitro fertilization techniques, a small number of spermatozoa (no more than six) are injected through the *zona pellucida into the perivitelline space (which surrounds the egg membrane). If fertilization subsequently occurs, the blastocyst is implanted in the mother's uterus.

succus *n.* any juice or secretion of animal or plant origin.

succus entericus (intestinal juice) the clear alkaline fluid secreted by the glands of the small intestine. It contains mucus and digestive enzymes, including *enteropeptidase, *erepsin, *lactase, and *sucrase.

succussion *n.* a splashing noise heard when a patient who has a large quantity of fluid in a body cavity, such as the pleural cavity, moves suddenly or is deliberately shaken.

sucralfate *n.* an aluminium-containing drug that forms a protective coating over the stomach or duodenal lining. Administered by mouth, sucralfate is used in the treatment of peptic ulcer. A fairly common side-effect is constipation. Trade name: **Antepsin**.

sucrase *n.* an enzyme, secreted by glands in the small intestine, that catalyses the hydrolysis of sucrose into its components (glucose and fructose).

sucrose *n.* a carbohydrate consisting of glucose and fructose. Sucrose is the principal constituent of cane sugar and sugar beet; it is the sweetest of the natural dietary carbohydrates. The increasing consumption of sucrose in the last 50 years has coincided with an increase in the incidence of dental caries, diabetes, coronary heart disease, and obesity.

suction *n.* the use of reduced pressure to remove unwanted fluids or other material through a tube for disposal. Suction is often used to clear secretions from the airways of newly born infants to aid breathing. During surgery, suction tubes are used to remove blood from the area of operation and to decompress the stomach (**nasogastric suction**) and the pleural space of air and blood (**chest suction**).

Sudan stains a group of azo compounds used for staining fats. The group includes **Sudan I**, **Sudan II**, **Sudan III**, **Sudan IV**, and **Sudan black**.

sudden infant death syndrome (SIDS, cot death) the sudden unexpected death of an infant less than two years old (peak occurrence between two and six months) from an unidentifiable cause. There appear to be many factors involved, the most important

of which is the position in which the baby is laid to sleep: babies who sleep on their fronts (the prone position) have an increased risk. Other factors increasing the risk include parental smoking, overheating with bedding, prematurity, and a history of SIDS within the family. About half the affected infants will have had a viral upper respiratory tract infection within the 48 hours preceding their death, many of these being due to the *respiratory syncytial virus.

SEE WEB LINKS
• Website of the Foundation for the Study of Infant Deaths: includes advice for professionals

Sudek's atrophy *see* REFLEX SYMPATHETIC DYSTROPHY. [P. H. M. Sudek (1866–1938), German surgeon]

sudor *n. see* SWEAT.

sudorific *n. see* DIAPHORETIC.

suffocation *n.* cessation of breathing as a result of drowning, smothering, etc., leading to unconsciousness or death (*see* ASPHYXIA).

suffusion *n.* the spreading of a flush across the skin surface, caused by changes in the local blood supply.

sugar *n.* any *carbohydrate that dissolves in water, is usually crystalline, and has a sweet taste. Sugars are classified chemically as *monosaccharides or *disaccharides. Table sugar is virtually 100% pure *sucrose and contains no other nutrient; brown sugar is less highly refined sucrose. Sugar is used as both a sweetening and preserving agent. *See also* FRUCTOSE, GLUCOSE, LACTOSE.

suggestion *n.* (in psychology) **1.** the process of changing people's beliefs, attitudes, or emotions by telling them that they will change. **2.** a thought or idea imparted to someone in a hypnotic state. *See also* AUTO-SUGGESTION.

suicide *n.* deliberately causing one's own death. A distinction is usually drawn between **attempted suicide**, when death is averted although the person concerned intended to kill himself (or herself), and *deliberate self-harm, when the harm is inflicted for reasons other than actually killing oneself. Under the Suicide Act 1961, suicide is not a criminal offence in the UK. However, it is a criminal offence for a person to aid, abet, counsel, or procure the suicide of another, although there have been a number of cases which have challenged this section of the

Act. Some have argued that doctors are in a position to make such deaths as painless as possible although physician-assisted suicide remains illegal in the UK (*see* ASSISTED SUICIDE). *See also* AUTONOMY.

sulcus *n.* (*pl.* **sulci**) **1.** one of the many clefts or infoldings of the surface of the brain. The raised outfolding on each side of a sulcus is termed a **gyrus**. **2.** any of the infoldings of soft tissue in the mouth, for example between the cheek and the alveolus.

sulfadiazine (sulphadiazine) *n.* a drug of the *sulphonamide group that is used to prevent the recurrence of rheumatic fever and (in combination with *pyrimethamine) to treat toxoplasmosis. It is administered by mouth or injection. In the form of **silver sulfadiazine** (Flamazine), it is applied as a cream to treat infected burns, leg ulcers, and pressure sores.

sulfamethoxazole (sulphamethoxazole) *n. see* CO-TRIMOXAZOLE, SULPHONAMIDE.

sulfasalazine (sulphasalazine) *n.* a drug that combines aminosalicylic acid and sulfapyridine (a drug of the *sulphonamide group), used in the treatment of ulcerative colitis, Crohn's disease, and rheumatoid arthritis (*see also* DISEASE-MODIFYING ANTIRHEUMATIC DRUG). It is given by mouth or in the form of suppositories. The most common side-effects are nausea, loss of appetite, and raised temperature. Trade name: **Salazopyrin**.

sulfinpyrazone (sulphinpyrazone) *n.* a *uricosuric drug given by mouth for the control of chronic gout. The main side-effects are nausea and abdominal pain; the drug may also activate a latent duodenal ulcer and it should not be taken by patients with impaired kidney function. Trade name: **Anturan**.

sulpha drug *see* SULPHONAMIDE.

sulphonamide (sulpha drug) *n.* one of a group of drugs, derived from sulphanilamide (a red dye), that prevent the growth of bacteria (i.e. they are bacteriostatic). Sulphonamides are effective against a variety of infections and were formerly widely used; because many of them are rapidly excreted and very soluble in the urine, they were particularly useful in treating infections of the urinary tract.

A variety of side-effects may occur with sulphonamide treatment, including nausea, vomiting, headache, and loss of appetite; more severe effects include *cyanosis, blood disorders, skin rashes, and fever. Because of increasing bacterial resistance to sulphonamides, and with the development of more effective less toxic antibiotics, the clinical use of these drugs has declined. Those still used include *sulfadiazine, *sulfasalazine, and sulfamethoxazole (combined with trimethoprim in *co-trimoxazole).

sulphone *n.* one of a group of drugs closely related to the *sulphonamides in structure and therapeutic actions. Sulphones possess powerful activity against the bacteria that cause leprosy and tuberculosis. The best known sulphone is *dapsone.

sulphonylurea *n.* one of a group of *oral hypoglycaemic drugs, derived from a *sulphonamide, that are used in the treatment of type 2 diabetes mellitus; they act by stimulating the islet cells in the pancreas to produce more insulin. The group includes *chlorpropamide, *glibenclamide, *gliclazide, and *tolbutamide. Side-effects, such as nausea, vomiting, and diarrhoea, are usually mild.

sulphur *n.* a nonmetallic element that is active against fungi and parasites. It is a constituent of ointments and other preparations used in the treatment of skin disorders (such as psoriasis).

sulphuric acid a powerful corrosive acid, H_2SO_4, widely used in industry. Swallowing the acid causes severe burning of the mouth and throat and difficulty in breathing, speaking, and swallowing. The patient should drink large quantities of milk or water or white of egg; gastric lavage should not be delayed. Skin or eye contact should be treated by flooding the area with water.

sumatriptan *n.* a *$5HT_1$ agonist that is effective in the treatment of acute *migraine and cluster headaches. It is administered by mouth, subcutaneous injection, or nasal spray. Possible side-effects include sensations of tingling and tightness, dizziness, drowsiness, fatigue, chest pain, and a rise in blood pressure. Trade name: **Imigran**.

sunburn *n.* damage to the skin by excessive exposure to the sun's rays, principally UVB (ultraviolet B), at wavelengths of 290–320 nm. Sunburn may vary from reddening of the skin to the development of large painful fluid-filled blisters, which may cause shock if they cover a large area (*see*

BURN). Fair-skinned red-haired people (Fitzpatrick skin phototype I) are more susceptible to sunburn than others. Severe sunburn in childhood is a risk factor for the development of malignant *melanoma and other skin tumours in later life.

sunitinib *n.* an inhibitor of multiple kinases (*see* PROTEIN KINASE, TYROSINE KINASE INHIBITOR) that blocks the action of *vascular endothelial growth factor. It is used for the treatment of advanced *renal cell carcinoma and of *gastrointestinal stromal tumour after disease progression or on intolerance to *imatinib. It is administered orally; its most common side-effects include fatigue, asthenia, gastrointestinal disturbances, hypertension, and bleeding. Trade name: **Sutent**.

sunstroke *n. see* HEATSTROKE.

super- *prefix denoting* 1. above; overlying. 2. extreme or excessive.

superciliary *adj.* of or relating to the eyebrows (supercilia).

superego *n.* (in psychoanalysis) the part of the mind that functions as a moral conscience or judge. It is also responsible for the formation of ideals for the *ego. The superego is the result of the incorporation of parental injunctions into the child's mind.

supererogation *n.* (in ethics) action that goes above and beyond what is morally necessary or required by duty. The extent to which an action must exceed that which is expected or required in order to be considered supererogatory is both debatable and debated. —**supererogatory** *adj.*

superfecundation *n.* the fertilization of two or more ova of the same age by spermatozoa from different males. *See* SUPERFETATION.

superfetation *n.* the fertilization of a second ovum some time after the start of pregnancy, resulting in two fetuses of different maturity in the same uterus.

superficial *adj.* (in anatomy) situated at or close to a surface. Superficial blood vessels are those close to the surface of the skin.

superinfection *n.* an infection arising during the course of another infection and caused by a different microorganism, which is usually resistant to the drugs used to treat the primary infection. The infective agent may be a normally harmless inhabitant of the body that becomes pathogenic when

other harmless types are removed by the drugs or it may be a resistant variety of the primary infective agent, such as *MRSA (*see also* METICILLIN).

superior *adj.* (in anatomy) situated uppermost in the body in relation to another structure or surface.

superior canal dehiscence syndrome (SCDS) a rare condition characterized by sound- or pressure-induced vertigo (*see* TULLIO PHENOMENON), hearing loss, *autophony, and a sense of fullness in the affected ear. It is associated with absence of the bone that normally lies over the superior *semicircular canal. Diagnosis involves computerized tomography and *vestibular evoked myogenic potential testing. Treatment involves surgery to repair the bony defect.

supernumerary *n.* (in dentistry) an additional tooth.

superovulation *n.* controlled hyperstimulation of the ovary to produce more follicles with oocytes. Usually induced by gonadotrophin preparations (e.g. *human menopausal gonadotrophin), it is performed in *in vitro fertilization and other procedures of assisted conception in order to improve the pregnancy rates. *See also* OVARIAN HYPERSTIMULATION SYNDROME.

supination *n.* the act of turning the hand so that the palm is uppermost. *Compare* PRONATION.

supinator *n.* a muscle of the forearm that extends from the elbow to the shaft of the radius. It supinates the forearm and hand.

supine *adj.* 1. lying on the back or with the face upwards. 2. of the forearm) in the position in which the palm of the hand faces upwards. *Compare* PRONE.

supine hypotension *see* AORTOCAVAL COMPRESSION.

supportive *adj.* (of treatment) aimed at reinforcing the patient's own defence mechanisms in overcoming a disease or disorder.

suppository *n.* a medicinal preparation in solid form suitable for insertion into the rectum or vagina. **Rectal suppositories** may contain simple lubricants (e.g. glycerin); drugs that act locally in the rectum or anus (e.g. corticosteroids, local anaesthetics); or drugs that are absorbed and act at other sites (e.g. analgesics, such as diclofenac). **Vaginal**

suppositories are used in the treatment of some gynaecological disorders (*see* PESSARY).

suppression *n*. **1.** the cessation or complete inhibition of any physiological activity. **2.** (in psychology) a *defence mechanism by which a person consciously and deliberately ignores an idea that is unpleasant to him.

suppressor gene a gene that prevents the expression of another (non-allelic) gene.

suppressor T cell a type of T *lymphocyte that prevents an immune response by B cells or other T cells to an antigen.

suppuration *n*. the formation of pus.

supra- *prefix denoting* above; over. Examples: **supraclavicular** (above the clavicle); **suprahyoid** (above the hyoid bone); **suprarenal** (above the kidney).

supraglottis *n*. that part of the *larynx that lies above the vocal folds and includes the *epiglottis.

supraorbital *adj*. of or relating to the area above the eye orbit.

supraorbital reflex the closing of the eyelids when the supraorbital nerve is struck, due to contraction of the muscle surrounding the orbit (orbicularis oculi muscle).

suprapubic catheter a catheter passed through the abdominal wall above the pubis, usually into a very enlarged bladder with urinary retention. Usually, suprapubic *catheterization is performed only if it is not possible to perform urethral catheterization.

supraregional specialty *see* CATCHMENT AREA.

suprarenal glands *see* ADRENAL GLANDS.

supraventricular tachycardia (SVT) a rapid regular heart beat that is usually due to a re-entry circuit between the atria and ventricles in the context of an *accessory pathway (*see* WOLFF-PARKINSON-WHITE SYNDROME). It is less commonly due to an ectopic focus in an atrium that is spontaneously discharging at a fast rate (atrial tachycardia).

supravital staining the application of a *stain to living tissue, particularly blood cells, removed from the body.

surfactant *n*. a wetting agent. **Pulmonary surfactant**, secreted by type II *pneumocytes, is a complex mixture of compounds (including lipids, protein, and carbohydrates) that prevents the air sacs (alveoli) of the lungs from collapsing by reducing surface tension. In its absence, as in the immature lungs of premature babies, *atelectasis and *respiratory distress syndrome will develop.

surgeon *n*. a qualified medical practitioner who specializes in surgery. *See* DOCTOR.

surgery *n*. the branch of medicine that treats injuries, deformities, or disease by operation or manipulation. *See also* CRYO-SURGERY, MICROSURGERY. —**surgical** *adj*.

surgical emphysema *see* EMPHYSEMA.

surgical neck the constriction of the shaft of the *humerus, below the head. It is frequently the point at which fracture of the humerus occurs.

surgical spirit methylated spirit, usually with small amounts of castor oil and oil of wintergreen: used to sterilize the skin, particularly before injections.

surrogate *n*. **1.** (in psychology) a person or object in someone's life that functions as a substitute for another person. In the treatment of sexual problems, when the patient does not have a partner to cooperate in treatment, a surrogate provided by the therapist acts as a sexual partner who gives service to the patient up to and including intercourse. According to psychoanalysts, people and objects in dreams can be surrogates for important individuals in a person's life. **2.** (in reproduction) *see* SURROGATE MOTHER.

surrogate mother a woman who becomes pregnant (by artificial insemination or embryo insertion) following an arrangement made with another party (usually a couple unable themselves to have children) in which she agrees to give the child she carries to that party when it is born. Surrogacy arrangements may be made through a specialist agency or privately and women who act as surrogates may be known or not known to the putative parents. Such an arrangement is made on the understanding that no payment is involved between either parties although reasonable expenses can be paid. Certain activities in connection with surrogacy are regulated by the Surrogacy Arrangements Act 1985: it is unlawful for any form of advertisement to be employed, and for commercial agencies to commission surrogate mothers. When the baby is born, a parental order (*see* SECTION 30 ORDER) under the *Human Fertilization and Embryology Act 1990 allows for the legal recognition of the commissioning party's parenthood status.

susceptibility *n.* vulnerability to disease. It is partly a reflection of general health and health-related behaviour but is also influenced by vaccination or other methods of increasing resistance to specific diseases.

suspensory bandage a bandage arranged to support a hanging part of the body. Examples include a sling used to hold an injured lower jaw in position and a bandage used to support the scrotum in various conditions of the male genital organs.

suspensory ligament a ligament that serves to support or suspend an organ in position. For example, the suspensory ligament of the lens is a fibrous structure attached to the ciliary processes (*see* CILIARY BODY) by means of which the lens of the eye is held in position.

sustentaculum *n.* any anatomical structure that supports another structure. —**sustentacular** *adj.*

Sutent *n. see* SUNITINIB.

suture **1.** *n.* (in anatomy) a type of immovable joint, found particularly in the skull, that is characterized by a minimal amount of connective tissue between the two bones. The cranial sutures include the **coronal suture**, between the frontal and parietal bones; the **lambdoidal suture**, between the parietal and occipital bones; and the **sagittal suture**, between the two parietal bones (see illustration). **2.** *n.* (in surgery) the closure of a

wound or incision to facilitate the healing process, using any of various materials. A wide variety of suturing techniques have been developed to meet the differing circumstances of injuries to and incisions in the body tissues (see illustration). **3.** *n.* the material – silk, catgut, nylon, any of various polymers, or wire – used to sew up a wound. **4.** *vb.* to close a wound by suture.

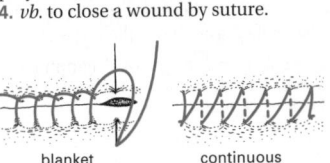
blanket   continuous

(skin)

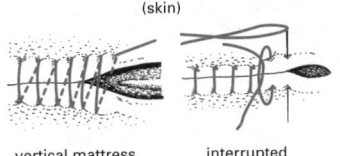
vertical mattress   interrupted

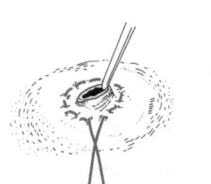
purse string (intestine)

Suture. Types of surgical suturing.

suxamethonium *n.* a depolarizing *muscle relaxant. It is administered by intravenous or intramuscular routes to produce rapid muscle relaxation for a brief period during surgery carried out under general anaesthesia. Trade name: **Anectine**.

Suzi *n. see* SUBZONAL INSEMINATION.

SVT *see* SUPRAVENTRICULAR TACHYCARDIA.

swab *n.* a pad of absorbent material (such as cotton), sometimes attached to a stick or wire, used for cleaning out or applying medication to wounds, operation sites, or body cavities. In operations, gauze swabs are used to clean blood from the site; such swabs are always carefully counted and contain a *radiopaque 'tag' to facilitate identification

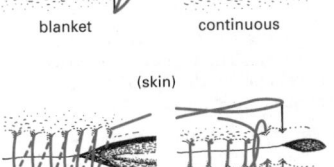
frontal bone
coronal suture
sagittal suture
parietal bone
lambdoidal suture
occipital bone

Suture. Sutures of the skull (internal surface of the vault).

should it by mischance remain in the body after operation.

swallowing (deglutition) *n.* the process by which food is transferred from the mouth to the oesophagus (gullet). Voluntary raising of the tongue forces food backwards towards the pharynx. This stimulates reflex actions in which the larynx is closed by the epiglottis and the nasal passages are closed by the soft palate, so that food does not enter the trachea (windpipe). Lastly, food moves down the oesophagus by *peristalsis and gravity.

Swan-Ganz catheter a catheter with an inflatable balloon at its tip, which can be inserted into the pulmonary artery via the right chambers of the heart. Inflation of the balloon enables indirect measurement of pressure in the left atrium. [H. J. C. Swan (1922–2005), US cardiologist; W. Ganz (20th century), US engineer]

sweat *n.* the watery fluid secreted by the *sweat glands. Its principal constituents in solution are sodium chloride and urea. The secretion of sweat is a means of excreting nitrogenous waste; at the same time it has a role in controlling the temperature of the body – the evaporation of sweat from the surface of the skin has a cooling effect. Therefore an increase in body temperature causes an increase in sweating. Other factors that increase the secretion of sweat include pain, nausea, nervousness, and drugs (*diaphoretics). Sweating is reduced by colds, diarrhoea, and certain drugs. Anatomical name: **sudor**.

sweat gland a simple coiled tubular *exocrine gland that lies in the dermis of the *skin. A long duct carries its secretion (*sweat) to the surface of the skin. Sweat glands occur over most of the surface of the body; they are particularly abundant in the armpits, on the soles of the feet and palms of the hands, and on the forehead.

swine influenza a disease of domesticated pigs, first seen in humans in early 2009, caused by H1N1, a strain of *influenza A virus. Very contagious, the World Health Organization has now declared it to be a pandemic strain in humans. Swine influenza is currently believed not to be as virulent as *avian influenza and it seems to be less severe than the virulent 1918 pandemic, with which it shares antigenic features.

sycosis *n.* inflammation of the hair follicles caused by infection with *Staphylococcus au-*

reus; it commonly affects the beard area (**sycosis barbae**) of men in their thirties or forties. The infection usually spreads unless treated by applying antibiotic ointments or giving antibiotics by mouth.

Sydenham's chorea a form of *chorea that mainly affects children and adolescents, especially females. It can occur some months after an infection caused by β-haemolytic streptococci (such as rheumatic fever or scarlet fever), causing uncontrolled movements of the muscles of the shoulders, hips, and face (hence the archaic name, **St Vitus' dance**). Formerly a frightening disease, it is now readily cured by antibiotics. [G. Sydenham (1624–89), English physician]

Symbicort *n. see* BUDESONIDE.

symbiosis *n.* an intimate and obligatory association between two different species of organism (**symbionts**) in which there is mutual aid and benefit. *Compare* COMMENSAL, MUTUALISM, PARASITE.

symblepharon *n.* a condition in which the eyelid adheres to the eyeball. It is usually the result of chemical (especially alkali) burns to the conjunctiva lining the eyelid and eyeball.

symbolism *n.* (in psychology) the process of representing an object or an idea by something else. Typically an abstract idea is represented by a simpler and more tangible image. Psychoanalytic theorists hold that conscious ideas frequently act as symbols for unconscious thoughts and that this is particularly evident in dreaming, in *free association, and in the formation of psychological symptoms. According to this theory, a symptom (such as difficulty in swallowing) might be a symbolic representation of an unconscious idea (such as a fantasy of oral intercourse). —**symbolic** *adj.*

symmelia *n. see* SIRENOMELIA.

symmetry *n.* (in anatomy) correspondence of form on either side of a plane or axis. Human bodies are symmetrical around the *sagittal plane.

sympathectomy *n.* the surgical *division of sympathetic nerve fibres. It is done to minimize the effects of normal or excessive sympathetic activity. Most often it is used to improve the circulation to part of the body; less commonly to inhibit excess sweating or to relieve the *photophobia induced by an abnormally dilated pupil of the eye.

sympathetic nervous system one of the two divisions of the *autonomic nervous system, having fibres that leave the central nervous system, via a chain of ganglia close to the spinal cord, in the thoracic and lumbar regions. Its nerves are distributed to the blood vessels, heart, lungs, intestines and other abdominal organs, sweat glands, salivary glands, and the genitals, whose functions it governs by reflex action, in balance with the *parasympathetic nervous system.

sympathin *n.* the name given by early physiologists to the substances released from sympathetic nerve endings, now known to be a mixture of *adrenaline and *noradrenaline.

sympathoblast *n.* one of the small cells formed in the early development of nerve tissue that eventually become the neurons of the sympathetic nervous system.

sympatholytic *adj.* opposing the effects of the sympathetic nervous system. *Guanethidine blocks the transmission of impulses along adrenergic nerves; it is used to treat high blood pressure. *Alpha blockers and *beta blockers are other kinds of sympatholytic drugs.

sympathomimetic *adj.* having the effect of stimulating the *sympathetic nervous system. The actions of sympathomimetic drugs are **adrenergic**: they act on alpha or beta *adrenoceptors. **Alpha-adrenergic stimulants** (**alpha agonists**) stimulate alpha receptors. They include *vasoconstrictors (e.g. *ephedrine, *phenylephrine, *metaraminol), used to treat nasal congestion and severe hypotension, and the selective α_2 agonists *apraclonidine and *brimonidine, which are used in the treatment of glaucoma. **Beta-adrenergic stimulants** (**beta agonists**) stimulate β_1 and/or β_2 adrenoceptors. β_2 agonists such as *salbutamol, *salmeterol, and *terbutaline relax bronchial smooth muscle and are used as *bronchodilators. Other β_2 agonists, including **ritodrine** (Yutopar), relax uterine muscle and are used in the treatment of premature labour (*see* TOCOLYTIC). β_1 agonists (e.g. *dobutamine) stimulate β_1 receptors in the heart and are therefore used for their *inotropic effects.

sympathy *n.* (in physiology) a reciprocal influence exercised by different parts of the body on one another.

symphyseal fundal height (SFH) a clinical assessment of fetal growth by measurement of the distance between the maternal pubic symphysis and uterine *fundus. This test has a low *sensitivity and high false-positive rate with significant inter- and intra-observer variation, and alone is unsuitable for diagnosis. If *intrauterine growth restriction is suspected, it is necessary to supplement this measurement with ultrasound biometric tests.

symphysiotomy *n.* the operation of cutting through the front of the pelvis at the pubic *symphysis in order to enlarge the diameter of the pelvis and aid delivery of a fetus whose head is too large to pass through the pelvic opening. This procedure is now rarely employed.

symphysis *n.* **1.** a joint in which the bones are separated by fibrocartilage, which minimizes movement and makes the bony structure rigid. Examples are the **pubic symphysis** (the joint between the pubic bones of the pelvis) and the joints of the backbone, which are separated by intervertebral discs (see illustration). **2.** the line that marks the fusion of two bones that were separate at an early stage of development, such as the symphysis of the *mandible. —**symphyseal** *adj.*

posterior longitudinal ligament — anterior longitudinal ligament

adjacent vertebrae

intervertebral disc

Symphysis between two vertebrae.

sympodia *n. see* SIRENOMELIA.

symptom *n.* an indication of a disease or disorder noticed by the patient himself. A **presenting symptom** is one that leads a patient to consult a doctor. *Compare* SIGN.

symptomatology (**semeiology**) *n.* **1.** the branch of medicine concerned with the study of symptoms of disease. **2.** the symptoms of a disease, collectively.

syn- (sym-) *prefix denoting* union or fusion.

synaesthesia *n.* a condition in which a secondary subjective sensation (often colour) is experienced at the same time as the sensory response normally evoked by the stimulus. For example, the sound of the word 'cat' might evoke the colour purple.

synalgia *n. see* REFERRED PAIN.

synapse *n.* the minute gap across which *nerve impulses pass from one neuron to the next, at the end of a nerve fibre. Reaching a synapse, an impulse causes the release of a *neurotransmitter, which diffuses across the gap and triggers an electrical impulse in the next neuron. Some brain cells have more than 15,000 synapses. *See also* NEUROMUSCULAR JUNCTION.

synarthrosis *n.* an immovable joint in which the bones are united by fibrous tissue. Examples are the cranial *sutures. *See also* GOMPHOSIS, SCHINDYLESIS.

synchilia (syncheilia) *n.* congenital fusion of the lips.

synchondrosis *n.* a slightly movable joint (*see* AMPHIARTHROSIS) in which the surfaces of the bones are separated by hyaline cartilage, as occurs between the ribs and sternum. This cartilage may become ossified in later development, as between the *epiphyses and shaft of a long bone.

synchronized cardioversion *see* CARDIOVERSION.

synchysis scintillans (asteroid hyalosis) tiny refractile crystals of cholesterol suspended in the vitreous humour of the eye. They usually cause no symptoms.

syncope (fainting) *n.* loss of consciousness due to a sudden drop in blood pressure, resulting in a temporarily insufficient flow of blood to the brain. It commonly occurs in otherwise healthy people and may be caused by an emotional shock, by standing for prolonged periods, or by injury and profuse bleeding. Recovery is normally prompt and without any persisting ill-effects. *See also* NEUROCARDIOGENIC SYNCOPE.

syncytiotrophoblast *n. see* TROPHOBLAST.

syncytium *n.* (*pl.* **syncytia**) a mass of *protoplasm containing several nuclei. Muscle fibres are syncytia. —**syncytial** *adj.*

syndactyly *n.* congenital webbing of the fingers. Adjacent fingers are joined along part or all of their length. They may be joined only by skin, or the bones of the fingers may be joined. Treatment is surgical separation of the fingers, and skin grafts may be required.

syndesm- (syndesmo-) *combining form denoting* connective tissue, particularly ligaments.

syndesmology *n.* the branch of anatomy dealing with joints and their components.

syndesmophyte *n.* a vertical outgrowth of bone from a vertebra, seen in ankylosing *spondylitis, *Reiter's syndrome, and *psoriatic arthritis. Fusion of syndesmophytes across the joints between vertebrae contributes to rigidity of the spine, seen in advanced cases of these diseases.

syndesmosis *n.* an immovable joint in which the bones are separated by connective tissue. An example is the articulation between the bases of the tibia and fibula (see illustration).

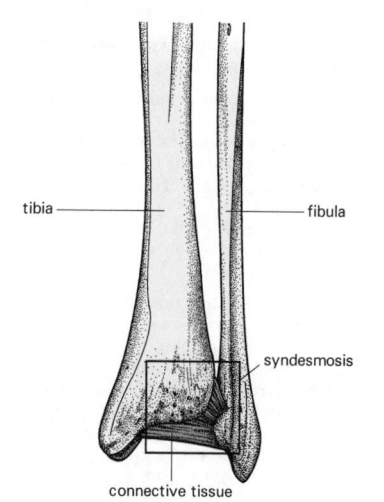

A syndesmosis.

syndrome *n.* a combination of signs and/or symptoms that forms a distinct clinical picture indicative of a particular disorder.

syndrome of inappropriate secretion of antidiuretic hormone (SIADH) a condition of inappropriately high plasma levels of ADH (*see* VASOPRESSIN) with associated water retention, dilutional *hyponatraemia, and the production of highly concentrated urine. Renal, adrenal, thyroid, and hepatic function are normal, as is the volume of circulating blood (euvolaemia). It is caused by a variety of pathological conditions, usually intrathoracic and intracerebral, and also by a number of drugs, including antidepressants, chemotherapy agents, and some of the older antidiabetic agents. The treatment involves fluid restriction, treatment (or removal) of the underlying cause (or drug), and, in severe cases, administration of *demeclocycline to reduce the effects of ADH on the kidney. Very rarely, hypertonic saline is given.

syndrome X *see* METABOLIC SYNDROME.

synechia *n.* (*pl.* **synechiae**) an adhesion between the iris and another part of the eye. An **anterior synechia** is between the iris and the endothelium of the cornea or the part of the sclera that normally hides the extreme outer edge of the iris from view. A **posterior synechia** is between the iris and the lens.

synechialysis *n.* surgical division or separation of *synechiae.

syneresis *n.* 1. contraction of a blood clot. When first formed, a blood clot is a loose meshwork of fibres containing various blood cells. Over a period of time this contracts, producing a firm mass that seals the damaged blood vessels. 2. (in ophthalmology) degenerative shrinkage of the vitreous humour due to ageing, which usually results in a *vitreous detachment.

synergist *n.* 1. a drug that interacts with another to produce increased activity, which is greater than the sum of the effects of the two drugs given separately. Some synergists may have dangerous effects, as when MAO inhibitors enhance the effects of antihistamine and antimuscarinic drugs. 2. a muscle that acts with an *agonist in making a particular movement. —**synergism** *n.*

synergistic gangrene gangrene of tissues produced by different bacteria acting together, usually a mixture of aerobic and anaerobic organisms. Particular forms are **Meleney's gangrene** (of the abdominal wall) and **Fournier's gangrene** (of the scrotal area). Synergistic gangrene has a pronounced tendency to spread along fascial planes, causing *necrotizing fasciitis.

syngeneic *adj.* describing grafted tissue

that is genetically identical to the recipient's tissue, as when the donor and recipient are identical twins.

synoptophore *n. see* AMBLYOSCOPE.

synostosis *n.* the joining by ossification of two adjacent bones. It occurs, for example, at the *sutures between the bones of the skull.

synovectomy *n.* surgical removal of the synovium of a joint. This is performed in cases of chronic synovitis, such as rheumatoid arthritis, when other measures have been ineffective, in order to reduce pain in the joint and prevent further destruction.

synovia (synovial fluid) *n.* the thick colourless lubricating fluid that surrounds a joint or a bursa and fills a tendon sheath. It is secreted by the synovial membrane.

synovial joint *see* DIARTHROSIS.

synovial membrane (synovium) the membrane, composed of mesothelium and connective tissue, that forms the sac enclosing a freely movable joint (*see* DIARTHROSIS). It secretes the lubricating synovial fluid.

synovioma *n.* a benign or malignant tumour of the synovial membrane. Benign synoviomas occur on tendon sheaths; malignant synoviomas (**synovial sarcomas**) may occur where synovial tissue is not normally found, e.g. in the oesophagus.

synovitis *n.* inflammation of the membrane (synovium) that lines a joint capsule, resulting in pain and swelling (arthritis). It is caused by injury, infection, or rheumatic disease. Treatment depends on the underlying cause; to determine this, samples of the synovial fluid or membrane are taken for examination.

synovium *n. see* SYNOVIAL MEMBRANE.

Syntometrine *n. see* ERGOMETRINE.

syphilide (syphilid) *n.* the skin rash that appears in the second stage of *syphilis, usually two months to two years after primary infection. Syphilides occur in crops that may last from a few days to several months. They denote a highly infectious stage of the disease.

syphilis *n.* a sexually transmitted disease caused by the bacterium *Treponema pallidum*, resulting in the formation of lesions throughout the body. Bacteria usually enter the body during sexual intercourse, through the mucous membranes of the vagina or urethra, but they may rarely be transmitted through wounds in the skin or scratches. Bacteria may also pass from an infected pregnant woman across the placenta to the developing fetus, resulting in the disease being present at birth (**congenital syphilis**).

The primary symptom – a hard painless ulcer (*chancre) at the site of infection – forms 2–4 weeks after exposure. Neighbouring lymph nodes enlarge about two weeks later. Secondary stage symptoms appear about two months after infection and include fever, malaise, general enlargement of lymph nodes, and a faint red rash on the chest that persists for 1–2 weeks. After months, or even years, the disease enters its tertiary stage with widespread formation of tumour-like masses (*gummas). Tertiary syphilis may cause serious damage to the heart and blood vessels (**cardiovascular syphilis**) or to the brain and spinal cord (**neurosyphilis**), resulting in *tabes dorsalis, blindness, and *general paralysis of the insane.

Treatment is with antibiotics, such as penicillin and doxycycline. Syphilis can be diagnosed by several blood tests. *Compare* BEJEL. —**syphilitic** *adj.*

syring- (syringo-) *combining form denoting* a tube or long cavity, especially the central canal of the spinal cord.

syringe *n.* an instrument consisting of a piston in a tight-fitting tube that is attached to a hollow needle or thin tube. A syringe is used to give injections, remove material from a part of the body, or to wash out a cavity, such as the ear canal.

syringobulbia *n. see* SYRINGOMYELIA.

syringoma *n.* multiple benign tumours of the sweat glands, which show as small hard swellings usually on the face (especially around the eyes), neck, or chest. Treatment is difficult.

syringomyelia *n.* a disease of the spinal cord in which longitudinal cavities form within the cord, usually in the cervical (neck) region. The centrally situated cavity (**syrinx**) is especially likely to damage the motor nerve cells and the nerve fibres that transmit the sensations of pain and temperature. Characteristically there is weakness and

wasting of the muscles in the hands with a loss of awareness of pain and temperature. An extension of the cavitation into the lower brainstem is called **syringobulbia**. Cerebellar *ataxia, a partial loss of pain sensation in the face, and weakness of the tongue and palate may occur. Syringomyelia is associated with an *Arnold-Chiari malformation and tumours of the spinal cord.

system *n.* (in anatomy) a group of organs and tissues associated with a particular physiological function, such as the *nervous system or *respiratory system.

systemic *adj.* relating to or affecting the body as a whole, rather than individual parts and organs.

systemic circulation the system of blood vessels that supplies all parts of the body except the lungs. It consists of the aorta and all its branches, carrying oxygenated blood to the tissues, and all the veins draining deoxygenated blood into the vena cava. *Compare* PULMONARY CIRCULATION.

systemic sclerosis a rare connective-tissue disease affecting many systems in the body, mainly in women (3–6:1) in their forties. Genetic and autoimmune factors are implicated. In the diffuse form of the disease, besides *scleroderma, there may be involvement of the lungs, with pulmonary *fibrosis; renal failure and gastrointestinal and myocardial disease also occur. The limited form is also called *CREST syndrome.

systole *n.* the period of the cardiac cycle during which the heart contracts. The term usually refers to **ventricular systole**, which lasts about 0.3 seconds. **Atrial systole** lasts about 0.1 seconds. —**systolic** *adj.*

systolic anterior motion (SAM) the state of the *mitral valve when it is abnormally pulled forward during ventricular contraction, a characteristic feature of *hypertrophic cardiomyopathy.

systolic dysfunction impairment of heart function due to reduced contraction of the left *ventricle. It is most commonly secondary to *cardiomyopathy or *myocardial infarction and may result in heart failure. *Compare* DIASTOLIC DYSFUNCTION.

systolic pressure *see* BLOOD PRESSURE.

T₃ T_3 *see* TRIIODOTHYRONINE.

T₄ T_4 *see* THYROXINE.

tabes dorsalis (locomotor ataxia) a form of neurosyphilis occurring 5–20 years after the original sexually transmitted infection. The infecting organisms progressively destroy the sensory nerves. Severe stabbing pains in the legs and trunk, an unsteady gait, and loss of bladder control are common. Some patients have blurred vision caused by damage to the optic nerves. Penicillin is used to arrest the progression of this illness. *See also* SYPHILIS, GENERAL PARALYSIS OF THE INSANE.

tablet *n.* (in pharmacy) a small disc containing one or more drugs, made by compressing a powdered form of the drug(s). It is usually taken by mouth but may be inserted into a body cavity (*see* SUPPOSITORY).

tabo-paresis *n.* a late effect of syphilitic infection of the nervous system in which the patient shows features of *tabes dorsalis and *general paralysis of the insane.

TAB vaccine a combined vaccine used to produce immunity against the diseases typhoid, paratyphoid A, and paratyphoid B.

tachy- *combining form denoting* fast; rapid.

tachyarrhythmia *n. see* ARRHYTHMIA.

tachycardia *n.* an increase in the heart rate above normal. **Sinus tachycardia** may occur normally with exercise or excitement or it may be due to illness, such as fever. *Arrhythmias may also produce tachycardia (**ectopic tachycardia**). *See* VENTRICULAR TACHYCARDIA, SUPRAVENTRICULAR TACHYCARDIA.

tachyphylaxis *n.* a falling-off in the effects produced by a drug during continuous use or constantly repeated administration, common in drugs that act on the nervous system.

tachypnoea *n.* rapid breathing.

tacrolimus *n.* a powerful *immunosuppressant administered orally or by intravenous infusion to prevent rejection of transplanted organs. Side-effects include gastrointestinal disturbances, tremor, headache, and liver and kidney impairment; it may have adverse effects on the heart. It is also used, in the form of an ointment, for the treatment for atopic *eczema. Trade names: **Advagraf, Prograf, Protopic**.

tactile *adj.* relating to or affecting the sense of touch.

tadalafil *n. see* SILDENAFIL.

taenia *n.* (*pl.* **taeniae**) a flat ribbon-like anatomical structure. The **taeniae coli** are the longitudinal ribbon-like muscles of the colon.

Taenia *n.* a genus of large tapeworms, some of which are parasites of the human intestine. The 4–10 m long beef tapeworm, *T. saginata*, is the commonest tapeworm parasite of humans. Its larval stage (*see* CYSTICERCUS) develops within the muscles of cattle and other ruminants, and people become infected on eating raw or undercooked beef. *T. solium*, the pork tapeworm, is 2–7 m long. Its larval stage may develop not only in pigs but also in humans, in whom it may cause serious disease (*see* CYSTICERCOSIS). *See also* TAENIASIS.

taeniacide (taenicide) *n.* an agent that kills tapeworms.

taeniafuge *n.* an agent, such as *niclosamide, that eliminates tapeworms from the body of their host.

taeniasis *n.* an infestation with tapeworms of the genus *Taenia*. Humans become infected with the adult worms following ingestion of raw or undercooked meat containing the larval stage of the parasite. The presence of a worm in the intestine may occasionally give rise to increased appetite, hunger pains, weakness, and weight loss. Worms are expelled from the intestine using various anthelmintics, including *niclosamide. *See also* CYSTICERCOSIS.

Tagamet *n. see* CIMETIDINE.

Takayasu's disease (pulseless disease) progressive occlusion of the arteries arising from the arch of the aorta (including those to the arms and neck), resulting in the absence of pulses in the arms and neck. Symptoms include attacks of unconsciousness (syncope), paralysis of facial muscles, and transient blindness, due to an inadequate supply of blood to the head. [M. Takayasu (1860–1938), Japanese ophthalmologist]

takotsubo syndrome sudden extensive damage to the left *ventricle that classically occurs following acute emotional shock. The clinical syndrome mimics acute *myocardial infarction, but no coronary artery is occluded and the extent of ventricular damage exceeds that supplied by any single coronary artery. The appearance of the left ventriculogram resembles a Japanese lobster pot, from which the name derives. The cause is unknown, and in most cases spontaneous recovery occurs.

tal- (talo-) *combining form denoting* the ankle bone (talus).

talc *n.* a soft white powder, consisting of magnesium silicate, used in dusting powders and skin applications. Talc used to dust surgical rubber gloves causes irritation of serous membranes, resulting in adhesions, if not washed off prior to an operation.

talipes *n. see* CLUB-FOOT.

talus (astragalus) *n.* the ankle bone. It forms part of the *tarsus, articulating with the tibia above, with the fibula to the lateral (outer) side, and with the calcaneus below.

tambour *n.* a recording drum consisting of an elastic membrane stretched over one end of a cylinder. It is used in various instruments for recording changes in air pressure.

Tamiflu *n. see* OSELTAMIVIR.

tamoxifen *n.* a drug used in the treatment of *breast cancer: it binds with hormone receptors in the tumour to inhibit the effect of oestrogens (*see* ANTI-OESTROGEN, SELECTIVE (O)ESTROGEN RECEPTOR MODULATOR). Tamoxifen is also used to treat female infertility as it induces ovulation. The drug is administered by mouth; side-effects include nausea, vaginal bleeding, facial flushing, tumour pain, and hypercalcaemia. Trade name: **Nolvadex-D**.

tampon *n.* a pack of gauze, cotton wool, or other absorbent material used to plug a cavity or canal in order to absorb blood or secre-tions. A vaginal tampon is commonly used by women to absorb the menstrual flow.

tamponade *n.* **1.** the insertion of a tampon. **2.** abnormal pressure on a part of the body; for example, as caused by the presence of excessive fluid between the pericardium (sac surrounding the heart) and the heart. *See* CARDIAC TAMPONADE.

tamsulosin *n.* a highly selective *alpha blocker taken by mouth to treat *lower urinary tract symptoms thought to be due to benign prostatic hyperplasia (*see* PROSTATE GLAND). Side-effects include retrograde ejaculation that is reversible on stopping the drug. Trade name: **Flomaxtra XL**.

tantalum *n.* a rare heavy metal used in surgery as it is easily moulded and does not corrode. For example, tantalum sutures and plates are used for repair of defects in the bones of the skull. Symbol: Ta.

tapetum *n.* **1.** a layer of specialized reflecting cells in the *choroid behind the retina of the eye. **2.** a band of nerve fibres that form the roof and wall of the lower posterior part of the *corpus callosum.

tapeworm (cestode) *n.* any of a group of flatworms that have a long thin ribbon-like body and live as parasites in the intestines of humans and other vertebrates. The body of a tapeworm consists of a head (**scolex**), a short neck, and a **strobila** made up of a chain of separate segments (**proglottides**). Mature proglottides, full of eggs, are released from the free end of the worm and pass out in the host's stools. Eggs are then ingested by an intermediate host, in whose tissues the larval stages develop (*see* PLEROCERCOID, CYSTICERCUS, HYDATID). Humans are the primary hosts for some tapeworms (*see* TAENIA, HYMENOLEPIS). However, other genera are also medically important (*see* DIPHYLLOBOTHRIUM, DIPYLIDIUM, ECHINOCOCCUS).

tapotement *n.* a technique used in *massage in which a part of the body is struck rapidly and repeatedly with the hands. Tapotement of the chest wall in bronchitic patients often helps to loosen mucus within the air passages so that it can be coughed up.

tapping *n. see* PARACENTESIS.

tardive dyskinesia a condition characterized by involuntary repetitive movements of the facial muscles and the tongue, usually resembling continued chewing motions, and the muscles of the limbs. It is associated with long-term medication with certain antipsychotic drugs, especially the *phenothiazines, and occurs predominantly in older patients.

target cell 1. a cell that is the focus of attack by antibodies, cytotoxic T cells, or natural killer cells or is the object of the action of a specific hormone. 2. (in haematology) an abnormal form of red blood cell (*erythrocyte) in which the cell assumes the ringed appearance of a 'target' in stained blood films. Target cells are a feature of several types of anaemia, including those due to iron deficiency, liver disease, and abnormalities in haemoglobin structure.

targeted agent (**targeted therapy**) a drug that interferes with specific molecular targets in the pathways involved in cancer cell growth and signalling, in contrast to *cytotoxic drugs that act primarily on rapidly dividing cells. It typically requires prolonged courses of treatment, and the anticancer action can be synergistic with chemotherapy. Many new drugs are being developed and are undergoing trials to determine optimal use. The *tyrosine kinase inhibitors include imatinib and *epidermal growth factor receptor inhibitors; multitargeted agents include *sorafenib and *sunitinib. The monoclonal antibodies include *rituximab, *trastuzumab, *cetuximab, and *bevacizumab.

target lesions *see* ERYTHEMA (MULTIFORME).

target organ the specific organ or tissue upon which a hormone, drug, or other substance acts.

tars- (tarso-) *combining form denoting* 1. the ankle; tarsal bones. 2. the edge of the eyelid.

tarsal 1. *adj.* relating to the bones of the ankle and foot (*tarsus). 2. *adj.* relating to the eyelid, especially to its supporting tissue (tarsus). 3. *n.* any of the bones forming the tarsus.

tarsalgia *n.* aching pain arising from the tarsus in the foot.

tarsal glands *see* MEIBOMIAN GLANDS.

tarsectomy *n.* 1. surgical excision of the tarsal bones of the foot. 2. surgical removal of a section of the tarsus of the eyelid.

tarsitis *n.* inflammation of the eyelid.

tarsoplasty *n. see* BLEPHAROPLASTY.

tarsorrhaphy *n.* an operation in which the upper and lower eyelids are joined together, either completely or along part of their length. It is performed to protect the cornea or to allow a corneal injury to heal.

tarsus *n.* (*pl.* **tarsi**) 1. the seven bones of the ankle and proximal part of the foot (see illustration). The tarsus articulates with the metatarsals distally and with the tibia and fibula proximally. 2. the firm fibrous connective tissue that forms the basis of each eyelid.

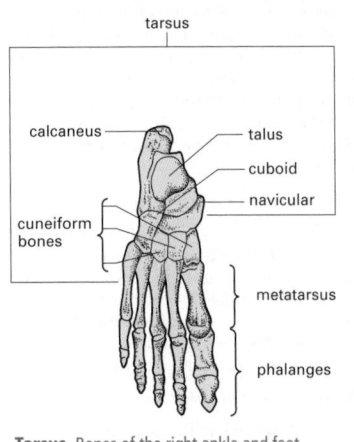

Tarsus. Bones of the right ankle and foot.

tartar *n.* an obsolete name for *calculus, the hard deposit that forms on the teeth.

taste *n.* the sense for the appreciation of the flavour of substances in the mouth. The sense organs responsible are the *taste buds on the surface of the *tongue, which are stimulated when food dissolves in the saliva in the mouth. It is generally held that there are four basic taste sensations – sweet, bitter, sour, and salt – but two others – alkaline and metallic – are sometimes added to this list.

taste buds the sensory receptors concerned with the sense of taste (see illustration). They are located in the epithelium that covers the surface of the *tongue, lying in the grooves around the papillae, particularly the circumvallate papillae. Taste buds are also present in the soft palate, the epiglottis, and parts of the pharynx. When a taste cell is stimulated by the presence of a dissolved substance impulses are sent via nerve fibres to the brain. From the anterior two-thirds of the tongue impulses pass via the facial nerve. The taste buds in the posterior third of the tongue send impulses via the glossopharyngeal nerve.

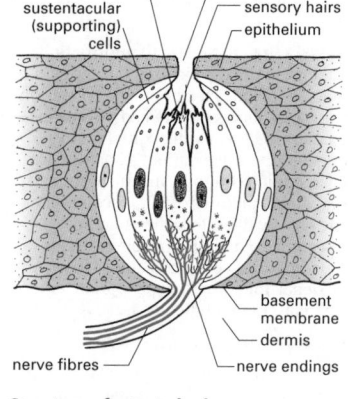

gustatory cells — pore
sustentacular (supporting) cells — sensory hairs
— epithelium
— basement membrane
— dermis
nerve fibres — — nerve endings

Structure of a taste bud.

taurine *n.* an amino acid that is a constituent of the *bile salt taurocholate and also functions as a *neurotransmitter in the central nervous system.

taurocholic acid *see* BILE ACIDS.

taxane *n.* any of a group of *cytotoxic drugs formerly extracted from a species of yew tree (*Taxus*) but now synthesized or produced by biotechnological methods. These drugs interact with tubulin, a protein involved in cell division, and have been found to exercise control on the growth of certain cancers, particularly breast and ovarian tumours. Taxanes include *docetaxel and *paclitaxel.

taxis *n.* (in surgery) the returning to a normal position of displaced bones, organs, or other parts by manipulation only, unaided by mechanical devices.

Taxol *n.* see PACLITAXEL.

Taxotere *n.* see DOCETAXEL.

Tay-Sachs disease (amaurotic familial idiocy) an inherited disorder of lipid metabolism (*see* LIPIDOSIS) in which abnormal accumulation of lipid in the brain leads to blindness, mental retardation, and death in infancy. The gene responsible for the disorder is *recessive, and the disease can now be largely prevented by genetic counselling in communities known to be affected (primarily Ashkenazi Jewish communities). [W. Tay (1843–1927), British physician; B. Sachs (1858–1944), US neurologist]

tazarotene *n.* see RETINOID.

TCC transabdominal cervical cerclage: *see* CERVICAL CERCLAGE.

T cell *n.* see LYMPHOCYTE, CYTOTOXIC T CELL, HELPER T CELL, REGULATORY T CELL, SUPPRESSOR T CELL.

TCP *Trade name.* a solution of halogenated *phenols: an effective *antiseptic for minor skin injuries and irritations. It may also be used as a gargle for colds and sore throats.

TCR T-cell receptor: an important component of the surface of T *lymphocytes, by which antigen is recognized.

TCRE *see* TRANSCERVICAL RESECTION OF THE ENDOMETRIUM.

Td/IPV a booster vaccine given to children between the ages of 13 and 18 years to top up immunity against tetanus, diphtheria, and polio. *See* IMMUNIZATION.

tear gas any of the several kinds of gas used in warfare and by the police to produce temporary incapacitation. Most tear gases produce stinging pain in the eyes and streaming from the eyes and nose. *See also* CS GAS.

tears *pl. n.* the fluid secreted by the lacrimal glands (*see* LACRIMAL APPARATUS) to keep the front of the eyeballs moist and clean. Tears contain *lysozyme, an enzyme that destroys bacteria. Irritation of the eye, and sometimes emotion, cause excessive production of tears. *See also* BLINKING.

technetium-99m *n.* an isotope of the artificial radioactive element technetium. It emits gamma radiation only, with no beta particles, at a convenient energy for detection by a *gamma camera and has a short half-life. For these reasons it is widely used in nuclear medicine as a *tracer for the examination of many organs (*see* SCINTIGRAM). Symbol: Tc-99m.

tectospinal tract a tract that conveys nerve impulses from the midbrain, across the midline as it descends, to the spinal cord in the cervical (neck) region. It contains important *motor neurons.

tectum *n.* the roof of the *midbrain, behind and above the *cerebral aqueduct. From the nerve tissue protrude two pairs of rounded swellings called the **superior** and **inferior colliculi**, which contain cells concerned with reflexes involving vision and hearing, respectively.

teeth *pl. n. see* TOOTH.

tegafur/uracil *see* FLUOROPYRIMIDINE, FLUOROURACIL.

tegmen *n.* (*pl.* **tegmina**) a structure that covers an organ or part of an organ. For example the **tegmen tympani** is the bony roof of the middle ear.

tegmentum *n.* the region of the *midbrain below and in front of the *cerebral aqueduct. It contains the nuclei of several cranial nerves, the *reticular formation, and other ascending and descending nerve pathways linking the forebrain and the spinal cord.

teichopsia *n.* shimmering coloured lights, accompanied by blank spots in the visual field (**transient scotomata**), often seen by sufferers at the beginning of an attack of migraine.

tel- (tele-, telo-) *combining form denoting* 1. end or ending. 2. distance.

tela *n.* any thin weblike tissue, particularly the **tela choroidea**, a folded double layer of *pia mater containing numerous small blood vessels that extends into several of the *ventricles of the brain.

telangiectasis *n.* (*pl.* **telangiectases**) a localized collection of distended blood capillary vessels. It is recognized as a red spot, sometimes spidery in appearance (*see* SPIDER NAEVUS), that blanches on pressure. Telangiectases may be found in the skin or the lining of the mouth or in the gastrointestinal, respiratory, and urinary tracts. The condition in which multiple telangiectases occur is termed **telangiectasia**. It may be seen as an inherited condition associated with a bleeding tendency (**hereditary haemorrhagic telangiectasia**: *see* OSLER-RENDU-WEBER DISEASE). Accessible bleeding telangiectases (e.g. in the nose) may be obliterated by cauterization.

telangiitis *n.* inflammation of the smallest blood vessels (*see* VASCULITIS).

teleceptor *n.* a sensory *receptor that is capable of responding to distant stimuli. An example is the eye, which is capable of de-

tecting changes and events at a great distance, unlike touch receptors, which depend on close contact.

telegony *n.* the unsubstantiated theory that mating with one male has an effect on the offspring of later matings with other males.

telemedicine *n.* the use of information technology in the diagnosis and treatment of patients. It includes telephone conversations between physicians or between physicians and patients; tele- or videoconferencing among members of a patient's health-care team; and **telepathology**, in which (for example) digital pictures of microscope slides can be sent by the Internet to a pathologist for a second opinion. Using telemedicine, a paramedic can access a consultant in an A and E department for the appropriate emergency treatment in difficult cases.

telencephalon *n. see* CEREBRUM.

teleradiology *n.* the process of transmitting and receiving medical images, to and from distant sites, using the telephone (or cable or satellite) network. This requires a dedicated broad-band link, such as an ISDN line, that has greater capacity for data transfer than standard telephone lines.

teletherapy (external beam radiotherapy) *n.* a form of *radiotherapy in which penetrating radiation is directed at a patient from a distance. Originally radium was used as the radiation source; today artificially produced X-rays are predominantly used. *See* LINEAR ACCELERATOR.

telmisartan *n. see* ANGIOTENSIN II ANTAGONIST.

telocentric *n.* a chromosome in which the centromere is situated at either of its ends. —**telocentric** *adj.*

telodendron *n.* one of the branches into which the *axon of a neuron divides at its destination. Each telodendron finishes as a terminal **bouton**, which takes part in a *synapse or a *neuromuscular junction.

telogen *n. see* ANAGEN.

telomere *n.* the end of a chromosome, which consists of repeated sequences of DNA that perform the function of ensuring that each cycle of DNA replication has been completed. Each time a cell divides some sequences of the telomere are lost; eventually (after 60–100 divisions in an average cell) the cell dies. Replication of telomeres is directed by **telomerase**, an enzyme consisting of RNA and protein that is inactive in normal cells. Its presence in tumours is linked to the uncontrolled multiplication of cancer cells.

telophase *n.* the final stage of *mitosis and of each of the divisions of *meiosis, in which the chromosomes at each end of the cell become long and thin and the nuclear membrane reforms around them. The cytoplasm begins to divide.

temazepam *n.* a *benzodiazepine used for the short-term treatment of insomnia and in *premedication before minor surgery. It is given by mouth; common side-effects include drowsiness, dizziness, and loss of appetite.

temoporfin *n. see* PHOTODYNAMIC THERAPY.

temozolomide *n.* an *alkylating agent used mainly for the treatment of *glioblastoma multiforme, either concurrently with radiotherapy or as a single-agent chemotherapy drug. It is taken by mouth. Trade name: **Temodal**.

temple *n.* the region of the head in front of and above each ear.

temporal *adj.* of or relating to the temple.

temporal arteritis *see* ARTERITIS.

temporal artery a branch of the external carotid artery that supplies blood mainly to the temple and scalp.

temporal bone either of a pair of bones of the cranium. The **squamous** portion forms part of the side of the cranium. The **petrous** part contributes to the base of the skull and contains the middle and inner ears. Below it are the *mastoid process, *styloid process, and zygomatic process (*see* ZYGOMATIC ARCH). *See also* SKULL.

temporalis *n.* a fan-shaped muscle situated at the side of the head, extending from the temporal fossa to the mandible. This muscle lifts the lower jaw, thus closing the mouth.

temporal lobe one of the main divisions of the *cerebral cortex in each hemisphere of the brain, lying at the side within the temple of the skull and separated from the frontal lobe by a cleft, the **lateral sulcus**. Areas of the cortex in this lobe are concerned with

the appreciation of sound and spoken language.

temporal lobe epilepsy *see* EPILEPSY.

temporo- *combining form denoting* **1.** the temple. **2.** the temporal lobe of the brain.

temporomandibular joint the articulation between the *mandible and the *temporal bone: a hinge joint (*see* GINGLYMUS).

temporomandibular joint syndrome a condition in which the patient has painful temporomandibular joints, tenderness in the muscles that move the jaw, clicking of the joints, and limitation of jaw movement. Stress, resulting in clenching the jaws and grinding the teeth, is thought to be a causal factor.

temsirolimus *n.* a *protein kinase inhibitor used for the treatment of advanced renal cell carcinoma. It targets a serine threonine kinase that regulates a signalling cascade controlling cell proliferation. It is administered by intravenous infusion; side-effects include hypersensitivity reactions (flushing, chest pain, breathlessness). Trade name: **Torisel**.

tenaculum *n.* **1.** a sharp wire hook with a handle. The instrument is used in surgical operations to pick up pieces of tissue or the cut end of an artery. **2.** a band of fibrous tissue that holds a part of the body in place.

tendinitis *n.* inflammation of a tendon. It occurs most commonly after excessive overuse but is sometimes due to bacterial infection (e.g. *gonorrhoea), or a generalized rheumatic disease (e.g. *rheumatoid arthritis or ankylosing spondylitis). Treatment is by rest, achieved sometimes by splinting the adjacent joint, and corticosteroid injection into the tender area around the tendon. Tendinitis at the insertion of the supraspinatus muscle is a frequent cause of pain and restricted movement in the shoulder. *See also* JUMPER'S KNEE, TENNIS ELBOW. *Compare* TENOSYNOVITIS.

tendinosis *n.* degeneration of a tendon, commonly associated with nodular thickening, that is due to atrophy and may eventually result in tendon rupture. It may occur with ageing or result from overuse or compromise of blood supply.

tendon *n.* a tough whitish cord, consisting of numerous parallel bundles of collagen fibres, that serves to attach a muscle to a bone. Tendons are inelastic but flexible; they assist in concentrating the pull of the muscle on a small area of bone. Some tendons are surrounded by **tendon sheaths** – these are tubular double-layered sacs lined with synovial membrane and containing synovial fluid. Tendon sheaths enclose the flexor tendons at the wrist and ankle, where they minimize friction and facilitate movement. *See also* APONEUROSIS. —**tendinous** *adj.*

tendon organ (Golgi tendon organ) a sensory *receptor found within a tendon that responds to the tension or stretching of the tendon and relays impulses to the central nervous system. Like stretch receptors in muscle, tendon organs are part of the *proprioceptor system.

tendon transfer plastic surgery in which the tendon from an unimportant muscle is used to replace the damaged tendon of an important muscle. A common tendon used is the palmaris longus tendon of the forearm.

tendovaginitis (tenovaginitis) *n.* inflammatory thickening of the fibrous sheath containing one or more tendons, usually caused by repeated minor injury. It usually occurs at the back of the thumb (**de Quervain's tendovaginitis**) and results in pain on using the wrists. Treatment is by rest, injection of cortisone into the tendon sheath, and, if these fail, surgical incision of the sheath.

tenecteplase *n. see* FIBRINOLYTIC, TISSUE-TYPE PLASMINOGEN ACTIVATOR.

tenesmus *n.* a sensation of the desire to defecate, which is continuous or recurs frequently, without the production of significant amounts of faeces (often small amounts of mucus or blood alone are passed). This uncomfortable symptom may be due to *proctitis, prolapse of the rectum, rectal tumour, or *irritable bowel syndrome.

tennis elbow a painful inflammation of the origin of the common extensor tendon on the lateral epicondyle of the *humerus, caused by overuse of the forearm muscles. Treatment is by rest, massage, and local corticosteroid injection. If the symptoms do not settle, surgery may be required. *See also* TENDINITIS. *Compare* GOLFER'S ELBOW.

teno- *combining form denoting* a tendon.

tenofovir disoproxil a reverse transcriptase inhibitor (*see* REVERSE TRANSCRIPTASE).

tenonectomy *n.* surgical removal of a portion of the *Tenon's capsule.

tenonotomy *n.* a surgical incision made into the *Tenon's capsule.

Tenon's capsule the fibrous tissue that lines the orbit and surrounds the eyeball. [J. R. Tenon (1724–1816), French surgeon]

tenoplasty *n.* surgical repair of a ruptured or severed tendon.

tenorrhaphy *n.* the surgical operation of uniting the ends of divided tendons by suture.

tenosynovitis (peritendinitis) *n.* inflammation of a tendon sheath, producing pain, swelling, and an audible creaking on movement. It may result from a bacterial infection or occur as part of a rheumatic disease causing *synovitis.

tenotomy *n.* surgical *division of a tendon. This may be necessary to correct a joint deformity caused by tendon shortening or to reduce the imbalance of forces caused by an overactive muscle in a spastic limb. *See also* SCISSOR LEG.

tenovaginitis *n. see* TENDOVAGINITIS.

TENS *see* TRANSCUTANEOUS ELECTRICAL NERVE STIMULATION.

tension-free vaginal tape (transvaginal tape, TVT) a relatively new surgical sling procedure for treating stress incontinence in women that uses a tape made of polypropylene mesh. The tape is inserted under the mid-urethra (rather than the bladder neck, as in a *pubovaginal sling), passing through the retropubic space on either side, and is fixed to the abdominal wall just internal to the pubic symphysis. The **transobturator tape (TOT)** procedure is similar, but in this technique a tunnel is created out to the *obturator foramen on either side, lessening the risk of vascular and bladder injuries. Tape procedures have lower morbidity rates than *colposuspension and have gradually replaced the latter as the surgical procedure of choice for treating female stress incontinence.

tensor *n.* any muscle that causes stretching or tensing of a part of the body.

tent *n.* **1.** an enclosure of material (usually transparent plastic) around a patient in bed, into which a gas or vapour can be passed as part of treatment. An **oxygen tent** is relatively inefficient as a means of administering oxygen; a face mask or intranasal oxygen are used where possible. **2.** a piece of dried vegetable material, usually a seaweed stem, shaped to fit into an orifice, such as the cervical canal. As it absorbs moisture it expands, providing a slow but forceful means of dilating the orifice.

tented diaphragm the radiological sign of a raised diaphragm, which is indicative of *peritonitis.

tentorium *n.* a curved infolded sheet of *dura mater that dips inwards from the skull and separates the cerebellum below from the occipital lobes of the cerebral hemispheres above.

terat- (terato-) *combining form denoting* a monster or congenital abnormality.

teratogen *n.* any substance, agent, or process that induces the formation of developmental abnormalities in a fetus. Known teratogens include such drugs as *thalidomide and alcohol; such infections as German measles and cytomegalovirus; and also irradiation with X-rays and other ionizing radiation. *Compare* MUTAGEN. —**teratogenic** *adj.*

teratogenesis *n.* the process leading to developmental abnormalities in the fetus.

teratology *n.* the study of developmental abnormalities and their causes.

teratoma *n.* a tumour composed of a number of tissues that are not usually found at that site and are derived from all three embryonic *germ layers. Teratomas most frequently occur in the testis and ovary (*see* DERMOID CYST), possibly derived from remnants of embryonic cells that have the ability to differentiate into many types of tissue; in most malignant teratomas, cells from all three *germ layers are present. **Malignant teratoma of the testis** is found in young men: it is more common in patients with a history of undescended testis. Like *seminoma, it frequently occurs as a painless swelling of one testis (pain is not a good indication that the swelling is benign). Treatment is by *orchidectomy avoiding an incision into the scrotum. The tumour can spread to lymph nodes, lungs, and bone, treatment of which may involve the use of chemotherapy drugs, such as vinblastine, bleomycin, cisplatin, and etoposide, with a high cure rate even in metastatic disease.

Teratomas often produce *alpha-fetoprotein, beta human chorionic gonadotrophin, or both; the presence of these substances (*tumour markers) in the blood is a useful indication of the amount of tumour and the effect of treatment.

teratospermia *n. see* OLIGOSPERMIA.

terbinafine *n.* an antifungal drug used to treat infections of the nails and ringworm. It is administered by mouth or topically; possible side-effects with oral treatment include nausea, abdominal pain, and allergic skin rashes. Trade name: **Lamisil**.

terbutaline *n.* a *bronchodilator drug: a short-acting beta agonist (*see* SYMPATHOMIMETIC) used in the treatment of asthma and other respiratory disorders characterized by reversible airways obstruction. It may be given by mouth, injection, or inhalation; common side-effects include nervousness and dizziness. Trade name: **Bricanyl**.

teres *n.* either of two muscles of the shoulder, extending from the scapula to the humerus. The **teres major** draws the arm towards the body and rotates it inwards; the **teres minor** rotates the arm outwards.

terlipressin *n.* a drug that releases *vasopressin over a period of hours. It is administered by intravenous injection to help to control bleeding from *oesophageal varices by constricting the small arteries in the intestinal tract. Trade name: **Glypressin**.

terminal dribble a *lower urinary tract symptom in which the flow of urine does not end quickly, but dribbles slowly towards an end. This must be distinguished from *postmicturition dribble, which occurs after voiding has been completed.

terpene *n.* any of a group of unsaturated hydrocarbons many of which are found in plant oils and resins and are responsible for the scent of these plants (e.g. mint). Larger terpenes include vitamin A, squalene, and the carotenoids.

tertian fever *see* MALARIA.

tertiary care the specialized services provided by centres equipped with diagnostic and treatment facilities not available at general hospitals. *Compare* PRIMARY CARE, SECONDARY CARE.

tertiary prevention reducing the impact of complications and progression of established disease. Examples include *cardiac rehabilitation following myocardial infarction, stroke rehabilitation, and screening people with diabetes for diabetic *retinopathy. In practice, the distinction between tertiary and *secondary prevention is often unclear. *See also* PREVENTIVE MEDICINE, PRIMARY PREVENTION.

TESA (testicular sperm aspiration) a technique used in the treatment of male infertility in which spermatozoa are removed by an incision into and aspiration from the testis. The sperm are then used to fertilize egg cells in vitro (*see* ICSI).

tesla *n.* the *SI unit of magnetic flux density, equal to a density of 1 weber per square metre. This unit is important in *magnetic resonance imaging (MRI). Most MRI scanners operate between 0.1 and 2.5 T, but some modern research scanners may go up to 7 T. Symbol: T.

testicle *n.* the *testis and its system of ducts (the vasa efferentia and epididymis) within the scrotum.

testicular feminization syndrome *see* ANDROGEN INSENSITIVITY SYNDROME.

testis *n.* (*pl.* **testes**) either of the pair of male sex organs that produce spermatozoa and secrete the male sex hormone *androgen under the control of *gonadotrophins from the pituitary gland. The testes of the fetus form within the abdomen but descend into the *scrotum in order to maintain a lower temperature that favours the produc-

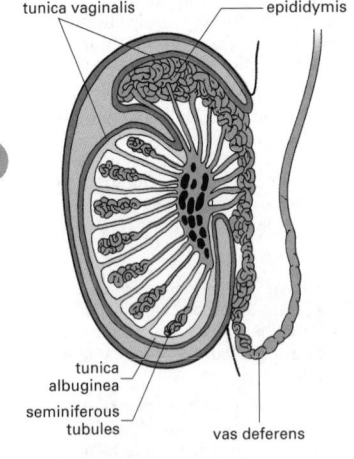

tunica vaginalis — epididymis

tunica albuginea

seminiferous tubules

vas deferens

Testis (longitudinal section).

tion and storage of spermatozoa. The bulk of the testis is made up of long convoluted **seminiferous tubules** (see illustration), in which the spermatozoa develop (*see* SPERMATOGENESIS). The tubules also contain *Sertoli cells, which may nourish developing sperm cells. Spermatozoa pass from the testis to the *epididymis to complete their development. The **interstitial (Leydig) cells**, between the tubules, are the major producers of androgens.

test meal a standard meal given to stimulate secretion of digestive juices, which can then be withdrawn by tube and measured as a test of digestive function. A **fractional test meal** was a gruel preparation to stimulate gastric secretion, whose acid content was measured. This has been replaced by tests using secretory stimulants. The **Lundh test meal** is a meal of oil and protein to stimulate pancreatic secretion, which is withdrawn from the duodenum and its trypsin content measured as a test of pancreatic function.

testosterone *n.* the principal male sex hormone (*see* ANDROGEN). Formed from **androstenedione** within the interstitial cells of the *testis, it is converted in target cells to *dihydrotestosterone, which mediates most of its actions. Preparations of testosterone are used for replacement therapy in males with testosterone deficiency; they can be administered orally, by intramuscular depot injection, or topically (in the form of skin patches or gels).

test-tube baby a colloquial name for a baby born to a woman as a result of fertilization of one of her ova by her partner's sperm outside her body. *See* IN VITRO FERTILIZATION.

tetan- (tetano-) *combining form denoting* 1. tetanus. 2. tetany.

tetanolysin *n.* a toxin produced by tetanus bacilli in an infected wound, causing the local destruction of tissues.

tetanospasmin *n.* a toxin produced by tetanus bacilli in an infected wound. The toxin diffuses along nerves, causing paralysis, and may reach the spinal cord and brain, when it causes violent muscular spasms and the condition of lockjaw.

tetanus (lockjaw) *n.* an acute infectious disease, affecting the nervous system, caused by the bacterium *Clostridium tetani*. Infection occurs by contamination of wounds by bacterial spores. Bacteria multiply at the site of infection and produce a toxin that irritates nerves so that they cause spasmodic contraction of muscles. Symptoms appear 4–25 days after infection and consist of muscle stiffness, spasm, and subsequent rigidity, first in the jaw and neck then in the back, chest, abdomen, and limbs; in severe cases the spasm may affect the whole body, which is arched backwards (*see* OPISTHOTONOS). High fever, convulsions, and extreme pain are common. If respiratory muscles are affected, a *tracheostomy or intubation and ventilation is essential to avoid death from asphyxia. Mortality is high in untreated cases but prompt treatment is effective. An attack does not necessarily confer complete immunity. Immunization against tetanus is effective but temporary. —**tetanic** *adj.*

tetany *n.* spasm and twitching of the muscles, particularly those of the face, hands, and feet. Tetany is usually caused by a reduction in the blood calcium level, which may be due to underactive parathyroid glands, rickets, or *alkalosis.

tetra- *combining form denoting* four.

tetracaine (amethocaine) *n.* a potent local anaesthetic applied as a gel to the skin before intravenous injections or the insertion of a cannula. It is also applied as eye drops before eye operations. Trade names: **Ametop, Minims Amethocaine Hydrochloride**.

tetracosactide (tetracosactin) *see* ACTH; SHORT SYNACTHEN TEST.

tetracyclines *pl. n.* a group of antibiotic compounds derived from cultures of *Streptomyces* bacteria. These drugs, which include *doxycycline, *oxytetracycline, and **tetracycline**, are effective against a wide range of bacterial infections. They are usually given by mouth to treat various conditions, including infections caused by *Chlamydia* species, respiratory-tract infections, and acne. Side-effects such as nausea, vomiting, and diarrhoea are fairly common. In addition, suppression of normal intestinal bacteria may make the patient susceptible to infection with tetracycline-resistant organisms. Tetracyclines should not be administered after the fourth month of pregnancy and their use should be avoided in children under 12 to prevent unsightly staining of the permanent teeth.

tetrad *n.* (in genetics) **1.** the four cells resulting from meiosis after the second telophase. **2.** the four chromatids of a pair of homologous chromosomes (*see* BIVALENT) in the first stage of meiosis.

tetradactyly *n.* a congenital abnormality in which there are only four digits on a hand or foot.

tetrahydrocannabinol *n.* a derivative of marijuana that has antiemetic activity and also produces euphoria. These two properties are utilized in the prevention of chemotherapy-induced sickness.

tetraiodothyronine *n. see* THYROXINE.

tetralogy of Fallot a form of congenital heart disease in which there is *pulmonary stenosis, enlargement of the right ventricle, a *ventricular septal defect, and in which the origin of the aorta lies over the septal defect. The affected child is blue (cyanosed) and frequently squats. The defect is corrected surgically. [E. L. A. Fallot (1850–1911), French physician]

tetraplegia *n. see* QUADRIPLEGIA.

tetrodotoxin *n.* puffer-fish toxin, one of the most powerful known nerve toxins with a mortality of about 50%. There is no known antidote.

thalam- (thalamo-) *combining form denoting* the thalamus. Example: **thalamolenticular** (relating to the thalamus and lenticular nucleus of the brain)

thalamencephalon *n.* the structures, collectively, at the anterior end of the brainstem, comprising the *epithalamus, *thalamus, *hypothalamus, and subthalamus, all of which are concerned with the reception and processing of information that enters from sensory nerve pathways.

thalamic syndrome a condition resulting from damage to the thalamus, often by a stroke, that is characterized by severe intractable pain and hypersensitivity in the area of the body served by the damaged brain region. It is extremely resistant to treatment.

thalamotomy *n.* an operation on the brain in which a lesion is made in a precise part of the *thalamus. It has been used to control psychiatric symptoms of severe anxiety and distress, in which cases the lesion is made in the dorsomedial nucleus of the thalamus, which connects with the frontal lobe. *See also* PSYCHOSURGERY.

thalamus *n.* (*pl.* **thalami**) one of two egg-shaped masses of grey matter that lie deep in the cerebral hemispheres in each side of the forebrain. The thalami are relay stations for all the sensory messages that enter the brain, before they are transmitted to the cortex. All sensory pathways, except that for the sense of smell, are linked to nuclei within the thalamus, and it is here that the conscious awareness of messages as sensations – temperature, pain, touch, etc. – probably begins.

thalassaemia (**Cooley's anaemia**) *n.* a hereditary blood disease, widespread in the Mediterranean countries, Asia, and Africa, in which there is an abnormality in the protein part of the *haemoglobin molecule. The affected red cells cannot function normally, leading to anaemia. Other symptoms include enlargement of the spleen and abnormalities of the bone marrow. Individuals inheriting the defective gene from both parents are severely affected (**thalassaemia major**), but those inheriting it from only one parent are usually symptom-free. Patients with the major disease are treated with repeated blood transfusions or bone marrow transplantation. The disease can be detected by prenatal diagnosis.

(⊕) SEE WEB LINKS

• Website of the UK Thalassaemia Society

thalassotherapy *n.* treatment by means of remedial bathing in sea water.

thalidomide *n.* a drug that was formerly used as a sedative. If taken during the first three months of pregnancy, it was found to cause fetal abnormalities involving limb malformation and was withdrawn as a sedative in 1962. Recently, however, thalidomide has been found to be effective in treating myeloma and severe reactions in leprosy. It appears to act in various ways, including as an immunomodulator, anti-inflammatory agent, and angiogenesis inhibitor. Side-effects include constipation, drowsiness, and (with long-term use) peripheral neuropathy. It should not be used in women who are pregnant or capable of becoming pregnant. Trade name: **Thalidomide Pharmion**.

thallium *n.* a leadlike element that has several dangerously poisonous compounds. The poison is cumulative and causes liver and nerve damage and bone destruction. The victim's hair is likely to fall out and does not grow again. Treatment is by administration of *chelating agents. Symbol: Tl.

thallium scan a method of studying blood flow to the heart muscle (myocardium) and diagnosing myocardial *ischaemia using an injection of the radioisotope thallium-201. Defects of perfusion, such as a recent infarct, emit little or no radioactivity and are seen as 'cold spots' when an image is formed using a *gamma camera and computer. Exercise may be used to provoke 'cold spots' in the diagnosis of ischaemic heart disease.

thallium-technetium isotope subtraction imaging a technique to image the parathyroid glands. Technetium is taken up only by the thyroid gland, but thallium is taken up by both the thyroid and parathyroid glands. *Digital subtraction of the two isotopes leaves an image of the parathyroid glands alone. It is an accurate technique (90%) for the identification of adenomas of the parathyroid glands secreting excess hormone.

theca *n.* a sheathlike surrounding tissue. For example, the **theca folliculi** is the outer wall of a *Graafian follicle.

theine *n.* the active volatile principle found in tea (*see* CAFFEINE).

thelarche *n.* the process of breast development, which occurs as a normal part of *puberty. Isolated premature breast development in girls is not uncommon and is almost always benign.

thenar *n.* **1.** the palm of the hand. **2.** the fleshy prominent part of the hand at the base of the thumb. *Compare* HYPOTHENAR. —**thenar** *adj.*

theobromine *n.* an alkaloid, occurring in cocoa, coffee, and tea, that has a weak diuretic action and dilates coronary and other arteries. It was formerly used to treat angina.

theophylline *n.* an alkaloid, occurring in the leaves of the tea plant, that has a diuretic effect and relaxes smooth muscle, especially of the bronchi (it is an *antimuscarinic drug). Theophylline preparations, particularly *aminophylline, are used mainly as bronchodilators to treat severe asthma attacks. Trade names: **Nuelin SA**, **Slo-Phyllin**, **Uniphyllin Continus**.

therapeutic index the ratio of a dose of a therapeutic agent that produces damage to normal cells to the dose that is necessary to have a defined level of anticancer activity. It indicates the relative efficacy of a treatment against tumours.

therapeutic privilege the entitlement of a doctor to withhold information from a patient when it is feared that disclosure could cause immediate and serious harm to the patient (e.g. because he or she is suffering from severe depression). In exceptional cases, the need to withhold information may be considered to override the requirement to obtain informed *consent before proceeding with treatment. In such a case therapeutic privilege could be used as a legal defence against the charge of *battery or *negligence. If doctors are intending to invoke the concept of therapeutic privilege they must be prepared to justify their decision. Furthermore, while it was once quite common for doctors to withhold bad news or upsetting information from patients for *paternalistic motives, it is now considered a breach of the patient's *autonomy and the ethicolegal justification for invoking therapeutic privilege where a patient has *capacity is, if it exists at all, extremely limited.

therapeutics *n.* the branch of medicine that deals with different methods of treatment and healing (**therapy**), particularly the use of drugs in the cure of disease.

therm *n.* a unit of heat equal to 100,000 British thermal units. 1 therm = 1.055×10^8 joules.

therm- (thermo-) *combining form denoting* **1.** heat. **2.** temperature.

thermoalgesia (thermalgesia) *n.* an abnormal sense of pain that is felt when part of the body is warmed. It is a type of *dysaesthesia and is a symptom of partial damage to a peripheral nerve or to the fibre tracts conducting temperature sensation to the brain.

thermoanaesthesia *n.* absence of the ability to recognize the sensations of heat and coldness. When occurring as an isolated sensory symptom it indicates damage to the spinothalamic tract in the spinal cord, which conveys the impulses of temperature to the thalamus.

thermocautery *n.* the destruction of unwanted tissues by heat (*see* CAUTERIZE).

thermocoagulation *n.* the coagulation and destruction of tissues by cautery.

thermography *n.* a technique for measuring and recording the heat produced by different parts of the body by using photographic film sensitive to infrared radiation. The picture produced is called a **thermo-**gram. The heat radiated from the body varies in different parts according to the flow of blood through the vessels; thus areas of poor circulation produce less heat. On the other hand a tumour with an abnormally increased blood supply may be revealed on the thermogram as a 'hot spot'. The technique was formerly used in the diagnosis of tumours of the breast (**mammothermography**) before the development of more sensitive techniques (*see* MAMMOGRAPHY).

thermoluminescent dosimeter (TLD) a radiation *dosimeter that utilizes the ability of activated sodium fluoride to luminesce in proportion to the radiation dose to which it is exposed when it is heated. It is now a common form of radiation dosimeter for personnel monitoring.

thermolysis *n.* (in physiology) the dissipation of body heat by such processes as the evaporation of sweat from the skin surface.

thermometer *n.* a device for registering temperature. A **clinical thermometer** consists of a sealed narrow-bore glass tube with a bulb at one end. It contains mercury, which expands when heated and rises up the tube. The tube is calibrated in degrees, and is designed to register temperatures between 35°C (95°F) and 43.5°C (110°F). An **oral thermometer** is placed in the mouth; a **rectal thermometer** is inserted into the rectum.

thermophilic *adj.* describing organisms, especially bacteria, that grow best at temperatures of 48–85°C. *Compare* MESOPHILIC, PSYCHROPHILIC.

thermophore *n.* any substance that retains heat for a long time, such as kaolin, which is often used in hot poultices.

thermoreceptor *n.* a sensory nerve ending that responds to heat or to cold. Such *receptors are scattered widely in the skin and in the mucous membrane of the mouth and throat.

thermotaxis *n.* the physiological process of regulating or adjusting body temperature.

thermotherapy *n.* the use of heat to alleviate pain and stiffness in joints and muscles and to promote an increase in circulation. *Diathermy provides a means of generating heat within the tissues themselves.

thiabendazole *n. see* TIABENDAZOLE.

thiamine *n. see* VITAMIN B₁.

thiazide diuretic *see* DIURETIC.

thiazolidinediones *pl. n.* a group of *oral hypoglycaemic drugs, including **pioglitazone** (Actos) and **rosiglitazone** (Avandia), used in the treatment of type 2 *diabetes mellitus. They act by reducing resistance of the body to its own insulin and may be taken alone or in combination with *metformin or a sulphonylurea. Thiazolidinediones should not be used in patients with heart failure or a history of heart failure.

Thiersch's graft *see* SPLIT-SKIN GRAFT. [K. Thiersch (1822–95), German surgeon]

thin membrane disease an inherited disease of the kidneys in which the glomerular basement membrane, which filters waste material from the blood, is too thin, allowing small amounts of blood to pass across it. This can be a cause of **benign familial haematuria** and thin membrane disease is a common finding in renal biopsy series where the procedure has been carried out as part of the investigation of *haematuria. Thin membranes are also found in other conditions, e.g. in some cases of *Alport's syndrome and *Berger's nephropathy.

thioguanine *n. see* TIOGUANINE.

thionamides *pl. n.* a group of chemically related compounds used as *antithyroid drugs. They exert their action on thyroid tissue by inhibiting the iodination of *thyroglobulin, which is an essential step in the manufacture of thyroid hormones.

thiopental (thiopentone) *n.* a short-acting *barbiturate. It is given by intravenous injection to induce general *anaesthesia. Possible complications of thiopental anaesthesia can include respiratory depression, laryngeal spasm, and thrombophlebitis. The drug is not used when respiratory obstruction is present.

thiophilic *adj.* growing best in the presence of sulphur or sulphur compounds. The term is usually applied to bacteria.

thioxanthene *n. see* ANTIPSYCHOTIC.

thorac- (thoraco-) *combining form denoting* the thorax or chest.

thoracentesis *n. see* PLEUROCENTESIS.

thoracic cavity the chest cavity. *See* THORAX.

thoracic duct one of the two main trunks of the *lymphatic system. It receives lymph from both legs, the lower abdomen, left thorax, left side of the head, and left arm and drains into the left innominate vein.

thoracic vertebrae the 12 bones of the *backbone to which the ribs are attached. They lie between the cervical (neck) and lumbar (lower back) vertebrae and are characterized by the presence of facets for articulation with the ribs. *See also* VERTEBRA.

thoracocentesis *n. see* PLEUROCENTESIS.

thoracoplasty *n.* a former treatment for pulmonary tuberculosis involving surgical removal of parts of the ribs, thus allowing the chest wall to fall in and collapse the affected lung.

thoracoscope *n.* an instrument used to inspect the *pleural cavity. —**thoracoscopy** *n.*

thoracotomy *n.* surgical opening of the chest cavity to inspect or operate on the heart, lungs, or other structures within.

thorax *n.* the chest: the part of the body cavity between the neck and the diaphragm. The skeleton of the thorax is formed by the sternum, costal cartilages, ribs, and thoracic vertebrae of the backbone. It encloses the lungs, heart, oesophagus, and associated structures. *Compare* ABDOMEN. —**thoracic** *adj.*

thought alienation a symptom of psychosis in which patients feel that their own thoughts are in some way no longer within their control. It includes *thought insertion, *thought withdrawal, and *thought broadcast. Any form of thought alienation is a *Schneiderian first-rank symptom, highly indicative of schizophrenia.

thought broadcast a symptom of psychosis in which the patient feels that his or her thoughts are being distributed into other people's thoughts. This is a *Schneiderian first-rank symptom, highly indicative of schizophrenia.

thought echo (echo de la pensée) a symptom of psychosis in which the patient has a hallucination of hearing aloud his or her own thoughts a short time after thinking them. Similar to the experience of thought echo is that of **Gedankenlautwerden**, in which the patients hear their own thoughts aloud at the time they think them. This was an original *Schneiderian first-rank symptom, but has been left out of most translations of Schneider's work into English.

thought insertion a symptom of psychosis in which the patient feels that thoughts are inserted into his or her own head by an outside force or agency. This is a *Schneiderian first-rank symptom, highly indicative of schizophrenia.

thought-stopping *n.* a technique of *behaviour therapy used in the treatment of obsessional thoughts. Attention is voluntarily withdrawn from these thoughts and focused on some other vivid image or engrossing activity.

thought withdrawal a symptom of psychosis in which patients believe that their own thoughts are being taken out of their head by an outside force. This is a *Schneiderian first-rank symptom, highly indicative of schizophrenia.

threadworm (pinworm) *n.* a parasitic nematode worm of the genus *Enterobius* (*Oxyuris*), which lives in the upper part of the human large intestine. The threadlike female worm, some 12 mm long, is larger than the male; it emerges from the anus in the evening to deposit its eggs, and later dies. If the eggs are swallowed and reach the intestine they develop directly into adult worms. Threadworms cause *enterobiasis, a disease common in children throughout the world.

3-D magnetic imager an instrument using magnetic technology to give a virtual image of an endoscope (especially a colonoscope) inside the body throughout the examination without using X-rays, which helps in the endoscope's steering. It uses an external antenna capturing the magnetic field generated by small coils built inside the endoscope. Trade name: **ScopeGuide**.

threonine *n.* an *essential amino acid. See also* AMINO ACID.

threshold *n.* (in neurology) the point at which a stimulus begins to evoke a response, and therefore a measure of the sensitivity of a system under particular conditions. A *thermoreceptor that responds to an increase in temperature of only two degrees is said to have a much lower threshold than one that will only respond to a change in temperature of ten degrees or more. In this example the threshold can be measured directly in terms of degrees.

thrill *n.* a vibration felt on placing the hand

on the body. A heart murmur that is felt by placing the hand on the chest wall is said to be accompanied by a thrill.

-thrix *combining form denoting* a hair or hairlike structure.

thromb- (thrombo-) *combining form denoting* **1.** a blood clot (thrombus). **2.** thrombosis. **3.** blood platelets.

thrombasthenia *n.* a hereditary blood disease in which the function of the *platelets is defective although they are present in normal numbers. The manifestations are identical to those of thrombocytopenic *purpura.

thrombectomy *n.* a surgical procedure in which a blood clot (thrombus) is removed from an artery or vein (*see* ENDARTERECTOMY, PHLEBOTHROMBOSIS).

thrombin *n.* a substance (*coagulation factor) that acts as an enzyme, converting the soluble protein fibrinogen to the insoluble protein fibrin in the final stage of *blood coagulation. Thrombin is not normally present in blood plasma, being derived from an inactive precursor, **prothrombin**.

thromboangiitis obliterans *see* BUERGER'S DISEASE.

thrombocyte *n. see* PLATELET.

thrombocythaemia *n.* a disease in which there is an abnormal proliferation of the cells that produce blood *platelets (*megakaryocytes), leading to an increased number of platelets in the blood. This may result in an increased tendency to form clots within blood vessels (thrombosis); alternatively the function of the platelets may be abnormal, leading to an increased tendency to bleed. Treatment is by radiotherapy, *cytotoxic drugs, *interferon, or drugs that inhibit *megakaryocyte maturation.

thrombocytopenia *n.* a reduction in the number of *platelets in the blood. This results in bleeding into the skin (*see* PURPURA), spontaneous bruising, and prolonged bleeding after injury. Thrombocytopenia may result from failure of platelet production or excessive destruction of platelets. —**thrombocytopenic** *adj.*

thrombocytosis *n.* an increase in the number of *platelets in the blood. It may occur in a variety of diseases, including chronic infections, cancers, and certain blood diseases and is likely to cause an increased tendency to form blood clots within vessels (thrombosis).

thromboembolism *n.* the condition in which a blood clot (thrombus), formed at one point in the circulation, becomes detached and lodges at another point. It is most commonly applied to the association of phlebothrombosis and *pulmonary embolism (**pulmonary thromboembolic disease**).

thromboendarterectomy *n. see* END-ARTERECTOMY.

thromboendarteritis *n.* thrombosis complicating *endarteritis, seen in temporal *arteritis, *polyarteritis nodosa, and syphilis. It may cause death of part of the organ supplied by the affected artery.

thrombokinase *n. see* THROMBOPLASTIN.

thrombolysis *n.* the dissolution of a blood clot (thrombus) by the infusion of a *fibrinolytic agent into the blood. It may be used in the treatment of *phlebothrombosis, *pulmonary embolism, and coronary thrombosis. *See also* TISSUE-TYPE PLASMINOGEN ACTIVATOR.

thrombolytic *adj.* describing an agent that breaks up blood clots (thrombi). Thrombolytic drugs are used to unblock arteries in the treatment of myocardial infarction. *See* FIBRINOLYTIC, TISSUE-TYPE PLASMINOGEN ACTIVATOR.

thrombophilia *n.* an inherited or acquired condition that predisposes individuals to *thrombosis. **Inherited thrombophilias** are established causes of systemic thrombosis due to defects in proteins involved in regulating *blood coagulation. Causes include *Factor V Leiden gene mutation, a *prothrombin gene mutation, deficiences in proteins C and S and antithrombin III, and hyperhomocysteinaemia (*see* HOMOCYSTEINE). —**thrombophilic** *adj.*

thrombophlebitis *n.* inflammation of the wall of a vein (*see* PHLEBITIS) with secondary thrombosis occurring within the affected segment of vein. Pregnant women are more prone to thrombophlebitis because of physiological changes in the blood and the effects of pressure within the abdomen. It may involve superficial or deep veins of the legs (the latter being less common in pregnancy than the former). Deep vein *thrombosis may precede *pulmonary embolism.

thromboplastin (tissue factor, Factor III, thrombokinase) *n.* a substance formed during the earlier stages of *blood coagulation. It acts as an enzyme, converting the inactive substance prothrombin to the enzyme *thrombin.

thrombopoiesis *n.* the process of blood *platelet production. Platelets are formed as fragments of cytoplasm shed from giant cells (*megakaryocytes) in the bone marrow by a budding process.

thrombosis *n.* a condition in which the blood changes from a liquid to a solid state within the cardiovascular system during life and produces a mass of coagulated blood (**thrombus**). Thrombosis may occur within a blood vessel in diseased states. Thrombosis in an artery obstructs the blood flow to the tissue it supplies: obstruction of an artery to the brain is one of the causes of a *stroke and thrombosis in an artery supplying the heart – *coronary thrombosis – results in a heart attack (*see* MYOCARDIAL INFARCTION). Thrombosis can also occur in a vein (**deep vein thrombosis**; *see* PHLEBOTHROMBOSIS), and it may be associated with inflammation (*see* THROMBOPHLEBITIS). The thrombus may become detached from its site of formation and carried in the blood to lodge in another part (*see* EMBOLISM).

thrombotic microangiopathy the formation of thrombi in arterioles and capillaries, leading to haemolytic anaemia and *thrombocytopenia. The term encompasses primary *haemolytic uraemic syndrome and *thrombotic thrombocytopenic purpura, as well as the microangiopathies that can complicate pregnancy (pregnancy-related haemolytic uraemic syndrome, *HELLP syndrome), *malignant hypertension, *scleroderma, *antiphospholipid antibody syndrome, organ transplantation, and cancer.

thrombotic thrombocytopenic purpura (TTP) a rare disorder of coagulation caused by deficiency or inhibition of *ADAMTS13, a protein that is responsible for breaking down von Willebrand factor (*see* VON WILLEBRAND'S DISEASE). This results in haemolytic *anaemia, *thrombocytopenia, and fluctuating neurological abnormalities. It is treated by *plasmapheresis.

thromboxane A$_2$ (TXA$_2$) a substance related to prostaglandins that is released by platelets activated by local tissue injury and promotes blood clotting and vasconstriction. *See* PLATELET ACTIVATION. *Compare* PROSTA-CYCLIN.

thrombus *n. see* BLOOD CLOT, THROMBOSIS.

thrush *n. see* CANDIDIASIS.

thym- (thymo-) *combining form denoting* the thymus.

thymectomy *n.* surgical removal of the thymus.

-thymia *combining form denoting* a condition of the mind. Example: **cyclothymia** (alternations of mood).

thymic aplasia failure of development of the *thymus, resulting in T-lymphocyte deficiency and compromised immunity.

thymidine *n.* a compound containing thymine and the sugar deoxyribose. *See also* NUCLEOSIDE.

thymine *n.* one of the nitrogen-containing bases (*see* PYRIMIDINE) occurring in the nucleic acid DNA.

thymitis *n.* inflammation of the thymus.

thymocyte *n.* a lymphocyte within the *thymus.

thymoma *n.* a benign or malignant tumour of the *thymus. It is sometimes associated with *myasthenia gravis, a chronic disease in which muscles tire easily. Surgical removal of the tumour may result in improvement of the muscle condition, but the response is often slow.

thymus *n.* a bilobed organ in the root of the neck, above and in front of the heart. The thymus is enclosed in a capsule and divided internally by cross walls into many lobules, each full of T lymphocytes (white blood cells associated with antibody production). In relation to body size the thymus is largest at birth. It doubles in size by puberty, after which it gradually shrinks, its functional tissue being replaced by fatty tissue. In infancy the thymus controls the development of *lymphoid tissue and the immune response to microbes and foreign proteins (accounting for allergic response, autoimmunity, and the rejection of organ transplants). T lymphocytes migrate from the bone marrow to the thymus, where they mature and differentiate until activated by antigen. —**thymic** *adj.*

thyro- *combining form denoting* the thy-

roid gland. Example: **thyroglossal** (relating to the thyroid gland and tongue).

thyrocalcitonin *n. see* CALCITONIN.

thyrocele *n.* a swelling of the thyroid gland. *See* GOITRE.

thyroglobulin *n.* a protein in the thyroid gland from which the *thyroid hormones (thyroxine and triiodotyrosine) are synthesized.

thyrohyoid *adj.* relating to the thyroid cartilage and hyoid bone. The **thyrohyoid ligaments** form part of the *larynx; contraction of the **thyrohyoid muscle** raises the larynx.

thyroid acropachy a rarely seen but well-documented alteration in the shape of the nails resembling *clubbing but unique to Graves' disease (*see* THYROTOXICOSIS). It is often associated with formation of new bone seen on X-rays of the hands and wrists, which is said to resemble bubbles along the surface of the bones.

thyroid antibodies autoantibodies against the thyroid gland, which cause *Hashimoto's disease. They are of two types: **microsomal**, against thyroid cytoplasm; and **anti-thyroglobulin**, against thyroid colloid (*see* THYROID GLAND).

thyroid cancer any malignant tumour of the thyroid gland, of which there are four main types: **papillary**, **follicular**, **medullary**, and **anaplastic**. These have characteristic presentations and degrees of malignancy, ranging from the papillary tumours, which tend to be relatively low-grade and in some cases can be treated by surgery and thyroxine suppression, to highly aggressive anaplastic tumours, which tend to present with locally advanced disease that is inoperable and unresponsive to radiotherapy or chemotherapy. *See also* HÜRTHLE CELL TUMOUR.

thyroid cartilage the main cartilage of the *larynx, consisting of two broad plates that join at the front to form a V-shaped structure. The thyroid cartilage forms the **Adam's apple** in front of the larynx.

thyroid crisis (thyroid storm) a life-threatening condition due to a severe worsening of previously undiagnosed or inadequately treated *thyrotoxicosis. It often follows infections, childbirth, nonthyroid surgery, or trauma but can occur without an obvious cause. The presenting features are a fever, severe agitation, nausea and vomiting, diarrhoea, and abdominal pains. An accelerated heart rate and irregularity of the heart rhythm can cause heart failure, and psychotic episodes or coma can result. Blood tests will reveal hyperthyroidism and may also show altered liver function, high blood sugar, high calcium levels, a high white blood cell count, and often anaemia. Treatment is with intravenous fluids, oxygen, antithyroid drugs (such as *carbimazole or *propylthiouracil), high-dose iodide solution (*see* LUGOL'S IODINE), high-dose steroids, and beta blockers. The patient must be cooled and given antipyretics, such as paracetamol. Any underlying cause must also be treated.

thyroidectomy *n.* surgical removal of the thyroid gland. In **partial thyroidectomy**, only the diseased part of the gland is removed; in **subtotal thyroidectomy**, a method of treating *thyrotoxicosis, the surgeon removes 90% of the gland.

thyroid gland a large *endocrine gland situated in the base of the neck (see illustration). It consists of two lobes, one on either side of the trachea, that are joined by an **isthmus** (sometimes a third lobe extends upwards from the isthmus). The thyroid gland consists of a large number of closed follicles inside which is a jelly-like **colloid**, which contains *thyroglobulin and the principal active substances that are secreted by the gland. The thyroid gland is concerned with regulation of the metabolic rate by the secretion of *thyroid hormone, which is stimulated by *thyroid-stimulating hormone from the pituitary gland and requires trace amounts of iodine. The *C cells of the thyroid gland secrete *calcitonin.

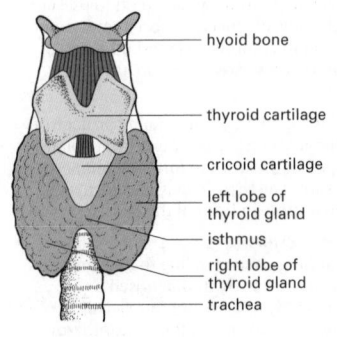

- hyoid bone
- thyroid cartilage
- cricoid cartilage
- left lobe of thyroid gland
- isthmus
- right lobe of thyroid gland
- trachea

Position of the thyroid gland.

thyroid hormone an iodine-containing substance, synthesized and secreted by the thyroid gland, that is essential for normal metabolic processes and mental and physical development. There are two thyroid hormones, *triiodothyronine and *thyroxine, which are formed from *thyroglobulin. Lack of these hormones gives rise to *cretinism in infants and *myxoedema in adults. Excessive production of thyroid hormones gives rise to *thyrotoxicosis.

thyroiditis *n.* inflammation of the thyroid gland. **Acute thyroiditis** is due to bacterial infection, and **subacute** (or **de Quervain's**) **thyroiditis** is caused by a viral infection. **Chronic thyroiditis** is commonly caused by an abnormal immune response (*see* AUTOIMMUNITY) in which lymphocytes invade the tissues of the gland. *See* HASHIMOTO'S DISEASE.

thyroid-stimulating hormone (TSH, thyrotrophin) a hormone, synthesized and secreted by the anterior pituitary gland under the control of *thyrotrophin-releasing hormone, that stimulates activity of the thyroid gland. Defects in TSH production lead to over- or under-secretion of *thyroid hormones.

thyroid storm *see* THYROID CRISIS.

thyroplasty *n.* a surgical procedure performed on the thyroid cartilage of the larynx to alter the characteristics of the voice.

thyrotomy *n.* surgical incision of either the thyroid cartilage in the neck or of the thyroid gland itself.

thyrotoxicosis *n.* the syndrome due to excessive amounts of thyroid hormones in the bloodstream, causing a rapid heartbeat, sweating, tremor, anxiety, increased appetite, loss of weight, and intolerance of heat. Causes include simple overactivity of the gland, a hormone-secreting benign tumour or carcinoma of the thyroid, and **Graves' disease** (**exophthalmic goitre**), in which there are additional symptoms including swelling of the neck (**goitre**) due to enlargement of the gland and protrusion of the eyes (**exophthalmos**). Treatment may be by surgical removal of the thyroid gland, *radioactive iodine therapy to destroy part of the gland, or by the use of drugs (such as *carbimazole or *propylthiouracil) that interfere with the production of thyroid hormones. —**thyrotoxic** *adj.*

thyrotoxic periodic paralysis a condition in which attacks of sudden weakness and flaccidity occur in patients with *thyrotoxicosis, seen most often in males of Asian descent. The attacks last from hours to days; they can be prevented by potassium supplements and subsequent treatment of the thyrotoxicosis.

thyrotrophin *n. see* THYROID-STIMULATING HORMONE.

thyrotrophin-releasing hormone (TRH) a hormone from the hypothalamus (in the brain) that acts on the anterior pituitary gland to stimulate the release of *thyroid-stimulating hormone. A preparation of TRH (**protirelin**) may be given by intravenous injection to test thyroid gland function and to estimate reserves of thyroid-stimulating hormone in the pituitary.

thyroxine (tetraiodothyronine, T₄) *n.* the principal hormone synthesized and secreted into the bloodstream by the thyroid gland (*see* THYROID HORMONE). Most of it is converted to a more metabolically active form, *triiodothyronine, within the peripheral tissues. Both hormones act to increase the basal metabolic rate. A preparation of thyroxine (**levothyroxine sodium**) can be administered by mouth to treat underactivity of the thyroid gland.

TIA *see* TRANSIENT ISCHAEMIC ATTACK.

tiabendazole (thiabendazole) *n.* an *anthelmintic used to treat *creeping eruption. It is administered orally and may cause vomiting, vertigo, and gastric discomfort.

tibia *n.* the shin bone: the inner and larger bone of the lower leg (see illustration). It articulates with the *femur above, with the *talus below, and with the *fibula to the side (at both ends); at the lower end is a projection, the medial *malleolus, forming part of the articulation with the talus. —**tibial** *adj.*

tibialis *n.* either of two muscles in the leg, extending from the tibia to the metatarsal bones of the foot. The **tibialis anterior** turns the foot inwards and flexes the toes backwards. Situated behind it, the **tibialis posterior** extends the toes and inverts the foot.

tibial torsion a normal variation in posture in which there is an in-toe gait due to mild internal rotation of the tibia. The condition is often apparent in infancy when the child starts walking and resolves spontaneously with time. Usually symmetrical, it is associated with normal mobility and is pain-free.

tibio- *combining form denoting* the tibia. Example: **tibiofibular** (relating to the tibia and fibula).

tic *n.* a repeated and largely involuntary movement (motor tic) or utterance (vocal tic) varying in complexity from a muscle twitch or a grunt to elaborate well-coordinated actions and repeated words or phrases. Simple tics occur in about a quarter of all children and usually disappear within a year. Tics most often become prominent when the individual is exposed to emotional stress. *See also* TOURETTE'S SYNDROME.

ticarcillin *n.* a *penicillin-type antibiotic that is used in combination with *clavulanic acid (as **Timentin**) to treat serious infections caused by *Pseudomonas* and *Proteus* bacteria. It is administered by intravenous infusion.

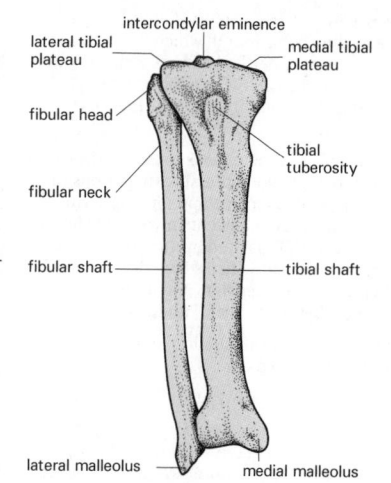

Right tibia and fibula.

tic douloureux *see* NEURALGIA.

tick *n.* a bloodsucking parasite belonging to the order of arthropods (the Acarina) that also includes the *mites. Tick bites can cause serious skin lesions and occasionally paralysis (*see* IXODES, AMBLYOMMA), and certain tick species transmit *typhus, *Lyme disease, and *relapsing fever. Diethyltoluamide (DEET) is used as a tick repellent. There are two families: Argasidae (soft ticks), which includes *Ornithodoros*, with mouthparts invisible from above and no hard shield (**scutum**) on the dorsal surface; and Ixodidae (hard ticks), including *Dermacentor*, *Haemaphysalis*, and *Rhipicephalus*, with clearly visible mouthparts and a definite scutum.

tick fever any infectious disease transmitted by ticks, especially *Rocky Mountain spotted fever.

Tietze's syndrome (costochondritis) a painful swelling of a rib in the region of the chest, over the junction of bone and cartilage. The cause is unknown and the condition usually resolves without treatment, but in some cases local injections of corticosteroids are required. [A. Tietze (1864–1927), German surgeon]

tilting-disc valve the most commonly used form of mechanical heart valve replacement.

time sampling (in psychology) a way of recording behaviour in which the presence or absence of particular kinds of behaviour is noted during each of several fixed prearranged periods of time. *See also* EVENT SAMPLING.

timolol *n.* a *beta blocker used in the treatment of high blood pressure (hypertension), angina, and glaucoma and for long-term prophylaxis after an acute myocardial infarction. It is administered by mouth or as eye drops or gel; side-effects include decreased heart rate, hypotension, and dizziness. Trade names: **Betim**, **Nyogel**, **Timoptol**.

tincture *n.* an alcoholic extract of a drug derived from a plant.

tinea *n. see* RINGWORM.

Tinel's sign a method for checking the regeneration of a nerve: usually used in patients with *carpal tunnel syndrome. Direct tapping over the sheath of the nerve elicits a distal tingling sensation (*see* PARAESTHESIA), which indicates the beginning of regeneration. [J. Tinel (1879–1952), French neurosurgeon]

tinnitus *n.* the sensation of sounds in the ears, head, or around the head in the absence of an external sound source. It can occur with any form of hearing loss or with normal hearing. It is thought to be due to a misinterpretation of signals in the central auditory pathways of the brain. The signals that are misinterpreted can arise in any part of the auditory system: the cochlea, cochlear nerve, or within the brain itself. Treatment includes the correction of any underlying condition, counselling, *cognitive behavioural therapy, relaxation techniques, sound therapy (*see* WHITE NOISE INSTRUMENT), and use of *hearing aids. A unified method of treatment that makes use of all of these components is referred to as *tinnitus retraining therapy.

tinnitus masker the former name for a *white noise instrument.

tinnitus retraining therapy (TRT) a method of treating *tinnitus based around a neurophysiological model of the condition. Developed by Pavel Jastreboff, it embraces various techniques, including explanation, counselling, relaxation techniques, and sound therapy.

tintometer *n.* an instrument for measuring the depth of colour in a liquid. The colour can then be compared with those on standard charts so that the concentration of a particular compound in solution can be estimated.

tinzaparin sodium *see* LOW-MOLECULAR-WEIGHT HEPARIN.

tioguanine (thioguanine) *n.* a drug that prevents the growth of cancer cells (*see* ANTIMETABOLITE) and is used in the treatment of leukaemias. It is given by mouth and commonly reduces the numbers of white blood cells and platelets. Other side-effects include nausea, vomiting, loss of appetite, and jaundice. Trade name: **Lanvis**.

TIPSS (transjugular intrahepatic portosystemic shunt) *see* PORTAL HYPERTENSION.

tissue *n.* a collection of cells specialized to perform a particular function. The cells may be of the same type (e.g. in nervous tissue) or of different types (e.g. in connective tissue). Aggregations of tissues constitute organs.

tissue culture the culture of living tissues, removed from the body, in a suitable medium supplied with nutrients and oxygen. **Tissue engineering**, in which skin, cartilage, and other connective-tissue cells are cultured on a *fibronectin 'mat' to create new tissues, is being explored for use in tissue grafting for patients with burns, sports injuries, etc.

tissue-type plasminogen activator (tPA, TPA) a natural protein, found in the body and now able to be manufactured by genetic engineering, that can break up a thrombus (see THROMBOLYSIS). It requires the presence of *fibrin as a cofactor and is able to activate *plasminogen on the fibrin surface, which distinguishes it from the other plasminogen activators, *streptokinase and *urokinase. tPAs include **reteplase** (Rapilysin) and **tenecteplase** (Metalyse), used to treat acute myocardial infarction, and *alteplase.

tissue typing determination of the *HLA profiles of tissues to assess their compatibility. It is the most important predictor of success or failure of a transplant operation.

titre n. (in immunology) the extent to which a sample of blood serum containing antibody can be diluted before losing its ability to cause agglutination of the relevant antigen. It is used as a measure of the amount of antibody in the serum.

titubation n. a rhythmical nodding movement of the head, sometimes involving the trunk. It is seen in patients with *parkinsonism and cerebellar disorders. Occasionally the use of this term is extended to include a stumbling gait.

TLD see THERMOLUMINESCENT DOSIMETER.

T lymphocyte n. see LYMPHOCYTE.

TMS see TRANSCRANIAL MAGNETIC STIMULATION.

TNF see TUMOUR NECROSIS FACTOR.

TNM classification a classification defined by the *UICC for the extent of spread of a cancer. T refers to the size of the tumour, N the presence and extent of lymph node involvement, and M the presence of distant spread (metastasis).

tobacco n. the dried leaves of the plant *Nicotiana tabacum* or related species, used in smoking and as snuff. Tobacco contains the stimulant but poisonous alkaloid *nicotine, which enters the bloodstream during smoking. The volatile tarry material also released during smoking contains carcinogenic chemicals (see CARCINOGEN).

tobramycin n. an *aminoglycoside antibiotic used to treat septicaemia and lower respiratory, urinary, skin, abdominal, and central nervous system infections. It is administered by intravenous or intramuscular injection or by inhalation. Kidney damage or hearing impairment may occur with high doses or prolonged use. Trade names: **Bramitob**, **Tobi**.

toco- (toko-) *combining form denoting* childbirth or labour.

tocolytic n. a pharmaceutical preparation used to treat preterm labour by stopping uterine contractions for long enough to allow administration of corticosteroids to enhance fetal lung maturity or to enable transfer to a unit with adequate neonatal facilities. Tocolytics include **atosiban** (Tractocile) and ritrodine (see SYMPATHOMIMETIC).

tocopherol n. see VITAMIN E.

tocophobia n. see TOKOPHOBIA.

toddler's diarrhoea a disorder of young children characterized by the passage of frequent loose, offensive, and bulky stools in which partially digested or undigested food may be visible (the 'peas and carrot' stool). There is no other definable abnormality and the children gain weight normally. Management consists of excluding other causes of diarrhoea and reassurance that the disorder is benign and self-limiting (it resolves by school age).

Todd's paralysis (Todd's palsy) transient paralysis of a part of the body that has previously been involved in a focal epileptic seizure (see EPILEPSY). [R. B. Todd (1809–60), British physician]

toko- *combining form. see* TOCO-.

tokophobia (tocophobia) n. a profound fear of childbirth. There are two types: **primary tokophobia**, which develops in adolescence and causes many women to avoid childbirth altogether; and **secondary tokophobia**, which occurs after a traumatic delivery and can stop a woman having another child. Women are more at risk from tokophobia if they have had any of the following: a history of rape or sexual abuse; harrowing memories of educational videos during adolescence; a history of depression; or experience of panic attacks.

tolbutamide n. a drug taken by mouth in the treatment of type 2 diabetes mellitus. It acts directly on the pancreas to stimulate insulin production and is particularly effective in elderly patients with mild diabetes (see SULPHONYLUREA). Side-effects may include headache and tinnitus.

tolerance *n.* the reduction or loss of the normal response to a drug or other substance that usually provokes a reaction in the body. **Drug tolerance** may develop after taking a particular drug over a long period of time. In such cases increased doses are necessary to produce the desired effect. Some drugs that cause tolerance also cause *dependence. *See also* GLUCOSE TOLERANCE TEST, IMMUNOLOGICAL TOLERANCE, TACHYPHYLAXIS.

tolterodine *n.* an *antimuscarinic drug taken by mouth to treat *detrusor overactivity giving rise to the *lower urinary tract symptoms of frequency, urgency, or urge incontinence. Trade name: **Detrusitol**.

toluidine blue a dye used in microscopy for staining basophilic substances in tissue specimens.

-tome *combining form denoting* a cutting instrument. Example: **microtome** (instrument for cutting microscopical sections).

tomo- *combining form denoting* **1.** section or sections. **2.** surgical operation.

tomography *n.* the technique of rotating a radiation detector around the patient so that the image obtained gives additional three-dimensional information. In plain film tomography the source of X-rays and the photographic film move round the patient to produce an image of structures at a particular depth within the body, bringing them into sharp focus, while deliberately blurring structures above and below them. In *computerized tomography (CT) this technique produces an image of a slice through the body at a particular level. The visual record of this technique is called a **tomogram**. *See also* DENTAL PANTOMOGRAM, OPTICAL COHERENCE TOMOGRAPHY, POSITRON EMISSION TOMOGRAPHY, SPECT SCANNING.

tomotherapy *n.* a type of radiotherapy in which the radiation is delivered in a slice-by-slice rotating method similar to a CT scan, which also allows daily *image-guided radiotherapy.

-tomy (-otomy) *combining form denoting* a surgical incision into an organ or part. Example: **gastrotomy** (into the stomach).

tone *n. see* TONUS.

tongue *n.* a muscular organ attached to the floor of the mouth. It consists of a **body** and a **root**, which is attached by muscles to the hyoid bone below, the styloid process

behind, and the palate above. It is covered by mucous membrane, which is continuous with that of the mouth and pharynx. On the undersurface of the tongue a fold of mucous membrane, the **frenulum linguae**, connects the midline of the tongue to the floor of the mouth. The surface of the tongue is covered with minute projections (**papillae**), which give it a furred appearance (see illustration). *Taste buds are arranged in grooves around the papillae, particularly the fungiform and circumvallate papillae. The tongue has three main functions. It helps in manipulating food during mastication and swallowing; it is the main organ of taste; and it plays an important role in the production of articulate speech. Anatomical name: **glossa**.

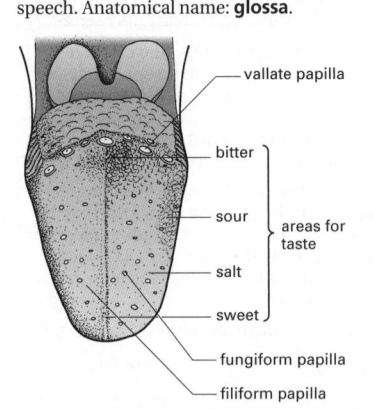

The tongue (upper surface).

tongue-tie *n.* a disorder of young children in which the tongue is anchored in the floor of the mouth more firmly than usual. No treatment is required unless the condition is extreme and associated with forking of the tongue, in which case surgical division of the tie may be necessary.

tonic **1.** *adj.* **a.** relating to normal muscle tone. **b.** marked by continuous tension (contraction), e.g. a tonic muscle *spasm. **2.** *n.* a medicinal substance purporting to increase vigour and liveliness and produce a feeling of wellbeing: beneficial effects of tonics are probably due to their placebo action.

tonicity *n.* **1.** the normal state of slight contraction, or readiness to contract, of healthy muscle fibres. **2.** the effective osmotic pressure of a solution. *See* HYPERTONIC, HYPOTONIC, OSMOSIS.

tonic pupil (Adie's pupil) a pupil that is dilated as a result of damage to the nerves supplying the ciliary muscle and iris. It reacts poorly to light but may constrict better for near vision, with slow redilation on refixation at a distance. The tonic pupil is sensitive to dilute 0.1% pilocarpine drops, which cause marked constriction but have little effect on a normal pupil. The tonic pupil may become miotic (*see* MIOSIS) over time.

tono- *combining form denoting* **1.** tone or tension. **2.** pressure.

tonofibril *n.* a tiny fibre occurring in bundles in the cytoplasm of cells that lie in contact, as in epithelial tissue. Tonofibrils are concerned with maintaining contact between adjacent cells. *See* DESMOSOME.

tonography *n.* the measurement and recording of intraocular pressure while the eyeball is subjected to pressure over a period of several minutes. It is used to assess aqueous outflow and diagnose glaucoma. *See* TONOMETER.

tonometer *n.* **1.** (ophthalmotonometer) a small instrument for measuring the pressure inside the eye. There are several types. The **applanation tonometer** measures the force required to flatten a known area of the cornea after a drop of local anaesthetic has made the cornea numb. A greater force is required when the pressure inside the eye is increased, and vice versa. The **Goldmann applanation tonometer** flattens a corneal area of 3 mm^2. **2.** an instrument for measuring pressure in some other part of the body. —**tonometry** *n.*

tonsillectomy *n.* surgical removal of the tonsils.

tonsillitis *n.* inflammation of the tonsils due to bacterial or viral infection, causing a sore throat, fever, and difficulty in swallowing. If tonsillitis due to streptococcal infection is not treated (by antibiotics) it may lead to *rheumatic fever or *nephritis.

tonsils *pl. n.* masses of *lymphoid tissue around the pharynx, usually referring to the **palatine tonsils** on either side of the *oropharynx. However, there is more tonsil tissue below the palatine tonsils, on the back of the tongue (the **lingual tonsils**), and small deposits around the openings of the *Eustachian tubes in the nasopharynx (the **tubal tonsils**). The tonsils are concerned with protection against infection. Together with the *adenoids, they form *Waldeyer's ring.

tonus (tone) *n.* the normal state of partial contraction of a resting muscle, maintained by reflex activity.

tooth *n.* (*pl.* **teeth**) one of the hard structures in the mouth used for cutting and chewing food. Each tooth is embedded in a socket in part of the jawbone (mandible or maxilla) known as the **alveolar bone** (or **alveolus**), to which it is attached by the *periodontal membrane. The exposed part of the tooth (**crown**) is covered with *enamel and the part within the bone (**root**) is coated with *cementum; the bulk of the tooth consists of *dentine enclosing the *pulp (see illustration overleaf). The group of embryological cells that gives rise to a tooth is known as the **tooth germ**.

There are four different types of tooth (*see* CANINE, INCISOR, PREMOLAR, MOLAR). *See also* DENTITION.

tooth extraction *see* EXTRACTION.

toothpaste *n.* a paste used for cleaning the teeth. It contains a fine abrasive and a suitable flavouring to promote use. Most toothpastes contain *fluoride salts, which help to prevent *dental caries. Some contain antimicrobials, to counteract dental *plaque, and whitening agents.

tooth wear a condition in which loss of tooth substance is excessive for the patient's age. It includes *attrition, *erosion, and *abrasion, but the cause is not always obvious.

topagnosis *n.* inability to identify a part of the body that has been touched. It is a symptom of disease in the parietal lobes of the brain. The normal ability to localize touch is called **topognosis**.

tophus *n.* (*pl.* **tophi**) a hard deposit of crystalline uric acid and its salts in the skin, cartilage (especially of the ears), or joints; a feature of *gout.

topical *adj.* local: used for the route of administration of a drug that is applied directly to the part being treated (e.g. to the skin or eye).

topical calcineurin inhibitors *see* CALCINEURIN INHIBITORS.

topiramate *n.* *see* ANTICONVULSANT.

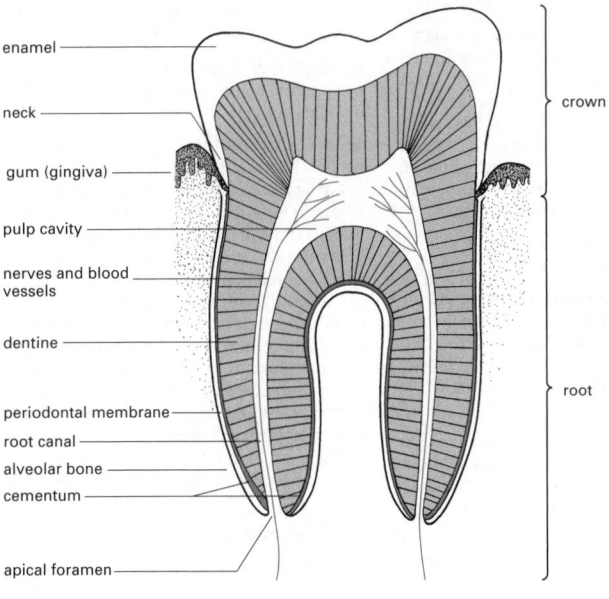

enamel

neck

gum (gingiva)

pulp cavity

nerves and blood
vessels

dentine

periodontal membrane

root canal

alveolar bone

cementum

apical foramen

crown

root

Section of a molar tooth.

topo- *combining form denoting* place; position; location.

topography *n.* the study of the different regions of the body, including the description of its parts in relation to the surrounding structures. —**topographical** *adj.*

topoisomerase inhibitor any one of a class of *cytotoxic drugs that work by blocking the action of topoisomerase enzymes, which promote the uncoiling of the DNA double helix, a necessary preliminary to replication. Topoisomerase I inhibitors include **irinotecan** (Campto), administered by intravenous infusion for treating advanced colorectal cancer (especially in combination with *fluorouracil); and **topotecan** (Hycamtin), given orally or by intravenous infusion for treating advanced ovarian cancer. Side-effects include delayed but severe diarrhoea and reduction in blood-cell production by the bone marrow. Topoisomerase II inhibitors include *etoposide and *doxorubicin.

topotecan *n. see* TOPOISOMERASE INHIBITOR.

Torkildsen procedure an operation in which a *shunt is created between the lateral *ventricle of the brain and the *cisterna magna to bypass a block of the cerebral *aqueduct and thus relieve *hydrocephalus. Originally this was achieved by means of an external indwelling catheter, but later techniques use an internal catheter, which reduces the risk of septic complications. [A. Torkildsen (20th century), Norwegian neurosurgeon]

torpor *n.* a state of sluggishness and diminished responsiveness: a characteristic of certain mental disorders and a symptom of certain forms of poisoning or metabolic disorder.

torsades de pointes a very dangerous form of *ventricular tachycardia characterized by a sinusoidal (twisting) pattern on the electrocardiogram due to a constantly shifting cardiac electrical vector (hence the French term, meaning 'twisting of points'). It is usually a side-effect of medication but may also occur in patients with severe deficiency of potassium or magnesium or inherited abnormalities of the cardiac electrical system. *See* LONG QT SYNDROME.

torsion *n.* twisting. Abnormal twisting of a testis within the scrotum or of a loop of bowel in the abdomen may impair blood and nerve supplies to these parts and cause severe damage.

torticollis (wryneck) *n.* an irresistible turning movement of the head that becomes more persistent, so that eventually the head is held continually to one side. This is a form of *dystonia; the spasm of the muscles is often painful. It may be caused by a birth injury to the sternomastoid muscle (*see* STERNOMASTOID TUMOUR). Relief may be obtained by cutting the motor nerve roots of the spinal nerves in the neck region or by injection of the affected muscles with *botulinum toxin.

toruloma *n.* a tumour-like lesion in the lungs resulting from *cryptococcosis.

torulosis *n. see* CRYPTOCOCCOSIS.

TOT transobturator tape. *See* TENSION-FREE VAGINAL TAPE.

totipotent *adj. see* STEM CELL.

Tourette's syndrome (TS, Gilles de la Tourette syndrome) a condition characterized by the simultaneous appearance of verbal and motor *tics within one year. Motor tics can be simple (eye rolling, flicking, incomplete movements) or complex (involuntary movements consisting of several components, mostly involving the arms). Verbal tics can be simple (grunts, throat clearing) or complex (uttering of words or, in 30% of patients, involuntary obscene speech). Rarely, the patient may also involuntarily repeat the words or imitate the actions of others (*see* PALILALIA). The condition usually starts in childhood and commonly improves with age. There is a strong hereditary element. Drug treatment and psychological support are sometimes helpful. [G. Gilles de la Tourette (1857–1904), French neurologist]

tourniquet *n.* a device to press upon an artery and prevent flow of blood through it, usually a cord, rubber tube, or tight bandage bound around a limb. Tourniquets are no longer recommended as a first-aid measure to stop bleeding from a wound because of the danger of reducing the supply of oxygen to other tissues (direct pressure on the wound itself is considered less harmful).

However, a temporary tourniquet to increase the distension of veins when a sample of blood is being taken does no harm.

tow *n.* the teased-out short fibres of flax, hemp or jute, used in swabs for cleaning, in *packs or *stupes for the application of poultices, and for a variety of other purposes.

Towne's projection a *posteroanterior X-ray film to show the entire skull and mandible. [E. B. Towne (1883–1957), US otolaryngologist]

tox- (toxi-, toxo-, toxic(o)-) *combining form denoting* 1. poisonous; toxic. 2. toxins or poisoning.

toxaemia *n.* blood poisoning that is caused by toxins formed by bacteria growing in a local site of infection. It produces generalized symptoms, including fever, diarrhoea, and vomiting. *Compare* PYAEMIA, SAPRAEMIA, SEPTICAEMIA.

toxic *adj.* having a poisonous effect; potentially lethal.

toxic epidermal necrolysis (TEN, Lyell's syndrome) a severe reaction to medications with a high mortality rate. Medications causing TEN include sulfonamides, anticonvulsants, antiretrovirals, and allopurinol. Widespread separation of the dead epidermal layer from underlying skin occurs, with consequent problems due to skin failure: impaired temperature regulation, infection risk, severe pain, etc. Mucous membranes are commonly affected, including the eyes (sometimes leading to blindness), mouth, and genitalia. Multi-organ failure may occur. Treatments include stopping the offending medication, good supportive nursing (usually in an ITU or HDU setting), antibiotics where appropriate, and intravenous immunoglobulin or ciclosporin.

toxicity *n.* the degree to which a substance is poisonous. *See also* LD$_{50}$.

toxicology *n.* the study of poisonous materials and their effects upon living organisms. —**toxicologist** *n.*

toxicosis *n.* the deleterious effects of a toxin; poisoning: includes any disease caused by the toxic effects of any substances.

toxic shock syndrome a state of acute *shock due to *septicaemia. The commonest cause is a retained foreign body (e.g. a tampon or IUCD) combined with the presence of staphylococci (*see also* STREPTOCOCCAL

TOXIC SHOCK SYNDROME). The condition can be life-threatening if not treated aggressively with appropriate antibiotics and supportive care (including fluid and electrolyte replacement).

toxin *n.* a poison produced by a living organism, especially by a bacterium (*see* ENDOTOXIN, EXOTOXIN). In the body toxins act as *antigens, and special *antibodies (**antitoxins**) are formed to neutralize their effects.

Toxocara *n.* a genus of large nematode worms that are intestinal parasites of vertebrates. *T. canis* and *T. cati*, the common roundworms of dogs and cats respectively, have life cycles similar to that of the human roundworm, *Ascaris lumbricoides. See* TOXOCARIASIS.

toxocariasis (visceral larva migrans) *n.* an infestation with the larvae of the dog and cat roundworms, *Toxocara canis* and *T. cati.* Humans, who are not the normal hosts, become infected on swallowing eggs of *Toxocara* present on hands or in food and drink contaminated with the faeces of infected domestic pets. The larvae, which migrate around the body, cause destruction of various tissues; the liver becomes enlarged and the lungs inflamed (*see* PNEUMONITIS). Symptoms may include fever, joint and muscle pains, vomiting, an irritating rash, and convulsions. Larvae can also lodge in the retina of the eye where they cause inflammation and *granuloma. The disease, widely distributed throughout the world, primarily affects children. Treatment is with mebendazole.

toxoid *n.* a poisonous material (toxin), such as that produced by tetanus and diphtheria agents, that has been rendered harmless by chemical treatment while retaining its antigenic activity. Toxoids are used in *vaccines.

Toxoplasma *n.* a genus of crescent-shaped sporozoans that live as parasites within the cells of various tissues and organs of vertebrate animals, especially birds and mammals, and complete their life cycle in a single host, the cat. *T. gondii* infects sheep, cattle, dogs, and humans, sometimes provoking an acute illness (*see* TOXOPLASMOSIS).

toxoplasmosis *n.* a disease of mammals and birds caused by the protozoan *Toxoplasma gondii*, which is usually transmitted to humans through ingesting undercooked meat or food or drink contaminated with the faeces of infected cats. Generally symptoms are mild (swollen lymph nodes and an influenza-like illness), but the disease can be serious in immunocompromised patients and requires treatment with a combination of *pyrimethamine and *sulfadiazine. Infection usually confers lifelong immunity. If acquired during pregnancy it can cause **congenital toxoplasmosis** in the unborn baby. Although most babies are unaffected or have very mild disease, some can have severe malformations of the skull and eyes or active infection in the liver. It can also cause stillbirth. Infection can be detected by blood tests in the mother; if the diagnosis is confirmed, the mother can be treated with spiramycin.

tPA (TPA) *see* TISSUE-TYPE PLASMINOGEN ACTIVATOR.

Tpot an acronym for *the pot*ential doubling time, the time taken for a tumour to double its cells in the absence of cell loss (i.e. by radiation). It is related to the rate constant for cell production (kP), where kP = log2/Tpot, and enables direct measurement of the rate of cell proliferation by tumours.

trabecula *n.* (*pl.* **trabeculae**) **1.** any of the bands of tissue that pass from the outer part of an organ to its interior, dividing it into separate chambers. For example, trabeculae occur in the penis. **2.** any of the thin bars of bony tissue in spongy *bone. **3.** the hypertrophied bands of bladder-wall muscle that are found in bladder outlet obstruction. —**trabecular** *adj.*

trabecular meshwork the tissue, located in the anterior chamber of the eye at the angle between the cornea and iris, that consists of a group of tiny canals through which aqueous fluid drains into *Schlemm's canal and exits the anterior chamber.

trabeculectomy *n.* an operation for glaucoma in which a part of the *trabecular meshwork is removed. This allows aqueous fluid to filter out of the eye under the conjunctiva, thus reducing the pressure inside the eye.

trabeculoplasty *n.* a method used to selectively destroy parts of the *trabecular meshwork and hence reduce intraocular pressure in the treatment of glaucoma. This may be achieved by means of a laser, as in **argon laser trabeculoplasty** (**ALT**; *see* ARGON LASER) and **selective laser trabeculoplasty** (**SLT**), in which a YAG laser is used to selectively target melanin within the pigmented trabecular meshwork cells to achieve lowering of the intraocular pressure.

trace element an element that is required in minute concentrations for normal growth and development. Trace elements include fluorine (*see* FLUORIDE), manganese, zinc, copper, *iodine, cobalt, *selenium, molybdenum, chromium, and silicon. They may serve as *cofactors or as constituents of complex molecules (e.g. cobalt in vitamin B_{12}).

tracer *n.* a substance that is introduced into the body and whose progress can subsequently be followed so that information is gained about metabolic processes. Radioactive tracers, which are substances labelled with *radionuclides, give off radiation that can be detected on a *scintigram or with a *gamma camera. They are used for a variety of purposes in *nuclear medicine. *See* MUGA SCAN, POSITRON EMISSION TOMOGRAPHY, SPECT SCANNING.

trache- (**tracheo-**) *combining form denoting* the trachea.

trachea *n.* the windpipe: the part of the air passage between the *larynx and the main *bronchi, i.e. from just below the Adam's apple, passing behind the notch of the *sternum (breastbone) to behind the angle of the sternum. The upper part of the trachea lies just below the skin, except where the thyroid gland is wrapped around it. —**tracheal** *adj.*

tracheal tugging a sign that is indicative of an *aneurysm of the aortic arch: a downward tug is felt on the windpipe when the finger is placed in the midline at the root of the neck.

tracheitis *n.* inflammation of the *trachea, usually secondary to bacterial or viral infection in the nose or throat. Tracheitis causes soreness in the chest and a painful cough and is often associated with bronchitis. In babies it can cause asphyxia, particularly in *diphtheria. Treatment includes appropriate antibacterial drugs, humidification of the inhaled air or oxygen, and mild sedation to relieve exhaustion due to persistent coughing.

trachelectomy *n.* radical removal of the cervix in cases of cervical cancer when the women have not completed childbearing.

tracheostomy (**tracheotomy**) *n.* a surgical operation in which a hole is made into the *trachea through the neck to relieve obstruction to breathing, as in diphtheria. A curved metal, plastic, or rubber tube is usu-ally inserted through the hole and held in position by tapes tied round the neck. It may be possible for the patient to speak by occluding the opening with his fingers. The tube must be kept clean and unblocked. Tracheostomy is also used in conjunction with artificial respiration, when it serves not only to secure the airway but also provides a route for sucking out secretions and protects the airway against the inhalation of pharyngeal contents. *See also* MINITRACHEOSTOMY.

tracheotomy *n. see* TRACHEOSTOMY.

trachoma *n.* a chronic contagious eye disease – a severe form of *conjunctivitis – caused by the bacterium *Chlamydia trachomatis*; it is common in some hot countries. The conjunctiva of the eyelids becomes inflamed, leading to discharge of pus. If untreated, the conjunctiva becomes scarred and shrinks, causing the eyelids to turn inwards so that the eyelashes scratch the cornea (*trichiasis); blindness can be a late complication. Treatment with tetracyclines is effective in the early stages of the disease.

tract *n.* **1.** a group of nerve fibres passing from one part of the brain or spinal cord to another, forming a distinct pathway, e.g. the spinothalamic tract, pyramidal tract, and corticospinal tract. **2.** an organ or collection of organs providing for the passage of something, e.g. the digestive tract.

traction *n.* the application of a pulling force, especially as a means of counteracting the natural tension in the tissues surrounding a broken bone (*see* COUNTERTRACTION), to produce correct alignment of the fragments. Considerable force, exerted with weights, ropes, and pulleys, may be necessary to ensure that a broken femur is kept correctly positioned during the early stages of healing. Traction is also used for the treatment of back pain by physiotherapists.

tractography *n.* a *magnetic resonance imaging technique using *diffusion tensor imaging to show the direction of the main nerve tracts in the brain and their connections.

tractotomy *n.* a neurosurgical operation for the relief of intractable pain. The nerve fibres that carry painful sensation to consciousness travel from the spinal cord through the brainstem in the spinothalamic tracts. This procedure is designed to sever the tracts within the medulla oblongata. *See also* CORDOTOMY.

tragus *n.* the projection of cartilage in the *pinna of the outer ear that extends back over the opening of the external auditory meatus.

tramadol *n.* an opioid analgesic (*see* OPI-ATE) used for the relief of moderate or severe pain. It is administered by mouth or injection and causes less respiratory depression, constipation, and likelihood of dependence than other opioids. Trade names: **Tramake, Zamadol, Zydol,** etc.

TRAM flap *t*ransverse *r*ectus *a*bdominis *m*yocutaneous *flap: a piece of tissue (skin, muscle, and fat) dissected from the abdomen and used to reconstruct the breast after mastectomy.

trance *n.* a state in which reaction to the environment is diminished although awareness is not impaired. It can be caused by hypnosis, meditation, catatonia, conversion disorder, drugs (such as hallucinogens), and religious ecstasy.

tranexamic acid a drug that prevents the breakdown of blood clots in the circulation (*fibrinolysis) by blocking the activation of plasminogen to form *plasmin, i.e. it is an **antifibrinolytic** drug. It is administered by mouth or intravenous injection as an antidote to overdosage by *fibrinolytic drugs and to control severe bleeding, for example after surgery or to treat menorrhagia. Possible side-effects include nausea and vomiting. Trade name: **Cyklokapron.**

tranquillizer *n.* a drug that produces a calming effect, relieving anxiety and tension. *Antipsychotic drugs (formerly known as **major tranquillizers**) have this effect and are used to treat severe mental disorders (psychoses), including schizophrenia and mania. *Anxiolytic drugs (formerly known as **minor tranquillizers**) are used to relieve anxiety and tension due to various causes.

trans- *prefix denoting* through or across. Example: **transurethral** (through the urethra).

transaminase *n.* an enzyme that catalyses the transfer of an amino group from an amino acid to an α-keto acid in the process of *transamination. Examples include *aspartate aminotransferase (AST), which catalyses the transamination of glutamate and oxaloacetate to α-ketoglutarate and aspartate, and *alanine aminotransferase (ALT),

converting glutamate and pyruvate to α-ketoglutarate and alanine.

transamination *n.* a process involved in the metabolism of amino acids in which amino groups ($-NH_2$) are transferred from amino acids to certain α-keto acids, with the production of a second keto acid and amino acid. The reaction is catalysed by enzymes (*see* TRANSAMINASE), which require pyridoxal phosphate as a coenzyme.

transcervical resection of the endometrium (TCRE) an operation, which is performed under local anaesthetic, in which the membrane lining the uterus (*see* ENDO-METRIUM) is cut away by a form of *electrosurgery using a *resectoscope, which is introduced through the cervix. Like *endometrial ablation, TCRE is used as an alternative to hysterectomy to treat abnormally heavy menstrual bleeding as it results in fewer complications and shorter stays in hospital.

transcoelomic spread a route of tumour *metastasis across a body cavity, such as the pleural, pericardial, or peritoneal cavity. Transcoelomic spread commonly occurs in advanced cancers of the lung, stomach, colon, ovary, and endometrium. It may be associated with the development of a malignant *effusion.

transcranial magnetic stimulation (TMS) stimulation of the brain by strong magnetic fields that induce electric currents in the underlying brain tissue. It is used as a research tool to discover more about the function of the brain. **Repetitive transcranial magnetic stimulation** (rTMS), consisting of a series of TMS pulses, is undergoing experimental trials in the treatment of psychiatric illnesses (especially depression), migraine, and tinnitus.

transcription *n.* the process in which the information contained in the *genetic code is transferred from DNA to RNA: the first step in the manufacture of proteins in cells. *See* MESSENGER RNA, TRANSLATION.

transcutaneous electrical nerve stimulation (TENS) the introduction of pulses of low-voltage electricity into tissue for the relief of pain. It is effected by means of a small portable battery-operated unit with leads connected to electrodes attached to the skin; the strength and frequency of the pulses, which prevent the passage of pain impulses to the brain, can be adjusted by the patient. TENS is used mainly for the relief of rheumatic pain.

transducer *n.* a device used to convert one form of signal into another, allowing its measurement or display to be made appropriately. For example, an *ultrasound probe converts reflected ultrasound waves into electronic impulses, which can be displayed on a TV monitor.

transduction *n.* the transfer of DNA from one bacterium to another by means of a *bacteriophage (phage). Some bacterial DNA is incorporated into the phage. When the host bacterium is destroyed the phage infects another bacterium and introduces the DNA from its previous host, which may become incorporated into the new host's DNA.

transection *n.* 1. a cross section of a piece of tissue. 2. cutting across the tissue of an organ (*see also* SECTION).

transfection *n.* the direct transfer of DNA molecules into a cell.

transferase *n.* an enzyme that catalyses the transfer of a group (other than hydrogen) between a pair of substrates.

transference *n.* (in psychoanalysis) the process by which a patient comes to feel and act towards the therapist as though he or she were somebody from the patient's past life, especially a powerful parent. The patient's transference feelings may be of love or of hatred, but they are inappropriate to the actual person of the therapist. **Countertransference** is the reaction of the therapist to the patient, which is similarly based on past relationships.

transferrin (siderophilin) *n.* a *glycoprotein, found in the blood plasma, that is capable of binding iron and thus acts as a carrier for iron in the bloodstream.

transfer RNA a type of RNA whose function is to attach the correct amino acid to the protein chain being synthesized at a *ribosome. *See also* TRANSLATION.

transformation zone the area of the *cervix of the uterus where the squamous epithelium, which covers the vaginal portion of the cervix, joins with the columnar epithelium, which forms the lining (endocervix) of the cervical canal.

transfusion *n.* 1. the injection of a volume of blood obtained from a healthy person (the **donor**) into the circulation of a patient (the **recipient**) whose blood is deficient in quantity or quality, through accident or disease. Direct transfusion from one person to another is rarely performed; usually packs of carefully stored blood of different *blood groups are kept in *blood banks for use as necessary. During transfusion the blood is allowed to drip, under gravity, through a needle inserted into one of the recipient's veins. Blood transfusion is routine during major surgical operations in which much blood is likely to be lost. 2. the administration of any fluid, such as plasma or saline solution, into a patient's vein by means of a *drip. *See also* AUTOTRANSFUSION.

transient ischaemic attack (TIA) the result of temporary disruption of the circulation to part of the brain due to *embolism, *thrombosis to brain arteries, or spasm of the vessel walls (*see* STROKE). The most common symptoms are transient loss of vision in one eye and weakness or numbness in one limb or part of a limb. Patients recover within 24 hours.

transillumination *n.* the technique of shining a bright light through part of the body to examine its structure. Transillumination of the sinuses of the skull is a means of detecting abnormalities.

transitional cell carcinoma a form of cancer that affects the **urothelium**, which lines the urinary collecting system of the kidney, ureters, bladder, and most of the urethra. It is the most common type of bladder cancer.

translation *n.* (in cell biology) the manufacture of proteins in a cell, which takes place at the ribosomes. The information for determining the correct sequence of amino acids in the protein is carried to the ribosomes by *messenger RNA, and the amino acids are brought to their correct position in the protein by *transfer RNA.

translocation *n.* (in genetics) a type of chromosome mutation in which a part of a chromosome is transferred to another part of the same chromosome or to a different chromosome. This changes the order of the genes on the chromosomes and can lead to serious genetic disorders, e.g. chronic myeloid leukaemia.

transmethylation *n.* the process whereby an amino acid donates its terminal methyl ($-CH_3$) group for the methylation of other compounds. Methionine is the principal methyl donor in the body and the donated methyl group may subsequently be involved in the synthesis of such compounds as choline or creatinine or in detoxification processes.

transmigration *n.* the act of passing through or across, e.g. the passage of blood cells through the intact walls of capillaries and venules (*see* DIAPEDESIS).

transobturator tape (TOT) *see* TENSION-FREE VAGINAL TAPE.

transoesophageal echocardiography (TOE) *see* ECHOCARDIOGRAPHY.

transplantation *n.* the implantation of an organ or tissue (*see* GRAFT) from one part of the body to another or from one person (the donor) to another (the recipient). Success for transplantation depends on the degree of compatibility between donor and graft: it is greatest for *autografts (self-grafts), less for *allografts (between individuals of the same species), and least for *xenografts (between different species; *see* XENOTRANSPLANTATION). Skin and bone grafting are examples of transplantation techniques in the same individual. A kidney transplant involves the grafting of a healthy kidney from a donor to replace the diseased kidney of the recipient: renal transplantation is the second commonest example of human transplant surgery using allografts (after corneal grafts – *see* KERATOPLASTY). Bone-marrow, blood-stem-cell, heart, heart–lung, pancreatic, and liver transplants are also very successful. A few patients have undergone laryngeal transplantation following *laryngectomy. Transplanting organs or tissues between individuals is a difficult procedure because the recipient's immune system perceives the transplant as a foreign object and rejects it. Special treatment (e.g. with *immunosuppressant drugs) is needed to prevent transplant rejection.

transposition *n.* the abnormal positioning of a part of the body such that it is on the opposite side to its normal site in the body. For example, it may involve the heart (*see* DEXTROCARDIA).

transposition of the great vessels a congenital abnormality of the heart in which the aorta arises from the right ventricle and the pulmonary artery from the left ventricle. Life is impossible unless there is an additional abnormality, such as a septal defect, that permits the mixing of blood between the pulmonary and systemic (aortic) circulations. Few of those untreated survive infancy and childhood, but the defect may be improved or corrected surgically. In **congenitally corrected transposition**, it is in fact the ventricles that are transposed rather than the great vessels. Thus the aorta arises from the right ventricle and the pulmonary artery from the left ventricle, as in uncorrected transposition, but in this case the blood flow in the systemic and pulmonary circulations follows the normal routes.

transrectal ultrasonography (TRUS) an *ultrasonography technique for examination of the prostate gland and seminal vesicles by placing an ultrasound probe through the anus to lie directly behind these structures in the rectum. Because of the close proximity of the probe, excellent detail is seen. The technique enables biopsies of the prostate to be taken in a systematic manner in the diagnosis of cancer. *See also* VESICULOGRAPHY.

transsexualism *n.* the condition of one who firmly believes that he (or she) belongs to the sex opposite to his (or her) biological gender. Children with such beliefs are treated with encouragement to engage in the activities appropriate to their biological sex and to work through their difficulties in psychotherapy. Adults with such beliefs can seldom be persuaded to change them; gender reassignment surgery, preceded by hormone treatment, is sometimes justifiable, to make the externals of the body conform to the individual's view of himself (or herself). *See also* GENDER IDENTITY DISORDER. —**transsexual** *adj., n.*

transthoracic impedance resistance to the flow of electricity through the heart muscle during *defibrillation due to the thoracic structures lying between the defibrillation paddles and the heart. These structures include the skin and soft subcutaneous tissues, the ribs and sternum, the lungs, and the pericardium. The best way to reduce the impedance, and thus to deliver the maximum available current to the heart, is to use defibrillation gel pads (*see* COUPLING AGENTS), to deliver the shock when the lungs are empty of air, or to press firmly down if using hand-held paddles. Transthoracic impedance is usually between 70 and 80 ohms.

transudation *n.* the passage of a liquid through a membrane, especially of blood through the wall of a capillary vessel. The liquid is called the **transudate**.

transuretero-ureterostomy *n.* the operation of connecting one ureter to the other in the abdomen. The damaged/obstructed ureter is cut above the diseased or damaged segment and joined end-to-side to the other ureter.

transurethral resection of the prostate (TURP) *see* RESECTION.

transurethral vaporization of the prostate (TUVP) a new technique that vaporizes (rather than resects) prostate tissue; it is associated with less bleeding during the procedure. TUVP is used to treat *lower urinary tract symptoms thought to be due to benign prostatic hyperplasia (*see* PROSTATE GLAND) or urinary retention.

transvaginal tape (TVT) *see* TENSION-FREE VAGINAL TAPE.

transvaginal ultrasonography *ultrasonography using a vaginal probe instead of an abdominal transducer. It allows the use of a higher frequency, thus providing superior resolution and therefore a more detailed anatomy of the female pelvis and an earlier and more accurate identification of fetal structures.

transverse *adj.* (in anatomy) situated at right angles to the long axis of the body or an organ.

transverse process the long projection from the base of the neural arch of a *vertebra.

transvestism (cross-dressing) *n.* dressing in clothes normally associated with the opposite sex, which may occur in both heterosexual and homosexual people. Cross-dressing may be practised by transsexuals (*see* TRANSSEXUALISM), in whom it is not sexually arousing. Other transvestites are fetishistic, and in these cross-dressing is sexually arousing and may lead to masturbatory or other sexual behaviour. Treatment may be by behavioural techniques, such as *aversion therapy, but is not always needed. *See also* SEXUAL DEVIATION. —**transvestite** *n.*

Trantas dots slightly elevated greyish-white dots consisting of clumps of degenerating eosinophils and epithelial cells, seen on the conjunctiva at the junction of the cornea and sclera in cases of allergic conjunctivitis. [A. Trantas (1867–1960), Greek ophthalmologist]

tranylcypromine *n. see* MAO INHIBITOR.

trapezium *n.* a bone of the wrist (*see* CARPUS). It articulates with the scaphoid bone behind, with the first metacarpal in front, and with the trapezoid and second metatarsal on either side.

trapezius *n.* a flat triangular muscle covering the back of the neck and shoulder. It is important for movements of the scapula and it also draws the head backwards to either side.

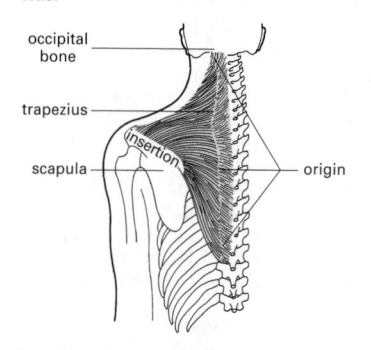

Left trapezius muscle.

trapezoid bone a bone of the wrist (*see* CARPUS). It articulates with the second metatarsal bone in front, with the scaphoid bone behind, and with the trapezium and capitate bones on either side.

trash foot a condition resulting from occlusion of the small arteries of the foot by atherosclerotic debris (*see* ATHEROMA). This occurs during abdominal aortic surgery or catheter manipulation, for example during coronary angiography. Clinically it presents with pain and eventually patchy ulceration and gangrene of the whole or part of the foot.

trastuzumab *n.* a *monoclonal antibody used to treat types of breast cancer that are positive for *HER2: the drug binds to these receptors on the tumour. It is administered by intravenous infusion; side-effects include damage to the heart, chills, fever, and allergic reactions. Trade name: **Herceptin**.

trauma *n.* 1. a physical wound or injury, such as a fracture or blow. **Trauma scores**

are numerical systems for assessing the severity and prognosis of serious injuries. 2. (in psychology) an emotionally painful and harmful event. *Post-traumatic stress disorder may follow an overwhelmingly stressful event, such as battle, assault, or serious injury. —**traumatic** *adj.*

traumatic fever a fever resulting from a serious injury.

traumatology *n.* accident surgery: the branch of surgery that deals with wounds and disabilities arising from injuries.

travel sickness *see* MOTION SICKNESS.

trazodone *n.* a drug, related to the tricyclic *antidepressants, that is used in the treatment of depression, particularly in agitated and anxious patients. It is administered by mouth; side-effects are milder than with tricyclic antidepressants. Trade name: **Molipaxin**.

Treacher Collins syndrome (**Treacher Collins deformity**) a hereditary disorder of facial development. It is characterized by underdevelopment of the jaw and zygomatic (cheek) bones and the precursors of the ear fail to develop, which results in a variety of ear and facial malformations. The ear abnormality may cause deafness. [E. Treacher Collins (1862–1919), British ophthalmologist]

treatment field *n.* (in radiotherapy) an area of the body selected for treatment with radiotherapy. For example, a **mantle field** comprises the neck, armpits, and central chest, for the radiotherapy of Hodgkin's disease. Radiation is administered to the defined area by focusing the beam of particles emitted by the radiotherapy machine and shielding the surrounding area of the body.

Treg cell *see* REGULATORY T CELL.

trematode *n. see* FLUKE.

tremor *n.* a rhythmical and alternating movement that may affect any part of the body. The **physiological tremor** is a feature of the normal mechanism for maintaining posture. It may be more apparent in states of fatigue or anxiety or when the thyroid gland is overactive. **Essential tremor** is slower and particularly affects the hands and arms when held out or holding a teacup. It can be embarrassing and inconvenient but it is not accompanied by any other symptoms. A

similar tremor may also occur in several members of one family and also in elderly people. Alcohol reduces the intensity of essential tremor. Treatment is with beta blockers, such as propanolol. **Primary orthostatic tremor** affects the legs when standing still, causing unsteadiness if the position is maintained. **Resting tremor** is a prominent symptom of *parkinsonism. An **intention tremor** occurs when a patient with disease of the cerebellum tries to touch an object. The closer the object is approached the wilder become the movements.

trench fever an infectious disease caused by the bacterium *Bartonella quintana* and transmitted by body lice (*Pediculus humanus corporis*). It was prevalent among soldiers during both World Wars and is now seen mainly in homeless people. Symptoms include variable fewer and persistent pain in the shins and other bones.

trench foot (**immersion foot**) blackening of the toes and the skin of the foot due to death of the superficial tissues and caused by prolonged immersion in cold water or exposure to damp and cold.

Trendelenburg position a special operating-table posture for patients undergoing surgery of the pelvis or for patients suffering from shock to reduce blood loss in operations on the legs. The patient is laid on his back with the pelvis higher than the head, inclined at an angle of about 45°. [F. Trendelenburg (1844–1924), German surgeon]

Trendelenburg's test (**Trendelenburg's sign**) a test for detecting dysfunction of the hip joint. Normally when a leg is lifted off the ground, the pelvis on the same side is raised by the hip abductor muscles on the other side. If these muscles cannot raise the pelvis against body weight, the pelvis will tilt downwards and the test is positive, indicating arthritis, paralysis of the muscles due to superior gluteal nerve injury, or other hip pathology (e.g. congenital hip dislocation). [F. Trendelenburg]

trephine *n.* a surgical instrument used to remove a circular area of tissue, usually from the cornea of the eye (in the operation of penetrating *keratoplasty) or from bone (for microscopical examination). It consists of a hollow tube with a serrated cutting edge. It is used during the preliminary stages of craniotomy.

Treponema *n.* a genus of anaerobic

spirochaete bacteria. All species are parasitic and some cause disease in animals and humans: *T. carateum* causes *pinta, *T. pallidum* *syphilis, and *T. pertenue* *yaws.

treponematosis *n.* any infection caused by spirochaete bacteria of the genus *Treponema. See* PINTA, SYPHILIS, YAWS.

trespass against the person *see* BATTERY.

tretinoin *n.* a *retinoid drug applied topically as a gel or lotion for the treatment of acne and sun-damaged skin; side-effects include redness and burning of the skin and increased sensitivity to sunlight. It is also taken by mouth to treat acute promyelocytic leukaemia; side-effects may include fever, breathlessness, flushing, headache, and fetal abnormalities (it should not be taken during pregnancy). Trade names: **Retin-A, Vesanoid**.

triad *n.* (in medicine) a group of three united or closely associated structures or three symptoms or effects that occur together. A **portal triad** in a portal canal of the liver consists of a branch of the portal vein, a branch of the hepatic artery, and an interlobular bile tubule.

triage *n.* a system whereby patients are evaluated and categorized according to the seriousness of their injuries or illnesses with a view to prioritizing treatment and other resources. In emergency situations it is designed to maximize the number of survivors.

triamcinolone *n.* a synthetic corticosteroid hormone that reduces inflammation but does not cause salt and water retention. It is used for treating a wide range of inflammatory and allergic conditions, including rheumatoid arthritis, eczema, psoriasis, and hay fever. It is administered by intramuscular or intra-articular injection, nasal spray, or topically; common side-effects include headache, dizziness, somnolence, muscle weakness, and a fall in blood pressure, particularly on the sudden withdrawal of treatment. Trade names: **Adcortyl, Kenalog, Nasacort**.

triamterene *n.* a potassium-sparing *diuretic that is given by mouth, usually in combination with a thiazide or loop diuretic, for the treatment of various forms of fluid retention (oedema). Common side-effects include nausea, vomiting, weakness, reduced blood pressure, and dry mouth. Trade name: **Dytac**.

triangle *n.* (in anatomy) a three-sided structure or area; for example, the *femoral triangle.

triangular bandage a piece of material cut or folded into a triangular shape and used for making an arm sling or holding dressings in position.

Triatoma *n.* a genus of bloodsucking bugs (*see* REDUVIID). *T. infestans* is important in transmitting *Chagas' disease in Argentina, Uruguay, and Chile.

triceps *n.* a muscle with three heads of origin, particularly the **triceps brachii**, which is situated on the back of the upper arm and contracts to extend the forearm. It is the *antagonist of the *brachialis.

triceps jerk a tendon reflex that acts at the level of the seventh cervical spinal nerve. With the elbow flexed and relaxed, the triceps tendon is struck just above the elbow, causing contraction of the triceps and extension of the elbow. This reflex is increased in upper *motor neuron lesions and absent in lower motor neuron lesions.

trich- (tricho-) *combining form denoting* hair or hairlike structures.

trichiasis *n.* a condition in which the eyelashes rub against the eyeball, producing discomfort and sometimes ulceration of the cornea. It may result from inflammation of the eyelids, which makes the lashes grow out in abnormal directions, or when scarring of the conjunctiva (lining membrane) turns the eyelid inwards. It accompanies all forms of *entropion.

Trichinella *n.* a genus of minute parasitic nematode worms. The adults of *T. spiralis* live in the human small intestine, where the females release large numbers of larvae. These bore through the intestinal wall and can cause disease (*see* TRICHINOSIS). The parasite can also develop in pigs and rats.

trichiniasis *n. see* TRICHINOSIS.

trichinosis (trichiniasis) *n.* a disease of cold and temperate regions caused by the larvae of the nematode worm *Trichinella spiralis*. Humans contract trichinosis after eating imperfectly cooked meat infected with the parasite's larval cysts. Larvae, released by females in the intestine, penetrate the intestinal wall and cause diarrhoea and nausea. They migrate around the body and may cause fever, vertigo, delirium, and pains in the limbs. The larvae eventually settle within cysts in the muscles, and this may result in pain and stiffness. The intestinal phase of the disease is treated with anthelmintics.

trichloracetic acid an *astringent used in solution for a variety of skin conditions. It is also applied topically to produce sloughing, especially for the removal of warts.

trichobezoar *n.* hairball: a mass of swallowed hair in the stomach. It may be the patient's own hair or animal hairs. *See* BEZOAR.

Trichocephalus *n. see* WHIPWORM.

trichoglossia *n.* hairiness of the tongue, due to the growth of fungal organisms infecting its surface.

trichology *n.* the study of hair.

Trichomonas *n.* a genus of parasitic flagellate protozoans that move by means of a wavy membrane, bearing a single flagellum, projecting from the body surface. *T. vaginalis* often infects the vagina, where it may cause severe irritation and a foul-smelling discharge (*see* VAGINITIS), and sometimes also the male *urethra; it can be transmitted during sexual intercourse. *T. hominis* and *T. tenax* live in the large intestine and mouth respectively. *See also* TRICHOMONIASIS.

trichomoniasis *n.* 1. an infection of the digestive system by the protozoan *Trichomonas hominis*, causing dysentery. 2. an infection of the vagina due to the protozoan *Trichomonas vaginalis*, causing inflammation of genital tissues with vaginal discharge (*see* VAGINITIS). It can be transmitted to males in whom it causes urethral discharge. Treatment is with *metronidazole.

trichomycosis *n.* any hair disease that is caused by infection with a fungus.

Trichophyton *n.* a genus of fungi, parasitic in humans, that frequently infect the skin, nails, and hair and cause *ringworm. *See also* DERMATOPHYTE.

trichorrhexis nodosa a condition in which the hairs break easily. It may be due to a hereditary condition or it may occur as a consequence of repeated physical or chemical injury. The latter condition may follow the use of heat or bleach on the hair or be caused by persistent rubbing.

Trichosporon *n.* a genus of fungi, parasitic in humans, that infect the scalp and beard.

trichotillomania *n.* a pathologically strong impulse that causes a person to persistently rub or pull out his or her hair, causing conspicuous hair loss. This is a disorder of impulse control.

trichromatic *adj.* describing or relating to the normal state of colour vision, in which a person is sensitive to all three of the primary colours (red, green, and blue) and can match any given colour by a mixture of these three. *Compare* DICHROMATIC, MONOCHROMAT.

trichuriasis *n.* an infestation of the large intestine by the *whipworm, *Trichuris trichiura*; it occurs principally in humid tropical regions. The infection is acquired by eating food contaminated with the worms' eggs. Symptoms, including bloody diarrhoea, anaemia, weakness, and abdominal pain, are evident only in heavy infestations. Trichuriasis can be treated with mebendazole.

Trichuris *n. see* WHIPWORM.

tricuspid atresia a rare form of congenital heart disease in which there is no communication between the right atrium and the right ventricle. Affected babies present with *cyanosis, breathlessness, particularly on feeding, and *failure to thrive. Diagnosis is by *echocardiography. Treatment involves surgical intervention, but the prognosis is often poor.

tricuspid valve the valve in the heart between the right atrium and right ventricle. It consists of three cusps that channel the flow of blood from the atrium to the ventricle and prevent any backflow.

tricyclic antidepressants (tricyclics) *see* ANTIDEPRESSANT.

tridactyly *n.* a congenital abnormality in which there are only three digits on a hand or foot.

trifluoperazine *n.* an *antipsychotic drug (a phenothiazine) used in the treatment of schizophrenia and other psychoses, severe anxiety, and severe nausea and vomiting. It is taken by mouth; common side-effects include drowsiness, dryness of mouth, dizziness, abnormal facial and body movements, and tremor. Trade name: **Stelazine**.

trifocal lenses lenses in which there are three segments. The upper provides a clear image of distant objects; the lower is used for reading and close work; and the middle one for the intermediate distance. Musicians sometimes find the middle segment useful for reading the score during performance.

trigeminal nerve the fifth and largest *cranial nerve (V), which is split into three main branches: ophthalmic, maxillary, and mandibular (see illustration). The motor fibres are responsible for controlling the muscles involved in chewing, while the sensory fibres relay information about temperature, pain, and touch from the whole front half of the head (including the mouth) and also from the meninges.

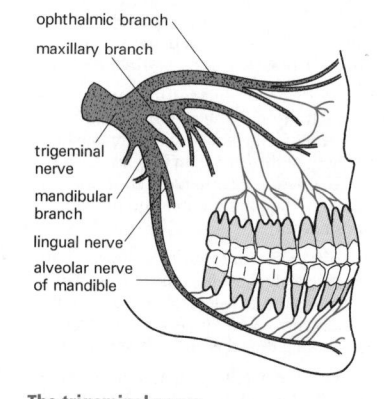

ophthalmic branch
maxillary branch
trigeminal nerve
mandibular branch
lingual nerve
alveolar nerve of mandible

The trigeminal nerve.

trigeminal neuralgia (tic douloureux) *see* NEURALGIA.

trigeminy *n.* a condition in which the heartbeats can be subdivided into groups of three. The first beat is normal, but the second and third are premature beats (*see* EC-TOPIC BEAT).

trigger finger an impairment in the ability to extend a finger, resulting either from a nodular thickening in the flexor tendon or a narrowing of the flexor tendon sheath. On unclenching the fist, the affected finger (usually the third or fourth) at first remains bent and then, on overcoming the resistance, suddenly straightens ('triggers'). Treatment is by incision of the tendon sheath or injection of steroid around the tendon.

triglyceride *n.* a lipid or neutral *fat consisting of glycerol combined with three fatty-acid molecules. Triglycerides are synthesized

from the products of digestion of dietary fat: they are the form in which digested fat is transported in the bloodstream (*see* CHYLO-MICRON). High concentrations of triglycerides in the blood predisposes to coronary heart disease (*see* HYPERTRIGLYCERIDAEMIA).

trigone *n.* a triangular region or tissue, such as the triangular region of the wall of the bladder that lies between the openings of the two ureters and the urethra.

trigonitis *n.* inflammation of the trigone (base) of the urinary bladder. This can occur as part of a generalized *cystitis or it can be associated with inflammation in the urethra, prostate, or cervix (neck) of the uterus. The patient experiences an intense desire to pass urine frequently; treatment includes the clearing of any underlying infection by antibiotic administration.

trigonocephaly *n.* a deformity of the skull in which the vault of the skull is sharply angled just in front of the ears, giving the skull a triangular shape. —**trigonocephalic** *adj.*

trihexyphenidyl (benzhexol) *n.* an *antimuscarinic drug that is used mainly to reduce muscle tremor and rigidity in drug-induced parkinsonism. It is taken by mouth; the most common side-effects are constipation, dry mouth, and blurred vision. Trade name: **Broflex**.

triiodothyronine (T$_3$) *n.* the most metabolically active of the *thyroid hormones, which is mostly formed in the tissues from *thyroxine. A preparation of triiodothyronine (*liothyronine sodium) is administered by mouth or injection for treating underactivity of the thyroid.

trimeprazine *n. see* ALIMEMAZINE.

trimester *n.* (in obstetrics) any one of the three successive three-month periods (the **first**, **second**, and **third trimesters**) into which a pregnancy may be divided.

trimethoprim *n.* an antibacterial drug that is active against a range of microorganisms; taken by mouth, it is used mainly in the treatment of chronic urinary-tract infections and respiratory-tract infections. Long-term treatment may cause anaemia due to deficiency of folate, with which the drug interacts (*see* DIHYDROFOLATE REDUCTASE IN-HIBITOR). Trimethoprim is also administered in a combined preparation with sulfamethoxazole (*see* CO-TRIMOXAZOLE) but is now more usually prescribed alone, because of the severity of the side-effects of co-trimoxazole. Trade name: **Trimopan**.

trimipramine *n.* a tricyclic *antidepressant drug that also possesses sedative properties. It is given by mouth for the treatment of depression. Common side-effects include drowsiness, dizziness, dry mouth, and a fall in blood pressure. Trade name: **Surmontil**.

trinitrophenol *n. see* PICRIC ACID.

triose *n.* a carbohydrate with three carbon units: for example, glyceraldehyde.

triple rhythm *see* GALLOP RHYTHM.

triple test **1.** (in *prenatal screening) a blood test that can be performed between the 15th and 20th weeks of pregnancy. Levels of *alpha-fetoprotein (AFP), *unconjugated oestriol (uE$_3$), and *human chorionic gonadotrophin (hCG) in the serum are computed with maternal age to determine the statistical likelihood of the fetus being affected by Down's syndrome or spina bifida. The **double test** is similar but omits measurement of uE$_3$. **2.** *see* INSULIN STRESS TEST.

triploid *adj.* describing cells, tissues, or individuals in which there are three complete chromosome sets. *Compare* HAPLOID, DIPLOID. —**triploid** *n.*

triptan *n. see* 5HT$_1$ AGONIST.

triquetrum (triquetral bone) *n.* a bone of the wrist (*see* CARPUS). It articulates with the ulna behind and with the pisiform, hamate, and lunate bones in the carpus.

trismus *n.* spasm of the jaw muscles, keeping the jaws tightly closed. This is the characteristic symptom of *tetanus but it also occurs less dramatically as a sensitivity reaction to certain drugs and in disorders of the *basal ganglia.

trisomy *n.* a condition in which there is one extra chromosome present in each cell in addition to the normal (diploid) chromosome set. A number of chromosome disorders are due to trisomy, including *Down's syndrome and *Klinefelter's syndrome. —**trisomic** *adj.*

tritanopia *n.* a rare defect of colour vision in which affected persons are insensitive to blue light and confuse blues and greens. *Compare* DEUTERANOPIA, PROTANOPIA.

trocar *n.* an instrument used combined with a *cannula to draw off fluids from a body cavity (such as the peritoneal cavity). It comprises a metal tube containing a removable shaft with a sharp three-cornered point; the shaft is withdrawn after the trocar has been inserted into the cavity.

trochanter *n.* either of the two protuberances that occur below the neck of the *femur.

troche *n.* a medicinal lozenge, taken by mouth, used to treat conditions of the mouth or throat and also of the alimentary canal.

trochlea *n.* an anatomical part having the structure or function of a pulley; for example the groove at the lower end of the *humerus or the fibrocartilaginous ring in the frontal bone (where it forms part of the orbit), through which the tendon of the superior oblique eye muscle passes. —**trochlear** *adj.*

trochlear nerve the fourth *cranial nerve (IV), which supplies the superior oblique muscle, one of the muscles responsible for movement of the eyeball in its socket. The action of the trochlear nerve is coordinated with that of the *oculomotor and the *abducens nerves.

trochoid joint (pivot joint) a form of *diarthrosis (freely movable joint) in which a bone moves round a central axis, allowing rotational movement. An example is the joint between the atlas and axis vertebrae.

Troisier's sign enlargement of the lymph node at the base of the neck on the left side (**Troisier's node**), which indicates metastatic spread from an abdominal malignant growth, usually a carcinoma of the stomach. [C. E. Troisier (1844–1919), French physician]

Trombicula *n.* a genus of widely distributed mites – the harvest mites. The six-legged parasitic larvae (chiggers) are common in fields during the autumn and frequently attack humans, remaining attached to the skin for several days while feeding on the lymph and digested skin tissues. Their bite causes intense irritation and a severe dermatitis. Various repellents, e.g. benzyl benzoate, can be applied to clothing. *Trombicula* larvae transmit scrub typhus in southeast Asia.

troph- (tropho-) *combining form denoting* nourishment or nutrition.

trophoblast *n.* the tissue that forms the wall of the *blastocyst. At implantation it forms two layers, an inner cellular layer (**cytotrophoblast**), which does not invade maternal tissue and forms the outer surface of the *chorion; and an outer syncytial layer (**syncytiotrophoblast**, or **plasmoditrophoblast**), which erodes the maternal tissue and forms the chorionic *villi of the placenta. *See also* GESTATIONAL TROPHOBLASTIC DISEASE.

trophozoite *n.* a stage in the life cycle of the malarial parasite (*Plasmodium*) that develops from a merozoite in the red blood cells. The trophozoite, which has a ring-shaped body and a single nucleus, grows steadily at the expense of the blood cell; eventually its nucleus and cytoplasm undergo division to form a *schizont containing many merozoites.

-trophy *combining form denoting* nourishment, development, or growth Example: **dystrophy** (defective development).

-tropic *combining form denoting* 1. turning towards. 2. having an affinity for; influencing. Example: **inotropic** (muscle).

tropical abscess (amoebic abscess) an abscess of the liver caused by infection with *Entamoeba histolytica*. *See* (AMOEBIC) DYSENTERY.

tropical medicine the study of diseases more commonly found in tropical regions than elsewhere, such as *malaria, *leprosy, *trypanosomiasis, *schistosomiasis, and *leishmaniasis.

tropical ulcer (Naga sore) a skin disease prevalent in wet tropical regions. A large open sloughing sore usually develops at the site of a wound or abrasion. The ulcer, commonly located on the feet and legs, is often infected with spirochaetes and bacteria and may extend deeply and cause destruction of muscles and bones. Treatment involves the application of mild antiseptic dressings and intramuscular doses of *penicillin. Skin grafts may be necessary in more serious cases. The exact cause of the disease has not yet been determined.

tropicamide *n.* an *antimuscarinic drug used in the form of eye drops to dilate the pupil so that the inside of the eye can more easily be examined or operated upon. Trade name: **Mydriacyl**.

tropocollagen *n.* the molecular unit of *collagen. It consists of a helix of three collagen molecules: this arrangement confers on the fibres structural stability and resistance to stretching.

troponins *pl. n.* a group of regulatory proteins found in muscle. Cardiac-specific forms (troponins T and I) may be detected in the blood between 4 hours and 14 days after heart muscle damage, and thus constitute highly sensitive and specific tests for the detection of *myocardial infarction.

trospium chloride an *antimuscarinic drug indicated for the treatment of overactivity of the bladder *detrusor muscle with symptoms of urge incontinence, urgency, and frequency. It is administered orally; the most common side-effects are dry mouth and constipation. Trade name: **Regurin**.

Trousseau's sign spasmodic contractions of muscles, especially the muscles of mastication, in response to nerve stimulation (e.g. by tapping). It is a characteristic sign of hypocalcaemia (*see* TETANY). [A. Trousseau (1801–67), French physician]

TRT *see* TINNITUS RETRAINING THERAPY.

truncus *n.* a *trunk: a main vessel or other tubular organ from which subsidiary branches arise.

truncus arteriosus the main arterial trunk arising from the fetal heart. It develops into the aorta and pulmonary artery.

trunk *n.* 1. the main part of a blood vessel, lymph vessel, or nerve, from which branches arise. 2. the body excluding the head and limbs.

TRUS *see* TRANSRECTAL ULTRASONOGRAPHY.

truss *n.* a device for applying pressure to a hernia to prevent it from protruding. It usually consists of a pad attached to a belt with straps or spring strips and it is worn under the clothing.

trust *n.* (in the NHS) a self-governing body that provides or commissions any of a range of health-care services, including *hospital, *community health, and mental health services. NHS trusts have their own boards and budgets and the freedom to provide services of their own selection (within legal and contractual frameworks). *See also* FOUNDATION TRUSTS, PRIMARY CARE TRUST.

trypanocide *n.* an agent that kills trypanosomes and is therefore used to treat infestations caused by these parasites (*see* TRYPANOSOMIASIS).

Trypanosoma *n.* a genus of parasitic protozoans that move by means of a long trailing flagellum and a thin wavy membrane, which project from the body surface. Trypanosomes undergo part of their development in the blood of a vertebrate host. The remaining stages occur in invertebrate hosts, which then transmit the parasites back to the vertebrates. *T. rhodesiense* and *T. gambiense*, which are transmitted through the bite of *tsetse flies, cause *sleeping sickness in Africa. *T. cruzi*, carried by *reduviid bugs, causes Chagas' disease in South America.

trypanosomiasis *n.* any disease caused by the presence of parasitic protozoans of the genus *Trypanosoma*. The two most important diseases are *Chagas' disease (South American trypanosomiasis) and *sleeping sickness (African trypanosomiasis).

trypsin *n.* an enzyme that continues the digestion of proteins by breaking down peptones into smaller peptide chains (*see* PEPTIDASE). It is secreted by the pancreas in an inactive form, trypsinogen, which is converted in the duodenum to trypsin by the action of the enzyme enteropeptidase.

trypsinogen *n. see* TRYPSIN.

tryptophan *n.* an *essential amino acid. *See also* AMINO ACID.

TSAB thyroid-stimulating antibody. TSABs are implicated in the causes of *thyroiditis.

T score a measure of bone mineral density used to evaluate the degree of bone thinning detected on *DEXA scanning. An individual's T score is the number of standard deviations above or below the mean reference value for young healthy adults. By convention, a score above –1 is considered normal, a score between –1 and –2.5 indicates **osteopenia**, and a score below –2.5 indicates *osteoporosis.

tsetse *n.* a large bloodsucking fly of tropical Africa belonging to the genus *Glossina*. Tsetse flies, which have slender forwardly projecting biting mouthparts, feed during the day on humans and other mammals. They transmit the blood parasites that cause *sleeping sickness. *G. palpalis* and *G. tachinoides*, which are found along river banks, transmit *Trypanosoma gambiense; G. morsitans*, *G. swynnertoni*, and *G. pallidipes*, which are found in savannah country, transmit *T. rhodesiense*.

TSH *see* THYROID-STIMULATING HORMONE.

T-sign *n.* an ultrasound diagnosis of monochorionicity at 10–14 weeks gestation: the intertwin membrane inserts directly into the placenta, forming a T-sign. *See* CHORIONICITY.

tsutsugamushi disease *see* SCRUB TYPHUS.

TTP *see* THROMBOTIC THROMBOCYTOPENIC PURPURA.

TTTS *see* TWIN-TO-TWIN TRANSFUSION SYNDROME.

tubal occlusion blocking of the Fallopian tubes. This is achieved by surgery as a means of *sterilization; it is also a result of *pelvic inflammatory disease.

tubal pregnancy *see* ECTOPIC PREGNANCY.

tube *n.* (in anatomy) a long hollow cylindrical structure, e.g. a *Fallopian tube.

tuber *n.* (in anatomy) a thickened or swollen part. The **tuber cinereum** is a part of the brain situated at the base of the hypothalamus, connected to the stalk of the pituitary gland.

tubercle *n.* 1. (in anatomy) a small rounded protuberance on a bone. 2. the specific nodular lesion of *tuberculosis.

tubercular *adj.* having small rounded swellings or nodules, not necessarily caused by tuberculosis.

tuberculide *n.* an eruption of the skin that arises in response to an internal focus of tuberculosis.

tuberculin *n.* a protein extract from cultures of tubercle bacilli, used to test whether a person has suffered from or been in contact with tuberculosis. In the **Mantoux test** a quantity of tuberculin is injected beneath the skin and a patch of inflammation appearing in the next 48–72 hours is regarded as a positive reaction, meaning that a degree of immunity is present.

tuberculoma *n.* a mass of cheeselike material resembling a tumour, seen in some cases of *tuberculosis. Tuberculomas are found in a variety of sites, including the lung or brain, and a single mass may be the only clinical evidence of disease. Treatment is by surgical excision, together with antituberculous drugs.

tuberculosis (TB) *n.* an infectious disease caused by the bacillus *Mycobacterium tuber-*

culosis (first identified by Koch in 1882) and characterized by the formation of nodular lesions (**tubercles**) in the tissues.

In **pulmonary tuberculosis** – formerly known as **consumption** and **phthisis** (wasting) – the bacillus is inhaled into the lungs where it sets up a primary tubercle and spreads to the nearest lymph nodes (the **primary complex**). Natural immune defences may heal it at this stage; alternatively the disease may smoulder for months or years and fluctuate with the patient's resistance. Many people become infected but show no symptoms. Others develop a chronic infection and can transmit the bacillus by coughing and sneezing. Symptoms of the active disease include fever, night sweats, weight loss, and the spitting of blood. In some cases the bacilli spread from the lungs to the bloodstream, setting up millions of tiny tubercles throughout the body (**miliary tuberculosis**), or migrate to the meninges to cause tuberculous *meningitis. Bacilli entering by the mouth, usually in infected cows' milk, set up a primary complex in abdominal lymph nodes, leading to *peritonitis, and sometimes spread to other organs, joints, and bones (*see* POTT'S DISEASE).

Tuberculosis is curable by various combinations of the antibiotics *streptomycin, *ethambutol, *isoniazid (INH), *rifampicin, and *pyrazinamide. Preventive measures in the UK include the detection of cases by X-ray screening of vulnerable populations and vaccination with *BCG vaccine of those with no immunity to the disease (the *tuberculin test identifies which people require vaccination). The childhood immunization schedule no longer includes BCG vaccination at 10–14 years of age; vaccination now targets high-risk groups, such as immigrants from countries with a high incidence of TB. There has been a resurgence of tuberculosis in recent years in association with HIV infection. The number of patients with multidrug resistant TB has also increased due to patients not completing drug courses. Many centres have introduced **directly observed therapy** (DOT), in which nurse practitioners watch patients taking their drugs or administer the drugs.

tuberose *adj. see* TUBEROUS.

tuberosity *n.* a large rounded protuberance on a bone. For example, there is a tuberosity at the upper end of the tibia.

tuberous (tuberose) *adj.* knobbed; having nodules or rounded swellings.

tuberous sclerosis (Bourneville's disease, epiloia) a hereditary disorder in which the brain, skin, and other organs are studded with small plaques or tumours; eye involvement includes retinal tumours (astrocytic *hamartomas), *coloboma, *papilloedema, optic nerve gliomas, and eyelid neuromas. Symptoms include epilepsy, learning difficulties, and behavioural disorders.

tubo- *combining form denoting* a tube, especially the Fallopian tube or Eustachian tube.

tuboabdominal *adj.* relating to or occurring in a Fallopian tube and the abdomen.

tubo-ovarian *adj.* relating to or occurring in a Fallopian tube and an ovary.

tubotympanal *adj.* relating to the tympanic cavity and the *Eustachian tube.

tubule *n.* (in anatomy) a small cylindrical hollow structure. *See also* RENAL TUBULE, SEMINIFEROUS TUBULE.

tubulointerstitium *n.* spaces around the kidney tubules containing cells and extracellular components. The tubulointerstitium is believed to influence many aspects of the development and functioning of the tubules and blood vessels of the kidney. —**tubulointerstitial** *adj.*

tubulovillous adenoma a type of polyp that arises in the colon and rectum and can undergo malignant transformation, usually over a period of years, although this can occur more rapidly in familial *polyposis syndromes.

tuftsin *n.* a tetrapeptide derived from IgG (*see* IMMUNOGLOBULIN), produced mainly in the spleen, that stimulates *neutrophil activity (phagocytosis). Levels of tuftsin are reduced after *splenectomy, resulting in diminished resistance to infection, especially by encapsulated organisms.

tularaemia (rabbit fever) *n.* a disease of rodents and rabbits, caused by the bacterium *Francisella tularensis*, that is transmitted to humans by deer flies (*see* CHRYSOPS), by direct contact with infected animals, by contamination of wounds, or by drinking contaminated water. Symptoms include an ulcer at the site of infection, inflamed and ulcerating lymph nodes, headache, aching pains, loss of weight, and a fever lasting several weeks. Treatment with chloramphenicol, streptomycin, or tetracycline is effective.

tulle gras a soft dressing consisting of open-woven silk (or other material) impregnated with a waterproof soft paraffin wax.

Tullio phenomenon dizziness induced by exposure to sound. It is seen in various conditions of the inner ear, including *Ménière's disease and *superior canal dehiscence syndrome. [P. Tullio (1881–1941) Italian biologist]

tumbu fly a large non-bloodsucking fly, *Cordylobia anthropophaga*, widely distributed in tropical Africa. The female fly lays its eggs on ground contaminated with urine or excreta or on clothing tainted with sweat or urine. The maggots are normally parasites of rats, but if they come into contact with humans they penetrate the skin, producing boil-like swellings (*see also* MYIASIS). The maggots can be gently eased out by applying oil to the swellings.

tumefaction *n.* the process in which a tissue becomes swollen and tense by accumulation within it of fluid under pressure.

tumescence *n.* a swelling, or the process of becoming swollen, usually because of an accumulation of blood or other fluid within the tissues.

tumid *adj.* swollen.

tumor *n.* swelling: one of the classical signs of *inflammation in a tissue, the other three being *calor (heat), *rubor (redness), and *dolor (pain). The swelling of an inflamed area is due to the leakage from small blood vessels of clear protein-containing fluid, which accumulates between the cells.

tumour *n.* any abnormal swelling in or on a part of the body. The term is usually applied to an abnormal growth of tissue, which may be *benign or *malignant. *Compare* CYST.

tumour-associated antigen a protein produced by cancer cells. Its presence in the blood can be revealed by means of a simple blood test, aiding the diagnosis of malignant melanoma and other cancers at their earliest – and most treatable – stages of development.

tumour-infiltrating lymphocyte (TIL) a lymphoid cell that can infiltrate solid tumours. Such cells can be cultured in vitro, in the presence of *interleukin 2, and have been used as vehicles for *tumour necrosis factor in gene therapy trials for cancer.

tumour marker a substance produced by a tumour that can be used to aid detection of the tumour and to monitor its size and the effects of treatment. An example is *alpha-fetoprotein, which is used to monitor treatment of malignant *teratomas. *See also* CA125, CA19-9, CARCINO-EMBRYONIC ANTIGEN, HUMAN CHORIONIC GONADOTROPHIN.

tumour necrosis factor (TNF) either of two proteins, TNF-α or TNF-β, that function as *cytokines. Produced by macrophages, monocytes, T lymphocytes, and various other cells, they mediate many responses, including inflammation, and have a marked action against tumour cells. Anti-TNF drugs (*see* CYTOKINE INHIBITOR) are used in the treatment of several disorders, especially rheumatoid arthritis.

Tunga *n.* a genus of sand fleas found in tropical America and Africa. The fertilized female of *T. penetrans*, the chigoe or jigger, burrows beneath the skin of the foot, where it becomes enclosed in a swelling of the surrounding tissues and causes intense itching and inflammation. Surgical removal of the fleas is recommended.

tunica *n.* a covering or layer of an organ or part; for example, a layer of the wall of a blood vessel (*see* ADVENTITIA, INTIMA, MEDIA). The **tunica albuginea** is a fibrous membrane comprising one of the covering tissues of the ovary, penis, and testis.

tunnel *n.* (in anatomy) a canal or hollow groove. *See also* CARPAL TUNNEL.

tunnel vision a visual-field defect in which only the central area of the *visual field remains. It occurs in advanced *glaucoma and is simulated by *aphakic spectacles.

turbinate bone *see* NASAL CONCHA.

turbinectomy *n.* the surgical removal or partial removal of one of the bones forming the nasal cavity (nasal conchae, or turbinate bones), performed in the treatment of nasal obstruction.

turgescence *n.* a swelling, or the process by which a swelling arises in tissues, usually by the accumulation of blood or other fluid under pressure.

turgor *n.* a state of being swollen or distended.

Turkel's needle a specially designed needle for purposes of transrectal prostatic biopsy.

Turner's syndrome (gonadal dysgenesis) a genetic defect in women in which there is only one X chromosome instead of the usual two. Affected women are infertile: they have female external genitalia but their ovaries fail to develop normally, resulting in absence of menstrual periods (*see* AMENORRHOEA). Characteristically they are short and have variable developmental defects, which may include webbing of the neck. [H. H. Turner (1892–1970), US endocrinologist]

TURP transurethral resection of the prostate: *see* RESECTION.

turricephaly *n. see* OXYCEPHALY.

tussis *n.* the medical name for **coughing.

TUVP *see* TRANSURETHRAL VAPORIZATION OF THE PROSTATE.

TVT *see* TENSION-FREE VAGINAL TAPE.

twin-peak sign *see* LAMBDA SIGN.

twins *pl. n.* two individuals who are born at the same time and of the same parents. **Fraternal** (or **dizygotic**) **twins** are the result of the simultaneous fertilization of two egg cells; they may be of different sexes and are no more alike than ordinary siblings. **Identical** (or **monozygotic**) **twins** result from the fertilization of a single egg cell that subsequently divides to give two separate fetuses. They are of the same sex and otherwise genetically identical; any differences in their appearance are due to environmental influences. All dizygotic twins and about one-third of monozygotic twins are **dichorionic** (i.e. they develop within separate chorionic membranes). About two-thirds of monozygotic twins are **monochorionic**, sharing a chorion. *See* CHORIONICITY. *See also* CONJOINED TWINS.

twin-to-twin transfusion syndrome (**TTTS**) a condition in which communicating vessels in the shared placenta of monochorionic **twins* (*see* CHORIONICITY) divert blood to one fetus (the recipient) from the other (the donor), resulting in one fetus with increased blood volume and one anaemic fetus. It complicates 15% of monochorionic twin pregnancies, and a system of ultrasound staging has been developed to assess

Twin-to-twin transfusion syndrome.

the severity of the syndrome. TTTS is associated with a high perinatal mortality rate. There is significant morbidity and poor neurodevelopmental outcome in surviving infants due to complications of the disease itself and the high preterm birth rate that invariably accompanies this condition. A range of treatments, including **amnioreduction and laser ablation of the communicating vessels, have led to an improvement in overall perinatal survival rates.

tylosis *n.* an extremely rare focal **keratosis occurring especially on the palms and soles. It occurs early in life and is inherited in an autosomal **dominant fashion. It is associated with oral leukokeratosis and with oesophageal cancer.

tympan- (tympano-) *combining form denoting* **1.** the eardrum. Example: **tympanectomy** (surgical excision of). **2.** the middle ear.

tympanic cavity *see* MIDDLE EAR.

tympanic membrane (eardrum) the membrane at the inner end of the external auditory meatus, separating the outer and middle ears. It is formed from the outer wall of the lining of the tympanic cavity and the skin that lines the external auditory meatus. When sound waves reach the ear the tympanum vibrates, transmitting these vibrations to the malleus – one of the auditory **ossicles in the middle ear – to which it is attached.

tympanites (meteorism) *n.* distension of the abdomen with air or gas: the abdomen is resonant (drumlike) on *percussion. Causes include intestinal obstruction, the *irritable bowel syndrome, and *aerophagy.

tympanogram *n.* the graphic record of a test of middle ear function carried out on a *tympanometer.

tympanometer *n.* an apparatus for testing the pressure in the middle ear and the mobility of the *tympanic membrane. It is used in the diagnosis of *glue ear. —**tympanometry** *n.*

tympanoplasty *n.* surgical repair of defects of the eardrum and middle ear ossicles. *See* MYRINGOPLASTY.

tympanotomy *n.* a surgical operation to expose the middle ear and allow access to the ossicles. It is usually performed by incising around the eardrum and turning it forwards.

tympanum *n.* the *middle ear (tympanic cavity) and/or the eardrum (*tympanic membrane).

typho- *combining form denoting* 1. typhoid fever. 2. typhus.

typhoid fever an infection of the digestive system by the bacterium *Salmonella typhi*, causing general weakness, headache, high fever, a rash (rose spots) on the chest and abdomen, chills, sweating, and in serious cases inflammation of the spleen and bones, delirium, and erosion of the intestinal wall leading to haemorrhage. It is transmitted through food or drinking water contaminated by the faeces or urine of patients or carriers. Often recovery occurs naturally but relapses are common. Treatment is usually with antibiotics, such as ciprofloxacin or ceftriaxone. Vaccines that provide temporary immunity are available. *Compare* PARATYPHOID FEVER.

typhus (spotted fever) *n.* any one of a group of infections caused by *rickettsiae and characterized by severe headache, a widespread rash, prolonged high fever, and delirium. They all respond to treatment with chloramphenicol or tetracyclines. **Epidemic**

typhus (also known as **classical** or **louse-borne typhus**) is caused by infection with *Rickettsia prowazekii* transmitted by lice. It was formerly very prevalent in overcrowded insanitary conditions (as during wars and famines), with a mortality rate approaching 100%. **Endemic typhus** (**murine** or **flea-borne typhus**) is a disease of rats due to *Rickettsia mooseri*; it can be transmitted to humans by rat fleas, causing a mild typhus fever. There are in addition several kinds of **tick typhus** (in which the rickettsiae are transmitted by ticks), including *Rocky Mountain spotted fever, and typhus transmitted by mites (*see* RICKETTSIAL POX, SCRUB TYPHUS).

tyramine *n.* an amine naturally occurring in cheese. It has a similar effect in the body to that of *adrenaline. This effect can be dangerous in patients taking *MAO inhibitors (antidepressants), in whom blood pressure may become very high. Cheese is therefore not advised when such drugs are prescribed.

Tyroglyphus *n. see* ACARUS.

tyrosine *n. see* AMINO ACID.

tyrosine kinase inhibitor any one of a class of drugs that interfere with cell growth in a variety of different ways by inhibiting the action of tyrosine kinases. This family of enzymes, which occur both within cells and as components of cell-membrane receptor sites, have an important role in cell division and cell growth. Many tumour cells have been shown to have both intracellular enzymes and extracellular receptor sites, and a variety of anticancer agents have been developed to inhibit enzyme activity at these sites. Among these drugs are *imatinib, **dasatinib** (Sprycel), and **nilotinib** (Tasigna), used for treating chronic myeloid leukaemia; *sunitinib, for treating renal cell carcinoma; and **erlotinib** (Tarceva), for treating pancreatic cancer and non-small-cell lung cancer. *See also* EPIDERMAL GROWTH FACTOR RECEPTOR.

tyrosinosis *n.* an inborn defect of metabolism of the amino acid tyrosine that causes excessive excretion of parahydroxyphenyl-pyruvic acid in the urine. Symptoms include fever, lethargy, irritability, and drowsiness.

ubiquinone *n.* a *coenzyme that acts as an electron transfer agent in the mitochondria of cells (*see* ELECTRON TRANSPORT CHAIN).

uE₃ *see* UNCONJUGATED OESTRIOL.

UGH syndrome **u*veitis associated with *glaucoma and **h*yphaema. This is an uncommon inflammatory condition occurring as a complication of intraocular lens *implants.

UICC Union international contre le cancer: an international body promoting cancer prevention and treatment. It produces respected texts on the most important types of cancer, particularly on tumour staging classifications.

UIP usual interstitial pneumonitis. *See* INTERSTITIAL PNEUMONITIS.

ulcer *n.* 1. a break in an epithelial surface. *See also* DENDRITIC ULCER. 2. a break in the skin extending to all its layers, or a break in the mucous membrane lining the alimentary tract, that fails to heal and is often accompanied by inflammation. Of the many types of skin ulcer, the most common is the **venous** (or **hypostatic**) **ulcer** of the leg, known incorrectly as a **varicose ulcer**, which is caused by increased venous pressure and usually occurs in older women. *See also* ARTERIAL ULCER, PRESSURE SORE.

For ulcers of the alimentary tract, *see* APHTHOUS ULCER, DUODENAL ULCER, GASTRIC ULCER, PEPTIC ULCER, STRESS ULCERS.

ulcerative colitis a condition causing inflammation and ulceration of the colon. *See* COLITIS.

ulcerative gingivitis acute painful gingivitis with ulceration, in which the tissues of the gums are rapidly destroyed. Occurring mainly in debilitated patients, it is associated with anaerobic microorganisms (*see* FUSO-BACTERIUM, BACTEROIDES) and is accompanied by an unpleasant odour. Treatment is with *metronidazole and a careful and thorough regime of oral hygiene supplemented with oxidizing mouthwashes. In the past ulcerative gingivitis has been called **Vincent's**

angina; in its severe form it is known as *noma.

ule- (ulo-) *combining form denoting* 1. scars; scar tissue. 2. the gums.

ulna *n.* the inner and longer bone of the forearm (see illustration). It articulates with the humerus and radius above and with the radius and indirectly with the wrist bones below. At its upper end is the *olecranon process and *coronoid process; at the lower end is a cone-shaped **styloid process**. —**ulnar** *adj.*

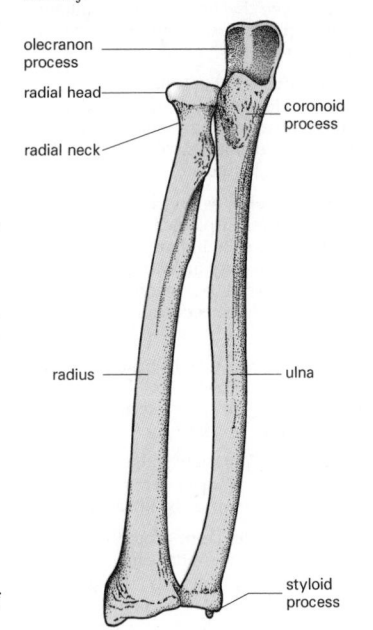

Right ulna and radius (front view).

ulnar artery a branch of the brachial artery arising at the elbow and running deep within the muscles of the medial side of the forearm. It passes into the palm of the hand, where it unites with the arch of the radial artery and gives off branches to the hand and fingers.

ulnar nerve one of the major nerves of the arm. It originates in the neck, from spinal roots of the last cervical and first thoracic divisions, and runs down the inner side of the upper arm to behind the elbow. In the forearm it supplies the muscles with motor nerves; lower down it divides into branches that supply the skin of the palm and fourth and fifth fingers.

ultra- *prefix denoting* 1. beyond. 2. an extreme degree (e.g. of large or small size).

ultracentrifuge *n.* a *centrifuge that works at extremely high speeds of rotation: used for separating large molecules, such as proteins.

ultradian *adj.* denoting a biological rhythm or cycle that occurs more frequently than once in 24 hours. *Compare* CIRCADIAN; NYCTOHEMERAL.

ultrafiltration *n.* filtration under pressure. In the kidney, blood is subjected to ultrafiltration to remove the unwanted water, urea, and other waste material that goes to make up urine.

ultramicroscope *n.* a microscope for examining particles suspended in a gas or liquid under intense illumination from one side. Light is scattered or reflected from the particles, which can be seen through the eyepiece as bright objects against a dark background.

ultramicrotome *n.* an instrument for cutting extremely thin sections of tissue (not more than 0.1 μm thick) for electron microscopy. *See also* MICROTOME.

ultrasonics *n.* the study of the uses and properties of sound waves of very high frequency (*see* ULTRASOUND). —**ultrasonic** *adj.*

ultrasonography (sonography) *n.* the use of *ultrasound to produce images of structures in the human body. The ultrasound probe sends out a short pulse of high-frequency sound and detects the reflected waves (echoes) occurring at interfaces within the organs. The direction of the pulse can then be moved across the area of interest with each pulse to build up a complete image. Scans may produce a single stationary image similar to a photograph (static) or multiple sequential images similar to a video (*real-time imaging). The ultrasound waves

are transmitted from – and echoes detected by – piezoelectric crystals contained within the scanning probe (*see* TRANSDUCER). As far as is known, there are no adverse effects from the use of ultrasound at diagnostic energies. Ultrasound waves are blocked by gas, as in the lungs and bowel, which can obscure underlying structures. The detail seen increases with the frequency of the ultrasound but the depth of penetration decreases. Ultrasonography is extensively used in obstetrics, including the diagnosis of pregnancy, assessment of gestational age, diagnosis of *malpresentations, ectopic pregnancies, and *hydatidiform moles, and detection of structural fetal abnormalities (*see also* TRANSVAGINAL ULTRASONOGRAPHY). It is also used to examine the abdominal organs, urinary tract, blood vessels, muscles, and tendons. More specialized techniques include *echocardiography, *transrectal ultrasonography (TRUS), **intraoperative ultrasound (IOUS)**, and endoscopic ultrasound examinations. *See also* DOPPLER ULTRASOUND.

ultrasound (ultrasonic waves) *n.* sound waves of high frequency (above 20 kHz), inaudible to the human ear. Ultrasound in the range 2–20 MHz can be used to produce images of the interior of the human body as the waves reflect off structures back to the probe (*see* ULTRASONOGRAPHY). Ultrasound waves have the advantage over X-rays of not being ionizing and are therefore much less harmful, particularly at energy levels used for diagnosis. The vibratory effect of ultrasound can also be used to break up stones in the body (*see* LITHOTRIPSY) and in the treatment of rheumatic conditions and cataract (*see* PHACOEMULSIFICATION). Ultrasonic instruments are used in dentistry to remove *calculus from the surfaces of teeth and to remove debris from the root canals of teeth in *root canal treatment. **High-intensity focused ultrasound** (*see* HIFU) can be used to destroy tissue, such as tumours. **Keepsake ultrasound** is the provision of ultrasound images of a fetus to the parents for nonmedical purposes; it is said by its proponents to help with bonding and to strengthen relationships in the family.

ultrasound marker the appearance, on *ultrasonography of a pregnant woman, of a feature suggesting an abnormality in the fetus. Such markers can be classified as major fetal structural abnormalities or minor ultrasound features called **soft markers**. The latter are usually transient and may resolve spontaneously, but they may indicate the risk of a serious chromosomal abnormality in the fetus. An example is increased nuchal translucency (*see* NUCHAL TRANSLUCENCY SCANNING).

ultraviolet radiation invisible short-wavelength radiation beyond the violet end of the visible spectrum. Sunlight contains ultraviolet rays, which are responsible for the production of both suntan and – on over-exposure – *sunburn. The dust and gases of the earth's atmosphere absorb most of the ultraviolet radiation in sunlight (*see* OZONE). If this did not happen, the intense ultraviolet radiation from the sun would be lethal to living organisms.

umbilical cord the strand of tissue connecting the fetus to the placenta. It contains two arteries that carry blood to the placenta and one vein that returns it to the fetus. It also contains remnants of the *allantois and *yolk sac and becomes ensheathed by the *amnion.

umbilical cord blood banked stem cells haemopoietic *stem cells collected from umbilical cord blood donated at birth, which can be stored indefinitely and used if a sibling or any other blood-compatible baby develops an illness (such as leukaemia) that could only be treated by cord-blood stem-cell transplantation. This facility is now available in the UK and the USA.

umbilical hernia *see* EXOMPHALOS.

umbilicus (omphalus) *n.* the navel: a circular depression in the centre of the abdomen marking the site of attachment of the *umbilical cord in the fetus. —**umbilical** *adj.*

umbo *n.* a projecting centre of a round surface, especially the projection of the inner surface of the eardrum to which the malleus is attached.

unciform bone *see* HAMATE BONE.

uncinate fits a form of temporal lobe *epilepsy in which hallucinations of taste and smell and inappropriate chewing movements are prominent features.

unconjugated oestriol (uE₃) a product of the placenta, levels of which are reduced in pregnancies affected by Down's syndrome. It is one of the markers used in *prenatal screening tests (*see* TRIPLE TEST).

unconscious *adj.* **1.** in a state of uncon-

sciousness. **2.** describing those mental processes of which a person is not aware. **3.** (in psychoanalysis) denoting the part of the mind that includes memories, motives, and intentions that are not accessible to awareness and cannot be made conscious without overcoming resistances. *Compare* SUBCONSCIOUS.

unconsciousness *n.* a condition of being unaware of one's surroundings, as in sleep, or of being unresponsive to stimulation. An unnatural state of unconsciousness may be caused by factors that produce reduced brain activity, such as lack of oxygen, *head injuries, poisoning, blood loss, and many diseases, or it may be brought about deliberately during general *anaesthesia. *See also* COMA.

uncus *n.* any hook-shaped structure, especially a projection of the lower surface of the cerebral hemisphere that is composed of cortex belonging to the temporal lobe.

undecenoic acid an antifungal agent, applied to the skin in the form of powder, cream, or aerosol spray for the treatment of athlete's foot. Trade name: **Mycota**.

undine *n.* a small rounded container, usually made of glass, for solutions used to wash out the eye. It has a small neck for filling and a long tapering spout with a narrow outlet to deliver a fine stream of fluid to the eye.

undulant fever *see* BRUCELLOSIS.

ungual *adj.* relating to the fingernails or toenails (ungues).

unguentum *n.* (in pharmacy) an ointment.

unguis *n.* a fingernail or toenail. *See* NAIL.

uni- *combining form denoting* one.

unicellular *adj.* describing organisms or tissues that consist of a single cell. Unicellular organisms include the protozoans, most bacteria, and some fungi.

unilateral *adj.* (in anatomy) relating to or affecting one side of the body or one side of an organ or other part.

union *n.* (in a fractured bone) the successful result of healing of a fracture, in which the previously separated bone ends have become firmly united by newly formed bone. Failure of union (**non-union**) may result if the bone ends are not immobilized or from

infection or bone diseases. *Compare* MALU-
NION.

Union international contre le cancer
see UICC.

unipolar *adj.* (in neurology) describing a
neuron that has one main process extending
from the cell body. *Compare* BIPOLAR.

unsaturated fatty acid a *fatty acid in
which one (**monounsaturated**) or many
(**polyunsaturated**) of the carbon atoms are
linked by double bonds that are easily split
in chemical reactions so that other substances can connect to them. These fats
occur in fish and plant-derived foods, and a
diet high in unsaturated fats is associated
with low serum cholesterol levels. *Compare*
SATURATED FATTY ACID.

uPM3 *see* PCA3.

UPPP *n. see* UVULOPALATOPHARYNGOPLASTY.

urachus *n.* the remains of the cavity of the
*allantois, which usually disappears during
embryonic development. In the adult it normally exists in the form of a solid fibrous
cord connecting the bladder with the umbilicus, but it may persist abnormally as a
patent duct. —**urachal** *adj.*

uracil *n.* one of the nitrogen-containing
bases (*see* PYRIMIDINE) occurring in the nucleic acid RNA.

uraemia *n.* the presence of excessive
amounts of urea and other nitrogenous
waste compounds in the blood. These waste
products are normally excreted by the kidneys in urine; their accumulation in the
blood occurs in kidney failure and results in
nausea, vomiting, lethargy, drowsiness, and
eventually (if untreated) death. Treatment
may require dialysis or transplantation.
—**uraemic** *adj.*

uran- (**urano-**) *combining form denoting*
the palate.

urataemia *n.* the presence in the blood of
sodium urate and other urates, formed by
the reaction of uric acid with bases. In *gout,
urataemia leads to deposition of urates in
various parts of the body.

uraturia *n.* the presence in the urine of
urates (salts of uric acid). Abnormally high
concentrations of urates in urine occur in
*gout.

urea *n.* the main breakdown product of
protein metabolism. It is the chemical form

in which unrequired nitrogen is excreted by
the body in the urine. Urea is formed in the
liver from ammonia and carbon dioxide in a
series of enzyme-mediated reactions (the
urea cycle). Accumulation of urea in the
bloodstream together with other nitrogenous compounds is due to kidney failure and
gives rise to *uraemia.

urease *n.* an enzyme that catalyses the hydrolysis of urea to ammonia and carbon
dioxide.

urecchysis *n.* the escape of uric acid from
the blood into spaces in the connective tissue.

ureter *n.* either of a pair of tubes, 25–30 cm
long, that conduct urine from the pelvis of
kidneys to the bladder. The walls of the
ureters contain thick layers of smooth muscle, which contract to force urine into the
bladder, between an outer fibrous coat and
an inner mucous layer. —**ureteral, ureteric**
adj.

ureter- (**uretero-**) *combining form denoting* the ureter(s). Example: **ureterovaginal**
(relating to the ureters and vagina).

ureterectomy *n.* surgical removal of a
ureter. This usually includes removal of the
associated kidney as well (*see* NEPHRO-
URETERECTOMY). If previous nephrectomy
has been performed to remove a kidney
that has been destroyed by *vesicoureteric reflux or because of a tumour of
the renal pelvis, subsequent ureterectomy
may be necessary to cure reflux into the
stump of the ureter or tumour in the ureter,
respectively.

ureteritis *n.* inflammation of the ureter.
This usually occurs in association with inflammation of the bladder (*see* CYSTITIS), particularly if caused by *vesicoureteric reflux.
Tuberculosis of the urinary tract can also
cause ureteritis, which progresses to *stricture formation.

ureterocele *n.* a cystic swelling of the wall
of the ureter at the point where it passes into
the bladder. It is associated with stenosis of
the opening of the ureter and it may cause
impaired drainage of the kidney with dilatation of the ureter and *hydronephrosis. If
urinary obstruction is present, the ureterocele should be dealt with surgically.

ureteroenterostomy *n.* an artificial communication, surgically created, between the
ureter and the bowel. In this form of urinary

diversion, which bypasses the bladder, the ureters are attached to the sigmoid colon (*see* URETEROSIGMOIDOSTOMY).

ureterolithotomy *n.* the surgical removal of a stone from the ureter (*see* CALCULUS). The operative approach depends upon the position of the stone within the ureter. If the stone occupies the lower portion of the ureter, it may be extracted by *cystoscopy, thus avoiding open surgery.

ureterolysis *n.* an operation to free one or both ureters from surrounding fibrous tissue causing an obstruction.

ureteroneocystostomy *n.* the surgical reimplantation of a ureter into the bladder. This is most commonly performed to cure *vesicoureteric reflux. The ureter is reimplanted obliquely through the bladder wall to act as a valve and prevent subsequent reflux. The operation is usually referred to as an **antireflux procedure** or simply **reimplantation of ureter**.

ureteronephrectomy *n. see* NEPHRO-URETERECTOMY.

ureteroplasty *n.* surgical reconstruction of the ureter using a segment of bowel or a tube of bladder (*see* BOARI FLAP). This is necessary if a segment of ureter is damaged by disease or injury.

ureteropyelonephritis *n.* inflammation involving both the ureter and the renal pelvis (*see* URETERITIS, PYELITIS).

ureteroscope *n.* a rigid or flexible instrument that can be passed into the ureter and up into the pelvis of the kidney. It is most commonly used to visualize a stone in the ureter and remove it safely under direct vision with a stone basket or forceps. Larger stones need to be fragmented before removal with an ultrasound or electrohydraulic *lithotripsy probe, lithoclast, or lasers. Ureteroscopy can also be used to visualize tumours in the ureter, and a flexible ureteroscope can be passed into the kidney to visualize and treat tumours or stones.

ureteroscopy *n.* the inspection of the lumen of the ureter with a *ureteroscope.

ureterosigmoidostomy *n.* the operation of implanting the ureters into the sigmoid colon (*see* URETEROENTEROSTOMY). This method of permanent urinary diversion may be used after *cystectomy or to bypass a diseased or damaged bladder. The urine is

passed together with the faeces, and continence depends upon a normal anal sphincter. The main advantage of this form of diversion is the avoidance of an external opening and appliance to collect the urine; the disadvantages include possible kidney infection and acidosis with long-term development of new tumours in 10% of cases.

ureterostomy *n.* the surgical creation of an external opening into the ureter. This usually involves bringing the ureter to the skin surface so that the urine can drain into a suitable appliance (**cutaneous ureterostomy**). The divided dilated ureter can be brought through the skin to form a spout, but ureters of a normal size need to be implanted into a segment of bowel used for this purpose (*see* ILEAL CONDUIT) to avoid narrowing and obstruction.

ureterotomy *n.* surgical incision into the ureter. The commonest reason for performing this is to allow removal of a stone (*see* URETEROLITHOTOMY).

urethr- (urethro-) *combining form denoting* the urethra.

urethra *n.* the tube that conducts urine from the bladder to the exterior. The female urethra is quite short (about 3.5 cm) and opens just within the *vulva, between the clitoris and vagina. The male urethra is longer (about 20 cm) and runs through the penis. As well as urine, it receives the secretions of the male accessory sex glands (prostate and Cowper's glands and seminal vesicles) and spermatozoa from the *vas deferens; thus it also serves as the ejaculatory duct.

urethritis *n.* inflammation of the urethra. This may be due to gonorrhoea (**specific urethritis**), another sexually transmitted infection, often infection with *Chlamydia trachomatis* (**nongonococcal urethritis, NGU**; or **nonspecific urethritis, NSU**), or to the presence of a catheter in the urethra. The symptoms are those of urethral discharge with painful or difficult urination (*dysuria). Treatment of urethritis due to infection is by administration of appropriate antibiotics after the causative organisms have been isolated from the discharge. Untreated or severe urethritis results in a urethral *stricture.

urethrocele *n.* prolapse of the urethra into the vaginal wall causing a bulbous swelling to appear in the vagina, particularly on straining. The condition is associated with previous childbirth. Treatment usually in-

u

volves surgical repair of the lax tissues to give better support to the urethra and the vaginal wall.

urethrography *n.* a technique for X-ray examination of the urethra. *Contrast medium is introduced into the urethra so that its outline and any narrowing or other abnormalities may be observed in X-ray images (**urethrograms**). In **ascending urethrography** contrast medium is injected up the urethra using a special syringe and penile clamp. In **descending urethrography** (or **micturating cystourethrography, MCU**), X-rays of the urethra can be taken during the passing of water-soluble contrast material previously inserted into the bladder in order to demonstrate disorders of micturition, particularly bladder emptying.

urethroplasty *n.* surgical repair of the urethra, especially a urethral *stricture. The operation entails the insertion of a flap or patch of skin from the scrotum or perineum into the urethra at the site of the stricture, which is laid widely open. The operation can be performed in one stage, although two stages are usual in the reconstruction of a posterior urethral stricture (*see* URETHROSTOMY). **Transpubic urethroplasty** is performed to repair a ruptured posterior urethra following a fractured pelvis. Access to the damaged urethra is achieved by partial removal of the pubic bone.

urethrorrhaphy *n.* surgical restoration of the continuity of the urethra. This may be required following laceration of the urethra.

urethrorrhoea *n.* a discharge from the urethra. This is a symptom of *urethritis.

urethroscope *n.* an *endoscope, consisting of a fine tube fitted with a light and lenses, for examination of the interior of the male urethra, including the prostate region. —**urethroscopy** *n.*

urethrostenosis *n.* a *stricture of the urethra.

urethrostomy *n.* the operation of creating an opening of the urethra in the perineum in men. This can be permanent, to bypass a severe *stricture of the urethra in the penis, or it can form the first stage of an operation to cure a stricture of the posterior section of the urethra (*urethroplasty).

urethrotomy *n.* the operation of cutting a *stricture in the urethra. It is usually performed with a **urethrotome**. This instru-

ment, a type of *endoscope, consists of a sheath down which is passed a fine knife, which is operated by the surgeon viewing the stricture down an illuminated telescope.

urge incontinence *see* INCONTINENCE.

urgency *n.* a *lower urinary tract symptom in which there is a compelling desire to pass urine immediately; this may or may not be associated with *incontinence (urge incontinence).

-uria *combining form denoting* **1.** a condition of urine or urination. Example: **polyuria** (passage of excess urine). **2.** the presence of a specified substance in the urine. Example: **haematuria** (blood in).

uric acid a nitrogen-containing organic acid that is the end-product of nucleic acid metabolism and is a component of the urine. Crystals of uric acid are deposited in the joints of people suffering from *gout.

uricosuric drug a drug, such as *probenecid or *sulfinpyrazone, that increases the amount of *uric acid excreted in the urine.

uridine *n.* a compound containing uracil and the sugar ribose. *See also* NUCLEOSIDE.

uridrosis *n.* the presence of excessive amounts of urea in the sweat; when the sweat dries, a white flaky deposit of urea may remain on the skin. The phenomenon occurs in *uraemia.

urin- (**urino-, uro-**) *combining form denoting* urine or the urinary system.

urinalysis *n.* the analysis of *urine, using physical, chemical and microscopical tests, to determine the proportions of its normal constituents and to detect alcohol, drugs, sugar, or other abnormal constituents.

urinary bladder *see* BLADDER.

urinary diversion any of various techniques for the collection and diversion of urine away from its usual excretory channels, after the bladder has been removed (*see* CYSTECTOMY) or bypassed. These techniques include *ureterosigmoidostomy and the construction of an *ileal conduit. **Continent diversion**, usually after cystectomy, may be achieved by constructing a reservoir or pouch from a section of small or large intestine or a combination of both. This can be emptied by catheterization via a small *stoma and has the advantage over an ileal conduit in not requiring a urinary drainage bag.

urinary tract the entire system of ducts and channels that conduct urine from the kidneys to the exterior. It includes the ureters, the bladder, and the urethra.

urination (micturition) *n.* the periodic discharge of urine from the bladder through the urethra. It is initiated by voluntary relaxation of the sphincter muscle below the bladder and maintained by reflex contraction of the muscles of the bladder wall.

urine *n.* the fluid excreted by the kidneys, which contains many of the body's waste products. It is the major route by which the end-products of nitrogen metabolism – *urea, *uric acid, and *creatinine – are excreted. The other major constituent is sodium chloride. Over 100 other substances are usually present, but only in trace amounts. Analysis of urine (*see* URINALYSIS) is commonly used in the diagnosis of diseases (for example, there are high levels of urinary glucose in diabetes and of ketone bodies in ketonuria); immunological analysis of urine is the basis of most *pregnancy tests.

urine output *see* VITAL SIGNS.

uriniferous tubule *see* RENAL TUBULE.

urinogenital (urogenital) *adj.* of or relating to the organs and tissues concerned with both excretion and reproduction, which are anatomically closely associated.

urinogenital sinus the duct in the embryo that receives the ureter and the Wolffian and Müllerian ducts and opens to the exterior. The innermost portion forms most of the bladder and the remainder forms the urethra with its associated glands. Part of it may also contribute towards the vagina.

urinometer *n.* a hydrometer for measuring the specific gravity of urine.

urobilinogen *n.* a colourless product of the reduction of the *bile pigment bilirubin. Urobilinogen is formed from bilirubin in the intestine by bacterial action. Part of it is reabsorbed and returned to the liver; part of it is excreted in the faeces (a trace may also appear in the urine). When exposed to air, urobilinogen is oxidized to a brown pigment, **urobilin**.

urocele *n.* a cystic swelling in the scrotum, containing urine that has escaped from the urethra. This may arise following urethral in-

jury. Immediate treatment is to divert the urine by suprapubic *cystotomy, local drainage of the swelling, and antibiotic administration.

urochesia *n.* the passage of urine through the rectum. This may follow a penetrating injury involving both the lower urinary tract and the bowel.

urodynamics *n.* the recording of pressures within the bladder by the use of special equipment that can also record urethral sphincter pressures. Simultaneously, abdominal pressure is usually recorded with a catheter in the rectum, vagina, or ileal conduit. It is an essential investigation in the study of urinary incontinence. In some men, urodynamic studies are necessary to determine if their *lower urinary tract symptoms are caused by bladder outlet obstruction or *detrusor overactivity.

urofollitropin *n. see* HUMAN MENOPAUSAL GONADOTROPHINS.

urogenital *adj. see* URINOGENITAL.

urogram *n.* an X-ray of the urinary tract or any part of it. It is usually obtained after the intravenous injection of a radiopaque substance, as in *intravenous urography, but the contrast medium can also be introduced percutaneously or, in the case of the bladder, transurethrally (for a **cystogram**; *see* CYSTOGRAPHY).

urography *n.* radiological examination of the urinary tract. This may involve the injection of radiopaque contrast material (*see* CYSTOGRAPHY, INTRAVENOUS UROGRAPHY, PYELOGRAPHY, URETHROGRAPHY). **CT urography** is increasingly used as an alternative to intravenous urography to demonstrate the presence of stones in the urinary tract; it involves a CT scan (*see* COMPUTERIZED TOMOGRAPHY), often without injecting any contrast material.

urokinase *n.* an enzyme produced in the kidney and also present in blood and urine that is capable of breaking up blood clots. It activates *plasminogen directly to plasmin, which dissolves blood clots (*see* PLASMINOGEN ACTIVATORS). Urokinase is administered by injection to treat deep vein thrombosis and pulmonary embolism. Trade name: **Syner-KINASE**.

urolith *n.* a stone in the urinary tract. *See* CALCULUS.

urology *n.* the branch of medicine concerned with the study and treatment of diseases of the urinary tract. —**urological** *adj.* —**urologist** *n.*

uroporphyrin *n.* a porphyrin that plays an intermediate role in the synthesis of *protoporphyrin IX. It is excreted in significant amounts in the urine in porphyria.

ursodeoxycholic acid a drug (a *bile acid) used to dissolve cholesterol gallstones and to treat primary biliary cirrhosis; it is administered by mouth. Side-effects are infrequent but include diarrhoea and indigestion. Trade names: **Destolit, Urdox, Ursofalk, Ursogal**.

urticaria (nettle rash, hives) *n.* an itchy rash resulting partly from the release of *histamine by *mast cells. This causes either short-lived itchy *weals, deeper swellings (angio-oedema), or both. Individual weals typically appear rapidly and resolve spontaneously within hours. **Acute urticaria** is common and represents an immediate response to such allergens as seafood or nuts; it has been linked with upper respiratory tract infections, although many cases remain unexplained. **Chronic urticaria** is not an allergic condition and may persist for years. **Angio-oedema** occurs when the weals involve the deeper levels of the skin, resulting in swelling of the lips, eyes, or tongue, which may constitute a medical emergency. Urticaria can be treated by taking antihistamines regularly, but sometimes immunosuppressant treatment is needed, especially in autoimmune subtypes. **Cholinergic urticaria** is a condition in which very small weals are brought on by heat, exercise, or emotion; treatment is with antihistamines, but other drugs, including danazol, may be used for severe cases.

usual interstitial pneumonitis (UIP) *see* INTERSTITIAL PNEUMONITIS.

uter- (utero-) *combining form denoting* the uterus. Examples: **uterocervical** (relating to the cervix (neck) of the uterus); **uterovaginal** (relating to the uterus and vagina); **uterovesical** (relating to the uterus and bladder).

uterine *adj.* of or relating to the uterus.

uterine artery embolization a method of embolizing the uterine artery under radiodiagnostic control (*see* EMBOLIZATION). It has been successful in controlling postpartum haemorrhage and can also be used in treating fibroids, correcting arterial or venous malformations of the genital tract, and terminating abdominal and cervical pregnancies.

uteroplacental insufficiency the most common cause of *intrauterine growth restriction, due to abnormalities in placental development and *trophoblast invasion. The exact cause may be unknown or due to a number of recognizable causes, e.g. preeclampsia, inherited *thrombophilias causing placental infarction or thrombosis, and systemic lupus erythematosus.

uterus (womb) *n.* the part of the female reproductive tract that is specialized to allow the embryo to become implanted in its inner wall and to nourish the growing fetus from the maternal blood. The nonpregnant uterus is a pear-shaped organ, about 7.5 cm long. It is suspended in the pelvic cavity by means of peritoneal folds (ligaments) and fibrous bands. The upper two-thirds of the uterus (body) is connected to the two *Fallopian tubes, and the narrower lower third (*cervix, or neck) projects at its lower end into the vagina. The uterus has an inner mucous lining (*endometrium) and a thick wall of smooth muscle (*myometrium). During childbirth the myometrium undergoes strong contractions to expel the fetus through the cervix and vagina. In the absence of pregnancy the endometrium undergoes periodic development and degeneration (*see* MENSTRUAL CYCLE). —**uterine** *adj.*

uterus didelphys (double uterus) a congenital condition resulting from the incomplete midline fusion of the two *Müllerian ducts during early embryonic development. The usual result is a double uterus with one or two cervices and a single vagina. Complete failure of fusion results in a double uterus with double cervices and two separate vaginae.

utilitarianism *n.* a consequentialist ethical theory holding that utility, or the greatest happiness, is morally important and should always be maximized. There are different definitions of utility but all relate to the consequences of actions as opposed to the intentions or principles behind them (*see* CONSEQUENTIALISM). Jeremy Bentham (1748–1832), the progenitor of utilitarianism, identified utility with pleasure and disutility with pain and argued that we should always act so as to maximize the former and minimize the latter. John Stuart Mill (1806–1873) refined the theory by distinguishing between lower and higher pleasures while contemporary theories tend to talk about maximizing preferences. As a result, utilitarianism is often divided into **act utilitarianism** (evaluating the consequences of action) and **rule utilitarianism** (evaluating the consequences of a generally accepted moral rule). Rule utilitarianism is sometimes said to be less problematic and more acceptable than act utilitarianism. However utility is defined, there is an obvious tension between maximizing utility for an individual and maximizing everyone's utility. —**utilitarian** *adj.*

utricle (utriculus) *n.* **1.** the larger of the two membranous sacs within the vestibule of the ear: it forms part of the membranous *labyrinth. It is filled with fluid (endolymph) and contains a *macula. This responds to gravity and relays information to the brain about the position of the head. **2.** a small sac (the **prostatic utricle**) extending out of the urethra of the male into the substance of the prostate gland.

uvea (uveal tract) *n.* the vascular pigmented layer of the eye, which lies beneath the outer layer (sclera). It consists of the *choroid, *ciliary body, and *iris. —**uveal** *adj.*

uveal tract *see* UVEA.

uveitis *n.* inflammation of any part of the uveal tract of the eye, either the iris (**iritis**), ciliary body (**cyclitis**), or choroid (**choroiditis**). Inflammation confined to the iris and ciliary body, which are commonly inflamed together, is called **anterior uveitis** or **iridocyclitis** (*see also* FUCHS' HETEROCHROMIC CYCLITIS); that confined to the choroid is termed **posterior uveitis**. In general, the causes of anterior and posterior uveitis are different; anterior uveitis (unlike choroiditis) is usually painful, with clusters of inflammatory cells (keratic precipitates) adhering to the inner surface of the cornea. All types may lead to visual impairment, and uveitis is an important cause of blindness. In most cases the disease appears to originate in the uveal tract itself, but it may occur secondarily to disease of other parts of the eye, particularly of the cornea and sclera.

Treatment consists of the use of drugs that suppress the inflammation, combined with measures to relieve the discomfort and more specific drug treatment if a specific cause of the uveitis is found. The drugs may be given as drops, injections, or tablets, often in combination.

uveoparotitis (uveoparotid fever) *n.* inflammation of the iris, ciliary body, and choroid regions of the eye (the uvea) and swelling of the parotid salivary gland: one of the manifestations of the chronic disease *sarcoidosis.

UVPP   *see* UVULOPALATOPHARYNGOPLASTY.

uvula *n.* a small soft extension of the soft palate that hangs from the roof of the mouth above the root of the tongue. It is composed of muscle, connective tissue, and mucous membrane.

uvulectomy (staphylectomy) *n.* surgical removal of the uvula.

uvulitis *n.* inflammation of the uvula.

uvulopalatopharyngoplasty (uvulopharyngopalatoplasty, UPPP, uvulovelopharyngoplasty, UVPP) *n.* a surgical operation to remove the uvula, part of the soft palate, and the tonsils in the treatment of snoring and *obstructive sleep apnoea.

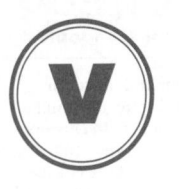

vaccination *n.* a means of producing immunity to a disease by using a *vaccine, or a special preparation of antigenic material, to stimulate the formation of appropriate antibodies. The name was applied originally only to treatment with vaccinia (cowpox) virus, which gives protection not only against cowpox itself but also against the related smallpox. However, it is now used synonymously with **inoculation** as a method of *immunization against any disease. Vaccination is often carried out in two or three stages, as separate doses are less likely to cause unpleasant side-effects. A vaccine is usually given by injection but may be introduced into the skin through light scratches; for some diseases (such as polio), oral vaccines are available.

vaccine *n.* a special preparation of antigenic material that can be used to stimulate the development of antibodies and thus confer active *immunity against a specific disease or number of diseases. Many vaccines are produced by culturing bacteria or viruses under conditions that lead to a loss of their virulence but not of their antigenic nature. Examples of live but attenuated (weakened) organisms in vaccines are those against measles, mumps, and rubella (the MMR vaccine) and tuberculosis. Other vaccines consist of specially treated toxins (*toxoids) or dead bacteria that are still antigenic. Precipitated toxoids are used against diphtheria and tetanus; dead organisms are used against cholera and typhoid. Extensive experimental study continues in the search for cancer vaccines, especially against melanoma and prostate cancer. *See* IMMUNIZATION.

vaccinia *n. see* COWPOX.

vaccinoid *adj.* resembling a local infection with vaccinia (cowpox) virus. A vaccinoid reaction is one of the possible results of vaccination against smallpox in individuals who already have partial immunity. The swelling, reddening, and blistering are considerably less than the so-called primary reaction that occurs after the inoculation of a person with no immunity against smallpox.

vacuole *n.* a space within the cytoplasm of a cell, formed by infolding of the cell membrane, that contains material taken in by the cell. White blood cells form vacuoles when they surround and digest bacteria and other foreign material.

vacuum extractor *see* VENTOUSE.

vagin- (vagino-) *combining form denoting* the vagina.

vagina *n.* the lower part of the female reproductive tract: a muscular tube, lined with mucous membrane, connecting the cervix of the uterus to the exterior. It receives the erect penis during coitus: semen is ejaculated into the upper part of the vagina and from there the sperms must pass through the cervix and uterus in order to fertilize an ovum in the Fallopian tube. The wall of the vagina is sufficiently elastic to allow the passage of the newborn child. —**vaginal** *adj.*

vaginal adenosis the presence of glandular tissue in or under the vaginal epithelium that undergoes squamous *metaplasia. It may be associated with intrauterine *diethylstilbestrol exposure. *See also* CLEAR-CELL CARCINOMA.

vaginal agenesis congenital absence of part or all of the vagina. *See* MAYER-ROKITANSKY-KÜSTER-HAUSER SYNDROME.

vaginectomy *n.* surgical excision of the vagina in cases of vaginal cancer.

vaginismus *n.* painful spasm of the muscles surrounding the vagina, usually in response to the *vulva or vagina being touched. Sexual intercourse may be impossible, and the condition may be associated with fear of or aversion to coitus. Other causative factors include vaginal infection and atrophic *vaginitis.

vaginitis *n.* inflammation of the vagina, which may be caused by infection (most commonly with **Trichomonas vaginalis*), dietary deficiency, or poor hygiene. There is often itching (*see* PRURITUS), increased vaginal discharge, and pain on passing urine. Vaginitis may indicate the presence of sexually transmitted disease. **Atrophic vaginitis** is postmenopausal thinning of the vagina caused by a reduction in the circulating levels of oestrogens. It is a common cause of vaginal dryness and postmenopausal bleeding.

vaginoplasty (colpoplasty) *n.* 1. a tissue-grafting operation on the vagina. 2. surgical reconstruction of the vagina, for example by using a loop of bowel brought through the *pouch of Douglas.

vaginosis *n. see* BACTERIAL VAGINOSIS.

vago- *combining form denoting* the vagus nerve.

vagotomy *n.* the surgical cutting of any of the branches of the vagus nerve. This is usually performed to reduce secretion of acid and pepsin by the stomach in order to treat a peptic ulcer. **Truncal vagotomy** is the cutting of the main trunks of the vagus nerve; in **selective vagotomy** the branches of the nerve to the gall bladder and pancreas are left intact. **Highly selective** (or **proximal**) **vagotomy** is the cutting of the branches of the vagus nerve to the body of the stomach, leaving the branches to the outlet (pylorus) intact: this makes additional surgery to permit emptying of the stomach contents unnecessary. Following surgery, patients may experience **postvagotomy diarrhoea** after a meal (*compare* DUMPING SYNDROME). Since the introduction of proton-pump inhibitors for the treatment of peptic-ulcer disease, these operations are rarely performed.

vagus nerve the tenth *cranial nerve (X), which supplies motor nerve fibres to the muscles of swallowing and parasympathetic fibres to the heart and organs of the chest cavity and abdomen. Sensory branches of the vagus carry impulses from the viscera and the sensation of taste from the mouth.

valaciclovir *n.* an antiviral drug used to treat *herpes infections. Like aciclovir, it is a *DNA polymerase inhibitor. Trade name: **Valtrex**.

valgus *adj.* describing any deformity that displaces the distal end of a limb away from the midline. *See* CLUB-FOOT (TALIPES VALGUS), HALLUX VALGUS, KNOCK-KNEE (GENU VALGUM). *Compare* VARUS.

validity *n.* an indication of the extent to which a measure (e.g. a clinical sign or test) is a true indicator of what it purports to measure (e.g. disease). Reduced validity can arise if the tests produce different results when conducted several times on the same person under identical conditions (i.e. **reduced reproducibility**, **reliability**, or **repeatability**). This may be because the same observer gets different results on successive occasions (**intraobserver error**) or because a series of different observers fail to obtain the same result (**interobserver error**). Such errors may arise because of a true difference in observation and/or interpretation or because of a preconceived notion (often unconscious) by the observer, which influences his or her behaviour. *Compare* INTERVENTION STUDY.

valine *n.* an *essential amino acid. *See also* AMINO ACID.

vallecula *n.* a furrow or depression in an organ or other part. On the undersurface of the cerebellum a vallecula separates the two hemispheres.

Valsalva manoeuvre an attempt by a person to exhale forcibly with a closed glottis while pinching the nose and keeping the mouth closed, so that no air exits through the mouth or nose, as when straining during a bowel movement or lifting a heavy weight. The resulting increased pressure transplants air through the Eustachian tube, thus equalizing the negative pressure in the middle ear. This manoeuvre can often relieve the ear pain associated with flying, which is usually associated with changes in pressure particularly occurring during takeoff and landing. [A. M. Valsalva (1666–1723), Italian anatomist]

valsartan *n. see* ANGIOTENSIN II ANTAGONIST.

value judgment a judgment of the worth, desirability, acceptability, or merit of something, as distinct from a claim about fact or neutral description.

valve *n.* a structure found in some tubular organs or parts that restricts the flow of fluid within them to one direction only. Valves are important structures in the heart, veins, and lymphatic vessels. Such a valve consists of two or three *cusps fastened like pockets to the walls of the vessel. Blood flowing in the right direction flattens the cusps to the walls, but when flow is reversed the cusps become filled with blood or lymph and dilate to block the opening (see illustration). *See also* AORTIC VALVE, MITRAL VALVE, PULMONARY VALVE, TRICUSPID VALVE.

V

(A)

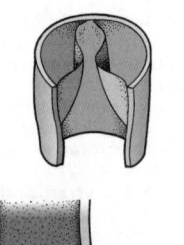

(B)

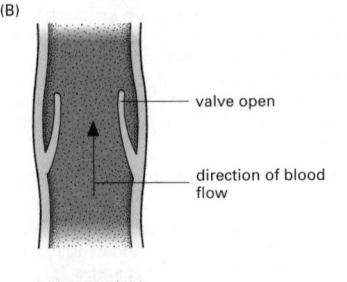

valve open

direction of blood flow

blood pressure closes valve so preventing backflow

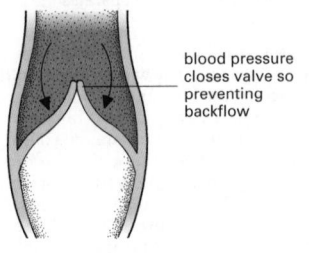

Valve. (A) Cut vein showing the two cusps of a valve; (B) action of a venous valve.

valvoplasty *n. see* VALVULOPLASTY.

valvotomy (valvulotomy) *n.* surgical cutting through a valve. The term is usually used to describe an operation to relieve obstruction caused by stenosed valves in the heart (*see* VALVULOPLASTY).

valvula *n.* (*pl.* **valvulae**) a small valve. The **valvulae conniventes** are circular folds of mucous membrane in the small intestine.

valvulitis *n.* inflammation of one or more valves, particularly the heart valves. This may be acute or chronic and is most often due to rheumatic fever (*see* ENDOCARDITIS).

valvuloplasty (valvoplasty) *n.* therapeutic dilatation of a narrowed heart valve. This used to be done by open heart surgery, but is now performed using balloon catheters threaded into the heart via the venous or arterial system (**balloon valvuloplasty**). It is most commonly used for treatment of *mi-

tral stenosis (using an Inoue balloon) or pulmonary stenosis, and occasionally used as a last resort for severe aortic stenosis.

vancomycin *n.* an antibiotic, derived from the bacterium *Streptomyces orientalis*, that is effective against most Gram-positive organisms (e.g. streptococci and staphylococci). Used for treating serious infections (including endocarditis and *MRSA) due to strains that are resistant to other antibiotics, it is usually administered by intravenous infusion but given by mouth for pseudomembranous colitis (*see* CLOSTRIDIUM). It usually has a low toxicity but may cause deafness and blood disorders. Vancomycin and teicoplanin (a related drug with similar uses) are known as **glycopeptide antibiotics**. Trade name: **Vancocin**.

van den Bergh's test a test to determine whether excess bilirubin in the blood is conjugated or unconjugated, and therefore whether jaundice in a patient is due to *haemolysis or to disease of the liver or bile duct. A sample of serum is mixed with sulphanilic acid, hydrochloric acid, and sodium nitrite. The immediate appearance of a violet colour is called a **direct reaction** and indicates that the jaundice is due to liver damage or obstruction of the bile duct. If the colour appears only when alcohol is added, this is an **indirect reaction** and points to haemolytic jaundice or a congenital unconjugated hyperbilirubinaemia (*see* GILBERT'S SYNDROME). [A. A. H. van den Bergh (1869–1943), Dutch physician]

vanillylmandelic acid (VMA) a metabolite of *catecholamines excreted in abnormal amounts in the urine in conditions of excess catecholamine production, such as *phaeochromocytoma. The measurement of VMA levels in a 24-hour urine sample is still used as a screening test for this condition, although this is being replaced by the direct measurement of urinary catecholamines. Urinary levels may be misleadingly high if foodstuffs with vanillin or the drug levodopa are taken before the test.

vaporizer *n.* a piece of equipment for producing an extremely fine mist of liquid droplets by forcing a jet of liquid through a narrow nozzle with a jet of air. Vaporizers are used to produce aerosols of various medications for use in inhalation therapy.

Vaquez-Osler disease *see* POLYCYTHAEMIA VERA. [L. H. Vaquez (1860–1936), French physician; Sir W. Osler (1849–1919), Canadian physician]

vardenafil *n. see* SILDENAFIL.

variable *n.* (in biostatistics) a characteristic (e.g. morbidity, lifestyle, or habit) relating to an individual or group. **Qualitative variables** are descriptive characteristics, such as sex, race, or occupation; **quantitative variables** relate to a numerical scale and are subdivided into **discrete variables**, found only at fixed points (e.g. number of children), and **continuous variables**, found at any point on a scale (e.g. weight).

variable positive airways pressure *see* BiPAP.

variance *n. see* STANDARD DEVIATION.

variant Creutzfeldt-Jakob disease (vCJD) *see* CREUTZFELDT-JAKOB DISEASE.

varicectomy *n. see* PHLEBECTOMY.

varicella *n. see* CHICKENPOX.

varices *pl. n. see* VARICOSE VEINS.

varicocele *n.* a collection of dilated veins in the spermatic cord, more commonly affecting the left side of the scrotum than the right. It usually produces no symptoms apart from occasional aching discomfort. In some cases varicocele is associated with a poor sperm count (*see* OLIGOSPERMIA) sufficient to cause infertility. Surgical correction or radiological embolization of the varicocele in such patients (**varicocelectomy**) usually results in a considerable improvement in the quality and motility of the sperm, but may or may not improve the number of pregnancies and live births thereafter.

varicose veins veins that are distended, lengthened, and tortuous. The superficial veins (saphenous veins) of the legs are most commonly affected; other sites include the oesophagus (*see* OESOPHAGEAL VARICES) and testes (*varicocele). There is an inherited tendency to varicose veins but obstruction to blood flow is responsible in some cases. Complications including thrombosis, *phlebitis, and haemorrhage may occur. Treatment includes elastic support and *sclerotherapy, but *avulsion (stripping), excision (*phlebectomy), or *endovenous laser treatment is required in some cases. Medical name: **varices**.

varicotomy *n.* incision into a varicose vein (*see* PHLEBECTOMY).

varifocal lenses (progressive lenses) lenses in which the power (*see* DIOPTRE) gradually changes from one prescription to the other and there is no dividing line on the lens between the different segments (*compare* MULTIFOCAL LENSES). The wearer can see clearly at any distance by raising or lowering the eyes.

variola *n. see* SMALLPOX.

varioloid 1. *n.* a mild form of smallpox in people who have previously had smallpox or have been vaccinated against it. 2. *adj.* resembling smallpox.

varix *n.* (*pl.* **varices**) a single *varicose vein.

varus *adj.* describing any deformity that displaces the distal end of a limb towards the midline. *See* BOW-LEGS (GENU VARUM), CLUBFOOT (TALIPES VARUS), HALLUX VARUS. *Compare* VALGUS.

vas *n.* (*pl.* **vasa**) a vessel or duct.

vas- (vaso-) *combining form denoting* 1. vessels, especially blood vessels. 2. the vas deferens.

vasa efferentia (*sing.* **vas efferens**) the many small tubes that conduct spermatozoa from the testis to the epididymis. They are derived from some of the excretory tubules of the *mesonephros.

vasa praevia an uncommon but potentially disastrous complication of delivery, occurring in about 1 in 5000 deliveries, when unprotected fetal vessels run across the *lower uterine segment and cervix in front of the presenting part of the fetus. It is associated with a velamentous insertion of the cord (where the umbilical cord inserts directly into the membranes rather than the placenta) and in cases with normal cord insertion when the vessels run between the two lobes of a bilobed placenta. Vessels unsupported by placental tissue or the umbilical cord can tear when the cervix dilates or the membranes rupture, causing rapid fetal haemorrhage. Immediate Caesarean section to save the baby from *exsanguination is indicated. Fetal mortality for cases not recognized before the onset of labour is very high; appropriate use of prenatal ultrasonography may prevent perinatal death.

vasa vasorum *pl. n.* the tiny arteries and veins that supply the walls of blood vessels.

vascular *adj.* relating to or supplied with blood vessels.

vascular endothelial growth factor (VEGF) a *growth factor made by both normal cells and their abnormal or malignant counterparts to stimulate new blood vessel formation (*see* ANGIOGENESIS). It can be targeted by a family of drugs known as *angiogenesis inhibitors, which include *bevacizumab.

vascularization *n.* the development of blood vessels (usually capillaries) within a tissue.

vascular system *see* CARDIOVASCULAR SYSTEM.

vasculitis (angiitis) *n.* (*pl.* **vasculitides**) a patchy inflammation of the walls of small blood vessels. It may result from a variety of conditions, including *polyarteritis nodosa, acute nephritis, and serum sickness. Symptoms include skin rashes, arthritis, *purpura, and kidney failure. In some cases treatment with cortisone derivatives may be beneficial.

vasculogenesis *n.* the formation of new blood vessels resulting from the directed migration and differentiation of angioblasts (precursor cells) into endothelial cells. The primitive vessels undergo further growth and remodelling by *angiogenesis. Although largely confined to the embryo, vasculogenesis has recently been shown to occur in adults from circulating angioblasts.

vas deferens (*pl.* **vasa deferentia**) either of a pair of ducts that conduct spermatozoa from the *epididymis to the *urethra on ejaculation. It has a thick muscular wall the contraction of which assists in ejaculation.

vasectomy *n.* the surgical operation of severing the duct (vas deferens) connecting the testis to the seminal vesicle and urethra. Vasectomy of both ducts results in sterility and is an increasingly popular means of birth control. Vasectomy does not affect sexual desire or potency.

vaso- *combining form. see* VAS-.

vasoactive *adj.* affecting the diameter of blood vessels, especially arteries. Examples of vasoactive agents are emotion, pressure, carbon dioxide, and temperature. Some exert their effect directly, others via the *vasomotor centre in the brain.

vasoactive intestinal peptide *see* VIP.

vasoconstriction *n.* a decrease in the diameter of blood vessels, especially arteries. This results from circulating vasoconstrictor hormones (e.g. *angiotensin I) or activation of the *vasomotor centre in the brain, which bring about contraction of the muscular walls of the arteries and hence an increase in blood pressure.

vasoconstrictor *n.* an agent that causes narrowing of the blood vessels and therefore a decrease in blood flow. Vasoconstrictor drugs are alpha agonists (*see* SYMPATHOMIMETIC): they are used to raise the blood pressure in disorders of the circulation, shock, or severe bleeding and to maintain blood pressure during surgery (e.g. *ephedrine, *metaraminol, *phenylephrine). Some vasoconstrictors (e.g. ephedrine, *xylometazoline) have a rapid effect when applied to mucous membranes and may be used to relieve nasal congestion. If the blood pressure rises too quickly headache and vomiting may occur. A vasoconstrictor is often added to local anaesthetic solutions used in dentistry to prolong their effectiveness.

vasodilatation *n.* an increase in the diameter of blood vessels, especially arteries. This results from local vasodilator hormones (e.g. *prostaglandins) or activation of the *vasomotor centre in the brain, which bring about relaxation of the arterial walls and a consequent lowering of blood pressure.

vasodilator *n.* a drug that causes widening of the blood vessels and therefore an increase in blood flow. Vasodilators are used to lower blood pressure in cases of hypertension. **Coronary vasodilators**, such as *glyceryl trinitrate, increase the blood flow through the heart and are used to relieve and prevent angina. Large doses of coronary vasodilators cause such side-effects as flushing of the face, severe headache, and fainting. **Peripheral vasodilators** affect blood flow to the limbs; they include *alpha blockers and some *calcium-channel blockers. Certain of the latter (e.g. *nifedipine) are used to treat conditions due to poor circulation, such as Raynaud's disease and intermittent claudication.

vaso-epididymostomy *n.* the operation of joining the vas deferens to the epididymis in a side-to-side manner in order to bypass an obstruction to the passage of sperm from the testis. The obstruction, which may be congenital or acquired, is usually present in the mid-portion or tail of the epididymis. Vaso-epididymostomy is therefore usually performed by anastomosing the head of the epididymis to a longitudinal incision in the lumen of the adjacent vas.

vasography *n.* X-ray imaging of the vas deferens. A contrast medium is injected either into the exposed vas deferens at surgery, using a fine needle, or by inserting a catheter into the ejaculatory duct (which discharges semen from the vesicle into the vas deferens) via an endoscope. The technique is used in the investigation of *azoospermia to look for blockages in the vas.

vasoligation *n.* the surgical tying of the vas deferens (the duct conveying sperm from the testis). This is performed to prevent infection spreading from the urinary tract and causing recurrent *epididymitis. It is sometimes performed at the same time as *prostatectomy to prevent the complication of epididymitis in the postoperative period.

vasomotion *n.* an increase or decrease in the diameter of blood vessels, particularly the arteries. *See* VASOCONSTRICTION, VASODILATATION.

vasomotor *adj.* controlling the muscular walls of blood vessels, especially arteries, and therefore their diameter.

vasomotor centre a collection of nerve cells in the medulla oblongata that receives information from sensory receptors in the circulatory system (*see* BARORECEPTOR) and brings about reflex changes in the rate of the heartbeat and in the diameter of blood vessels, so that the blood pressure can be adjusted. The vasomotor centre also receives impulses from elsewhere in the brain, so that emotion (such as fear) may also influence the heart rate and blood pressure. The centre works through *vasomotor nerves of the sympathetic and parasympathetic systems.

vasomotor nerve any nerve, usually belonging to the autonomic nervous system, that controls the flow of blood through blood vessels by its action on the muscle fibres within their walls or its action on the heartbeat. The *vagus nerve slows the heart and reduces its output, but sympathetic nerves increase the rate and output of the heart and increase blood pressure by causing the constriction of small blood vessels at the same time.

vasomotor symptoms subjective sensations experienced by women around the time of the *menopause, often described as explosions of heat (hot flushes), mostly followed by profuse sweating and sometimes preceded by an undetermined sensation with waking at night. Objective signs are sudden reddening of the skin on the head, neck, and chest and profuse sweating. Physiological changes include peripheral vasodilatation, *tachycardia with normal blood pressure, and raised skin temperature with normal body temperature.

vasopressin (antidiuretic hormone, ADH) *n.* a hormone, released by the pituitary gland, that increases the reabsorption of water by the kidney, thus preventing excessive loss of water from the body. Vasopressin also causes constriction of blood vessels. Synthetic vasopressin (Pitressin) is administered by injection or intravenous infusion to treat *diabetes insipidus and to control bleeding from *oesophageal varices by restricting arterial blood flow to the liver.

vasopressor *adj.* stimulating the contraction of blood vessels and therefore bringing about an increase in blood pressure.

vasospasm *n. see* RAYNAUD'S DISEASE.

vasotomy *n.* a surgical incision into the vas deferens (the duct conveying sperm from the testis). This is usually undertaken to allow catheterization of the vas and the injection of radiopaque contrast material for X-ray examination (*see* VASOGRAPHY), to test for patency of the duct in patients with *azoospermia.

vasovagal *adj.* relating to the action of impulses in the *vagus nerve on the circulation. The vagus reduces the rate at which the heart beats, and so lowers its output.

vasovagal attack excessive activity of the vagus nerve, causing slowing of the heart and a fall in blood pressure, which leads to fainting. *See* SYNCOPE.

vasovasostomy *n.* the surgical operation of reanastomosing the vas deferens after previous vasectomy: the reversal of vasectomy, undertaken to restore fertility.

vasovesiculitis *n.* inflammation of the *seminal vesicles and *vas deferens. This usually occurs in association with *prostatitis and causes pain in the perineum, groin, and scrotum and a high temperature. On examination the vasa and seminal vesicles are thickened and tender. Treatment includes administration of antibiotics.

V

vastus *n.* any of three muscles (**vastus intermedius**, **vastus lateralis**, and **vastus medialis**) that form part of the *quadriceps muscle of the thigh.

vault prolapse prolapse of the *fornix (vault) of the vagina, which occurs at the time of hysterectomy (vaginal or abdominal) when the superior vaginal support mechanism is disrupted. It can be surgically corrected.

VCE *see* VIDEO CAPSULE ENDOSCOPY.

vCJD *see* CREUTZFELDT-JAKOB DISEASE.

vector *n.* 1. an animal, usually an insect or a tick, that transmits parasitic microorganisms – and therefore the diseases they cause – from person to person or from infected animals to human beings. Mosquitoes, for example, are vectors of malaria, filariasis, and yellow fever. 2. an agent used to insert a foreign gene or DNA fragment into a bacterial or other cell in *genetic engineering and *gene therapy. Viruses, especially retroviruses, are often used as vectors: once inside the host cell, the virus can replicate and thus produce copies (*clones) of the gene.

vegetation *n.* (in pathology) an abnormal outgrowth from a membrane, fancied to resemble a vegetable growth. In ulcerative endocarditis, such outgrowths, consisting of *fibrin with enmeshed blood cells, are found on the membrane lining the heart valves.

vegetative *adj.* 1. relating to growth and nutrition rather than to reproduction. 2. functioning unconsciously; autonomic.

vegetative state the clinical condition of unawareness of the self or the environment. The patient breaths spontaneously and has a stable circulation and sleep/wake cycles. It results from extensive damage to the cerebral cortex and thalamus while the brainstem and hypothalamus remain intact. The commonest causes are traumatic brain injury (e.g. road-traffic accidents) and cardiopulmonary arrest. Conditions that mimic the vegetative state include the psychiatric state of *catatonia and the **locked-in syndrome**, resulting from damage to the brainstem, in which the patient is conscious but unable to speak or make any movements of the body except for blinking and upward eye movements. *See also* PERSISTENT VEGETATIVE STATE.

VEGF *see* VASCULAR ENDOTHELIAL GROWTH FACTOR.

vehicle *n.* (in pharmacy) any substance that acts as the medium in which a drug is administered. Examples are sterile water, isotonic sodium chloride, and dextrose solutions.

veil of ignorance a hypothetical state, advanced by the US political philosopher John Rawls, in which decisions about social justice and the allocation of resources would be made fairly, as if by a person who must decide on society's rules and economic structures without knowing what position he or she will occupy in that society. By removing knowledge of status, abilities, and interests, Rawls argued, one could eliminate the usual effects of egotism and personal circumstances on such decisions. Rawls maintained that any society designed on this basis would adhere to two principles: the **principle of equal liberty**, which gives each person the right to as much freedom as is compatible with the freedom of others, and the **maximin principle**, which allocates resources so that the benefit of the least advantaged people is maximized as far as possible. Rawls's exposition, and the maximin principle in particular, have proved widely influential in discussions of welfare provision and, especially, the allocation of medical resources.

vein *n.* a blood vessel conveying blood towards the heart. All veins except the *pulmonary vein carry deoxygenated blood from the tissues, via the capillaries, to the vena cava (see illustration opposite). The walls of veins consist of three tissue layers, but these are much thinner and less elastic than those of arteries (see illustration below). Veins contain *valves that assist the flow of blood back to the heart. Anatomical name: **vena**. —**venous** *adj.*

A vein (transverse section).

velamen (velamentum) *n.* a covering membrane.

Velcade *n. see* BORTEZOMIB.

vellus *n.* the fine hair that occurs on the body before puberty is reached.

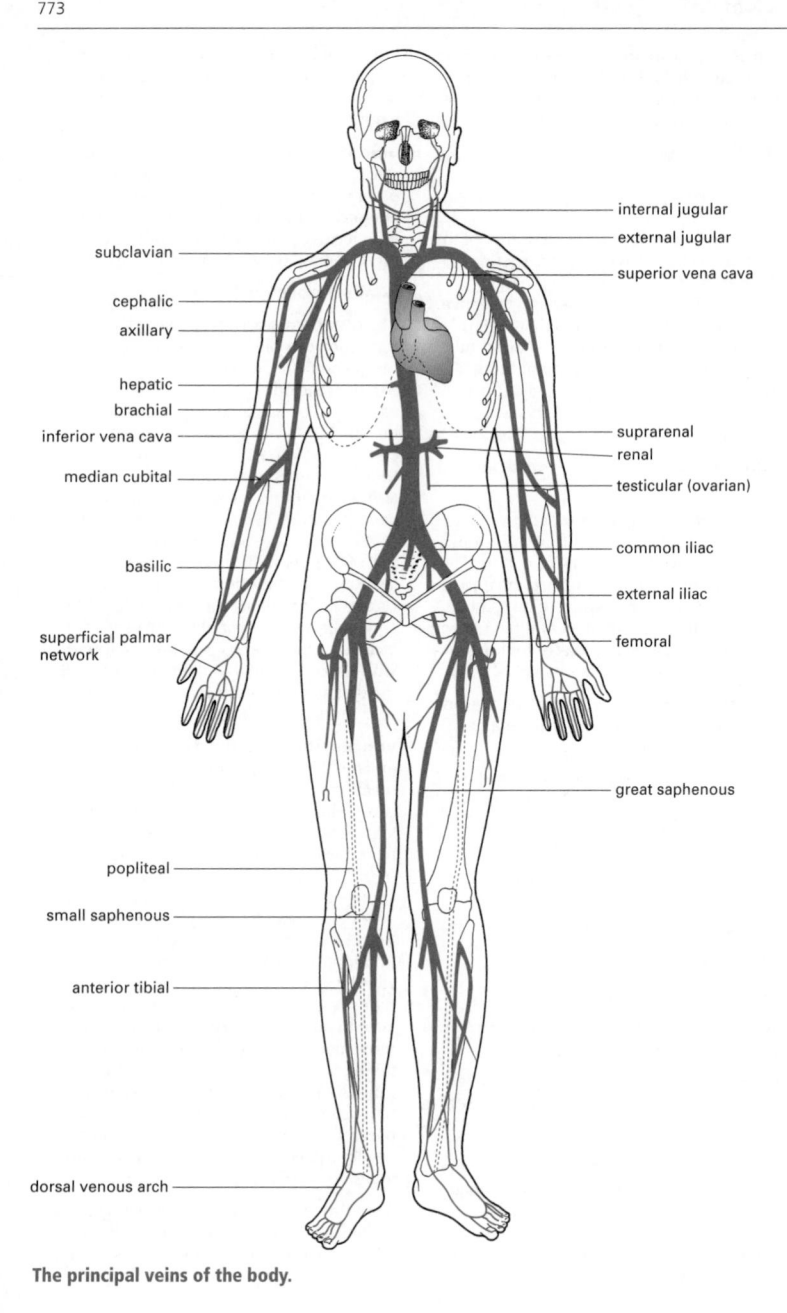

subclavian

cephalic

axillary

hepatic

brachial

inferior vena cava

median cubital

basilic

superficial palmar
network

popliteal

small saphenous

anterior tibial

dorsal venous arch

internal jugular

external jugular

superior vena cava

suprarenal

renal

testicular (ovarian)

common iliac

external iliac

femoral

great saphenous

The principal veins of the body.

velum *n.* (in anatomy) a veil-like covering. The **medullary velum** is either of two thin layers of tissue that form part of the roof of the fourth ventricle of the brain.

VEMP *see* VESTIBULAR EVOKED MYOGENIC POTENTIAL TEST.

vena *n.* (*pl.* **venae**) *see* VEIN.

vena cava (*pl.* **venae cavae**) either of the two main veins, conveying deoxygenated blood from the other veins to the right atrium of the heart. The **inferior vena cava**, formed by the union of the right and left common iliac veins, receives blood from parts of the body below the diaphragm. The **superior vena cava**, originating at the junction of the two innominate veins, drains blood from the head, neck, thorax, and arms.

vene- (veno-) *combining form denoting* veins.

veneer *n.* a facing of *composite resin or *porcelain applied to the surface of a tooth to give improved shape and/or colour. The tooth requires minimal preparation and the facing is retained by enamel that has been treated by the *acid-etch technique. Veneers are a more conservative way of treating discoloured teeth than by *crowns.

venene *n.* a mixture of two or more *venoms: used to produce antiserum against venoms (**antivenene**).

venepuncture (venipuncture) *n.* the puncture of a vein for any therapeutic purpose; for example, to extract blood for laboratory tests. *See also* PHLEBOTOMY.

venereal disease (VD) *see* SEXUALLY TRANSMITTED DISEASE.

venesection *n. see* PHLEBOTOMY.

venlafaxine *n. see* SNRI.

veno- *combining form. see* VENE-.

venoclysis *n.* the continuous infusion into a vein of saline or other solution.

venography (phlebography) *n.* imaging of the anatomy of veins in a particular region of the body. Traditionally a *radiopaque contrast medium is injected into a vein and X-ray photographs (**venograms**) taken as the medium flows towards the heart. Damage, obstruction, or abnormal communication with other vessels can be demonstrated. A common usage is in demonstrating deep vein *thrombosis in the legs. Increasingly ultrasound is now used, both with colour Doppler (*see* DOPPLER ULTRASOUND) and *compression venography. *See also* ANGIOGRAPHY.

venom *n.* the poisonous material produced by snakes, scorpions, spiders, and other animals for injecting into their prey or enemies. Some venoms produce no more than local pain and swelling; others produce more general effects and can prove lethal.

venosclerosis *n. see* PHLEBOSCLEROSIS.

venous thromboembolism (VTE) the formation of a blood clot in a vein, which may become detached and lodged elsewhere. It includes deep vein thrombosis (*see* PHLEBOTHROMBOSIS) and *pulmonary embolism. VTE has been the leading direct cause of maternal death since the first CEMACH report was published in 1985 (*see* MATERNAL MORTALITY RATE). Pregnancy causes a hypercoagulable state and venous stasis in the lower limbs, which increases the risk of VTE six-fold. Surgery (e.g. Caesarean section) and immobility further increase this risk, as do inherited *thrombophilias. There should be a low threshold of investigation (*see* DOPPLER ULTRASOUND) and treatment with *low-molecular-weight heparin until the diagnosis is confirmed or excluded. *See also* THROMBOEMBOLISM.

ventilation *n.* 1. the passage of air into and out of the respiratory tract. The air that reaches only as far as the conducting airways cannot take part in gas exchange and is known as **dead space ventilation** – this may be reduced by performing a *tracheostomy. In the air sacs of the lungs (alveoli) gas exchange is most efficient when matched by adequate blood flow (*perfusion). Ventilation/perfusion imbalance (ventilation of underperfused alveoli or perfusion of underventilated alveoli) is an important cause of *anoxia and *cyanosis. 2. the use of a *ventilator to maintain or support the breathing movements of patients. Invasive ventilation involves the insertion of an endotracheal tube (*see* INTUBATION), through which air is blown into the lungs; patients need to be paralysed and anaesthetized. This need can be eliminated by using techniques of *noninvasive ventilation.

ventilation-perfusion scanning (V/Q scanning) a nuclear medicine technique in which two different isotopes are used, one inhaled (usually *xenon-133 or *krypton-

81m), to examine lung ventilation, and one injected, to examine lung perfusion. In *pulmonary embolism, the area of lung supplied by the blocked artery is not being perfused with blood – a perfusion defect – but has normal ventilation. This technique is highly sensitive for pulmonary embolism.

ventilator *n.* **1.** a device to ensure a supply of fresh air. **2.** (**respirator**) equipment that is manually or mechanically operated to maintain a flow of air into and out of the lungs of a patient who is unable to breathe normally. **Positive-pressure ventilators** blow air into the patient's lungs; air is released from the lungs when the pressure from the ventilator is relaxed (*see* BiPAP, NIPPY, NONINVASIVE VENTILATION). **Negative-pressure ventilators** are airtight containers in which the air pressure is decreased and increased mechanically. This draws air into and out of the patient's lungs through the normal air passages. The original devices, known colloquially as **iron lungs**, had a seal around the neck and enclosed the whole body except the head. They have been replaced by **cuirass ventilators**, which work on a similar principle but enclose the chest only; there may be a role for these in adults and children with claustrophobia.

ventouse (**vacuum extractor**) *n.* a device to assist delivery consisting of a suction cup that is attached to the head of the fetus: traction is then applied slowly. Introduced in 1954, it is widely used and has now virtually replaced rotational obstetric forceps.

ventral *adj.* relating to or situated at or close to the front of the body or to the anterior part of an organ.

ventricle *n.* **1.** either of the two lower chambers of the *heart, which have thick muscular walls. The left ventricle, which is thicker than the right, receives blood from the pulmonary vein via the left atrium and pumps it into the aorta. The right ventricle pumps blood received from the venae cavae (via the right atrium) into the pulmonary artery. **2.** one of the four fluid-filled cavities within the brain (see illustration). The paired first and second ventricles (**lateral ventricles**), one in each cerebral hemisphere, communicate with the third ventricle in the midline between them. This in turn leads through a narrow channel, the **cerebral aqueduct**, to the fourth ventricle in the hindbrain, which is continuous with the spinal canal in the centre of the spinal cord.

*Cerebrospinal fluid circulates through all the cavities. —**ventricular** *adj.*

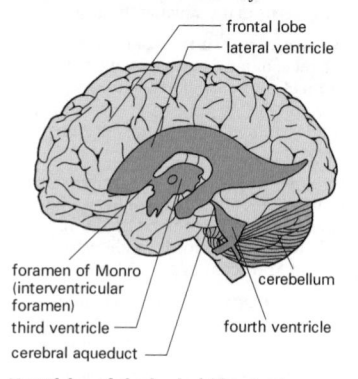

Ventricles of the brain (side view).

ventricul- (**ventriculo-**) *combining form denoting* a ventricle (of the brain or heart).

ventricular fibrillation (**VF**) *see* FIBRILLATION.

ventricular folds *see* VOCAL FOLDS.

ventricular septal defect (**VSD**) a defect of the heart, usually congenital but occasionally acquired due to damage following *myocardial infarction, in which there is a hole in the partition (septum) separating the two ventricles (*see* SEPTAL DEFECT). In 25% of patients there are other defects present. 50% of VSDs close spontaneously. If the hole is large, blood is diverted to the lungs at a greater pressure than usual and *pulmonary hypertension can occur, which becomes irreversible and progressive (*Eisenmenger reaction). Early surgical intervention can prevent this.

ventricular tachycardia (**VT**) a dangerously fast beating of the heart stemming from an abnormal focus of electrical activity in the *ventricles. The electricity does not pass through the heart along the usual channels and as a result the contraction of the heart muscle is often not as efficient as normal, which can result in a sudden drop in blood pressure or even *cardiac arrest. Left untreated it will prove ultimately fatal. *See also* ARRHYTHMIA, TORSADES DE POINTES.

ventriculitis *n.* inflammation in the ventricles of the brain, usually caused by infection. It may result from the rupture of a cerebral abscess into the cavity of the ventricle or from the spread of a severe form of *meningitis from the subarachnoid space.

ventriculoatriostomy *n.* an operation for the relief of raised pressure due to the build-up of cerebrospinal fluid that occurs in *hydrocephalus. Using a system of catheters, the fluid is drained into the jugular vein in the neck.

ventriculography *n.* X-ray examination of the ventricles of the brain or heart after the introduction of a contrast medium. This procedure has been largely made redundant by CT and MRI scanning.

ventriculoscopy *n.* observation of the ventricles of the brain through a fibre-optic instrument. *See* ENDOSCOPE, FIBRE OPTICS.

ventriculostomy *n.* an operation to introduce a hollow needle (cannula) into one of the lateral ventricles (cavities) of the brain. This may be done to relieve raised intracranial pressure, to obtain cerebrospinal fluid from the ventricle for examination, or to introduce antibiotics or contrast material for X-ray examination.

ventro- *combining form denoting* 1. ventral. 2. the abdomen.

ventrofixation *n. see* VENTROSUSPENSION.

ventrosuspension (ventrofixation) *n.* surgical fixation of a displaced uterus to the anterior abdominal wall. This may be achieved by shortening the round ligaments at their attachment either to the uterus or to the abdominal wall.

venule *n.* a minute vessel that drains blood from the capillaries. Many venules unite to form a vein.

verapamil *n.* a *calcium-channel blocker used in the treatment of essential hypertension, angina, and supraventricular arrhythmia. It is administered by mouth or intravenous injection; side-effects may include constipation, nausea, and hypotension. Trade names: **Cordilox**, **Securon**, **Univer**, **Vertab**.

vermicide *n.* a chemical agent used to destroy parasitic worms living in the intestine. *Compare* VERMIFUGE.

vermiform appendix *see* APPENDIX.

vermifuge *n.* any drug or chemical agent used to expel worms from the intestine. *See also* ANTHELMINTIC.

vermis *n.* the central portion of the *cerebellum, lying between its two lateral hemispheres and immediately behind the pons and the medulla oblongata of the hindbrain.

vermix *n.* the vermiform *appendix.

vernal conjunctivitis *conjunctivitis of allergic origin, often associated with hay fever or other forms of *atopy.

Verner-Morrison syndrome *see* VIPOMA. [J. V. Verner (1927–), US physician; A. B. Morrison (1922–), Irish pathologist]

vernier *n.* a device for obtaining accurate measurements of length, to 1/10th, 1/100th or smaller fractions of a unit. It consists of a fixed graduated main scale against which a shorter vernier scale slides. The vernier scale is graduated into divisions equal to nine-tenths of the smallest unit marked on the main scale. The vernier scale is often adjusted by means of a screw thread. A reading is taken by observing which of the markings on the scales coincide.

vernix caseosa the layer of greasy material which covers the skin of a fetus or newborn baby. It is produced by the oil-secreting glands of the skin and contains skin scales and fine hairs.

Verres needle a specialized cannula that is used to insufflate the peritoneal cavity with carbon dioxide in order to establish a *pneumoperitoneum prior to the insertion of *trocars during laparoscopic surgery.

verruca (plantar wart) *n.* (*pl.* **verrucae**) *see* WART.

verrucous carcinoma an *indolent preinvasive wartlike carcinoma typically of the oral cavity, associated with chewing tobacco, and vulva.

version *n.* a manoeuvre to alter the position of a fetus in the uterus to facilitate delivery. *See* CEPHALIC VERSION, PODALIC VERSION.

vertebra *n.* (*pl.* **vertebrae**) one of the 33 bones of which the *backbone is composed. Each vertebra typically consists of a **body**, or **centrum**, from the back of which arises an arch of bone (the **vertebral** or **neural arch**) enclosing a cavity (the **vertebral canal**, or **foramen**) through which the spinal cord passes. The vertebral arch bears one **spinous process** and two **transverse processes**, providing anchorage for muscles, and four **articular processes**, with which adjacent vertebrae articulate (see illustration). Individual vertebrae are bound together by ligaments and *intervertebral discs. —**vertebral** *adj*.

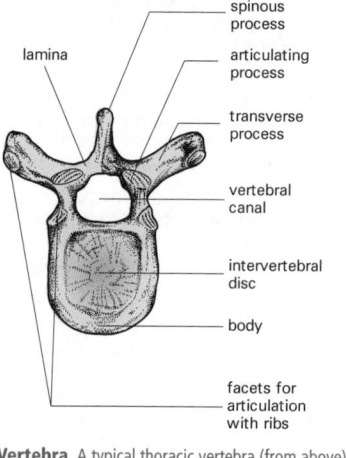

spinous
process

lamina

articulating
process

transverse
process

vertebral
canal

intervertebral
disc

body

facets for
articulation
with ribs

Vertebra. A typical thoracic vertebra (from above).

vertebral column *see* BACKBONE.

verteporfin *n. see* PHOTODYNAMIC THERAPY.

vertical banded gastroplasty *see* GASTROPLASTY, STOMACH STAPLING.

vertical transmission 1. (**mother-to-child transmission**) transmission of an infection, such as HIV, hepatitis B, or hepatitis C, from mother to fetus via the placental circulation. 2. (in population genetics) inheritance of an allele or condition from either the father or mother.

vertigo *n.* a disabling sensation in which the affected individual feels that either he himself or his surroundings are in a state of constant movement. It is most often a spinning sensation but there may be a feeling that the ground is tilting. It is a symptom of disease either in the *labyrinth of the inner ear or in the *vestibular nerve or its nuclei in the brainstem, which are involved in the sense of balance. *See also* BENIGN PAROXYSMAL POSITIONAL VERTIGO.

very low-density lipoprotein (VLDL) a *lipoprotein that is the precursor of *low-density lipoprotein (LDL). Containing triglycerides and cholesterol, it is produced in the liver and circulates in the bloodstream, where its triglycerides are hydro-

lysed to free fatty acids by *lipoprotein lipase. The remaining lipoprotein becomes progressively denser and richer in cholesterol to form LDL.

vesical *adj.* relating to or affecting an anatomical bladder, especially the urinary bladder.

vesicant *n.* an agent that causes blistering of the skin.

vesicle *n.* 1. a very small blister in the skin, often no bigger than a pinpoint, that contains a clear fluid (serum). Vesicles occur in a variety of skin disorders, including eczema and herpes. 2. (in anatomy) any small bladder, especially one filled with fluid. —**vesicular** *adj*.

vesico- *combining form denoting* the urinary bladder. Example: **vesicovaginal** (relating to the bladder and vagina).

vesicofixation *n. see* CYSTOPEXY.

vesicostomy *n.* the surgical creation of an artificial channel between the bladder and the skin surface for the passage of urine. It is sometimes combined with closure of the urethra.

vesicoureteric reflux the backflow of urine from the bladder into the ureters. This is due to defective valves (which normally prevent reflux). Infection is conveyed to the kidneys, causing recurrent attacks of acute *pyelonephritis and scarring of the kidneys in childhood. Children with urinary infection must be investigated for reflux by *cystoscopy; if the condition does not settle with antibiotic therapy corrective surgery must be performed.

vesicovaginal fistula an abnormal communication between the bladder and the vagina (*see* FISTULA) causing urinary incontinence. This may result from surgical damage to the bladder during a gynaecological operation (e.g. hysterectomy) or radiation damage following radiotherapy for pelvic malignancy. In developing countries it is often caused by necrosis associated with prolonged obstructed labour.

vesicular breathing *see* BREATH SOUNDS.

vesiculectomy *n.* surgical removal of a *seminal vesicle. This operation, which is rarely undertaken, may be performed for a tumour of the seminal vesicles.

V

vesiculitis *n.* inflammation of the seminal vesicles. *See* VASOVESICULITIS.

vesiculography *n.* any technique for imaging the seminal vesicles. This used to be performed by injecting a contrast medium into the vas deferens during *vasography. More commonly direct injection is now performed during *transrectal ultrasonography (TRUS), enabling sperm to be sampled at the same examination. Injected contrast medium or dye should be seen draining into the vas deferens to the bladder if there is no blockage. *Magnetic resonance imaging is a good technique for imaging the seminal vesicles with no radiation exposure. Both these techniques are useful for investigation of patients with *azoospermia.

vessel *n.* a tube conveying a body fluid, especially a blood vessel or a lymphatic vessel.

vestibular evoked myogenic potential test (VEMP) a test used to measure the response of the *saccule. It is used in the diagnosis of *superior canal dehiscence syndrome), *Ménière's disease, and other disorders of the inner ear.

vestibular glands the two pairs of glands that open at the junction of the vagina and vulva. The more posterior of the two are the **greater vestibular glands (Bartholin's glands)**; the other pair are the **lesser vestibular glands**. Their function is to lubricate the entrance to the vagina during coitus.

vestibular nerve the division of the *vestibulocochlear nerve that carries impulses from the semicircular canals, utricle, and saccule of the inner ear to the brain, conveying information about the body's posture and movements in space and allowing coordination and balance.

vestibular schwannoma a slow-growing benign tumour arising on one of the *vestibular nerves. It is also known as an **acoustic neuroma**, but this is a misnomer as the tumour arises from *Schwann cells rather than nerve cells and on a vestibular nerve rather than the cochlear (acoustic) nerve. Symptoms include hearing loss, tinnitus, and imbalance and there is an increased prevalence of the tumour in patients who have *neurofibromatosis type II. Diagnosis is by MRI scan and treatment is not always required. In those cases where treatment is necessary, this may be by surgery, radiotherapy, or *gamma knife.

vestibule *n.* (in anatomy) a cavity situated at the entrance to a hollow part. The vestibule of the ear is the cavity of the bony *labyrinth that contains the *saccule and *utricle – the organs of equilibrium. —**vestibular** *adj.*

vestibulocochlear nerve the eighth cranial nerve (VIII), responsible for carrying sensory impulses from the inner ear to the brain. It has two branches, the *vestibular nerve and the *cochlear nerve.

vestigial *adj.* existing only in a rudimentary form. The term is applied to organs whose structure and function have diminished during the course of evolution until only a rudimentary structure exists.

VF ventricular *fibrillation.

viable *adj.* capable of living a separate existence. The legal age of viability of a fetus is 24 weeks, by virtue of the Abortion Act 1967 (as amended), but some fetuses now survive birth at an even earlier gestational age due to advances in neonatal medicine and technologies. The treatment of very premature neonates can raise issues of *personhood, *quality of life, and resource allocation. —**viability** *n.*

Viagra *n. see* SILDENAFIL.

Vibramycin *n. see* DOXYCYCLINE.

vibrator *n.* a machine used to generate vibrations of different frequencies, which have a stimulating effect when applied to different parts of the body. A vibrator may also be used to loosen thick mucus in the sinuses or air passages.

Vibrio *n.* a genus of Gram-negative motile comma-shaped bacteria widely distributed in soil and water. Most species are saprophytic but some are parasites, including *V. cholerae*, which causes *cholera.

vibrissa *n.* (*pl.* **vibrissae**) a stiff coarse hair, especially one of the stiff hairs that lie just inside the nostrils.

vicarious *adj.* describing an action or function performed by an organ not normally involved in the function. For example, **vicarious menstruation** is a rare disorder in which monthly bleeding occurs from places other than the vagina, such as the sweat glands, breasts, nose, or eyes.

video- *combining form denoting* the use of

a video camera to view and record moving images. *See* VIDEOFLUOROSCOPY.

video capsule endoscopy (VCE) an investigation for visualizing the intestinal lining (mucosa). A small capsule containing a miniature digital video camera is swallowed by the patient and then moves along in the intestine passively with peristalsis. Various capsules are available for investigation of oesophageal, small-intestinal, and colonic disorders. The commonest in use is the small-intestinal capsule, for investigation of obscure gastrointestinal bleeding, recurrent iron-deficiency anaemia, suspected Crohn's disease or coeliac disease, and suspected small-intestinal tumours.

videofluoroscopy *n.* the technique of viewing and recording real time X-ray investigation using a video camera (*see* REAL-TIME IMAGING). This enables the moving images to be reviewed at a later time, by individual frames or in slow motion.

videokeratography *n. see* CORNEAL TOPOGRAPHY.

videokymography *n.* a method of studying the vibration of the *vocal folds of the *larynx using high-speed digital photography. *See* LARYNGEAL STROBOSCOPY.

video-otoscope *n.* a small *endoscope connected to a digital camera for examining the outer ear and eardrum.

vigabatrin *n. see* ANTICONVULSANT.

villus *n.* (*pl.* **villi**) one of many short finger-like processes that project from some membranous surfaces. Numerous **intestinal villi** line the small *intestine. Each contains a network of blood capillaries and a *lacteal. Their function is to absorb the products of digestion and they greatly increase the surface area over which this can take place. **Chorionic villi** are folds of the *chorion (the outer membrane surrounding a fetus) from which the fetal part of the *placenta is formed. They provide an extensive area for the exchange of oxygen, carbon dioxide, nutrients, and waste products between maternal and fetal blood. *See also* ARACHNOID VILLUS, CHORIONIC VILLUS SAMPLING.

VIN *see* VULVAL INTRAEPITHELIAL NEOPLASIA.

vinblastine *n. see* VINCA ALKALOID.

vinca alkaloid one of a group of *antimitotic drugs (*see also* CYTOTOXIC DRUG) derived from the periwinkle (*Vinca rosea*). Vinca al-

kaloids are used especially to treat leukaemias and lymphomas; they include **vinblastine** (Velbe), **vincristine** (Oncovin), and **vindesine** (Eldisine), which are administered intravenously. **Vinorelbine** (Navelbine), which can be administered intravenously or orally, is used in the treatment of advanced breast cancer and *non-small-cell lung cancer. Vinca alkaloids are highly toxic; side-effects include *myelosuppression, peripheral neuropathy, and severe irritation at the injection site.

Vincent's angina an obsolete term for *ulcerative gingivitis. [H. Vincent (1862–1950), French physician]

vincristine *n. see* VINCA ALKALOID.

vinculum *n.* (*pl.* **vincula**) a connecting band of tissue. The **vincula tendinum** are threadlike bands of synovial membrane that connect the flexor tendons of the fingers and toes to their point of insertion on the phalanges.

vindesine *n. see* VINCA ALKALOID.

vinorelbine *n. see* VINCA ALKALOID.

VIP (vasoactive intestinal peptide) a peptide hormone and neurotransmitter found widely throughout the central nervous system and the gastrointestinal tract. It has numerous actions, including vasodilatation of blood vessels in the gut, reduction of acid secretion by the stomach, and enhanced secretion of electrolytes into the small bowel.

VIPoma *n.* a usually malignant tumour of islet cells of the pancreas that secretes large amounts of *VIP. This results in severe watery diarrhoea ('pancreatic cholera' or the **Verner-Morrison syndrome**), with loss of potassium and bicarbonate and a low level of stomach acid. The treatment is surgical removal of the tumour.

viraemia *n.* the presence in the blood of virus particles.

viral pneumonia an acute infection of the lung caused by any one of a number of viruses, such as *respiratory syncytial virus, adenovirus, influenza and parainfluenza viruses, and enteroviruses. It is characterized by headache, fever, muscle pain, and a cough that produces a thick sputum. The pneumonia can often occur with or subsequent to a systemic viral infection. Treatment is by supportive care, but antibiotics are administered if a bacterial infection is superimposed.

virilism *n.* the development in a female of male secondary sexual characteristics, such as increased body hair, muscle bulk, and deepening of the voice.

virilization *n.* the most extreme result of excessive androgen production (*hyperandrogenism) in women. It is characterized by temporal balding, a male body form, muscle bulk, deepening of the voice, enlargement of the clitoris, and *hirsutism. Virilization in prepubertal boys may be caused by some tumours (*see* LEYDIG TUMOUR).

virology *n.* the science of viruses. *See also* MICROBIOLOGY.

virtue ethics a theoretical approach that stresses the characteristics of a person rather than rules or consequences. Certain qualities are believed to be inherently moral and therefore desirable. In medical ethics, the traits of a 'good doctor' provide the moral compass by which to assess professional practice.

virulence *n.* the disease-producing (pathogenic) ability of a microorganism. *See also* ATTENUATION.

virus *n.* a minute particle that is capable of replication but only within living cells. Viruses are too small to be visible with a light microscope and too small to be trapped by filters. They infect animals, plants, and microorganisms (*see* BACTERIOPHAGE). Each consists of a core of nucleic acid (DNA or RNA) surrounded by a protein shell. Some bear an outer lipid capsule. Viruses cause many diseases, including the common cold, influenza, measles, mumps, chickenpox, herpes, AIDS, polio, and rabies. *Antiviral drugs are effective against some of them, and many viral diseases are controlled by means of vaccines. —**viral** *adj.*

viscera *pl. n.* (*sing.* **viscus**) the organs within the body cavities, especially the organs of the abdominal cavities (stomach, intestines, etc.). —**visceral** *adj.*

visceral arch *see* PHARYNGEAL ARCH.

visceral cleft *see* PHARYNGEAL CLEFT.

visceral pouch *see* PHARYNGEAL POUCH.

viscero- *combining form denoting* the viscera.

viscodissection *n.* a surgical technique in which a *viscoelastic material is used to dissect and separate layers of tissue.

viscoelastic material any gel-like material used in ophthalmic surgery to help maintain the shape of ocular tissues as well as lubricate and minimize trauma. It is commonly used in intraocular surgery, such as cataract surgery.

viscus *n.* *see* VISCERA.

visual acuity sharpness of vision: the degree to which a person is able to distinguish and resolve fine detail. The essential requirements are a healthy retina and the ability of the eye to focus incoming light to form a sharp image on the retina. Acuity of distant vision is often expressed as a Snellen score (*see* SNELLEN CHART); acuity of near vision as a Jaeger score (*see* JAEGER TEST TYPES).

visual field the area in front of the eye in any part of which an object can be seen without moving the eye. With both eyes open and looking straight forward it is possible to see well-illuminated objects placed anywhere in front of the eyes, although the eyebrows and eyelids reduce the extent of the field somewhat. This is the **binocular visual field**. With only one eye open the field is **uniocular** and is restricted inwards by the nose. If the object is small or poorly illuminated it will not be seen until it is moved closer to the point at which the eye is actually looking, i.e. nearer to the centre of the visual field. Similarly, coloured objects are not seen so far away from the centre as are white objects of the same size and brightness. This is because the retina is not uniformly sensitive to light of different colours or intensities (*see* ROD, CONE): retinal sensitivity increases towards its centre (the *macula). Thus, while there is an absolute visual field beyond which things cannot be seen, no matter how large or bright they are, a relative field exists for objects of different brightness, size, and colour. The most common visual field loss is due to *glaucoma. *See also* PERIMETER.

visual pathway *see* OPTIC NERVE.

visual purple *see* RHODOPSIN.

visual reinforcement audiometry (visual reinforced audiometry, VRA) a behavioural test of hearing for children aged approximately 6 to 30 months in which the subject sits between two calibrated loudspeakers. A sound is generated from one loudspeaker. Children who turn towards the sound are rewarded by brief illumination of a toy adjacent to the loudspeaker. Older children can be tested with headphones, rather than using the loudspeakers, to enable each ear to be tested separately. The test can be adapted for use with older subjects who have learning disabilities.

vital capacity the maximum volume of air that a person can exhale after maximum inhalation. It is usually measured on an instrument called a **spirometer**.

vital centre any of the collections of nerve cells in the brain that act as governing centres for different vital body functions – such as breathing, heart rate, blood pressure, temperature control etc. – making reflex adjustments according to the body's needs. Most lie in the hypothalamus and brainstem.

Vitallium *n.* trade name for an alloy of chromium and cobalt that is used in instruments, prostheses, surgical appliances, and dentures.

vital signs signs that a patient is alive, on which are based a commonly performed set of measurements used internationally as a general baseline in medicine and surgery. These include measurements of *body temperature (T), *blood pressure (BP), heart rate (HR; *see* PULSE), and *respiratory rate (RR) and can also include assessment of consciousness using the *Glasgow Coma Scale (GCS) and of **urine output** (UO, in millilitres per hour).

vital staining (intravital staining) the process of staining a living tissue by injecting a stain into the organism. *Compare* SUPRAVITAL STAINING.

vital statistics *see* BIOSTATISTICS.

vitamin *n.* any of a group of substances that are required, in very small amounts, for healthy growth and development: they cannot be synthesized by the body and are therefore essential constituents of the diet. Vitamins are divided into two groups, according to whether they are soluble in water or fat. The water-soluble group includes the vitamin B complex and vitamin C; the fat-soluble vitamins are vitamins A, D, E, and K. Lack of sufficient quantities of any of the vitamins in the diet results in specific vitamin deficiency diseases.

vitamin A (retinol) a fat-soluble vitamin that occurs preformed in foods of animal origin (especially milk products, egg yolk, and liver) and is formed in the body from the pigment β-*carotene, present in some vegetable foods (for example cabbage, lettuce, and carrots). Retinol is essential for growth, vision in dim light, and the maintenance of soft mucous tissue. A deficiency causes stunted growth, *night blindness, *xerophthalmia, *keratomalacia, and eventual blindness. The recommended daily intake is 750 μg retinol equivalents for an adult (1 μg retinol equivalent = 1 μg retinol or 6 μg β-carotene).

vitamin B any one of a group of water-soluble vitamins that, although not chemically related, are often found together in the same kinds of food (milk, liver, cereals, etc.) and all function as *coenzymes. *See* VITAMINS B$_1$, B$_2$, B$_6$, B$_{12}$, BIOTIN, FOLATE, NICOTINIC ACID, PANTOTHENIC ACID.

vitamin B$_1$ (thiamine, aneurine) a vitamin of the B complex that is active in the form of **thiamine pyrophosphate**, a coenzyme in decarboxylation reactions in carbohydrate metabolism. A deficiency of vitamin B$_1$ leads to *beriberi. Good sources of the vitamin are cereals, beans, meat, potatoes, and nuts. The recommended daily intake is 1 mg for an adult.

vitamin B$_2$ (riboflavin) a vitamin of the B complex that is a constituent of the coenzymes *FAD (flavine adenine dinucleotide) and *FMN (flavine mononucleotide). Riboflavin is therefore important in tissue respiration. A deficiency of riboflavin causes a condition known as *ariboflavinosis, which is not usually serious. Good sources of riboflavin are liver, milk, and eggs. The recommended daily intake for an adult is 1.3–1.6 mg.

vitamin B$_6$ (pyridoxine) a vitamin of the B complex from which the coenzyme *pyridoxal phosphate, involved in the transamination of amino acids, is formed. The vitamin is found in most foods and a deficiency is therefore rare.

vitamin B$_{12}$ (cyanocobalamin) a vitamin of the B complex. The form of vitamin B$_{12}$ with coenzyme activity is **5-deoxyadenosyl cobalamin**, which is necessary for the synthesis of nucleic acids, the maintenance of *myelin in the nervous system, and the proper functioning of *folate, another B vitamin. The vitamin can be absorbed only in the presence of **intrinsic factor**, a protein secreted in the stomach. A deficiency of vitamin B_{12} affects nearly all the body tissues, particularly those containing rapidly dividing cells. The most serious effects of a deficiency are *pernicious anaemia and degeneration of the nervous system. Vitamin B_{12} is manufactured only by certain microorganisms and is contained only in foods of animal origin. Good sources are liver, fish, and eggs. The daily recommended adult intake is 3–4 µg.

vitamin C (ascorbic acid) a water-soluble vitamin with *antioxidant properties that is essential in maintaining healthy connective tissues and the integrity of cell walls. It is necessary for the synthesis of collagen. A deficiency of vitamin C leads to *scurvy. The recommended daily intake is 30 mg for an adult; rich sources are citrus fruits and vegetables (the main source of the vitamin in the British diet is potatoes).

vitamin D a fat-soluble vitamin that enhances the absorption of calcium and phosphorus from the intestine and promotes their deposition in the bone. It occurs in two forms: **ergocalciferol** (**vitamin D_2, calciferol**), which is manufactured by plants when the sterol ergosterol is exposed to ultraviolet light, and **cholecalciferol** (**vitamin D_3**), which is produced by the action of sunlight on 7-dehydrocholesterol, a sterol widely distributed in the skin. A deficiency of vitamin D, either from a poor diet or lack of sunlight, leads to decalcified bones and the development of *rickets and *osteomalacia. Good sources of vitamin D are liver and fish oils. The recommended daily intake is 10 µg for a child up to five years and 2.5 µg thereafter. Vitamin D is toxic and large doses must therefore be avoided.

vitamin E any of a group of chemically related fat-soluble compounds (**tocopherols** and **tocotrienols**) that have *antioxidant properties and are thought to stabilize cell membranes by preventing oxidation of their unsaturated fatty acid components. The most potent of these is α-**tocopherol**. Good sources of the vitamin are vegetable oils, eggs, butter, and wholemeal cereals. It is fairly widely distributed in the diet and a deficiency is therefore unlikely.

vitamin K a fat-soluble vitamin occurring in two main forms: **phytomenadione** (of plant origin) and **menaquinone** (of animal origin). It is necessary for the formation of *prothrombin in the liver, which is essential for blood clotting, and it also regulates the synthesis of other clotting factors. A dietary deficiency does not often occur as the vitamin is synthesized by bacteria in the large intestine and is widely distributed in green leafy vegetables and meat.

vitelliform degeneration (Best's disease) degeneration of the *macula of the eye that is inherited as a dominant characteristic and usually starts in childhood. There is widespread abnormality of retinal pigment epithelium (*see* RETINA) with the accumulation of a yellowish material, especially in the macular area.

vitellus *n.* the yolk of an ovum.

vitiligo *n.* a common disorder in which symmetrical white or pale *macules appear on the skin. The face and extremities (including the genitalia) are commonly affected. It is more conspicuous in darker skin types. Vitiligo is an *autoimmune disease and may occur with other such diseases (e.g. thyroid disease or *alopecia areata). It is usually progressive, although spontaneous repigmentation may occur. Treatment with potent topical corticosteroids, topical *calcineurin inhibitors, or phototherapy may be effective. Cosmetic camouflage may be necessary if treatments are unsuccessful.

vitrectomy *n.* the removal of the whole or part of the vitreous humour of the eye. **Anterior vitrectomy** is removal of the front portion of the vitreous humour. Vitrectomy is often required to remove a nonresolving vitreous haemorrhage and also as a part of surgical procedures on the retina, including repair of a detached retina.

vitreous detachment the separation of the *vitreous humour from the underlying retina. This is a normal ageing process, but it is also more common in such conditions as diabetes and severe myopia. It can sometimes cause a tear in the retina and lead to *retinal detachment.

vitreous humour (vitreous body) the transparent jelly-like material that fills the chamber behind the lens of the eye.

vitrification *n.* a process in which eggs or embryos in vitro are preserved by being dehydrated, treated with an antifreeze chemical, and then flash-frozen with liquid nitrogen. They instantly become converted into a glassy material without the formation of ice crystals, which can damage the genetic material, seen with slower forms of freezing.

vitritis *n.* inflammation within the vitreous humour of the eye.

viviparous *adj.* describing animal groups (including most mammals) in which the embryos develop within the body of the mother so that the young are born alive rather than hatch from an egg. —**viviparity** *n.*

vivisection *n.* a surgical operation on a living animal for experimental purposes.

VMA *see* VANILLYLMANDELIC ACID.

vocal folds (vocal cords) the two folds of tissue which protrude from the sides of the *larynx to form a narrow slit (glottis) across the air passage (see illustration). Their controlled interference with the expiratory air flow produces audible vibrations that make up speech, song, and all other vocal noises. Alterations in the vocal folds themselves or in their nerve supply by disease interferes with phonation.

root of the tongue
epiglottis
vocal fold (true vocal cord)
ventricular fold (false vocal cord)
glottis
larynx

The vocal folds.

vocal fremitus *see* FREMITUS.

vocal resonance the sounds heard through the stethoscope when the patient speaks ("ninety nine"). These are normally just audible but become much louder (**bronchophony**) if the lung under the stethoscope is consolidated, when they resemble the sounds heard over the trachea and main bronchi. Vocal resonance is lost over pleural fluid except at its upper surface, when it has a bleating quality and is called **aegophony**. *See also* PECTORILOQUY.

vocational training a period of supervised training for dentists and doctors in general practice before they are allowed to work independently in NHS practice.

volar *adj.* relating to the palm of the hand or the sole of the foot (the **vola**).

Volkmann's contracture fibrosis and shortening of muscles due to inadequate blood supply, which may arise from arterial injuries or *compartment syndrome. Sites most commonly involved are the forearm, hand, leg, and foot and the condition may result in clawing of the fingers or toes. It may be a complication of fractures, vascular surgery, or using a tight bandage or plaster cast. [R. von Volkmann (1830–89), German surgeon]

volsellum (vulsellum) *n.* surgical forceps with clawlike hooks at the ends of both blades.

volt *n.* the *SI unit of electric potential, equal to the potential difference between two points on a conducting wire through which a constant current of 1 ampere flows when the power dissipated between these points is 1 watt. Symbol: V.

voluntary *adj.* 1. describing a decision or action taken freely, i.e. without coercion or undue pressure. *Consent must be voluntary if it is to be legally valid. *See also* AUTONOMY. 2. under the control of *striated muscle.

voluntary admission (informal admission) entry of a patient into a psychiatric hospital with his (or her) agreement. *Compare* COMPULSORY ADMISSION.

voluntary muscle *see* STRIATED MUSCLE.

volvulus *n.* twisting of a part of the digestive tract, usually leading to partial or complete obstruction and often reducing the blood supply, causing gangrene. A volvulus may untwist spontaneously or by manipulation, but surgical exploration is usually performed. **Gastric volvulus** is a twist of the stomach, usually in a hiatus *hernia. **Small-intestinal volvulus** is twisting of part of the bowel around an *adhesion. **Sigmoid volvulus** is a twist of the sigmoid colon, usually when this part of the colon is particularly long. **Compound volvulus** (or **ileosigmoid knotting**) involves both the small and the large bowel.

vomer *n.* a thin plate of bone that forms part of the nasal septum (*see* NASAL CAVITY). *See also* SKULL.

vomica *n.* 1. an abnormal cavity in an organ, usually a lung, sometimes containing pus. 2. the abrupt expulsion from the mouth of a large quantity of pus or decaying matter originating in the throat or lungs.

vomit 1. *vb.* to eject the contents of the stomach through the mouth (*see* VOMITING). 2. *n.* the contents of the stomach ejected during vomiting. Medical name: **vomitus**.

vomiting *n.* the reflex action of ejecting the contents of the stomach through the mouth. Vomiting is controlled by a special centre in the brain that may be stimulated by drugs (e.g. *apomorphine) acting directly on it; or by impulses transmitted through nervous pathways either from the stomach (e.g. after ingesting irritating substances or in stomach diseases, such as peptic ulceration or pyloric stenosis), the intestine (e.g. in intestinal obstruction), or from the inner ear (in motion sickness). The stimulated vomiting centre sets off a chain of nerve impulses producing coordinated contractions of the diaphragm and abdominal muscles, relaxation of the muscle at the entrance to the stomach, etc., causing the stomach contents to be expelled. Medical name: **emesis**.

von Hippel-Lindau disease an inherited syndrome in which *haemangioblastomas, particularly in the cerebellum, are associated with renal and pancreatic cysts, *angiomas in the retina (causing blindness), cancer of the kidney cells, and red birthmarks. [E. von Hippel (1867–1939), German ophthalmologist; A. Lindau (1892–1958), Swedish pathologist]

von Recklinghausen's disease 1. a syndrome due to excessive secretion of *parathyroid hormone (hyperparathyroidism), characterized by loss of mineral from bones, which become weakened and fracture easily, and formation of kidney stones. Medical name: **osteitis fibrosa**. 2. *see* NEUROFIBROMATOSIS. [F. D. von Recklinghausen (1833–1910), German pathologist]

Von Rosen's sign *see* BARLOW MANOEUVRE. [S. Von Rosen, Swedish orthopaedic surgeon]

von Willebrand's disease an inherited disorder of the blood that is characterized by episodes of spontaneous bleeding similar to *haemophilia. It is due to a variety of abnormalities of the **von Willebrand factor**, a glycoprotein necessary for *platelet activation. This results in a bleeding tendency. The most common type of von Willebrand's disease is inherited as an autosomal *dominant trait; some types are inherited as autosomal

*recessive traits. [A. von Willebrand (1870–1949), Swedish physician]

voxel *n.* short for 'volume element', the volume of tissue in a body that is represented by a *pixel in a cross-sectional image. It depends on the slice thickness of the original scan.

vPAP (variable positive airways pressure) trade name for a brand of ventilator that delivers air to the lungs at different levels of pressure. *See* BiPAP.

VRA *see* VISUAL REINFORCEMENT AUDIOMETRY.

VSD *see* VENTRICULAR SEPTAL DEFECT.

VT *see* VENTRICULAR TACHYCARDIA.

VTE *see* VENOUS THROMBOEMBOLISM.

vulnerability *n.* a position of relative disadvantage, which requires a person to trust and depend upon others. In a medical context, all patients are vulnerable to an extent and some may be particularly so owing to impaired decision-making abilities or social position. Any *exploitation of a vulnerable person is considered contrary to medical ethics. There is increasing interest in the vulnerabilities of health-care professionals themselves and the evidence for compassion fatigue, burnout, and *ethical erosion is strong. A number of commentators have argued that the most effective therapeutic relationships occur when both the patient and clinician are aware of their own humanity because they have each experienced being vulnerable. A number of specific services and support groups have been established to help doctors and other health-care professionals in difficulty. —**vulnerable** *adj.*

vulsellum *n. see* VOLSELLUM.

vulv- (vulvo-) *combining form denoting* the vulva.

vulva *n.* the female external genitalia. Two pairs of fleshy folds – the **labia majora** and **labia minora** – surround the openings of the vagina and urethra and extend forward to the clitoris (see illustration). *See also* VESTIBULAR GLANDS. —**vulval** *adj.*

vulval cancer a relatively rare gynaecological cancer, most common in the elderly. The most common symptom is longstanding itch, but vulval pain, discharge, and bleeding have also been reported. Surgery is the primary treatment, with wide excision by radical *vulvectomy and regional *lymphadenectomy. Radiotherapy and chemotherapy can also be used.

vulval intraepithelial neoplasia (VIN) premalignant disease of the vulva, which has histological features and terminology similar to those of *cervical intraepithelial neoplasia (CIN). Viral aetiological factors, such as HPV, are thought to be involved. The most common presenting symptom is itch, but VIN may be asymptomatic and detected only during treatment of preinvasive or invasive lesions of the cervix or lower genital tract.

vulval vestibulitis pain on entry or touch of the vulva, with redness of the *vestibular glands, tenderness on pressure, and dyspareunia. The pain, which is localized, is described as a severe burning sensation;

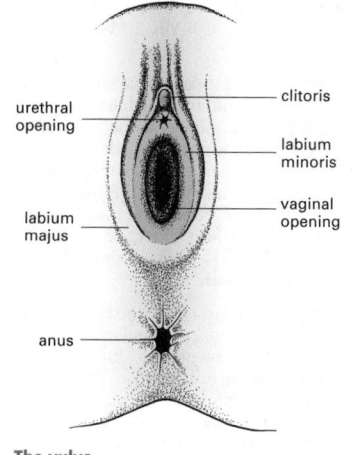

The following labels appear on the figure:
- clitoris
- urethral opening
- labium minoris
- labium majus
- vaginal opening
- anus

The vulva.

itching is not usually a feature (*compare* VULVITIS). The condition seems to be more common in premenopausal Caucasian women with a history of anxiety and related disorders. See also VULVODYNIA.

vulvectomy *n.* surgical removal of the external genitals (*see* VULVA) of a woman. **Simple vulvectomy** involves excision of the labia majora, labia minora, and clitoris and is carried out for a nonmalignant growth. **Radical vulvectomy** is a much more extensive operation carried out for a malignant growth, e.g. cancer of the vulva. It involves wide excision of the labia majora and minora and the clitoris in addition to complete removal of all regional lymph nodes on both sides. The skin covering these areas is also removed, leaving an extensive raw area that is allowed to heal by *granulation.

vulvitis *n.* inflammation of the vulva, which is often accompanied by intense itching (*see* PRURITUS).

vulvodynia *n.* unexplained vulval pain, often coupled with sexual dysfunction and psychological disorder, which is often described by the patient as a burning stinging sensation and/or rawness. **Cyclic vulvodynia** occurs in relation to menstruation or coitus and is thought to be due to changes in vaginal pH that make the vulva more susceptible to infection. **Essential** (or **dysaesthetic**) **vulvodynia** is thought to be due to an altered perception of cutaneous pain, like postherpetic *neuralgia. Treatment of essential vulvodynia is with tricyclic antidepressants at night, biofeedback, vestibulectomy, cognitive behavioural therapy, topical capsaicin cream, lignocaine gel, and good skin care.

vulvovaginitis *n.* inflammation of the vulva and vagina (*see* PRURITUS, VAGINITIS).

V

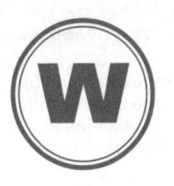

Waardenburg's syndrome an inherited form of deafness accompanied by a characteristic white forelock of hair and multiple colours within the irises of the eyes. It is inherited as an autosomal *dominant disease, i.e. the children of an affected parent have a 50% chance of inheriting the disorder, although severity is variable. The gene responsible has been identified. [P. J. Waardenburg (1886–1979), Dutch ophthalmologist]

wafer *n.* a thin sheet made from moistened flour, formerly used to enclose a powdered medicine that is taken by mouth.

WAGR syndrome *W*ilms' tumour (*see* NEPHROBLASTOMA), *a*niridia, *g*enitourinary abnormalities, and mental *r*etardation: a condition due to a deletion of part of the short arm of chromosome 11.

waiter's-tip deformity *see* ERB'S PALSY.

waiting list a list of the patients awaiting admission to hospital after having been assessed either as an out-patient or on a *domiciliary consultation involving a specialist. In general the patients are offered places in the order in which their names were placed on the list, but in certain circumstances (e.g. if the condition is potentially dangerous or painful) the consultant may recommend urgent or even immediate admission. One of the variables recorded in relation to hospital admissions is the length of time between the name being placed on the list and the patient being admitted (**waiting time**). General practitioners may also request **direct admission** (immediate) for urgent cases who have not been seen by the consultant; such admission may be arranged by phone with the consultant or his or her deputy, or via the accident and emergency department of the hospital.

Waldenstrom's macroglobulinaemia (lymphoplasmacytic lymphoma) a type of low-grade relatively slow-growing non-Hodgkin's *lymphoma characterized by enlarged lymph nodes and high levels of abnormal IgM (*macroglobulin) in the blood (*see* MACROGLOBULINAEMIA). [J. G. Waldenstrom (1906–96), Swedish physician]

Waldeyer's ring the ring of lymphoid tissue formed by the *tonsils. [H. W. G. von Waldeyer (1836–1921), German anatomist]

walking distance the measured distance that a patient can walk before he or she is stopped by pain in the muscles, usually the calf muscles, or breathlessness. It is a useful estimate of the degree of impairment of the blood supply. *See* CLAUDICATION.

Wallerian degeneration degeneration of a ruptured nerve fibre that occurs within the nerve sheath distal to the point of severance. [A. V. Waller (1816–70), British physician]

warfarin *n.* an *anticoagulant used mainly in the prevention and treatment of deep vein thrombosis and pulmonary embolism and to prevent embolism in other patients at risk. It is given by mouth. The principal toxic effect is local bleeding, usually from the gums and other mucous membranes, and the drug should be avoided during pregnancy. Warfarin has also been used as a rat poison. Trade name: **Marevan**.

wart *n.* a benign growth on the skin caused by infection with *human papillomavirus (a few of the many serotypes are *oncogenic). **Common warts** are firm horny papules, 1–10 mm in diameter, found mainly on the hands. Most will clear spontaneously within two years. **Plantar warts** (or **verrucae**) occur on the soles and are often tender. **Plane warts** are flat and skin-coloured – and therefore difficult to see; they are usually found on the face and may be present in very large numbers. **Anogenital warts** are frequently associated with other genital infections (*see* CONDYLOMA). Treatment of warts is with OTC (over-the-counter) remedies, such as lactic and salicylic acids; *cryotherapy with liquid nitrogen is also effective. Curettage and cautery is very occasionally used, as well as immunotherapy with diphencycloprop-enone.

Warthin's tumour (adenolymphoma) a tumour of the parotid salivary glands, containing epithelial and lymphoid tissues with

787

cystic spaces. [A. S. Warthin (1866–1931), US pathologist]

Wassermann reaction formerly, the most commonly used test for the diagnosis of *syphilis. A sample of the patient's blood is examined, using a *complement-fixation reaction, for the presence of antibodies to the organism *Treponema pallidum*. A positive reaction (WR+) indicates the presence of antibodies and therefore infection with syphilis. [A. P. von Wassermann (1866–1925), German bacteriologist]

water bed a bed with a flexible water-containing mattress. The surface of the bed adapts itself to the patient's posture, which leads to greater comfort and fewer pressure sores.

waterbrash *n.* a sudden filling of the mouth with dilute saliva – this often accompanies dyspepsia, particularly if there is nausea – or with acid or bitter fluid in patients with *heartburn.

water-deprivation test a test for *diabetes insipidus in which fluid and food intake is withheld completely for (usually) 24 hours, with regular measurement of plasma and urinary *osmolality and body weight. Normally (and in a person with psychogenic *polydipsia) the output of *vasopressin will be increased in order to concentrate the urine as the plasma osmolality rises; correspondingly, the urine osmolality also rises and its volume diminishes. In a patient with diabetes insipidus, however, the urine osmolality will remain low and of high volume while the patient steadily dehydrates. The test must be abandoned if the patient loses 3% of body weight.

Waterhouse-Friderichsen syndrome acute haemorrhage in the adrenal glands with haemorrhage into the skin associated with the sudden onset of acute bacteraemic *shock. It is usually caused by meningococcal septicaemia (*see* MENINGITIS). [R. Waterhouse (1873–1958), British physician; C. Friderichsen (20th century), Danish physician]

Waters' projection a *posteroanterior X-ray film to show the maxillae, maxillary sinuses, and zygomatic bones. [C. A. Waters (1888–1961), US radiologist]

watt *n.* the *SI unit of power, equal to 1 joule per second. In electrical terms it is the energy expended per second when a current

of 1 ampere flows between two points on a conductor between which there is a potential difference of 1 volt. 1 watt = 10^7 ergs per second. Symbol: W.

Watzke-Allen sign a test used in the diagnosis of a macular hole in the retina. A thin line of light is projected over the macula with a *slit lamp and the patient is asked to report on its appearance. A line appearing broken may indicate a macular hole.

weal (hive) *n.* a transient swelling, confined to a small area of the skin, that is characteristic of *urticaria and also occurs due to *dermographism.

weaning *n.* the process of gradually introducing nonmilk feeds to an infant, which is generally recommended between four and six months of age. This is when the gastrointestinal and renal tracts are mature enough to handle the variety of foods ingested.

weber *n.* the *SI unit of magnetic flux, equal to the flux linking a circuit of one turn that produces an e.m.f. of 1 volt when reduced uniformly to zero in 1 second. Symbol: Wb.

Weber's test a hearing test in which a vibrating tuning fork is placed at the midpoint of the forehead. A normal individual hears it equally in both ears, but if one ear is affected by conductive *deafness the sound appears louder in the affected ear. If one ear has a sensorineural deafness the sound appears louder in the unaffected ear. [F. E. Weber (1832–91), German otologist]

web space the soft tissue between the bases of the fingers and toes.

Wechsler scales standardized scales for the measurement of *intelligence quotient (IQ) in adults and children. They are administered by a chartered psychologist. *See* INTELLIGENCE TEST. [D. Wechsler (1896–1981), US psychologist]

Wegener's granulomatosis an autoimmune disease predominantly affecting the nasal passages, lungs, and kidneys, characterized by the formation of necrotizing *granuloma in addition to pulmonary *vasculitis. It is associated with the presence of antineutrophil cytoplasmic antibodies (*ANCA). Untreated, the disease is usually fatal, but it can be controlled (sometimes for years) with steroids, cyclophosphamide, and azathioprine. [F. Wegener (1907–90), German pathologist]

Weil-Felix reaction a diagnostic test for typhus. A sample of the patient's serum is tested for the presence of antibodies against the organism *Proteus vulgaris*. Although this relatively harmless organism is not the cause of typhus, it possesses certain antigens in common with the causative agent of the disease and can therefore be used instead of it in laboratory tests. Typhus is suspected if antibodies are found to be present. [E. Weil (1880–1922), German physician; A. Felix (1887–1956), Czech bacteriologist]

Weil's disease *see* LEPTOSPIROSIS. [A. Weil (1848–1916), German physician]

Weiss ring a ringlike opacity on the posterior vitreous surface, arising as a result of a posterior *vitreous detachment. It is seen as a ring-shaped *floater.

Welch's bacillus *see* CLOSTRIDIUM. [W. H. Welch (1850–1934), US pathologist]

Werdnig-Hoffmann disease a hereditary disorder – a severe form of *spinal muscular atrophy – in which the cells of the spinal cord begin to die between birth and the age of six months, causing a symmetrical muscle weakness. Affected infants become floppy and progressively weaker; respiratory and facial muscles become affected. Children usually die by the age of 20 months from respiratory failure and there is no treatment. *Genetic counselling is required for parents of an affected child as each of their subsequent children has a one in four chance of being affected. [G. Werdnig (1844–1919), Austrian neurologist; J. Hoffmann (1857–1919), German neurologist]

Wermer's syndrome *see* MENS. [P. Wermer, US physician]

Werner's syndrome a rare genetic disorder resulting in premature ageing that starts at adolescence. Growth may be retarded and affected individuals may suffer from a thin skin, arterial disease, leg ulcers, and diabetes. Treatment is limited to the management of complications, such as diabetes. The gene responsible codes for an enzyme involved in the mechanisms of DNA replication and repair, which in affected individuals is defective. [C. W. O. Werner (1879–1936), German physician]

Wernicke's encephalopathy mental confusion or delirium occurring in combination with paralysis of the eye muscles, *nystagmus, and an unsteady gait. It is caused by a deficiency of vitamin B_1 (thiamine) and is most commonly seen in alcoholics and in patients with persistent vomiting or an unbalanced diet. Treatment with thiamine relieves the symptoms. [K. Wernicke (1848–1905), German neurologist]

Wertheim's hysterectomy a radical operation performed for cervical cancer, in which the uterus, Fallopian tubes, ovaries, upper vagina, broad ligaments, parametrium, and regional lymph nodes are removed. [E. Wertheim (1864–1920), Austrian gynaecologist]

Western blot analysis a technique for the detection of specific proteins. After separation by *electrophoresis, the proteins are bound to radioactively labelled antibodies and identified by X-ray. *Compare* NORTHERN BLOT ANALYSIS, SOUTHERN BLOT ANALYSIS.

West Nile fever a viral disease caused by the West Nile virus (a *flavivirus), which is spread by the *Culex pipiens* mosquito. It causes encephalitis, with influenza-like symptoms, enlarged lymph nodes, and a bright red rash on the chest and abdomen. In patients with a weakened immune system (such as the elderly) it can progress to convulsions, coma, and paralysis.

wet-and-dry bulb hygrometer *see* HYGROMETER.

Wharton's duct the secretory duct of the submandibular *salivary gland. [T. Wharton (1614–73), English physician]

Wharton's jelly the mesoderm tissue of the umbilical cord, which becomes converted to a loose jelly-like *mesenchyme surrounding the umbilical blood vessels.

wheeze *n.* an abnormal high-pitched (sibilant) or low-pitched sound heard – either by the unaided human ear or through the stethoscope – mainly during expiration. Wheezes occur as a result of narrowing of the airways, such as results from *bronchospasm or increased secretion and retention of sputum; they are commonly heard in patients with asthma or chronic bronchitis.

whiplash injury a soft-tissue injury of the neck resulting from a sudden jerking back (hyperextension) of the head and neck, usually following a rear-end motor vehicle collision. It is associated with muscle, tendon, and ligament tears and inflammation in the front of the neck, which causes pain and stiffness. The possibility of fractures and other serious spinal injuries should be excluded by X-ray or MRI. Treatment includes analgesics, NSAIDs, a soft surgical collar, and physiotherapy. Symptoms occasionally last for many months or years.

Whipple's disease a rare disease, occurring commonly (but not exclusively) in males, in which absorption of digested food in the intestine is reduced. As well as symptoms and signs of *malabsorption there is usually abdominal pain, skin pigmentation, and arthritis. Diagnosis is usually made by small-intestinal biopsy (duodenal or *jejunal biopsy) demonstrating the presence of PAS-positive (*see* PERIODIC ACID–SCHIFF REACTION) macrophages containing the causative microorganism, *Tropheryma whipplei*. The disease usually responds to a prolonged course of antibiotics. [G. H. Whipple (1878–1976), US pathologist]

Whipple's operation *see* PANCREATEC-TOMY. [A. O. Whipple (1881–1963), US surgeon]

Whipple's triad a combination of three clinical features that indicate the presence of an *insulinoma: (1) attacks of fainting, dizziness, and sweating on fasting; (2) severe hypoglycaemia present during the attacks; (3) relief from the attacks achieved by administering glucose. [A. O. Whipple]

whipworm *n.* a small parasitic whiplike nematode worm, *Trichuris trichiura* (*Trichocephalus dispar*), that lives in the large intestine. Eggs are passed out of the body with the faeces and human infection (*see* TRICHURIA-SIS) results from the consumption of water or food contaminated with faecal material. The eggs hatch in the small intestine but mature worms migrate to the large intestine.

whistle-blowing *n.* expressing concerns about the professional performance of a member of staff, team, or organization. NHS trusts are required to have a whistle-blowing policy that sets out the procedures to be followed by those who wish to raise questions about an aspect of professional practice. Such policies must accord with the Public Interest Disclosure Act 1998, which protects whistle-blowers from being penalized. *See also* PUBLIC INTEREST DISCLOSURE.

Whitaker's test a direct percutaneous renal infusion test to investigate obstruction of the ureter causing *hydronephrosis. [R. Whitaker (20th century), British urologist]

white blood cell *see* LEUCOCYTE.

white fat *see* BROWN FAT.

white finger the pale waxy appearance of a finger resulting from spasm of the vessels of the finger. It occurs in *Raynaud's disease but can also be attributed to the long-term use of vibrating equipment (**vibration white finger**). In the latter case, it is a source of compensation claims.

white matter nerve tissue of the central nervous system that is paler in colour than the associated *grey matter because it contains more nerve fibres and thus larger amounts of the insulating material *myelin. In the brain the white matter lies within the grey layer of cerebral cortex; in the spinal cord it is between the arms of the X-shaped central core of grey matter.

white noise instrument a device, resembling a small hearing aid, that produces sounds of many frequencies at equal intensities and is used in the treatment of tinnitus. It was formerly known as a **tinnitus masker**.

whitlow *n. see* PARONYCHIA.

WHO *see* WORLD HEALTH ORGANIZATION.

whoop *n.* a noisy convulsive drawing in of the breath following the spasmodic coughing attack characteristic of *whooping cough.

whooping cough an acute highly infectious disease usually caused by the bacterium *Bordetella pertussis*, primarily affecting infants and often occurring in epidemics. After an incubation period of 1–2 weeks there is a catarrhal stage, in which the infant has signs of an upper respiratory tract infection; transmission is through droplet spread. This is followed by an irritating cough that gradually becomes paroxysmal within 1–2 weeks. The paroxysms are followed by a characteristic *whoop and vomiting. In the very young the classical whoop may not develop and instead the paroxysms may be followed by periods of *apnoea. The illness can last 2–3 months, giving it the name 'the cough of 100 days' in some countries. Infection can be complicated by bronchopneumonia, weight loss due to repeated vomiting, *bronchiectasis, and convulsions due to *asphyxia or bleeding into the brain tissue. Minor complications include subconjunctival haemorrhage, *epistaxis (nosebleed), facial *oedema, and ulceration of the tongue.

W

*Immunization against the infection was introduced in the UK in the 1950s and offers protection. An attack usually confers lifelong immunity. Despite good vaccine coverage resulting in the current low levels of disease, whooping cough is still a significant cause of illness and death in the very young. Medical name: **pertussis**.

Widal reaction an *agglutination test for the presence of antibodies against the *Salmonella* organisms that cause typhoid fever. It is thus a method of diagnosing the presence of the disease in a patient and also a means of identifying the organisms in infected material. [G. F. I. Widal (1862–1929), French physician]

Williams syndrome a hereditary condition, caused by a defect (a *deletion) in chromosome 7, marked by a characteristic 'elfin' facial appearance (including large eyes, a wide mouth, and small chin), *hypercalcaemia, short stature, mental retardation, and *aortic stenosis. Most affected children are highly sociable and have unusual conversational ability, using a rich and complex vocabulary. The condition can be diagnosed prenatally. [J. C. P. Williams (20th century), British physician]

Williams vulvovaginoplasty a surgical technique of vaginal reconstruction, with the formation of a pouch between the urethra and rectum.

Wilms' tumour *see* NEPHROBLASTOMA. [M. Wilms (1867–1918), German surgeon]

Wilson's disease an inborn defect of copper metabolism in which there is a deficiency of *caeruloplasmin (which normally forms a nontoxic complex with copper). The free copper may be deposited in the liver, causing jaundice and cirrhosis, or in the brain, causing mental retardation and symptoms resembling *parkinsonism. There is a characteristic brown ring in the cornea (the **Kayser-Fleischer ring**). If the excess copper is removed from the body by regular treatment with *penicillamine both mental and physical deficits tend to improve. Medical name: **hepatolenticular degeneration**. [S. A. K. Wilson (1878–1936), British neurologist]

windigo psychosis a delusion of having been transformed into a windigo, a mythical monster that eats human flesh. It is often quoted as an example of a culture-specific syndrome (confined to certain North American Indian tribes).

windowing *n.* a technique of image manipulation commonly used in *cross-sectional imaging to manipulate a *grey scale image. Typically there is too much data obtained in a scan to see on a single image: the radiologist therefore chooses the window level centred on the density of the tissue of interest and a window width wide enough to include the densities of all the tissues that need to be seen. Tissues denser than this window usually appear white, and tissues darker appear black. Sometimes several different images of the same scan are required at different window settings to see adequately all the necessary detail (for example, window settings to observe the lung are different from those for the bones or the soft tissues in the chest on CT). *See also* HOUNSFIELD UNIT.

windpipe *n. see* TRACHEA.

wisdom tooth the third *molar tooth on each side of either jaw, which erupts normally around the age of 20 years.

Wiskott-Aldrich syndrome a rare *sex-linked recessive disorder characterized by eczema, *thrombocytopenia, and deficiency in the immune response (*immunodeficiency). It is caused by a decrease in the amount of **Wiskott-Aldrich syndrome protein** (**WASP**: a protein occurring in lymphocytes, platelets, and other cells) due to a mutation in the *WASP* gene.

witch hazel (hamamelis) a preparation made from the leaves and bark of the tree *Hamamelis virginiana*, used as an *astringent, especially for the treatment of sprains and bruises.

withdrawal *n.* 1. (social withdrawal) (in psychology and psychiatry) the removal of one's interest from one's surroundings. 2. *see* COITUS INTERRUPTUS. 3. *see* THOUGHT WITHDRAWAL.

withdrawal symptoms *see* DEPENDENCE.

Wohlfahrtia *n.* a genus of nonbloodsucking flies. Females of the species *W. magnifica* and *W. vigil* deposit their parasitic maggots in wounds and the openings of the body. This causes *myiasis, particularly in children.

Wolff-Chaikoff effect the inhibition of thyroid hormone production by administration of large doses of iodide. This occurs at a critical dosage level below which the addition of iodide to an iodine-deficient individual results in increased production of thyroid hormone. The effect is transient in individuals with normal thyroids but may persist in thyroiditis; it can be utilized medically to induce a hypothyroid state, for example in patients with *thyroid crisis (*see* LUGOL'S IO-DINE). [L. Wolff (1898–1972), US cardiologist; I. L. Chaikoff (20th century), US physiologist]

Wolffian body *see* MESONEPHROS. [K. F. Wolff (1733–94), German anatomist]

Wolffian duct *see* MESONEPHROS.

Wolff-Parkinson-White syndrome a congenital abnormality of heart conduction caused by the presence of an *accessory pathway of conduction between the atria and ventricles (*see* ATRIOVENTRICULAR BUN-DLE). It results in premature excitation of one ventricle and is characterized by an abnormal wave (**delta wave**) at the start of the QRS complex on the electrocardiogram. The accessory pathway predisposes the patient to episodes of fast heart rate (*supraventricular tachycardia) due to the rapid self-sustaining circulation of an electrical impulse from the atria to the ventricles and back again (a re-entry circuit). Emergency treatment is in the form of drugs that temporarily block the re-entry circuit. Permanent destruction of the accessory pathway by *radiofrequency ablation is usually curative. [L. Wolff; Sir J. Parkinson (1885–1976), British physician; P. D. White (1886–1973), US cardiologist]

Wolfram syndrome (DIDMOAD syndrome**)** a rare syndrome consisting of a combination of *diabetes insipidus, *diabetes mellitus, *optic atrophy, and *deafness.

womb *n. see* UTERUS.

Wood's light ultraviolet light filtered through a nickel oxide prism, which causes fluorescence in skin and hair affected by some fungal and bacterial infections and is therefore useful in diagnosis. For example, *erythrasma fluoresces coral pink, while scalp ringworm caused by *Microsporum* species fluoresces green. [R. W. Wood (1868–1955), US physician]

woolsorter's disease *see* ANTHRAX.

word blindness *see* ALEXIA.

working tax credit a benefit payable to working people with a low income. There are four categories of eligibility: a person responsible for a child; a disabled person; a

person who is aged over 50, has recently started work, and was receiving certain benefits before starting work; and a person aged over 25 and working more than 30 hours per week.

World Health Organization (WHO**)** an international organization working to improve global public health. Membership is open to all countries, and the member states are divided into six regions; the United Kingdom is part of the WHO European Region. Health issues are discussed and policies evolved mainly through topic-specific working groups. WHO staff are seconded by invitation to advise countries on solving public health problems (especially infectious disease control). WHO handles information on the internationally *notifiable diseases, publishes the *International Classification of Diseases, and awards fellowships to enable health staff from poorer countries to obtain further training.

SEE WEB LINKS
• WHO website: links to a comprehensive database of international health statistics

worm *n.* any member of several groups of soft-bodied legless animals, including flatworms, nematode worms, earthworms, and leeches, that were formerly thought to be closely related and classified as a single group – Vermes.

wormian bone one of a number of small bones that occur in the cranial sutures.

wound *n.* a break in the structure of an organ or tissue caused by an external agent. Bruises, grazes, tears, cuts, punctures, and burns are all examples of wounds.

woven bone immature bone, in which the collagen fibres are arranged haphazardly and the cells have no specific orientation. It is typically found in the early stages of fracture healing, eventually being replaced by mature *lamellar bone.

wrist *n.* 1. the joint between the forearm and hand. It consists of the proximal bones of the *carpus, which articulate with the radius and ulna. 2. the whole region of the wrist joint, including the carpus and lower parts of the radius and ulna.

wrist drop paralysis of the muscles that raise the wrist, which is caused by damage to the *radial nerve. This may result from compression of the nerve against the humerus in the upper arm or from selective damage to the nerve, which is a feature of *lead poisoning.

wryneck *n. see* TORTICOLLIS.

Wuchereria *n.* a genus of white threadlike parasitic worms (*see* FILARIA) that live in the lymphatic vessels. *W. bancrofti* is a tropical and subtropical species that causes *el-ephantiasis, lymphangitis, and chyluria. The immature forms concentrate in the lungs during the day. At night they become more numerous in the blood vessels of the skin, from which they are taken up by blood-sucking mosquitoes, acting as carriers of the diseases they cause.

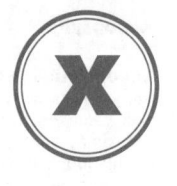

xanthaemia (carotenaemia) *n.* the presence in the blood of the yellow pigment *carotene, from excessive intake of carrots, tomatoes, or other vegetables containing the pigment.

xanthelasma *n.* yellow *plaques occurring symmetrically around the eyelids. It is quite common in elderly people and of no more than cosmetic importance, but in some cases it may be a manifestation of disorders of fat metabolism (hyperlipidaemia). The plaques may be removed surgically or by careful use of saturated trichoracetic acid.

xanthine *n.* a nitrogenous breakdown product of the purines adenosine and guanine. Xanthine is an intermediate product of the breakdown of nucleic acids to uric acid.

xanthinuria *n.* excess of the purine derivative *xanthine in the urine, usually the result of an inborn defect of metabolism. It is both rare and symptomless.

xantho- *combining form denoting* yellow colour.

xanthochromia *n.* yellow discoloration, such as may affect the skin (for example, in jaundice) or the cerebrospinal fluid (when it contains the breakdown products of haemoglobin from red blood cells that have entered it).

xanthoma *n.* (*pl.* **xanthomata**) a yellowish skin lesion associated with any of various disorders of lipid metabolism. There are several types of xanthomata. **Tuberous xanthomata** are found on the knees and elbows; **tendon xanthomata** involve the extensor tendons of the hands and feet and the Achilles tendon. Crops of small yellow papules at any site are known as **eruptive xanthomata**, while larger flat lesions are called **plane xanthomata**.

xanthomatosis *n.* the presence of multiple xanthomata in the skin. *See* XANTHOMA.

xanthophyll *n.* a yellow pigment found in green leaves. An example of a xanthophyll is **lutein**.

xanthopsia *n.* yellow vision: the condition in which all objects appear to have a yellowish tinge. It is sometimes experienced in digitalis poisoning.

X chromosome the sex chromosome present in both sexes. Women have two X chromosomes and men one. Genes for some important genetic disorders, including *haemophilia, are carried on the X chromosomes; these genes are described as *sex-linked. *Compare* Y CHROMOSOME.

Xeloda *n. see* CAPECITABINE.

xeno- *combining form denoting* different; foreign; alien.

xenodiagnosis *n.* a procedure for diagnosing infections transmitted by insect carriers. Uninfected insects of the species known to carry the disease in question are allowed to suck the blood of a patient suspected of having the disease. A positive diagnosis is made if the disease parasites appear in the insects. This method has proved invaluable for diagnosing Chagas' disease, using reduviid bugs (the carriers), since the parasites are not always easily detected in blood smears.

xenogeneic *adj.* describing grafted tissue derived from a donor of a different species.

xenograft (heterograft) *n.* a living tissue graft that is made from an animal of one species to another of a different species. For example, attempts have been made to graft animal organs into humans. *Bioengineering techniques are now available to produce animals whose *MHC is compatible with that of another species. *See also* XENOTRANSPLANTATION.

xenon-133 *n.* a radioactive isotope that has a half-life of about five days and is used in ventilation scanning of the lungs in nuclear medicine (*see* VENTILATION-PERFUSION SCANNING). It gives off beta particles, which are responsible for the relatively high radiation dose compared to *krypton-81m. Symbol: Xe-133.

xenophobia *n.* excessive fear of strangers and foreigners. *See* PHOBIA.

Xenopsylla *n.* a genus of tropical and sub-tropical fleas, with some 40 species. The rat flea, *X. cheopis*, occasionally attacks humans and can transmit plague from an infected rat population; it also transmits murine typhus and two tapeworms, *Hymenolepis nana* and *H. diminuta*.

xenotransplantation *n.* the *transplantation of organs from one species into another. Experimental work into the feasibility of transplanting pig organs into human beings is under way. It includes the genetic manipulation of pig embryos to produce animals whose organs produce a human cell-surface protein and would therefore not be rejected at transplantation.

xero- *combining form denoting* a dry condition.

xeroderma *n.* a mild form of the hereditary disorder *ichthyosis, in which the skin develops slight dryness and forms branlike scales. It is common in the elderly. **Xeroderma pigmentosum** is a rare genetically determined disorder (*see* GENODERMATOSIS) in which there is an inherited defect in the *DNA repair mechanism in the skin, which corrects ultraviolet radiation damage; this leads to multiple skin cancers. Affected individuals must avoid exposure to sunlight.

xerophthalmia *n.* a progressive nutritional disease of the eye due to deficiency of vitamin A. The cornea and conjunctiva become dry, thickened, and wrinkled. This may progress to *keratomalacia and eventual blindness.

xeroradiography *n.* X-ray imaging produced by exposing an electrically charged plate and then dusting it with a fine blue powder. The powder is then transferred to paper. This technique has been superseded by *computerized radiography.

xerosis *n.* abnormal dryness of the conjunctiva, the skin, or the mucous membranes. Xerosis affecting the conjunctiva is due to changes in the membrane itself, which becomes thickened and grey in the area exposed when the eyelids are open.

xerostomia *n. see* DRY MOUTH. *Compare* PTYALISM.

xiphi- (**xipho-**) *combining form denoting* the xiphoid process of the sternum. Example: **xiphocostal** (relating to the xiphoid process and ribs).

xiphisternum *n. see* XIPHOID PROCESS.

xiphoid process (**xiphoid cartilage**) the lowermost section of the breastbone (*see* STERNUM): a flat pointed cartilage that gradually ossifies until it is completely replaced by bone, a process not completed until after middle age. It does not articulate with any ribs. Also called: **ensiform process** or **cartilage**, **xiphisternum**.

X-linked disease *see* SEX-LINKED.

X-linked lymphoproliferative syndrome (**XLP syndrome, Duncan's disease**) a hereditary disorder of the immune system caused by a defective *sex-linked gene carried on an *X chromosome. There is uncontrolled proliferation of B-*lymphocytes in response to infection by the Epstein-Barr virus, which can lead to fulminating hepatitis or lymphoma. This condition is due to a defect in a gene, *SAP*, which encodes a signalling molecule found in the cytoplasm of cells.

XLP syndrome *see* X-LINKED LYMPHOPRO-LIFERATIVE SYNDROME.

Xolair *n. see* OMALIZUMAB.

X-rays *pl. n.* electromagnetic radiation of extremely short wavelength (beyond the ultraviolet), which pass through matter to varying degrees depending on its density. X-rays are produced when high-energy beams of electrons strike matter. They are physically indistinguishable from gamma rays, produced during radioactive decay. Both are used in diagnostic *radiology (*see* RADIOGRAPHY, NUCLEAR MEDICINE) and in *radiotherapy. Great care is needed to avoid unnecessary exposure, because the radiation is harmful to all living things (*see* IONIZATION, RADIATION SICKNESS). Heavy elements, such as lead and barium, tend to stop X-rays and can be used to shield people from unwanted exposure to ionizing radiation.

X-ray screening the use of an image intensifier to produce *real-time imaging during an X-ray examination on a TV monitor. It is widely used in angiography and *interventional radiology to guide procedures. *See* VIDEOFLUOROSCOPY.

xylene (**dimethylbenzene**) *n.* a liquid used for increasing the transparency of tissues prepared for microscopic examination after dehydration. *See* CLEARING.

xylometazoline *n.* a *sympathomimetic

drug that constricts blood vessels (*see* VASO-CONSTRICTOR). It is applied topically (in the form of drops or a spray) as a nasal decongestant for the relief of the common cold and sinusitis. Toxic effects are rare, but the congestion may worsen transiently when treat-ment stops. Trade names: **Otradrops**, **Otraspray**, **Otrivine**.

xylose *n.* a pentose sugar (i.e. one with five carbon atoms) that is involved in carbohydrate interconversions within cells. It is used as a diagnostic aid for intestinal function.

X

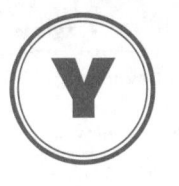

YAG laser a type of *laser whose active medium is a crystal of yttrium, aluminium, and garnet. It is used for cutting tissue, for example in lens *capsulotomy or *iridotomy. Specialized types (e.g. the *holmium:YAG laser) are used for various specific purposes.

yawning *n.* a reflex action in which the mouth is opened wide and air is drawn into the lungs then slowly released. It is triggered by drowsiness, fatigue, or boredom.

yaws (pian, framboesia) *n.* a tropical infectious disease caused by the spirochaete *Treponema pertenue* in the skin and its underlying tissues. Yaws occurs chiefly in conditions of poor hygiene. It is transmitted by direct contact with infected persons and their clothing and possibly also by flies of the genus *Hippelates*. The spirochaetes enter through abrasions on the skin. Initial symptoms include fever, pains, and itching, followed by the appearance of small tumours, each covered by a yellow crust of dried serum, on the hands, face, legs, and feet. These tumours may deteriorate into deep ulcers. The final stage of yaws, which may appear after an interval of several years, involves destructive and deforming lesions of the skin, bones, and periosteum (*see also* GANGOSA, GOUNDOU). Yaws, which commonly affects children, is prevalent in hot humid lowlands of equatorial Africa, tropical America, the Far East, and the West Indies. It responds well to antibiotics.

Y chromosome a sex chromosome that is present in men but not in women. It carries the **SRY** (sex reversal on Y) gene, which encodes a protein (**testis-determining factor**, or **SRY protein**) that switches the default female pathway of embryonic development to the male pathway by initiating testis formation. *Compare* X CHROMOSOME.

yeast *n.* any of a group of fungi in which the body (mycelium) consists of individual cells, which may occur singly, in groups of two or three, or in chains. Yeasts reproduce by budding and by the formation of sexual spores (in the case of the perfect yeasts) or asexual spores (in the case of the imperfect yeasts). Baker's yeast (*Saccharomyces*) ferments carbohydrates to produce alcohol and carbon dioxide and is important in brewing and breadmaking. Some yeasts are a commercial source of proteins and of vitamins of the B complex. Yeasts that cause disease in humans include *Candida*, *Cryptococcus*, and *Malassezia*.

yellow fever an infectious disease, caused by an *arbovirus, occurring in tropical Africa and the northern regions of South America. It is transmitted by mosquitoes, principally *Aëdes aegypti*. The virus causes degeneration of the tissues of the liver and kidneys. Symptoms, depending on severity of infection, include chill, headache, pains in the back and limbs, fever, vomiting, constipation, a reduced flow of urine (which contains high levels of albumin), and *jaundice. The more serious cases may prove fatal, but recovery from a first attack confers subsequent immunity. The disease is treated by fluid replacement and can be prevented by vaccination.

yellow spot *see* MACULA (LUTEA).

Yersinia *n.* a genus of aerobic or facultatively anaerobic Gram-negative bacteria that are parasites of animals and humans. *Y. pestis* causes bubonic *plague; *Y. enterocolitica* causes intestinal infections.

yolk (deutoplasm) *n.* a substance, rich in protein and fat, that is laid down within the egg cell as nourishment for the embryo. It is absent (or nearly so) from the eggs of mammals (including humans) whose embryos absorb nutrients from their mother.

yolk sac (vitelline sac) the membranous sac, composed of mesoderm lined with endoderm, that lies ventral to the embryo. It is one of the *extraembryonic membranes. Its initially wide communication with the future gut is later reduced to a narrow duct passing through the *umbilicus. It probably assists in transporting nutrients to the early embryo and is one of the first sites where blood cells are formed.

yttrium-90 *n.* an artificial radioactive isotope of the element yttrium used in *radiotherapy.

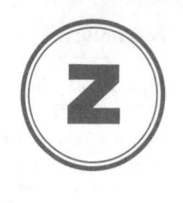

zafirlukast *n. see* LEUKOTRIENE RECEPTOR ANTAGONIST.

zaleplon *n. see* HYPNOTIC.

zanamivir *n.* an antiviral drug that acts by inhibiting the action of *neuraminidase in viruses. This enzyme destroys the receptor sites on the surface of the host cells. Zanamivir is used for the treatment of influenza A and B. To be effective, the drug must be taken within 48 hours of the onset of symptoms. Administered by inhalation, it is liable to cause tightening of the bronchial tubes and this may be dangerous in people with asthma. Trade name: **Relenza**.

Zantac *n. see* RANITIDINE.

zein *n.* a protein found in maize.

zidovudine (AZT) *n.* a *reverse transcriptase inhibitor used in the treatment of AIDS and HIV infection. The drug slows the growth of HIV infection in the body, but is not curative. It is administered by mouth or intravenously in combination with other *antiretroviral drugs; the most common side-effects are nausea, headache, and insomnia, and it may damage the blood-forming tissues of the bone marrow. Trade name: **Retrovir**.

Ziehl-Neelsen stain an acid-fast *carbol fuchsin stain used specifically for identifying the tubercle bacillus. [F. Ziehl (1857–1926), German bacteriologist; F. K. A. Neelsen (1854–94), German pathologist]

Zieve's syndrome a combination of severe *hyperlipidaemia, haemolytic *anaemia, and *jaundice seen in susceptible individuals drinking alcohol to excess. [L. Zieve (1915–), US physician]

zinc *n.* a *trace element that is a cofactor of many enzymes. Deficiency is rare with a balanced diet but may occur in alcoholics and those with kidney disease; symptoms include lesions of the skin, oesophagus, and cornea and (in children) retarded growth. Symbol: Zn.

zinc oxide a mild *astringent used in various skin conditions, usually mixed with other substances. It is applied as a cream, ointment, dusting powder, or as a paste, often in the form of an impregnated bandage.

zinc sulphate a preparation used in the treatment of proven zinc deficiency. It is administered by mouth or injection. Trade name: **Solvazinc**.

zinc undecenoate (zinc undecylenate) an antifungal agent with uses similar to those of *undecenoic acid.

zoledronic acid (zolendronate) a *bisphosphonate drug that is used to treat Paget's disease and malignant *hypercalcaemia and is also establishing a role in treating bone metastases, both in terms of symptom relief and preventing bone fractures. It is administered by intravenous infusion. Trade names: **Aclasta**, **Zometa**.

Zollinger-Ellison syndrome a rare disorder in which there is excessive secretion of gastric juice due to high levels of circulating *gastrin, which is produced by a pancreatic tumour (*see* GASTRINOMA) or an enlarged pancreas. The high levels of stomach acid cause diarrhoea and peptic ulcers, which may be multiple, in unusual sites (e.g. jejunum), or which may quickly recur after *vagotomy or partial *gastrectomy. Treatment with proton-pump inhibitors, by removal of the tumour (if benign), or by total gastrectomy is usually effective. [R. M. Zollinger (1903–92) and E. H. Ellison (1918–70), US physicians]

zolmitriptan *n. see* 5HT$_1$ AGONIST.

zolpidem *n. see* HYPNOTIC.

zona pellucida the thick membrane that develops around the mammalian oocyte within the ovarian follicle. It is penetrated by at least one spermatozoon at fertilization and persists around the *blastocyst until it reaches the uterus. *See* OVUM.

zonula *n. see* ZONULE.

zonule (zonula) *n.* (in anatomy) a small band or zone; for example the **zonule of**

Zinn (**zonula ciliaris**) is the suspensory ligament of the eye. —**zonular** *adj.*

zonulolysis *n.* dissolution of the suspensory ligament (**zonule of Zinn**) of the lens of the eye by means of an enzyme solution, which facilitates intracapsular removal of a lens affected by cataract. This technique is not used for modern cataract surgery.

zoo- *combining form denoting* animals.

zoonosis *n.* an infectious disease of animals that can be transmitted to humans. *See* ANTHRAX, AVIAN INFLUENZA, BRUCELLOSIS, CAT-SCRATCH DISEASE, COWPOX, GLANDERS, Q FEVER, RIFT VALLEY FEVER, RABIES, RAT-BITE FEVER, TOXOPLASMOSIS, TULARAEMIA, TYPHUS.

zoophobia *n.* excessively strong fear of animals. *See* PHOBIA.

zopiclone *n. see* HYPNOTIC.

zotepine *n. see* ANTIPSYCHOTIC.

zwitterion *n.* an ion that bears a positive and a negative charge. Amino acids can yield zwitterions.

Zyban *n. see* BUPROPION.

zygoma *n. see* ZYGOMATIC ARCH, ZYGOMATIC BONE.

zygomatic arch (**zygoma**) the horizontal arch of bone on either side of the face, just below the eyes, formed by connected processes of the zygomatic and temporal bones. *See* SKULL.

zygomatic bone (**zygoma**, **malar bone**) either of a pair of bones that form the prominent part of the cheeks and contribute to the orbits. *See* SKULL.

zygote *n.* the fertilized ovum before *cleavage begins. It contains both male and female pronuclei.

zygotene *n.* the second stage of the first prophase of *meiosis, in which the homologous chromosomes form pairs (bivalents).

zym- (**zymo-**) *combining form denoting* 1. an enzyme. 2. fermentation.

zymogen *n. see* PROENZYME.

zymology *n.* the science of the study of yeasts and fermentation.

zymolysis *n.* the process of *fermentation or digestion by an enzyme.

zymosis *n.* 1. the process of *fermentation, brought about by yeast organisms. 2. the changes in the body that occur in certain infectious diseases, once thought to be the result of a process similar to fermentation. —**zymotic** *adj.*

zymotic disease an old name for a contagious disease, which was formerly thought to develop within the body following infection in a process similar to the fermentation and growth of yeast.

Z

Appendices

1. SI units

TABLE 1.1 **Base and supplementary SI units**

Physical quantity	Name of unit	Symbol for unit
length	metre	m
mass	kilogram	kg
time	second	s
electric current	ampere	A
thermodynamic temperature	kelvin	K
luminous intensity	candela	cd
amount of substance	mole	mol
*plane angle	radian	rad
*solid angle	steradian	sr

*supplementary units

TABLE 1.2 **Derived SI units with special names**

Physical quantity	Name of unit	Symbol for unit
frequency	hertz	Hz
energy	joule	J
force	newton	N
power	watt	W
pressure	pascal	Pa
electric charge	coulomb	C
electric potential difference	volt	V
electric resistance	ohm	W
electric conductance	siemens	S
electric capacitance	farad	F
magnetic flux	weber	Wb
inductance	henry	H
magnetic flux density (magnetic induction)	tesla	T
luminous flux	lumen	lm
illuminance (illumination)	lux	lx
absorbed dose	gray	Gy
activity	becquerel	Bq
dose equivalent	sievert	Sv

TABLE 1.3 Decimal multiples and submultiples to be used with SI units

Submultiple	Prefix	Symbol	Multiple	Prefix	Symbol
10^{-1}	deci	d	10^{1}	deca	da
10^{-2}	centi	c	10^{2}	hecto	h
10^{-3}	milli	m	10^{3}	kilo	k
10^{-6}	micro	μ	10^{6}	mega	M
10^{-9}	nano	n	10^{9}	giga	G
10^{-12}	pico	p	10^{12}	tera	T
10^{-15}	femto	f	10^{15}	peta	P
10^{-16}	atto	a	10^{16}	exa	E
10^{-21}	zepto	z	10^{21}	zetta	Z
10^{-24}	yocto	y	10^{24}	yotta	Y

TABLE 1.4 Conversion of units to and from SI units

From	To	Multiply by
in	m	0.0254
ft	m	0.3048
sq in	m^2	0.00064516
sq ft	m^2	0.092903
cu in	m^3	0.0000164
cu ft	m^3	0.0283168
l(itre)	m^3	0.001
gal(lon)	m^3	0.0045609
gal(lon)	litres	4.5609
lb	kg	0.453592
$g\,cm^{-3}$	$kg\,m^{-3}$	1000
lb/in^3	$kg\,m^{-3}$	27679.9
mmHg	Pa	133.322
cal	J	4.1868
m	in	39.3701
cm	in	0.393701
cm^2	sq in	0.155
m^2	sq in	1550
m^2	sq ft	10.7639
m^3	cu in	61023.6

TABLE 1.4 (cont.)

From	To	Multiply by
m^2	sq ft	10.7639
m^3	cu in	61023.6
m^3	cu ft	35.3146
m^3	l(itre)	1000
m^3	gal(lon)	219.969
kg	lb	2.20462
$kg\,m^{-3}$	$g\,cm^{-3}$	0.001
$kg\,m^{-3}$	lb/in^3	0.0000363
Pa	mmHg	0.0075006
J	cal	0.238846

Temperature conversion

°C (Celsius) = $5/9(°F - 32)$

°F (Fahrenheit) = $(9/5 \times °C) + 32$

2. Biochemical reference values for blood

(B = whole blood; P = plasma; S = serum)

TABLE 2.1 Everyday tests

Determination	Sample	Reference range
Alcohol		
legal limit (UK)	B or P	<17.4 mmol/l
Albumin	P	35–50 g/l
in pregnancy	P	25–38 g/l
Ammonia	B	<40 µmol/l
α-Amylase	P	25–180 somogyi units/dl
Anion gap $(Na^+ + K^+) - (HCO_3^- + Cl^-)$	P	12–16 mmol/l
Bilirubin	P	3–17 µmol/l
Bicarbonate (see also Table 2.2)	P	22–28 mmol/l
Calcium		
ionized	P	1.0–1.25 mmol/l
total	P	2.12–2.65 mmol/l
total in pregnancy	P	1.95–2.35 mmol/l
Chloride	P	95–105 mmol/l
Cholesterol (see also Table 2.6)	P	3.9–7.8 mmol/l
Copper	P	12–26 µmol/l
Creatinine	P	70–150 µmol/l
in pregnancy	P	24–68 µmol/l
Digoxin		
children	P	2.0–3.0 nmol/l
adults	P	1.0–2.0 nmol/l
Glucose (fasting)	P	3.0–5.0 mmol/l
Glycated haemoglobin (HbA_{1C})	B	5–8%
Iron		
male	S	14–31 µmol/l
female	S	11–30 µmol/l
total iron-binding capacity (TIBC)	S	45–75 µmol/l

TABLE 2.1 (cont.)

Determination	Sample	Reference range
Lactate		
venous	B	0.5–2.2 mmol/l
arterial	B	0.5–1.6 mmol/l
Magnesium	P	0.75–1.05 mmol/l
Osmolality	P	278–305 mosm/kg
Phosphate (inorganic)	P	0.8–1.45 mmol/l
Potassium	P	3.5–5.0 mmol/l
Protein (total)	P	60–80 g/l
Sodium	P	135–145 mmol/l
Troponin I	P	<0.2 ng/ml
Troponin T	P	<0.1 ng/ml
Urea	P	2.5–6.7 mmol/l
in pregnancy	P	2.0–4.2 mmol/l
Urea nitrogen (BUN)	P	1.16–3.12 mmol/l
Uric acid		
male	P	210–480 μmol/l
female	P	150–390 μmol/l
in pregnancy	P	100–270 μmol/l
Zinc	P	6–25 μmol/l

TABLE 2.2 **Blood gases**

Measurement	Reference range
Anion gap	12–16 mmol/l
Arterial CO_2 (P_{aCO_2})	4.7–6.0 kPa
Mixed venous CO_2 (P_{vCO_2})	5.5–6.8 kPa
Arterial oxygen (P_{aO_2})	12.0–14.5 kPa
Mixed venous oxygen (P_{vO_2})	4.0–6.0 kPa
Newborn arterial oxygen	5.3–8.0 kPa
H^+ ion activity	36–44 nmol/l
Arterial pH	7.35–7.45 pH units
Bicarbonate	
arterial – whole blood	19–24 mmol/l
venous – plasma	22–28 mmol/l
cord blood	14–22 mmol/l

TABLE 2.2 (cont.)

Measurement	Reference range
Base excess	± 2 mmol/l
Carboxyhaemoglobin	
non-smoker	<2%
smoker	3–15%
toxic at:	>15%
coma at:	>50%

TABLE 2.3 **Diagnostic enzymes**

Enzyme	Sample	Reference range
Acid phosphatase		
total	S	1–5 U/l
prostatic	S	0–1 U/l
Alkaline phosphatase	P	80–250 U/l
Alanine aminotransferase (ALT)	P	5–35 U/l
α-Amylase	P	25–180 somogyi units/dl
Angiotensin-converting enzyme (ACE)	S	21–54 U/l
Aspartate aminotransferase (AST)	P	15–42 U/l
Creatine kinase (CK)		
male	P	24–195 U/l
female	P	24–170 U/l
Gamma-glutamyl transferase (GGT)		
male	P	11–51 U/l
female	P	7–35 U/l
Lactate dehydrogenase (total)	P	240–525 U/l

TABLE 2.4 Hormones

Hormone	Sample	Reference range
Adrenaline (epinephrine)	P	0.03–1.31 nmol/l
ACTH	P	3.3–15.4 pmol/l
Aldosterone		
recumbent	P	100–450 pmol/l
midday	p	2-fold increase of recumbent level
Angiotensin II	P	5–35 pmol/l
Antidiuretic hormone (ADH)	P	0.9–4.6 pmol/l
Calcitonin		
male	P	<100 nmol/l
female	P	<30 nmol/l
Cortisol		
00.00 h	P	80–280 nmol/l
09.00 h	P	280–700 nmol/l
Follicle-stimulating hormone (FSH)		
follicular phase	P or S	0.5–5.0 U/l
ovulatory peak	P or S	8–15 U/l
luteal phase	P or S	2–8 U/l
postmenopause	P or S	> 30 U/l
male	P or S	0.5–5.0 U/l
Gastrin		
male + female (>60 yr)	P	<50 pmol/l
female (16–60 yr)	P	<38 pmol/l
Glucagon	P	<50 pmol/l
Growth hormone	P	<20 mU/l
Human chorionic gonadotrophin	S	<5 U/l
Insulin (fasting)	P	<15 mU/l
Insulin C-peptide (fasting)	P	<0.4 nmol/l (undetectable in hypoglycaemia)
Insulin-like growth factor-1 (IGF-1)	P	0.52–3.4 kU/l
Luteinizing hormone		
premenopausal	P or S	6–13 U/l
follicular phase	P or S	3–12 U/l
ovulatory peak	P or S	20–80 U/l
luteal phase	P or S	3–16 U/l
postmenopause	P or S	>30 U/l
male	P or S	3–8 U/l

TABLE 2.4 (cont.)

Hormone	Sample	Reference range
Noradrenaline	P	0.47–4.14 mmol/l
17-β-oestradiol		
follicular phase	P	75–260 pmol/l
mid-cycle	P	370–1470 pmol/l
luteal phase	P	180–1100 pmol/l
male	P	<220 pmol/l
Parathyroid hormone (intact)	P	0.9–5.4 pmol/l
Pancreatic polypeptide	P	<200 pmol/l
Progesterone		
male	P	<5 nmol/l
female postovulation	P	15–77nmol/l
follicular (newborn)	P	<3 nmol/l
17-Hydroxyprogesterone	P	7–16 nmol/l
Prolactin		
male	P	<450 U/l
female	P	<600 U/l
Renin activity	P	
recumbent		1.1–2.7 pmol/ml per hr
erect after 30 min		3.0–4.3 pmol/ml per hr
Somatostatin	P	30–166 pmol/l
Testosterone		
male	P or S	9–42 nmol/l
female	P or S	1–2.5 nmol/l
Thyroid-stimulating hormone	P	0.5–5.5 mU/l
Thyroid-binding globulin	P	13–28 mg/l
Triiodothyronine (T_3)	P	1–3 nmol/l
Free T_3	P	3.3–8.2 pmol/l
Thyroxine (T_4)	P	70–140 nmol/l
Free T_4	P	9–25 pmol/l
Vasoactive intestinal peptide (VIP)	P	<30 pmol/l

TABLE 2.5 **Proteins and immunoproteins**

Protein/immunoprotein	Sample	Reference range
Albumin	P	35–50 g/l
α_1-Antitrypsin	S	107–209 mg/l
Complement		
C3		65–190 mg/dl
C4		15–50 mg/dl
Caeruloplasmin	S	16–60 mg/dl
C1 esterase inhibitor	S	15–35 mg/dl
C-reactive protein (CRP)	S	<10 mg/l
Ferritin	S	14–200 µg/l
Fibrinogen	P	2–4 g/l
D-dimer	S	<500 µg/l
Haptoglobins	S	0.6–2.6 g/l
Immunoglobulins		
IgG	S	6.0–13.0 g/l
IgA	S	0.8–3.0 g/l
IgM	S	0.4–2.5 g/l
IgE	S	<120 kU/l
β_2-Microglobulin	S	<3 mg/l
Thyroid microsomal antibodies		
male	S	<1/400
female (<44 yr)	S	<1/400
female (>44 yr)	S	<1/6400
Total protein	P	60–80 g/l
β_1-Transferrin	S	1.2–2.0 g/l

TABLE 2.6 **Lipids and lipoproteins**

Lipid/lipoprotein	Sample	Reference range
Cholesterol	P	3.9–7.8 mmol/l
ideal upper limit		5.2 mmol/l
acceptable upper limit		6.5 mmol/l
Triglyceride (fasting)	P	0.55–1.90 mmol/l
Nonesterified (free)	S	
fatty acids (NEFA)		
male		0.19–0.78 mmol/l
female		0.06–0.9 mmol/l
Lipoproteins (as cholesterol)		
low-density (LDL)	S	1.55–4.4 mmol/l
ideal upper limit		3.4 mmol/l
acceptable upper limit		4.2 mmol/l
high density (HDL)	S	0.8–2.0 mmol/l
ideal (male)		>0.9 mmol/l
ideal (female)		>1.2 mmol/l
Total cholesterol/HDL	S	
ideal		<5 ratio

TABLE 2.7 **Vitamins**

Vitamin	Sample	Reference range
Vitamin A		
(retinol)	S	
male		1.06–3.35 µmol/l
female		0.84–2.95 µmol/l
β-carotene	S	
male		0.01–6.52 µmol/l
female		0.019–2.93 µmol/l
Vitamin B		
Thiamine (B_1)	P	>40 nmol/l
Riboflavin (B_2)	S	100–630 nmol/l
Pyridoxine (B_6)	P (EDTA)	20–120 nmol/l
Vitamin B_{12}	S	138–780 nmol/l
Folate	S	12–33 µmol/l
red blood cell folate	B	500–1300 µmol/l
Vitamin D metabolites		
25-(OH) D	S	17–125 nmol/l
1,25-$(OH)_2$ D_3	S	50–120 pmol/l
Vitamin E (a–tocopherol)	S	11.5–35 µmol/l

TABLE 2.8 Tumour markers

Tumour marker	Sample	Reference range
Alpha-fetoprotein (AFP)	S	<10 kU/l
Carcino-embryonic antigen (CEA)	S	<10 µg/l
Neuron-specific enolase (NSE)	S	<12 µg/l
Prostate-specific antigen (PSA)	S	<4 µg/l
Human chorionic gonadotrophin (hCG)	S	<5 IU/l
CA125	S	<35 U/ml
CA19–9	S	<33 U/ml

3. Biochemical reference values for urine

Determination	Reference range
Aldosterone	10–50 nmol/24 h
Albumin	<80 mg/24 h
α-Aminolaevulinic acid	9.9–53.4 µmol/24 h
Amylase	
secretion rate	1–17 somogyi U/h
clearance	0.01–0.04 of creatinine clearance value
Arginine	1.3–6.5 µmol/mol creat
Ascorbic acid	34–68 µmol/l
Calcium	2.5–7.5 mmol/24 h
Catecholamines	<2.6 µmol/24 h
Chloride	110–250 mmol/24 h
Copper	0.47–0.55 µmol/l
Cortisol	60–1500 nmol/l
	<280 nmol/24 h
Creatinine	
male	9.0–17.0 mmol/24 h
female	7.5–12.5 mmol/24 h
pregnancy	8.0–13.5 mmol/24 h
Glucose	0.06–0.84 mmol/l
Homovanillic acid (HVA) – adults	<43 µmol/24 h
Hydroxyindoleacetic acid (5-HIAA)	16–73 µmol/24 h
Hydroxymethylmandelic acid (HMMA)	16–48 µmol/24 h
Iron	<1.8 µmol/24 h
Lead	<0.4 µmol/l
β_2-Microglobulin	4–370 µg/l
Magnesium	3.3–4.9 mmol/24 h
Osmolality	350–1000 mosm/kg
Oxalate	<450 µmol/24 h
Phosphate (inorganic)	15–50 mmol/24 h
Porphyrins	
coproporphyrin	50–350 nmol/24 h
porphobilinogen	0.9–8.8 µmol/24 h
uroporphyrin	0–49 nmol/24 h
Potassium	20–60 mmol/l
	40–120 mmol/24 h

3. (cont.)

Determination	Reference range
Protein	<120 mg/24 h
pregnancy	<300 mg/24 h
Sodium	50–125 mmol/l
	100–250 mmol/24 h
Urea	250–500 mmol/24 h
Uric acid	<5.0 mmol/24 h
pregnancy (except late)	<7.0 mmol/24 h
Urobilinogen	<6.7 μmol/24 h
Vanillylmandelic acid (VMA)	<35 μmol/24 h
Zinc	2.1–11.0 μmol/24 h

4. Biochemical reference values for faeces

Determination	Reference range
Fat (on normal diet)	<7 g/24 h
Nitrogen	70–140 mmol/24 h
Urobilinogen	67–473 µmol/24 h
Coproporphyrin	<0.46 nmol/g dry weight
Protoporphyrin	<2.67 µmol/24 h
Protoporphyrin	£0.11 nmol/kg dry weight
Total porphyrin	
(ether soluble)	10–200 nmol/g dry weight
(ether insoluble)	0–24 nmol/g dry weight

5. Biochemical reference values for cerebrospinal fluid

Determination	Reference range
Glucose	3.3–4.4 mmol/24 h
Protein	0.15–0.40 g/l
Chloride	122–128 mmol/l
Lactate	<2.8 mmol/l

6. Haematological reference values

Measurement	Reference range
haemoglobin	(male) 13.5–18.0 g/dl (female) 11.5–16.0 g/dl
packed cell volume or haematocrit (PCV)	(male) 0.40–0.54 l/l (female) 0.37–0.47 l/l
red cell count	(male) $4.5–6.5 \times 10^{12}$/l (female) $3.9–5.6 \times 10^{12}$/l
mean cell volume (MCV)	81–100 fl
mean cell haemoglobin (MCH)	27–32 pg
mean cell haemoglobin concentration (MCHC)	32–36 g/dl
reticulocyte count absolute count	0.8–2.0 per cent $25–100 \times 10^9$/l
total blood volume	70 ± 10 ml/kg
plasma volume	45 ± 5 ml/kg
red cell volume	(male) 30 ± 5 ml/kg (female) 25 ± 5 ml/kg

white cell count
    neutrophils
    lymphocytes
    eosinophils
    basophils
    monocytes
	$4.0–11.0 \times 10^9$/l
	$2.0–7.5 \times 10^9$/l
	$1.3–3.5 \times 10^9$/l
	$0–0.44 \times 10^9$/l
	$0–0.10 \times 10^9$/l
	$0.2–0.8 \times 10^9$/l

platelet count	$150–400 \times 10^9$/l
bleeding time	1–9 min
coagulation time	5–11 min
thrombin time	10–15 s
prothrombin time	10–14 s
activated partial thromboplastin time	35–45 s
fibrinogen concentration	1.6–4.2 g/l
fibrinogen titre	normal – up to 1/128
erythrocyte sedimentation rate	(male) 0–10 mm (female) 0–15 mm
cold agglutinin titre at 4°C	less than 64

7. Paediatric reference values

Determination	Sample	Reference range
Alkaline phosphatase	P	
<1 year		30–250 IU/l
1–14 years		150–570 IU/l
>14 years		80–250 IU/l
Ammonia	P	
newborn		64–107 µmol/l
0–2 weeks		56–92 µmol/l
>1 month		21–50 µmol/l
Aspartate aminotransferase	P	
1–3 years		20–60 IU/l
4–6 years		15–50 IU/l
Bicarbonate	P	
infants		18–22 mmol/l
older children		20–26 mmol/l
Bilirubin	P	
first week of life		100–200 µmol/l (total)
after first week of life		2–14 µmol/l (total)
and throughout childhood		0–0.4 µmol/l (direct)
Calcium	P	
1–3 weeks		1.9–2.85 mmol/l
3 weeks and above		2.12–2.65 mmol/l
β-Carotene	S	
<1 year (upper limit falls with age up to 3½ years)		1.3–6.3 µmol/l
3½ years onwards		1.9–2.8 µmol/l
Creatinine	P	
cord blood		57–100 µmol/l
2 weeks–6 years		33–61 µmol/l
6 years–10 years		39–70 µmol/l
>12 years		49–81 µmol/l
Creatinine clearance	P	
3–13 years		94–142 ml/min per 1.73m^2
Creatine kinase (CK)	P	
neonates		75–400 U/l
infants 3–12 months		10–145 U/l
children 1–15 years		15–130 U/l
Gamma-glutamyl transferase (GGT)	P	
0–1 month		12–271 U/l
1–2 months		9–159 U/l

7. (cont.)

Determination	Sample	Reference range
2–4 months		7–98 U/l
4–7 months		5–45 U/l
7–12 months		4–27 U/l
1–15 years		3–30 U/l
Glucose (fasting)	S	
cord		2.5–5.3 mmol/l
premature/low birth wt		1.1–3.3 mmol/l
neonates		1.67–3.3 mmol/l
1 day		2.2–3.3 mmol/l
1–7 days		2.8–4.6 mmol/l
>7 days		3.3–5.5 mmol/l
Total protein	P	
1st month		51 g/l (mean)
1st year		61 g/l (mean)
1–6 years		61–78 g/l
7–16 years		66–82 g/l
Immunoglobulins		
IgG	S	
cord		5.2–18.0 g/l
0–2 weeks		5.0–17.0 g/l
2–6 weeks		3.9–13.0 g/l
6–12 weeks		2.1–7.7 g/l
3–6 months		2.4–8.8 g/l
6–9 months		3.0–9.0 g/l
9–12 months		3.0–10.9 g/l
1–2 years		3.1–13.8 g/l
2–3 years		3.7–15.8 g/l
3–6 years		4.9–16.1 g/l
6–9 years		5.4–16.1 g/l
9–12 years		5.4–16.1 g/l
12–15 years		5.4–16.1 g/l
IgA	S	
cord		0.00–0.02 g/l
0–2 weeks		0.01–0.08 g/l
2–6 weeks		0.02–0.15 g/l
6–12 weeks		0.05–0.4 g/l
3–6 months		0.1–0.5 g/l
6–9 months		0.15–0.7 g/l
9–12 months		0.20–0.7 g/l
1–2 years		0.3–1.2 g/l
2–3 years		0.3–1.3 g/l
3–6 years		0.4–2.0 g/l

7. (cont.)

Determination	Sample	Reference range
6–9 years		0.5–2.4 g/l
9–12 years		0.8–2.8 g/l
12–15 years		0.8–2.8 g/l
IgM	S	
cord		0.02–0.2 g/l
0–2 weeks		0.05–0.2 g/l
2–6 weeks		0.08–0.4 g/l
6–12 weeks		0.15–0.7 g/l
3–6 months		0.20–1.0 g/l
6–9 months		0.40–1.6 g/l
9–12 months		0.60–2.1 g/l
1–2 years		0.50–2.2 g/l
2–3 years		0.50–2.2 g/l
3–6 years		0.50–2.0 g/l
6–9 years		0.50–1.8 g/l
9–12 years		0.50–1.9 g/l
12–15 years		0.50–1.9 g/l
Lactate	P (venous)	0.5–2.2 mmol/l
	P (arterial)	0.5–1.6 mmol/l
	B	0.5–1.7 mmol/l
Phosphate (inorganic)	P	
newborn		1.20–2.78 mmol/l
young children		1.29–1.78 mmol/l
girls 15 years		0.9–1.38 mmol/l
boys 17 years		0.83–1.49 mmol/l
(from 7 years levels fall steadily to reach adult levels at 15–17 years)		
Potassium	P	
newborn		up to 6.6 mmol/l
>1 month–6 years		4.1–5.6 mmol/l
boys 7–16 years		3.3–4.7 mmol/l
girls 7–16 years		3.4–4.5 mmol/l
Sweat sodium		10–40 mmol/l
Sweat chloride		0–50 mmol/l
Thyroid-stimulating hormone (TSH) (outside neonatal period)	S	0.5–5.0 mU/l
Uric acid	P	
childhood		0.06–0.24 mmol/l
boys 16 years		0.23–0.46 mmol/l
girls 16 years		0.19–0.36 mmol/l

8. Medical certificates

(commonly used forms)

www.dwp.gov.uk

SC2

Self-certification form used by an employee to provide their employer with details of sick absences of four or more consecutive days (SC1 for unemployed or self-employed).

Med 3

Required only after seven days of self-certification.

Med 5

Used when evidence for incapacity for work needs to be provided retrospectively.

Med 4

Requested by the DWP (Department of Work and Pensions) when a patient has been receiving a Med 3 certificate for more than 28 weeks.

Med 6

Issued to notify the DWP if the exact diagnosis has not been entered on forms Med 3, 4, or 5, as it may be harmful for the patient and/or employer to know the diagnosis. A full report is then requested by the DWP.

RM7

Sent to the DWP to request an independent assessment usually earlier than 28 weeks in instances where Med 3 certificates are being issued but the patient's incapacity for work is doubtful.

DS1500

Issued when a person suffering from a potentially terminal illness (defined by Social Security legislation) where death as a consequence of the illness "can reasonably be expected within six months." This allows rapid access to claiming disability living allowance (DLA) and attendance allowance (AA) under "special rules."

9. Baby milk formulas

(standard formulations)

Whey-dominant

Sometimes called first milks and often display the number 1.

Milupa	Aptamil First
Cow & Gate	First Infant Milk
Hipp	Hipp Organic Infant Milk
HJ Heinz	Nurture Newborn
SMA Nutrition	SMA Gold

Casein-dominant

Also referred to as second milks and display the number 2.

Milupa	Aptamil Extra Hungry
Cow & Gate	Infant Milk For Hungrier Babies
HJ Heinz	Nurture Hungry Baby
SMA Nutrition	SMA White

Follow-on milks

Suitable from six months of age and are higher in some nutrients, notably iron; often labelled number 3.

Milupa	Aptamil Follow-on
Cow & Gate	Follow-on Milk for babies six months+
Cow & Gate	Good Night Milk
Hipp	Hipp Organic Follow-on Milk
Hipp	Hipp Organic Good Night Milk – 6 months+
Hipp	Hipp Organic Growing Up Milk ' 10 months+
HJ Heinz	Nurture Growing Baby Follow-On
SMA Nutrition	SMA Progress

10. Street names for illicit drugs

www.talktofrank.com

Illicit drug	Slang/street names
	(can vary around the country and with differing forms of the drug)
amphetamines	speed, phet, Billy, whizz, sulph, base, paste, dexies
amyl nitrites	poppers, ram, thrust, rock hard, kix, TNT, liquid gold
cannabis	bhang, black, blast, blow, blunts, Bob Hope, bush, dope, draw, ganja, grass, hash, hashish, hemp, herb, marijuana, pot, puff, Northern Lights, resin, sensi, sinsemilla, shit, skunk, smoke, soap, spliff, wacky backy, weed, zero.
	Some names are based on where it comes from: Afghan, homegrown, Moroccan, etc.
cocaine and crack	powder cocaine: coke, Charlie, C, white, Percy, snow, toot.
	crack (a smokeable form of cocaine): rocks, wash, stones, pebbles, base, freebase
Ecstasy	E, pills, brownies, Mitsubishi's, Rolex's, Dolphins, XTC
gases, glues, and aerosols	thinners, volatile substances
GHB (gammahydroxybutyrate)	GHB, GBH, liquid Ecstasy
heroin	brown, skag, H, horse, gear, smack
ketamine	green, K, special K, super K, vitamin K
khat	khat, quat, qat, qaadka, chat
magic mushrooms	magic mushrooms, liberties, magics, mushies, liberty cap, shrooms, Amani, agaric
LSD (lysergic acid diethylamide)	acid, blotter, cheer, dots, drop, flash, hawk, L, lightening flash, liquid acid, Lucy, microdot, paper mushrooms, rainbows, smilies, stars, tab, trips, tripper, window.
	Sometimes LSD is known by the pictures on it, e.g. strawberries
Tranquillizers	jellies, benzos, eggs, norries, rugby balls, vallies, moggies, mazzies, roofies, downers

11. Online medical resources

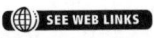

Recent years have seen a proliferation of online medical resources, ranging from specialist databases to sites offering advice and information to patients and their families. The following is a selection of authoritative, quality-controlled sites that provide free information on essential topics. These resources are widely used by health-care professionals but in most cases are freely accessible to the general public. To access any of these websites, go to the dictionary's web page at http://www.oup.com/uk/reference/resources/med, click on **Web links** in the Resources section, go to **Appendix web links**, and then click through to the relevant site.

- Anatomy Atlases: annotated images of human anatomy, including cross-sections and microscope plates.

- Bandolier: evidence-based health-care information for professionals and consumers. Includes lifestyle advice.

- BBC Health: basic advice on illnesses and conditions, healthy living, etc.

- BestTreatments: provides doctors and patients with the latest research evidence about the effectiveness of thousands of treatments. Developed by the British Medical Journal in partnership with NHS Direct.

- British Medical Journal: full text of all articles from January 1997 is now available free online.

- British Nutrition Foundation: independent evidence-based advice on healthy eating. Includes recipes.

- Cancersource: a US site providing a range of resources for oncology professionals and advice and support for patients.

- Children First for Health: a child-centred resource providing age-appropriate health information (including first-person accounts) for children, teenagers, and their families. Provided by the Institute of Child Health and Great Ormond Street Hospital.

- Cinahl (Cumulative Index to Nursing and Allied Health Literature): a bibliographic database for nursing and allied health care.

- ClinicalTrials: an online registry of research trials organized by the US National Institutes of Health. Many health-care journals now demand that trials of therapeutic interventions are registered at ClinicalTrials as a prerequisite for publication.

- Cochrane Collaboration: systematic evidence-based reviews of health-care interventions; mainly for professionals, but with plain-language summaries for laypeople.

- Directgov: a UK government website providing information on common illnesses, healthy living, and local health services (including waiting lists and performance tables).

• Dr Foster: information on the availability and quality of UK health care: includes guides to hospitals, consultants, birth units, and complementary practitioners.

• eMedicine: a clinical knowledge database for professionals.

• eMedicine Health: comprehensive first-aid and emergency advice for laypeople.

• Free Information Centre: provides numerous links to medical and nursing resources.

• Healthtalkonline: award-winning charity website providing information on conditions and treatment choices, together with patients' accounts of their experiences.

• International Centre for Nursing Ethics: links to various resources, including the archives of Nursing Ethics.

• Internet Mental Health: a US site that describes the most common mental disorders and their usual treatments.

• Intute Med Hist: a catalogue of free resources relating to the history of medicine and related sciences.

• Intute Medicine: a gateway site for medical education and research.

• KidsHealth: an award-winning site providing parents with information about children's health issues from before birth to adolescence. Provided by the Nemours Foundation.

• Medicines.org: up-to-date information on most medicines currently available in the UK: developed by the Medicines Information Project in partnership with NHS Direct.

• MentalWellness: information about bipolar disorder, schizophrenia, and general mental health for patients and families.

• National Drugs Helpline: online resources include an A–Z of the most common drugs with their appearance, effects, health risks, and legal status. Also offers help and support, including a 24-hour confidential advice service.

• NetDoctor: a comprehensive resource for health-care consumers featuring A–Z listings of conditions, interventions, medicines, and support groups.

• NHS Direct Online: information on common illnesses and treatments, self-help advice, and details of local hospitals, doctors, pharmacies, etc.

• NHS Evidence (formerly the National Library for Health): a gateway to a wide range of online resources, including specialist libraries and journals; mainly for professionals, but with many areas accessible to the public.

• Obgyn: news and research in the field of women's health: mainly for professionals, but with no restrictions on access.

• Patient UK: comprehensive information on conditions and treatments, healthy living, and patient support groups.

• Psycinfo: a database of psychological literature provided by the American Pyschological Association.

- PubMed: a freely accessible search engine run by the US National Institutes of Health that accesses citations from MEDLINE, the US National Library of Health's bibliographic database.

- studentBMJ: an online journal for medical students provided by the BMJ. There is a searchable archive of all articles published since 2000.

- Teenage Health Freak: advice and information for teenagers, including Dr Ann's Virtual Surgery.

- Transcultural Nursing: an introduction to cultural diversity in nursing, together with case studies.

- UK Centre for the History of Nursing and Midwifery: links to archives and other resources for the study of nursing history worldwide.

- UK Foundation of Nursing Studies: provides links to general and specialist sites of interest to nurses.

- Women's Health Information: covers pregnancy, infertility, reproductive health, and other issues in women's health.

12. Abbreviations and symbols

Abbreviations

ABG	arterial blood gas
A&E	accident and emergency department
AC	(in prescribing) ante cibum (before food)
ADR	adverse drug reaction
AE	air entry
AF	anterior fontanelle
AMT	abbreviated mental test
AP	anteroposterior
APC	argon plasma coagulation
ATSP	asked to see patient
AVPU	alert, verbal (responses present), pain (responses present), unresponsive
AXR	abdominal X-ray
BD	bis die (twice daily)
BIBA	brought in by ambulance
BiPAP	bilevel positive airways pressure
BMI	body mass index
BNO	bowels not opened
BO	bowels opened
BP	blood pressure
BS	bowel sounds; breath sounds
Bx	biopsies
CA	cancer
CABG	coronary artery bypass graft
CAPD	chronic (or continuous) ambulatory peritoneal dialysis
CAT	computerized (axial) tomography
CBT	cognitive behavioural therapy
CCF	congestive cardiac failure
CFA/UIP	cryptogenic fibrosing alveolitis/usual interstitial pneumonitis
CI	contraindication
CKD	chronic kidney disease
CN	cranial nerves
CNS	central nervous system
C/O	complaining of
COC(P)	combined oral contraceptive (pill)
COPD	chronic obstructive pulmonary disease
CPAP	continuous positive airways pressure
CRT	cardiac resynchronization therapy
CSU	catheter stream urine
CT	computerized tomography
CTPA	computerized tomographic pulmonary angiogram
CVS	cardiovascular system

CVVH	continuous venovenous haemofiltration
CXR	chest X-ray
D&V	diarrhoea and vomiting
DCBE	double-contrast barium enema
Ddx	differential diagnosis
DH	drug history
DIB	difficulty in breathing
DIPJ	distal interphalangeal joint
DKA	diabetic ketoacidosis
DNA	did not attend
DM	diabetes mellitus
DN	district nurse
DPH	Director of Public Health
Dx	diagnosis
E&D	eating and drinking
EBM	expressing breast milk
ECG	electrocardiogram
ECHO	echocardiogram
ECT	electroconvulsive therapy
ED	emergency department; erectile dysfunction
EDD	estimated date of delivery
EEG	electroencephalogram
EF	ejection fraction
eGFR	estimated glomerular filtration rate
ENT	ear, nose, and throat
EPAU	early pregnancy assessment unit
EPS	electrophysiological study
ESM	ejection systolic murmur
ESRF	end-stage renal failure
ETOH	ethanol/alcohol
ETT	exercise tolerance test
EUA	examination under anaesthesia
EUM	examination under microscope
FB	foreign body (see Blood tests below)
FH	family history; fundal height
FHH	fetal heart heard
FM	fetal movements
FNA	fine-needle aspiration
FOB	faecal occult blood
FROEM	full range of eye movements
FROM	full range of movement (see Symbols, numbers, and diagrams below)
GA	general anaesthetic
GAHS	Glasgow alcoholic hepatitis score
GB	gall bladder
GCS	Glasgow Coma Scale
GI	gastrointestinal

GIS	gastrointestinal system
GORD	gastro-oesophageal reflux disease
HDU	high-dependency unit
HH	hiatus hernia
HNPU	has not passed urine
HONK	hyperosmolar non-ketosis
HPC	history of presenting complaint
HS	heart sounds
HVS	high vaginal swab
Hx	history
I&D	incision and drainage
ICD	implantable cardiovertor/defibrillator
ICU	intensive care unit
IDA	iron-deficiency anaemia
IM	intramuscular
IP	in-patient
IPAA	ileal pouch anal anastomosis
ISQ	in status quo (unchanged)
ITU	intensive therapy unit
IUCD	intrauterine contraceptive device
IV	intravenous
IVI	intravenous infusion
Ix	investigations
J.A.C.C.O.L.	jaundice, anaemia, clubbing, cyanosis, oedema, lymphadenopathy
JVP	jugular venous pressure
K 6/28	menstrual cycle (e.g. menstruation lasting 6 days, occurring every 28 days)
KUB	kidneys, ureters, and bladder
LA	local anaesthetic
LIF	left iliac fossa
LKKS/LKS	liver, kidney, kidney, spleen/liver, kidney, spleen
LLL	left lower lobe (of lung)
LMP	last menstrual period
LN	lymph node
LOC	loss of consciousness
LOS	lower oesophageal sphincter
LRTI	lower respiratory tract infection
L(U)SCS	lower (uterine) segment Caesarean section
LUTS	lower urinary tract symptoms
LVF	left ventricular failure
LVH	left ventricular hypertrophy
Mane	(in prescribing) in the morning
MC&S	microscopy, culture, and sensitivities
MCPJ	metacarpal phalangeal joint
MELD	model end-stage liver disease
MI	myocardial infarction

Muct.	micturition
MMSE	Mini-Mental State Examination
MRI	magnetic resonance imaging
MSE	mental state examination
MSU	midstream specimen of urine
MTPJ	metatarsal phalangeal joint
MUA	manipulation under anaesthesia
MVP	mitral valve prolapse
MW	midwife
Mx	management
N	normal
NAD	nothing abnormal detected
NBM	nil by mouth
NDM	neurodevelopmental
NICU	neonatal intensive care unit
NIPPV	noninvasive (or nasal) intermittent positive-pressure ventilation
NKA	no known allergies
NKDA	no known drug allergies
Noct.	nocturia
Nocte	(in prescribing) at night
NSTEMI	non-S–T elevation myocardial infarction
OC&P	oocytes, cysts, and parasites
OCD	obsessive–compulsive disorder
OD	overdose; (in prescribing) omni die (daily)
O/E or OE	on examination
OGTT	oral glucose tolerance test
OM	(in prescribing) omni mane (in the morning)
ON	(in prescribing) omni nocte (at night)
OP	out-patient
OPD	out-patient department
ORIF	open reduction, internal fixation
PA	posteroanterior
PC	presenting complaint; (in prescribing) post cibum (after food)
PCA	patient-controlled analgesia; percutaneous coronary angioplasty
PCI	percutaneous coronary intervention
PEFR	peak expiratory flow rate
PEG	percutaneous endoscopic gastrostomy
PERL	pupils equal and reactive to light
PERLA	pupils equal and reactive to light and accommodation
PICU	paediatric intensive care unit
PIPJ	proximal interphalangeal joint
PMH	past medical history
PN	percussion note
PND	paroxysmal nocturnal dyspnoea; postnasal drip
PNS	peripheral nervous system; postnasal space (nasopharynx)
PO	per os (by mouth)

POP	plaster of Paris; progestogen-only pill
PP	peripheral pulses
PR	per rectum
PRN	(in prescribing) pro re nata (as required)
PSH	past surgical history
PSM	pansystolic murmur
Pt	patient
PU	passing urine
PUO	pyrexia of unknown origin
PV	per vaginum
QDS	quarter die sumendus ([to be taken] four times a day)
ROM	range of movement
RR	respiratory rate
RS	respiratory system
RT	radiotherapy
RUL	right upper lobe (of lung)
RUQ	right upper quadrant (of abdomen)
Rx	therapy (or treatment)
SC	subcutaneous
SCBU	special care baby unit
S/E	side-effect
SEMS	self-expanding metal stent
SH	social history
SI	sexual intercourse
SL	sublingual
SLR	straight leg raise
SMI	severe mental illness
SOB	shortness of breath
SOBOE	shortness of breath on exertion
SOS	in an emergency
SPECT	single photon emission computing tomography
SR/ROS	systems review/review of systems
Stat	(in prescribing) statim (immediately)
STEMIS–T	elevation myocardial infarction
T	temperature
TB	tuberculosis
TCI	to come in (to hospital)
TDS	ter die sumendus ([to be taken] three times a day)
TEMS	transanal endoscopic microsurgery
Ti	tinnitus
TIA	transient ischaemic attack
TM	tympanic membrane
TOE	transoesphageal echocardiography
TOP	termination of pregnancy
TPP	time, place, person
TPRS	tone, power, reflexes, sensation

Ts&As	tonsillectomy and adenoidectomy
TTA	to take away (drugs)
TTO	to take out (drugs)
TVF/VF	tactile vocal fremitus/vocal fremitus
TWOC	trial without catheter
UGIB	upper gastrointestinal bleed
UGT	urogenital (or urinogenital) tract
UIP	usual interstitial pneumonitis
UO	urine output
UPSI	unprotected sexual intercourse
URTI	upper respiratory tract infection
USS	ultrasound scan
UTI	urinary tract infection
VBL	variceal band ligation
V/Q	scan ventilation-perfusion scan
VR	vocal resonance
WNL	within normal limits
XR	X-ray

Abbreviations for blood tests

Blood test requests

FBC	full blood count
U+E	urea and electrolytes
LFT	liver function tests
GGT	gamma-glutamyl transferase
TFT	thyroid function tests
ESR	erythrocyte sedimentation rate
CRP	C-reactive protein
HbA1c	glycated haemoglobin
OGTT	oral glucose tolerance test

Blood test results

FBC:

Hb	haemoglobin
MCV	mean corpuscular volume
WBC	white blood cell count
PLTS	platelets

U+E:

Na	sodium
K	potassium
Urea	urea
Cr	creatinine
eGFR	estimated glomerular filtration rate

LFT:

ALP	alkaline phosphatase
ALT	alanine aminotransferase
AST	aspartate aminotransferase
Bili	bilirubin
GGT	gamma-glutamyl transferase

TFT:

TSH	thyroid-stimulating hormone
T4	thyroxine

THE DELAWARE

by

HARRY EMERSON WILDES

Illustrated by
Irwin D. Hoffman

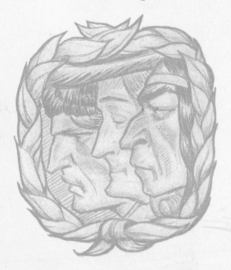

FARRAR & RINEHART
INCORPORATED

New York   *Toronto*

To

R. W. W.

Contents

Illustrations

THE DELAWARE

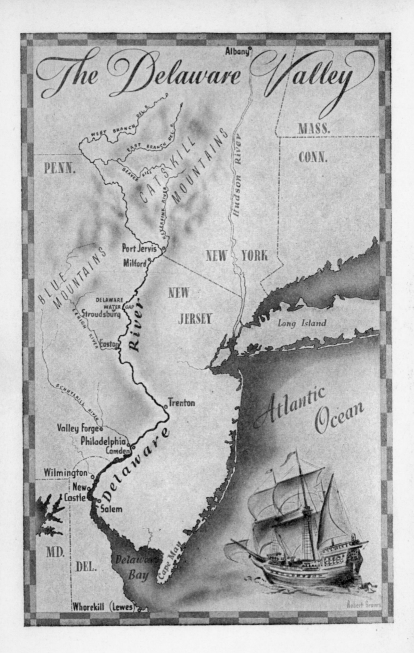

The Delaware Valley

I

Down the River

NOBODY really knows where the Delaware rises. Scores of white-water trout streams, fed from icy springs among the Catskills, race through the hemlock forests where Cooper's Leatherstockings roamed. Almost any one of these innumerable brooks could easily be taken as a source.

Every settler on the upper Delaware will tell you, therefore, that the river starts from his own springhouse or from his barnyard pool. The more imaginative claim that three great rivers—the Delaware, the Susquehanna, and the Hudson—all spring from rugged Mine Hill in lower Schoharie County. One longbow monopolist insists that from the west eaves of his farmhouse the rain drains to the Susquehanna, the east roof sends its water to the Delaware, while storms that pelt against the northern wall trickle off to the Schoharie and come in time into the Hudson.

The lack of unanimity about the sources of the Delaware is typical; the river is a controversial stream. The Mine Hill protagonists fight unending war with those who think the river comes from marsh-bordered Mayham Pond or with the partisans of triangular Potter Hill, which looms over Stamford reservoir and Utsayantha Lake, or with those benighted folk who hold that Grand Gorge across the Moresville Range is a more likely origin. But all agree in opposing those purists who insist that a turbulent mountain creek twisting about the bases of high precipices is in no sense a river, and that the Delaware does not, in fact, exist until the East Branch meets the West Branch far to the south at Hancock on the Pennsylvania line. For thus to dismiss the myriad brooks would mean the loss of superb scenery, of colorful tradition, and of unique personality from the valley of the Delaware. The upper portions of those branches, formed by the confluence of mountain streams, symbolize in large degree the spirit of the river. Wild-flowing torrents, rivulets which never knew a master, rushing treacherously from rock to waterfall, calm suddenly as they merge with the Delaware. The river winding quietly and smoothly over its wide bed, with few sharp bends and virtually no rapids, offers level bottom lands well fit for farms where men may live in peace and happiness.

So, the river exerted its civilizing influence. To its lower reaches came dreamers and visionaries looking for a new heaven upon earth; bands of mystics, shy and unconventional, came seeking refuge from religious persecution. But other men came too, lured by the riches of the valley, misreading the Delaware's mild pacifism—swashbucklers and rebels, mutineers and gangsters, violent newcomers who scorned the ways of peace and who sought to prosper by chicanery and cunning. These, too, the Delaware accepted, soothed them and imposed upon them dignity and order.

In early days the people could not take full advantage of the river's opportunities. The Indians were fishermen, netting millions of fine, fat shad that swarmed upstream each spring; but few of them were sailors. There was no need to venture on the water while the open woods afforded easy trails. When Europeans came to settle in the valley, they, too, were quite content to stay on shore, trading and growing their crops, without a hankering for navigation. The river was too winding and the winds blew much too hard for sailing ships to be of value. Philadelphia was a harbor, and a safe one; indeed, until the opening of the Erie Canal, it was the busiest port of the nation. But above the colonial capital the river was not crowded.

Britain's naval needs first led to a full use of the river. Shipbuilders on the lower Delaware, making brigs and sloops and small three-masted snows for the West Indian trade, offered markets for the loggers of the Catskills and for the husky raftsmen who floated timber downstream to the Philadelphia yards. Lumber, therefore, was the first great industry to unify the people of the Delaware, and to bind all the settlers on the stream into a co-operative commonwealth. Lumber in the early days provided the common interest that in later years was supplied by iron, coal, and farm produce.

One might even use the lumber industry as the thread on which to string the story of the river from early times to the times with which we are familiar. To see the river through the eyes of raftsmen floating logs downstream to market is to view the river as the early settlers saw it. The type of man developed by the rough, vigorous demands of timbering stood in contrast with the types characteristic of the lower Delaware. For the rich, easily cultivated farms that lay on either side of the stream were settled by placid, unaggressive people who loved books and shrank from rough reality. Quakers, who sought the "inner light," and Mennonites, who fled from war, were typical of those who came to live along the Delaware. Had it not been for the river and its timber, these would have given the tone to Pennsylvania history.

Yet the river did not breed a race of puny, introspective intellectuals; it called, especially on the upper reaches, for hardihood and physical vigor. Men in the Catskill forest lands rose long before dawn, tilled the river-bottom fields, cared for their stock, and then went up into the hills to log the pines and shape up ships' masts. They cut and hauled till sun had set, ate hasty suppers of salt pork and beans and boiled potatoes, and after dark finished up their evening farm chores. The weak, the timid, and the infirm were early weeded out.

The raftsmen, too, were brawny rivermen, powerful with their huge sweeps, wise in their knowledge of the shifting channels. Long before the Revolution had begun, shrewd Dan Skinner, admiral of the raft fleet, and Josiah Parks, his obstreperous bosun, were rafting 80-foot pine logs from the Catskill foothills down to Philadelphia and walking back upstream through the untracked forests with their pockets full of gold. When Dan became too old to act as "ironman," or steersman of the raft, he organized his timber trust that ruled the logging industry.

The industry was rightly his by virtue of invention and discovery. Old Dan had been a sailor on one of the Connecticut schooners that carried fish and grain to the West Indies and, when he trekked from New England across New York to the Delaware, his eye was caught by the unlimited supply of tall pine trees that would make good masts for sailing ships. No agent of the Royal Navy had gone through the forests to mark off the better trees with the king's broad arrow mark of reservation; no speculator from the Quaker colony below had bought the woodland cheap to hold for higher prices. Old Dan, together with loud-mouthed Josiah, monopolized the field. When neighbors asked to share the industry, Old Dan allowed them entry, but he charged his fee. No man could be a steersman on a Skinner raft unless he paid to Dan and to Josiah two full bottles of good liquor; no apprentice was allowed to serve as forehand, fending the raft from rocks on either side, unless the tribute price of one large bottle was first paid.

The returns were well worth the small initiation fee, for the admiral's men were handsomely rewarded in pay and perquisites. Perhaps they had to be well paid to compensate them for their heavy labor. Swerving the long rafts about the dreaded "P'int" where violent Beaver Kill enters the East Branch, rounding the hairpin turn at Peas Island, running the swirling eddies that swung the rafts in circles, took a swelling biceps and an unrelenting watchfulness.

Dan Skinner knew the task and, what is more, he knew the art of handling men. Each raft, before it entered the U-turn at Peas Island, tied up to receive its store of rum sufficient to make each raftsman drunk. Then, sending his happy men forward through the danger zone, where they would pole and push the logs, often while wading in cold water up to the waist and shoulders, Dan Skinner prepared a second rum supply to greet them after they emerged. Each Skinner raftsman knew that Peas Island was a place for heavy labor, but he knew also that Peas Island was the spot where he would get drunk twice. Instead of shirking the hard work, he looked forward to the crisis with gleeful anticipation.

Storage houses were set up wherever overnight haltings were anticipated. Each day's labor, rafting through the deep gorges of the upper branches of the stream, was capped by revelry and, though the tangled forest land boasted few settlements, the men were seldom lonely, nor ever discontented with their lot.

Near Hancock, the towns become more frequent, though their names, perhaps, betray the primitive development of the upper region. Barkaboon and Pakatakan, Touchmenot and Cobble, the Knob and the Devil's Backbone identify the larger mountains; Clabber and Hungry Hollow, Nobody Station and Slow and Easy, Wolf Hollow and Hog Hollow indicate that settlements are none too prosperous amid the folded valleys that lie back from the stream. And there are towns named China and Michigan, Texas and Damascus, not far from Nineveh, Arabia, and Galilee, to show that even in the wilderness men dream of far-off places, while in the midst of a wide, unsettled section without even one-room schools one hamlet boasts the name of Harvard.

Below Hancock, the raftsman's task was somewhat less exacting. The Delaware, broad and united, flows gently in the shadow of sheer cliffs, so bold, so rugged, and so perpendicular that the steersman, standing with his long oar to guide the logs along the proper channel, is dwarfed to insignificance. Dan Skinner's men were under orders to tie up for the night, liquorless, that they might start next morning, fresh and rested, for the passage of Long Eddy, for the swift run about Coshecton Hill, and for the passage through the Dreamer Islands, where rafts were almost sure to ground. Once past these danger spots, once south of "Lackawack," where the rapid Lackawaxen flows into the Delaware, once over dreaded Minisink ford, where whirlpools swung many a raft onto the rocks, carousing was allowed, to celebrate the safe voyage. The inns that lay below the Lackawack and Minisink were noisy with the songs and boasts and riotings of raftsmen.

A few new rafts now joined the fleets that Admiral Dan Skinner forwarded to Philadelphia. Above Port Jervis, the last New York settlement, the pines and hemlocks were innumerable, and loggers profited by cutting masts and by stripping hemlock bark for tanneries. South of Port Jervis the timber changed in character. New Jersey's Kittatinny Mountains and the foothills of the Poconos in Pennsylvania are crowned by oaks and maples which, though brilliant and spectacular in late September with their gold and crimson leaves, were of slight use to Dan Skinner and his raftsmen friends.

The rafts moved southward steadily, beneath ridges where rhododendron and laurel bloomed, past fields of gray-green buckwheat, toward Milford and the Water Gap. There was solemn ceremony to be observed at the three-mile sheer cliff that forms the west shore of the Delaware near Milford, in honor of the legendary Brink who fell headlong from the top into the river, among the rocks, and lived to tell the tale. The raftsmen, arriving at Brink's tavern, toasted his astonishing good luck, and each spring when the first raft arrived the crews hauled a barrel of red paint to the cliff summit and let the contents trickle down the rock. The huge red stain was always pointed out to wide-eyed new raftsmen as Brink's blood.

Two tall hills, Mt. Tammany in New Jersey and Mt. Minsi on the Pennsylvania shore, guard the river at the Water Gap, where the Delaware breaks through the Blue Ridge chain. Near here, as every raftsman had been told by Admiral Dan Skinner, lived old Tom Quick, Indian hunter and the admiral's good friend. The news of Tom's exploits was Dan Skinner's one real outside interest. Steersmen were invariably enjoined to report Tom's latest score.

In revenge for the time when hostile Indians, angered at white encroachments, had driven the whites from settlements in the interior and when a score of

farmers, including Tom Quick's father, were drowned
by Indians in the thin-ice river near Death Eddy, south
of Milford, Tom had sworn to kill an even hundred
redskins. In the years before his ambition was much
publicized, his totals mounted swiftly. Later, when all
the river from Philadelphia up to the Schoharie country
was following his progress, the notches on his gunstock
grew more slowly. Just after he had killed his ninety-
ninth—by an ambush not worthy of the man-to-man
conflicts in which his first victims had been worsted—
Tom Quick was taken with pneumonia. He grew delirious; then calming suddenly, he climbed from his bunk
and fell upon his knees before the doctor, begging him
"for humanity's sake" to bring in one more Indian so
that old Tom Quick might carry out his vow. He died
before accomplishing his life's ambition.

South of the Water Gap the river widens, though
sentinel hills still hem it in on both sides. For thirty
miles the Delaware flows placidly, with only a rift or
two, until, at Easton, it meets its second tributary, the
rapid Lehigh, from the coal fields to the west.

Those of Dan Skinner's men who were convoying
hardwood logs ceased their rafting here. Easton saw-
mills cut up the oaks, the chestnuts, and the hemlocks
into building timbers. Some of this lumber was shipped
on the roads that led to New York and to the interior
of Pennsylvania; some of it was used for building
houses for the large numbers of folk settling in Bethlehem, where the steel plants flourished, and in Philips-
burg, across the Delaware. The admiral's crews, however, were not at all concerned with the disposal of their
logs; to them, the river front of Easton was a place for
jubilee. According to the terms of Skinner's contracts,
raftsmen were entitled to a thoroughgoing spree, with
all bills paid for liquor and for lodging, for hearty

eating, and for entertainment of a more licentious nature. If their voyage ended here, the debauch would be a celebration to be well remembered; if, more fortunately, they were logging 80-foot pines to the shipyards, there would be a second, and even more elaborate, Philadelphia jubilation.

The worst was over now; the river below Easton was a friendly, though shallow, stream. Beyond the rocky bluffs of Hockamixon Hill, or past Baldpate, which belied its name, were fertile farms. Backbreaking labor was unnecessary in these lower counties—crops were bounteous and farmers enjoyed wealth and leisure. Folk along the Delaware had time to think, to dream, and to experiment. Rough men from the upper reaches of the river were astonished that life could be so rich and pleasant.

They rode their rafts through regions that were to become famous in colonial and Revolutionary history, past the earth-colored covered bridge which led to the old-time Stockton Inn, past Coryell's Ferry, where the scenery was of breath-taking beauty, though not, of course, so wild and mountainous as the Catskills, past Washington's Crossing, where the glorious victory of Trenton was prepared, past Trenton itself (where now the gilt-domed capitol stands watching over the long, low barracks where Hessian soldiers were surprised).

From Trenton southward, geologists declare, the wide, slow Delaware is in reality a long arm of the sea. Now that the last, eight-foot falls are passed, tidewater flows as far north as the town itself. The raftsmen might relax, as the ever-broadening Delaware runs on past Burlington, site of an early Quaker settlement, along Philadelphia's interminable and unkempt water front, beyond low-lying Camden on the Jersey shore, to the shipyards where the logs were fashioned into masts.

The rivermen had finished their tasks; the long-awaited spree could be enthusiastically enjoyed. Then, following the footsteps of their admiral, they plodded home again, upstream, trudging the long miles to the Catskills, pausing at each inn to lighten the contents of their pockets and to renew, at their own expense, the delights of tavern fellowship.

More thrifty men, however, continued a journey down the Delaware, shipping as deckhands on the packets that sailed round the Jersey coast to New York harbor. They saw the sluggish Schuylkill join the Delaware, just south of Philadelphia, and they sailed past the thriving town of Chester, where Penn had made initial settlement. From the river, the spire of New Castle courthouse was visible, though the larger portion of that pretty colonial town was hidden from a shipboard view, nor was New Jersey's Salem, land of peace where Hollanders and Swedes had lived, sufficiently close for casual observation. The raftsmen would see little of the lower Delaware, particularly when the river suddenly expands into a broad thirty-mile bay. Usually the little ships slipped by fashionable Cape May point into the Atlantic before the loggers were aware that they had left the river.

The sudden disappearance of the river, like its spontaneous rising, made an endless topic for debate. As no one knew the true source of the stream, so no one definitely knew just where the river ended. It vanished suddenly, with the quiet modesty that is so typically Delawarean. Raftsmen, beating up the Jersey coast, argued hotly as to when the river had become the bay; even after they had transshipped to the Hudson River boats that would bear them northward to a point at which they might debark for their hike overland to the Catskills, they were discussing the Delaware's peculiarities.

For the Delaware is a gentle river, gracious and inviting; its charms are never-ending; and, surely, those who see its glories never can forget the river's beauty. Yet frequently it gives a false impression to a casual observer. Sedulously the stream and the folk who settle on its shores play down their virtues, frowning on all words and deeds that seem like boasting. Cardinal among the principles of good form, stressed, indeed, by the example of the river, is that no gentleman is self-assertive and that it is far preferable to retreat from common view than to court popular acclaim. If other sections of the land, unused to self-effacement, accept the river and its people at a false valuation, the loss is not the Delaware's.

2

"The Pleasantest River"

Explorers Off-Course

CERTAINLY Henry Hudson had no license to be sailing off America in the summer of 1609. According to the calculations of the Amsterdam Chamber of the Dutch East India Company, the 80-ton *Halve Maen,* which Hudson's English tongue insisted on calling the *Half Moon,* should have been bucking ice floes near Novaya Zemlya in the Arctic Ocean, searching for a northeast passage from Holland to the Orient. It was for such a voyage that the Dutchmen were paying Hudson his princely fee of almost $320, not for a trip westward to America. Hudson was thousands of miles off-course.

The disobedience was not deliberate. Hudson had sailed forth in good faith and, after a month of voyaging along the Norwegian coast, had safely doubled North Cape. Then, though June was not yet over, he met with fogs and cold, and his crew, fearing a winter of snow and ice floes, clamored for a return to warmer latitudes. Their unanimity, it should be noted, was their first agreement upon any point since the *Halve Maen* had left Holland, for those eighteen Dutch and English sailors, quarreling over nationality and language, had made it anything but a happy ship. Hudson had thus far prevented open fighting, but now that his men were agreed upon returning he knew that to continue on the northeast journey would spell mutiny and disaster. He gave orders to turn about.

Less than six weeks had passed since the *Halve Maen* left Holland, so Hudson dared not return at once to Amsterdam. Those thrifty Dutch merchants who had guaranteed his $320 would never have paid so huge a sum for an abortive voyage; they must have some evidence that exploration had been actually undertaken.

Luckily, Hudson had private information. His old friend Captain John Smith, the friend of Pocahontas, had sent him letters and descriptive maps about Virginia. With these as partial guide, Hudson struck across the Atlantic to see if he could find a northwest passage. His sailors could not complain of cold in a summer voyage to America, nor would his Amsterdam patrons object in the event of his success. Should the trip prove disappointing, the merchants would be no angrier than they would be over his abandonment of the Novaya Zemlya quest.

The Atlantic was almost as hostile as the Arctic. For a month or more, the little *Halve Maen* faced fierce gales. By the time she sighted Newfoundland the foremast had been cut away and the sails were ripped to ribbons. For six weeks the ship lay rocking off the Grand Banks while the sailors made repairs. Then, in August, 1609, the *Halve Maen* sailed away, reaching down the coast to the Virginia Capes, thence north again, nosing into waterways that might seem to lead into the interior. On the twenty-eighth he entered a fair stream which, with pardonable exaggeration, he described as "one of the finest, best and pleasantest rivers in the world." For seven hours he explored its banks, enjoying the soft land breezes that brought the perfume of sweet shrubs and summer flowers, marveling at the "great white birds, cat-headed and with owl like bodies," trembling, no doubt, at the sight of rattle-snakes "with heads like those of dogs and bodies thick as Dutch beer-barrels" which hung head down from the forest trees. There is a certain lack of exactitude, per-haps, in the Dutch description of the fauna of the neigh-borhood, but there is no doubt that the *Halve Maen* men admired the scene.

But Hudson dared not tarry, lest his employers criticize his lack of zeal in searching for a route to Asia. As soon as the swiftness of the current and the sand deposits at the bends made it clear that he had found a river, rather than a strait, he came out, set sail along the coast of what is now New Jersey, and sought his waterway anew. He had, however, tarried long enough to give the Dutch a valid claim to the river which he had been the first to enter. Less than a week later he entered the Hudson.

A year went by before another white man came. This time it was an Englishman, Sir Samuel Argall, vice-governor of Virginia, and he, like Hudson, came with-out authority. Just why Argall, sent to the Bermudas to fetch hogs to feed Virginia's cavaliers, was coming home from Cape Cod with a load of fish is mysterious, and why, when Virginia was starving, he should pause to look about him at new territories is a matter for con-jecture, but such were the circumstances under which the Argall ship appeared. Sir Samuel knew the ameni-ties of life well enough to name the northern cape of the river's mouth in honor of Baron De la Warr, the man whose orders he ignored.

The name, thus fastened to a cape, was soon trans-ferred to a river and a bay. Baron De la Warr had never seen, and never was to see, the place that bore his name; indeed, he was but nine months in America, but that brief time was filled with incident. It was De la Warr's opportune arrival in Virginia that saved the settlement, for the colonists were already embarked upon their ships for home when he arrived at Jamestown. He rescued the settlers from starvation, fortified the little town against attack, reorganized the colony, and made possible the continuance of English rule upon the continent. Preferably, perhaps, his name should fittingly have been attached to some landmark closer to Virginia, but the region of the Delaware is proud to honor his memory.

No doubt, it was just as well for the great river to be called the Delaware, for that name, at least, has euphony and is immeasurably more pleasant than the titles which might have been applied. The Indians had called the stream Poutaxat, Makiriskitton, Makarish-Kisken and Whitituck; the Dutch referred to it as either the Zueydt or South River, to distinguish it from the North River at New Amsterdam, or as the Nassau. Some called it Prince Hendrick's or Prince Charles's River; the Swedes, with less imagination, termed it simply New Sweden Stream, and, for a brief moment, there was talk of naming it Godyn's Bay, in honor of a later patron.

The Delaware, to be sure, has always had difficulties with its nomenclature. Not even the most erudite philologists can explain the origin of the name, St. Jones' Creek, on which the town of Dover stands, for, though all agree that St. Jones is no corruption of St. John, they bog down on further explanation. The St. Pink Creek near Trenton is comparatively easy, since the Indian name was Assunpink, but neither causes half the trouble that is stirred by a small stream that lies near Lewes at the entrance of the bay.

The conflict here dates back to 1614 when Cornelis Jacobsen Mey, of Hoorn in Holland, took the ship *Fortune* down the Jersey coast. Wholly ignorant of Argall's Cape De la Warr, Mey called the sandy spit that separates the ocean from the bay by his own name. The present summer resort, Cape May, preserves the sound, though not the spelling. The southern tip of land, across the bay, he dubbed Cape Cornelis, and, to a beach to the south, a strip of sand which from the sea appears to be a long cape, he gave the name Hindlopen, after a village of his native province. Cape Cornelis soon assumed, and misspelled, the false cape's name, and now is always called Cape Henlopen.

Misnamed Whorekill

Evidently Mey was homesick. Following the patterns set by all explorers, he called his creeks and capes by good familiar names. A little stream, which flowed into the bay a mile or two above Cornelis, he honored by the name of his own native village, the pleasant town of Hoorn. At virtually the same time, certainly within a week or so, another homesick Hollander, Wilhelm Cornelis Schouten, was naming the farthest tip of South America after the same Dutch town.

But Schouten's Cape Horn did not cause the same confusion that was stirred by Mey's creek, the Hoornkill. Lazy English vocal cords soon made a most unfortunate corruption of the sound. To every Britisher the stream became the Whorekill and, to the anger of true Delawareans, a logical interpretation was provided to explain the twisted name. The Indians who dwelt along the stream, the amateur philologists explained, were generous in offering their maidens to the white arrivals.

Old Samuel Smith, first historian of the settlements

along the Delaware, accepted the plausible explanation. Indeed, in his *History of the Colony of New Caesaria, or New Jersey,* he went a full stride farther. Flatly, in telling of the Hoornkill, he describes it as "the Whorekill, or Harlot's creek." Not for him were the frenzied arguments that Whorekill was a lazy man's corruption of a noble name. The long and bitter rivalry between the Jerseymen and Delawareans may date from this unfounded slur.

Of all this, however, Mey was ignorant. He and most of his fellow navigators went home to Holland to spin enthusiastic stories of the beauties of the Delaware. Meanwhile, they left their friend Cornelis Hendricksen to take his little yacht *Onrust,* or *Restless,* on further explorations.

The *Onrust* had a pleasant history. A tiny 16-ton ship, about the same as those small oyster boats that operate today along the Delaware, she was the first vessel built in North America. Her first skipper, Adrian Block, had made her in 1613 on an island off Rhode Island which he christened for himself. The *Onrust* explored Long Island Sound, and then went south to make a survey of the Delaware. Hendricksen took soundings, drew charts, traded with the Indians for sable, otter, mink, and bear skins, went hunting in the vast oak forests, and gloried in a country which, he said, had a climate just like Holland's.

How far the *Onrust* actually explored is not now certain, though from his vague reports to Amsterdam it seems that Hendricksen must have come at least as far upstream as the present site of Philadelphia. He found, he said, three rivers emptying into the Delaware, and though the Dutch idea of a river often was sufficiently elastic to include what we would call a creek, it is quite likely that he came beyond the Schuylkill's mouth.

Certainly the *Onrust* sailed as far as Christina Creek, the place where Wilmington now stands, for there we know that Hendricksen went ashore to meet the Indians. And there he underwent a most surprising shock, for he was greeted in good Dutch by friends whom he had thought long dead. Three Hollanders who had gone north along the Hudson, months ago, were captives living with the Minquas.

Their story added greatly to the Dutch knowledge of geography. The men had gone upstream to Albany and thence, following the Mohawk River and Schoharie Creek, had wandered through a fertile farming region to the sources of the Delaware. They did not know the rivers by these names, nor had they any knowledge where the streams might lead them; intrepidly tracing down the waterways in the shadow of high infertile hills, they found the river growing wider, swifter, and increasingly alluring. Then, at last, somewhere near the picturesque Water Gap, they had been taken prisoner by the Indians and brought down to where they met Hendricksen.

The men were ransomed and set free, and from their stories Hendricksen compiled reports of the resources of the region that did more to further Dutch enthusiasm for establishing a colony along the Delaware than had any previous accounts. The explorations of the men gave, moreover, to the Netherlands a clear-cut claim by virtue of discovery of the entire valley of the Delaware.

Unluckily, Holland was in no position to take advantage of her claims. After a long war with Spain, she had acquired her independence but only on condition that she should not, at least until the close of 1621, interfere with Indies trade. Holland's hands were temporarily tied.

Within two months after the expiration of the twelve years' truce, a charter was issued to the Dutch West India Company to trade with the Americas. Few private corporations have ever been endowed with such tremendous sweep of power. Not only did the charter grant a trade monopoly for Africa, the two Americas, and the Pacific, but the company could colonize and govern, administer the courts, conclude alliances, and make war. The States-General pledged themselves to fight for the West India Company's defense, gave it an outright gift of sixteen warships and a million guilders, and asked, as its return, the right to name one delegate among the nineteen officers and to be allowed the formality of issuing the formal declarations of hostilities.

Again the chief attention of the Dutch was centered on the Hudson, though Captain Mey, the newly appointed resident governor, was impressed by Hendricksen's reports of the riches of the Delaware. He had at his disposal some thirty Walloon colonists, Belgian Protestants who had fled from Spanish persecution, to be distributed among the new Dutch forts. Some he sent to Fort Orange, now called Albany; some were shipped to the Connecticut; a few, at Mey's particular desire, were ordered to begin a colony along the Delaware.

These three or four families, whose names should certainly have been preserved, were the first white settlers to live along the Delaware. They came in 1623 and built a brick house at the Whorekill, but they had little real support from the officials at New Amsterdam. For some strange reason, the troops assigned for their defense were ordered to go upstream to build their fort, and so the poor Walloons, living near the capes, had no protection except that accorded by a fort some ninety miles away.

The homesick Hollanders had no imagination. Their forts, whether on the Hudson or on the Delaware, bore exactly the same names. They had, too, in the main, the same history.

Fort Nassau, the log stronghold built on a point of rocks on the east bank of the Delaware opposite the southern part of where Philadelphia was to stand, served slight strategic function. Directly across from the outlet of the Schuylkill, it would be important in the years to come to control the fur trade of that tributary, but in 1623 the little swamp-surrounded point of rock was useless. Mey hoped, probably, to start a colony far up the river at the head of navigation, but this, too, was distant, and the Walloons who were to settle there were homesick and frightened. The colonists, therefore, went back to New Amsterdam; the fort, irregularly occupied, was used chiefly by the Indians as a lodging house when they expected trading ships to call. The first colonizing was a failure.

The Dutch had not made a promising start; the plans of Sweden, beautiful on paper, were even less successful. The great Gustavus Adolphus, meditating on the European turmoils, dreamed of a New World colony along the Delaware "where the laborer should reap the fruit of his toil, where the rights of conscience should be inviolate, and which should be open to the whole Protestant world." He thought of it as "an asylum for the persecuted of all nations, a place of security for the honor of the wives and daughters of those who were flying from bloody battlefields, and from homes made desolate by the fire and sword of the persecutor." No slaves should burden that soil, for "they labor with reluctance and soon perish." It was an excellent forecast of the plans which William Penn was half a century later to put into execution, but when Gustavus Adolphus saw his vision, in 1624, the times were not yet ripe. Hostilities with Poland, followed by Swedish intervention in the Thirty Years' War, put an end to any thought that Sweden might send out a colony. He did, however, grant a charter to a Swedish South Company for exclusive trade and in it stressed not only the financial gains that might be made, but the missionary possibilities to be exploited.

Luckless Zwaanendael

For eight years after the collapse of the Walloon experiment, no colonizers settled on the Delaware, but in the decade of the 1630's interest revived. English, Swedes, and Dutch almost simultaneously remembered the Delaware's advantages.

The Hollanders were first to come. Two patroons from New Netherlands, Samuel Blommaert and Samuel Godyn—hence Godyn's Bay as one of the names of the Delaware—had purchased from the Indians a tract of land extending from the present southern boundary of Delaware thirty-two miles northward. To clinch their title, they asked David Pietersen De Vries, of Hoorn, to plant a settlement, to grow tobacco, and to hunt for seals and whales. De Vries could not then emigrate, though he went later to the Delaware, but he directed an expedition under Gilles Hossett which settled on the Whorekill in 1631, at a place called "Zwaanendael," the place of swans. There are no swans native to the Delaware, but wild geese were plentiful and probably the Hollanders were shaky in their ornithology.

The fate of Zwaanendael is quite as picturesque as

that of the more publicized "Lost Colony" of Roanoke, though more actual details are known. Hossett made friends with the Indians, going even to the extent of buying once again the land on which the little settlement was standing, and Zwaanendael became a trading post where Dutch and Indians consorted freely. In return for "small beer" which the Dutch brewed from the maize and from persimmons, the Indians brought sturgeon, fresh speared from the river, or carried venison and turkeys to the colonists. Both Dutch and Indians feasted happily on six-inch oysters and on the flocks of partridges and pigeons which abounded.

Hossett was so happy that he planned for the extension of the colony on the opposite Cape Mey. Sailing over the ten-mile stretch of water between the points of land, he bargained with the Indians for the sale of twelve square miles of territory at the south tip of New Jersey. This, too, was in the name of Godyn and Blommaert, for, though the hoped-for whaling had not proved profitable, Zwaanendael gave every promise of prosperity.

The simple, friendly Dutchmen, with their instinct for good order, could not, however, impress upon the Indians the Dutch idea of sovereignty nor teach the meanings of a sacred symbol. Loyally, Hossett posted on a pillar a plate of tin bearing the coat of arms of "the High and Mighty Lords, States-General of the Free, United Netherlands." He made a ceremonious occasion of the placing of the pillar, greeting it with a salute of guns; he caused the garrison to prepare a solid Dutch feast of fish, and cheese, and ham, and fowls, "with cabbage set around," with good Dutch beer to drink, with boiled fruit puddings for desserts, and strips of smoked shad and sturgeon to revive a flagging appetite.

But the Indians were not appreciative of the symbol. Soon one chief, whose name is not preserved, pried off the tin plate to make himself a pipe. The garrison was horrified, and so expressed their indignation that the astonished Indians, who still felt awe toward white men, were worried how the Hollanders might be appeased.

At this point the story varies. According to one version, the Indians, to regain the friendship of the whites, sacrificed their thoughtless chief and brought his corpse as an atonement to the Dutch. By another, and far more probable account, the angry Hossett put the man to death. Whatever the facts, the rest is certain. The Indians, recovering from their superstitious reverence of whites, fell upon the garrison to seek revenge. Every Hollander was killed. So thorough was the massacre that no less than twenty-five arrows were shot into the body of a huge chained mastiff. Then the Indians gleefully butchered the Dutch cattle and held a great triumphal feast. Next year, when De Vries came to view the colony, he found "the ground bestrewed with heads and bones of murdered men."

De Vries, undaunted, sought the explanation. He fired a cannon to attract any possible survivor; when this failed to bring response, he slipped upstream to find some Indians. He found them shy and not disposed to talk, but by the lavish gifts of "duffels, bullets, hatchets, and some Nuremberg toys" he won their confidence and heard the story of the fate of Zwaanendael.

It was, he found, no isolated experience. Some of his Indian guests were wearing jackets of an English cut. By skillful questioning, sweetened by the distribution of more gifts, he drew out their confession that they had but recently attacked and killed the crew of a small English sloop. He later learned that this had been dispatched by the Virginians to explore the Delaware.

The colony at Zwaanendael was not revived. De Vries sailed back to Holland in midsummer of 1633. But the colony existed long enough to make a permanent mark on the map of the United States. The fact that Dutchmen lived at Zwaanendael along the Whorekill was the means of making Delaware a separate colony and an independent state.

3

"Where Birds Sing Matins"

Albion Knights

SIR EDMUND PLOWDEN does not rate even a
footnote in the formal histories, and that is a pity, for
this gay, romantic Irishman brought new and more engaging color to the Delaware. Fired by the medieval
myth of St. Brendan's seven years of wandering in the
"Promised Land of the Saints," forty days' sail westward from the Irish coast, Sir Edmund not unnaturally
confused the Delaware with Brendan's veritable paradise. He begged a patent for this "fairest country that
a man might see, where angels in the guise of birds
sang matins, prime and evensong and all such service
as Christian men delight to hear," where all the trees
were thick with luscious fruit, "where it was always
day and temperate, and neither hot nor cold."

The Stuart kings, ignorant of geography and careless of detail, were never niggardly. Though James I
had granted all the land between the 38th and 41st
degrees of latitude to the London and Plymouth companies, and though, by deed of 1632, Charles, his son,
had granted almost precisely this same land to Cecil
Calvert, second Lord Baltimore, the Plowden application found a favorable hearing. The happy Irishman
received a deed to all the land that lay between Cape
Mey and Sandy Hook, westward indefinitely from the
Atlantic. If his deed was genuine, Sir Edmund Plowden
would be sole possessor of what is now New Jersey,

Pennsylvania, Delaware, and points west as far as San Francisco.

Evidently even Charles had qualms about the legality of his lavish grant, for, as in the case of his patent to Lord Baltimore, he carefully excluded from the gift all areas which had been previously cultivated by any Christian state. The luckless Zwaanendael settlement, indubitably Dutch and, as such, unquestionably Christian, was thus omitted from their ownership, but all the remaining, unsettled area was given in full fee to both proprietors. The man who first made settlement, apparently, would gain clear title to the Delaware.

There is other evidence that Charles was not at ease in his donations. Baltimore received his grant from Charles as king of England; Plowden's charter was approved by Charles as Irish sovereign, and seemed to require no loyalty to London. Sir Edmund's territory, indeed, was looked upon as Ireland's overseas dominion, not as British territory.

Plowden had never visited America, but his imagination, elaborating the Brendan story, was unlimited. He visioned his possession as a realm where lush meadows of red clover alternated with fertile fields of fat, black soil. Honeysuckle perfumed all the air; forests were alive with abundant game that could be shot from open doorways; rivers were almost solidly stocked with delicious fish and oysters. There was no warfare in this land, the Irishman asserted, for all the neighbors welcomed new arrivals. Had not St. Brendan's men been entertained right royally by cultured monks who gratified each slightest wish? Even Indians were kind.

Perhaps the natives were kindly by compulsion. In Plowden's land—for some inexplicable reason an Irish dependency was named New Albion!—dwelt twenty-three great kings. These, he said, were destined to conversion by the sword if they refused the faith. And, as an earnest of determination, his Albion Knights, the settlers on the Plowden patent, each carried as a talisman a medal on a ribbon. An open Bible and a crown were thereon embossed, a hand menacingly grasped a dagger, and around these symbols ran a ring of decapitated Indian heads. One chief alone among the twenty-three remained alive on this Plowden medal, evidently as a reward for his complaisance in accepting Plowden's rule.

To Albion Knights the picture may have been alluring, but Plowden offered yet other benefits. He wished to see his semi-independent barony in all the glittering panoply of European courts. Each of the Plowden children—there were eighteen in all—became a nobleman or a great lady and each was promised an elaborate retinue of gentlemen and maids in waiting. Other titles were provided for all who would make quick, extensive settlement. Those who came earliest, indeed, might have the privilege of dwelling next to Plowden, the great lord of a twenty-four mile manor near what is now the town of Salem. More dilatory settlers must be content to live far up the Delaware, near that vast American Mediterranean Sea from which, said Plowden, the river flowed. Yet even these, though distant from Plowden's refulgence, could make a brave showing, for each would float downstream to Plowden's court in decorated barges that would shame Cleopatra. All this he set forth in a real-estate promotion brochure which, he said, was written by "Beauchamp Plantagenet, blood-relative of kings."

Unhappily for the Delaware's color, Plowden never carried out his plan; his home cares were too pressing. About the time that he had planned to sail to his New Albion, in 1634, his wife Mabel, mother of the eighteen offspring, brought suit against him, alleging that the gallant knight whipped her unmercifully. Evidence is not lacking that the charge was true, but there were other reasons for what Plowden called a persecution. Only recently, perhaps to win more favor from the Irish, Plowden had shifted his religion and the parish vicar, angered at apostasy, seconded Mabel's accusations. Instead of settling with his nobles in New Albion, therefore, Plowden went to jail. Only after he was freed, and after Mabel had divorced him, was the harassed knight free to visit his supposed estate.

This, too, had sad and serious aftermath. Lord Baltimore contested the Plowden deed, alleging that Charles I could not, even as king of Ireland, regrant lands which had already been conveyed by him, as king of England. The Virginians also protested that the deed was false. Some were cynical enough to add that Plowden's trip abroad was not wholly voluntary; that he was, in fact, transported for failure to pay Mabel her alimony. The Salemites refused to greet him as their lord and, when Plowden went to inspect New Albion, a rebellious crew, resenting his lordly mannerisms, marooned him on a lonely island, sick, naked, and without provisions. He died of exposure. His Albion Knights, bereft of leadership, sank back into obscurity.

Three Angry Dutchmen

New settlers were soon to pour into the valley. The time was not yet ripe for Englishmen, and Hollanders were still too dazzled by their seemingly complete monopoly of Oriental trade, but farther north in Europe the Swedes were looking longingly across the seas. As early as 1623, Willem Usselinx of Antwerp had unfolded plans for a colony of religious refugees along the Delaware, but Gustavus Adolphus had been obliged, because war demands were far too pressing, to postpone consideration of the scheme. However, Usselinx was undismayed. Returning to Holland, he enlisted the support of Samuel Blommaert, the Whorekill man, and of Peter Minuit, he who had bought Manhattan from the Indians. The three joined forces to persuade the Swedes to start a colony.

Unquestionably, the three Dutchmen were moved by anger and by vengeful motives. Samuel Blommaert, embittered at the way Holland had ignored his Whorekill losses, burned with desire to show up the stupidity of his former associates. So wrought up was he that he took the cash paid him by the Dutch West India Company for his holdings at Zwaanendael and at Cape Mey and poured it into the coffers of the Swedish colonizing company. He told his partners what he knew about the Delaware and made clear to them the methods followed by the Netherlanders. And it was Blommaert who had persuaded Peter Minuit to join the Swedish group.

Not that shrewd, dynamic Peter Minuit needed much encouragement. He, too, was angry at the Dutch, for enemies had charged that he had stolen Dutch West India Company funds and had stirred up discord at New Netherlands. Minuit, the "Midnight Man" who proudly adopted the bat as his personal totem, flamed with indignation at the unfairness, ingratitude and unbearable highhandedness of the West India Company directors. He eagerly embraced the opportunity of joining forces with the Swedes to break up the trade of his old associates and himself chipped in one-eighth of the 24,000-guilder capital stock of the Swedish enterprise.

Usselinx, the suave promoter, Blommaert, the administrator and financier, Minuit, the skilled fieldworker, made excellent teammates. Backed by the full support of Sweden, they dispatched an expedition which left Europe in the closing days of 1637.

The opportunity glowed golden for the Swedish crown. At home, the nation faced serious social difficulties. Finns were roving into Sweden, mocking every effort at control. Accustomed to the limitless forests of their own land, they burned down Sweden's trees to make rude clearings, killed off wild game, and, by the diabolic charms of witchcraft, so the Swedes superstitiously maintained, brought disease, disaster, and dismay wherever they went.

Queen Christina's advisers maintained that the Delaware was perfect for such as these. The Finns, with their delight in hunting, would find the river well suited to their temperament. To rid Sweden of their menace, and to populate the colony across the seas, Finns were rounded up for deportation. With them were sent debtors, criminals, and military slackers not wanted in the mother land.

Evidently Sweden had a broad interpretation of deportable offenses. One trooper, who climbed a monastery wall for the mysterious design of chopping down six apple trees and two sweet cherries, chose emigration as a substitute for hanging, though either alternative seems unduly harsh. A man who "shot some elk" was hustled to the Delaware. Married men, found guilty of adultery, evidently a rare crime in Sweden, were shipped overseas where women were extremely scarce and where, presumably, their Don Juan tendencies would find no scope. The Swedes were far more anxious to colonize their new possession than they were to mete out punishment to fit the crime.

Few of the folk thus hurried to America were vicious or decadent; the worst that could be said of them was that they were ill-adjusted or that their folkways did not conform precisely to the pattern of the time. Unlike the criminal colonies sent out by other nations to other remote settlements, the Swedish emigrants were men of whom the nation could expect successful enterprise. The forest destroyers were the type of men to clear out sites for farms and towns; the hunters could employ their prowess to preserve their fellows from starvation; even the warlocks of the Finns could use their magic to bring winds to sail the ships and to put spells, if necessary, on the Indians. Once in America, these Finns forgot their wizardry; only on occasion did a warped old man or some malignant crone wreak vengeance by illicit means. There was less of this than in godly Massachusetts.

The trip was not enjoyable. Crowded to the gunwales with passengers and soldiers, packed to the danger point with cargoes of supplies including a heavy load of axes, mirrors, toys, and cheap brass chains to trade for furs, the two Swedish ships which made up Minuit's expedition butted slowly through the sea. Sickness broke out; food ran low; always there was fear lest some chance spark fall into the ton and a half of powder stored within the hold. Before the Swedes came to America, the black bat ensign which Minuit kept flying at the masthead seemed a harbinger of grief.

Not till spring came to the Delaware was there relief from suffering. Then, just as the shad and sturgeon runs began, and when the river was alive with Indian canoes towing grapevine nets to snare the fish, while the very air was fresh and fragrant with the scent of spicy blossom, the two ships stood into the bay. Both banks were dotted with the lodges of the Minquas, where squaws in bright-colored garments were tending fires of smoldering hickory to smoke the catch for winter use. The land seemed prosperous and blooming. The grateful Swedes asserted that this was earthly paradise.

But early names along the Delaware have been short-lived. Paradise Point, the first landing place of Minuit, no longer finds its name on the map. Near by, however, is a stream that still bears its Swedish title. In memory of loved parents, home in distant Sweden, a broad, smooth-flowing waterway was called the Morderskill, or Mothers' Creek. Modern tongues distort this fine remembrance of the filial love of early settlers into the Murderkill, and legends are invented to explain the meaning of the name.

Evidently the Minuit adventurers expected better boons than paradise, for they embarked again upon their little ships to sail still farther up the river. Minuit, planning to avoid the crowded regions where the Minquas pitched their lodges, steered for the point of rocks where Hendricksen had met the three lost Dutchmen. There, on the little creek which in honor of the reigning Swedish queen, the twelve-year-old daughter of Gustavus Adolphus, he named Christina Creek, a colony was established. It was within the present bounds of Wilmington.

Forest-destroying Finns

It was to be, in large degree, a Finnish town. Worrying over plans for his new city, where his black bat flag would fly, Minuit had realized that his colony could endure only by reliance upon the Finns. Those wild marauders who loved to chop down trees, and whose delight was hunting, must feed the people with the fresh meat so sorely needed after three long months of salted food and they must house the settlement against the rigors of the weather. The Swedes were river people and they were fine farmers, but the pioneers were Finns. The Finnish mode of living, foreign as it was to Sweden, was precisely what the Delaware required.

Almost as soon, therefore, as his ships were moored, Minuit sent colonists and soldiers to their duties, some to palisade the site, in case the Indians proved less friendly than they seemed, others to begin the planting, still others, and among them all the Finns, to cut the trees for building houses.

The forest destroyers cut logs of even lengths for walls, notching them at the corners so that the transverse logs might lie close at the joints. Well chinked with stone and yellow clay, ceiled inside with planking like a ship, and sometimes weatherboarded for additional protection, these Finnish one-story cabins were weathertight and, when heated by their huge clay-plastered chimneys, were warm in wintertime. Later, as leisure gave the opportunity, small windows could be cut so that light might enter through oiled-paper panes, plank bedsteads would be cleated to the corners of the cabin, tables and three-legged stools could be built of ax-smoothed slabs, turned bark side under. But in the first days of the settlement there was no time for luxury. Minuit's settlers slept on piles of grass or of dry leaves to keep themselves from the packed earth floor and, if their cabins were so large as to boast a half-story attic, they climbed aloft on pegs driven deep into the logs. When all were comfortably housed, the larger families would build a shed, with sloping roof and open often on one side, for storage purposes or as a sort of summer kitchen, and some might go so far as to clapboard the hut with slabs of softwood, but white pine was not abundant in the valley of the Delaware and such

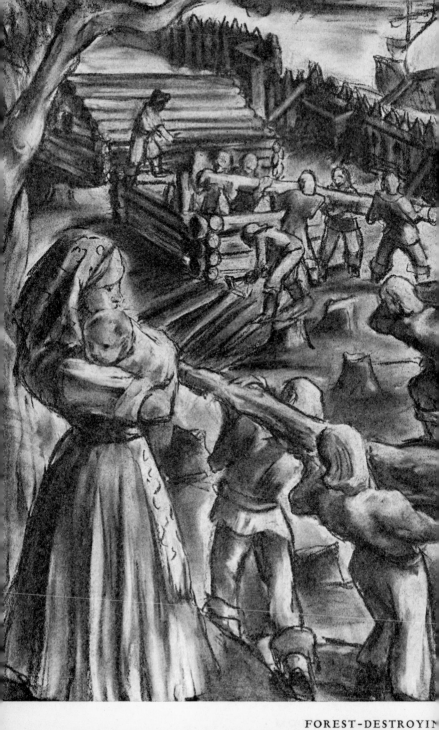

FOREST-DESTROYIN

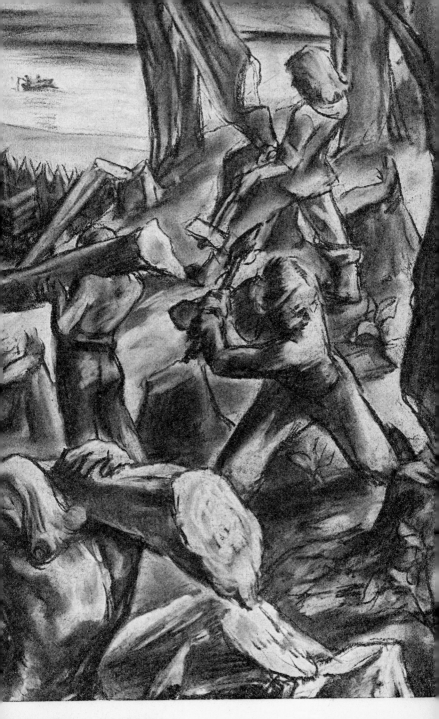

INNS BUILD FREEDOM

touches were luxuries that frugal Swedes and Finns did not think fitting. The quarters were cramped; entrance through the slab door swung on leather hinges necessitated that even medium-sized Finns must duck their heads; but few complained of hardship.

So began in America the construction of the log cabin, the typical frontier dwelling that was to be the symbol of a pioneering people, the house that was to spread westward from the Delaware to all the nation. Built on the pattern of the Finns, selected by the Swedes as best suited of all houses for newcomers in the wilderness, the log cabin has come to be distinctively American. From such houses as the Finns first built near Wilmington have come men whom a democratic and progressive nation honors for hardihood, integrity, and wisdom.

Happily, the Indians were less hostile than Minuit had feared; instead, as always during the Swedish residence on the Delaware, the natives were friendly and co-operative. From them the settlers learned how to make moccasins; in return, the Swedes gave lessons to the squaws in the fashioning of furs to keep out winter cold and in more effective ways of sewing leather clothes for summer use. Settlers fortunate enough to have wives enjoyed the comfort of linens, for flax grew luxuriantly after the colonists were well established. And after the sheep became numerous some settlers wore heavy woolen underclothes which were warm and durable, even if not ornamental.

Their food was on the hearty side. Four meals a day of solid and substantial meats, lightened possibly by peas and beans and turnips, provided energy for the day's muscular exertions. Swigs of rum and water gave stimulation at odd moments, while at noon the indispensable "meridian," a rum punch built of fresh spring water, sugar, lemon juice, and spirits, whetted the appetite for food. On winter evenings a similar rum punch, warmed by toasted bread floating on its surface or heated by a red-hot poker plunged hissingly into the bowl, made living more endurable.

The Swedes were not limited to such plain beverage. Their "manatham" of small beer, rum, and sugar, their "tiff" or "flip" of manatham with a slice of toast or bit of buttered bread floating on the surface, their "hätt-pät" of warmed beer and rum, their "sampson" of hot rum and cider, their "sillibub," or "oelost," of fresh warm milk and wine and water, and their mulled rum, hot, with eggs and allspice afforded ample opportunity for varying their customary fare. The eggnogg which they first brought into the valley of the Delaware has long remained a favorite for Eastertime and for the formal calls on New Year's Day.

They were not solely dependent on their liquor, however, for enjoyment. More pleasant to the Swedes, and to the "roving Finns," were the huge log *bastu,* the steam bathhouses set along the riverbanks.

The bastu was a well-sealed hut, provided with a huge stone fireplace, and with two bunks built along the walls. Before the bathers came, a roaring fire was kindled, and when the bathhouse was so hot that none but Swedes could possibly endure the heat, the guests were bidden to attend. Naked, they lay on the upper bunk, perspiring freely, while the women who attended them poured water on the red-hot stones to fill the bastu with steam. Then the bathers crawled closer, lying full length on the rough boards of the lower platform, while they flagellated themselves with bundles of birch branches or were scrubbed roughly by the bath attendant. This done, the hardy pleasure seekers hastened out of doors, to plunge into the river or roll naked in the snow.

It was a Spartan life, but it was a peaceful group and, on the whole, a happy one. For all their heavy drinking they were sober, for hard, rough work eliminates the evils of excessive alcohol, and what hard labor could not do, the pastor's regulations might accomplish. Any man who came drunk into the church was fined forty shillings and was ordered to perform some public penance. The court records do not show that many had to pay.

Three other ordinances might be mentioned here because they so well became a region to be famous later for its Bethlehem Bach Choir and for the Philadelphia Symphony. What other pioneer community, in this or any other land, ever passed a law that ordered harsh-voiced citizens to stand mute or "sing softly"? Has any other settlement provided a five-shilling fine for such a sin as "untimely singing"? And who but Swedes would ever dream of issuing a law forbidding folk "to sing as if they were calling cows"? These Swedes were people of aesthetic sensibility.

But clouds again were gathering. The Dutch, re-occupying the old Fort Nassau, whence Minuit, while in the Dutch employ, had ordered troops away, came threateningly to demand that Sweden leave the Delaware. Minuit ignored the protest and defied the Dutch to put him out. He was warlike in his gestures and well settled at Christina. The Netherlanders went off muttering dire threats, but carefully remained on their side of the river.

This was Minuit's last service on the Delaware. Now that he had built his fort, bought land from the Indians within a space of six blazed trees, arranged his colonists, and scared off the Dutch, he set sail for the island of St. Kitts to trade his produce for tobacco. While there, a hurricane sprang up, and Minuit was killed. The Swedish colony had lost its most dynamic force.

The English, too, were now renewing their interest in the Delaware. The Yankee folk settled in New Haven were evidently discontented with their situation. Scarcely had they settled in the shadow of West Rock before they looked about for better habitation. They chose the Delaware as their promised land.

Two captains, George Lamberton and Nathaniel Turner, were dispatched in 1640 on the Delaware adventure. They settled on the eastern bank, at Varken's Kill, or Salem Creek, and since the river lay between them and the Swedes, the garrison of Christina gave a benevolent approval. The Englishmen, according to the Swedish point of view, would keep the Dutch amused and would allow the Swedes to colonize the western land in peace.

The Dutch behaved according to the Swedish wish. An expedition sent down from Fort Nassau ordered Lamberton away, and since his little force of twenty families was suffering from pleurisy and there seemed some question whether Plowden was not, after all, the rightful owner, the New Havenites withdrew.

But the consequences were not at all consistent with Swedish plans. Connecticut, always hankering for the Delaware, returned, in anticipation of the moment "when God shall so inlarge the English plantations in Delaware as that they shall grow the greater part of the jurisdiction . . . that the governor may be constantly there." Lamberton bought land from the willing Indians at the mouth of the Schuylkill, and then sent letters to the Swedes demanding that they clear out of English territory.

4

The Swedish Dictators

Big Belly Printz

Lamberton sent his letters to the wrong person. A new Swedish governor had come in February, 1643, a huge, irascible cavalryman who had the powers of a dictator and would stand no nonsense. John Bjornsson Printz, 400-pound mercenary whom the awed Indians at once nicknamed "Big Belly," who swore like a trooper and was not above either the major or the minor vices, was blustering at Christina. To order him, the master of all land between Cape Henlopen and Trenton Falls, to leave the country of his sovereign queen was to challenge Jove himself.

Printz acted quickly. Scarcely had he set foot on shore before he demanded that his troops parade for an inspection. His practiced military eye was shocked at what he saw, but he was not dismayed. To their astonishment, his men were drilled within a scant inch of their lives until such time as the exacting Printz was satisfied.

Nor did this hardy veteran of Austrian, Brunswicker, and Danish armies like the defenses that had been prepared. In their supposedly free time between drills, the soldiers cut great hemlock logs to make new forts against "our evil neighbors, especially the English." At Varken's Kill, directly opposite the English stronghold, Printz set up Fort Elfsborg, with eight guns, to command the river. Every ship that sought to mount

the Delaware was now commanded to drop anchor and
to crave the Swedish leader's permission to go farther.
Even poor De Vries, who might be supposed to have
undergone sufficient humiliation in the remembrance
of Zwaanendael, was compelled to bow to Printz's alien
orders.

A second, and stronger, fort went up on Tinicum,
a marshy island at the river's bend, due west of Nassau
and just south of Lamberton's location on the Schuylkill. This site, christened now New Gothenburg, was
chosen as the capital, and on it, after drills were satisfactory and forts had been made impregnable, Big Belly
Printz proposed to build a palace that would as completely overshadow other buildings as he himself was
greater than all other men.

But first he had to settle with the Yankees. Learning that Lamberton's yacht was lying quietly at anchor
halfway between Elfsborg and Christina, Printz issued
a polite request that Lamberton come for a call. When
the Connecticut leader came to New Gothenburg, anticipating at least a banquet, Printz put him into
irons. Two other Yankees, John Thickpenny and John
Woolen, who accompanied their leader, were also jailed.

Big Belly's object was to find out what Lamberton
was doing, and his methods were peculiar. Himself accustomed to drink prodigiously, he plied the Lamberton
assistants with strong liquor, drinking glass for glass
with them to make them friendly. When they were
gloriously drunk, and Printz still craftily sober, he
pressed them to confess that Lamberton and they were
plotting to incite an Indian rebellion, that Lamberton
was trading illegally, and that the English had no right
to any land upon the Schuylkill or at Varken's Kill.

The ordeal by liquor did not work, perhaps because
the two assistants had nothing to confess. Printz then

ordered Lamberton to trial and, by a curious proceeding whereby the prosecution offered all the testimony, judged the admissibility of evidence, and dictated what the court should finally decide, ordered that all English should depart except those who took the oath of loyalty to Sweden. Lamberton was not released until he paid a fine of beaver skins and listened to a scathing lecture from his conqueror.

Both Lamberton and Printz would have been amazed to learn that three centuries later another Lamberton would be mayor of a city of two million people on the Delaware.

The Englishmen were beaten, though all knew that the rebuff was temporary and that they would return in force. The Dutch, at Nassau across the Delaware, also were troublesome. Poor Printz, with but eighty able-bodied men at his command, was only too aware that crisis was at hand.

His first hope was that Sweden would dispatch an expeditionary force. With two hundred soldiers, Printz wrote home, he could "break the necks of everyone upon the river." But Sweden paid no heed to his appeal; engrossed in her internal troubles, she ignored the Delaware. Not a ship, not a trooper, not a pound of war materials, and not a word of any sort came to the colony for twenty-eight interminable months.

Failing men, Printz put his faith in fortresses. On Lamberton's old site he erected Nya Korsholm, a blockhouse to secure the Schuylkill's mouth and to prevent Dutch or Yankees from interfering with the rich trade in beaverskins on that river. To guard the trail by which the Indians came down from the interior, he built a mighty citadel, Vasa, where little Cobbs' Creek joins the larger Darby Creek. This Vasa, or, as the Indians called it, Karakung, was a powerful log fort "capable of defense by four or five men, well-supplied with shot and powder." A quarter of a mile beyond, Printz built a water mill, called Molndal, first gristmill in the area.

Now he was at liberty to cultivate refinements. To make a proper palace for a man who must put up a bold front because his power was so weak, Big Belly Printz conscripted labor to erect a vast two-story mansion built of bricks and logs. Characteristically, he picked the highest, healthiest site for his own residence, where cooling breezes blew all summer and from which he might command a perfect view of all approaches by both land and water. Here, in his palace-fortress, were windows made of honest Swedish glass, and ovens and huge fireplaces. Here was a library, too, with literary contents worth a full $200 and here were pearls and jewelry for Madame Printz, valued at six times the worth of the books. The inventories showed also that Madame Governor had costumes that had cost $800 and underthings amounting to $200 more. Big Belly, as was just and right, had formal clothing that, so far as cost was reckoned, far outshone his lady's fripperies, but there is no mention of any underthings for him whatever.

Printz Hall was a magazine for stores, as well as residence and sanctuary. Three thousand pounds of salt pork and a quarter of a ton of salted beef, a tiny cache of some 560 pounds of smoked ham and bacon, 80 pounds of cheese, and 200 pounds of lard were kept as a reserve against emergencies. And lest the Dutch or English besiege Printz Hall and try to force submission, he kept malt and hops on hand to make Dutch beer and a hundred pounds of candles to provide illumination.

It was a pity then that careless Swen Vass, a gunner set as sentry to keep watch on a bitter cold November night in 1645, built himself a fire so high that it got out of control. Printz Hall went up in flames; only the dairy was preserved. Big Belly Printz was forced to spend a freezing winter with the common people. It was small compensation to look forward to pleasant spring sailing on the Delaware, in the first pleasure ship ever built for yachting in America. Meanwhile, he arrested Vass, convicted him of willful destructiveness, and sent him home in irons to be punished. A new gubernatorial palace was immediately begun.

In writing of his woes, Printz was mindful of the needs of his subordinates. As reward for himself he asked that twenty farms be given him and that his salary be raised. Then, as an afterthought, he added that his colony was well and happy. There was no sign, he said, that gold or salt or silkworms could be relied upon as a resource, but wine grapes and whales were plentiful, lacking only men who understood the business. Some twenty-eight of his men, though they had oxen and cows in plenty, were not content—they wanted women. Send them, Printz demanded, buxom Swedish girls, with plaited yellow hair. It is sad to report that this requisition, like the call for troops, was quietly ignored.

Where men are making money, women will follow of their own volition. Hearing that the colonists were prospering, for all Sweden rang with the report that Printz's men had cleared a profit of 10,000 florins in a year, the good ship *Katt* (named after Pussy) sailed in July, 1649, with much-needed cargo: eighteen cannons, powder, lead and muskets, seventy "forest-destroying Finns" and other emigrants, together with a bevy of assorted ladies who craved pioneering. Printz's requisition was in a fair way of being honored, though the girls had volunteered to try life in the colonies and had not been drafted into service.

The *Katt's* history is tragic. Caught, with all sails standing, in a hurricane, the ship was wrecked sixteen miles off Puerto Rico. No lives were lost, but every article of value was either sunk by the storm or stolen by the Spaniards. The men were forced to beg for means of livelihood; the women were commandeered. One girl, the most attractive of the lot, was retained by the governor in his own household; the others, after two years' servitude, were shipped away from the island in a tiny bark.

Their freedom was but brief. Next morning, off the Virgin Islands, they were seized with shouts by Frenchmen who insisted, "Women are needed in this country for our soldiers in the forts." They were robbed again of what little goods they had acquired, tortured to disclose the whereabouts of more, and were then distributed about the Virgin Islands, forbidden under pain of death from association with each other. Four men of the seventy escaped; none of the women survived the series of catastrophes.

Meanwhile, the colony, cut off from home support, weakened by the drills and building work demanded by Big Belly Printz, and nervous because of constant fear of Dutch attack, was losing its morale. Printz, the men said, was treating them as slaves, demanding that they work for him at Printz Hall and on his great plantations without pay, refusing to allow them to trade with the Indians, though he himself was filling his warehouse with bargain beaverskins; Big Belly, they alleged, was brutal, avaricious, and unjust. "At no time," the colonists complained had they been "secure as to life and property." A petition of eleven charges signed by almost all the colonists except the soldiers, was presented to him, pleading that he change his ways.

Printz was furious, of course. He arrested Anders Johnson, leader of the opposition, tried him for treason, and ordered him to be executed. Two days later, Big Belly issued a formal denial of each charge, branded his enemies as rebels, and dared them to continue their complaints. They held their peace, but so strong was the undercurrent that, as Printz confessed, there were not thirty men in all New Sweden whom he dared to trust. He feared he might be murdered. Hastily he departed for Sweden, leaving Johan Papegoja, his son-in-law, to govern in his stead.

The Swedes had reached, and passed, their highest peak. Neglected by the crown, torn by internal dissension, they were an easy prey for any strong attacker. A belated Swedish ship, surviving rough weather, a dysentery epidemic, a threatened attack by three Turkish slavers, and a hurricane, limped into port to bring assistance, but the aid came much too late. Pieter Stuyvesant, the new Dutch governor of New Amsterdam, was ready to reduce all enemies of Holland on the Delaware.

A Dutch armada of seven ships, carrying some six hundred men, appeared in 1655 before the Swedish forts. The defenders, vastly outnumbered and so poorly supplied that there were less than two rounds of ammunition for each soldier, gave up without a battle. The very day that Charles X, king of Sweden, captured Warsaw from the Poles, his empire in New Sweden fell. The Delaware was Dutch.

Again the names were changed. Christina, which we now know as Wilmington, became Altenae, or Altoona; Fort Casimir was renamed Nieuew Amstel; the Delaware, which Sweden always called New Sweden Stream, was now the Zueydt.

For the first time in its history the river lost its

independence, for even in the palmiest New Sweden days the Delaware had been, in point of fact if not of right, self-governing. Sweden had not cared, in the pressure of its other interests, to keep too tight a rein on its colony. But now, with Dutch control, the river sank into a mere dependency, first of the city of New Amsterdam and then, when Manhattan paid its debts to Hollanders who had lent it money, of the city of Amsterdam itself. The Delaware became a suburb of the Netherlander capital, ruled by the city authorities of that flourishing commercial center.

The Delaware takes little pride in the short period of Dutch control. Undoubtedly, as part of Amsterdam alone and not of the United Provinces, it might have argued that the valley was an independent area, beyond control by Holland to whom it owed no actual allegiance; certainly as an integral portion of the capital, this suburb made Amsterdam the largest city in the world, perhaps the largest in point of area that ever had existed. But the settlers of the Delaware were not engaged in sterile reasoning. The fact remained that they were now dependent on alien absentees, who knew little and seemed to care less about their fate. The Delaware was not happy to run second to either of the Amsterdams.

When word came, after eight years of Dutch rule, that again Englishmen were looking greedily upon the Delaware, the riverfolk were not too greatly angered. Already the colony had shrunk in size; nowhere did Dutch writs run more than eight miles distant from the forts. A visit by young Charles Calvert, heir to Lord Baltimore, was made occasion for a ceremonial reception where strong Swedish beer, such as Calvert never tasted in his Maryland domains, flowed lavishly in welcome.

Calvert had come to call attention to the Maryland demand for all the river that "lay beneath the fortieth parallel of north latitude," but, though he pressed his claim with vehemence, there was a stronger English claim to the river and the bay. Charles II, restored to the English throne, needed lands to pay his debts; he held a hatred for the Dutch and he desired that England should be master of the lands that lay between New England and the southern provinces.

The Merry Monarch granted patents to the New World lands that brought new claimants to the Delaware. On March 12, 1664, he gave his brother, later to be King James II, title to New England, New Jersey, and New York. Evidently he regarded his grandfather's charter to Lord Baltimore as still a valid grant, for the west shore of the Delaware was not included in the gift, nor was Maryland transferred. James, however, seems to have assumed that he was entitled to control the Dutch settlements along the river as an appendage of New Amsterdam. He paid no heed to the fact that New Amsterdam had, in point of law, no rights along the Delaware.

The Swedes, so meek when Hollanders descended on their land, were anxious now to regain their old status. Always they had feared the English more than the Dutch, and now that British rule was fastened on them a small section of the Swedish diehards rose to win their freedom. For some six months in 1669, the flat, fertile plains on the west bank of the stream were in rebellion.

The Long Finn

Marcus Jacobsen, self-styled "the Long Finn," knew all the tricks that are employed by good political manipulators. As plain Marcus Jacobsen he could win few followers, for he was born of servile stock and had been noted only as a petty criminal. Robberies in England and in Maryland had given him a certain reputation as a desperado, but had caused the better class to shun his company. As the Long Finn he was not respectable.

Jacobsen proceeded to invent an ancestry for himself. In Sweden there was a famous family, the Koenigsmarks, whose men had military genius and whose women were sought far and wide as consorts of the European rulers. Jacobsen, far off along the Delaware, claimed that he, too, was a Koenigsmark, the son of Sweden's leading general. He had come, he said, to lead the Swedes to glory.

Even at that distant date, the lure of pure blood was effective. The Long Finn, whose authentic ancestry was mixed Lapp and Finn and Swedish blood, stressed the duty of allowing only pure-blood folk to rule. The Long Finn urged his followers to deal with none but Swedes; he tried to keep the Indians from contact with the colony, except as slaves and furnishers of beaver; he handicapped the English and the Dutch in order that his Swedes might dominate the land. Illiterate and fuzzy-minded, the Long Finn shouted demands that the Swedes tear up the treaties which subjected them to alien conquerors. In sentences that rasped the ears, he cried out that the world owed justice to a people beset on every side by enemies.

He was an irredentist, demanding that, no matter where the Swedes should settle, their residences should be added to the Swedish crown. Those former residents of the river valley who had fled to Maryland to escape the Dutch, or had gone north along the Schuylkill, or inland along the creeks to set up new homes in unsettled land, must all be brought under Sweden's protecting blue and gold. The Long Finn preached that for any foreigners to rule the Swedes in any portion of America would violate the sacred rights of Swedish supermen.

Tall, powerful, and handsome, outstandingly blond even in a settlement of Nordics, this Long Finn attracted followers. Most helpful was the aid of Pastor Lars Lock, who used his pulpit as a sounding board for Long Finn propaganda. In Lock's long sermons the deeds of Jacobsen seemed divinely sanctioned, obedience to his decrees was stressed as a religious duty. Lock's arguments on the Long Finn's behalf were extraordinarily potent among people who were devout churchfolk, accustomed to accept the comments of a cleric as of supernatural origin. Lars Lock, "trumpeter to the cause," promised that those who perished in the fight against the Long Finn's foes would win a special glory.

The program sounds peculiarly modern in these days of dictatorship, for the Long Finn anticipated almost every political device employed by current totalitarians. Three centuries ago the Long Finn was employing methods now familiar to the Germans and Italians.

Luckily for Britain, this Long Finn was something of an ascetic, else he might have been entrapped by the cleverness of a woman. Armegot Printz, battling Amazon, daughter of Big Belly and America's first feminist, was herself ambitious to be boss. Disdaining her small husband, Papegoja, as a weakling and a coward, Armegot refused to bear his name but insisted, long before the time of Lucy Stone, that she retain her maiden name. Living in her giant father's Printz Hall on Tinicum, she refused to yield to British law, declined to pay her taxes, declared her independence of Englishmen, of Dutchmen, and of Swedes as well. On Jacobsen's dramatic entrance into the colony, the powerful Armegot exerted all her charm to win him to her train, but when he proved too independent, she withdrew her blessing. Had Armegot and Jacobsen remained united in their efforts, the pair would probably have ruled the river.

Johan Anderssen, a gunner nicknamed Stalkofta, or the Steelcoat, and John Coleman, wirepuller from behind the scenes, were members of the inner circle. Each had secret motives. Just as Armegot wished to recover Big Belly's brewery and to regain his pleasure yacht, so Anderssen and Coleman, none too successful farmers, coveted the estates of Englishmen. The Steelcoat, it was whispered, looked lecherously at lovely ladies and dallied with the thought that he could have a harem. His trim, gold-laced uniform, especially designed to set off his best features and to divert attention from a certain physical peculiarity, was always glittering where the women of the colony were wont to congregate. It was, in fact, his longing for the wives of other men that first caused his fellows to band together for the overthrow of Jacobsen's intrigue.

Coleman's English name was an effective mask to hide the plotters' purposes. He, as it happened, was a Finn, but Englishmen were not familiar with the quirks of Finnish nomenclature, and assumed that he was truly British. Coleman was permitted to gather armament enough to fit out a private army for the Long Finn's use. Powder, shot, and guns were stored in large sufficiency, and some, the rumors said, were given to the Indians, whose language Coleman spoke.

Nothing less than a blood purge of the foreigners would satisfy ambitious Jacobsen. He called a meeting to stimulate his men. Mounting a table, when the group was comfortably drunk, he spoke of Swedish sufferings. In his high-pitched, hysterical voice he reminded them how Britain had refused to aid the Swedes in colonizing the river valley and how, by force and guile, the English were now masters of the land. He told them, too, how base-born foreigners, monopolizing trade and currency, profited at the expense of honest Swedes. Then, without the shadow of a fact to prove his claim, he said that out of sight of land, at sea beyond the capes, a Swedish fleet lay waiting for a signal to sail up the Delaware to liberate them from bondage. That signal, said the Long Finn, would be the massacre of every alien.

Perhaps this beer-hall Putsch might have been effective had not huge Armegot been present. The only woman in the hall, she emerged from self-imposed retirement to make open boast that, if the Long Finn won, she would regain the lands which Peter Kock, one of the pro-British colonists, had taken from her father in his absence. Somewhat drunken, both by beer and by heady oratory, she waved a knife with which she would start the slaughter.

Kock saw his danger. While from tables at the ends of the room, big Armegot and the Long Finn were urging their blood purge, Kock grabbed the knife and ran from the room. The Long Finn, sensing treachery, jumped from his tabletop to catch the traitor. Kock got outside, slammed the door, leaned his weight against it, and yelled for help. The Long Finn pushed the door part open. Kock slashed the Long Finn's wrist, but could not stop him from escaping. The Long Finn rushed into the woods, followed by the English troops who had been waked by Kock's loud calls.

Jacobsen was captured in the forests. The vengeance imposed upon him was severe. For five long winter months, until the governor was free to come down from New York, the Long Finn lay in an un-heated cell. By court decision, he was sentenced to be hanged, but the governor, desiring to show "clemency and mercy," commuted the death penalty to two hundred lashes "severely laid on" from a cat-o'-nine-tails. Then, after a giant R, for rebel, had been branded on his cheek, the prisoner was sent in irons to Barbados to be sold into slavery. His followers lost half their property in fines. They were accounted lucky to escape so easily. Thereafter, until the Revolution, there was no talk of rebellion against British rule.

5

Terrestrial Canaan

Strawman Fenwick

THE Swedes and Dutch fought boundary disputes by blood-curdling threats in paper proclamations;
the Stuart Restoration introduced them to the pleasures
of the law courts. Anxious to repay their friends for
services during the lean days of Cromwell, both Charles
II and his brother James, Duke of York, made lavish
grants of lands and perquisites, without regard to charters previously granted. In consequence, land titles on
the Delaware, once almost crystal clear, grew murky
and unfathomable. The legendary skill of Philadelphia lawyers has been sharpened in the effort to make
sense of the conflicting claims.

The east bank of the Delaware, from the head of
the river to Cape May, was the chief territory in contention. Three months after James received the title,
he transferred the entire area to John, Lord Berkeley,
the same man who had once himself arranged to convey
exactly the same territory to Plowden and his Albion
Knights—and to Sir George Carteret, admiral and privy
councilor. In honor of the island home from which
the Carterets had come, he called the land New
Caesarea, or New Jersey. It was, as all agreed, a more
euphoneous and more pleasant title than New Canary,
the first name proposed. Then, to make the deed more
sound, the duke sailed off with four ships and a hundred
heavy guns to put New Netherlands and the Delaware

under British rule. The fleet reached Nieuew Amstel on the last day of September, 1664, surprised the fort, killed three Dutch watchmen, raised the British flag, and sold his prisoners into slavery. Once again the town's name was changed, this time to New Castle; Altenae assumed the English name of Willing's Town, or Wilmington.

Just why the duke deeded New Jersey to his friends is not clear, for neither of them wanted territory on the Delaware. Both Berkeley and Carteret were already well rewarded by vast estates in Carolina, and neither of them had the slightest wish to voyage to their new domains. They promptly sold out their claims; Carteret disposed of his share, the east Jersey area, to a syndicate of twelve, among whom was William Penn; Lord Berkeley, preferring the London fleshpots to the Jersey wilderness, sold what he called New West Jersey, bordering the Delaware, to one John Fenwick, Quaker and reformed cavalryman.

Or so he said, for the story is fantastic. Major Fenwick was a straw man acting for a London brewer, Edward Byllynge, one of Berkeley's closest friends. Byllynge, deep in debt, had made a hurried deal to defraud his creditors and he trusted Fenwick to return the land when bankruptcy was safely passed. Fenwick was to have one-tenth for his share in the illegal enterprise.

But Fenwick had his troubles too. Like Byllynge, he was broke, but two good Quaker friends, John Eldridge, tanner, and Edmund Warner, poultryman, advanced him a hundred pounds to help him sail to Jersey. As security for their loan, Fenwick handed them a mortgage-deed for the land promised him by Byllynge. Scarcely had he left the English coast, before his friends foreclosed upon his colony and sold homestead lots in New West Jersey. Even though they may have been wholly unaware that all the land was legally in Byllynge's name, the Eldridge-Warner business principles were highly questionable.

Poor Fenwick had a moment's peace when he arrived on the Delaware. In April, 1675, on the banks of Varken's Kill, near the abandoned Fort Elfsborg, he called together a great council of the Indians. There, under the famous Salem Oak, he purchased Indian rights to his tenth of New West Jersey and, uniquely among the founders of new settlements, he stipulated that the Indians might peaceably remain upon the lands as long as they desired to stay. His Quaker colony of Salem, land of peace, never had complaint or quarrel with the natives.

For the most part Salem belied its name, so far as Fenwick was concerned. His life was one of worry and contention. Sir Edmund Andros, governor of the Duke of York's possessions, had never been informed of any change in ownership. Now, hearing that a stranger had arrived demanding the privilege of governing New Jersey, Andros thought only that usurpers had invaded his master's realm. He immediately dispatched a company of troops, out of the hundred soldiers that he had to guard New York against attack, to bring the interloper to New York in chains.

Their methods were direct. When Fenwick failed to heed the warrant of the governor, the soldiers beat him severely and, after he again refused to go with them to New York, they fired on him with guns and pistols. By Fenwick's own graphic story, which may not be completely accurate, the soldiers took point-blank aim at him, at a distance of four yards, with a gun "laden with many swan shot." They fired at him, said Fenwick, with two bullets from a pistol from a point but two feet distant from his head. Each time, however, the Andros emissaries missed their target.

Fenwick then took refuge in his house but it was surely not his castle. At midnight the troops burst open the door, seized the sleeping colonist, and took him to New York. There Fenwick was imprisoned, awaiting Andros's autocratic pleasure, for twenty-seven months until, in August, 1677, word came from James to let the man go free.

Again Fenwick went to Salem and there, waiting for him, was his false friend John Eldridge. The bedeviled colonizer, forgetting his mature Quaker principles, reverted to his cavalryman youth. He punched Eldridge in the nose and was at once arrested by the vigilant Andros soldiery. Back he went to New York and was again imprisoned. Soon thereafter the Duke of York stepped in to settle difficulties by abolishing Fenwick's claims to rule. In December, 1683, Fenwick died, leaving a will in which he named William Penn as one of his executors.

"None Here That Wants"

The Fenwick controversy failed to halt the settlement of other sections of New Jersey. John Ogilby, lord deputy of Ireland and a friend of Berkeley and Plowden, wrote a book in which he lauded the New Jersey shores. "If there be any terrestrial paradise to be had by any People, especially of any inferior rank, it must," he wrote, "certainly be here. . . . If there be any terrestrial Canaan, 'tis surely here, where the Land floweth with Milk and Honey."

The ship *Shield*, filled with Quaker passengers who were allured by Ogilby's promises, came to the Delaware in December, 1678. They dared not settle on the west bank, which was not in Berkeley's grant; they called at Salem, but the Fenwick titles were too much in dispute for them to make a permanent settlement. The ship stood up the Delaware, the first to venture high up that stream.

At Coaquanock, on the west bank, just above the confluence with the Schuylkill, they saw high bluffs topped with a spruce forest. As the *Shield* came tacking round a bend, close in to shore, its rigging tangled in the trees. Sailors set to work to disengage the spars, while passengers had leisure to examine the shores. One among them said, "This would be an excellent place for a town, if only it were on the Jersey side." The chance comment proved an admirable forecast; within four years the site was chosen as the place for Philadelphia to be founded.

The *Shield* sailed on still farther, to a place where wide, level plains gave promise of fertility, where creeks afforded access to the hinterland, and where a good-sized island offered protection against winter ice floes and spring freshets. Here the *Shield* was moored, and here Burlington was founded.

The plan of government, largely drawn by William Penn, was most farsighted. By a charter, called "Concessions and Agreements," the fundamental guarantees of liberty were granted. The rights of religious freedom, of free speech, and of petition, of trial by jury, and of the supremacy of fundamental charters over statutes were assured to colonists. Capital punishment was made illegal, even in the case of traitors. A popular assembly, serving for a year and holding open sessions, made all laws, with no veto to declare them invalid. Imprisonment for debt, that bane of England, was not permitted in the Burlington settlement. Byllynge,

Eldridge, Penn, and Warner, the guiding spirits of the colony, were wholly accurate when they declared, "We lay a foundation for after ages to understand their liberty as men and Christians, that they may not be brought in bondage . . . for we put the power in the people." These Concessions and Agreements are well called "the broadest, sanest, and most equitable charter draughted for any body of colonists up until this time."

Certainly the little colony flourished. Within a few months, the settlers were writing home in happiness: "Here wants nothing but people. There is not a poor body in the province, nor that wants; here is abundance of provisions; pork and beef at two pence a pound; fish and fowl plenty: Oysters I think would serve all England: . . . Cyder good and plenty, for one penny per quart: Good drink that is made of water and molasses, stands in about two shillings per barrel, wholesome like our eight shilling beer in England: Good venison plenty, brought us in at eighteen pence the quarter: Eggs at three pence per dozen: Vines, walnuts, peaches, strawberries, and many other things plenty in the woods."

Just why so calm and contented a colony should have need of laws against evildoers seems difficult to fathom, but the Assembly thought legislation necessary. To issue challenges, a matter alien to the Quakers, would incur six months' imprisonment in the new log jail, with a 10-pound fine to boot; no persons were to wear "pocket pistols, skeins, stilladers, daggers or dirks or other unusual weapons, save officers and strangers travelling upon lawful errands."

Honoring one's parents was a duty in New Jersey by the laws approved by the Assembly. "Undutiful children, smiting or cursing their father or mother, except provok'd thereunto for self-preservation . . .

should be punished with death." No child, evidently of whatever age, nor any servant, should presume to marry without consent of elders unless the banns were published long before. No person, irrespective of his age or sex, should "revel" after nine at night unless he was prepared to spend the night in jail. New Jersey's self-governing Assembly did not trust its people so freely as Penn might have wished, but the proprietaries had no right to veto any laws.

Twelve Mile Circle

Inspired by the success of Burlington, anxious to assist his fellow Quakers, William Penn petitioned for land whereon to plant another colony dedicated to political and religious freedom. His father, Admiral Sir William Penn, had lent about £16,000 to Charles II and had not pressed the needy monarch for repayment. To liquidate the debt, following the admiral's death, Penn proposed that territory on the Delaware be granted him, between the 40th and 42nd parallels, westward from the river five degrees.

As prices were then running, Penn's suggestions were welcome, for Penn, by canceling the debt, was paying at the rate of about a dollar per square mile for unexplored woodlands. In addition, he agreed to give a yearly tribute of two beaverskins and to grant as royalty to Charles one-fifth the value of any precious metals discovered in the province. Charles II did not know that this twenty per cent royalty on gold and silver would be a negligible sum, but neither did William Penn when he agreed to make the payments.

Lord Baltimore was not enthusiastic over Penn's request. The Maryland proprietor warmly argued that the entire west bank of the river belonged to him by virtue of his charter; even after Penn had founded Philadelphia, Lord Baltimore insisted that the town belonged to Maryland.

Nor was the Duke of York too pleased at having Penn for neighbor. In his three lower counties on the Delaware, held as an appendage of New York, the duke possessed a strategic post from which to control the trade of both New West Jersey and Pennsylvania. His agents clapped a ten per cent transport tax on all produce shipped on the river, but the Duke of York preferred that the Delaware's commerce be subordinated to New York interest. The establishment of a flourishing trade center on the upper river was far from pleasing.

Just how the duke was finally persuaded to transfer his land in Delaware to Penn is not entirely clear. Penn, it is known, went personally to appeal to James to ask him to agree to Charles II's grant of Pennsylvania, but what arguments were used has never been reported. They must have been potent, for James at first consented to have Penn receive some land, starting "at a point on a circle twelve miles north of New Castle," and then turned over his three lower counties to the Quaker.

The Twelve Mile Circle, thus created, produced legal complexities lasting to this day. Why it was originally drawn, at a twelve-mile radius from New Castle courthouse, is still a mystery, unless, as seems most probable, the Duke of York desired to keep the Quakers at a good, safe distance from his seat of government. Why, after the cession of the three lower counties to William Penn, the Circle was not replaced by a more reasonable straight line is equally obscure. It does not, like most boundaries, follow creek or crest of hill, it does not perpetuate the limits of ancient farms nor does it mark the course of ancient roads. The Twelve Mile Circle is as wholly artificial as any frontier ever drawn.

Moreover, it was not drawn accurately. Years after the first survey, more careful study made by better engineers disclosed slight variations, nothing of importance, to be sure, but just enough to throw calculations all askew.

Again, it was the Pennsylvania-Maryland boundary that was affected. By all calculations the line, as later drawn by Mason and Dixon, should have touched the Twelve Mile Circle; instead, a little wedge of land was found to lie between Maryland and Pennsylvania. By custom for years past, that land had been a part of Delaware; a state legislator living on the square mile or so of territory had, it is reported, voted to keep slavery in Delaware and his side had triumphed by a one-vote margin. When, in the late nineteenth century, surveyors running a more accurate Twelve Mile Circle, announced that this wedge was in Pennsylvania, the few residents revolted and demanded that they remain Delawareans. Again a slight adjustment was made in the running of the line. By flattening the circle at its top, enough compensation was afforded Pennsylvania to make up for loss of the small wedge. But all this was many years past the life time of William Penn.

Other, and far more important, boundary disputes arose from the duke's light gesture of keeping Quakers at a distance. If the Circle bounded Delaware and Pennsylvania, did it also mark the line between New Jersey and the three lower counties? Drawn at the time of the Fenwick controversies, when ownership to New West Jersey was in doubt, it might perhaps be possible that James, Duke of York, as overlord of both banks of the Delaware, intended to take over jurisdiction of the Fenwick lands. The Circle, if prolonged across the Delaware, would carve a huge slice out of Jersey, including all of Salem.

No one, in all probability, took such an extreme argument seriously, but Delaware was hotly to contend that, by this Twelve Mile Circle, she was entitled to ownership of all the river contained within its area, up to low-water mark on the Jersey shore. New Jersey, with equal heat, replied that no man in his senses would suppose that anyone would draw a boundary elsewhere than in the middle of a stream, or, at the most, midway of the channel. It was a long-drawn battle of skilled lawyers, carried, for more than a century, as Case No. 1 on the docket of the United States Supreme Court.

The matter was important, involving the right to fish for shad and sturgeon, which yielded hauls worth many thousand dollars, and it included the right to tax the wharves which had been pushed out beyond low-water mark on the Jersey shore. The output of the mighty Dupont plants at Carney's Point and Penns' Grove and the control of two important ferries, the only ones across the river south of Chester, were vitally affected by the court's decision. And the contest has not closed; while in 1924 a decision was handed down granting Delaware's contention, the Jersey experts are still clamoring for a reopening of the suit.

All this, one pauses to reflect, because a royal duke, more than a quarter of a millennium ago, idly thought a circle's arc would make a pretty boundary.

6

Penn's Holy Experiment

The Frame of Government

Poor William Penn is well-nigh a forgotten man; though many a Delaware valley institution takes his name to add gravity and weight by Penn's reputation, his authentic personality is now almost unknown. There is no juice in those conventional biographies which stress his sober qualities; official artists, who have depicted him when he was old and tired and spiritually exhausted, have done him a disservice. William Penn ranks now with the dry-as-dusts; he has been desiccated by well-meaning adulation.

To do him justice, William Penn was colorful and gay, hospitable and fond of worldly pleasure. He liked the luxuries of dress, especially the flowing periwigs that gave him curls that fell upon his shoulders and the sheer silk hose that well set off his calves. He drove to town behind a pair of spirited, blooded horses, consorted with lively company at tables that bore the best of food and drink; he sang a pleasant ballad and he danced with suppleness enough to make his capers long remembered. The handsome, dark-eyed young proprietor kept up with the latest modes; he watched the fashions closely that his beaver hat might possess "the true mayoral brim"; he flashed his silver buckles as he strode the sunny streets. Penn was a living proof that high ideals do not depend on blue-nosed Puritanism and that a governor who takes great pains to start a vineyard and a brewery may be wise and virtuous and, withal, remarkably efficient.

That Pennsylvania is the only state to bear its founder's name was none of William Penn's design. He struggled hard against the title, preferring to call his grant New Wales or, failing that, Sylvania, but the king was adamant. Desiring to honor the memory of Admiral Penn, Charles II insisted that the province be called Penn's Woods, or Pennsylvania. William Penn, the son, though he offered a twenty-guinea bribe to the engrosser of the charter to delete the Penn, "lest it should be looked on as a vanity in me," could not veto the king's command. To Penn's chagrin the charter, granted March 4, 1681, bears the name Pennsylvania, heavily emphasized with red-ink underscoring.

The three pages of strong parchment, fancifully illuminated with heraldic devices and bearing upon the first page a well-executed portrait of the king, made William Penn the "true and absolute proprietor" of his province, subject only to the proviso that all laws made there must be submitted within five years to the king for his approval. Within a month thereafter, Penn was promising to purchasers who would agree to pay ten cents an acre for blocks of 5,000 acres: "You shall be governed by laws of your own making, and live a free, and, if you will, a sober and industrious people. I shall not usurp the right of any, or oppress his person. God has furnished me with a better resolution, and has given me the grace to keep it." In this, he was thoroughly sincere; no one ever questioned his integrity, though certain of his agents were at times a bit too zealous in their salesmanship.

Probably the founder had learned much from his experiences with the colony at Burlington; certainly the "Frame of Government" for Pennsylvania was not so liberal as that provided in New Jersey. Moreover, events in Great Britain had not been favorable to extreme democracy, and Penn, though always a staunch believer in liberty and popular control, was politician enough to trim his sails to the prevailing winds. Had he been stiff-necked in such matters, he might not have won his charter. There would be, in the future, ample opportunity to grant additional concessions when the time grew favorable.

In Pennsylvania, therefore, Penn set up a government by landowners, administered by a governor himself or a deputy named by him for an indefinite term, and subject in every instance to proprietary control. The real power lay in the governor, who, aided by a council of seventy-two chosen for a seven years' term, prepared bills for submission to a general assembly and asked for its approval or rejection. The lower house elected annually, had power neither to debate nor to amend. Alteration in this Frame of Government was to be made only by the governor's consent and by approval of at least six-sevenths of both the Council and the General Assembly.

The Frame left much to be desired, so far as popular control is concerned; perhaps it was not wholly in accord with the generous promises made when Penn received his charter. But there are other clauses which redeem the Frame, such provisions as those protecting Pennsylvania against taxation not levied by vote of the Assembly, against star-chamber procedure, and against corruption on the part of officeholders. Penn's insistence upon the "virtuous education of youth," upon liberty of worship "for all who believe in God," and upon honest administration of justice was a century in advance of contemporary England.

The Frame was Pennsylvania's constitution and,

as such, dealt chiefly with broad principles. It is note-worthy, however, that included in the fundamental law were prohibitions of certain social sins. Swearing, lying, drunkenness, drinking of healths, obscenity, stage plays, cards, dice, masks, revels, and bullbaiting were specifically forbidden. So too, was any other deed out-lawed which might "excite the people to rudeness, cruelty, looseness and irreligion."

Penn had no fear that this Frame might too tightly circumscribe the freedom of his wards. He was con-vinced that "Any Government is free to the people under it, whatever be the Frame, where the laws rule and the people are a party to the laws."

The Half-faced Camp

The first arrivals to be brought to Pennsylvania under this new Frame came with Captain Smith in the ship *John and Sarah* late in 1681. They found no houses ready on the site provided for them at the high bluffs of Coaquanock, so they dug holes in the cliff, or hol-lowed out natural caves. Propping the roofs with trunks of fallen trees, building chimneys of stone and clay, these "half-faced camps" afforded shelter for the new arrivals. And one at least, the cave called "Penny Pot" provided a safe birthplace, for John Key, born here, carried the nickname "the First-Born" for all the eighty-five years of his life.

William Penn himself arrived, with a hundred Quaker friends from Sussex, on the 300-ton ship *Welcome* in October, 1682. He called first at New Castle, produced his deeds from James, Duke of York, and took possession, by the solemn delivery of "turf and twig and water and soyle," of the Delaware and its west bank. At Upland, now called Chester, the thirty-eight-year-old founder first touched Pennsylvania soil. Pausing here to issue a decree calling an election for the Council and Assembly, he went farther up the river to view the site for the new settlement which he proposed to call Philadelphia, city of Brotherly Love.

The little stream, Dock Creek, upon whose low and sandy beach Penn landed early in November, has long vanished from the Philadelphia scene. Like so many other creeks that in Penn's time cut their way across the grassy meadows and through the huckleberry patches, threading the dense oak woods of Philadelphia, Dock Creek has been arched over. The watercourse is part of Philadelphia's ancient sewer system.

Penn approved the site, and liked the products of his province. "The soil is good," he wrote a friend in England, "air serene and sweet from the cedar, pine and sassafras, with a wild myrtle of great fragrance. I have had better venison, bigger, more tender, and as fat as in England. Turkeys of the wood I had of forty and fifty pounds weight. Fish in abundance, especially shad and rock. Oysters are monstrous for bigness. In the woods are divers fruits, wild, and flowers that for colour, largeness and beauty, excel." He later was to like the peaches too,—"one may have them by bushels for little"—and, said he, "they make a pleasant drink." The Pennsylvania peach brandy, even then, was a beverage that could win friends.

Gabriel Thomas, who accompanied Penn and was to write an appreciation of the province that would put "Beauchamp Plantagenet" and John Ogilby both to shame as propagandists, was equally enthusiastic: "Though this country has made little noise in story, or taken up but small room on maps . . . I could say much in praise of this sweet tract of land. The air here is delicate, pleasant and wholesome; the heavens serene and rarely overcast. There are very fine thriving gardens and orchards. The gardens abound in grapes, tulips, pinks, carnations, roses, lilies, not to mention those that grow wild in the fields . . . There are strawberries, raspberries, peaches, pears, quinces, cherries, currants, watermelons, muskmelons and other fruits. In the woods there is abundance of red deer, wild animals for food, profit and game, and the sea is full of oysters, fish and delicious sea food."

Even the unpredictable Pennsylvania climate, with its extremes of heat and cold, seemed pleasant to the founder. Sharp, frosty weather continued almost constantly after the *Welcome's* arrival, but Penn enjoyed the winter. It was not, he proudly said, "foul, thick, black weather, as our northeast winds in England, but a sky as clear as in summer and the air dry, cold, piercing and hungry; yet I remember not that I wore more clothes than in England." The summer heat, which can sometimes be tropical and muggy, won his praise.

Every prospect pleased him, and, for a space, his colony dwelt in a perfect peace. The Assembly, held at Upland in December, 1682, approved his Frame, and, with the guidance of the Council, passed laws to put it into complete effect. Political and religious freedom were accorded to all who professed belief in God and who observed the Christian Sunday, a grant which, in the complete absence of atheists and Jews, gave liberty to all the colonists. Some punishments were made more rigorous than Penn might have wished, such as condemning adulterers to life imprisonment for their second offense or making polygamy punishable by hard labor for life, but, on the whole, the Assembly and the Council followed enlightened Quaker ideas of penology.

For the first year or two both Pennsylvania and the three lower counties of Delaware enjoyed halcyon days.

St. Tammany of Shackamaxon

Penn was particularly careful to cultivate good relations with the Indians. He looked on them not only as aborigines toward whom civilized white men owed social responsibility, but also as a race peculiarly set apart for Quaker friendship. To Penn, as to most of the other Quakers of the province, the Indians were a chosen people. Their swarthy skin, "the make of their figures," their religious observances, combined to convince the Quakers that the Indians were the true descendants of the Ten Lost Tribes of Israel. "They observe new moons; they offer their first fruits to a Maneto, or supposed Deity, whereof they have two, one, as they fancy, above (good); another below (bad); and have a kind of feast of tabernacles, laying their altars upon twelve stones, observe a sort of mourning twelve months, customs of women, and many other rites."

The chain of proof to link the Hebrews and the Indians was weak, indeed, but Quakers were not scientific anthropologists. Superficial similarities were quite enough to satisfy the curious and so, perhaps, to give to the Lenni-Lenape, the natives of the Delaware, a status of importance. Penn was proud that within his province he possessed the scions of the ancient Israelites; because of this, no doubt, he gave them far more generous treatment than even his warm, fair-minded, character had hitherto judged necessary. When, as Brother Onas, he was adopted by the tribe, Penn's pride was filled to overflowing. He repaid the honor by donating to the Lenni-Lenape a camping ground on which chiefs coming down to Philadelphia might always tether their horses and pitch their tents. The site, now smoothly cemented over, is still reserved in central Philadelphia, an open oasis, complete with hitching posts for ponies, in the fashionable Walnut Street shopping district. No Indian, it is sad to note, has camped there for a generation.

Prior to Penn's arrival, his agents had already purchased land along the Delaware, paying for it 350 fathoms of white wampum, a score each of blankets, guns, coats, shirts, and stockings, 40 axes and an equal number of scissors, 200 knives and a double-handful of fishhooks. To celebrate the sale, the Indians were to have 17 gallons of rum, together with much beer and cider, with 200 small glasses to drink it from; in addition, they were to get 300 guilders in small coins to jingle in their pockets. The arrangements were quite finished, but Penn desired to ratify the purchase by a formal conference in person with the Lenni-Lenape chiefs.

Penn's proposal delighted the Indians. The tribe, it may be said, was in disgrace, for brother Indians looked down upon the Lenni-Lenape as weak and ineffectual, and as a people subject to the mighty Iroquois Confederacy. In scorn, the Five Nations who comprised that great confederation referred to the Delawares as "women" and, though they courteously called them "grandfathers" in token of their longer residence, the Iroquois had slight regard for Delaware achievements. To have William Penn single out the Lenni-Lenape for special honor restored self-respect to Indians who dwelt along the Delaware.

In 1683, therefore, Penn and his Quaker Council met the great chiefs of the Lenni-Lenape. Customarily, the site is said to be at Shackamaxon, then half a mile above the city, near the riverbank. There, under a great tree, the famous Penn Treaty Elm, everlasting and unbroken faith was pledged between the white men and the Indians. The treaty was so rigorously observed, during the Quaker rule in Pennsylvania, that Voltaire referred to it as one "never sworn to, and never broken." Penn's statue, on top of the Philadelphia City Hall—one of the few statues of the founder in any portion of Penn's domain—faces Shackamaxon.

Later scholarship has questioned whether Shackamaxon really was the site of Penn's great treaty, but that such a council met and that a lasting understanding was agreed upon is indisputable. The wampum belt that sealed the ceremony is preserved by the Historical Society of Pennsylvania. With more ample justice, critics also doubt the accuracy of the famous painting of the scene, made by the Quaker artist, Benjamin West, court painter to George III, for West included numerous anachronisms in his canvas. At thirty-nine, William Penn was surely not a corpulent old man in broad-brimmed hat and snuff-colored, shadbelly coat. Rather, by contemporary evidence, he was agile and athletic, fond of leaping and dancing in the Indian assemblies, given to a nice taste in hats and wigs.

Tradition varies, too, concerning the precise date on which the famous treaty was concluded. West's unhistoric painting, showing trees in full summer leaf, follows the accepted date of June 23rd; other legends name May Day as the time when the Indians and Quakers proclaimed their lasting friendship. All reports are in accord, however, on the personality of the leading figure among the Indians.

This chief, destined to become more famous as the years elapsed, was Tammany, or Tamend, whose name means affable, and who was described as "in the highest degree endowed with wisdom, virtue, prudence, charity, meekness, hospitality; in short, with every good and noble qualification that a human being may possess." So friendly was he and so pleased with William Penn, that at the famous conference he sold Penn lands for "so much wampum and other goods as Penn shall please to give."

Tammany in later years became a patron figure not only of the folk along the Delaware, but of the whole United States. His votaries, on May Day of each year, paraded through the city streets with bucktails in their hats, to voice their scorn of all aristocrats. St. Tammany, sanctified by the proletariat, was set up in contrast to the well-born Englishmen, who honored their St. George, and the Welsh and Scots, who praised St. David and St. Andrew. To many of the revolutionists against the British, St. Tammany was a sacred symbol of freedom, justice, and fair dealing. The Great Saint of the Bucktails, whose grave is by a spring some distance west of Doylestown, north of Philadelphia, was made the democratic patron. When parties rose in free America, St. Tammany was widely hailed as leader of the Jeffersonians.

Penn's haste to have his province quickly peopled brought in a diverse population. English-speaking Quakers, who made up the first migration, were soon outnumbered by later immigrants. Soon after the Shackamaxon Treaty, versatile young Francis Daniel Pastorius, master of seven languages, learned as a professor in law, theology and science, medicine, agriculture, history and poetry, land agent and religious leader, came with a band of Germans to set up a community, at Germantown, five miles from Philadelphia. It was the origin of a settlement that was to have enormous influence, from which the first protest against slavery was to issue, in 1688, and which was to be, for a brief period after the Revolution, the capital of the United States. Pastorius settled here to form an earthly paradise where, surrounded by his scores of beehives, he might write a veritable encyclopedia of all knowledge.

Such men were closely kin to Penn in social-mindedness. Like Penn, these pacifistic Germans hated war and strove for peace and justice. Living in a distant settlement, with almost complete self-government, they asked only for the right to lead their own lives quietly.

Especially, they prized isolation. At Germantown laws forbade newcomers to buy land until they had been properly introduced and found acceptable. No private citizen was to entertain a transient guest and none, except an approved traveler, was to be admitted to an inn after nine-o'clock curfew. Pastorius was fearful of all strangers, remembering, no doubt, the anarchy and chaos of the postwar Germany from which his friends had fled. Later, when the friendliness and peace of the Delaware settlements was more thoroughly appreciated, these isolation laws were canceled.

Responding to Penn's plea for population, twenty-three ships, laden with Germans, Welsh, and Englishmen, entered Philadelphia harbor within a year after the city was established. Not all were pacifists, nor Quakers, but all were heartened and inspired by Penn's widely publicized desire "to afford asylum to the good and oppressed of every nation": "I aimed," he said, "to frame a government which might be an example. I desired to show men as free and happy as they could be."

7

Shattering an Ideal

Testy Judge More

Not even the governor could pull Nick More out of bed at seven in the morning. Everyone, including the governor, was well aware that anyone who bothered Judge More's rest would get a scathing tongue-lashing that would sear the skin away. The old chief justice, stubborn and irascible, insisted on his ease.

The governor, however, had been put in an embarrassing position. Penn had sent him to be intermediary between the popular Assembly and the proprietary officers, and Penn expected him to act with justice and diplomacy toward both groups. The task was hard, indeed, especially when More swore at the Assembly, cursing it for its stupidity, damning it for passing "cursed laws," and scorning its authority. Even staid, slow-minded Quakers could not stand an unlimited amount of More's haughty arrogance; the popular Assembly, taking mean advantage of More's absence from the session, called upon the governor to remove Chief Justice More from office.

But More, for some unfathomable reason, stood in well with William Penn. There was, it seems, no reason why he should, for certainly Chief Justice Nicholas More was not cut from the same high-principled patterns as the founder. Nicholas More voted "no" to everything that the Assembly wanted and was the antithesis of William Penn.

Sometimes high idealists, naïvely accepting others at their own face value, eagerly believing that all men are as selfless as themselves, are fooled through their own optimism. Certainly the founder was deceived in Nicholas More. Incapable of guile himself, Penn could not realize that those who spoke fair words were sometimes tricksters, if not charlatans. He trusted Nicholas More so much that the man was sent to Pennsylvania with instructions that made him almost a master of the province, for More was simultaneously named to be chief justice, councilman, assemblyman, and speaker.

Such was the powerful figure whom the Assembly, by unanimous vote of all members present, called upon the governor to dismiss from office. It was a ticklish moment for the governor: if he obeyed the Assembly's wish, he might antagonize the founder; if he failed to heed the vote of the Assembly, he might himself be subject to impeachment for neglect of duty.

His decision was an inspiration. Anxious to observe the proper legal forms, the governor made matters as difficult as possible. The Assembly would, he said, be granted opportunity to press its charge against Chief Justice More provided they could get him into court at seven in the morning.

The Assembly, also, was to bring along Chief Justice More's official records as evidence of their complaints, but here it struck another snag. More flatly refused to surrender any documents to those he called "persons of seditious spirit." In fact, he said, there were no records, a whopping lie to which his loyal clerk, Patrick Robinson, nodded an assent. Then, when Robinson was taken to another room and was told that if there were no records all the court officials could be clapped in jail, the clerk broke down and admitted that More had really kept some minutes of proceedings, though they were written in a Latin shorthand "which no person could read but More himself, no, not even an angel from Heaven."

Robinson was worthy of his dictatorial master. Like Nicholas More, he scorned the whole Assembly as a group of windbags. When John White, leader of the anti-More proceedings, blustered to compel the clerk to disclose the secrets of the courts, Pat Robinson turned on his heel and stalked away. Ten minutes later, he came back with the sheriff, seized White, and locked him up. The Assembly, outraged at the affront to its dignity, called for troops to get its leader out of prison. By threats and force, the legislators freed White from his cell.

Robinson remained undaunted. When White had gone home that night, Robinson again joined forces with the sheriff. They broke down John White's door, dragged him from his bed, and cast him into jail again. When seven o'clock came, and the hearings were to be held on the motion to impeach Chief Justice More the Assembly leader was still in prison.

More also was absent, nor were his Latin shorthand minutes available as evidence. The Council and the governor, secretly relieved, dismissed the charges, though the Assembly had prepared in haste a three-page accusation charging More of twisting testimony, of badgering juries, and of "using severall contemptuous and derogatory expressions." These were not looked upon as sufficiently damning to justify removing More from office.

The failure of this first impeachment trial in American history, and the overriding of the Assembly's wishes, widened the breach between the branches of the proprietary government. Had Penn been present, his soothing personality and his quiet tact would certainly have brought some proper compromise, but Penn was still in England, fighting charges that he was a "self-devoted slave to despotism," a rebel plotting to restore the Stuarts, and an insolvent debtor. Not until 1699 was Penn able to get back to the Delaware.

He found his colony materially prosperous but politically disordered. The three lower counties, jealous of the more rapid progress of the upper section, were clamoring for freedom. Pennsylvania, they declared, was Penn's pet because he held proprietary rights to it while they, less closely linked, were treated as stepchildren. To keep the peace, Penn recognized the secession of the province of Delaware. He gave the new colony its own legislature, though he continued to assign his agents as governors of both Delaware and Pennsylvania.

Drabness Disappears

Penn did not sense that, underneath the calm serenity of Quaker life, a revolution was beginning. Costumes were blossoming. Girls were brave in display of black velvet petticoats, embroidered with gold and silver, under their gold and purple gowns. Green silk stockings and fine morocco shoes were common. Staider Quaker ladies, who dared not indulge in color, did much with silk and lace and hidden ribbons. And if they could not flaunt the powdered periwigs of English maids in waiting nor ape the huge wire-stiffened "frontages" that were veritable muslin pagodas, they could slant their demure bonnets in a way to shock the sober graybeards.

The days were passing, too, when men wore dove-gray, knee-length coats. Young bloods, seeking nattier, more modern styles, were gay in satins, deep-laced, with gold and silver ornaments. Crimson and sky blue, salmon, cinnamon, and plum gave color to the drawing rooms; to the horror of the older Friends, small swords were glistening. Parents grumbled, as in the everlasting way of outraged age, but style could no more be controlled than Canute's sea.

The old regime was dying on the Delaware. Disciplines, developed in the days when Quakers were comparatively carefree, proved ill-adapted for governing a province overseas. Friends who had in England cheerfully evaded cares and had pleasantly picked to pieces the policies of overlords were now confronted by reality. Like every opposition come to power, they soon learned that administration is both a headache and an art. Pacifism was possible on an island where a strong navy and a well-trained veteran army held off invasion, but nonresistance would spell death on the frontier. The Quakers found that it was much easier passively to submit in England to a dominant group of determined Presbyterians and Anglicans than to try in America to rule them by nonviolent coercion.

Not only was the revolution visible in clothes; virtually all the ways of life along the river were affected. Fine foods and little luxuries were seen in richer Quaker houses. Gracious living supplanted the traditional plain fare. As fathers gained more worldly wealth, the Quaker homes were made more livable. Penn's manor on the Delaware, his great estate at Pennsbury, became a model for the better city houses. Costly silver, chastely ornamented in that simple style which sometimes is a boast of wealth, fine porcelains, rich tapestries, and heavy rugs appeared in Quaker homes. Few Philadelphians could match the gorgeous twelve-oared barge in which the proprietor was wont to travel, as befits a governor, when he came down the Delaware, but rank deserves some perquisites, and Philadelphians preferred to keep their splendor within doors.

Even in modes of speech the transformation could be traced. While the use of "thee" and "thou" remained, caution was now displayed to use these Quaker pronouns only with one's fellow Quakers. Toward all others, the once scorned "you" might be employed, though always with a certain overtone which, in less well-bred folk, might be construed as aristocratic condescension. Little Quaker boys, effectively forbidden to use evil language toward their playmates, mildly cursed their friends by calling them "You *you*."

Eventually, to be sure, the breakdown of discipline would have its terrible effect upon the Quaker sect. Even in the early days of Queen Anne's reign certain of the weaker Friends had swung far from orthodox tradition and the more prosperous were creeping back, unobtrusively, into the arms of the forgiving Church of England. More were to follow; in time, the sons of the proprietor were to give up their Quakerism and become Episcopalians.

The apostates were a minority, but a minority that was to strengthen with the years. While the Quakers were dividing, their opponents waxed in power. That very openhandedness with which the Quakers welcomed all the peoples of the earth brought in great waves of immigrants, not all of whom were of the same high caliber as Penn's comrades of the *Welcome*.

Contempt for law and order was increasing. The ordinances were being disregarded. Tobacco smoking in the streets, once regarded as peculiarly heinous, had become so common, in spite of fines supposed to be laid against it, that even the highly placed were guilty. Luke Watson, one of the county justices, dared to smoke while court was in session, and when remonstrance by his brother judges was of no avail, he was fined fifty pounds of tobacco. Even this did not restrain his appetite. On the same day a second fine of a hundred additional pounds of tobacco had to be imposed.

The courts were evidently having trouble in maintaining proper decorum. William Bradford swore in their presence and was reprimanded; Thomas Hasellum was fined for "singing and making a noise," though the records do not say whether this was one or two offenses; Thomas Jones, a hardened character who would not keep the peace, stuck spurs into the legs of bailiffs who annoyed him, and kicked the sheriff in the mouth. His crime had been "cursing the justices at a horrible rate."

More grievous sins were committed. Three men debased the coinage and were punished by having to replace each counterfeit found in the province with a good coin of standard silver. One Robert Roman practiced geomancy and had his mystic library confiscated. Pirates were reported off Cape Henlopen; there were rumors that good Quaker citizens were agents for the infamous Captain Kidd.

Piracy was particularly abhorred. As soon as Kidd's presence was discovered, the Assembly passed a law forbidding trade with every port of bad repute. Among the measures passed was one interdicting trade with "Madagascar and Natoll." The Assembly, it seems, had no notion where "Natoll" might lie, but the measure was adopted on vague rumor that it lay near Madagascar.

Not even jails were safe. Two men arrested for piracy were reported to be strolling around Philadelphia. Wroth at the laxity, the Assembly called in the warden of the prison. His reply to questioning was illuminating. "They never go out of jail," he said, "without my leave and a keeper, which, I think, may be allowed in hot weather."

The people were not blending. Half a century after Penn's arrival, the population was not homogeneous; indeed, it was growing more diverse. New England, and Virginia, by rigid regulation of both church and state, had kept a kind of uniformity among their residents; the Delaware settlements were but a hodgepodge of nationalities, of religions, and of languages. More than a thousand Welsh and Swedes still used their native speech; the Hollanders, though a trifle more elastic of tongue, conversed together in Dutch; Palatines knew nothing but Low German. The Assembly sessions were often Babel towers of strange jargon.

We praise today, and rightly, the Quaker toleration, but there many then thought the Quaker methods a mistake. Persecution is not pretty, and the people of the Delaware are pleased that there was never any bigotry on that stream, but it is possible that Quakers might have been a bit more rigid in their regulations. Instead of stepping to the fore to give some guidance to the divergencies that were appearing, Quakers drew themselves into a sort of shell. Faced with the problem of discordant minorities, they showed an etiquette that betrayed the feminine shyness of those who wanted to be loved but dared not display their eagerness. Inwardly passionate to be helpful, the Quakers, burdened by a reserve that hardened into formalism, were more stiff than courteous, more cold than welcoming. The immigrants, misconstruing this shyness, regarded Friends as either too weak to take a hand or as too snobbish to be bothered.

Thanks to the tolerant spirit, the new arrivals caused but slight concern. Those German pacifists, the Mennonites, Moravians, and strange Schwenkfelders were akin to Quakers in belief. All held similar concepts of righteousness; none were meddlesome in the affairs of others; none would bear aggressive arms, nor would any take an oath. At first all were quiet, peaceful folk who moved sedately to frontiers, not to grab the land from Indians, but for the purer purpose of seeking sanctuary from the world.

Some were odd-appearing, it is true, like the vegetarian Dunkers whose black beards hung raggedly over their long white gowns, who abhorred worldliness—some of them thought buttons sinful—and communed with spirits. Rough mountaineers, fled from war-torn Germany, drifted aimlessly along the city streets, wide-eyed and wondering, their wooden clogs clattering noisily on the cobbles. There was no spring to their step, for these were sickly, half-starved refugees worn down by weeks of hardship. Tricked into giving their slender resources for a portion of their passage money, promising to work for seven years to pay off the remainder, these unfortunates had undergone unbelievable privations. Many of those who started had already perished from ship fever; many more had starved to death. One shipload came to Pennsylvania after feeding for a week on nothing but the ship's rats. Now that they had come to the promised land where all was peace and plenty, they found themselves almost in slavery to the "soul-drivers" who had bought their time.

Not all the river residents sought inward light by silent meditation as did the Dunkers, the Moravians, the Quakers, and the Mennonites. Not all the settlers were dreamy mystics who sought salvation in the wilderness. Not all the people of the Delaware agreed that private contemplation could bring each mortal into a direct and personal knowledge of God's will. The Quaker theory that a man might win perfection on this earth and free himself completely of all sin was heresy to certain of the settlers.

Raw-boned, red-haired Scotch-Irishmen, blustering and quick to fight, most certainly no converts to passive resistance, poured into the valley of the Delaware, though most of them tarried no longer than to enjoy a spree or two before pressing onward to the free frontier. Delicate-looking, though tough and hardy, Welshmen took up lands just west of Penn's fair, green, country town, where they began a century of protest that they had been brought to Pennsylvania under false pretenses. The clamor of the Welsh for their rights continued long beyond the Revolution, though they checked their indignation against Penn for long enough to fire a shot or two against their ancient enemies, the English.

These, certainly, were no mystics. Few German Lutherans, Welsh Baptists, or Scotch-Irish Presbyterians were convinced of the desirability of full liberty of conscience. Not even all the Anglican communicants, for all their cherished breadth of mind, were anxious to defend another's point of view.

The Quakers were in difficulties. So long as the Delaware had been peopled by the righteous, the magistrates had had slight trouble in their governing; now that the colony was filling with materialistic folk who came for gain and not primarily for God, the gentle admonition of mild Quaker officers had little weight. New evils were arising. Excited horsemen celebrated the semiannual fairs by racing down the crowded city streets; swearing, strictly outlawed by city ordinance, was prevalent; lotteries were being started; within the very prison walls a rumshop was discovered. But these could be the target for legislation and could be controlled, if not prevented. Even though the Quaker strength was lessening, and though the more liberal-minded city sophisticates were coming into more and more importance, there was slight fear that Pennsylvania would become another Restoration England.

The fundamental problem was more serious. Although in theory the valley of the Delaware was a Quaker commonwealth where Penn was sole proprietor, yet, by his very liberality, the non-Quakers had assumed aggression. Imbued by the passion of religious wars in Europe, many of them sought to correct the evils which they thought inherent in the Quaker rule. Even to the tolerant Church of England folk, the Quakers were anathema; full, they said, of "many notions, of wicked and damnable principles."

Against such criticism, the Quaker armory was weakest. Trained as a minority of holiness, the Quakers glorified the right of independent thought; peace-loving, they abhorred the use of force. Europe marveled at the temerity of men who set up a realm where speech was free and where the ruling powers scorned to crush opponents. True to their principles, though they knew that their opponents fought with no spiritual swords, the helpless Quakers could do little but watch the growth of violent insubordination.

The Hot Church Party

Serious disturbance was afoot in Pennsylvania. Through errors of the Quaker magistrates, the first petition for a Church of England parish was not only denied, but was answered by the jailing of the Anglicans who had ventured to present the plea. It was the first, and the only important, violation of religious freedom, and it drew heavy condemnation from the proprietor and from all right-thinking Friends. The mistake was remedied at once. Christ Church was established; but the angry Anglicans were never wholly reconciled.

There was, no doubt, much cause for complaint. By Quaker doctrine, the Delaware could never be defended. No militia could be sent against the Indians, no guns set up to keep off pirates, no safety could be guaranteed against the ill-disposed. Not even civil justice would be possible, the churchmen reasoned, for, if oaths were illegal, there could be no fear of supernatural intervention when a witness lied on the stand. Fraud, perjury, and chicane would be unrestrained.

The Anglicans, soon dubbed the "Hot Church party," had other reasons for their hatred of the Friends. Judge Robert Quarry, head of the Admiralty Court, and as such the special agent of the throne, saw deep into the future. From his experience as royal governor of Carolina, and from his simultaneous service on the councils of five different provinces, he realized the inefficiency and wastefulness of local rule. Ultimately, he foresaw, the scattered colonies must all unite; failing this, he hoped as a preliminary step to merge Pennsylvania, Delaware, New Jersey, and New York into one great province, lying between the unified regions of New England and the South. The Hot Church party seemed an excellent agency to further his design.

Colonel Quarry was an able propagandist. In his reports to London, he recited not only the bare bones of admiralty practice, but added, for the ear of Queen Anne, all the other numerous incidents which smacked to him of treason. Cleverly, he secured Queen Anne's permission to insist that, while the Quaker scruples as to oaths should be religiously observed, all other litigants, and all officers, should swear the customary loyalty.

This was a master stroke, for the Quakers were

thereby hung upon the horns of a dilemma. If, as representatives of the proprietor, they would not give the
oath to others, then they were ineligible for Queen
Anne's service; indeed, they put themselves, so far as
scarlet-robed Colonel Quarry was concerned, among the
traitors to the realm. But if, forswearing their Quaker
principles, they gave the oaths as Anne commanded,
they ran the risk of being read out of Quaker meeting.
There was the easier way of letting others hold the
offices, but then they played directly into Quarry's
hand for thus the Hot Church party legally assumed
the running of the province. Penn would have advised
that Quakers quietly ignore the law, on the constitutional ground that Queen Anne had no right to issue
such decrees, but Penn was not in Pennsylvania, and the
officials had to make their own decisions.

The transfer of New Jersey from a proprietary to
a royal colony furthered Quarry's scheme. He and his
Hot Church friends, supported by the ablest lawyers,
assumed the leadership of what they carefully called the
Popular party, and invited the support of all non-
Quaker groups. It was another master stroke, for thus
the hot-blooded frontiersmen who thought the Quakers
cowards, the militant Protestants who wanted no free
thought for others, the imperialists who preferred a
British Empire to a set of scattered semi-independent
proprietorships, and all disgruntled people of the Delaware would be united.

Had Colonel Quarry been successful in thus amal-
gamating every anti-Quaker faction, the Penn experiment could not have long endured. Nor was it wholly
Quarry's fault that he did not succeed. His sniping was
so accurate, his propaganda so effective, that William
Penn was on the point of selling out his rights. If only
he could be rid of Quarry, Penn declared, he would

resign his charter to the crown, provided only that he be reimbursed for the £12,000 expended on the province.

At this point the Quakers had two great strokes of luck. One, most unhappy in every other respect, was the illness of the founder, making him for a time incapable of conducting his affairs. Negotiations for the sale of Pennsylvania were postponed indefinitely. The other, and perhaps decisive, factor was the personality of the man who would, if Quarry's scheme succeeded, take over the administration of the river.

Unhappily for Quarry's Hot Church crowd, the royal representative was not a winsome character. As governor of New Jersey and New York, Edward Hyde, Lord Cornbury, had made himself disliked. His graft, his drunkenness, even his misrule might easily have been overlooked, but there was another element in the Cornbury character which repelled the people. Any other royal governor might have welded the discordant groups whom Quarry courted, but Cornbury was impossible. Not even the resourceful Colonel Quarry could deodorize the man.

Lord Cornbury, cousin to Queen Anne, was blessed with an extraordinary facial resemblance to his sovereign. With such advantages, it was not difficult for him to believe that, as personal representative of the monarch, he owed a duty to her subjects to let them gaze upon her image. On pleasant evenings, therefore, the eccentric governor strolled on the ramparts of his residence to act the role of queen.

His performance was highly realistic. Gowned in rich, green silk, with bands of golden patterns appliquéd about the broad circumference of the dress, with a flounce of gold lace looped back to show a lace-fringed underskirt, Lord Cornbury played the queen. His stomacher, gold banded like the skirt, was stiff and high, the full sleeves laced below the elbow as a match for his high lace frontage headdress. Long streamers hanging from the frontage fluttered in the summer breezes. He was a veritable image of a royal queen.

The strait-laced burghers did not like the masquerade, nor did they approve his pinchpenny device of making callers pay admission to his presence. And when Cornbury announced himself as hostile to the Presbyterian beliefs, the cumulative opposition to his rule became intense. Delaware and Pennsylvania would have none of him. The Hot Church party plans collapsed.

Quarry's machinations were thereby halted for a time, but discord was not ended. So long as Penn and his sons remained good Quakers, the governors and appointed officers administered the Delaware in Quaker fashion, though the upcountry Scotch-Irish regularly returned anti-Quaker members to the legislatures. Bickerings and misunderstandings marked the progress of the province, while canny Quakers, sensing that a union of their foes would wrest control from the proprietors, carefully played one minority against another.

Such was the situation when, in 1699, Penn returned from England after a fifteen years' absence. He set himself to try to bring back peace. Living in his stately manor house at Pennsbury, on a wide creek off the Delaware above the site of Burlington, he did his best to preserve his province.

Now that King James was gone, more freedom could be granted. The old necessity for compromise was no longer felt, but at the same time it seemed desirable for Penn to tighten his own grip upon the government, lest conflicting interests destroy the great experiment.

The Frame of Government was modified. A new

council of ten men, replacing the former unwieldy
group of seventy-two, was created, and Penn reserved
the right to dismiss any of them at his pleasure. This
was a desperate device to keep control in Quaker hands,
and it was destined to cause continued opposition down
to the Revolutionary War. But Penn believed that his
principles of freedom would be unaffected and that his
beloved tolerance for religious difference, his prized
freedom of speech and thought, and the rights of individual liberty would remain. He hoped that the melt-
ing-pot experiment, anticipatory of a more national
assimilation of diverse races and of strange ideas, would
continue to move forward to success.

Penn was happy during his two-year stay at Pennsbury; in spite of constant bickering with his officials,
affairs ran smoothly. No less than nineteen councils
with the Indians were held there to cement good relations between the province and the savages. But in the
autumn of 1701 Penn was called away again. Strong
demands in England for the abolition of all proprietary
governments demanded his attention. The Penn family,
including the newborn John Penn, "the American,"
went back to England. Penn was never to return.

From London, Penn sent young John Evans, brilliant Welsh courtier, to act as governor. With him
came William Penn, Jr., only son of Penn's first marriage. The partnership was not a happy one for Pennsylvania, for Evans was more devoted to royalism than
to Quakerism, and neither he nor young Penn was as
grave and dignified as sober Quakers wished.

Evans was sure that Quakers were pretenders. He
did not credit their sincerity in their aversion to war
preparations. On one occasion, desiring to procure a
grant of money for defense, he bribed some New Castle
acquaintances to send word that twelve French priva-

teers were heading up the river. Then, riding through the Philadelphia streets, sword drawn, he summoned the inhabitants to defend themselves. Panic spread throughout the city. Many Quakers threw their plate and other valuables into the wells; others took to their boats to flee up the creeks for safety. None of them abandoned pacifistic principles.

Worse scandal spread when Penn and Evans were caught in a raid on an inn. The watch, drawn by a midnight fracas, burst into the tavern to suppress disorder. Young Penn tried to shoot the officers. He was badly beaten in the affray, but the governor quashed all proceedings against the disturbers of the peace. He also protected Penn against moralists who objected to his association with his "half wife," Lady Jenks, who rode with him on fox hunts "in men's clothes." The open flouting of good morals by Penn, the governor, and Lady Jenks caused much grief to the Quakers and to the founder. The errant governor was recalled to England. Young William followed, and soon died.

8

"To Keep the Quakers Quiet"

Young Ben Franklin

ON A Sunday morning in October, 1723, a tired and lanky boy, dirty-faced and with his working clothes stuffed out with shirts and stockings, strolled wide-eyed up Market Street in Philadelphia. Young Ben Franklin, seventeen years old, and already a poet, a printer, and a good newspaperman, had come to the town where he was henceforth to be famous.

He found the little, tree-shaded Philadelphia, which Penn had planned to be a fair, green, country town, growing to maturity; its straight, too-narrow streets, cutting each other at uncompromising right angles, were filled with strangers like himself. New people were arriving: some, like himself, on the packets that brought visitors from New York and the north; others, riding into the city over the rough trails that led south, came to take up jobs as carpenters and masons, farmers and lumbermen. Every ship poured in a load of immigrants, from England, from Ulster, and from Germany. Philadelphia, as Franklin saw the city, was a cosmopolitan metropolis, a busy site of arts and crafts, of trades and manufacture.

He came in contact, too, with diplomats and politicians. Such men as Johann Conrad Weiser, who knew more about the Iroquois than any other man alive, bustled into town to talk with old Shikellamy, the ambassador of the Five Nations. Agents of the French and even of the Spanish paid fleeting calls on the Pennsylvania governor, seeking, no doubt, to allay Quaker fears at foreign encroachments close to Pennsylvania's borders. Messengers raced back and forth to carry letters to the administrators of New Jersey and New York. The Philadelphia streets were bustling places.

Had Franklin come a decade earlier he would have gained a readier acceptance. Now that the population was so swelled, residents had no time for such fine courtesies as in the past. Strangers were no longer warmly welcomed on arrival. Even within Philadelphia's own social circles times had changed. Fathers of brides felt no necessity for entertaining wedding guests for two full days, nor for providing them with abundant meals or serving them strong punch at quarter-hour intervals. For all his stress on thrift, Ben Franklin would have relished these old-time customs.

Frivolity and worldliness, unknown, according to the carping old graybeards, in the time of William Penn, had taken hold of Philadelphia. Up in Boston the young printer had been told that Philadelphia was a place of gravity and decorum; instead, he found a thrilling town where young men were learning to speak French, where dancing was encouraged, and where light music was to be heard in every fashionable drawing room. Wealth had brought leisure, and leisure had given birth to culture, if not to sophistication.

None of this, however, was available to ambitious young apprentices, nor even to those who had already won a reputation in Boston journalism. Franklin, not in the least envious of the socially elect, sought outlet for his energies. Practically minded, motivated by that healthy curiosity that sends the world ahead, the young printer delved deep into experiment. Gathering about him a society of like-minded youths, some apprentices, others young businessmen, a few enterprising scholars, Franklin made himself the center of a dynamic circle. He himself invented a new stove, better and more economical than any that had preceded it; he built an artificial arm and hand to help him reach a longer distance without rising from his comfortable armchair; he formed a club, the Junto, "for mutual improvement," which was at once "an intelligence office and star chamber, a business protective union and an inquisition, a gossip club and a propagator of political opinion, a whispering gallery and a society of savants." Though young Ben Franklin was not a member of the inner circle of society, he soon knew more than any of his contemporaries about what was really happening in Pennsylvania. His Junto would, in time, become the American Philosophical Society, the most learned of American associations.

The insatiable Franklin energy was inexhaustible. Through his inspiration, Philadelphia gained a circulating library, a fire company, and a college, but what was more than all the material organizations acquired through Franklin's leadership, it won a point of view. Quakers, who had once considered isolation the most desirable type of life, now learned that social intercourse is civilizing. The city, under Franklin's steady pressure, gained a reputation for humanitarian ideals; it started hospitals and revolutionized the care of poor folk and demented persons; it instituted social betterments. Philadelphia became mature, largely under Franklin's skillful tutelage.

Lonely John Bartram, who loved strange plants, won recognition now that Franklin praised his efforts, and Philadelphians who once smiled to think of Bartram's wanderings subscribed a fund to make it possible for him to travel. Local physicians and lawyers were widely recognized as masters of their art; Philadelphians proudly pointed out that when there was a great case in New York, like Peter Zenger's trial for libel, only Philadelphia could provide a lawyer wise enough to be entrusted with the case.

The Franklin spirit made the town a happy settlement, proud of its free speech, proud of its experiments in science, pleased with its intellectual leadership. There was disappointment, to be sure, that culture had not spread beyond the city's limits, but missionary work would soon be undertaken there.

Witchcraft and Murder

Outside the city, the province was not peaceful. A succession of bad winters and burning summers, coupled with epidemics of smallpox and ship fever brought in, it was alleged, by overcrowded immigrant vessels, produced discontent. Frontiersmen felt themselves neglected by the city people. Countrymen, though they disregarded laws requiring them to pay for land, and stirred up trouble with the Indians, complained that Quaker legislators paid no heed to their appeals.

Riotous hillmen, deep in debt, fell ready victims to that siren craze which always captivates the poor. Almost spontaneously, from several quarters, came loud demands for paper money. Lobbyists poured down to threaten the Assembly, causing so much disturbance and terrifying the lawmakers so continuously that the Riot Act was read against them. Two of the chief troublemakers were compelled to crave forgiveness on their knees, but the Assembly, still shaking, passed a bill to issue some £30,000 in paper money.

The episode was the first instance of a pressure

group at work along the Delaware. Despite the humiliation of the two ringleaders, the appeal was so successful that thereafter the threat of direct action was consistently employed.

The Delaware was no longer calm; a period of violence followed. Not even the most brutal punishments, reluctantly applied by legislators who lamented the necessity, restrained the criminals. Public lashings at the whipping posts no longer stemmed the crime wave. More drastic punishments seemed necessary.

The case of Catherine Bevan of New Castle shocked the whole community. Convicted of murdering her husband, she was condemned to death by hanging. To make the penalty more terrifying, the gallows was placed over a huge pile of logs. But through the carelessness of her executioners the fire was built so high that the flames burned the ropes before the hanging was completed. Catherine fell, while yet alive, into the burning pyre. No one dared attempt to rescue her.

This was an outstanding tragedy, but its awful ending failed to halt the criminals. At Trenton three men were hanged for poisoning six people, including Judge William Trent, the founder of the village. So common was the talk of executions that a five-year-old boy, who had overheard his elders, played hangman and strangled himself by a rope hung on the palings of the garden fence.

There were lesser evils too. The calm of summer evenings and of Sundays was being shattered. Negro slaves, white servants, and adolescent youths congregated on the courthouse steps. When work was done, they brought their milk pails and improvised a crude town band; they sang, and played their boisterous games. Some shouted, screamed, and cursed in their excitement. They gambled recklessly.

It was impossible to keep the Quaker quiet. Neither Quaker theory of noninterference with individual liberty nor Quaker practice of allowing free self-expression could cope with the emergency. The Friends spoke long in meeting, condemning noise and tumult, but the culprits were not members of the Quaker groups and the testimonies had little influence. The legislators then passed a curfew law making the evenings a bit more quiet, but the pleasant days of Quaker peace were gone.

Such was the state of the fair, green country town when John Penn, the American, returned in 1734 to the Delaware. There was little sign of change as he set foot at New Castle. The town still chattered nervously of Catherine Bevan's fate, but there was more talk of crops and markets and of the wished-for prosperity. As soon as he reached the Schuylkill's shore, however, Penn felt the difference. Thirteen shots, fired from the shining six-pounders set up to defend the town, sounded a salute that would never have been heard in his father's time. John Pass had cast the balls; it was good practice for an ironfounder who later was to have a hand in the recasting of a great state bell. The State House wherein that Liberty Bell was soon to hang was only just completed.

The Walking Purchase

The guns were preliminary to a gala welcome. Cavalcades of well-fed citizens, many of them Quakers who would once have set their faces firmly against display, rode out to meet the son of William Penn. Councils gave a splendid and impressive dinner, against the protests of those who felt that £40 was far too much to spend on a banquet.

Upcountry men agreed with those who criticized

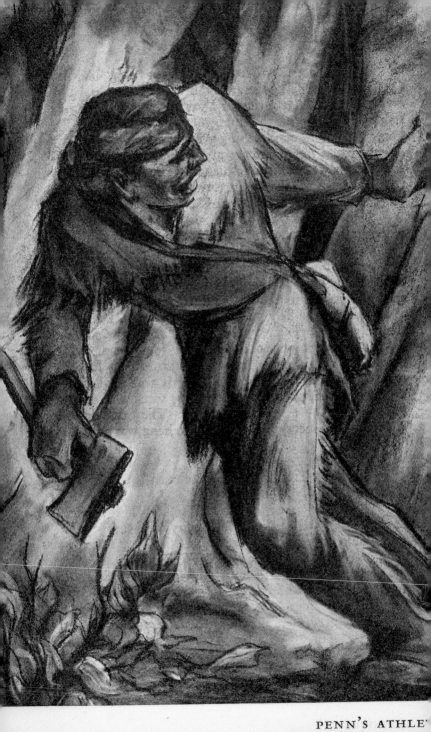

PENN'S ATHLET

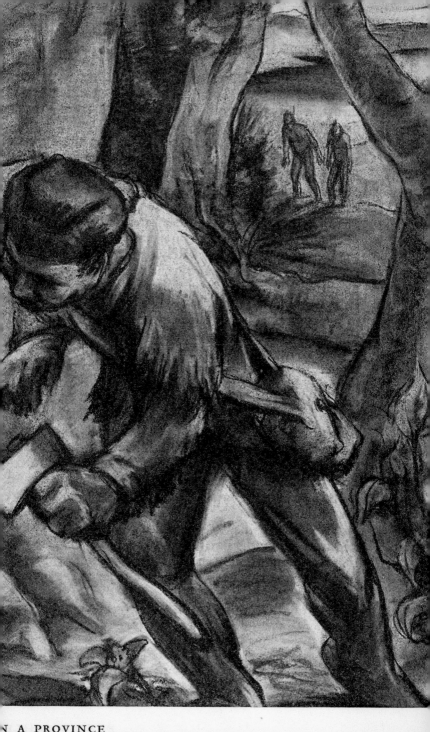

the sycophantic Councils. Scotch-Irish settlers angrily demanded that the Penns protect the frontier settlements, and that more land be purchased from the Indians.

Controversy rages to this day about the episodes which followed. The dominant Six Nations argued firmly that the Delawares, "that tribe of women," had no further land to sell; with equal fervor the latter insisted that they were masters of the stream. Thomas Penn, knowing that the Delawares were much more pliable than the pugnacious northern Indians, defended the Delaware contention. Relying on the Indian reverence for his father's memory, the resourceful proprietor produced a copy of a deed whereby, he said, his father Onas had purchased all the land "as far as a man can go in a day and a half." Its authenticity was doubtful then, and still remains mysterious; in any case, a copy of a deed is never final proof; but, after three years of intense persuasion, Penn convinced the Delawares that they should accept it as a valid contract. He agreed to defend the grant against all challengers.

All was ready for official measurements. The "Walking Purchase" was to be made in the fall of 1737. There was a difference in point of view, however, as to the methods to be used. According to Indian interpretation, a friendly party of whites and Indians would set out, strolling leisurely in gentlemanly fashion, until thirty-six hours had elapsed. There would be frequent rests for food and smoking, and the day would be limited to the time the sun was visible. Their estimate was that the grant would thus embrace about thirty miles of land along the river, reaching about as far as the present site of Easton.

Thomas Penn had other views. He combed the colony for young and wiry woodmen. Selecting Ed-

ward Marshall, James Yates, and Solomon Jennings as
the best athletes to be found, he trained them well and
ordered them to make themselves thoroughly familiar
with the route. They were instructed secretly to blaze
a trail through the woods, and to clear it of all under-
brush. He promised a reward of five pounds in money
and a gift of five hundred acres to the man who went
the farthest distance.

At dawn of the appointed day, a group of whites
and Indians collected at the starting line. Some of
Penn's friends were on horseback and were, he said, to
ride along the route to see that everything was fairly
done; the Indians were on foot. At the proper signal,
all started off. Penn's experts walked at a quick but
reasonable pace until they got beyond the sight of those
who remained behind. Then, when none but the Indian
walkers and the three athletes were left, they quickened
their gait, walking so rapidly, and so nearly running,
that the Indians protested. The Delawares, winded and
exhausted, fell behind and out of sight. Two of the
Indians, attempting to keep up, collapsed, but none of
the whites slackened speed. With their accompanying
horsemen, the three athletes rushed forward.

Twenty miles beyond the starting point a group,
gathered to see the walkers pass, marveled on the speed
with which the men had marched and on their freshness
after so long a walk. Only the Indians suspected that
the men might have ridden for a part of the distance.

Even though he may have had such help, Jennings
could not stand the strain. Before the end of the first
day he was exhausted. Yates and Marshall pushed ahead
until dusk made the blazed trail impassable, but they
were up to start again before the dawn. Yates fell into
a stream, too tired to rise. Marshall pulled him out and

waited until the horsemen overtook the runners; then he, the last of the selected three, rushed on ahead. At noon, the end of the thirty-six hour journey, Marshall fell full-length upon the ground, grasping a sapling as the limit of Penn's claim. Instead of the anticipated thirty miles, he had covered sixty-five, an average for each hour that he walked of more than three and a half miles uphill over rough, forest paths. The record would not be a shameful one on modern scientific tracks.

The Delawares were far from pleased at such an outcome. They were angry, too, that Marshall had not run along the river. He had struck into the country, finishing near the present site of Mauch Chunk in the coal region, and the boundary was drawn from there northeastward to the Delaware. When the Indians protested that such had never been the plain intention of the so-called deed, the Pennsylvanians sent word to the Six Nations to come down and force the Delawares to move away. This, too, was a clear violation of agreements, for there had been arrangements that no Indian would be dislodged as a consequence of the Walking Purchase. The Penns thus lost valuable Indian allies. The Delawares, forcibly removed from their old river, slowly wandered west to the Wyoming valley.

Far from being an abode of peace, the Delaware saw other quarrels. The valley became known as the center of riot, war, and insurrection.

Great Fish Fight

The long succession of disorders began along the Schuylkill. The cause was traceable to a too-successful business enterprise. Envious and less skilled neighbors sought to break down a smoothly operating trust. At

Valley Forge the residents had begun a large-scale fishing business which monopolized the shad.

Each spring the fat fish, most toothsome of the sea food of the colonies, swam up the rivers in vast shoals. Seldom could they be caught by hook and line, but the rivermen snared them with nets of cord or grapevine. Innumerable of these nets were spread at scores of narrow places in the water.

Now farsighted fishermen invented better methods. Instead of stringing flimsy nets, never long enough or strong enough to stop the shad from breaking through, they fenced the stream. Close-barred racks were built from shore to shore and a deep pool was cleared away below the obstacle.

Upon the arrival of the shad the entire populace of Valley Forge, mostly on horseback, hurried to the river-bank bearing large bushes, stakes, long-handled shovels, and a variety of other tools with which they beat the river. Wading and riding upstream they screamed and shouted to scare the fish, raked the bottom of the river, and drove every shad well up into the pool below the fence. The fish ascending to spawn were caught in such huge numbers that they literally forced each other out of water. A pole could not be thrust into the stream without striking shad. Tens of thousands were thus captured without difficulty. The work of gutting them, salting them for winter use, and packing them in barrels went on continuously. The Valley Forge community had sufficient fish to last them for a year.

The upstream fishermen were not amused, but, like true Pennsylvanians, they preferred peace to war. Because in America there is always pious hope that legislation can work wonders, they twice drew up petitions to the Assembly to outlaw fishing fences. Twice they were successful in their pleas, but each time Valley Forge, anticipating the rebels who were to winter there, refused to honor the decrees. Probably on the sole ground that the Assembly favored the fish fence prohibition, the governor upheld the objection. He allowed racks to be built so high that navigation was impossible.

Twice more the Assembly issued solemn ordinances, but again the governor interfered. Then in 1736 the legislature, bowing to the executive, reversed its stand and said that fences were permissible, but this time the governor demanded that they be condemned. In matters such as these the important element was never the population, nor even the fish, but always the schoolboy squabbles between the governors and legislatures.

By 1738 the upstream people, starved for shad, resorted to direct action. Under the leadership of Timothy Miller, they collected their canoes and floated downstream just before the fish were due. Few Valley Forgers were on hand, and the angry invaders cut away the fences. Some were rescued, but when the Miller navy interfered with salvage work the Valley Forgers called for help. Launching their own canoes, they fought against invasion. Miller's thumb was broken by a club, and then the other invaders fled. The aroused defenders chased them into the shallow Perkiomen Creek, drove the canoes aground, and captured every warship, while the upstream heroes fled into the woods.

The fish fight was not over with this initial repulse. Legal experts were called in, and they declared that upstreamers had just cause for grievance. Two constables, accompanied by three canoes of henchmen, went to destroy the fences a second time. Two hundred Valley Forgers, "very rude and abusive," mustered for defense. In quavering voice the constables read their warrants, commanding them in the king's name to keep the peace. But, like their grandsons forty years later, the Valley

Forge defenders "damned the King's laws and the law-makers," cursed the constables, and clubbed three oarsmen into the river. They then took the offensive, offering to pay five pounds just to get a crack at Admiral Tim Miller. Lest their posse succumb to silver bullets, the constables withdrew in haste.

The Quaker spirit was undismayed, however. Compromise prevailed. The fences were allowed to stay, provided only that they be low enough to let canoes pass, and that an opening be left for some few shad to swim upstream. Thereafter the Miller navy served only peaceful purposes of commerce.

Faker and Evangel

Though all knew that the compromise was but a truce, the Delaware valley jubilated as though Armageddon had been won. Restraints were breaking down; the people celebrated madly. The beginnings were innocent enough, as quiet family parties wandered through the streets to view the newcome camel, first of its species to be seen along the Delaware, or as they let their tastes run riot in their clothes and furnishings. And then came two men who brought warmth and color to the picture, two men of most divergent views.

First was the glamorous and wholly inexplicable Sheik Sidi, Emir of Syria, who rode into Philadelphia without advance publicity. He knocked at the door of the State House, and silently held forth a note purporting to be written by the New York governor, in which Sheik Sidi, whom the note called Shedid Alhazar, "appeared to us here to be a gentleman, whatever else he might be besides." It was a dubious introduction at best, but royalty was rare, and the Pennsylvanians were willing to accept him at face value. No one could understand a word that Sidi said, nor could Sidi converse with anyone. Banquet followed banquet in his honor, entertainments were elaborate, and Sidi, by his smiles, signified his full content. And then, by some mysterious spontaneity, doubts began to burgeon. No words were ever spoken to the sheik but he sensed that he had stayed his time. He wandered off to Barbados, taking with him the silver offerings for which he had not asked but which had been collected for him by the sentient Quakers. It was Philadelphia's first experience with needy noblemen, and undoubtedly was worth the hundred pistoles that the Friends subscribed.

The Moslems supposedly shun the use of liquor, but Sidi was broad-minded. The gilded youth discovered in him a taciturn, but most absorbent, guide. Never in the past of Pennsylvania had there been a violent objection to punch and rum and cider, but after Sidi's meteoric social course, drinking ceased to be an avocation. From now on, in the tavern slang, men became "as dizzy as a goose." They "took Hippocrates' elixir"; their "heads were filled with bees"; they "walked by starlight"; enthusiastically, "they ate their opium."

It was a fitting time, then, for the Reverend George Whitefield to arrive. In tones that were sweet-voiced but so powerful that listeners two miles away could not escape, the fiery young British evangelist awakened Philadelphia to a consciousness of sin. Himself a graduate of dissipation, so he said, he knew the pitfalls of the taverns; as a youthful wastrel, he declared, he was a proper guide to bring young men back to righteousness.

Whether because of his message or because he staged a first-class show, raging and denunciating on his improvised platform on Society Hill, Whitefield drew tremendous audiences. Fifteen thousand listeners, virtually the entire population of the city, crowded round him to watch his small eyes shoot sparks at the "slothful shepherds and dumb dogs" who manned the city's pulpits. He drew forth money contributions from skeptics such as Franklin, who had gone to hear the man through curiosity alone and had resolved to keep his money in his pockets. Through the force of his scintillating sermons, enlivened by his vigorous dramatics on the platform, the dancing schools, the taverns and the concert halls were closed. Philadelphia was luxuriating in reform.

But old James Logan, chief justice of the province and Penn's close companion, shrewdly saw that the Whitefield fervor was a temporary phase. The Delaware, as we now know by looking backward from our modern times, is given to the following of emotional hysterias. Regularly, as though observing the dictates of a graph, the valley falls victim to evangelism. No doubt the net result is good; quite possibly the people benefit by regular soul purgings; unquestionably the experience is refreshing.

Whitefield's moral teachings faded as he moved to triumphs elsewhere; his lessons were forgotten, when the fickle people scented gains that were both material and immediate. Declaration of war against Spain in 1741 brought visions of legitimatized piracy in the West Indies, and over strong Quaker opposition interest turned toward battle. Seven companies of soldiers were recruited in the former Quaker colonies for war in Cuba. The lovely *Tartar* privateer, finest and largest ship yet built along the Delaware, stood full-sail under a gentle breeze, to raid the Spanish Main.

Her fate was sad and sudden. Just why a new ship should capsize in a comparative calm has never been completely understood, but the *Tartar* overturned.

All but three of her adventurers were drowned in Delaware Bay within easy sight of shore. The Quakers said, of course, that war was sinful and that the Lord had little love for those who wished their fellows ill, but the Quaker explanation was not generally liked. Nor, it should be added, did the *Tartar's* fate discourage other privateers.

There was sufficient conflict left at home these days, particularly in politics. For all the exhortations of George Whitefield, the times were most unhappy even for those who sought their glories in the skies. Deaths had risen by 280 per cent above the figures of the year before. War, pestilence, and famine, fires, bitter cold, and the influx of unrestricted immigration caused discontent and rioting. The citizens, compensating for their emotional debauch in Whitefield's time, now sought scapegoats for their sufferings.

Many of the inhabitants considered the Quakers and the Germans responsible for the distress. The former would not grant sufficient funds for protecting the province properly against attack or for levying a necessary war, and they were kill-joys who opposed clean fun; the latter, it was said, had brought in fever from the Palatine. In the election that was coming in October, 1742, the anti-Quaker faction undertook to wipe away the influence of both hated groups.

In some degree, the situation was precisely what has been observed when Quarry and his Hot Church party sought to win the province; in actuality, the times had changed. The Penns had turned from Quakerism to the Church of England; the governor now represented the proprietary interest rather than the popular. The Quaker-dominated Assembly fought against the Penns and was allied with the frontier on everything except the question of defense.

The governor's group, now called the Gentlemen's party, sought to win the Germans from their stanch alliance with the Quakers. Failing to divide the opposition, it was prepared to carry the election by more drastic means. The Country party, as the Quaker-German alliance was now called, was equally prepared to guard its old majorities.

Paradoxical as it may appear, the election in pacifist Pennsylvania was decided by the stronger weapons. The Gentlemen enlisted seventy sailors who came with clubs to beat off German voters from the polls. The Country party, chiefly Quakers and nonresistant Germans, took possession of the stairs up which each voter had to pass to cast his ballot. Each side used violence against the other, but, as the Country party held strategic advantages, the election trended steadily toward Quaker-German victory. As a last resort, the Gentlemen attacked the Country guards on the stairs, only to be driven off with the loss of fifty of the sailors taken prisoner. The battle was a sweeping victory for Pacifists against Gentlemen. The governor was so completely overwhelmed that for the rest of his four years in office he accepted calmly the dictation of the Country legislature.

But the Assembly could not consolidate its gains. When, relying on its conquest of the governor, it sought to impose restrictions on the Scotch-Irish frontier, the results were less happy. Surveyors sent out to map out frontier farms and to compel the squatters to pay purchase price or rent were driven from the scene. Neither the governor nor the Assembly dared proceed further with the scheme.

9

The Skies Darken

The Brimstone Rain

Two hundred and forty-two Indian chiefs came, singing serenades, to ask for peace at Lancaster in 1744, but the skies were darkening. Obviously the Quaker-dominated Assembly would vote no funds for war; equally obviously, conflict was not distant.

Down at Salem, Irishmen were threatening to "cut the throats of Quakers in their beds," but that romantic rising to support Bonnie Prince Charlie's pretensions to the throne was mostly tavern talk, soon ended when the four ringleaders had their ears nipped at the pillory in a December frost. But there really was war on the horizon, for New Jersey, now a royal colony, was sending troops to fight the French at Louisburg and voices in Pennsylvania were demanding that the Quakers help.

Local politicians, foreseeing trouble, dodged responsibility. Twice in 1745 men elected to be mayor of Philadelphia flatly refused to serve, though their refusals cost them £30 apiece in fines; the third man chosen left town rather than be forced into the office. The Board of Aldermen, electors of the mayor, found themselves reluctantly obliged not only to pay a salary to a man to take the job, but also to forgo the formal dinner which, by custom, mayors had to tender to the board.

When French and Spanish privateers, relying on the Quaker pacifism, actually came up the bay to fire on Salem and New Castle, the strain was at last too much for even Quakers to endure. True to their principles, the legislators would not vote appropriations for munitions; instead, they set aside £4,000 to be expended for the royal use in buying bread and meat and grain. Franklin and his prowar fellows gave a liberal construction to the phrase, as the Assembly no doubt intended, and bought "black grain," or powder, with the funds.

It was, in one sense, the end of Quaker isolation, though the money granted for munitions was insufficient. James Logan, among other Friends, at last admitted the necessity of war in self-defense and, at Ben Franklin's solicitation, urged that the narrow channels of the Delaware be fortified. No less than 39 cannons, fifteen of them 28-pounders, were hauled overland from Boston. A hundred companies of volunteers, the "Association Regiments," were formed as a militia, and, though it rained brimstone on the fourth of May, as a symbol of heavenly displeasure at the armament, the populace in general approved proper preparation. Action, it was felt, was necessary; prices, because of wartime, had climbed so high that wheat, at 6 shillings a bushel, was at twice its proper level, and beef, at 43 shillings per hundredweight, was costly beyond all due proportion. Depredations by privateers on the sea and by profiteers at home must not be endured, even if the price was to be the end of pacifism.

The Quakers did not minimize the ill effects of war. Too many eager young lads who had set forth for Cuba or for Louisburg came home as hardened veterans addicted to the curses of the camp. Demobilized soldiers, unwilling to settle down to farm routine, turned highwaymen, infesting the provincial roads and making travel dangerous. Respect for law diminished;

vice grew fashionable.   Sidi was triumphant, and Whitefield was forgotten.

According to the moralists, whose figures may have been exaggerated, one house in every ten was now a dramshop, selling liquor at a price so low that even redemptioners and adolescents could drink freely. Gambling houses vitiated the morals of the young.   The settlements which once had merited the compliments of Europe for their virtue seemed almost as sinful as the Old World slums.

Civic pride went down too.   No longer were housewives scrubbing down the steps and sweeping streets before their houses; instead, they threw dirt and filth into the roadway, piling up the gutters two feet deep with refuse, providing a paradise for innumerable stray dogs that ran at large to snap at horses, kill sheep, and scare the cattle.   With the coming of the summer heat, the fear of rabies brought new terrors to the unhappy city.

Responsibility for the breakdown of morale is not wholly to be placed on the aftermath of war, nor, despite the vigorous accusings of the royalists, are the proprietary rulers to be saddled with the blame.   The fault lay in the social composition of the folk along the Delaware, where four parties, all of approximately the same strength, contended for the mastery.   Where churchmen and Quakers, Germans and Scotch-Irish lived in mutual suspicion, where none were willing to co-operate except on terms of special privilege, and where laws passed by an Assembly were almost certain to be vetoed by a governor or canceled by a king, good government was sorely handicapped.

Civic honesty was below par and chicanery was common at the polls as in the Bloody Election between Pacifists and Gentlemen.   More frequently, there was wholesale purchasing of votes. Sheriffs and coroners were chosen by electors who spent the whole day tapping free kegs set up by candidates. Unregistered voters, marshaled from the ships in port, were herded to the polls to cast their ballots. Snap elections, set for a time when country citizens could not conveniently come into town, or after they had gone back home at dusk, guaranteed control to city politicians. There is an ominous note in the 1748 minutes of the Councils, that the £100 salary paid to the mayor should be stopped, because "the business of the mayoralty had grown more profitable."

Ordinary crime-prevention methods were of slight avail against such deep-grained evils. For highway robbery and cruder crimes, the whipping post was sometimes a deterrent. The pillory and stocks, placed full in the public eye, where culprits could be seen and where the youth might pelt them with unpleasant eggs and overripe vegetables, were ready against misdemeanants. The sheriff, armed with his "delicate pocket scissors," clipped the ears of petty thieves. But none of these devices was efficient for the guarantee of better government.

Indian Revenge

There was a special need for civic betterment because the safety of the settlements was more than usually in danger. Enemies were pouring into Pennsylvania and were threatening New Jersey. Indians, angered at the trickery of the Walking Purchase and resenting the reversal of the founder's pacifistic plans, were muttering that they must be revenged. The upper reaches of the Delaware were terror-stricken.

The young Penns, whose agents preferred legalistic

smartnesss to strict justice, intensified the anger of the savages. Realizing that the rapid growth of population necessitated much more ground than had been justly purchased, the Penns bilked Indians of lands. Although they knew full well that the Delawares denied the claim of other Indians to any part of Pennsylvania, the Penns began to dicker with the Iroquois and other tribes of the Six Nations. At Albany, in 1754, a deal was made whereby the Penns "bought" from the Iroquois all rights to lands in Pennsylvania west of the Susquehanna River. That the Delawares claimed exclusive title to that land was of slight concern to the proprietors. If they, using methods which would not in the light of modern morals bear deep scrutiny, could buy a title from a group of drunken Indians, the bargain was well worth the risks involved. John Penn, and his associates, among whom was Benjamin Franklin, came home from Albany with a title in their pockets. The entertainment and the bribes had cost £500, but the Penns had more than doubled the extent of land over which the Iroquois acknowledged Pennsylvania's sway.

Outraged Delawares, insisting that neither the Iroquois nor any other of the Six Nations owned a foot of land in western Pennsylvania, protested that the sale was void and, when they learned that not only had the ground been sold beneath their feet but that they were now to be pushed out of Pennsylvania, rose in arms. These Delawares, who once had been Penn's friends, and whose solemn treaty, "never sworn to and never violated," had been faithfully observed, allied themselves with France. Pennsylvania, once the most peaceful of the provinces, heard the war whoops sound.

Braddock's disaster, worst of all defeats suffered on American soil by British arms, gave a signal for the Delawares to wreak their vengeance. The first blow fell upstate, near what is now Sunbury. The Indians ravaged an entire settlement, killing and capturing twenty-five whites. This misfortune, as Richard Peters, secretary of the Council and one of the Albany negotiators, sadly noted, "was the first inroad ever made upon the province since its first settlement." It is noteworthy that that massacre took place on the very line of the Albany Purchase.

Penn's famous peace with Tammany was now completely shattered. Other onslaughts followed swiftly. The blaze of burning houses, and of barns stored with autumn harvests, illumined every section of the north and west frontiers. Berks County, on the Schuylkill, Northampton, on the Lehigh and the Delaware, were terror-stricken. Raiders were discovered in sight of Reading and within twenty miles of Easton.

Of all the people who deserved protection, the gentle Moravians ranked high. Missionaries to the Indians, ever eager to assist them as friends and mediators, interested, quite as much as Quakers, in promoting peace and toleration, the Moravians were unaggressive souls. Unarmed and unsuspecting, they dwelt in semi-communistic fashion in the wilderness.

Yet these were victims of barbaric massacre. As sixteen of them sat at their evening meal at Gnadenhutten in late November, 1755, a band of Indians approached stealthily. A sudden barking of the dogs betrayed the coming of outsiders. A sixteen-year-old lad who opened the door to welcome the arrivals met a volley of rifle shots. Four men were killed outright as they sat at table; seven others were murdered as they fled. The house was burned, the meetinghouse was wrecked, the barns, with forty head of cattle, were destroyed.

Here, too, as at Sunbury, there was a rude sort of

justice in the place picked for the Indian revenge. As Sunbury was on the frontier violated by the Albany Purchase, so Gnadenhutten was close by the spot to which the runner Edward Marshall had carried the limits of the Walking Purchase. Gnadenhutten, near the present site of Lehighton on the upper reaches of the Lehigh, was not far removed from that small sapling which Marshall grasped as he fell exhausted at the end of his long journey.

The Gnadenhutten massacre was but one in a long series of atrocities. Fire and slaughter ravaged the frontiers of what was once a pacifistic province. Hundreds of houses were destroyed, scores of settlers were scalped and slain; many, without respect for age or sex, were carried off as prisoners or subjected to unheard-of tortures. As Conrad Weiser, interpreter and agent to the Indians, frantically reported to the governor, "This country is in a dismal condition. It can't hold out long. Consternation, poverty, confusion everywhere."

The Dutch Mob

Outside the larger settlements, the frontier counties were depopulated. Hundreds of frightened farmers rushed into towns to seek safety. But this heightened the distress, for the summer had been severely dry and crops were small. Some portions of Berks County, where Indian attacks were numerous, were so severely sun-scorched that the corn was yielding but a bushel to the acre. The small towns, crowded by refugees, could not supply sufficient food.

Frantic messages were sent to the Assembly, appeals that seemingly could not be disregarded by anyone in authority. Breathless express riders, racing down to

Philadelphia from Lancaster and York, from Berks and from Northampton, gasped almost simultaneous pleas for help. And the Assembly temporized!

The reasons for delay were both cynical and silly. The governor, remembering that at the previous elections Germans had been voting steadily to fasten Quaker domination on the province, refused to interfere. The churchmen and Scotch-Irish Presbyterians accused the upstate Germans, those whose relatives were massacred, of pro-French and pro-Indian connections! Steadfast support, by pacifist Moravians and Mennonites, of non-militant administration was cited as proof that these unfortunates were plotting in the interests of France. The crucifixes worn by ardent Moravian Protestants were seen as proof that the Moravians were seeking to deliver Pennsylvania to the pope.

There were financial reasons, too, for the reluctance of the administration to relieve the sufferers. The Quaker Assembly, now well-nigh converted to a militant defense, desired to lay a tax on land wherewith to purchase arms. But this was difficult, because the heirs of Penn insisted that their lands should be exempt from any such taxation. Agreement was impossible when merchants demanded a high tax on land, when owners of rich plantations clamored for an excise, and when debtors insisted on emission of a paper currency. Instead of reaching an immediate decision for the protection of the suffering upstate Germans, the Assembly conducted a hot economic argument.

Frontier patience, never strong, snapped quickly when debate was offered in the place of aid. Mindful of the manner in which, a generation earlier, the hill-folk lobbied for cheap money, the upstaters resolved to march on Philadelphia. Governor Morris suddenly learned that "a body of five hundred Dutch from

Berks" were on their way to terrorize the legislature, and that two thousand Chester County farmers—a section heretofore deemed stanchly Quaker—were also on the march. Apprehensive that the mob "will be productive of mischief," the governor pleaded for a quick decision. But the Assembly would not be hurried.

Three days after the governor's warning, the vanguard tramped into the city. Philadelphia, anticipating riot, was alarmed, but sent the sheriff out to halt the march. Politely, as though in total ignorance of all the happenings, he asked the strangers what they wished. The "Dutch Mob" gave no answer, but took the sheriff prisoner and made him guide them to the governor's mansion. Morris, in his turn, seemed sympathetic. He would willingly assist them, but the fault lay wholly with the legislators. He himself, he said, had just received a letter from the Penns, wherein the young proprietors were offering to grant £5,000 for the purpose of defense against the Indians. The Assembly, Morris said, would not co-operate.

Morris was not entirely candid in the matter. He did not tell the Dutch Mob that the letter talked of wholly different affairs. He did not say that the money had been sent to help defray the bills of Braddock and that the remittance had arrived too late. On his own responsibility he diverted the funds from what the Penns desired to what was really needed for proprietary interests. In point of fact, he might have added, the £5,000 donated by the Penns was a somewhat larger sum than would have been exacted from them had their lands been taxed.

The Dutch Mob hurried on to the Assembly. Like Morris, but with less success, that body tried to shift responsibility, accusing the governor of causing the delay. But, with the promise of the £5,000, the march-ers were impatient of buck passing. They must have a militia law immediately to provide an army for defense.

The Assembly yielded. At a special night session it drafted a bill to meet the Dutch Mob's needs. By a suspension of the rules, the measure was passsed hurriedly and sent to the governor. Within twelve hours the bill was enacted into law. The Dutch Mob was victorious.

Or, at least, it seemed so. More calm and careful scrutiny of the legislation disclosed that shrewd Quaker legislators had inserted jokers that gave less than was desired. No Quaker could be drafted into service, nor could a conscientious objector be required even to contribute money for defense. The troops empowered were not to be subjected to any campaign that lasted longer than three days, nor were they to be garrisoned at any place for more than three weeks' time. No boy less than twenty-one years of age could be enlisted, nor were any troops to be retained in service for more than eleven consecutive months.

The bill, though better than nothing, was a disappointment to its advocates. Morris, however, rejoiced, for the Germans, disillusioned at their Quaker allies, deserted in large masses to his party. The Scotch-Irish, too, were loud in their approval of the Morris action in contributing so large a sum for defense of the frontiers. The governor's party grew amazingly in power and prestige, and, to consolidate its strength, demanded more concessions from the legislature.

Continuation of the massacres gave ample argument for a stronger frontier policy. Two weeks after the passsage of the mild Militia Act, a silent German funeral procession came down to Philadelphia, carrying the corpses of new victims of Indian assaults.

Round and round the State House, where the Assembly was in session, the cortege passed, poignantly illustrating the effect of mistaken gentleness in dealing with the Indians. Seventy-eight more whites were scalped and dead; forty villages were burned; the scalp yells of Indians were heard at placid Nazareth and Bethlehem, in the very center of Moravian communities.

Tedyuscung's Yearlong Spree

The Quakers were still reluctant to abandon their cherished principles of peace and, since all but eight of the thirty-six members of the Assembly were under Quaker influence—largely elected, it should be recalled, by German votes—it was impossible to secure a definite declaration of war against even proved marauders. The Assembly did, however, pass a bill providing for the setting up of frontier forts, a string of wooden blockhouses, each garrisoned by half a hundred men, along the mountain crests from the Delaware to the Susquehanna and thence southward to the Maryland line. Benjamin Franklin was commissioned as a colonel to raise a regiment to build the forts in Northampton County, including Fort Allen on the site of Gnadenhutten.

By the strong insistence of the Governor's party, aided by the new German and Scotch-Irish allies, resistance was intensified against the Indians. They, in turn, made war more desperately. A new chieftain, Tedyuscung, a Jersey-born chief of the Delawares, assumed command, to the renewed distress of the Moravians, for Tedyuscung, known to them as Brother Gideon, was one of their most prized Indian converts. Diplomat, as well as warrior, Tedyuscung enhanced the prestige of his

Delawares, insisting on their independence of the Six Nations and demanding that all treaties signed by the latter should be disregarded, so far as they affected Delaware privileges.

Pennsylvania answered by a decree which must have sorely shocked the shade of William Penn. Instead of relying upon peaceful methods of persuasion, Governor Morris ordered that a bounty should be paid for every Indian scalp. One hundred and thirty pieces of eight, an amount equal to about the cost of sixty gallons of rum, were offered for the scalp of every Indian, man, woman, or child over twelve years of age. For every female captive and for every child under twelve taken prisoner the same amount was offered.

The rule was drastic, but it brought results. Within three months Tedyuscung was asking for peace, provided only that the Delawares be recognized as independent of their Six Nations overlords and that the Walking Purchase be canceled. The new governor, William Denny, was equally insistent on the matter of the Walking Purchase, denying flatly that injustice had been done. Relying on the support of the Six Nations, he refused the claim of Tedyuscung to be leader of the tribe. Though Tedyuscung had already gone out among his people to give the "peace halloo" whereby hostilities would be suspended, the conferences proved abortive.

The commissioners played on Tedyuscung's weakness. Conrad Weiser and the other Pennsylvania delegates saw to it that the chief was drunk every day. They kept demanding that he recede from his opposition to the Walking Purchase, but for more than fifteen months, during which time, according to the Pennsylvanians, he was seldom sober, he managed to defend his stand. Finally, in October, 1758, a conference with all

the Indians, including ten tribes, came to a conclusion
that the Walking Purchase would be ratified by Indians
if the province would deed back the land supposedly
acquired at Albany. New Jersey was to pay $1,000 to
extinguish Indian claims to territory in that colony.

Even now, however, Tedyuscung would not yield.
When plans to force him from the leadership could not
be carried out, despite the combined efforts of Nickas,
the Mohawk chieftain, Tagashata, sachem of the
Senecas, Governors Bernard of New York and Denny
of Pennsylvania, the province was compelled to buy
him off. In 1762 the Pennsylvanians paid Tedyuscung
£400 to withdraw his objections to the Walking Purchase. A year later he was burned to death when Indian enemies set his house on fire while he lay in a
drunken stupor.

More valiant in his opposition than any other Indian in the Delaware valley since the time of gentle
Tammany, Tedyuscung is remembered to this day by
a large statue high on a hill above the Wissahickon. His
deeds are not generally known, however, for the pedes-
tal bears only his name.

10

White Savages

The Paxtang Boys

"A<small>NOTHER STEP</small>," cried Captain Loxley, "and you die! We want no rebels here."

The hand that held the match close to the touchhole of the small brass cannon trembled; Loxley's face was flushed. His dingy, tarnished regimentals sat illfitting on his spindly frame; his weapons were not burnished bright; his colors were not gleaming in the sun. Nor was Captain Benny Loxley happy to be placed in this position, though, as a loyal soldier of the king, he was determined to maintain the peace. No ruffians from the Lancaster frontier could take possession of the city while he remained alive. Major General Thomas Gage had placed him in command of Philadelphia and little Captain Loxley was resolved to guard his trust. He waved his sword again weakly, motioned to his *mohairs*, men-in-mufti volunteers, and called upon the horsemen to draw rein or die.

The mounted butchers were aghast at the reception. Trotting happily toward Philadelphia on the narrow, rutted road that led from Germantown, their thoughts had been of peace and happiness, of beer at the Blue Anchor, of long churchwarden pipes, of drinking songs and gossip. To mounted butchers on a city holiday, the Loxley ultimatum was a shock.

But Loxley had good reason for alarm. These festive mounted butchers were not warriors, and certainly had no rebellious motives, but there were other men who, rumor said, were rushing to town to slaughter all the Quakers and kill the garrison. Loxley let the butchers pass, while he and his mohairs waited for the rebels.

Philadelphia waited too, in bright illumination all night long. By Loxley's orders every window showed a lighted candle; every watchman carried a bright lantern on his rounds. The doughty warrior, whose post close to the courthouse and the tavern had been a social center rather than a camp, fearing ambush in the dark, was on his guard against surprise.

Well might he be alarmed when two thousand murderers, the dreaded Paxtang Boys, were on the march for Philadelphia. Impatient at the Quaker pacifism, tired of the way the Penns, the governors, and the Assembly had truckled to the Indians, angered at the cowardice of cityfolk, these Paxtangs from the Susquehanna, headed by bloody Lazarus Stewart, had sworn to shoot, to knife, and to destroy "red vermin." They thoroughly approved Lord Jeffrey Amherst's plan to spread smallpox among the savages by giving them infected blankets; they heartily endorsed the wish of Colonel Henry Bouquet to track down Indians by using bloodhounds.

Philadelphia was their present target, for there was the seat of government and there lived Quaker legislators who were squandering the taxes in gifts to savages while not a shilling was voted to protect the distressed frontiers. Paxtangs were convinced that Quakers cared more for the welfare of the Indians than for the whites; some thought, indeed, that Quakers were allied with Frenchmen to destroy the British rule. If Philadelphia could be captured, Stewart and the Paxtangs thought, the province would be safe against red savagery and Quaker cowardice.

Violence alone would turn the trick, for at the game of politics the Paxtangs were but amateurs. Pennsylvania's Assembly was a hand-picked group of Quaker sympathizers. Philadelphia and the adjacent Quaker areas in Bucks and Chester counties chose twenty-six assemblymen; five frontier counties, taken all together, had but ten. On any bill that might come up for vote, the Quaker partisans would have a two-to-one majority, and more.

Finding legal methods hopeless, Stewart and the Paxtangs went on the warpath. Firm in the belief that every Indian was at heart pro-French, the Paxtangs shot at sight. Taking Tom Quick as their hero, they slaughtered even sleeping girls and helpless children. A young hysterical lieutenant, scouting seven friendly Indians on a lonely road, killed them as they walked peaceably to church. To own scalps taken from an Indian was a mark of merit with the Paxtang Boys.

The Indians were helpless to resist. Bewildered by the white man's legal arguments, tricked by shrewd pettifoggers who misinterpreted the treaties, deceived by men whom they had every wish to trust, the Indians were baffled at the cause of the uprisings. They had resented Weiser's cleverness in keeping Tedyuscung drunk until the Indian would grant the land that white men coveted; they had been angered at the Walking Purchase; when, in addition to these injuries, the white invaders murdered squaws and children, the Indians could no longer be restrained.

Panic raged on the Pennsylvania frontier. Following the Paxtang precedent, the warriors made indiscriminate attacks. Twenty-three white settlers were scalped; scores of others fled in fear. Terror-stricken men and women, from isolated clearings, ran, half clothed and unarmed, to shelter in the towns. Distant clearings were deserted; outlying farms were left untenanted. The Indians, rushing onward to wreak vengeance on their persecutors, found only empty houses. These they burned; the smoke from blazing buildings curled constantly within sight of the frightened towns where women huddled with their children.

The Paxtangs gave no heed to what had caused this vengeful rising. To them, the angered Indians seemed devilish; even those who once had been friendly were now classed as treacherous and hostile. Any red man caught by any Paxtang was immediately murdered.

The innocent Moravians stirred Paxtang wrath, for these white missionaries, who wore a crucifix identical with that of Quebec Catholics, were charged with being spies of France. This was the period of the French and Indian War, when feeling against France ran high, and when frontiersmen, angry at French aid to Indians, smelled treachery and treason in those who would not shoot to kill. The Moravians, moreover, had been moving freely among the savage villages, preaching to the Indians and laboring to teach them how to prosper.

Conestoga Massacre

No one, surely, could have been more peaceful than a tiny tribe of Conestogas, living on a little tract assigned to them by William Penn. Basketmakers and bowl carvers, fishermen and farmers, they lived a quiet life, peddling their wares in near-by Lancaster.

These Conestogas drew upon themselves the Paxtang fury. Day after day, they muttered threats against the Conestoga camp, charging that these Indians had harbored raiders and were guilty of incredible massacre. Word of the threats reached the ears of governor John Penn, nephew of "the American," but he pigeonholed the letters as of no importance. His nonchalance convinced the Paxtangs that they had no cause to fear his intervention.

Scotch-Irish Paxtang township gaily celebrated its first great "victories." Toward Christmastime, in 1763, half a hundred Paxtang militiamen had ridden down to Lancaster to enjoy a spree. There they had heard of the small Conestoga camp from which, they were informed, the men were absent. At dawn one cold December morning, while the few remaining Indians were sleeping soundly, the Paxtangs rode to camp to kill the savages. Six Indians were shot to death; two Conestogas only managed to escape.

Frightened, the Indians took refuge in the county jail at Lancaster. Fourteen Conestogas huddled in the courthouse yard trembled for their lives but trusted in the hope that a small company of regulars, garrisoned near by, would guard them from a second raid. They stood, frozen with fear, while Lazarus Stewart, shouting from outside the yard, threatened that he would "kill the Conestoga vermin in their nest."

Christmas passed safely, while Stewart and his Paxtangs rioted in glee, but, as soon as Christmas Day had passed, the Paxtangs came again upon the town. Ignoring the regulars, who seemed strangely unconcerned, the Paxtangs took possession of the town, seized the workhouse warden, robbed him of his keys, and broke into the jail. The troops stood idle as the Paxtang Boys, with rifles, knives, and tomahawks, massacred the refugees. Then, cheering for their exploits, the Paxtangs rode home as heroes.

Pennsylvania was horrified, but no one took efficient action. John Penn put the blame on the Assembly; the legislators charged that Penn had been remiss. Each wondered why the troops had been so unconcerned and why the local magistrates were so inactive. There was no fitting answer to any of the questions, but neither was there any action. Franklin, to be sure, drew up a bill to bring the Paxtangs into court, but the bill was left to languish in committee while the Assembly concerned itself with a consideration of last year's deficits. No Paxtang Boy was ever brought to trial.

Indeed, the Paxtangs took the initiative. They demanded, arrogantly, that the Assembly mend its ways. Knowing that his fellows would never execute a Paxtang for the murder of a Conestoga, Stewart himself demanded that he go to trial at once before a jury of his neighbors. He boasted of his actions.

"What I have done," he said, "was done for the security of hundreds of settlers on the frontiers. The blood of a thousand of my fellow creatures called for vengeance. Let me be tried where prejudice has not prejudged my case. Let my brave rangers, who have stemmed the blast nobly and never flinched, have an equitable trial. They were my friends in the hour of danger; to desert them now were cowardice. What remains now is to leave our cause with our God—and our guns."

Oddly enough, Stewart, thus confident of acquittal if tried in his home county, and thus truculently warning of violence to come, insisted that he, himself, had shed no Indian blood.

Jittery John Penn

John Penn was jittery with fear. The Paxtangs, glorying in their murders, had taken law into their own

hands and were looking now for further victims. At
Philadelphia, they had heard, a little group of a hundred
and forty Indians, converts of the pacifist Mennonites,
were seeking refuge. Stewart had demanded that these
Moravian Indians be delivered up for execution. Penn
had refused to yield the refugees, and he had heard that
Paxtang Boys, immensely increased by frontiersmen
sympathizers, were moving to attack the capital.

Penn wavered. First he thought that he had better
put the Indians on an island in the middle of the Delaware, to keep them safe against a Paxtang raid. Then
he worried whether this was safe, for, after all, the
angry two thousand Paxtangs might defeat Ben Loxley's
little corps of troops and sack the city. A ship was just
about to sail for England and Penn wondered if he
might not send the Indians to London. The skipper,
not at all anxious to transport a savage cargo, slipped
anchor and sailed away at night.

Penn's next hope was to pass the buck to someone
else. Though he was aware that Loxley's force was
small, he weakened his defenses by detaching a High-
lander company, the only regulars in town, to shepherd
the Moravian converts into New York. The Indians
were compelled to march in haste across New Jersey so
that Philadelphia's hands would be completely clear of
anyone to whom the Paxtangs might object. But the
New Yorkers saw no reason for accepting danger;
promptly upon the arrival of the Scots troops and the
Indians, New York ordered that the refugees return to
Philadelphia. They had a long and wearied march back
to their Pennsylvania barracks, facing what might be
certain masssacre.

At last Penn resolved to match the Paxtang violence with force. He read the Riot Act, demanded that
the Asssembly authorize resistance, and called a thou-

sand men—the mohairs—to the colors. Cannons were quickly wheeled in place; the alarm bell rang; the city waited for attack.

But Lazarus Stewart was a clever leader. Instead of coming into town by the expected way, where Loxley had drawn up artillery, he led the Paxtangs by a roundabout approach. There were no heavy guns commanding the rutty road that led from Germantown; Loxley hastily hauled up a minor piece to train on the road.

Diplomacy succeeded where force might fail. As soon as the excited mounted butchers brought word to John Penn that the Paxtangs were at last arrived, he sent three clergymen to halt the march. A Presbyterian divine, he thought, might soothe the wild Scotch-Irishman; a Lutheran was picked to calm the Pennsylvania Germans who had joined the Paxtang army; an Anglican was named to represent the better city elements. All three were charged with the responsibility of reasoning with the raiders.

Fluent talkers all, the clergymen held up the Paxtang march. Cleverly they tangled Lazarus Stewart in theological arguments, mingling their insistence that the Paxtangs bow to the appointed civil leaders with vague praise of Captain Ben Loxley's military prowess. They gained the Paxtang consent to wait another day before taking over the capital.

Next day John Penn and the Assembly, for once working in unison, sent out more hard-boiled diplomats, Franklin among others. These, too, dilated upon the hopelessness of trying to attack the city, alleging, with more vehemence than truth, that each citizen was armed with sword and gun, and that even the pacifist Quakers were in arms against the Conestoga murderers. The Paxtangs, much impressed by the high standing of the diplomats, agreed to stop their march, provided the

Assembly, which Franklin said was eager to see the light, would consider their grievances. Franklin assured them that the Assembly would do whatever was needed to assure the Paxtang Boys of justice. It was a safe promise.

Then, as an afterthought perhaps, the Paxtangs asked another boon. They hoped that Penn would grant the privilege of letting "some of their shabby gang come through the city." Penn did so, but he took the precaution of having the Paxtangs come into town by a most circuitous route that would take them past the artillery that had been parked in the wrong places.

Ten days later the Assembly finally got around to considering the Paxtang grievances. It took three weeks to make up their minds to approve a bill for voluntary military service in the event that a similar crisis should ever come again. Meanwhile, John Penn had sent his inconvenient Moravian Indian refugees back to their old homes on the frontier. Thereafter they might get along with Paxtang Boys as best they could. Luckily for them, the Paxtangs had had enough adventure to content them for the moment.

Yankee Aggression

Royal Double-dealing

CONNECTICUT still craved the Delaware. Nat
Turner and George Lamberton, returning to New
Haven with glowing tales of fertile fields and rich resources, excited Yankee cupidity. The restless New
Englanders, hankering, no doubt, for lands where winters were less rigorous, looked on the Delaware as their
rightful sphere of influence.

Legally, they seemed to have an airtight claim to
much of Pennsylvania. In 1662, Charles II, magnani-
mous because of his recent restoration to the Stuart
throne, had given to Connecticut all land from Narra-
gansett Bay westward to the Pacific, excepting such territory "then possessed or inhabited by any other Christian prince or state." The exception, a usual prudent
clause in royal charters, thus excluded the Dutch New
Netherlands from Connecticut control, but gave the
northern third of what is now Pennsylvania to the New
Havenites.

But Charles was overgenerous. When William
Penn applied for land nineteen years later, the merry
monarch granted the same territory to the Quakers.
Ordinary citizens who tried a trick like that, disposing
of the same property to two different people at two different times and pocketing the proceeds, would fall
afoul of law, but kings are different. At least, the
Stuart kings had broader privileges. Certainly Charles II

had no qualms of conscience. As absolute monarch he assumed the right to give away the nation's land and, if he so desired, to take it back again. The king, so far as land grants were concerned, could do no wrong, for legally the title to all territory was vested in the throne. All that Charles was doing, if his lawyers were correct, was to allow his favorites to lease the use of ground, and if he was moved to cancel leases already made to the New Havenites, he felt himself within his rights, particularly as Connecticut had never made a move to take advantage of its Pennsylvania opportunities.

He was, in fact, an old hand at this business of Indian giving. He had canceled land deals in Virginia and in New York. And at this moment he was bothered by the lamentations of Lord Baltimore, who was insisting that Charles was giving to the Quakers land already set aside to be a part of Maryland.

This latter controversy was particularly engaging. If the nobleman was correct in his contention, Penn's capital at Philadelphia would be a part of Maryland, but if Penn's counterclaims, based on a later gift from Charles, was valid, Baltimore would become a Pennsylvania town. Not even this pretty situation, however, worried the reckless Charles; it was a matter for the English jurists and for court officials, and they chewed the matter over for some eighty years. Then, when Lord Baltimore and William Penn were long since dead and everyone was wearied with the matter, it was at last decided to leave decision to the experts.

Two English surveyors, Charles Mason and Jeremiah Dixon, were called in to draw a boundary line, to begin at a point on the Twelve Mile Circle, thirty-one miles west of the Delaware and fifteen miles south of the Philadelphia city limits, and to run due west to the Pennsylvania boundary. It was a four-year job to cut through the forest but the line then drawn has grown into what is probably the most famous boundary in America. This Mason and Dixon's line, in future years, would mark off North from South, divide the slave states from the free, separate the aristocratic plantation people from the enterprising individualism of small farm owners. From Jeremiah Dixon's name, shortened and familiarized, would come the nickname Dixie. Such, at least, is the Delaware version; there are other explanations, hinging upon the "dix" printed upon Louisiana $10-notes, but these we loyal Delawareans refuse to credit.

The Pennsylvania-Maryland dispute could be settled peaceably, but no such good fortune attended the Connecticut dispute. Yankees were evidently more aggressive folk than Marylanders, and William Penn, the pacifist, was succeeded by more worldly heirs. Therefore, when Connecticut settlers came into the region of the Delaware to claim privileges granted them back in 1662, the young Pennsylvania proprietors were prepared to fight. For half a century violence and bloodshed marred the peaceful story of the Delaware. Long military campaigns—the so-called Pennamite Wars—were waged to settle the dispute.

Penn's heirs had taken few chances. Though they were well assured that they had legal title to their province, on the current theory that the last grant was the valid one, they were at pains to bolster up their claim. As early as 1736 they had bought an option from the Indians for all lands not already actually purchased from the aborigines. And when the Indians, following Charles II's royal lead, sold that same land to Connecticut, the Penns were wroth. Nor could the Indians see clearly where they had erred, for to the Indians land sales meant merely a license to free use of ground on

equal terms with every other user. They had no understanding of fee simple ownership, nor any clear conception of an option. All that the 1736 arrangements implied was that the foolish Pennsylvanians had been kind
enough to hand out presents lavishly with no demand
for an immediate return.

The Penns were in a delicate position; obliged to
argue that a later grant by Charles II was legitimate,
they had to insist that a second sale by Indians was
wholly wrong. Their lawyers squirmed adroitly, while
Connecticut attorneys imposed derisive objections, but,
deviously and with infinite cunning, the Penns made
out a prima facie case. Luckily for them, the Connecticut deeds showed erasures in strategic spots, but the
chief Pennsylvania weapon was the absolutist power of
the Stuart kings. Old William Penn, had he been living
to hear how his descendants defended royal privilege,
would have been aghast.

For two generations the matter was an academic
problem. So long as neither province sought to make a
settlement in the disputed area, ownership was not a
pressing question. Neither the arrival of Connecticut
explorers on the upper Delaware nor the chartering, in
1753, of a colonizing Susquehanna Company, roused the
Penns' anxieties. Nor was Pennsylvania much concerned in 1762 when Indians destroyed a little Yankee
settlement, massacred twenty farmers, burned the crude
huts and stole ripened crops. The tragedy, to Pennsylvania, seemed unfortunate, but, after all, the New
Havenites were interlopers not entitled to defense.

But when, in February, 1769, forty Connecticut
farmers came down into the valley of Wyoming, the
most fertile section of the disputed territory, to build
a blockhouse which, from their numbers, they called
Forty Fort, the Penns were alarmed. Much of upper

Pennsylvania was unfitted to colonial requirements, being mountainous and forested and far removed from markets, but Wyoming was a veritable paradise. A valley twenty-one miles wide, well watered by the Susquehanna, which at that point is close to the Delaware, Wyoming was rich in grain and game. The Penns were themselves interested in making settlement on those fertile fields and had but recently sent three henchmen to the valley to protect their legal rights. Ten private soldiers went along to fight, if necessary, any aliens who might make incursion. If the Yankees were again preparing to attack the Pennsylvania territory, as they had twice invaded the valley of the Delaware, the Penns would be on guard.

Pennamite Wars

The three Pennsylvanians were particularly chosen for their official status. Captain Amos Ogden, New Jersey trader and Indian fighter, came as a military expert to reconnoiter the defenses of the valley; Charles Stuart, a surveyor, mapped the region; John Jennings, sheriff of Northampton County and as such the personal representative of Governor John Penn, embodied law and order. It should be noted carefully that the three men came as deputies of the proprietors and in no sense as agents of the province. The area in question was not owned by Pennsylvania, nor by any private citizen of that colony; the only interested parties were the young proprietors. Not until the Revolution wiped out the proprietary claims was the province intimately concerned in the progress of the Pennamite Wars.

In large degree, the Connecticut invaders also were without official sanction. Their colony, to be sure, had granted a charter to the Susquehanna Company, but had then ostentatiously withdrawn official sanction for the actions of the colonizers. When Captain Zebulon Butler, veteran of the French and Indian War, and hero of the capture of Havana, led his forty pioneers into Wyoming, he came as the land agent of the Susquehanna Company, and not as a Connecticut official.

Geography was a determining factor of this private quarrel. Butler, following the trail marked out in 1615 by the Dutch wanderers whom Hendricksen had found at Christina Creek, came from the Hudson to the upper Delaware. He had not, however, pursued the river all the way. Arriving at the big bend at Coshecton, he had struck across comparatively low ground, through grazing country filled with lakes, until, crossing the Moosic Mountains, he went downstream again, guided by the Roaring Brook and Lackawanna River, to Wyoming.

The Pennsylvania route was somewhat easier. Penn's men came up the Delaware to Easton, thence by way of the Lehigh past Allentown and the Gnadenhutten site, northwest over the "Warriors' Route" to come into the valley by the southern pass. The Pennsylvanians had the additional advantage of being able, by a short detour over rolling hills, to climb the high Penobscot Knob and so to scout the situation before the Yankees knew danger was at hand.

For all their advantage in terrain, the Pennsylvanians were caught in a precarious position. Ten warriors were helpless against the forty from Connecticut. The veteran Captain Butler soon shut them up within the walls of an impromptu fort.

But Ogden was undismayed. His guile was greater than his military strength. Suggesting a discussion, he asked three Yankee leaders to come within the fort, and then, confronted them with Jennings, sheriff of the county. Connecticut, despite its free thought in religion, was a slave to law and order, and when the three saw legal warrants for their custody they agreed to go down to the county seat at Easton to answer Penn's ejectment suit. No doubt, they thought that any judge would gladly recognize the priority of Yankee rights.

A strange procession threaded down the narrow trail that wintry February. Captain Ogden and the sheriff, conducting three prisoners, led the van, accompanied, at a short distance, by the remaining thirty-seven soldiers of Connecticut. They came to Easton, and the sheriff turned them over to the court. The judge at once released them under bail to keep the peace. Immediately, the forty fighters started back to occupy their little Forty Fort.

No sooner had they got back to their homes than Jennings was upon them with another warrant, and once again they tramped down through the snow to Easton. Again they were released on bail to keep the peace and, once again, both little armies trudged back to Wyoming to take up their old positions.

Evidently, Jennings grew tired of crossing the Blue Mountains in the snow, or else his posse mutinied at meaningless arrests, because the Yankees were allowed to live in peace until the spring came. By May, when he returned undaunted to attempt a third arrest, he found the Yankees reinforced, waiting in a new blockhouse which they called Fort Durkee, in honor of the leader of the reinforcement. But Major John Durkee, innkeeper and justice of the peace, was much too modest to accept the honor. He preferred to name the new stockaded blockhouse for two steadfast Englishmen who championed the rights of colonists. These patrons were

John Wilkes and Colonel Isaac Barre, and from them the new town of Wilkes-Barre got its name.

Captain Ogden waited until he, too, had larger forces; then, with two hundred soldiers and a four-pound cannon, he marched to the attack. In September, when the crops were ripe, he hurried from Penobscot Knob to fall upon the unsuspecting Yankees. He captured them without a shot, again by waving a new warrant from his friend the sheriff. He sent Durkee down to Philadelphia—evidently he was tired of having Easton judges turn the Yankees loose—and ordered all the other Connecticut intruders to go home. First, however, he compelled them to complete the harvests, that the Pennsylvania soldiers might take home the booty.

So far the laurels lay with Ogden, who had thrice dislodged the Yankees without spilling a drop of blood. But the situation was to turn. No sooner had the all-victorious commander returned to Philadelphia than the persistent Connecticuts came back. This time they were but ten in number, but as allies they had forty Scotch-Irish Pennsylvanians, part of the Paxtang Boys, under the leadership of Lazarus Stewart. Connecticut had bribed them with the promise of a township. Wyoming was again in Yankee hands.

Ogden liked his leisure about as well as any man alive, but he had no time to savor the delights of Philadelphia. Once more he traveled the old Warriors' Route to Wyoming only to find, as usual, when he scouted from Penobscot Knob, that he was again outnumbered. More Yankees were arriving every day.

He took no overt action. With a careless unconcern he strolled down to his stronghold, spread his men as though they were at peace, and waited for results. And his reward was quick, for Yankees walked up to his fort, thinking it to be their own, entered, and were at once arrested.

This time, however, he was not at liberty to send them down to court. In any case, the shipping of his prisoners was but an empty gesture, for even Durkee, once in irons at Philadelphia, was now free and on the march. Durkee attacked the Ogden fort, and though he was repulsed with the loss of one man dead—the first casualty in the Pennamite Wars—he surrounded Ogden, set fire to the blockhouse, and compelled the crafty soldier to surrender. Connecticut had won, and for five months Wyoming was at peace.

The peacefulness was not to last. On the September equinox in 1770 Ogden was back again, with a hundred and forty soldiers who, quietly and with precision, surprised and captured every Yankee. Only at Fort Durkee was there resistance, and this was short and ineffectual. Several Connecticut men were killed, the rest were taken prisoner. Down at Easton, the county jail was filled to bursting; once more, because they had committed no offense against others than the Penns, the Yankees were released.

Again the Ogden rest was shattered; again the Paxtang Boys came down. The old routine was followed yet another time. Ogden rushed up from Philadelphia, drove out the Yankees for the fifth expulsion, but this time, learning from his previous experience, he waited in Wyoming.

His action was unlucky for him. Within three months, Zeb Butler arrived with a new and more efficient Yankee army, and settled down to starve the Pennsylvanians into complete submission.

But Ogden was undaunted. At midnight, he slipped from his fortress, rushed naked to the river, carrying his clothing bundled in his hand, and dived nto the water. Swimming in the darkness on his back, with only his nostrils above-water, he managed to escape the Yankee watchers. Then, safely beyond the limits of the Connecticut outposts, he came to shore, put on his dripping clothing, and ran toward Philadelphia. He covered a hundred and twenty miles in three days' time, and returned with a small force of men.

This relief came too late. Connecticut also had added troops. Ogden held out until August, 1771, and was then obliged to bow to larger armies. The Penna-mite War was over. Connecticut had won.

A year later the Connecticut Assembly formally annexed Wyoming, gave it the new name of Westmore-land, and added it to Litchfield County. Durkee was sent to Hartford as assemblyman. The crowning blow was dealt when Connecticut had the consummate au-dacity to demand that the Penns pay £40,000 as damages.

The Penns, however, would not recognize the Yan-kee right to rule, much less pay any such amount. They laid their plans craftily for a renewal of the war. Real-izing that their weakness lay in lack of popular support, they widened interest in Wyoming by selling land at an extraordinarily low rate to settlers. The purchasers, of course, were gambling on the Penns' eventual success, for, if the Yankees held a legal title, then the Penns had nothing to convey. But if the Penns prevailed, the cheap farms in rich Wyoming were unquestionably good bargains.

When the Pennamite Wars resumed in 1775, Con-necticut was astonished at the huge Pennsylvania forces that appeared. On Christmas Day, seven hundred Pennsylvania soldiers, well armed, equipped with a field piece and a flatboat navy, appeared on the river. But there was one drawback to this strength; the mighty

Amos Ogden had been displaced. Dr. William Plunkett, a surgeon of the French and Indian War, was in command.

The Plunkett Expedition had set forth without the blessing of the Continental Congress. Now that warfare had begun with Britain, the Congress pleaded that the colonies abandon internecine strife, and that all efforts be turned toward winning recognition for the common cause. But Pennsylvania had a larger view. The time seemed ripe to drive away the Yankees and to win for Pennsylvania complete control of all the province. The thought may not have been absent that a final blow might well be struck to end proprietary rule as well.

Zeb Butler ended Plunkett's hopes. Catching the new leader in an ambuscade, Butler's smaller army drove the Pennsylvanians out. The short, unfortunate Second Pennamite War was over almost before it had begun. Connecticut retained control of Wyoming and the regions to the west.

The Pennsylvanians now obeyed the Continental Congress. For the remainder of the Revolutionary War no new efforts were begun to renew the war against Connecticut. Wyoming was soon to suffer more severely than any other section of the state, but not at Pennsylvania's hands.

12

"The Last Refuge of Virtue"

Tamoc Caspipina

Modern society sees itself in mirrors which, if neither accurate nor flattering, are at least informative. The gossip columnist, the commentator, the realistic novelist, lay bare the inner secrets of communities. The small details of social history, those minutiae which are, to sociologists, far more revealing than the formal acts of kings and warriors, are ruthlessly exposed.

So, too, the Delaware, uniquely among other eighteenth century areas, was privileged. Though the weekly papers of the time were stodgy journals, packed with politics, heavy with commercial news, and filled with solemn correspondence from almost every center other than their own, the Delaware had less formal publicists. Gazettes, in regions where each man knew his fellows intimately, ignored personalities, but private diaries and letters from contemporaries expose the foibles and the little idiosyncrasies that differentiate one culture from another.

The Delaware was favored by three men, excellent reporters, who saw the valley from different points of view. The Reverend Jacob Duché, a social analyst, anticipated later scientists by producing a sort of Philadelphia Survey. Under the pseudonym of Tamoc Caspipina—an acrostic drawn from the initial letters of his title as "The assistant minister of Christ Church and St. Peter's in Philadelphia in North America"—

Duché reported on the city's physical appearance and
on its welfare agencies. The squint-eyed eccentric
whose rich and honeyed speaking voice made him a
magnetic orator, wrote twenty letters praising the civic
spirit of the Delaware, approving the city's gridiron
plan, which, he said, was patterned after that of Baby-
lon, and pleading for extension of the educational facilities. Tamoc Caspipina's identity was at first well kept
Almost everyone along the Delaware was suspected of
having written the searching series of letters which were
so eagerly read.

Duché did well to keep his secret, for at times his
pen dripped acid criticism. Instead of heaping praise
upon the city for its excellent police that made riots rare
(except at election time), and instead of giving lavish
enthusiasm to the hospital and to the well-run workhouse, Caspipina attacked the city's architectural mon-
strosities. He lamented the bad taste which spoiled the
wide and noble High Street by building a row of sham-
bles down the center; he had nothing but scorn for the
dilapidated old courthouse, with the scummy duck-
pond that lay just beneath its northern windows; he
urged better buildings, and much better teachers, for
the college.

He hated, too, a growing tendency which he believed would make the Delaware excessively bluestock-
ing. Fashionable Philadelphia, he protested, took many
of its pleasures seriously. Men and women thronged
Dr. Benjamin Rush's drawing room to hear his popular
talks on chemistry, but failed to follow up their interest when that volatile experimenter finished. Once or
twice a year the college set aside a week for lectures,
"for the entertainment of the curious," open to all who
chose to pay the half-dollar daily fee, but Caspipina
charged, and rightly, that the crowds went just to listen,

ot to think. He worried that both the Library Com-
any of Philadelphia, at its rooms in Carpenters' Hall,
nd the General Circulating Library, a cheaper institu-
on at the Green Lamp, were patronized by too many
ho sought only the very latest books.

There was, of course, little choice for readers.
hose who had finished Oliver Goldsmith's four-volume
History of England and Samuel Smith's *History of the
Province of New Caesarea, or New Jersey* were per-
orce obliged, if they liked history, to take up the only
ther available new work, Anthony Benezet's *Historical
Account of Guinea,* with its powerful arguments
gainst the slave trade. Sermons were always procura-
le, and so were such practical works as the six parts
f Gale's *Complete Surveyor* and Dr. William Cadogan's
Treatise on Gout, but for the lover of lighter reading,
he circulating libraries offered little more than Richard
Cumberland's Drury Lane comedy, *The West Indian,*
r, very occasionally, a scrap of verse by "the surprising
African poetess," Phillis Wheatley. When, in November, 1773, copies of John Hawkesworth's *Voyages and
Discoveries in the Southern Hemisphere* arrived on the
Delaware, the three volumes were eagerly read. For
weeks thereafter conversation was studded with reference to the travel logs of Commodore John Byron, who
found the Falkland Islands. Samuel Wallis and Captain Carteret, explorers of the Pacific, were household
names, while the immortal Captain Cook, whose works
Hawkesworth edited, became a popular hero. One of
Philadelphia's better known coffeehouses, the Queen of
Otaheite, was christened in honor of the great adven-
turer's discoveries.

Tamoc Caspipina was appalled at Philadelphia's
failure to appreciate her local genius, the internationally
famous botanist, John Bartram. The self-taught sci-

entist had built up by the lower ferry a seven-acre gar
den laboriously reclaimed from Schuylkill-flooded
marshlands. It was the first botanical garden in Amer
ica. The slim and active Bartram had traveled u
the rivers of America, especially along the Delaware, th
Schuylkill, the Susquehanna, the Potomac, and th
James, to gather strange specimens of plants, to collec
fossils, and to learn geology. Then, coming home t
his small estate, he had hybridized his plants, and pub
lished his discoveries.

All Europe knew of Bartram's scientific work
Linnaeus, indeed, was fond of calling him "the world'
greatest natural botanist"; the Edinburgh Society
awarded him, in 1773, its gold medal for "advancemen
of the arts"; the English crown was paying him ar
annual pension of £50. A few years earlier the Phila
delphians had taken a collection to send him roaming
through the middle provinces, and even to East Florida
to gather specimens.

But Bartram's popularity had waned. His earnes
propaganda for abolition of slavery and his emphasi
on equal rights were not well received. Even his fellow
Quakers had disowned him; they said John Bartram wa
too worldly in his scientific interests.

Caspipina recognized that John Bartram lacked the
advertising touch. Because William Young was more
cocksure and vocal than his seventy-year-old master
Young seemed to Philadelphians to be a greater man.

Young had won his start by methods which were
questionable. As a neighbor, he had been allowed to
wander freely through the Bartram gardens. John
Bartram's open-handed hospitality admitted Young to
family meals, where the master, his Negro assistants,
travelers, and guests all dined at one long table. Young
listened carefully to all the information he could pick

up. With this smattering of science as his education,
he gathered seeds and plants from Bartram's garden,
made them into packets, and sent them, together with
self-laudatory letters, to the king and queen, and to
various high-placed members of the British aristocracy.

Queen Charlotte, accepting Young at his own face
value, sent for him to come to London. She financed
his study under British teachers, and, when his education was complete, granted him a yearly pension of
£300, six times the Bartram stipend. He returned to
Philadelphia with the title of "botanist to the queen."

On his return, the royal honors caused Young to
be received as master of his science; Bartram was secondary in importance. The older botanist, who hated
litigation and sought to live in peace with all the world,
refused to tell how Young had won his reputation. He
refrained, too, from criticizing Young's ornate pamphlet, beautifully printed at Paris, which purported to
describe the treasures to be found in Young's nonexistent garden. Such Philadelphians as cared to ride long
distances to see Young's estate were loath to criticize the
queen's own botanist. To one German scientist who
had the temerity to ask where Young kept his unusual
specimens, the bombastic Young replied, "The absence
of rare plants from this spot means nothing; all America, field or forest, is my garden."

To Tamoc Caspipina's joy, Young's leadership was
not lasting. A greater charlatan appeared, in the person of a Kingsessing quack who put forth an elixir
known as the American Balsam. For three-and-six a
bottle, this cure-all guaranteed to tone the stomach, end
rheumatism, dissolve gallstones, cure tuberculosis, raise
low spirits, strengthen the brain, aid the memory, and
prevent barrenness. Young's fame, for all his wealth

of imagination, dwindled in comparison with the reputation of so sovereign a remedy.

Dragons for Scandal

A second critic, Alexander Mackraby, wrote of
Philadelphia pleasures. The residents, he said, "are
dragons for politicks and scandal; they drink too much.
Taverns and coffee houses are almost as frequented as
at London."

Mackraby evidently enjoyed himself. He described
with gusto a midnight escapade, when young officers
exhilarated by their wine, went forth with the regimental band of clarinets and horns, hautboys and bas-
soons, to play under the window of the current toast,
though Mackraby himself seems to have gained nothing
but a heavy cold for his exertions. He thoroughly approved of whist, perhaps because he usually won, and
he regretted that the town was so dull that there were
few plays or public entertainments where he might
meet the girls. He had to go to church to strike up an
acquaintance with the beauties. He liked the sleighing,
too, when girls and men set out, preceded by fiddlers on
horseback, to an out-of-town roadhouse, where they
might dance and sing and romp, eat and drink and
"kick away care" from morning until night.

"You can have no idea," he wrote his friends in
England, "of the state of the pulse seated with pretty
women, mid-deep in straw, your body armed with furs
and flannel, clear air, bright sunshine and spotless sky,
horses galloping, every feeling turned to joy and jollity."

There seemed to be, Mackraby thought, a lack of
loyalty along the Delaware. On St. George's Day,
always a time of merriment for loyal Britons, he could

ind but twenty native Englishmen to celebrate the
feast. But the small band did their best. They met at
a tavern, stuffed themselves with roast beef and plum
pudding, "got drunk, pour l'honneur de St. George,"
and then, wearing their badges proudly, they went to
the play, where they made all the audience sing "Rule,
Britannia," "Britons, Strike Home," and "God Save the
King." It was a special triumph, because Mackraby had
been hearing too much talk of independence.

For ten years before the Declaration of Independence was signed, the Delaware had been muttering
against British rule. The press blazed with hostile
comments against the monarch. His filial devotion to
his mother was mocked. "It has been observed," the
Pennsylvania Packet wrote, "that the French king, an
old man, is governed by a young woman, while the k—
of —, a young man, is governed by an old woman."
The blanks were cautiously left unfilled.

The royalists were singularly oblique in their reply,
for they seem to have misconstrued the *Packet's* implied
libel. "The King," they answered, "is remarkable temperate, seldom indulging himself in more than four
glasses of wine at dinner." They also added, though the
point had seemingly not been raised, "He wears a wig
because his hair is thin." The boy prince, George Augustus Frederick, later to be George IV, was too much
even for good loyalists to explain away. Antiroyal accusations that the Prince of Wales was cursed with
"turbulence and positiveness of temper" were answered
by assurances that the fault might possibly be cured.
His tutor, it was explained, had resorted "to confining
him at times three days together in a small room without any amusement or attendance."

Respect for the monarch was growing thinner;
submission to authority was waning. The shocking ex-

hibition of bad manners between the two Penn brothers, John and Richard, who refused to speak a civil word to each other even at a public ceremonial, destroyed the last vestige of loyalty to the proprietors.

Palinurus Peeper

Such goings-on gave rise to a new phase of journalism. For the first time in America a gossip columnist broke into public print. Philadelphia read the revelations of a Walter Winchell. One "Palinurus Peeper," the "Pennsylvania Spy," announced a keyhole column.

Palinurus promised to spare no one in his castigations of society. "I shall introduce myself by some means or another into the various scenes of public as well as domestic life," he boasted. "I am not only admitted as a visitor among the principal families of the city and country but have likewise the honor of being enrolled among the members of several respectable corporations, as well as private clubs." The idea of a member of the American Philosophical Society, for so he professed himself, acting as a Broadway columnist has a certain refreshing air!

"From the Coffee House and the New Tavern I expect abundant matter." Without a smile, he went on to hope, "The political, commercial, literary and religious interests of the Province will there, no doubt, be learnedly discussed by many a knot of grave and sensible freeholders." His expectations were well rewarded. Bars have always been the center for much heated argument, though few but Palinurus Peeper would describe the orators as "knots of grave, respectable freeholders."

He promised also to give candid comments on the

theater and other entertainments and to review the writings and to discuss the personalities of "the literati who meet Thursday evenings at the Golden Fleece." He invited letters from his readers and encouraged them to give him leads which he might follow.

The "Pennsylvania Spy" had ample material afforded him. The popularity of Ellenor Fitzgerald, who set up a millinery shop in the very same Green Lamp where the library flourished was a case in point. Her cleverness in fashioning feminine accessories and especially in so washing and "stoving" silk stockings that they were equal to new won her an enviable trade. No woman left the library without a call on the ambitious little lady, but that was only to be anticipated. What was more astonishing was that the library gained immediate increasing popularity with men and that so few of them passed by without at least a pleasant glance in her direction.

Ellenor was piquant too, but, like all ladies of her time, she dared not advertise her wit too freely lest she be misunderstood. She it was, some suspected, who wrote a famous letter to the *Pennsylvania Packet* analyzing local beaux. Her advice to young girls may be almost as applicable today as it was when it appeared.

"All young women," the letter said, "should look upon the men in general with a penetrating eye. Nature has furnished them with a strong desire of insinuating themselves into our favor and, in return, has furnished us with more art and cunning.

"I think the men may be very well divided into three sorts; the rattle, the honest lover, and the sober, sly deceiver. The first is like a dog that barks much, but is not apt to bite; the second (like our honest bulldog), won't hurt you if you let them alone, and may be of service to you, if you take them for your defence;

but the third will creep to your heels before you are aware of him, and will certainly bite you if he can.

"The cool, temperate deceiver is by much the most dangerous of the whole pack. These are the worst sort of poisonous creatures, for they are of a pleasing countenance. Never give these modest underminers the least encouragement, but either crush them, or fly from them.

"I will give you some marks by which you may be the better able to distinguish them. They are always over-furnished with officiousness and assiduity and pretended friendship and modesty and honor. . . . They have a sigh ready, or tears if necessary, and their knees are so supple that they are ever ready to bend to you. They can tremble, too, before they speak.

"Beware of all men, but chiefly of those who are most extravagant in your praises."

It was excellent advice and, had it been followed, would have robbed Palinurus Peeper of rich material, but whether Ellenor learned her facts from the gentlemen who came to get books at the library or whether she had wider contacts cannot now be learned. Certainly there were ample opportunities, despite poor Mackraby's wails, for a clever, pretty young girl to "take the measure of the men."

Palinurus had much ground to cover. The Delaware had learned to make small talk and to enjoy the social graces. Newfangled barrel organs, exactly like the king's, were making merriment, though their repertoire was limited to four tunes: "Coronation Anthem," "Lovely Nancy," "Cruel, Tyrant Love," and "Rule, Britannia." There were dances where the young folk might assemble. Crusty Caspipina dyspeptically complained that such goings-on engendered jealousies and backbiting, that the girls were too devoted to their dress, and that the men, by dancing until eleven, were made unfit for work next day. In spite of these criticisms, the dances proved popular.

Palinurus covered races and reported concerts. He went to see jugglers, such as Saunders at the Bunch of Grapes, and praised the star for exhibiting a "clean conveyance, without descending to the low tricks of cups and balls and ribbons." Like all the other men, he stood agape to see the marvelous equestrian Faulks, "rider without a peer" who stood upon the saddle of a trotting horse, playing gaily on a horn. He was amazed when Faulks lay on his back across the saddles of two gallopers, and he applauded when the rider raced a horse around a track, jumping back and forth across the animal.

Other sports, unhappily, were beyond the pale of Palinurus. Fox hunting, cockfighting, and boxing were socially acceptable, but Palinurus did not think them news. He was too far removed from the backwoods region to report the gouging contests where men leaped upon a fallen foe, dug their knees into the adversary's chest, grabbed handfuls of hair, and pressing their thumbs upon the eyeballs of the victim, tried to start them from their sockets.

Nor did he mention bundling which, supposedly a New England custom, was common to the settlements of Pennsylvania Dutch. Tamoc Caspipina had observed the practice and had wondered that it was devoid of evil consequence, but Caspipina had supposed that the "cold, slow, indolent disposition" of Pennsylvanians might provide the explanation, though he added loyally that the Delaware was "the last refuge of virtue." He disagreed with Ellenor. Along the Delaware, he said, "gallant adventures are little known and still less practiced." After a long and arduous research, he gave as his solemn conclusion that "Philadelphia has only two unfaithful wives." Unhappily, he did not give their names.

Marriage by Lottery

It would be unjust to rob the Delaware of its unique contributions to the art of marriage. Far up the valley, near Bethlehem and Nazareth, the calm Moravians who lived their useful lives in communistic peace took seriously the old adage that marriage is a lottery. Because in early life the two sexes lived apart, with slight opportunity for making acquaintances, the youths were handicapped in choosing sweethearts. When a young Moravian, therefore, felt that he was ready to assume responsibility he asked his minister for guidance. Usually he was instructed to draw up a list of girls who he hoped might listen to his suit. Then, if his application was approved, the elders, after careful consultation with the matron of the virgins, prepared a drawing of the lots. Two slips of paper were prepared, one bearing the word "Yes" and the other reading "No." These were inserted in a Bible, with a short, blank end extending from the tight-closed volume. If the young man drew the slip marked "Yes" he could propose to the first name on his list; if the slip was negative, he tried his luck again. For lads who loved but one girl, and who submitted one name only, a luckless draw was sad indeed.

More often the young man had lived so far removed from any girls that he had no choice at all. In such case the ministers, assisted by the matrons, drew up a list of candidates for the lad to accept as his own. Then, indeed, his marriage was a lottery.

The scheme was not so heartless as the bare recital

might suggest. No girl was under any compulsion to accept the verdict of the lot. She could refuse a call until such time as Mr. Right appeared to claim her hand. If, when Mr. Right pulled forth his slip, he found it "No," she had no recourse but to await another applicant. So strong was the belief in the supernatural guidance of the Bible that few lucky ladies turned the young men down. History fails to record that marriage among the Moravians was any less successful than where headstrong boys and girls followed their free, untrammelled will.

West Jersey, also, had a custom of its own. Whenever a man died, leaving his widow so burdened by debts that she could not pay them off, she was obliged, if so be she was lucky enough to find a second spouse, to marry in her shift. Thus, abandoning all her clothes and other property to her creditors, she passed through an obvious bankruptcy and started life anew.

A Jersey bride, moreover, had a special privilege made hers by solemn covenant. Whenever a couple was about to marry, a never-failing article in the marriage contract assured her of "the free and unmolested exercise of the right to do the whitewashing." Why the guarantee was made, or when it began to be assured, is lost in the hazes of antiquity, but no Jersey maiden failed to insist upon her special perquisite.

Possibly the more fashionable young men along the Delaware were, in the days just prior to the Revolution, above mere manual labor. The gilded youth, swinging far away from the simple Quaker precedents, were captivated by the macaroni craze.

The macaronis, cultural descendants of the beaux and bloods who formerly were social leaders at the British court, were cut from the same cloth as the dudes and jitterbugs of later days. Taking their name from

gay young blades who came home from the Grand
Tour with exaggerated ideas of European sophistication
and who, to symbolize their travels, dined on a dish of
macaroni, these ultramodernists went to extremes in
modishness, effeminacy, and refinement.

The old-line conservatives detested the macaroni.
"He is," wrote one outraged divine, "the buffoon and
baboon of our times. His mind is wholly set upon cuts
and slashes, knots and roses, patchings and pinkings,
jaggings and taggings, borderings and brimmings, half-
shirts, half-arms, yawning breasts, gaping knees, arith-
metical middles, geometrical sides, mathematical waists,
musical heels and logical toes." The macaroni costume
—a great knot of artificial hair fastened at the nape of
the neck, a very small cocked hat, tight-fitting clothes,
and a huge walking stick with long tassels—drew jeers
from the rougher classes, especially when the macaroni
added the effeminate touch of an umbrella to ward off
the rain, but the fashion obsessed the valley. David
Ramsay, graduating from the College of Philadelphia
Medical School in 1773, took the macaronis as the topic
for his commencement speech and seriously traced their
origin and growth. Even the sedate clergy came, in
time, to copy macaroni modes. Dr. William Currie,
crusty Anglican parson of St. David's Church, paid
formal parish calls in macaroni garb.

> The priest that once with rose and band,
> With formal wig, and hat in hand,
> Sagacious phiz that might demand,
> A bow from any tony;
> Behold him now all debonaire,
> With tiny hat and tortured hair,
> And while he prattles to the fair,
> He shews the macaroni.

For all their affected, mincing, "French" ways, the macaronis did exert a certain healthful influence on contemporary manners. Living in the days of six-bottle men, they opposed excessive drinking. In times when social life was decadent, they respected virtue; instead of using the violent, heavy oaths then customary, they swore only with such mild imprecations as "May I be deaf at the concert." General speech and writing was weighted down by involved classicisms and by tortured sentences, but the macaronis, "sworn foes of learning," preferred simplicity of style. Their behavior certainly left much to be desired by standards of the present day; their practice of thrusting an opera glass into a lady's face and simpering, and being then "pruddigisly enteerteen'd" with her confusion, was not appealing, but these worse phases of their manners did not long endure. By the outbreak of the Revolution, little was left of macaronism but the memory, and the lines in "Yankee Doodle"

> He stuck a feather in his cap
> And called it macaroni.

Of such material Palinurus Peeper built his primitive gossip column. He was, however, too far in advance of his time. The Delaware residents were unused to frank writing. Either the vulnerable members of the community waved their horsewhips too openly or the editor feared libel suits, for the "Pennsylvania Spy" soon ceased to make his revelations. One fine morning saw the *Pennsylvania Packet* devote his column to enthusiastic praise for "the work of Providence in making Pennsylvania happy"; thereafter Palinurus peeped no more.

It was a pity, for good copy was about to come.

A spring had been discovered within a block of the State House. Careful examination "by different Gentlemen of the medical Faculty," among them the ubiquitous Benjamin Rush, proved that the water "exceeded in strength any chalybeates yet known in the province." Rush wrote a testimonial which made the new-found fountain seem "a universal nostrum." Society flocked to take the waters, though they gagged at its disagreeable taste, and several sufferers, drinking it for various disorders, praised it for its curative properties.

Not until much later was it learned that the spring had no medical values whatever, and that the strange flavor, which Rush and his coterie of scientific men had said was due to healthful minerals, was caused by drainage from the outhouses through which the "spring" had coursed.

Palinurus would have reveled in the story.

13

Aflame for Freedom

The Cohansey Tea Party

To TELL the story of the Delaware during the trying times after 1774 is to recite the complete history of the Revolutionary War. The valley was the center of colonial defense, the heart of American resistance, the mainspring of democratic opposition to royal tyranny. At times when the South seemed to falter, when New England was suspected of being lukewarm in the cause, the three provinces of New Jersey, Delaware, and Pennsylvania kept liberty alive.

Here independence was proclaimed, at the State House that henceforth is forever known as Independence Hall; here the news of freedom was proclaimed, by peals from what has ever after been called the Liberty Bell; here statesmen gathered to affirm their resolution and, in the Continental Congress, to direct the conduct of the war. Here the new nation was created and here the Constitution was drawn up. No other section of the nation may boast of so continuous or so magnificent a record of constructive progress.

More actual war was seen in the valley of the Delaware than in any other region; more great battles were fought—at Trenton, Princeton, Brandywine, Germantown, and Monmouth; more winter camps were made and more privations undergone. The names of Valley Forge, of Whitemarsh, and of Morristown, for that long camp extended through New Jersey almost to the riverbank, recall the awful ordeals which the tattered army underwent.

The Delaware's firm resistance to taxation without representation was well known to all the other colonies, and to England. The crisis was met when the East India Company sought to land taxed tea in America, against the protest of the provinces. Early in the summer of 1773 the residents along the Delaware made their position clear. In letters to London they warned that, if the tea was sent, both ships and cargoes might be burned. When this notice was ignored, a Philadelphia mass meeting, held in the State House yard, unanimously resolved that the tax could not be countenanced, that "it had a direct tendency to render assemblies useless and to introduce arbitrary government and slavery," and that "whoever shall directly or indirectly aid or abet in unloading, receiving or vending the tea . . . is an enemy to his country." The resolutions were dispatched to other provinces for their guidance. A Boston town meeting, three weeks later, endorsed the Philadelphia action and adopted similar resolutions.

This publicity probably deprived the Delaware of the opportunity of taking the first decisive step against the landing of the tea. The pilots were on the lookout for the tea ship *Polly*, an "old, black ship, commanded by short, fat Captain Ayres." They threatened to put a halter round his neck, to dump ten gallons of liquid tar upon his head, and, over that, to lay the feathers of a dozen wild geese. Ayres, warned of the Delaware's opposition, sailed with caution and with undue delay, waiting to see if brother skippers, bound to other ports from which no danger was expected, would meet a more agreeable reception. He did not come into the Delaware until Christmas Day.

Meanwhile, on November 28th, other tea ships,

which had left in company with the *Polly* and had sailed
in convoy with it across the whole Atlantic, had arrived
at Boston.   Three days later another vessel put in at
Charleston, but Ayres remained at sea.   The Charleston
people, giving the tea ship forty-eight hours' grace,
compelled it to go back to England; Boston, after waiting eighteen days, dumped the tea into the harbor.

The news of Boston's Tea Party came to Philadelphia on Christmas Eve.   Fancifully dressed masqueraders—the famous Philadelphia Mummers—were rev-
eling in the streets, their gorgeous costumes, bright with
color and glittering with spangles, representing every
character of fairyland and legend.   From house to house
they went, reciting doggerel explanatory of their fantastic disguises, and demanding Christmas "dole."   The
waits, too, were strolling through the city, singing carols
and asking for donations for their Christmas boxes.
Within the houses, citizens were decorating drawing
rooms with holly, mistletoe, and laurel; the Christmas
tree, recently brought to the Delaware by German immigrants, was ready for Kris Kringle to arrive and place
his gifts beneath it.

Amid these preparations the bells of Christ
Church, which had all afternoon and evening been
pealing merry melody, suddenly rang out in wilder,
more excited tones.   The watch called out that news
had come.   An express courier, riding down from Boston, brought word of the Tea Party.   The city jubilated to celebrate the Bostonian defiance.

It was Captain Ayres' good fortune that, after such
long waiting, he should choose this time to bring his
cargo into port.   Early Christmas morning the *Polly*
came into the river.   The Delaware felt cheated that
Ayres had come so late and thus deprived them of the
opportunity of leading colonial resistance, but, both

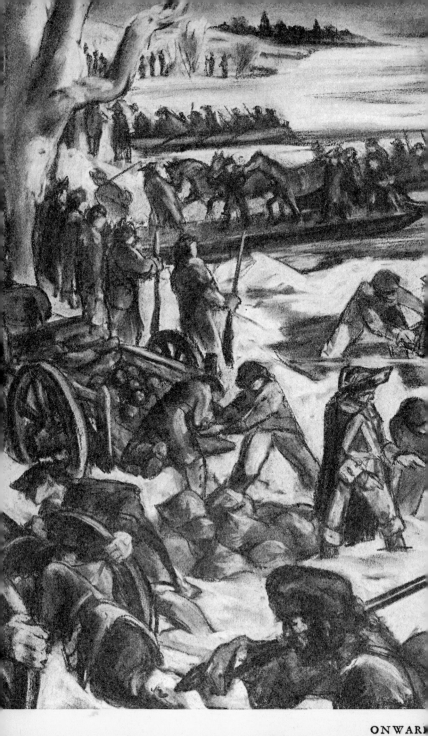

ONWAR

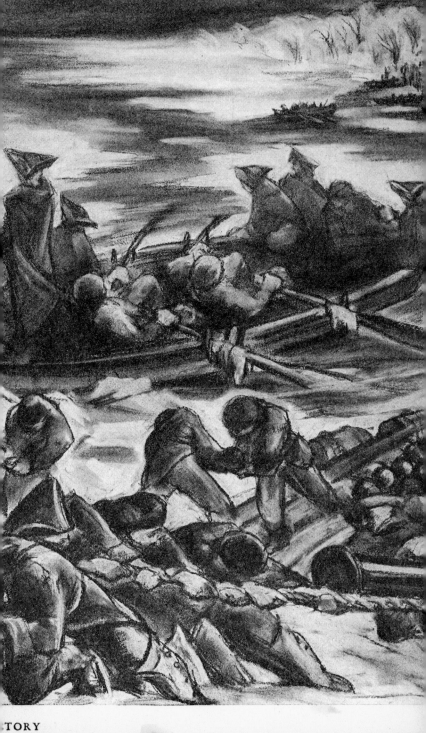

because of Christmas spirit and because the drastic action at Boston had made the message clear enough, sharp action was not now deemed necessary. A mass meeting of eight thousand citizens decreed that Ayres might stay one day, to buy his necessary stores and to refill his water butts, but that he must then return to England with his tea.

A later skipper, trusting that the Delaware might have moderated in its resolution, was not so well received. When the brig *Greyhound* slipped into small Cohansey Creek, just where the bay narrows to become the river, to land its taxed tea after nightfall, a belated tea party was held. Farmers of the district, marshaled by their clergymen, broke into the barn where Captain James Allen had smuggled his unwanted cargo. They dragged the chests into the fields, heaped them into a wide, tall pile, and set the tea afire. The farmers danced about the burning chests, shouting their defiance to a Parliament that laid taxation without allowing colonists their proper representation.

Though all the group was known, and though Allen hired two of the best Philadelphia lawyers to bring the men to justice, not one participant was ever punished. Delaware and New Jersey lawyers gave their services for the defense; a jury of the district, some of them, no doubt, close friends of the raiders, failed to find sufficient evidence. Even their weak neighbor, Henry Stacks—"Tea Stacks"—who had first filled all his pockets with the smuggled tea before he dragged chests to the pyre, was thoroughly exonerated. He never, however, lived down the nickname which he earned that night.

Owing to Ayres's irresolution, Boston had anticipated the Delaware in overt resistance to the tax on tea, and thereby drew down upon herself the first strong penalties. By successive acts of Parliament, the Boston harbor was shut to commerce, the right of free speech was limited, freedom of election was suspended, troops were quartered in private houses. The laws were aimed at Boston only, but they might have been, with equal logic, directed against Philadelphia, which inspired and stimulated the resistance.

The Continental Congress

Boston's troubles found a sympathetic ear in Philadelphia; the Delaware was afire with fury and resentment. Lawyer John Dickinson, owner of a trenchant pen, wrote blistering letters "from a Pennsylvania Farmer" to point out the evils of the British policy, and, though he hoped still for conciliation, to suggest that force would be the final outcome. Charles Thomson, called by the Indians "the man who tells the truth," was, as John Adams wrote, "the very life of the cause of liberty." Thomas Mifflin, once a macaroni, poured out his wealth to organize resistance. Even the "broadbrims" had men like Timothy Matlack who organized the "Fighting Quakers" to oppose British tyranny. Such were the men who rode out, accompanied by the town militiamen, to greet the hundred delegates who came to hold a Continental Congress.

Carpenters' Hall, the meeting place of the First Continental Congress, was not the most desirable assembly hall in Philadelphia. The three-story brick structure, built four years before by members of the Carpenters' Guild, stood somewhat isolated from the busy section of the town. Its graceful white steeple, half hidden by a gable at the foot of a narrow alley, was scarcely visible above the rooftops of surrounding houses.

It was, however, the best place available. The State House was already fully occupied by the provincial legislature and by various committees active in organizing intercolonial affairs. The new-built City Tavern, finest of American inns, was deemed too small for delegates of eleven provinces, though its owner generously offered to throw his large clubrooms into one great hall if the congressmen accepted his hospitality. Carpenters' Hall, however, seemed preferable, for its well-stocked library would be ready for immediate consultation, its long entry gave delegates a chance to stretch their legs at indoor exercise, and its committee rooms allowed opportunity for private conversation. Some delegates thought, too, that the selection of a guildhall would invite desired support from artisans and tradesfolk who might be suspicious of the lawyers and politicians in a more formal meeting place.

Unhappy news greeted the delegates on their arrival. Confused accounts from Boston implied that General Thomas Gage had fired into the city and that women and children had been killed in the bombardment. The Delaware was in a frenzy. All but the orthodox Quakers clamored for reprisals and, had it not been for a speedy contradiction of the false report, thousands of men would have marched off to help New England.

Philadelphia showed warm hospitality to its guests. Five hundred delegates and city notables gathered at an elaborate banquet, at which thirty-two toasts were drunk, beginning with tributes to the king and queen and ending with a compliment to John Hancock, the Massachusetts leader who was slated to be president of Congress.

There is no need here for a detailed account of the proceedings of the Continental Congress. It met, September, 1774, to canvass the situation. "We go to the Congress at nine," wrote John Adams to his wife, "and there we stay, most earnestly engaged in debates upon the most abstruse mysteries of state, until three in the afternoon. Then we adjourn, and go to dine with some of the nobles of Philadelphia at four o'clock, and feast upon ten thousand delicacies, and sit, drinking Madeira, claret or burgundy, till six or seven, and then go home, fatigued with business, company, and care. I shall be killed with kindness in this place." Seven weeks after the sessions started, in October, 1774, the delegates finally adopted an "American Association," binding the provinces not to export goods to England, and neither to import nor to use any taxed British commodities. They recommended, also, that representatives be chosen for a second Continental Congress to be held in May.

This new group also met under trying circumstances. A month before the delegates convened, news had arrived that British troops had fired on minutemen at Lexington and Concord. This time the reports were true. The valley of the Delaware was now resolved to fight. In every county, troops were hurriedly enrolled and twice a day were being drilled in military rudiments. Many of the younger Quakers donned cockades and uniforms, much to the horror of the stricter Friends. For this violation of their nonresistant faith, "Fighting Quakers" were read out of meeting. Many, however, rushed to join Joseph Cowperthwaite's Quaker Blues, or John Cadwalader's silk-stocking company of Greens. The Greens, perhaps, were rather the more popular, for the suave and polished Colonel Cadwalader, who knew well how to handle men, set out each afternoon huge demijohns of good Madeira for his men to drink when drill was done. More than two thousand soldiers were in training within a month after Lexington was fought. John Adams wrote admiringly, "So sudden a formation of an army never took place anywhere." Troops poured into Philadelphia.

Captain Jonathan Caldwell's Delawareans, recruited at this time, came north prepared to fight or play. They brought with them two gamecocks, hatched from the eggs of a small, lean, steel-blue hen, which, they insisted, could outfight any other birds. The cocks were never beaten, and when the time for battle came, the Delawareans rushed into action shouting, "We're sons of the Blue Hen, and we're game to the end." The Caldwell troops were known, thereafter, as the Blue Hen's Chickens, and Delawareans ever since have proudly borne the same nickname.

Patriots along the Delaware more than did their part to form, equip, and maintain an army. The river itself was fortified, a fleet of shallow-draft row galleys was provided, fire rafts were built to send against the enemy when British ships appeared, a chevaux-de-frise, a spiked barricade, was sunk across the channel. The defenses were sufficient to keep the upper river clear of hostile ships for almost two years' time.

Caesar Rodney's Ride

No story of the Delaware would be complete without at least a mention of the drama that accompanied the adoption of the Declaration of Independence. How the members of the Second Continental Congress schemed and debated in their sessions at the famous hip-roofed Independence Hall is known to every schoolboy; how the colonies were divided over the advisability of openly proclaiming that independence which they all desired is common information; but the means by which a unanimity was finally assured is seldom known beyond the basin of the Delaware.

Not all the colonies were ready to proclaim their freedom when, on June 7, 1776, Richard Henry Lee of Virginia brought up a resolution for severing the provinces from English rule. The middle colonies particularly were undecided, partly, as in New York's instance, for commercial reasons, partly, like Maryland, because their royal governor, horse-loving Robert Eden, was beloved, partly also, no doubt, because some larger landowners were content with British rule or because the Quakers were averse to any measure that would provoke violence.

When Lee's resolution was first offered, neither the advocates of instant independence nor the more conservative representatives who favored freedom at some later day were ready for a vote. Each group preferred to wait until more colonies were in accord. A three weeks' postponement was arranged, with Lee's resolution to be acted upon not earlier than July 1st.

During the interval each faction canvassed the delegates. In most of the provinces, a safe majority was counted in the resolution's favor, but each vote would be important, especially in the case of little Delaware whose delegation was divided. One representative, Thomas McKean, was hot for instant freedom; another, George Reed, of New Castle, thought haste was inadvisable. The vote of Delaware would thus be cast, since each colony voted as a unit, on how the third man acted. He, Brigadier General Caesar Rodney, was not in Philadelphia. He had been excused some time before to go to the lower reaches of the river to help put down a threatened Tory rising.

McKean, knowing that the vote was set for July 1st, dispatched a rider to bring Rodney back. When the messenger found him, he was already returning. Only a few hours remained before the vote on independence would be taken.

Rodney, "slender as a reed," took horse immediately. Though he was past middle age and already suffering from the painful cancer which was to cause his death, he rode without unnecessary halt. Up the King's Road from Dover, through the flat, fertile fields of Delaware, splashing across the shallow creeks, and riding after dark in the ten-mile stretch of Blackbird Forest, he pressed on toward Philadelphia. For thirty miles he rode through lonesome country in the night, changing horses whenever he came to any inn, but stopping for neither meals nor sleep. He passed through New Castle, the Nieuew Amstel of the Dutch, whistled to the ferryman to hurry him across the Christina that he might ride on to Wilmington. Then, ever northward, he galloped forward, waiting impatiently to be ferried over the Brandywine, for the footbridge was too narrow for a horse, crossing the rising land that led him to the ancient blacksmith shop on Penny Hill. The creek at Naaman's, close to the Twelve Mile Circle line that marked the Pennsylvania boundary, was little hindrance, though Rodney wished that he had time to share a bowl of Tom Robinson's famous punch and to chat a bit with Sally, Tom's sparkling sister whose wit was captivating. But Rodney had no time to tarry, except to borrow one of Tom's good horses; he clattered northward, through Chester, clumping over the bridges that spanned the four deep creeks that lay above, skirting the low, unhealthy marshes that lay along the river. By late afternoon he was climbing, slowly now for the

Robinson horse was spent, up the rough steep hill from whose stony summit he would see the Schuylkill.

The way was easy now, but time was short. The sun was well down in the sky as Rodney splashed over the "floating bridge" whose plank walk, laid on lashed logs, sank beneath the weight, but the bridge was firm enough to let horse and rider pass to the eastern bank. Only a mile or two of good hard road remained.

McKean, meanwhile, was exhausting every possible device of parliamentary tactics to delay voting on the resolution. New York, as friends of independence knew, could not be counted on; Edward Rutledge felt uneasy lest South Carolina waver in her support; Pennsylvania, too, was doubtful. Of the nine Pennsylvania delegates, only three—John Morton, James Wilson, and Benjamin Franklin—were sure to vote for independence; two men were definitely hostile to the resolution; two more, as everyone was well aware, would not attend a session of the Congress. All depended on the way in which two undecided delegates would vote. If Franklin could persuade these two uncertain men, John Dickinson and Robert Morris, to refrain from voting "No," the small minority of three enthusiastic independence advocates would thus outweigh the two determined loyalists. While McKean was busy with his dilatory tactics, waiting for Rodney to arrive, Franklin was pleading with Dickinson and Morris to vote "Yes" or, at the worst, sit silent and Rutledge was persuading his fellow Carolinians to stand firm in their support.

By late afternoon of the hot, muggy day the delegates were grown impatient. Small, black flies, so bothersome in the Pennsylvania summer, were biting vigorously through the thin silk stockings of the weary statesmen; it was long past the usual dinner hour; cries were constant that the matter come at last to vote.

Much had been accomplished. By wearing down the resistance of two sick members of his delegation, Rutledge had won back the Carolina vote; New York, though unwilling to go on record as favoring separation, agreed to cast no vote; Franklin won the same promise from Robert Morris, the canny merchant, and from John Dickinson, the cautious lawyer. Pennsylvania, thus, was safe. Only Delaware was left to mar a seeming unanimity, but, now that so much time had passed without a word from Rodney, the independence men abandoned hope that Delaware would favor freedom. Reluctantly, they let the question come before the house.

Charles Thomson, the pious, scholarly secretary of the Continental Congress and one of the warmest partisans of liberty, rose to his feet to call the roll. He polled Connecticut and, as a thunderous "Yes" resounded, the friends of freedom cheered; the first step toward freedom had been taken. Then Thomson called on Delaware, second state in alphabetic order.

Tom McKean turned slowly toward John Hancock, the presiding officer, to say that Delaware could not agree and that the delegation was divided. Beneath his cold, proud vanity he felt a bitter disappointment that his own state, alone among the thirteen, was thus about to go on record; he could not understand why Caesar Rodney, so ardent in the cause of independence, had failed to answer to his plea.

Scarcely had he uttered his first words, however, before commotion broke into the chamber. Behind McKean a door burst open, and a slender, breathless figure, with face pale as ashes, rushed upon the floor. Half a hundred startled statesmen, taken by surprise, swung suddenly about, some clapping their hands to their sword hilts, some raising their arms to shield their faces against attack, still others shouting a protest against the violation of the council hall. It was Caesar Rodney, who, after eighty miles of hasty riding, had arrived at last. Delaware was safe for freedom; McKean could add his state to those which stood for independence.

14

Britons Can Be Beaten

Trenton and Princeton

THE states were free, but every omen indicated that the little nation would not long maintain its liberty. British forces, striking south from New York toward the Delaware, swept all before them. Washington's small army, racked by hunger and disease, lay shivering in the biting December cold, seemingly unable to resist. The recent capture of General Charles Lee, whom many thought the ablest leader of the Continental camp, caused some of the more timorous to slip away, hoping to avoid the death or imprisonment that seemed to many of them inevitable. In New Jersey the rebels were on the run; Delaware and Pennsylvania, once happily remote from danger, feared imminent invasion. Sir William Howe and Lord Cornwallis, with ample troops, were resting at Trenton, prior to an attack in force on Philadelphia.

Washington gained an inkling of the British plans. Because the brass-capped Hessian mercenaries, the marauders of the countryside, were homesick for their fatherland, the British leaders attempted to console them with a feast. Christmas, at Trenton, was to be observed in customary German style, with extra rations of roast goose, if foragers could find sufficient fowls, with extra gills of rum, and, if all went well, with the beloved German Christmas tree, tinseled and gay with lights, set up in the long low Hessian barracks close to the riverbank. The customary sentry guards need not, the British reasoned, be so numerous as usual, for Washington's small force, encamped upon the west shore of the Delaware, from Trenton up to Coryell's Ferry, seemed helpless to move. The Hessians might, the British thought, celebrate their Christmas feast in perfect safety. Washington could take no possible advantage of the relaxed Hessian vigilance.

Thus the setting was perfect for an American surprise attack, especially as Washington had three full days in which to lay his plans. If he could throw his men across the stream, to fall upon the Hessians in the night, he would be able to wreak fearful havoc on the celebrating mercenaries.

The Delaware was difficult to cross, however. Huge ice boulders, piled high in wild confusion on the shore, blocked access to the river. Even if the troops were gathered on the banks, rough ice, far too treacherous to bear a soldier's weight, stretched out for yards into the stream and a swift and swirling midstream current carried jagged ice floes. To cross at Trenton for direct assault on the enemy positions would be suicidal; the noise of Continentals crashing through the ice would waken every Hessian.

Nine miles up the river was a long and narrow island, lying diagonally across the western half of the stream. Here the banks were low and level; ice floes were less numerous. Sheltered by the lee of the long island, the Delaware was less tightly frozen; blocks of ice were not so large nor nearly as numerous; the current was more leisurely. Here, at McKonkey's Ferry, Washington concentrated twenty-four hundred men. He set them scouring the western bank for miles north and south to gather whatever skiffs and boats might be available. By midnight on Christmas he planned to set his men across the Delaware.

The task was certainly not easy, but he had among his men a regiment of seasoned sailors. Colonel John Glover's Marblehead fishermen, accustomed to the management of small boats in choppy New England seas, made light of the task of ferrying the troops across the Delaware. Safe in the knowledge that no enemy could spy successfully across the river in the thick weather of a late December day, they chopped away the ice that cluttered up the shore, hacked out a wide harbor for their boats, cut open a passage toward midstream. They dared not cross the river to prepare a suitable harbor on the Jersey side, for spies and enemy patrols would thus discover what movements were afoot, but the soldiers first to cross at night would be expected to clear away approaches while the boats were going back for reinforcements.

To their delight, the Marblehead fishermen, who expected nothing but flimsy rowboats to be rounded up along the Delaware, were supplied with 60-foot double-ended craft used, in peaceful times, to carry iron from upstream furnaces to Philadelphia. Scouts had found these great Durham boats hidden away in little creeks or beached on the shore above Coryell's and had run them down the river for Washington to use as transports. In happier times, husky, bearded boatmen, conspicuously dressed in bright red shirts, bawling lusty chanteys, poled the Durhams forward, each man running to the bow along a platform from the stern, planting the spike end of his 20-foot pole against the stony river bottom, and walking down a cleated runway to the stern. Great sails flew when wind was fair and when the course was straight downriver, but not even Marblehead fishermen could use the sails to cross the stream.

With transports such as these, the task of ferrying the army over three hundred yards of water was less difficult. Between midnight and three o'clock in the morning of December 26th, the troops were safely set across to Jersey. Then, pausing for a short space to form his men into two divisions, Washington gave orders to advance. So accurate was his planning that five hours later one section, marching down the river road under command of Nathanael Greene, fell upon the outposts of the enemy exactly the same time that the second section, hurrying along the Scotch road with hotheaded John Sullivan, attacked the same posts from the opposite side. By nightfall the Continentals were back in their camps on the Pennsylvania side with a thousand prisoners and scores of guns and cannons.

The victory at Trenton restored American morale. Lee's capture was forgotten; Washington's strategy was hailed as equal to that of any of the great soldiers of the past. Men who had been ready to desert, or who had been insistent that they would leave the service just as soon as their short periods of enlistment had expired, resolved to stay with the army. The proof that trained Hessians could be defeated and that land invasion could be beaten back revived the confidence of the Continental army. Washington, to be sure, was back across the Delaware, but only to prepare a new attack. Three days later he returned to Jersey, took up quarters in recaptured Trenton, and prepared to take up the offensive.

Cornwallis almost took him by surprise. With a superior army, the British general marched down from New Brunswick to the St. Pink, or Assunpink, Creek; the van of the invading forces reached Trenton itself

by four o'clock in the afternoon of January 2nd.
Washington, learning through his efficient secret service that the enemy was greatly superior in numbers,
made one of the most daring moves in all the war.
Marching silently by night, with muffled cannon wheels
and shrouded hoofs of cavalry horses, he rode around
the British army, fell upon it at dawn in the rear, at
Princeton, and crushed three regiments. He lost his
able general, Hugh Mercer, who was clubbed down in
the fighting and then stabbed with seven bayonet
thrusts, but central and south New Jersey were recovered. The movement was, as Horace Walpole said,
"a prodigy of generalship."

Two mementos have remained of these great victories. One, a well-deserved tribute, is the naming of
the central county of New Jersey, where Trenton and
Princeton are located, after the unfortunate General
Mercer. The other, well-intentioned but historically
incorrect, is the famous painting, by Emanuel Leutze,
German-born artist, of "Washington Crossing the
Delaware." Like West's picture of Penn's Treaty, it
contains more inaccuracy than artistic virtues, but it
does commemorate a triumph of the Revolutionary
War. Leutze, like most people, would have been astonished to learn that Washington himself considered the
second crossing of the Delaware, following the Battle
of Trenton, as more arduous than the midnight transit.
There was, as Washington wrote to Congress, more ice,
more hardship, and more difficulty than he had experienced on his way to fight the Hessians.

Spy Mania

The victories relieved the Delaware of imminent
invasion, but the valley still was apprehensive. The

enemy had come too close for comfort; fear of its return could not be readily dismissed. Citizens were jittery and, because they were alarmed, saw new menaces in every shadow. Each man suspected that his neighbor was a secret British agent. Any resident who faltered in enthusiasm or questioned the wisdom of the governing authorities was set down as a traitor. Unusual behavior proved intended treason. Each stranger seemed to spy.

There was good ground to question the loyalty of a few people. British sympathies, always strong among the landed gentry and the wealthier commercial groups, were never wholly absent, and some men were unquestionably ready to betray the Continental cause. James Molesworth, for example, clerk in the Philadelphia mayor's office, accepted British bribes to find the secret passage through the five spiked rows of chevaux-de-frise. Until that channel was revealed, British sailors knew, no man-of-war could penetrate the maze, and, if there were no warships to support attack, assaults on Philadelphia would, as Trenton proved, be wholly futile. Molesworth agreed to find some pilots who could bring the British fleet upstream.

Only ten men knew the secret courses, but three of these, the traitor thought, were men who might be bought. He had authority to offer them £500 apiece, with the promise of commissions in the Royal Navy, but Molesworth thought he knew a more effective lure. Two pretty Irish girls agreed to use their charms to win the pilots over. Molesworth counted on them to extract the secret of the channel; he, then, could pocket the greater portion of the bribes.

Sally O'Brien and Abigail McKay played their parts well and won the pilots' confidence, but when the questions as to how to pass the sunken barricades grew too definite, and when Molesworth was too constantly in their company, the men became suspicious. They waited until Molesworth came into the open with his plans, accepted £50 in golden guineas from him, and then told the whole story to the city watch. Molesworth was arrested and tried for treason; next day he was hanged. The women were imprisoned.

This was a clear-cut case, wherein the victim was unquestionably guilty. But there were other instances in which the patriots' shattered morale led them to see treachery where little fact was proved. Outspoken critics of the Revolution, blunt men who spoke their minds too freely, were assailed as traitors. Caustic Robert Dove, who entertained his friends with sharp satiric verses and with caricatures etched in malice, was soon suspected of disloyalty. Dr. Abraham Chovet, master anatomist whose wax models of internal organs were marvels of their kind, fell under the ban because his quarrelsome, profane sarcasms cut too close to the quick of certain sensitive statesmen. Eighty other so-called Tories were jailed, banished, or, like Chovet, pledged to keep the peace.

The Quakers were especially unfortunate. Their principles were stanchly pacifist and they professed unwillingness to aid the war in any way. To angry patriots the policy of nonresistance spelled only treason; the frequent "testimonies" at the Quaker meetings seemed invariably hostile to the cause of freedom. Many indignant rebels were convinced that Quakers were in secret correspondence with the British to betray the Revolution. The spy fever grew so hot that orders were drawn up to jail the Quaker leaders.

Fear of a new invasion by the British intensified the hatred. To prevent these nonresistants' giving aid to the English cause, the Pennsylvania government,

nce wholly Quaker, commanded that the more impor-
ant Quakers be deported from the state. Many of
hem, chiefly old men unaccustomed to privation, were
packed in springless wagons, drummed out of Philadelphia, and hurried under guard to the mountains of
Virginia. For eight winter months, while the British
were at Philadelphia and the Continental Army was at
Valley Forge, the Quakers were kept in exile. They
were not permitted to return until the English Army
was well out of the Delaware region.

Former leaders did not escape persecution. The
long antagonism to proprietary rule now culminated in
attacks on the Penns for their alleged pro-British sympathies. John Penn, the prewar governor, and all his
officials, some forty in all, were arrested; their property
was confiscated. The goods of every Tory were forfeit
to the state. Even the College of Philadelphia, whose
trustees were chiefly Revolutionary sympathizers, suffered because its head, Dr. William Smith, had long
warred on the popular Assembly. The college was
suspended; its charter was annulled.

The college was luckier than its fellow victims.
Two years after the suppression a new charter was
authorized, allowing the institution to resume its work
as the University of Pennsylvania, and giving to it as
endowment a large amount of confiscated Tory property. Not until a dozen years had passed was justice
done to many who had been robbed of their estates.
The Penns completely lost all rights to the province
which the founder had begun.

The persecutions went far toward undermining the
general respect for government. Conservatives were
outraged and, though unable to express their feelings
openly, lukewarm in their support. Even many Whigs
turned away from full co-operation with a radical gov-

ernment which some thought to be "truly ridiculous." "Not one of the laws of the Assembly," one disillusioned patriot wrote, "is regarded; no courts are open; no justice is administered. . . . I question if any man of tolerable merit would accept the government of Pennsylvania." The state was drifting into the position which Delaware occupied when ten men successively declined to act as delegates, and two men refused the governorship.

The stage was being set for violent conflict between the radical party, largely made up of frontiersmen, and the advocates of more cautious evolutionary progress. But while fear of Britain was so strong civil struggle was suspended. Not until the Revolution had been won did the two contending groups come into active opposition.

Betsy Ross

But the story of the period is not just one sad tale of fear and tribulation. There is a pleasant legend of the times, which, though probably not firmly founded on historic fact, should certainly be mentioned. While the Delaware was nervous with anticipation of a new attack, and while the people were excitedly accusing one another of sedition, the new flag of the nation was created.

The tradition tells how Robert Morris, George Ross, and General George Washington called upon the seamstress Betsy Ross to have her make the Stars and Stripes basing the pattern on the Washington coat of arms, and how she then taught them to cut five-cornered stars by single slashes of the scissors. The legend was never in wide currency until a century had passed, and is today upheld chiefly by the Betsy Ross descendants, but it contains truth enough to allow it a continued hearing.

Certainly there was a girl called Betsy Griscom, and much was known of her. Her skill at needlework was generally praised; her devotion to Quaker principles was a model to young girls. Her breathless elopement with young John Ross, upholsterer from New Castle, had caused much gossip and resulted in her being read out of meeting. The tragic death of Ross, by the explosion of some powder he was guarding on the wharves, had left the girl a widow at twenty-four, but she carried on his business and was prospering.

Among her clients was the Pennsylvania navy, which wanted some flags to place on the row galleys on the river. These white banners, with green pine trees in the center and bearing the legend "An Appeal to Heaven," were flying in full view of all Philadelphia. It was on this account, says family tradition, that the three men came to her to have her make the Stars and Stripes, particularly as George Ross was her husband's elder brother.

But there are other facets which detract a trifle from the story about Betsy Ross. George Washington, the central figure of the tale, had little time to spend in Philadelphia. His army was in northern Jersey, straining every nerve to keep close watch on redcoats in New York, and it is doubtful whether he was long enough at the capital to pay a call on the upholsterer. Nor is it certain that George Ross was any too well pleased with Betsy's actions, for gossip closely linked the widow of only a year with another suitor and the Ross clan felt that she was not evincing proper sorrow. There is no account of payment for this flag ever being made to Betsy Ross, though account books show a careful record for the pine-tree ensigns, and historians have hesitated to put their seal on the Betsy Ross affair.

Whoever made the flag, it is certain that the Stars and Stripes were officially adopted as the national flag on June 14, 1777. It is also true that on the very next day energetic Betsy Ross was married once again, this time to Captain Joseph Ashbrook, the swain to whom the Ross family objected.

Within two months the Stars and Stripes saw action. Howe's British force, landing after a long detour from New York up the Chesapeake, fell on Philadelphia in the rear. He met a small detachment of nine hundred Pennsylvania horse and seven hundred Marylanders and Blue Hen's Chickens at Cooch's Bridge, in Delaware. The site, the records state, was near Iron Mountain, but the name must be accepted with reserve since the highest land in all the state of Delaware is but four hundred feet above sea level. The American force, led by General "Scotch Willie" Maxwell, was heavily outnumbered; the rebel arms were far inferior to those of Howe's well-equipped veterans, but the fight was stubbornly maintained. Eventually, when Howe brought up artillery, the rebels were dislodged after losing thirty killed and wounded. The Stars and Stripes had undergone its first engagement. Brandywine followed in a week, and then, successively, came Paoli and Germantown, the fearful winter at Valley Forge, followed by the rising triumphs of the rebel cause.

Wooden Grenadier

Betsy Ross's story may be doubted, but there is no question of the truth of Sally Wister's innocent adventures. The happy sixteen-year-old, deceptively demure, flirted outrageously with the American soldiers, from Maryland's red-faced General William Smallwood down to the lowliest subaltern.

Troopers, immaculate in blue and scarlet, caused her a moment's terror when they rode up to her house near Germantown. But when she found they were not British her fears subsided. She was more chagrined over being surprised in her everyday green dress than worried about any harm that might befall her. And when she and her cousin Priscilla learned that the advancing troops had chosen her father's house as the Smallwood headquarters, and that the staff would spend the greater portion of their time close by, her joy was great. "When we were alone," she told her diary, "our dress and lips were put in order for conquest, and the hopes of adventures gave brightness to each before passive countenance."

The coming of the general with six slim aides, accompanied by a guard of soldiers, crowding the yard and house with glittering military equipment, thrilled even a sedate Quaker maiden who, one would think, abhorred all thoughts of war. That evening there was too much bustle for the men to notice Sally, even in her most feminine chintz dress, but Smallwood expected to remain indefinitely. "I am going to my chamber to dream," she said, "of bayonets and swords, sashes, guns and epaulets."

Major Benjamin Stoddard, nineteen-year-old nephew of the general—bashful, manly, and later to be secretary of the navy under two presidents—was Sally's first concern. He would not glance at her, though Sally smiled her prettiest and was so charming that she wondered how even a stoic could resist her. "But still, I won't despair. Who knows what mischief I yet may do?" The next time, she resolved, she would put on her grown-up silk-and-cotton gown made without an apron; meanwhile she cast her glance on homesick Lieutenant Lee, who longed to be home in tidewater Virginia. To Sally's scarce-concealed dismay, young Lee would talk of nothing but the fried hominy and turkey hash of old Virginia!

Major Tilly was much more responsive. The presence of the girls excited him; he chattered a steady stream, boasting of his bravery, telling of his valor. He spoke so fast that he rarely managed to complete a sentence, but broke off to start a new and often wholly irrelevant topic. He had the same trick even with his flute, for he would not play a single tune to its completion, but would pipe a phrase or two, then start again, and look up eagerly for Sally's approval. She detested him; she vowed that she would have revenge upon this chatterer for all her disappointments.

Her opportunity came soon. On the evening following the troops' arrival, Sally and Priscilla went strolling down the road by moonlight. Horsemen were heard; the girls were fearful that the riders might be British.

"Let's run!" Priscilla cried.

"Oh, no," objected Sally. "It's better to be heroines. Let's take no notice of them."

The horsemen trotted closer. The girls, as Quaker maidens should, walked on deliberately, their eyes demurely downcast on the road. One man dismounted, threw his reins to an attendant, and bowed politely. It was Major Stoddard. Sally was delighted, but she showed no sign of pleasure. Other officers came up; a gay group strolled on slowly.

Now that the ice was broken, Stoddard proved a perfect beau. Quite recovered from his shyness, he chaffed the girls about their fears.

"What, Miss Sally, would you do if the British were to come?"

"Do? Why, I'd be frightened just to death."

But Stoddard had a better notion for her. "Why not run up the stairs and hide behind that figure on the landing? It's realistic enough to frighten even me." He was speaking of a life-size wooden image of a British grenadier that had been made for amateur theatricals.

"What, sir," said Sally, "are our officers so craven that they run away to hide behind a redcoat officer? Where's your courage? Major Tilly, I am sure, would have no fear. There, sir, is a man of bravery."

Stoddard, knowing Tilly's braggadocio, resented Sally's slur.

"Suppose," said he, "we try it out on him? Face Major Tilly with this grenadier, and we shall see how brave he is."

Sally giggled at the thought. In the dim candle-lighted hall, the wooden figure would appear to be a live British soldier. She and Stoddard told the others of their plan. The group hurried to the Wister house. Stoddard lugged the grenadier to a dark corner just inside the entrance; then he stood behind it. The other officers went into the drawing room to tell Tilly that they had met a messenger on the road who was inquiring for his quarters. Then, after a few moments had elapsed, the girls sent a servant to knock on the door to tell the officers that someone wished to speak to Major Tilly. The Negro was instructed to stand back and thus to throw a deeper shadow on the wooden grenadier.

Tilly came out laughing, and stepped into the entry. As he passed the bowing servant, a bass voice thundered:

"Are any rebels here?"

Tilly wheeled toward the door, saw the grenadier, and fled. Not waiting for a second word, he dashed through the yard and leaped the fence. The conspirators watched him stumble into the plowed field that lay across the lane. Stoddard, convulsed with laughter, tried to call him back.

Two hours elapsed before the braggard major dared come home. His hair had come untied and was hanging in strings on his shoulders; his uniform was splashed with mud. The girls and officers were waiting for him. He wore a shamefaced grin.

"Why, Mr. Tilly," Stoddard asked, "where *have* you been?"

Tilly's smile disappeared. "You go to the devil," he growled, but bowing to the girls, he begged their pardon for his "indecency," and soon joined the laugh on himself.

"Well, certainly," wrote Sally in her diary, "these military folk will laugh all night. Such screaming I never did hear."

15

King of the Marches

BRANDYWINE was lost. Two powerful British armies, converging on Washington in a pincer movement through the fog, caught the patriot army in a trap. By nightfall on September 11, 1777, despite the brave resistance of Anthony Wayne, the only active Pennsylvania general, of John Sullivan, and of the newly arrived La Fayette, the Americans were forced to retreat.

Philadelphia lay open to the British, but Washington's faith was not shaken. To lose the capital was a calamity, but one which might be borne. If, by a quick, hard march toward the munitions centers near the Schuylkill, the Continentals could refill their pouches, stock themselves with guns and ammunition, recruit more men, and take possession of the roads that led from Philadelphia into the interior, they could successfully besiege the British force. Under such conditions, Washington foresaw, a redcoat occupation of the capital might even work to the American advantage.

He ordered Wayne to march at daybreak by a circuitous route and, avoiding traveled roads, capture the highways leading from the city. Wayne was to move rapidly, and so far as possible secretly, telling of his purpose to no one but his immediate aides. By noontime he had come to the wide road that ran westward from the city. His men, still tired from their long fighting, began to grumble. Even Patrick Anderson and Adam Hubley, always the most loyal of his followers, were restless and unhappy.

"Where are we off to now?" a subaltern complained. "Looks like we're headed for the Indian country."

"Home, I hope," said Pat. "I know the way this Great Road runs. It strikes out through Blockley into Merion, where the Welshmen live, goes past Wayne's place near General Paoli Inn. Takes me home to Valley Forge if we go far enough."

"Hope it's a better road than this trail we've been walking," a Jerseyman growled. "My feet are sore with all these stones. Is Pennsylvania built of rocks?"

"You're on a good road now," Pat Anderson replied. "Best one we have. Goes out as far as Lancaster. You'll see more pack trains here in one day than Jersey ever saw. They come down from the mountains with pig iron and whisky. You never saw so much whisky in all your life."

"I know the stuff," said Jersey, "and I wouldn't drink it. We get better liquor at home. Our lightning costs a lot of money; you can't buy it for a shilling a gallon the way you buy your rum or that whisky you've been speaking of; but lightning's worth the difference. One drink of that——"

"Stop talking about drinking," Hubley interrupted. "You won't get a chance to drink on this Great Road. These Welshmen won't give a drink to any soldier. I told the Council of Safety about them just last spring. The innkeeping robbers charged soldiers two shillings for a meal, and not a good meal either. They even tried to make us pay for sleeping on the taproom floor."

"They'll not do that again," said Bill George of the

Philadelphia Militia. "The Council sent them word to stop. My brother Jesse saw to that; he's one of the enforcing agents."

"Yes, he did," Hubley called. "And then what happened? Every one of them pulled their signs down and closed the inns. From Bill Stadleman's Black Horse, up here on the edge of Merion, there wasn't an inn open for miles. Mifflin was so angry that he talked of making them open up by force."

"Mifflin's just talking," interjected Anderson. "That man talks more and does less than any other general. He should have been a lawyer. It's a good thing for the army that he lost his temper last month and quit the service. When he was commissary general he wasted army money just the same way that he threw away his own. Stadleman got two hundred pounds to keep open. We've some careless officers in this army of ours, but Mifflin was the worst of all."

"But Brother Jesse says that Washington is coaxing Mifflin to come back. The general wishes to improve the commissariat."

"With Mifflin? He's too poor a stick. It's Mifflin's fault that we're hungry now. We'll need a better man than handsome Tommy Mifflin if we're to get enough to eat."

The conversation ceased. Before the army was a knot of men, waiting hat in hand for its approach. A group of well-dressed citizens stood beneath a big sycamore, at Eaglefield, a mile above the Middle Ferry. Wayne halted. The men approached politely. The general motioned to them to speak.

"Sir," the strangers' leader said, "this is my friend, Baron William Warner, the owner of the Castle which you see upon the hill. These other gentlemen are citizens of our State-in-Schuylkill, and I am Samuel Morris, the governor—"

"You are what?" asked Wayne. "Governor? Of the State-in-Schuylkill? I fear I do not understand. This is the commonwealth of Pennsylvania. The governor is Thomas Wharton. You cannot mean—"

"Tom is my friend, general, as well as my superior. The State-in-Schuylkill is evidently new to you. We are a social club. We call ourselves the Fishing Society of the State-in-Schuylkill, and Governor Wharton is among our members. Nearly every citizen of our society is now engaged in patriotic service; there are but a few of us left here, but we desire to offer you an invitation to come with your staff to dinner at the Castle."

"Thank you, Mr. Morris, you are kind. We cannot stay, for we are ordered to press on to Merion. But your State-in-Schuylkill is interesting. I must confess that it is new to me. And, pardon me, but I have never heard of any Baron Warner. If he is a newcomer to our cause, I hope he will accept my thanks. We stand in great need of such men."

"But I'm as firm a Pennsylvanian as you are, general. The title is by courtesy. I lend my land to these brave fishermen and in return they pay me annual rent of one fresh perch per year. They give me their first fish and I consume it while they plank their shad. I'm truly sorry that you cannot stay to dine. We barbecue a pig and we broil beef in better style than any other kitchen in the commonwealth."

"We do it all ourselves," said Morris. "Our State-in-Schuylkill is truly democratic. When we were formed, on May Day of seventeen-thirty-two, we swore an oath to be an independent commonwealth. We did it half in jest and half in earnest, but we did declare that British writs would never run within our Castle.

Our governors, our legislators, our sheriffs, coroners, and judges make our rules. Our State-in-Schuylkill is so convinced that men are equal and that men are free that we dispense with servants. We don our aprons and straw hats and live a day or two each week as Rousseau wants all men to live. It is indeed a sorrow to us that you cannot stay."

The general thanked the State-in-Schuylkill once again, the officers waved greetings, and the men raised cheers as Wayne's troops moved on. It seemed a happy omen for the march, but the good impression was not to be permanent. Under a swinging sign that promised "Entertainment for Man and Beast," another delegation waited. Its dozen members were thin-lipped and glowering. Hubley and Bill George identified the leaders. They were near-by innkeepers. Jacob Wyncoop of the Rose and Crown was there, together with Bill Stadleman of the Black Horse, beneath whose sign the men were gathered, and Tony Tunis, of the Ordinary, was beside them.

"We warned the Council not to send more robbers," shouted Stadleman's rough voice. "We want no traitors here."

Wayne was nonplused. He was accustomed to strange greetings, hostile or friendly, but the charge of robbery was new. Sitting stiffly in the saddle, he demanded explanation.

Colonel John White's Georgians, it appeared, had stormed through Blockley a week or so before, scattering destruction and dismay. The township people, welcoming the militiamen as friends, had been maltreated. According to Stadleman, they had abused travelers at the inns, robbed houses and barns, stolen the stock, and even cut down standing timber. When Stadleman protested they threatened to set fire to all the houses, damned Congress, and declared that they would never fight against the king.

But Wayne had heard something of the men confronting him. Wyncoop and Tunis were loyal, but there were evil rumors current of the Black Horse and its landlord. It was a wild place, where travelers were reported to have been poisoned for their money. Still, the fellow must be placated for the sake of the others who would follow his lead. So Wayne assured the delegation that his regiment harbored no Georgians, only loyal and law-abiding Pennsylvanians. Stadleman bowed and scraped and assured the general that everything was quite all right and that the tavernkeepers would be pleased to be of service.

The old Lancaster road was crowded. Residents had never known such throngs. Heavy Conestoga wagons, blazing in their coats of bright red and brilliant blue, had rumbled in the past along the rutty, dusty trail, but never in great numbers. More frequently the passers-by were horsemen or foot travelers plodding beneath heavy packs. In former years there had been herdsmen driving geese to market, shooing the fowls along at a rate of perhaps a mile an hour with long poles to which red-flannel flappers had been tied. There had been drovers too, shouting their cattle down the road to slaughter. But neither herdsmen nor drovers had been along the Lancaster road for weeks. The loss from foraging soldiers had been too heavy. The arrival of Wayne's men, though only a portion of the army, was a memorable affair in the history of this narrow wagon road.

Wayne was now near home; his tannery and farm lay just across the ragged cornfields where the shocks still stood, beyond the chestnut woods that lay along the creek, over the meadowland where his prize cattle grazed. But he could not leave his men, though he was almost certain that the British, worn out by the Brandy-wine engagement, had halted to recuperate. But chaplains were less urgently needed; he granted a short leave of absence to his friend and neighbor, pastor David Jones.

Davy rode off from the army to the old stone house where his wife Anne and the children were clustered on the long, wide porch that faced the road. The coming of the Continentals had been rumored, but he had sent no word of his arrival. The children shrieked with glee as he flung himself from his horse and ran up to the steps.

Nothing had been harmed. Neither British patrols nor Tory raiders had as yet appeared near Waynesborough. Friendly neighbors, anxious for news of the general and of the popular young preacher, whose famous sermon, "Defensive War in a Just Cause Sinless," was so well known by hearsay and by printed broadside, had been attentive to the family. The larder was filled; there was even a seven-pound loaf of sugar just arrived as a gift from the parishioners.

The old two-story house was comforting this raw and windy night. The great fireplace at the far end of the room blazed cheerfully, though Pastor Davy noticed that the chimney draft had not been fixed and that wood smoke still puffed out into the room to add more blackness to the hand-hewn beams. This was a matter he must make right as soon as the war was over. But now he dined, on the savory stew remaining from the children's meal. Anne made him a dessert of batter cakes of flour, eggs, and milk, baked in a frying pan with lard and sprinkled with crumbs from the great sugar loaf. Had she known that he was coming, she kept insisting, she could have had his favorite wheat-flour dumplings with his meat, she would have fixed him vegetables, she would have made a proper pudding rich with suet and dripping. But now he must be satisfied with chocolate from one of his cherished china bowls.

The loyal congregation ruined the pastor's plan of starting early in the morning to overtake the army. Word had spread throughout the neighborhood that Davy Jones was back. Almost at daybreak the parishioners were riding to the pastor's home. Older men with clothes bearing silver buttons, their heavy riding coats thrown open to show the embroidered waistcoats, dismounted heavily, and doffed their beaver hats as they approached the house. Some came on foot, swinging their silver-mounted canes, escorting silk-gowned wives and daughters who displayed their silk gloves and Irish linens. The shortage of young men was apparent; this part of Pennsylvania had sent its boys into the army.

It was a handsome group of stocky, delicately featured, blue-eyed blonds. This small settlement of Baptists contained few of the dark-complexioned people who lived across the Schuylkill in the other part of the Welsh Tract. These Radnor folk insisted proudly that their small bones and slender frame, their sharp, well-cut features and their light, or auburn, hair were proof of their descent from Welsh aristocrats. They were not descended from the serfs; they were not the offspring of farm hands and yeomen; these were true "bonheddig" people, pure Cymric on both sides, men whose pedigrees ran back, untainted by alien blood, to the ancient times when Gwynedd, the White Land, had mastered most of Britain.

Pastor David Jones kept no sacred parlor for special social ceremony. The pastor received his guests under the carved mantelboard, in front of the pictured tiles that lined the big fireplace. The appointments were familiar. The tall clock and the corner cupboard filled with the china coffee service, the hinged tea table and the high-back rush-seat chairs, the candles in their silver sticks against the waxed wainscotting, the hardwood floors, smoothed by the holystone and sanded in Anne's favorite designs, were similar in style to the furnishings of other homes in the well-to-do community. The men and women were not here to inspect the household goods but to pay their respects to the pastor who had unexpectedly returned.

Not until after the noonday meal of solid and substantial fare was he free to resume his army duties, but even then he pottered round the lawns, poking with his stick at places where he thought fruit trees might be planted. In later years the Jones mansion was to be surrounded by a huge orchard, for Davy Jones put trees wherever he could dig a hole. There was to come a time, after the Revolution was over, when doggerel would sing of Pastor Davy, in old-fashioned cue, cockade, knee breeches, and silver buckles:

Munching his apples, pears and plums,
To the squeak of his fiddle, fife and drums.

These times, of course, were far in the future. In September, 1777, it was his immediate duty to return to the Continental Army. But getting there was difficult. During his stay at home, while clouds were thickening and drizzle was beginning, the British had been marching. Scouts appeared; breathless riders shouted that battle lines were forming on the ridges. Davy realized that he must take a wide detour to escape capture.

It was lucky that he delayed no longer. A few moments after his departure, while some of his parishioners still lingered at his home, green-uniformed

Queen's Rangers rode up to the house demanding Davy's surrender. When they discovered that he had managed to escape, the Rangers, angry at missing the redoubtable pastor on whose head Howe had set a price, wrecked the house, carrying off the silver, the handsome "chocka-lete" bowls, sixteen pairs of stockings, and the prized loaf of sugar.

16

Sturdy Friends of Freedom

THE next few weeks were filled with heartbreak for the Continentals. Wayne, hiding in the woods near the General Paoli Inn, waiting for a chance to fall upon the British by surprise, was himself unexpectedly attacked by Major General Sir Charles Grey and the crack Black Watch. Through Tory treachery and the failure of sentries to give timely warning of the British advance, the Black Watch bayonets killed two hundred Americans before Wayne could form his men into a battle line. He managed to withdraw his guns to safety.

The Paoli Massacre was but the first of the disappointments that befell the Continental arms. Washington, hurrying north to the munitions centers to refill his chests, was hard pressed by the British and forced away before his task was finished. General Howe, threatening the arsenals at Reading, compelled the Americans to make lengthy countermarches to protect their stores and then, when Washington had been decoyed far to the north, the clever Englishman raced back to capture Philadelphia without a battle.

Luckily, the Continental troops were left in regions friendly to the Revolution. Upstate Pennsylvania, largely settled by peaceful, enterprising German immigrants, was probably the one region in America where independence burned most brightly. Washington arrived among them at the time when their harvests were fresh-gathered and their barns were bursting with supplies.

These German settlers were sturdy friends of freedom. Mennonites and Schwenkfelders, Moravians and Lutherans, were to a man devoted to the cause of liberty, and so widespread was their reputation in this regard that even in pre-Revolutionary days men moved down to Pennsylvania from the Dutch settlements of New York to find freedom that was not elsewhere to be so easily secured.

Graduates of the best Swiss and German universities, the pastors of these backwoods regions promoted culture unsurpassed in other portions of the colonies. Franklin knew of them and catered to their tastes; more than half the books that issued from his press were German volumes for the upstate homes. The two Christopher Sowers, Pennsylvania publishers who fought for social reform and abolition of the slave trade, found ready markets for new books. The elder Sower printed the Bible in German for these people forty years before any printer in America brought out an English version. John and Andrew Krauss, before they reached their twentieth year, planned, designed, and built the first pipe organs ever made in the Americas.

Such were the people to whose protection the Americans were hurrying. Once across the Schuylkill, the Continental Army could rely upon ample stores of food and clothing. Each hausfrau, said the Pennsylvania officers, would bake the troops an ovenful of rich, dark rye bread, the kind that screeched as the knife cut through the crust. Shoes and blankets would be instantly available.

One young lieutenant was unimpressed. "I was here," said Jim McMichael, "two months ago. I know the country. I went from Bethlehem to Reading and met only one person who could talk English. They thought me a barbarian because I couldn't speak their German, but they appeared to me like so many dumb brutes. I did talk Latin to them till I found that they knew less of that than they did of English. So, I concluded, to my own satisfaction, that they were devoid of all the qualities that make for happiness—unless, of course, they are content to mix only with others as ignorant as themselves."

"You don't know the Muhlenbergs," protested Anderson. "They are an amazing clan. I've known them now for thirty years. The old man, Henry Melchior Muhlenberg, came out to Trappe when I was twenty-three. He seemed a little fellow then, too thin and scraggly to endure the kind of life he had to live, but he was stronger than we thought. The folks across the river didn't know that he was coming; they hadn't sent for him. He walked alone to Trappe, over those thirty miles of almost unbroken country, swimming the creeks because he did not know the fords, and when he got there the people laughed at him. But not for long. He settled down to preach, and those sermons of his were the finest things that had been heard in Pennsylvania. He's the pride of the community right now. Talks to them in four different languages, especially in Latin."

"German, isn't he? One of those Dutch fellows that you have up here."

"Came over when he was thirty. Told me once that he picked Pennsylvania because he could not find a place to preach in the East Indies. Took up an eight-year-old call for a preacher that the Pennsylvania folks had forgotten that they ever sent. That's why he had so hard a time to get accepted here."

"He's the father of the general, I suppose, but," interrupted Jim McMichael, "I don't see how that makes him so remarkable. You said it was an amazing clan. Why so? They're just preachers, aren't they?"

"Oh, yes, they're preachers. All the men. Six boys, all strapping big and every one of them's a preacher. Big John the general is the oldest. He's the chap who went to Germany to go to school and who ran away when his German guardian tried to bind him out to be a grocer. The Muhlenbergs don't like to trade.

"They don't?" asked Caleb North. "That's curious. Their grandfather, old Conrad Weiser from up Reading way, was the biggest Indian trader in the province. That Weiser family, father, mother, and all fifteen of the youngsters talked Indian oftener than they talked German. Those Weisers liked to trade. It's mighty odd that these Muhlenbergs don't like to dicker."

"Father, maybe, taught them to be scholars. Folks who wear spectacles don't seem to do so well at business."

"The Weisers did," continued North. "Old Conrad was the finest scholar that you ever saw. Had a complete law library in his backwoods cabin up there at Womelsdorf. Sent down to Philadelphia for an organ. Old Conrad said he had to have a music room. Music in a frontier cabin! Do you have that sort of thing up your way, Jim?"

"We fight Indians up in Paxtang, we don't give concerts for them. But Pat here said the Muhlenbergs were something special and all I see is that they're preachers who don't trade. What's so remarkable about the Muhlenbergs? Except this funny shaped church of theirs—"

"That funny church, as you are pleased to call it, my Paxtang friend," interrupted the silent Charles

Willson Peale, "is the only one of its kind in all these states. That gambrel roof, the triangular apse, the strange windows in the gallery, the ax-hewn timbers framed with tenons and dowels, is an architectural masterpiece. You don't know it, but this is a German-rural style of architectural design, and one of the very few works of art outside Philadelphia in all this commonwealth of yours. People will be coming here for generations after you are dead to look at this little jewel."

The soldiers were silent. The outburst was unprecedented from Peale and, if all the truth is to be told, the soldiers probably had no notion of what the artist was talking about. Pat Anderson was the first to regain his tongue.

"Yes, they're all preachers, but the Muhlenbergs are more than that. The old man is a doctor and a lawyer, and if he put his mind to it he could be the biggest businessman in Pennsylvania. He can handle men. That soft, dignified, tenor voice of his can make you do anything he asks. Fred, the man, you know, who sent the letter to Big John rebuking him for mixing revolutionary ideas in his sermons, just came back here from New York. He was pastor of the Old Swamp Church over there. He's the writer and the politician in the family; he'll go far if we succeed. You and I fight the wars and then fat Fred comes in and runs the government. You watch Fred Muhlenberg. Gotthilf, who has a temper like a fiery furnace, knows more about the plants and trees near here than anyone else I ever met. He goes walking all over the county, walked once to Lancaster, they tell me, and he knows every blade of grass between Lancaster and the ocean. That boy talks five different languages, including Greek. I'll bet you fellows never even heard of Greek. Oh yes, indeed, those Muhlenbergs are brilliant."

"Well, if you went to church more, you'd know about this Augustus Church you're seeing," added one of the Pennsylvania Germans. "We call this place the shrine of Lutheranism. If you could read that dedicatory stone over the main entrance, you'd see why. It says, if I can still read my Latin: 'Under the auspices of Christ, Henry Melchior Muhlenberg with his Council,' and it gives the names of six, as you see, 'erected from the very foundation this building dedicated by the Society of the Augsburg Confession. A.D. 1743.' This church is famous, too, because it has one of the first pipe-organs ever built in any country church, because it had a long schoolhouse where Muhlenberg used to teach, and because this little stone annex is the place where the first charity school in the province was located. Ben Franklin and Conrad Weiser, Provost Smith of the university, and Governor James Hamilton all came up here to supervise the school. This Trappe church is an extremely important place for us Lutherans."

"It will be important for us too, maybe," said Jim. "A place like this makes a good hospital. If the redcoats cross the river, this Trappe church, with all these fancy trimmings Peale talks about, will be crowded with the wounded. We'll burn those old carved doors for campfires."

Anderson, during the later moments of the conversations, had been called aside by one of the general's green-ribboned aides. He nodded vigorously as he listened to the instructions that the aide was evidently giving. Then, turning to his friends, he told them to go off to find their quarters. He, it seems, had orders to report to Washington at once.

"Does that mean the British are near here?" Mc-Michael asked the aide. It was a question that strict military discipline should not have permitted, but the aide was young and none too strict. "It means," said he, "that if you go over to that hilltop and look west you'll see the redcoats at Valley Forge. Our couriers report that they are moving up the river in the direction of Reading."

"Conrad Weiser's country," said North. "Muhlenberg will wish to hear of this. I'll go over to the parsonage to tell him what is happening."

Pat's mission was to guide the general to a convenient vantage point where Washington might look across the river to the British camp. It was a welcome duty, for Anderson was anxious to get a glimpse at his own acres just across the stream to see if reports were true that Hessians were encamped along the three-mile stretch of road that lay between Valley Forge and the mouth of Pickering Creek. Spies had brought him word that the brass-capped, mustaschioed mercenaries were smashing down doors and breaking locks open by thrusting bayonets into the keyholes. At his own house, Anderson was told, whooping Hessians drove cattle and sheep into the parlor to be butchered. At William Fussell's Fountain Inn at Phoenixville, "the high-water mark of British invasion in Pennsylvania," they took every movable object. Mary Fussell had attempted to save her curtains by wrapping them beneath her dress, but the laughing Hessians threw her to the floor and unwound the draperies to make flowing togas for themselves.

Sixteen-year-old Becky Havard had a somewhat similar experience. After the long-continued rains that marked September every farm housewife used the first clear day for washing. From an excited Negro slave,

Becky heard the terrifying news that Hessians were arriving. She rushed out to her clothesline, stuffed half-dry washing into her basket, and carried it to safety. Then she went back for a second load but, just as she was unpinning a sheet, a Hessian trooper shouldered through the gate. He grinned and pointed to her sheet. She could not understand a word he said, but she was certain what he wanted. She pulled the sheet to free it from the line; the Hessian pulled against her from the other side. He was much stronger than the girl, but he was laughing so heartily that Becky was about to draw the whole sheet to her side. The Hessian then drew his sword and slashed the taut sheet through the middle. Suddenly it ripped apart. He pranced heavily away, waving his flag of victory, as Becky fell flat on the ground, weeping in impotent anger.

Fight Them with Pie

By comparison with mercenaries any army might have seemed a group of Galahads. In the 1777 campaign the Britishers were not seriously resented by the farmers through whose land they passed. So long as England paid well for provisions and so long as her commanders kept the soldiers well in hand, Pennsylvania civilians found little fault.

Neither gentle dealing nor meticulous paying for commandeered provisions could, of course, remove all fears from the populace. Knowing that they were included in Britain's black books for their political or military deeds, many "disaffected rebels" were in terror. Howe sent out punitive expeditions to arrest them; officers were instructed to capture them at almost any cost.

Among the men thus sought was Zebulon Potts, a fighting Quaker, who had raised a company of militia and had fought at Brandywine. A British force was sent to take him prisoner. Zebulon hastily fled. Only his wife and children were at home when the British called there.

Martha Potts was nimble-witted and resourceful. "You, John, take the silver to the spring. Scrape up the sand in the bottom of the springhouse, and hide the silver under it. They'll break down the springhouse door but they'll never think to poke their bayonets into the bottom. Then run and warn the neighbors. And, Tom, you drive the cattle to the woods. Get them deep inside where they'll be safe. Hurry."

"There is no time," objected Tom. "The troops are almost here. The cows will stray. The British will hear them and shoot us."

"No, they won't. These men make too much noise marching. They won't take time to hunt through woods. Let me take care of them. You go and drive the cattle. I can keep the soldiers here a little while. I'll feed them pie."

Martha knew that there was not much time to lose. She rushed to the pantry, pulled down her doughboard, and hurriedly mixed dough. Luckily her fruit preserves had not been put away. She hastily floured pans to have the time that would be taken up by greasing, covered the bottoms with her dough, poured in some fruit, and, omitting all the careful niceties, thrust her tarts quickly into the oven. The tarts would not be perfect; the dough was badly mixed and not well rolled; the crust was sure to burn. But Martha knew that hungry men would not be too particular and hoped that appetizing smells from cooking fruit would cause the first arrivals to delay until the baking was complete. Meanwhile her cattle would be safe, her silver hidden, and her neighbors warned.

Fortunately more time was taken up by the British searching for some neighbor to guide their columns. Nearly half an hour passed before the troops arrived. The column halted. A young captain strode up the path. He knocked with his riding crop. Martha shook the flour from her fingers, hastily wiped her face, grabbed chubby five-year-old Ann close in her arms, and fumblingly opened the door.

"Mercy!" she gasped. "Do not harm my little baby. I am defenseless here. Take what you want and go away. I'm not a soldier. Please let me go."

"Madam, we do not war on women. We are looking for your husband. Where is the damned rebel?"

"He is not here. He has gone away. He hasn't been home for a week. Don't damn Zebulon. He tries to keep the peace. He is a constable. He doesn't want to fight."

"Where is he?"

"I don't know. He didn't tell me. Maybe he will come back soon. I'll tell him that you came. But, please, you must not stay. You'll frighten my little Annie. She is so young, so helpless. We haven't harmed anyone. Please go away. I must finish up my work. It's baking day."

"Baking day? Are you baking?"

"Yes. I've tarts in the oven now. Can't you smell them? They are almost done. Please go away. I must look after them."

The aroma of the cooking fruit was irresistible. Much of the tantalizing smell, as the efficient cook well knew, was due to overfilling of her pans. Piecrust and fruit had spilled in her haste to get her tarts into the oven. In happier times she would have rushed to rescue

as much as she could but now she waited, knowing that
soldiers who had fared so long on hardy camp food
would be beguiled by sweets. Meanwhile Tom and
Johnnie would be finishing their tasks.

The plot succeeded. The captain lingered. His
men stood at ease along the road. With leisurely deliberation Martha drew her tarts. None of them was
good. All were burned about the edges; the crusts stuck
to the bottom of the pans; the pastry broke in bits. At
any other time she would have wept with disappointment, scraped the pans and thrown the messes to the
pigs, but now she smiled and showed her baking to the
captain.

"They are not good," she said. "I was too nervous
when I heard your army coming. I didn't know that
you would be so polite. Won't you wait until I bake
some more?"

No young British captain, far from home and on
the march since daybreak through a hostile countryside,
was likely to be finicky about a pie. He called his
fellow officers. They greedily spooned up the broken
tarts. Luckily they were too hot for the burned crust
to taste too bitter. The officers thanked Martha for
her consideration, wished that all the rebel ladies were
as thoughtful, and politely took their leave.

Not a cow was lost, the silver was secure, and
Zebulon was safe. Martha made some better pies as
celebration.

"Never argue with a man," she said. "Feed him
pies and he will help you."

Zebulon was temporarily out of danger, but there
was no certainty when the British might return. Howe
set a price upon his head to induce the neighbors to
denounce the rebel. Possibly the British general hoped
that Friends who had expelled him from the meeting

for his "strenuosity" might be bribed into surrendering him for British punishment. He was, of course, mistaken. The Friends did not approve of Zebulon's military activity, but they were beyond the thought of treachery. They agreed that if the British came by night they would warn their neighbor by throwing pebbles on his roof. On one occasion Zebulon was so close to capture that he was obliged to hide under a barrel in the woodshed. In return for their watchfulness he, as the official commissioner of Washington for the neighborhood, provided them with passes certifying to their loyalty and allowing them, when necessary, to pass safely through the insurgent lines.

David Beats King George

Not only families active in the rebel cause were dismayed by the approach of British columns. No home in the neighborhood was safe against invasion; no group was certain that its peace would be preserved. The approach of redcoats, in spite of Howe's promises and of the distribution of his gold, was always an occasion for alarm.

The experience at the home of Henry Rittenhouse was typical of those in hundreds of farm homes throughout the colonies. The homestead lay in the path of British advance on the capital. Once the British passed the Fatland Ford the troops were certain to march by the house and, it was sure, to stop and make investigations.

The Rittenhouse boys, living on the family farm across the Schuylkill, were terror-stricken. They were certain that the British were on their way to kill the family because two older brothers were serving in the

militia regiment. Young David, twelve-year-old name-
sake of the famous astronomer, was full of his responsibility as temporary male head of the clan.

"I'll take care of you, mother. Don't you fret.
Joe is big enough to help me protect you and Baby
Henry."

"I'm sure you will, dear," his mother answered
absently, as she hurried to hide the family treasure.

David kept careful watch along the road to scout
the coming of the redcoats. Immediately on spying
dust clouds in the distance he rushed back breathlessly.

"Mother, they're coming! Get me the gun and
give Joe a butcher knife. We'll keep them out."

Nothing, Mrs. Rittenhouse well knew, was more
fraught with danger. There was no reasoning with him
in this emergency; some substitute adventure had to be
provided to sublimate his energy.

"No," she said. "It's better for you boys to be
safe. The army will need soldiers in the future. The
British will not hurt me, but they might take you
prisoner if you fight them. You could not help me if
you were in jail. You and Joe take Henry down to
the glen and stay there until they go. I'll ring the
farm bell when it's safe again. We'll tell your big
brothers how you saved the lives of three men for Washington's next army. That is the most patriotic action
you can do."

David was convinced and rushed to keep his
brothers safe for future fighting. But all the time that
he was in the glen he kept alert to see that no redcoat
captured his strategic defense positions.

Before the British troops arrived, Mrs. Rittenhouse
had added worries. The kitchen door burst open and
fifteen-year-old Mary Curry, daughter of her nearest
neighbor, rushed in, gasping with fright.

"Oh, Mrs. Rittenhouse, Ma sent me to hide our spoons and I saw the soldiers coming up the road and I can't get back and I've still got the spoons. Oh, what shall I do?" Mary was sobbing hysterically.

"Hush, child, there's no time to cry. Get in there and hide with your spoons." She pushed the frightened girl into the kitchen closet, then, straining with all her force, she shoved a large corner cupboard along the wall so that the hiding place was completely covered. When the British entered her kitchen, Mrs. Rittenhouse, with trembling fingers, was knitting on a stocking.

The men searched the house for food and valuables, muttering angrily because so little was to be found. "Open this door," they gruffly called when they found the corner cupboard locked. "There's nothing there," she answered, but she moved to get the key. Before Mrs. Rittenhouse could hand the key to the intruders, a soldier crashed the doors with an ax, smashing crockery and scattering spices about the floor.

Mary, in her dark recess, almost choked when she threw her forearm across her mouth to keep from screaming. She could not know that the door to her closet was hidden from the redcoats' sight and that she was entirely safe.

The British went off grumbling. Swiftly Mrs. Rittenhouse released the girl and sent her home still clutching the silver spoons. She rang the big farm bell and watched the boys come racing home, their faces glowing with excitement.

"Mother," said David, "I saved my whole army from capture. I'll bet you any other general would be proud of a record like that. And, look, they left an ax behind them. We drove them off and captured their baggage, didn't we? Old George Third will find that he can't beat the Rittenhouses."

17

The Darkest Days

Philadelphia Falls

Breathless horsemen, dashing into town at dawn, brought the rumor that redcoats had been seen within the city limits. In an hour Philadelphians were on the move. Church bells, already loaded into carts in readiness, were hauled away toward Allentown and Bethlehem. Congress, pausing only for a brief, excited session, voted hastily to adjourn to meet again at Lancaster as soon as possible. Carts and carriages, horsemen and pedestrians, clogged all roads westward. Only Tories stayed within the city.

It was a false alarm; the British were nowhere near the capital. Howe, indeed, was waiting patiently, some twenty miles away, to hear the news of Grey's surprise attack on Wayne's men at Paoli. Not for another week did Lord Cornwallis lead his grenadiers down Second Street to camp the troops on fashionable Society Hill. Ten days elapsed before the occupation was complete.

Their rule was courteous, but firm. By orders of the British commander, no persons were to be molested, nor was any property to be confiscated without payment. But, as invariably happens in military occupation, enforcement of instructions was not strictly supervised.

Theoretically looting was a capital offense and a man or two were hanged for stealing, but thieving went on continuously under the guise of "borrowing." Mrs.

Henry Drinker lost her blankets by verbal requisition of a soldier who professed the action was "by General Howe's special orders"; Mary Pemberton was robbed of her best bedclothes and, in addition, of six dozen bottles of her cherished Madeira. Foragers took provisions, paying for them by receipts calling for but one-tenth the amount actually taken away. Billeting officers went about the streets, chalking the names of officers on the doors of houses, and commanding the inhabitants to move away.

Such actions are probably unavoidable when hostile armies occupy a city, and Philadelphians might have taken them with good grace had not the British insisted on requiring menial tasks. Leading citizens received commands to sweep the streets, to clean their chimneys, and to carry off the refuse. They resented, too, the drinking, gaming, and other habits of the British officers and, when they protested, were aghast to hear that English leaders contemplated burning every patriot house within a four-mile radius of the city.

Prices rose fantastically in the first days of the occupation. Traditional history, taught in all the schools, declares that redcoats lived in luxury all winter, while Washington was starving at Valley Forge, but the true fact is that the American design of keeping Howe bottled up in Philadelphia worked admirably. Few supplies could come in from the countryside so long as American patrols kept watch over roads entering the town and, for the first few weeks of British occupation, the Delaware was closed to British navigation. Good beef, normally selling at fourpence a pound, shot up to two shillings within two weeks after Howe's arrival, and by the middle of November cost seven shillings sixpence. No butter was available; firewood, once obtained almost for the asking, brought twenty shillings a cord, and the army was obliged to cut it from the woods at Center Square.

False tradition also blackens the memory of Pennsylvania patriots by charging them with selling food to redcoats rather than to their own Continental soldiers, when the fact is clear that no supplies could be procured for either army. When two contending forces, each of more than ten thousand men, scour a farming area for weeks on end, burning what they cannot eat or transport in their wagons, little provision will be left for later comers. Such was the case in fertile Pennsylvania, which, since the end of August, had been called upon to feed the entire armed forces of both England and America. When winter came storehouses were completely empty, barns contained no cattle, the copious harvests of the autumn had been consumed.

By late November, however, the batteries defending the Delaware had been reduced and the invading British Army could draw food from other sources. Supply ships from the north, from the West Indies, even from the mother country, sailed up the Delaware to relieve the British famine. Howe and his men were now well fed, though even with these resources forage for the cavalry was scarce.

Valley Forge

At Valley Forge the patriots were in distress. The near-by countryside was clear of food, and while ample stocks existed in the farmlands of interior Pennsylvania, transportation troubles prevented bringing meat and flour to the camp. Except for a few weeks in the early winter, the weather was not unduly cold, but there were constant rains, rendering the roads hub-deep in mud and, since horses were few and hard to come upon, supply trains were at a standstill. On more than one occasion the Continental forces were reduced to less than quarter rations; there were times when flour barrels were completely empty and not a pound of meat could be secured.

Sickness ravaged the camp; medicines were lacking; adequate hospitals could not be maintained. Surgeons worked incessantly, by rushlight candles well into the night, with heavy saws and long unsterilized shears to make emergency operations. Under such conditions Washington dared attempt no major battles lest his wounded die of gangrene or lockjaw. Often he had too few soldiers fit for service to assign for necessary guard duty or for proper scouting.

Yet the soldiers, ill fed, sick, and clad in tattered rags, did not despair. Again and again they overcame hardships that might have been considered overwhelming. At Germantown they even dared a direct assault on the well-fortified British lines, failing of success only because Sullivan's division moved on too hastily in a fog and got out of touch with its supporting troops. Had Sullivan been lesss successful in advancing, had General Adam Stephen not become confused, had bookish General Henry Knox not clung too closely to the textbook laws of war, the little, battered Continental Army might have won a major battle. That Washington lost Germantown is only incidental; the important point is that a broken, ill-supplied, almost demoralized American force came within an inch of hurling back the best-trained veterans of England. Washington's generalship, his timing, and his leadership were as superb as they had been at Trenton.

By springtime, through the splendid work of Major General Baron Frederick William Steuben, formerly of

Frederick the Great's Prussian army, the Continental troops were disciplined into a coherent army. Through the helpful aid of France, the men were well supplied with guns and munitions; medical supplies were adequate; foodstuffs were again rolling into camp. The thirteen colonies, which early in the fall had seemed discordant units, sniping viciously at each other quite as much as they were warring against England, were again united; morale had been restored. It is no exaggeration to declare that, at Valley Forge, an army had been brought into existence. Indeed, it is only just to point out that the Revolutionary War was really won at Valley Forge.

Howe at Philadelphia was almost unaware of the great change that had occurred in rebel fortunes. His secret service had been poor; his news about the Continental Army had been faulty. He himself was in disgrace at home; his failure to reduce the colonies into submission had led to his recall to face a parliamentary investigation.

Before he left for home, however, his officers, grateful for the entertainments which he had allowed, prepared one final jubilation. In mid-May, 1778, a lavish Meschianza, a pageant of extraordinary proportions, was arranged by André and Captain John Montresor, his aide.

The Meschianza

Philadelphia Tories were the special guests of army officers on this occasion. Decorated barges, escorted on either side by flatboats bearing the regimental bands, carried the participants from the upper limits of the city along the water front to Robert Wharton's country seat, just south of Philadelphia. There they landed, amid salutes from all the warships in the river, and, preceded by massed bands, walked through a double line of grenadiers to the rope-lined lawn where the tournament was held. Two pavilions, one for partisans of the Blended Rose and the other for supporters of the Burning Mountain, flanked the field. On front benches of each stand seven Philadelphia ladies, dressed in Turkish costumes, sat, with trophies in their turbans, to reward their favored cavaliers.

Distant trumpets announced the coming of the knights. Seven champions, mounted on gray horses, dashed into the tilting field, and riding the circuit, paused before their ladies in salute. Their herald then proclaimed a challenge, in the name of the Knights of the Blended Rose, declaring that the damsels of their choice excelled all others in wit, beauty, and accomplishment.

The challenge was immediately accepted. A trumpet call was heard. Another herald entered, followed by the black and orange knights. They, too, rode about the lawn, drew up before their ladies, and saluted. Then the knights received their lances from attendant esquires, fixed their shields upon their left arms, and gracefully saluting their opponents, wheeled their horses, and galloping against each other, shivered their spears against the hostile shields.

In second and third encounters, the knights rode against each other, discharging pistols in the air; a fourth engagement was with swords. Then, finally, two chiefs fought a furious duel, with blunt and buttoned weapons, until the marshal of the Meschianza rushed between them to declare that all the ladies were now satisfied with proofs of love and valor, and "as they prized the future favors of their mistresses, that they should instantly desist from further combat."

The "Turkish" ladies, with their knights and guests, now left the field, walking under triumphal arches on which the regimental colors were displayed, and entered the Wharton mansion. Carpeted stairs led them into a spacious hall paneled in Siena marble, where refreshments were served. Here the knights, kneeling, received their favors. A ball followed, in a pale-blue and rose-pink drawing room, where eighty-five mirrors reflected the innumerable wax lights provided for illumination. Fireworks were displayed at intervals throughout the evening.

At midnight the dance was interrupted. A splendid supper for four hundred guests was served by slaves in Oriental costumes and silver collars. A thousand candles, mirrored by half a hundred tall pier glasses, brilliantly lighted the glittering scene. The festivities continued until dawn.

The Meschianza created a furor in Philadelphia. Never before had there been so elaborate a spectacle. Later hosts, determined not to be surpassed in extravagance, took the fete as a model for their entertainments.

The more conservative citizens, however, frowned upon the costumes which flouted all traditions of decency. The dignified chief justice of the state, Edward Shippen, learning that his daughters were to wear towering, jeweled headdresses, in the extreme British fashion, with spangled shoes, lace-edged veils, and white silk overdresses, open from the waist to show their under robes, and wide pink sashes, flatly ordered the young girls to stay at home. Three of the knights, therefore, had been obliged to ride in honor of substitute ladies. The brokenhearted Shippen girls wept all night long.

Baiting Tories

Two weeks later the Continental troops came back to Philadelphia. They found the city in a state of turmoil. Patriotic leaders who had fled the town upon the coming of the British now returned, demanding that the Tories be condemned for treason; those who had remained in Philadelphia were hot with anger against men like John Roberts and Abraham Carlisle who had served the enemy as civilian officers. Charges of treachery were rife; citizens denounced each other; men who had been docile under British rule were vehement in their demands for vengeance.

Washington's choice as military governor was unfortunate. To honor his trusted general, Benedict Arnold, and to give his friend an opportunity to recuperate from wounds, he had appointed Arnold to supreme command of the nation's capital. Arnold not only allowed the Tory-baiters full license in their hunt for traitors, but approved the sentences whereby Roberts and Carlisle were sent to death. He took advantage of the general confusion to make himself dictator of the city and to gratify "his own ill-regulated passion for luxurious display." Later, when the commonwealth of Pennsylvania launched formal charges against him for fraud and peculation, Arnold was convicted on charges that he had used his official position for his private profit.

The precautions brought no peace, and fears increased that disaffected Tories still lurked undiscovered. The grand jury issued formal warnings that the wives of British emissaries were forwarding intelligence to redcoat leaders and that they were spreading "poisonous, errroneous and wicked falsehoods" against the

Continental cause. The spy hunt spread to include all those who sold goods at more than the price which purchasers thought reasonable. Eventually, the militia declared war on everyone who opposed an ultrademocratic government.

Lawyers were particularly suspect; even those like James Wilson who had signed the Declaration of Independence. Because he thought the Pennsylvania constitution ought to have a double house like England's Parliament, a militia band, armed with muskets and fixed bayonets, marched on the Wilson house. Gunfire broke out, both from the street and from a terrified group which had taken refuge in the building. General Thomas Mifflin, formerly quartermaster general of the army, Colonel William Grayson, once Washington's aide-de-camp and now member of the Board of War, Colonel James Chambers, one of the earliest Pennsylvania volunteers, and Captain Allen McLane, the army's best scouting officer, were among the thirty men besieged within "Fort Wilson."

As the angry militiamen approached the Wilson house, Mifflin threw open a window to urge the mob not to use violence, but he was answered by a musketry volley which killed a comrade and shattered every pane of glass on the street side of the house. Two attackers battered down the door with heavy sledges, caught Chambers by the hair and pulled him downstairs, wounding him with bayonets. Other mob members ran to the arsenal for cannons to fire against the walls. Three men were killed, several were wounded in the fighting.

Governor William Reed was ill with fever. He got up from his sickbed and rushed to the scene, pistol in hand, his knee-buttons unfastened, his boots down. With him came two white-uniformed horsemen, whom the crowd mistook for Frenchmen. Word spread that the army was approaching; the mob scattered. The Tories, hitherto in hiding, again came forth and paraded the streets, insulting the advocates of independence and setting up a cannon at the corner of two principal streets. They vanished again when the City Troop appeared. It was the last time British sympathizers dared show themselves in arms in Philadelphia, and for eleven years thereafter the ultrademocratic faction ruled throughout the state of Pennsylvania.

18

Drink, Dine and Dance

MAJOR PHILIP PANCAKE was in ecstasy; his plans for the gala Fourth of July parade were working perfectly. John Durant, the printer, clad as Mercury in a white dress and red ribbons, with garlands of fresh red and blue flowers round his head, could flap the wings he wore at head and foot. Frank Serre had found a way to spread an elegant pair of lady's corsets so that they could be seen in their magnificence; George Freytag's stocking makers, each with his golden crown, blue starred, floated a pair of huge blue stockings in the brisk south wind.

No such celebration ever had been staged before in these United States, thought Major Philip Pancake, marshal of the Federal Procession, nor, in all probability, would such a gala jubilee be held again. Pancake had worked incessantly to bring the brewers into line with ears of barley in their hats and hop vines twining round their waists. He had had a difficult time persuading the fifty-eight glovemakers to don their buckskin breeches and wear hats with deer-tails dangling, but they had come around to Pancake's way of thinking and were waiting now, each with his golden fleece in his hand. Dick Porter's tallow chandlers, gay in blue aprons decorated with a silver dove, were waiting too, holding their olive branches and, to Philip Pancake's great delight, they brought along a thirteen-branched silver candlestick, with thirteen silver stars about the base. It was most fitting that the great procession should be spectacular, for this parade would mark a double holiday, commemorating both the twelfth anniversary of the nation's freedom, and the recent acceptance by New Hampshire, two weeks before, of the new and improved Constitution of the United States. Ever since sunrise, when a full peal of bells from Christ Church steeple greeted the happy day, the town had been agog with expectation. Even the ships in harbor were decked out with flags of friendly nations, France, Holland, Sweden, Prussia, and Morocco, and each ship floated a huge white banner, golden lettered with the name of one of the free states. Thousands of citizens, pouring in from the interior, lined the three-mile route awaiting Major Pancake's extravagant display. He and his twelve white-frocked attendants waited impatiently for the nine white-plumed directors who, promptly at nine-thirty, would give their signal through their speaking trumpets for the great procession to begin.

The cavalcade was well worth waiting for. From the moment the City Troop of Light Dragoons cleared a passageway for grave Thomas FitzSimons, riding Rochambeau's old horse in symbolic celebration of the French alliance, down to the very end of the three-hour pageant there were thrills galore. The Pennsylvania Supreme Court justices, in their robes of office, sitting in their eagle-shaped chariot, drew huge applause; the Admiralty Court, headed by merry Francis Hopkinson, song writer and jurist, was envied for its originality, for Hopkinson, carrying a gold anchor on a green silk ribbon, was accompanied by his marshal, Clement Biddle, who had a green-ribboned silver oar, and by his registrar, James Read, whose hat was decorated by a silver pen and whose great green baize bag, bulging with parchments, had the word "Admiralty" embroidered in large silver letters on its side.

These were but preliminary to the procession's masterpiece, the grand Federal Edifice, popularly known as Franky's New Roof in memory of Benjamin Franklin's clever statesmanship. A carriage drawn by ten white horses bore the splendid building, a great Greek temple, whose dome was supported by thirteen Corinthian columns and whose frieze was decorated by thirteen golden stars. But, as the Federal Edifice grew closer, spectators saw that there was symbolism in its building, for three of the thirteen columns were deliberately left unfinished as a sign that, as yet, three states had failed to ratify the document. Yet there was promise in the symbolism too, for above the dome was fixed a cornucopia, a horn of plenty, from which fruits and grain and all the riches of the earth were pouring down.

The best part of the party was yet to come. Richard Peters, a gentleman farmer who was noted for his wit but who in his graver moments was a solemn judge, marched forward with a corps of farmers, going through the motions of plowing up the soil, of sowing seed along the city streets, of reaping bumper crops. Peter Wallace Gallaudet, the merchant and father of the man who was to give great blessings to the deaf, came carrying a golden beehive. Behind him moved the manufacturers, carding cotton, spinning thread, and weaving suits of working jeans in what was called the federal rib. Nor were they, even on this festal day, averse to using propaganda, for they bore a mighty banner, of thirty-seven kinds of cloth bordering a regulation national flag, to which they fastened streamers calling for a high protective tariff. This portion of the great procession was not unanimously popular, as Major Philip Pancake had foreseen, but the manufacturers had been insistent on the matter and the parade officials, most of whom were Federalists and sympathizers of the Hamilton fiscal program, had not heeded Pancake's protests.

The brewers, too, were using the golden moment for self-advertisement. Alien settlers, many of them French refugees from strife-torn Martinique, were trying to induce Americans to drink more wine, to the detriment of the Delaware valley's flourishing beer and cider business. Ten brewers, therefore, loaded hogsheads of beer, ale, and porter on a dray and improvised a chant "Home brew'd is best" as they walked on under a banner reading "Proper drink for Americans."

Commercialism was absent from the other sixty exhibits. Joe Rice's sailmakers, to be sure, kept pointing to their motto "May industry be rewarded," which some thought a subtle plea for higher wages, but the white-leather aproned coopers were more innocuous with "Love as brethren." Dave Rose's brickmakers, marching under a green silk banner, pointed out "It was found hard in Egypt, but we find it easy," but the blacksmiths, boasting no banner at all, drew most attention. As their nine-horse float rolled onward, Jack Mingle and his helper Chris Keyser demonstrated Biblical texts by literally beating swords into plowshares and sickles to show that America's new constitution stood for peace.

No one stopped to count the actual number of paraders, though the total must have mounted into the thousands. Every member of each of sixty-odd trades and professions was in line, together with every officeholder, all the faculties and student bodies of the schools and colleges, members of the bar, "the clergy of the different Christian denominations, with the rabbi of the Jews, walking arm in arm," the soldiers and physicians. The coroner rode in state on horseback, side by side with the sheriff; twenty watchmen, "with their flams decorated and in their proper dress," strolled past crying "Ten o'clock and a glorious starlight morning," to honor the ten states that had approved Franky's New Roof; the printers, bearing a blue-and-silver eagle and a huge scroll tied with blue silk binding, scattered copies of Francis Hopkinson's new ode in both an English and a German version. Only the country people could have been left along the streets to watch the great procession, but they were numerous enough, some estimates ranging as high as seventeen thousand.

In early afternoon, when the procession had arrived at William Hamilton's Bush Hill estate, a grand collation was served. Tables, shaded by huge canvas awnings, stood in a gigantic circle on the Bush Hill lawn, surrounding the great Federal Edifice. A feu de joie of three rounds of musketry, three volleys of artillery, and three cheers from the assembly greeted this new, and last, phase of the party. Then the company went to dinner, to consume an infinite amount of cold meats, desserts and cakes. In deference to the opinions of the brewers, who outnumbered the twelve distillers in the parade, no spirits were distributed, nor were any of the hated foreign wines permitted. The only drinks were porter, beer, and cider, but there was ample provision of each of these. No participant left Bush Hill with his thirst unslaked.

Market of Brothers

Independence was assured; wartime sacrifices were no longer necessary; taut nerves relaxed along the Delaware. Now that freedom had been won, patriots who had strained to win the war surrendered to the luxuries. The valley of the Delaware became, in the words of Richard Henry Lee, "an attractive scene of debauchery and amusement." General Nathanael Greene saw in the middle states dissipations far more flagrant than those in other sections of the land. "When I was in Boston last summer," he said, "I thought luxury was very predominant there; but they are no more to compare with those now prevalent in Philadelphia than an infant babe to a full-grown man. I dined at one table where there were a hundred and sixty dishes."

Those who bewailed the passage of the good old times, when Quaker simplicity had prevailed, believed that the British occupation of the city had accustomed citizens to ideas of self-indulgence and extravagance. After the evacuation, however, Americans had forgotten the Spartan disciplines of Valley Forge. Tory ladies were at first excluded from all entertainment, but when Benedict Arnold, military commandant of the city, set a precedent by asking Peggy Shippen, one of the Meschianza belles, to be his partner at a ball, the boycott ended. Mary White Morris, sister of the Anglican bishop and wife of Robert Morris, indignantly complained, "Even our military gentlemen are too liberal to make any distinction between Whig and Tory ladies. If they make any, it is in favor of the latter."

Relief from war tension showed itself in various relaxations from the former stricter codes. Drinking, discouraged since the macaroni days, increased, especially among the women. At a cold collation in Martha Washington's honor, eighty celebrants emptied forty-five huge punch bowls, together with twenty-two bottles of assorted liquors and two bottles more of "crab cider." Fashion called for ladies to wear more jewelry, though men were restricted to the new French fad of wearing two watches, one on each side of the waistcoat, connected by a silver chain from which dangled seals or keys or brightly colored stones. Washington's cream-colored four-horse coach, originally imported for Richard Penn, inspired a rivalry in gilded, painted carriages.

More entertainments were given. Engraved invitations were not yet known, but liveried servants moved from house to house delivering playing cards, whose backs bore written requests for the recipients to come to dances or to dinners.

Food was plentiful now; the markets were full to overflowing. Twice weekly, thrifty German farmers drove their carts to town, loaded down with grain and fruit and vegetables. Besides the customary beef and pork and mutton, the citizens might dine on bear or venison, raccoon, opossum, pigeon, or wild turkey. Prices were extremely low, with beef at fourpence per pound and veal, lamb, or fowl at even less, and hunger was unknown. It was cheering to hear the Christ Church bells ring out their octaves as the market carts approached, and then to see the huge appetizing piles of produce, and the handsome, hand-woven baskets of fresh fruits.

To foreigners, accustomed to the piercing cries, the shouts, the quarrels of European market places, the immaculately kept Philadelphia meat and produce stands were always fascinating. The quiet calm, the absence of bickering for better price, the law and order of the markets were surprising. Brissot de Warville, who visited the Delaware in 1788, was overwhelmed by such peacefulness.

"You would say," he wrote, "that it was a market of brothers, that it was a rendezvous of philosophers, of the pupils of the silent Pythagoras, for silence reigns without interruption. . . . This is the astonishing effect of habit, a habit inspired by the Quakers who planted morals in this country."

Not all the visitors were as much impressed by Philadelphia's quietness. All was tranquil in the narrow, shaded streets; the lantern-swinging night watch who passed along the city's brick pavements, calling the hours and the state of the weather, found few stragglers astir. The forty thousand residents who crowded Philadelphia in the first days of the republic kept carefully indoors. Strangers fortunate enough to be invited into the homes found lavish entertainment.

Inhibitions had been shattered; the city folk were gay. Now it was possible for anyone to speak his mind with freedom, to criticize even the all-puissant Congress if he chose, to mock the failings of the statesmen. One merry jape that went the rounds turned on the inability of Congress to fix a permanent capital; when it was proposed to set up a mounted statue of George Washington, the wits suggested that the horse be hollow. There, they said, the congressmen might live, rolling from town to town within the statue, and if, as certainly would happen, there were secret documents that must be filed away from prying eyes, the private papers could be hidden in the horse's private parts.

Shocking the French

Even the French diplomats, fresh from the frivolities of Versailles, were shocked at some of the excesses. The Delaware gambled hard, at whist or loo or billiards; it was not uncommon for a gentleman, or even for a lady, to lose several hundred dollars at a sitting. Now that macaroni restraint was gone, young men came to fancy themselves as "hearty fellows," whose hallmark was the ability to be drunk on many a successive night. At stag dinners in the taverns it was no uncommon practice for the master of the feast to turn the key upon the sober, compelling them to stay till all were heavily intoxicated. At any meal whatever, in formal dining rooms, at city taverns, or in lonely rural inns, no man could eat his meal without constant interruption from his fellows, whether friends or strangers, who insisted that he join them in a toast.

The practice of compulsory drinking, for no one could refuse without giving serious affront, robbed drunkenness of any social sting. The cultured Frenchmen, knowing well that men who drank too much would be forever banned from the society of ladies, were astonished that no such restraint was found among the gentry of the Delaware.

Dancing was more acceptable to French taste, but this, like other social graces, had been carried to extremes. The people danced at every opportunity, even at the quiet, graceful teas which now replaced the former four o'clock meat-and-pudding dinner. Here, again, the Versailles courtiers were rather at a loss, for balls in France were light, though formal, but along the Delaware the dances were rigidly arranged. "Dancing," the Marquis de Chastellux wrote wonderingly home, "is said to be the emblem of gaiety and love; here it seems to be the emblem of legislation, and of marriage; of legislation, inasmuch as places are marked out, the country dances named, and every proceeding provided for, calculated and submitted to regulation of marriage, as it furnishes each lady with a partner, with whom she dances the whole evening without being allowed to take another."

De Chastellux was, however, pleased to learn that if, by social law, no man might change his partner during a whole evening, the hospitality along the Delaware was friendly to the foreigner. Custom required that strangers be rewarded with the handsomest young ladies. Lovely Anne McCall Willing, acknowledged social leader of the town, the pretty Shippen sisters, and attractive brown-eyed Mary Vining, who spoke French so musically and with such vivacity that Frenchmen lost their hearts, were invariably dancing partners for eligible alien visitors.

The patterns were set by the very highest circles. When Philadelphia was the capital, the president gave afternoon levees. The general, carefully garbed in plain black velvet, with pearl-colored waistcoat and silver buckles, received his callers in the large state dining room. Holding in his hand his yellow gloves and his cocked hat, his long sword in its shiny white leather scabbard by his side, Washington bowed gravely to each arrival. Promptly at a quarter past three, fifteen minutes after the levee was opened, the doors were closed against more visitors, the men ranged in a circle, and the president moved slowly about, chatting briefly with each guest. Then he returned to his original position, and, as each man took his leave, he bowed politely, and the levee was over.

Lady Washington's receptions were less formal. Twice a week, while Congress was in session, she gave her "routs" in her upstairs drawing room. The Shippen girls, and Anne Willing, who married William Bingham, richest merchant of the city, the Allens, and the Chews, the Cadwaladers and Biddles and the other famous Philadelphia families attended; members of Congress and their wives paid their respects; and, toward the close of each reception, the president arrived, without his sword and hat and gloves, for here, in Martha Washington's apartments, he was not the host but a simple gentleman.

The Washingtons were not always on parade, however. Their hospitality shone brightest at their small, informal gatherings. At breakfast, for example, they entertained their guests in pleasant simplicity. Martha made the tea and coffee at the table. One servant, and he without a livery, served sliced tongue, dry toast, and bread and butter. There was no form, no ceremony; a silver hot-water urn and tableware alone betrayed the family's wealth. Meals like these gave no possible excuse to antifederalist "Demoncrats" to inveigh against the royal family's wanton luxury.

The Court Party

The wealthy, and especially the Binghams, were anathema to many. Mrs. William Bingham was the darling of society, but she was also bitterly attacked for wastefulness. Her great three-acre estate, with its exotic orange trees set out in tubs about her garden in the very heart of Philadelphia, roused envy among the underprivileged. The marble stairway which led upstairs to wide ballrooms, hung with French wallpaper and decorated by expensive Italian paintings, or to attractive drawing rooms, soft with English carpets and upholstered crimson-and-gold furniture, was deemed too gorgeous for a simple Quaker town. The lesser houses, unable to keep pace with Bingham's fortune, often spent beyond their means to follow Bingham's style.

The group that gathered round the Binghams, the so-called "court party," was undeniably distinguished.

Old Benjamin Chew, courteous and dignified, Chief
Justice Edward Shippen, and Robert Morris lent suavity
of manner and authority of speech to the court party's
formal dinners. The Federalist political leaders, who
administered the government, were always to be found
at the dinners, balls, and entertainments of this important clique.

Among the foreigners who thronged the capital,
Wilmington's Mary Vining was a special favorite. The
royal courts of France and England and the principali-
ties of Germany knew of her personality through enthusiastic report carried to Europe by Chateaubriand
and Lafayette, by the Viscount de Noailles, the Comte
de Ségur, and a host of others.

The foreign group, centering about the alien lega-
tions, was a second social set, and to it came colorful
figures. Talleyrand, tall and sallow, his potbellied body
seemingly perched on little sticks, came to live in Philadelphia for a time, fascinating dinner parties with his
sparkling conversation, repelling them with his atrocious
table manners. For Talleyrand, resting his elbows on
the table, cut his meat into small pieces, pierced them
with his fork until the prongs were full, then thrust
the mass within his mouth, closed his teeth, pulled out
the fork, and chewed noisily, talking steadily all the
time. Louis Philippe came too, a dignified, dark-eyed
young man with deep-sunk eyes, who tried to marry one
of Bingham's daughters. He was refused because, Bingham said, "If you resume your rightful place, you will
become too great for her; and if you do not so succeed,
you are not good enough." There were other foreign
notables, like Alexander Baring, later Lord Ashburton,
who did marry one of Bingham's girls, the Duc de la
Rochefoucault, author of a famous book on travels in
America, and Kosciuszko, whose name Americans could

neither pronounce nor spell. Later there would come
the Marquis d'Yrujo, the Spanish minister, to marry the
celebrated beauty Sally McKean, daughter of the justice
who had once summoned Caesar Rodney to his side.

The world of literature, of art, and of fashion gathered here at Philadelphia. At Oellers' Inn, where always
were available great bowls of ice-cooled rum punch and
pineapple flavored to give a specially appealing savor,
or at Gray's Gardens, four miles from the city on the
Schuylkill banks, Charles Brockden Brown, young head
of Philadelphia's Belles Lettres Club discoursed on the
progress of his latest novel. Robert Proud, the first
historian of Pennsylvania, forgot his academic chores
and talked of bygone days, and Judge Richard Peters
cracked his everlasting puns. David Rittenhouse, Dr.
William White, first Episcopalian bishop in America,
Dr. Rush, who like his older friend Ben Franklin knew
everything, and Francis Hopkinson, who turned off
clever verses faster than most men could write poor
prose, might also grace a gathering. In these last two
decades of the eighteenth century Philadelphia reached
the zenith of its fame.

19

Riot and Pestilence

God's retribution, warned the righteous, must someday fall upon the people for their luxury, frivolity, and waste. Idleness and dissipation, together with the drift away from strict codes of conduct, must soon call down a rain of death.

The Delaware paid no heed to prophecy. Instead, it plunged more deeply into gaiety. Young folk danced and chattered lightheartedly; they sang, even in the streets; they cultivated pleasure, and gave no thought to warnings. Long-faced prudes who thought all laughter sinful pointed to omens of ill. In January, 1793, mumps were more prevalent than usual; a blustery, wet May canceled the promise of a pleasant early spring. Heavy colds were common; scarlet fever raged. All these, the superstitious said, were caused by Philadelphia's disregard of simple ways of life.

The year grew worse. Rain fell almost constantly in summer, leaving pools of water in the swampy fields that lay about the city. Mosquitoes bred in unprecedented numbers. The air was hot and humid.

August brought calamity. Scores of Philadelphians fell sick with fever, headache, and sore throat; their eyes were bloodshot and their pulses quick. It was a strange disease for which physicians, uncertain of their diagnosis, could do no more than prescribe the usual bloodlettings and give the customary doses of Peruvian bark.

But neither these nor blisters applied to neck, head, and limbs effected cure, though doctors kept their patients drunk with brandy and warm with blankets dipped in vinegar. Patients grew no better; indeed, after four days of treatment, temperatures fell alarmingly, the skin turned lemon-yellow, there was severe nosebleeding and black vomit. Then the doctors knew for certain what the ailment was. Dreaded yellow fever had arrived; before a week had passed, the victims died.

Philadelphia was terror-stricken. Many fled to higher land, distant from the swamps. Germantown was crowded with refugees. Thomas Jefferson was pleased to find a cot in the corner of a taproom and did not grudge the $8 that he had to pay for such accommodation. More than a third of the 45,000 inhabitants deserted the capital.

Within the city those who could not flee were panicky. Some were certain that the plague was meant as spiritual scourge to call the people back to better ways of living; others, certain that the fever had been brought by French exiles from Santo Domingo, clamored for a massacre of those who had infected Philadelphia; a smaller group, of doctors, was convinced that sacks of damaged coffee, rotting on the wharves, had putrefied and caused the sickness; still others laid the blame on bad air emanating from the swamps.

Nobody knew how to check the fever. Bonfires burned all day and all night to purify the air and, because the doctors thought gunpowder was a good preventive, rifles snapped incessantly. Revolutionary cannon, dragged from the arsenals, were hauled up and down the streets, and were fired as often as they could be loaded. Within the houses, terrified people burned niter; men, women, and children puffed huge "segars"

whose smoke, it was believed, was proof against con-
tagion. Some trusted in the power of garlic as a specific
against infection, and went about chewing the weed,
with big bunches of it in their pockets, hats, belts, and
shoes, and bundles of it strapped to their skin. Others
wore camphor bags and drank tar water, mixed with
myrrh and pepper.

The city meeting places were deserted. Churches,
coffeehouses, offices, and all resorts where people once
had congregated were lonely places. Friends avoided
one another; even doctors, on their rounds to dash
buckets of cold water over their patients in a desperate
attempt to reduce the fever, refused to draw too close
to the sufferers. They placed ten-grain calomel pills
and fifteen grains of jalap within the patient's reach
and told the victim to take the dose.

Sick folk who stayed at home fared better than
those who went into the hospitals, for during the first
days of the epidemic no proper care was provided. City
officials, commandeering the big home of William Hamilton at Bush Hill during the time the owner was away
from the city, set up an emergency ward, but they
could find no proper staff. Street women, pressed into
service as nurses, turned Bush Hill into a brothel, ban-
queting on the food provided for the sick. Patients
were not washed, nor were they fed; Bush Hill became
a filthy charnel house.

Stephen Girard, mariner, financier, and merchant,
assumed responsibility for a task that no other Philadelphian dared attempt. Himself the victim of ill fortune, for the only woman he ever loved was hopelessly
insane, he volunteered to take full charge of Bush Hill
and to transform it from a murder den into a place
for cure. For two months Girard and his assistant,
Peter Helm, cared for the sick, visiting their houses,

carrying out the victims, driving them in his own carriage to Bush Hill. He cleaned out the incompetent nurses, procured efficient doctors, enlarged the wards, insisted on proper food, and saw to it that medicines were regularly given.

When, in November, cooler weather came the epidemic ceased, after four thousand sufferers had died. The frightened exiles returned; gradually the neighbor cities, Baltimore, Trenton, and New York, allowed communication with the stricken town; Albany ceased to fire on ships from Philadelphia. Normal life was again possible.

McKean Builds a Machine

Danger of disease was past, but an ugly aftermath remained. William Cobbett was convinced that patients had been sacrificed through ignorance. In vicious articles, written under the pseudonym of Peter Porcupine, the irascible English pamphleteer, master of mudslinging, called Dr. Rush a quack who killed the sick by calomel and bleeding. Rush had written, Porcupine alleged, self-laudatory letters to the press praising his own skill. According to Cobbett, he had forged a series of testimonials to increase his reputation.

Rush promptly sued for libel, called witnesses to defend his character, among them Chief Justice Thomas McKean, and asked for damages. The case dragged slowly through the courts. Eventually it reached the highest bench, where Tom McKean decided that the claim was fully justified. He granted Rush $5,000, the largest libel award ever granted up to that time in America.

Cobbett, naturally, was furious. In a pamphlet

called the "Rush Light" he violently attacked McKean for acting both as witness and as judge. He branded Pennsylvanians as "the most malicious and cowardly race in existence." He damned them all to hell and hoped that Rush would bleed them all to death. Then Cobbett fled to England.

Dual duty was, of course, no novelty to cold-blooded Tom McKean. For almost half a century he had been an officeholder, and for six years of that time had acted as official of two states simultaneously. To one who had been both Delaware assemblyman and congressman, and at the same time Pennsylvania's chief justice, there was no bar against his judging a case in which he had been witness for the prosecution.

Connoisseurs of conflict may bewail the flight of Cobbett, for a war of Billingsgate between McKean and Peter Porcupine would certainly have been Homeric. Tom McKean was quick with violent invective, and he was not tactful in his methods. Elected as governor of Pennsylvania, he rose to answer a congratulatory speech by damning everyone who had opposed him. As Grand Sachem of Pennsylvania's Tammany, he promised that he would throw out of office every man who did not do exactly what he ordered. He introduced the "spoils system" into politics along the Delaware, and by appointing twelve close relatives to office, at a yearly cost of $30,000 to the state, he established what his enemies called a "royal family."

McKean's vote-getting machine, supported by patronage and by lavish use of the pork barrel, set a pattern for Pennsylvania politics. Later leaders, copying his model, built up political organizations that could put Tweed to shame. The energetic, domineering governor was America's first professional boss.

He was unbeatable by ordinary methods. His opponents tried in vain to vote him out of office, only to learn that officeholders and recipients of state funds would go to any length to keep their jobs. Then, despairing of defeating him at the polls, the good-government crowd tried to impeach him on the ground that he had vetoed too many acts of the legislature. McKean contemptuously dismissed the efforts, and scorned the "geese" and "clodhoppers" who tried to dislodge him. Finally, despairing of getting rid of him by any other method, the anti-McKean faction boomed the stubborn governor for the second place on the Jefferson ticket. McKean was not to be allured even by the vice-presidency; he stayed in office as governor of Pennsylvania until 1808, though in later years he was so paralyzed that he could not sign his name.

Hot Water War

Quite possibly Pennsylvania required a dogmatic, uncompromising ruler. The turbulent state, scarcely recovered from the Whisky Rebellion in the western counties, was once more threatened by revolt. Pennsylvania Germans in the east, like the Scotch-Irish west of the mountains, were aggrieved. A national direct property tax, laid by Congress in anticipation of a possible war with France, was violently resented.

Presidential arrogance, rather than disloyalty, lay at the basis of the trouble. Pennsylvania Germans, thoroughly devoted to the nation, resented the high-handed methods used by the Federalists to put down Democratic opposition. None of them were aliens, nor were any of them seditious, but the national administration, by its stringent Alien and Sedition Laws and its harsh repression of all criticism, treated them as

subject peoples. When in 1798 a federal law provided
that all lands and dwelling houses be assessed to pay
a graduated tax, the upstate Pennsylvania German:
voiced a violent objection.

John Fries, Bucks County auctioneer, took down
his Revolutionary sword from above the fireplace,
clapped on an old three-cornered hat with a broken
white feather, whistled to his dog "Whiskey," and made
the tavern rounds protesting at the house tax law. At
each stopping place, the nervous, black-eyed Fries called
for the erection of "liberty poles" on which he raised
defiant streamers against tyranny, and five-striped flag:
to represent the eastern counties which he hoped to
raise against the government. He taught a battle cry
"Dämm de President, dämm de Congress, dämm de
Arischdokratz," and as he raced about the countryside
a little force of fifty determined men rallied to his side.

The Pennsylvania German counties were a bedlam.
Each tavern was a center for noisy, demonstrating rebels, hallooing, cursing and swearing, denouncing John
Adams, the house tax, and the assessors who were
charged with the enforcement of the laws. Drum:
pounded; fifes squealed; rifle shots, fired by energetic
farmers practicing their gunnery, cracked constantly.

Poor Cephus Childs, one of those suspected of
friendliness to the new law, wrote home that he could
not make head or tail of the commotion. "They
damned the house tax and the stamp act, and called
me a 'stampler'; they damned the Alien and Sedition
laws, and finally all the laws, the government, and all
the laws the present government had made. They
damned the Constitution, also. They did not mention
what Constitution, whether of this State or of the
United States. They damned the Congress, and damned
the President, and all the friends to government, be-

cause they were all Tories, as none were friends to the present government but the Tories. They said they would not have the government, nor the President, and they would not live under such a damned government; 'we will have Washington'; others said 'No, we will have Jefferson, he is a better man than Adams; huzza for Jefferson.' "

So general was the uproar that, before many days had passed, John Fries was claiming ten thousand men; moreover, he boasted, George Washington himself was coming to assist the rising with a force of twenty thousand troops! Insubordination was so prevalent that local officials threw up their hands in helpless dismay, and called for state militia. These, too, were unsuccessful, and after the rebels had broken into the jail at Bethlehem to free those prisoners arrested for opposing the unpopular tax law the state appealed for federal assistance. Strutting proudly at the head of his small army, now a hundred and fifty strong, John Fries defied the nation. His small dog barked approval; the tricolored cockades of the riflemen nodded their willingness to fight against the whole force of the United States.

Five hundred New York regulars, aided by two thousand Jersey militiamen, with artillery drawn from Lancaster, Carlisle, and Harrisburg, marched by presidential order to suppress the rising. The countryfolk watched them sullenly, offering no resistance, but refusing to give aid in any form. The Fries force melted away, though Fries himself kept issuing warnings that his men would shoot the legs from under any Federals who dared to enter the rebellious region. More effective opposition, however, still remained. Whenever government agents knocked on the doors, irate housewives, leaning from their upper windows, emptied kettlefuls of boiling water on the visitors. The "Hot Water War" went on, though infantrymen made military occupation of the Pennsylvania German counties.

A lucky speech brought peace that force could not procure. Brigadier General William McPherson, issuing a proclamation of amnesty to all who would surrender, told the loungers in a tavern that the insurrection was absurd. The tax, said he, was too small to be regarded seriously, particularly as it was a "soak-the-rich" affair.

"The poor man, whose house and lot do not exceed two acres, has no tax to pay, and, if it were worth $500, the tax is but a dollar. The rich man, with a house rated at $1,000, has to pay three times as much, for the tax operates progressively to the most costly house and opulent people. Hereby, my fellow citizens, you must be convinced that an opposition to this tax is not only contrary to the Constitution, the laws, and every principle of good government, but, in itself, is inconsistent and ridiculous."

McPherson's speech cooled down the angry Pennsylvania Germans, and the revolt subsided. Fries, accompanied only by the little black Whiskey, fled to the swamps, to hide himself within a deep briar patch until the troops withdrew. McPherson's men, scouring the country, found no trace of him, though they searched each house and barn and beat the bushes thoroughly. As they were about to leave the swamp, excited little Whiskey barked too loud and Fries was found.

The rebel leader, tried for treason, was condemned to death, but President Adams, against the advice of his whole Cabinet, granted him a pardon. Federalists thought him ungrateful when, in spite of presidential clemency, he campaigned among his Pennsylvania German neighbors in violent objection to an Adams re-election.

20

Wise Men Take No Chances

Lord High Admiral

Poor John Fitch was drunker than a lord. No one could doubt that he was drunk. All evening long he had been drinking rum, drinking it straight, without a chaser, strong, aromatic Barbados rum. John Fitch was drunk.

Maybe he was crazy too, as well as drunk. Certainly his angry mutterings were far from being sensible. No one in his senses, drunk or sober, would accuse upright Dr. Franklin, now almost eighty, of stealing scientific ideas from a youngster, even if one stretched a point to call John Fitch's absurd notions "scientific." Who but a crazy man would ever hope to push a boat upstream against both wind and tide by force of steam? But Fitch was muttering that good Ben Franklin was desirous of gaining "the honor" for himself. Honor, indeed.

Of course, it might have been that John Fitch had a touch of sun. All afternoon he'd spent out there on the glasslike Delaware, broiling in the burning heat, pottering with that small skiff of his, trying to make the fool thing go. He'd gone out in the morning with such proud boasts that those buckets on the endless chain than ran on rollers could be made to dip into the water and that the skiff would move straight up the Delaware. It had been fun to watch him for a while and notice his singing change to silence, and then to hear him start to curse when he became convinced that his engine could not work. The idlers had enjoyed themselves, calling out advice, telling him to man the oars, to hoist his shirt for a sail, to blow the skiff upstream, to step into the water and push the boat himself, but the jeers had palled in time, and the idlers had wandered off to more exciting spectacles. Who would stand on a muddy riverbank to watch a crazy inventor sitting in a skiff when there were horses racing only half a mile away?

John Fitch had stayed all day, that fiery July Thursday in 1786, and his skiff had not moved a single inch. No one expected that it would. The wise men of the American Philosophical Society had told him, almost a year before, when he showed them a little brass model that he had sailed in Joe Longstreth's meadow brook up in Southampton township, that the idea was not practical. Congress, over in New York, had listened, none too patiently, to his excited talk, and then had turned him off without a single sentence of encouragement. George Washington, down at Mount Vernon, had not been impressed; the Pennsylvania legislature soothed the scrawny, black-eyed inventor, but cannily refused to vote him any help. A few compassionate businessmen, to be sure, had chipped in their subscriptions to the steamboat scheme, but that was more as a left-handed charity than from any real conviction that the crazy plan would ever really work.

Small wonder, then, that Fitch sat drinking rum and muttering that he was bedeviled by bad luck. Ever since that Sunday afternoon in April, 1785, when old man Sinton's shining one-horse chair had splattered his best broadcloth suit with mud, unhappy John Fitch had been obsessed with this idea of a carriage or a ship moved by steam. He never had been lucky, anyway.

He had tried a dozen trades from potash making to silversmithing, and every one had brought him failure. All he had to show for all his labor was a limping leg, caused by the rheumatism caught while surveying in the Ohio wilderness. There was nothing left for him, thought Fitch, but dreariness; he'd have to spend the rest of his life peddling hand-drawn maps of that enormous swampy Northwest waste, and who would want to buy them?

John Fitch drank alone that night, muttering to his rum, shunned by other patrons in the dingy tavern. Next day, he tried in vain to work again upon his skiff, but his fingers were all thumbs; his brain was cloudy. Disgusted with the skiff, with his idea of steam, and most of all disgusted with himself, he knocked off early, dragged himself back to his small attic room, and turned in for some needed sleep.

By midnight he was wide awake, his brain boiling with a new discovery. The endless chain, he saw, was wrong; it made the buckets strike the water at too great an angle; the power was all lost in banging at the surface of the water and in pulling buckets out again. What he really needed, John Fitch clearly saw, was oars or paddles. Three sets of paddles, dangling on each side like an ancient Roman galley, could be made to move in unison, like Indians canoeing, and they would push the boat ahead. John Fitch slept no more that night; he sat before his desk, candles guttering on either side of him, and drew his plans for a new and improved steamship.

This time, he was resolved, it would be a vessel of some size, capable of carrying a paying load of passengers and freight. He had a good steam engine, with a cylinder a foot in diameter, and he would build a boat to match the engine. There would, he thought, be no question of the engine's being wrong in principle, for Harry Voight, the watchmaker, would take care of the mechanical details; if only he could figure out the angle at which those paddles should be fixed and could work out their proper size, the steamboat problem would be solved.

Now there was no advance publicity and no ungrounded boasting; indeed, if anything, John Fitch was careful to make understatements even to himself. He doubled the number of his paddles, putting six to a side; he made careful plans to give his boat the minimum resistance to the water; he checked his engine carefully, and tried it out innumerable times. Then, on an August Wednesday in 1787, he invited the whole Constitutional Convention to adjourn its sessions for the afternoon to watch a trial trip on the Delaware.

Washington stayed home that afternoon, but almost every other member came out to take a place on the specially reserved wharf to watch the steamboat start. Mooring lines were cast off; eager volunteers poled the boat away from shore. Proudly John Fitch, standing at the helm, signalled to Harry Voight to turn on the power.

With unearthly clanks and clangor, with creaks and unexpected hisses of escaping steam, the first successful steamship in the world moved slowly up the Delaware. The Fitch experiment was working; the crowd, even the dignified members of the Constitutional Convention, cheered heartily, though they thought it still merely an amusing toy. It never, they said, can carry enough cargo to justify the cost of operation.

Progress at the rate of five miles per hour was,

however, much too rapid for the flimsy craft. The boiler exploded. Voight and Fitch worked desperately to beach the boat before it burned or sank. Skeptics on the shore were more than ever certain that steamships were impractical.

But Fitch had proved that steam would move a vessel, and he had witnesses to prove that his small ship had triumphed over wind and tide. He went again to see the legislatures, to ask them, without subscribing a single penny to the venture, if they would grant him an exclusive right to operate steamships on the rivers of their states for fourteen years. Delaware, New York, New Jersey, Pennsylvania, even distant Virginia, voted him a monopoly for steamboat traffic. Fitch was able, too, to collect subscriptions from a few rich men who, before, had been reluctant to throw away their money. A larger, better boat, forty-five feet long, with a bigger engine, was now built, but Fitch, always itching to experiment, moved the paddles from the vessel's side to make a new device, "like three or four snow shovels," on the stern.

This ship worked too. By July, 1788, Fitch began a regular passenger service on the Delaware between Philadelphia and Burlington. Again, the first trip was a social triumph. Crowds watched the vessel steam away from Philadelphia, saw it move upstream at the tremendous speed of seven miles an hour. At Point-no-Point, near Bridesburg, the farmers halted their wheat harvest to watch the ship steam by. Men cheered; women waved their aprons; young lads put out in sharpies to row beside the noisy craft, while exultant John Fitch shouted thanks for their congratulations. At Dunk's Ferry in Bucks County, close by the Long-streth farm where Fitch had made his early model,

Revolutionary cannon fired salutes under the direction of old man Sinton, whose flying chair had stirred the envious John Fitch to thoughts of easier and swifter travel.

It was a gala trip to Burlington, and those who crowded the green slopes to watch the uncouth monster puff itself to shore were thrilled at the great novelty. They, too, were cheering, but they were dismayed to see the ship, while yet in midstream off the wharf, drop anchor while the helmsman ran quickly to the center of the craft. Then came a most tremendous roar; the boiler had exploded. Fitch had not been quick enough to help his fireman colleague draw the fires.

No one was hurt, and the ship was brought safely to shore. Fitch had amply proved his argument that steam navigation was feasible, though his efforts thus far had cost a boiler for each trip.

By May 1790, the Lord High Admiral of the Delaware, as wags now nicknamed John Fitch, prepared another, and still larger, vessel for the service. He piloted his ship to Burlington and Chester, to Gray's Ferry on the Schuylkill and to Wilmington, with no other breakages than a couple of cracked "axles" and a splintered paddle or two. Nearly three thousand miles of passenger traffic were completed in the summer season, though the vessel made no profit. Fuel costs were greater than the gross receipts. Philadelphia capital was more than ever certain that steamships were nothing more than noisy, smoky playthings. When, therefore, the great ship burned, following its grounding in a gale, the canny businessmen would sink no money in replacements. John Fitch, left with "not a penny for soft soap," much less the thousands that he needed for a steamer, gave up his attempts on the Delaware.

The Doubting Delaware

Oliver Evans had much the same experience. As early as 1787, while Fitch was tinkering with ships, Evans talked about a carriage that needed no horses but moved by its own steam. He, too, found no support in Congress, and met nothing but derision when he asked the Delaware legislature to advance his aim. He could not even get a patent for his steam carriage plan. Evans, more energetic and less broody than John Fitch, went straight to the people with his scheme. A descendant of the rebellious Steelcoat of the Long Finn insurrection, he sought no surcease in the rum bowl; instead, he told the public what he thought of its stupidity.

"The time will come," he said to jeering audiences, "when people will travel in stages moved by steam engines at fifteen to twenty miles an hour. A carriage will leave Washington in the morning, breakfast at Baltimore, dine at Philadelphia, and sup at New York on the same day. . . . Posterity will not be able to discover why the legislature or Congress did not grant the inventor such protection as might have enabled him to put in operation these great improvements."

Neither the smoking steamship, puffing loudly up the river and breaking some essential machinery on each trip, nor Evans's clanking motor carriage convinced the Delaware that a new era was at hand. Conservatives saw little future in newfangled modes of travel. Steam transportation seemed an interesting toy which might divert the public for a time but would never prove commercially profitable. Their attention turned, instead, to wilder theorists who thought that man might travel through the air.

The Delaware had already had experience with an ambitious aviator. For several months one Peter Carnes "of Bladensburg, Virginia," had been papering the town with handbills to proclaim his aerostat balloon which, he predicted, would sail freely through the skies. But when Carnes finally arrived, and filled his silk balloon with hot air from a furnace fastened underneath, the aerostat rose but a scant twelve feet before it struck a wall and threw the navigator out. Relieved of Carnes's weight, the balloon rose high, but the furnace set the silk afire. The great bag soared flaming over Philadelphia.

Now, about the time when Fitch and Evans were asking for financial aid, a second aeronaut, François Blanchard, arrived in town. He was a greater showman than his brother inventors. He called upon the president to ask a passport certifying to any peoples of the world where he might land that he had gone by air from the United States, and then, when excitement ran high, he summoned all the town to watch him start for the unknown. Acid and iron filings were to fill his big balloon with gas.

Blanchard stepped into his spangled chariot, suspended from the varnished yellow silk bag, as a band played and cannons were discharged. He cut the ropes that held him to the ground. Up shot the balloon, Blanchard waving a tricolor in one hand and an American flag in the other, while the long white feathers in his new cocked hat danced merrily in the breeze. He crossed the Delaware on that first flight but he was never able to repeat his trip. His gas balloon was uncontrollable; he could not predict his destination. The president's official passport, admitting him to strange and unknown lands, was never necessary.

The Delaware enjoyed the party, but was disin-

clined to pay for it. Blanchard, protesting that he had
sunk $3,000 in preparing for his flight, asked for help.
No more than $500 was subscribed. The inventor left
the city in dusgust.

Go West, Young Man!

New interests challenged attention. Throughout
the eighteenth century statesmanship and science, culture and the learned arts, had flourished in the valley of
the Delaware; society shone more brilliantly than elsewhere in America. But now that the nation's capital
was moved to its new seat among Potomac swamps,
drawing with it the glittering alien attachés and luring
away the cream of the sophisticated, residents in the
Delaware area turned to new activities.

Alert young men saw opportunities for progress in
the West. The new lands of Kentucky and Ohio, rich
and undeveloped, attracted those who could not live a
static life. Restless boys who saw slight chance to
better their condition in the settled Delaware valley
struck out for the West. Long caravans of Conestoga
wagons, blue bodied and with red-painted wheels, rumbled out of Philadelphia along the new-built turnpike
toward Lancaster to seek the virgin farm lands that lay
beyond the Alleghenies. Countless other youths went
by horse or stage; some walked, pushing their scanty
store of goods on wheelbarrows or carrying their possessions on their backs.

Like every other tide of emigration, this steady
westward stream bore with it men of most diverse
ability. The misfits and the discontents who could not
find happiness amid the keen competition of the settled
eastern seaboard, adventurers who gambled that the

West would yield a better profit than the calm and settled Delaware, mingled with many mystics who sought Utopia beyond the mountains and with eager lads who yearned to carve out empires for themselves. Their spiritual ancestors had come, moved by similar ambitions, to settle on the Delaware.

To some degree, this draining off relieved the Delaware of serious social problem. Dynamic youths who find no legal opening are sometimes wont to drift to crime, but once these highly metabolic folk find wholesome outlet for their energy they make a most desirable portion of the population. The Delaware gained added peace by their departure; the West acquired good colonists.

The Delaware lost potential troublemakers, but it also lost some color. Those enterprising emigrants were largely men who, properly adjusted, could have brought innovation and a certain unconventional distinction. They left behind them staider folk, too calm or too content to leave, too timorous to take a chance or too sedate, men whose imaginations kept within complacent bounds. In consequence, the valley of the Delaware assumed a steadiness of disposition, a tranquillity of tone. Social atmosphere grew older; conventionality was often worshiped as a fetish. In years to come it would be said that Philadelphia, worse than being politically corrupt, was contented. Friends of the Delaware saw in the peacefulness of social life a calm reflection of the patterns of the river, a cool, quiet, unemotional quality prized by the Quakers and their pacifistic allies.

The river remained unperturbed. Life always had been rich and pleasant; well-bred people always courteous and kind. Energetic, pushing folk might leave the Delaware, but the solid, well-contented residents could carry on their quiet well-worn ways. Young men in skin-tight trousers and polished boots whose sharp-pointed toes were linked by silver chains to whited tops, their hair tucked up behind with small combs of tortoise shell or unobtrusively queued, were not dismayed to find that progress passed them by. Philadelphians had never liked the bustle of prosperity.

Girls in high headdresses, narrow-skirted gowns, and tight-sleeved bodices of soft, clinging blue or white or yellow went gaily on their social rounds. The theater was at its height; Charles Willson Peale's remarkable museum, where every known American animal stood lifelike in its proper habitat, vied with Rickett's Circus as a place of popular resort.

Some social circles tried to live in emulation of their former grandeur. Looking back today, after the passage of a century and a half, one sees that there was something hectic in the effort to pursue past glory. A few leaders lost something of their old fastidiousness; in the wild hope of snaring foreign social lions, they sometimes welcomed strangers indiscriminately. La Rochefoucauld, familiar with the Philadelphia of the past, now thought that people of the Delaware gave teas and dinners for any alien of any country, any class, or any character, without much real investigation of his merits. They welcome everyone, he said, "philosopher, preacher, man of letters, prince or dentist, wit or idiot." But, he added, "after the first warm rapture, the stranger may be dropped."

Better Philadelphians were never guilty of such frenzies. Instead, the true inner group retreated rather within itself, becoming introspective and aloof. Birth gave prestige, not wealth; intellectual achievement outranked business and finance. The Delaware was making the most of those qualities which it had been permitted to retain.

21

Mary Vining

THE tall white-haired woman moved slowly forward from the gloomy parlor, holding to her toothless mouth a dainty cambric handkerchief. Her dark eyes, still as warm as they had been a quarter century before when they had captivated officers of three gallant armies, twinkled at her nephew.

"Come here, my little rogue," she teased, "and you may kiss my hand. You will be glad to do so, for prince's lips have touched it."

The boy shrank back. This was a new Aunt Mary, quite unlike the shy woman who had long sat secluded in the shadows and who, even in her tight-shaded parlor, wore a veil to shield her from the sun. He had never heard her speaking English. The few times she had spoken to him during the ten years of his life, she had used French, which was musical and cadenced but quite different from the French his governess had taught him. In fact, Mademoiselle had confided in him that his aunt's French dated from before the time when the Revolution had upset the Versailles court. Never in all his years of living in the same tree-shaded house had he seen his Aunt Mary move from her apartment.

Why she was vivacious now was a mystery to young John Vining, but boys of ten do not attempt to solve the strange behavior of their elders. He could not know that Mary Vining's strange seclusion was the talk of Wilmington, that her refusal to set foot outside the door was in fulfillment of a vow taken long ago that she would not look again upon a man. Not even in these later days did she see her close friend Governor John Dickinson. The little boy kissed her hand, catching the odd scent of Aunt Mary's French perfume, and then fled hastily into the sunlight.

Mary sighed, and turned back to her parlor. Her steps were dragging now, as they always seemed to drag these days; her shoulders melted from their temporary squareness. She sank into the depths of her big chair, where once the gallant soldier, Anthony Wayne, had sat admiring her. Her little dream was ended; now she knew, as Mary Vining always knew on every other day but this, that she was lonely and deserted. On this one day, the New Year, birthday of her lover Anthony, she tried each year to bring back youth. For this New Year was yet another anniversary of that unhappy day on which she once had waited longingly for Wayne to come home to their wedding.

Mary Vining was the cousin of the famous Caesar Rodney, gay, vivacious, and brilliant. She dominated every social circle. Neither Anne Bingham, nor any of the Shippen sisters, nor the magnificent Walcott girl, who was the toast of all New England gentlemen, nor any of the Chew family possessed Mary Vining's zest for conquest. British officers, smitten by her beauty, dared court-martial for one last look at her, and rode through the rebel lines to Wilmington the night before the English left Philadelphia. Young diplomats from France came eagerly to see the fascinating person of whom their own vivacious queen spoke jealously. Louis Philippe, who hoped someday to be king, charming Lafayette, and dashing Francisco Miranda, Venezuelan patriot, were at her feet, together with half a hundred brilliant men of Pennsylvania and Delaware. No woman of the Delaware had ever known such adulation.

Perhaps that admiration had been too great, for Mary Vining herself confessed that she was spoiled by too much praise. Perhaps there was no man, except Wayne, to match her versatility and charm, unless it was her young brother, John Vining, congressman and "Pet of Delaware." But if she stood too high among the people of her time, she suffered tragically for it.

Few among her former intimates knew that, for twenty years, Mary Vining nursed a hopeless love. Dashing Mad Anthony Wayne, Beau Brummel of the Revolution, met her at a ball a few short months before he forced his way up Stony Point, and he and Mary fell irrevocably in love. But Wayne was married to an ailing wife, and had two children. He was responsible, moreover, for the financial support of both his mother and his wife's mother, and his ancestral farm at Waynesborough, twenty miles from Philadelphia, was not profitable. If he had tried to cast aside his responsibilities, the stringent social code of the time would have made him an outcast.

Wayne threw himself into the task of organizing an effective army. His was an arduous assignment, for as a Pennsylvanian he was charged with three men's work. His state had made serious mistakes in naming as his superiors men who neither could nor would perform their duties. Yet, under the strict military etiquette so cherished by the Revolutionary officers, Wayne could not act in controvention of their orders. Throughout the greater portion of the war Wayne was only a brigadier, but he shouldered the responsibilities of the two major generals who outranked him.

Even after the Revolution had been won Wayne

was not free to give all his attention to his own desires. The task of clearing up the work in Georgia, the administration of a large, but dilapidated, plantation which had been given him in recognition of his success, his political activities down south, all claimed his time. When these were, at last, settled Wayne was drafted into the war against the western Indians. Then, when Wayne was forty-eight and Mary thirty-seven, the ailing Polly Wayne died of her long illness. The general was off on the frontier, winning for the nation the vast Northwest Territory. Not for three years more was he free to come back home.

He and Mary Vining were at once engaged. Mary was enthusiastically happy for the several weeks that Wayne was home on furlough. They played together and visited their friends; they chatted eagerly about their plans for marriage. Wayne could stay only a short time in Philadelphia; although he had removed the menace of the Indians by winning Fallen Timbers, he had to go west again to make a final treaty. When he left Philadelphia for the army, in May, 1796, it was agreed that he and Mary should be married upon his return at Christmastime.

But when Christmas came Mad Anthony was dead. A sharp appendicitis pain, mistaken for a gout attack, had been poorly cared for and, while Wayne was hurrying home to marry Mary, he had died, ten days before Christmas.

Mary had hoped to spend her Christmas in Wayne's company. His letters said that he would be home and that he wished to entertain his friends at dinner. Mary undertook to make arrangements, though she knew that travel from the frontier was uncertain and that the dinner might possibly have to be postponed. She sent out tentative invitations to their mutual friends, but warned them that no recent news had come from Wayne. When Christmas drew closer, with no letter to announce his near arrival, she canceled the arrangements, but looked forward the more eagerly to New Year's Day. That holiday would be Wayne's fifty-second birthday; she hoped that it might also be their wedding day.

But as gunshots were fired, and rockets, squibs, and India crackers were set off, in the ancient fashion of the Delaware to celebrate the coming of another year, a courier arrived. He brought the news that Wayne was dead. There had been no inkling of his illness, nor any message of the homeward journey since he had promised to be home by Christmas Day.

The shock was too great to be borne. A fat and pleasant Irish immigrant, Jane Mauthrell, calling on the Vining servants, saw Mary slump down to the floor. She ran in to help, and mothered the brokenhearted beauty. She was so comforting that she remained thereafter a fixture in the Vining household.

The Willows, Mary's Wilmington home, stood in a shaded yard well back from the road. For more than a quarter century the brooding woman kept herself within the grounds in strict seclusion. On only three occasions during these twenty-five years did Mary Vining emerge from what she called her "living tomb." She stayed indoors, listening to Jane Mauthrell's reading of the Bible. At times she worked on a history of the Revolutionary War which she had planned to write with Wayne; more often she brooded over the "worked mahogany chairs" in which Wayne had sat, or polished the great chased silver coffee pot he had liked.

Her three emergences were bitter disappointments. Once, urged strongly by her devoted friend John Dickinson, the farmer-lawyer who had been the governor of both Delaware and Pennsylvania, she tried to overcome her grief and to resume her social life. Ten years had passed since she had last been seen in public, and her beauty, once so glamorous, was gone. Her cheeks were sallow; her eyes less bright; the great mass of jet-black hair was now lusterless and gray. The curved mouth had become a thin straight line, and there were gaps where teeth had fallen out.

Mary was poignantly conscious of the change. All through the dinner she kept a handkerchief close to her lips, so that she might hide her mouth when any of the diners turned toward her. Her sunken, yellowed cheeks were smothered beneath rouge and powder; her voice, once musical and charming, was flat and toneless on the rare occasions when she spoke. The experiment of dining out was not repeated.

The second journey from the Willows was more tragic still. A year or two after the Dickinson dinner, in 1809, Mary journeyed up to Philadelphia to be present at the reinterment of Wayne's remains. A first burial, hastily made at Erie by the army, was far away from Wayne's beloved Old St. David's, where Parson William Currie once had ruled. Wayne's son Isaac brought back the remains for burial in the family plot. Mary Vining, heavily swathed in black, drove with Caesar Augustus Rodney, nephew and heir of her cousin, the rider, to be present at the ceremonies. She spoke to no one, visited none of her former friends, paid slight heed to the changes that had taken place.

Twelve years later, Mary Vining died, on the eve, Jane Mauthrell said, of yet a third emergence. For Mary in her solitude had learned the consolations of religion and was about to be received into the Episcopalian faith. Two days before her confirmation was to occur she died, on Good Friday, 1821. On Easter Sunday she was buried, and in the fashion of the time, six young girls in white carried her coffin to the grave.

The aftermath reflects no credit on the manners of the time. For years Wilmington had whispered gossip concerning Mary Vining's self-imposed seclusion. Few of the younger folk had ever seen her face and the six pallbearers were unacquainted with her except through chattered rumor.

Betsy Montgomery, self-appointed historian of Wilmington, was unable to restrain her curiosity. Though she had never known Miss Vining and had never seen her alive, Betsy believed that she was justified in breaking down the guarded secrets. For her *Reminiscences of Wilmington* she wanted to know exactly what the Willows house was like, what kind of life Miss Vining had led, and how the famous beauty looked in death. She virtually forced her way into the house, over the protests of Jane Mauthrell, pushed her way to the coffin, and peered inside. Jane was not anxious to make a scene but insisted so earnestly that Betsy come away that the historian caught only a glimpse of the age-ravaged face of an old woman who had been, half a century before, a Revolutionary belle. When she came to write her book, she revenged herself upon Mary Vining's long-time companion; Jane Mauthrell's name was completely missing from the Montgomery story.

Jane was determined that no similar incident should occur. At the funeral the pallbearers wore linen scarfs, three feet in length, swathed about their bonnets and pinned beneath their chins. As further precaution, the coffin lid was tightly screwed down before the young girls came to carry Mary Vining to her grave. The mystery that had surrounded her while living remained with her in death.

22

The Delaware Renaissance

SAMUEL F. B. MORSE came late; his telegraph was half a century behind the times. As early as 1809 shipping men were sending telegraphic signals on the Delaware.

Jonathan Grout, a foreign trader, deserves the credit for invention of the telegraph. Reading of European scientific progress, he learned that quick electrical communication was feasible. If six or eight wires were strung and current were sent through them, signals could be sent by various combinations of breaking connections. Grout told the then existing Chamber of Commerce of his ideas and, through it, gained permission from the Pennsylvania legislature to use Reedy Island, then state-owned property, as a telegraph terminus.

The scheme worked well. Messages announcing the arrival of incoming ships were sent by wire forty-five miles to Philadelphia. For three years, till the outbreak of the War of 1812, the Grout telegraph system operated successfully.

Shipping ceased upon the outbreak of war. Traders, already suffering seriously from the effects of Jefferson's embargo policies, closed their doors. Ships lay rotting at the wharves; seamen were idle; commerce died completely. There was no need for Grout's telegraph, for no vessels were arriving in the river. Moreover, British guns were a constant threat. As soon as war broke out, an English squadron bottled up the bay. The Delaware was helpless to resist. Unfortified little Lewes, at the site of ancient Whorekill, was particularly vulnerable. Two hundred and forty British cannons covered the small town, where only a handful of old men, veterans of the Revolution, were available for defense. Yet Lewes won glory where towns of greater magnitude failed sadly.

Probably the British were inefficient in their efforts to attack the little town. Angered at the refusal of the settlement to collect twenty bullocks for provisioning the blockaders, the British opened fire. For twenty-two hours, the entire English Fleet bombarded the town. Eight hundred shells were fired, but the aim was so atrocious that the total casualties were a dog, a hen, and one milk can. Not a single human being was even scratched by the continued fire. No effort was made to land troops, and when the bombardment ceased the British vessels sailed away, without the bullocks they had sought.

When the War of 1812 was over, swift-moving steamships came so rapidly that revival of the telegraph seemed unnecessary. A new invention, too, was prospering so greatly that it seemed likely to supplant both ships and telegraph. This was the railroad. Begun in the same year as Grout's telegraph, it was proving its usefulness. Thomas Leiper, an enterprising Scottish-born sergeant of the silk-stockinged City Troop, had laid oak scantlings in the Bull's Head tavernyard for use as an experimental track. When it worked well, Leiper built a larger railroad, from his quarries on Crum Creek three-quarters of a mile to deep water on the Delaware. For eighteen years he hauled his stone on this early road until, finding that rail transport was more expensive han water carriage, he dug a canal to take the railroad's place.

Leiper's success led to more ambitious plans. Progressive Jersey businessmen revived the Evans scheme of railroad building. They drafted plans for the construction of a road to link tidewater on the Delaware, perhaps at Trenton or Camden, with deep channels on the Raritan, at Amboy or New Brunswick. They asked a charter and received it, but once the license was in hand, in 1815, the promoters found it difficult to raise sufficient capital. Their line, the Camden and Amboy, was not built for sixteen years.

Meanwhile, Philadelphia mine owners built the first long railway in America. In 1828 William and Maurice Wurts, anxious to cut the costs of hauling anthracite, began the Delaware and Hudson line from Carbondale to Honesdale. To pull their coal carts, they imported from England the "Stourbridge Lion." This was the first locomotive to operate in the United States.

The highly touted Stourbridge Lion proved a disappointment. In hauling its first heavy load the engine crashed through the light wooden rails on which the freight train was to run. But when the track was strengthened the locomotive worked efficiently. Soon thereafter a seventeen-mile New Castle and French-town line, connecting the Delaware with the head of the Chesapeake, offered regular passenger service. Time of travel between Baltimore and Philadelphia was thereby reduced, though many shook their heads in doubt whether wooden rails fastened on stone sleepers would be sufficiently strong to guarantee safety when trains ran as fast as ten miles an hour.

The Delaware now knew that railroad transportation was feasible, but there were other means of travel which conservatives preferred. The folk along the river

had always been water-conscious; from the time of
Swedish settlement, canoes and skiffs had been employed
in journeying. Though the Wurtses and Leiper showed
that engines could be made to run, the Delaware was
not anxious to hazard life on experiments.

The Pennsylvania Canal

People frowned on using steam for transportation,
but they were enthusiastic over conventional ideas. The
canal-building fever which possessed the nation in the
first part of the nineteenth century raged along the
Delaware.

The valleys of the Delaware, the Lehigh, and the
Schuylkill are rich in tributaries. Small creeks are
numerous; many of them offer natural passages through
mountain ranges. From early days settlers of the area
had dreamed that canals, connecting river systems,
would open the interior to easy trade. Penn had
planned a waterway to run across the colony from the
Delaware to the Susquehanna. After the Revolution,
when the riches of the West were better known, Pennsylvanians had visions of a great canal to link the Delaware with the Ohio, perhaps with the Great Lakes.

"The time will come," wrote an enthusiast to Governor Thomas Mifflin, "when canals shall pass through
every vale, wind round every hill, and bind the whole
country in one bond of social intercourse."

Certainly the state was optimistic about its abilities. Pennsylvania is crossed by two wide mountain
ranges, but engineers believed that canals could readily
be dug to link Philadelphia with Pittsburgh by water
level routes. When this proved to require enormous expense a fantastic project was begun. The shallow, stony

Schuylkill was dredged, far above Reading, and a narrow creek was widened to carry canalboats farther west.

Then a railroad track was built, its ends extending to the water's edge. The loaded barge was hoisted on a flatcar and portaged over the first range of mountains to a point where navigation could be resumed in a small creek leading to the Susquehanna. Thus the railroad, instead of complicated locks, lifted canalboats over two mountain ranges to the Ohio River.

Men capable of realizing such a vision ought, by rights, to be entitled to reward. Pennsylvania's magnificent conception, one of the major engineering feats of nineteenth century American history, deserved to prosper, if only for its audacity. But geography was hostile. The plan was feasible and the rail-and-water combination involved no insoluble problem, but the costs of operation were enormous. New York's Erie Canal, using the Hudson and the Mohawk and cutting through a fairly level territory, carried goods at cheaper rates. Western trade, which once had rumbled through Philadelphia on Conestoga wagons, now flowed in Erie barges to New York.

The Delaware's economic life was dislocated. Business interests suffered as commerce went by routes that detoured Philadelphia. Traffic on the Delaware diminished. More important, young men, ambitious to succeed, deserted to Manhattan. Again the Delaware was drained of aggressive, enterprising leaders.

Canals and deepened rivers helped, however, to prevent complete collapse. Western wheat could not be profitably handled, but coal, mined along the Lehigh and the upper Schuylkill, could readily be floated down to market. Millions were appropriated to dredge the Schuylkill, Lehigh, and Delaware rivers, to cut canals connecting navigable streams, to build locks and dams, and to provide port facilities. Before the waterways were dug, the freight per ton of coal from Pottsville to Philadelphia, a distance of approximately ninety miles, had cost $28; by river and canal, the charge dropped to one-ninth of that sum.

New Jersey and Delaware followed the Pennsylvania lead. A barge canal from Trenton to the Raritan took coal to New York harbor at a greatly diminished rate and did away with the necessity for towing boats along the treacherous New Jersey coast. The Delaware and the Chesapeake were linked, thus making inland navigation possible from New York and Philadelphia to Baltimore and Washington.

Not only did mining sections prosper, but other industries were aided. Scattered iron furnaces, operated hitherto by charcoal and limited in output because of difficult transport, now grew into large-scale enterprises. Small mills, once dependent on water power, developed into large factories. The valleys of the Lehigh, Schuylkill, and Delaware became centers of enormous industry. Pennsylvania took rank as the leading industrial state.

New occupations came, to supplant the farmers, financiers, and city merchants of the past. Matthias Baldwin, a pious jeweler who spent his evenings tinkering with model engines, gave up "making gewgaws" for the Woolworth Brothers to start a locomotive factory. Though Southerners refused to buy his engines because they hated his abolitionist ideas, the locomotives made in Philadelphia were known throughout the nation. John Roebling began at Trenton the manufacture of wire rope for use as hawsers on canalboats, but soon enlarged his plant to make all types of fabricated steel. In time he was to crown his work by building the great Brooklyn Bridge. At Philadelphia, William Cramp founded a shipbuilding plant which grew into the largest and best equipped shipyard of America. Cotton, carpet, and woolen mills, kilns for porcelain and pottery, glass blowing and silk weaving, gained a new prosperity.

Farther down the Delaware, the introduction of the coal and iron age enlarged the scope of Eleuthère Irénée du Pont's powder mills near Wilmington. A royalist refugee from France, he had come to the United States with letters to Thomas Jefferson. He planned to start a factory near Washington, but when he examined the Potomac site he concluded that "the country, the people, the location are all worthless," and chose, instead, a site along the Brandywine. Work began in a small log cabin, "amid the rocks and rattlesnakes," but with the coming of power machinery the powder mills developed into an enormous enterprise. Du Pont was widely honored for his refusal, in 1831, to sell munitions for spot cash to the South Carolina nullification leaders. "The destination of this powder being obvious," he declared, "we think it right to decline. When our friends in the South will want powder for peaceful purposes, we shall be happy to serve them." Again, at the outbreak of the war with Mexico, du Pont declined to sell munitions to President Santa Anna. "However unjust our proceedings may be," the company replied, "and however shameful our invasion of Mexican territory, we cannot make powder to be used against our own country."

The Delaware Peach

The Delaware's industrial development caused changes also in its agriculture. For years the farms had not been profitable. Unscientific tillage, especially the failure to rotate crops and the insufficiency of fertilizer, had mined the soil of necessary minerals. Many farmers left their lands to move to virgin acres in the West; once rich fields along the Delaware were left uncultivated.

Now that green towns and pleasant villages, where every home possessed its kitchen garden, were giving way to crowded cities, demand for food increased. Almost simultaneously, Jersey farmers found that marl, an excellent natural enricher of the soil, lay close at hand. Mixed with the worn-out earth, marl restored fertility. New Jersey turned into a vast truck patch, from which New York and Philadelphia bought their vegetables.

Rapid growth of railways and canals hastened this process. Huge amounts of western wheat, grown on cheap but fertile farms, competed with the more expensive eastern grains. Jerseymen and Pennsylvanians, driven from wheat markets, found profit in dairying, poultry raising, and meat production.

In Delaware, more remote from city markets than was much of Jersey, a solution was discovered in growing fruit. Always, since the days of Penn, Delaware peaches were famous, though in early years they were used chiefly for making a powerful, but pleasant, brandy. About the time of the Industrial Revolution, Major Philip Reybold set out several hundred acres of budded Crawford peaches, and shipped two hundred baskets of fresh fruit to city markets. The experiment was highly profitable. Within a few years central Delaware was one great orchard.

Scientific knowledge was insufficient, however. Peaches are a tender crop, easily blighted by inattention, frost, or parasites. The "yellows," a disease no one then knew how to treat, ravaged the orchards. Later research showed that yellows can be prevented by proper sprayings, but the discovery came too late. Delaware's peach orchards had been wrecked; peaches were replaced by hardy apple trees, which required less nursing.

New Jersey's orchards were set out at a later date, after scientific spraying had been developed; the Jersey fruit was, therefore, less affected by the yellows, the San Jose scale, and other blights which ravaged Delaware. South Jersey in particular continued as a leading fruit-producing area. Its vineyards yielded wines which many connoisseurs ranked among the best American vintages.

Growth of industry along the river wrecked a flourishing New Jersey occupation. The fisheries had been renowned for scores of years. Shad and sturgeon, perch and herring, swimming upstream with the tide, were carried by the current close to the Jersey shore. Each spring the Jersey fishermen set nets half a mile or more in length. On one occasion sixty thousand fish were caught in a day's haul.

Cheap food was thus available. Before the Industrial Revolution, an alewife, the Delaware herring, sold for twopence; a shad cost but a penny more. Salt fish, barreled for winter use, was marketed for three farthings a pound. The shovel-nosed sturgeon, useful for making a cheap grade of caviar, were then so plentiful that they could be counted by dozens at a time. Penn complained that they leaped into the air, endangering small skiffs.

This abundance disappeared. Upstream factories poured their wastes into the Delaware; acids from the tanneries, sewage from the cities, and oils from mills poisoned the stream. Fish ceased to spawn in such vast numbers in the valley of the Delaware. Fishermen who once had dipped out, by hand seines, three thousand catfish in a single night found that the species had almost vanished. Only the oyster industry, carried on in South Jersey fresh-water coves protected from pollution, remained; the other fisheries dwindled in importance.

Thus, the economic life along the Delaware was modified by coal and iron and high-speed transportation. But other than material changes affected daily life. The Delaware assumed another mode of living; people of strange races came to settle in the valley, bringing with them new ideals. Almost in self-defense against an alien influence, the Delaware took refuge in a standard uniformity of culture, abandoning its boasted individuality. The river was no longer a unique and special stream.

23

The World of Fashion

CONTEMPORARY country journals reflect the prejudices of the day. Indignant protests against carpenters who would not work for less than seventy-five cents a day and who, even at that exorbitant rate, refused to labor longer than eleven hours at a stretch, were followed by scathing ridicule of those who thought the red love apple, or tomato, good to eat. Old Robert Gibbon Johnson, wealthiest citizen of Salem County, founded agricultural societies to push his tomato hobby. To make the vegetable popular, he started county fairs, on models which he said came down from Fenwick's time. Not, however, until 1820, when he dared to eat a prize tomato publicly on the courthouse steps, would cautious South Jersey accept as edible the vegetable that is now its largest crop.

Editors exuded civic pride. When a young Salem County athlete walked forty miles between dawn and sunset of one day the local press was jubilant because a record had been set, and when the county raised an ox so huge that it bid fair to yield a ton of dressed beef joy was unrestrained. The ox, polished, manicured, and beribboned, was taken on a special steamboat to be butchered. All the forty miles from Salem to Philadelphia a band played, and at each small town along the way attention was drawn to Salem County's triumph.

Elijah Brooks, editor of the *Salem Messenger,* was

275

unique in his profession. Elections bored him. Shouting politicians, especially those who went about in black silk vests on which a head of Jackson had been printed, failed to bestir his interest. In making brief announcement that a state election would be held, Brooks editorialized in a despondent vein:

"The election will probably be conducted without any other object than personal promotion. To get a legal right to sit and yawn, stretch one's limbs and sleep away a month or two in the State House at Trenton is the height of some men's ambition. How silly it is to persevere and suffer through all the torturing rains of anxious hopes and glory just to attain the privilege of exposure to public opinion and to say 'Aye' to a proposition to dig a ditch through a salt marsh and to say 'Nay' to a petition for a law to preserve oyster beds."

In national elections he was even less concerned. Suppressing all details, he wrote, "There was so much lack of interest in this election that we forego publishing the returns." Two weeks later, after public sentiment had flared so high against his censorship that talk was heard of starting a rival to the *Messenger*, Brooks changed his mind. "There appears," he said, "to be a demand that the returns be published." He denounced those who could think of such "a base, inhuman thing" as establishing a competitive newspaper.

Brooks's ire was not confined to politicians. He disliked soldiers, especially those stationed at the near-by garrison, and called them "desperadoes from that den of iniquity, Fort Delaware." He opposed river steamers, predicting that they would harm local industry. "The farmers will take their butter, cheese and eggs away and buy groceries and dry goods, and we will have nothing to eat." He warred on noisy camp meetings. "If," an editorial declared, "it is the purpose of these worshippers to avoid hell, they certainly raise enough of it here first."

He went too far, however, when he criticized the Baptists. Learning that they had chopped holes in the creek ice that they might practice immersion, Brooks wondered why there had been need for haste; he speculated as to what sins had been committed serious enough to require a winter ceremony. Angry Baptists canceled their subscriptions, withdrew their advertising, and refused to patronize the paper until Brooks apologized. The editor, facing bankruptcy, "regretted his untimely remarks and believed that the rite of baptism should be administered whenever the hungering soul demanded." A few months later, after Brooks had printed the rumor of a rival's death with an editorial note "Good! This is the best news we have heard yet," the colorful newspaperman withdrew from Salem.

His departure into lands unknown left a void in local journalism. His comments on the story of the roving Delaware elephant would surely have been entertaining. Nearly all the valley swallowed the report that, in 1837, a circus, in ferrying across the river, lost an elephant in the dark, and that the big animal, homesick no doubt for Delaware, "took a rowboat from the shore and rowed back to Wilmington." The startling gem of early press-agentry would undoubtedly have evoked a scintillating and devastating editorial from Elijah Brooks.

Sports reporting missed him too, when Brooks left New Jersey much too soon to cover its famous 94-round, bare-knuckle boxing match for the bantam-weight championship in which the winner earned a purse of $150 while the loser fought for glory only. So widespread was the fame of this encounter that a second fight was staged a month later. Five tugs came

down the river from Philadelphia, bearing some six
hundred fans to watch Walker and Weedon fight a
light-heavyweight encounter. The contest started at
dawn. For ten rounds scarcely a blow was struck, but
from the eleventh to the seventieth Weedon played a
constant tattoo on his opponent's eyes. Walker was
completely blinded, but the fight continued until, in
the seventy-sixth round, he was kneed in the belly.
Walker dropped dead; the fight fans, terrified, hurried
to their tugs and steamed away. Weedon, the conqueror, won no prize whatever for his boxing; instead,
he was arrested and sentenced to a six-year term in jail.

The Salem fights, while long and bloody, lacked
the glamour of a boxing match across the river. Two
Philadelphia boxers, unable to stage a match at home
because of strict antiprize-fight laws, were taken down
to the Twelve Mile Circle at the point where Pennsylvania, Maryland, and Delaware meet. Boxing was
illegal in all three states, but the promoters hoped to
evade the law by operating on disputed land. At daybreak the contest started on Chester County soil, but the
sheriff soon arrived. The boxers, stepping a few yards
off, continued the fight in Delaware territory until
the New Castle authorities hurried to the scene. Then,
barred from both Pennsylvania and Delaware, the con-
testants moved again, to finish their struggle in Maryland. The sheriffs of both Chester County and New
Castle, according to the gleeful tales told by spectators,
sat in their own bailiwicks and watched the progress of
the fight.

Few worthy people participated in such pleasures.
Fighting was ill-bred, beneath the notice of prominent
folk. Following the free and uninhibited democracy of
Jacksonian days, the valley had grown socially conscious and correctly formal. Though the Delaware

never returned to the unbending etiquette of pre-Revolutionary days, conduct became subject to rigid rules.
Tobacco-chewing young men who hoped someday to
gain such affluence as would enable them to drive in
two-horse barouches to country seats along the river
fronts assiduously cultivated good manners; simpering
young ladies, packing their nightcaps in their carpet
satchels, resolved to study carefully Miss Leslie's *Behaviour Book* to avoid committing social blunders.

Avoid the Painted Face

Following some rules was easy. Any girl could
remember that she must not wear her black silk mitts
to breakfast, for that custom was quite obsolete, and
that she should not eat salt fish at any public table lest
she discommode her neighbors by its odor. It was not
hard to bear in mind Miss Leslie's strict injunction that
"no lady looks worse than when gnawing a bone" and
that "nothing should be sucked or gnawed in public,"
not even corn bitten from the cob or melon nibbled
from the rind. No girl would pick her teeth in public,
though custom allowed fashionable European ladies to
do so, nor was it correct to rock on the porch.

Miss Leslie, dictator of fashion on the Delaware,
went on to make life more difficult. She warned against
acquaintances who, by their crass behavior, showed their
lack of breeding. Women with painted faces or white
kid gloves were dangerous. "Such persons," Miss Leslie
warned, "have frequently the assurance to try to be
very sociable with respectable ladies who are travelling
alone. Keep aloof from them always." Ladies of over
thirty-five, who did not wear the elegant but simple
caps appropriate to age, were doubtful too. To the

social arbiter, such figures were "pitiable objects" who "scarcely look respectable." Every man, of course, was dangerous, especially if he prolonged his evening calls beyond a seasonable hour. "If he seems inclined to do so," Miss Leslie warned, "there is nothing amiss in hinting to him that it is past ten o'clock."

"By-the-by," the etiquette dictator added in a postscript, "unless he is a relation, let no young lady address a gentleman by his christian name. It is a familiarity which he will not like."

Men also were circumscribed in action. Cecil Hartley, the Delaware's authority on masculine affairs, surrounded swains with strict restraint. Beginning with his morning ablutions, when, we are told, "a sponge bath can do little harm and almost always some good," the young man walked a straight and narrow path. He should not shave, for "the person who invented razors libelled nature and added a fresh misery to the days of man." Rather should he grow a mustache and a beard, provided only he does not wax the points into needle sharpness. "If a man wear the hair on his face which nature has given him, in the manner that nature distributes it, keeps it clean and prevents its overgrowth, he cannot do wrong."

Coarse flannel next the skin was de rigueur, but rough hairshirts were even better, Hartley preached. They act, he said, "as a shampooer, and with perpetual friction soothe the surface of the skin, and prevent the circulation from being arrested at any one point of the body." Outside shirts were less important, though young men were advised, in case they dressed for dinner, that they should also change their shirts at night.

A hundred rules were laid down for men to follow, many of which are still as applicable as ever in the past. Rule 53, however, is a dandy:

"Never enter a room, in which there are ladies, after smoking, until you have purified both your mouth, teeth, hair, and clothes. If you wish to smoke just before entering a salon, wear an old coat and carefully brush your hair and teeth before resuming your own."

Slang, too, was taboo. Hartley's portrait of a bounder showed a "cove" who wore a "tile" instead of a hat, wrapped a "choker" round his neck in lieu of a proper cloth, and who dressed "like a regular brick." Such a cad, no doubt, might have a pocketful of "tin," of "rhino," or "the ready," and might "hang out" in a respectable home, but polite society would cut him dead. The slang addict was far beyond the social pale.

Society along the river was in process of refinement, thanks to the dozen books on etiquette published in the post-Jacksonian decade, but material conveniences were little changed. City water, for example, was not plentiful. Though Nicholas Roosevelt had contracted, as early as 1804, to supply Philadelphia with abundant water, he had begged to be released from carrying out his pledge. City Councils, learning that Roosevelt had lost nearly $50,000 on a steam-engine project, excused him from fulfilling his water obligations. Until late in the 1850's pumps at street intersections served many families.

When water had to be laboriously lugged in buckets, to be heated in wash boilers on the wood-burning kitchen range, daily bathing was a luxury which few could boast. Saturday night scrubbings, when all the family, beginning with the youngest, took turns in using the same water, were customary functions. Cleanliness was difficult when water was scarce.

High-speed transportation and refrigeration now abolish seasonal limitations, but prior to the Civil War the Delaware was dependent on such foods as it could grow or such as could stand slow freighting. Today's ubiquitous canned commodities were not in common use until the postwar period. Many families, therefore, lived the greater portion of the year on salt meat and cabbage, beans and bread, washed down by the beer for which Philadelphia has been famous since William Penn's arrival. Fresh meat was frequently available, though its appearance, hung on hooks or racks above the pavements with no screens to keep off dust and flies, was scarcely reassuring. Milk was plentiful and cheap, but it was sold from open twenty-gallon cans. Not until the World War had been fought did all river communities require sanitation in such matters.

Gas was coming into common use but whale oil was the usual household illuminant. Cape May and Wilmington sent out their whaling fleets to free themselves from economic dependence on New England, and some of the more daring sailors took the opportunity to sail around the world when they had finished hunting in the South Pacific. Wilmington, indeed, used her whaling fleet as a reformatory agency. Young men who drank too much—and they were regrettably numerous in mid-nineteenth century days—were shanghaied, with the connivance of their parents, for a three years' whaling cruise around the Horn.

Just how the Jefferson Temperance Society of Wilmington got the notion that a whaler was a wholesome, nonalcoholic sanitarium is not entirely clear. Certainly the bucko mates of Sag Harbor ships could have disillusioned the polite and trusting folk who ran the Wilmington establishment. New England knew full well that whalers were sometimes steeped in sin, what with liquor, lovely and loose ladies of the South Sea islands, and all the other illicit joys in which hard-bitten seafolk sought surcease from the perils of the waves. Nor is there information now available to show how well the Delaware roués fared when they arrived at sailors' rendezvous. It is a sociological loss that whaling stopped so soon, for it would be helpful to compare the luck of Wilmington's dry whalers with the success of more normal vessels in the trade.

24

The Battle-Axes

PENNSYLVANIA did not discover love, but it tried hard to make the passion modern. Just a century ago, when all the rest of the United States was sinking into prim Victorian conventionality, ambitious Pennsylvanians experimented with an ultramodern, stream-lined version of companionate marriage.

The story has been secret for almost a century, for Pennsylvanians are modest folk who hate to blow their bugles. When other people burst with pride at their achievements, Pennsylvanians stand quietly aside and make no counterclaim. Salem may get the credit for a witchcraft mania, but there was witch delusion on the Delaware ten years before the Massachusetts madness, and even in enlightened 1940 Philadelphia murderers excused themselves in open court by pleas that they were "hexed." Connecticut may take honors for inventing bundling—that eighteenth century substitute for buggy rides and parking—but Pennsylvanians have long bundled efficiently and well. Nor does Pennsylvania shout its claims for the invention of the steamboat, the telegraph, or the motorcar, though all these first rose along the banks of the Delaware.

Even the latter-day cult of nudism found early devotees along the Delaware. Long before the Revolution, a group called Rogerines, named from their founder, scandalized the populace by running about

naked, and by professing a life of "primitive inno-
cence." An Englishman, traveling near Bristol on the
Delaware, reported that "in this county, they go into
churches and other religious meetings, where they dance
about in an extraordinary manner, Billy to Betty, and
cry out constantly, 'Who can do as we do and yet be
pure and undefiled?'" The Briton assured his friends
that this had happened, but delicately advised a friend
to whom he wrote of the occurrence, "Pray do not read
this to any women."

For these pioneering efforts in the field of invention and social behavior, Pennsylvanians do not bother
to claim special recognition. But as to love the state
cannot keep silent; love is a Pennsylvania patent. While
other states, in the curious decade of the 1840's, were
playing with new varieties of reformed religion, while
there was spiritualistic fervor that took the form of
violent camp meetings, while politics were being revolutionized by the hard-cider barrel, locofocos, and the
agitation for women's rights, the people in the valleys
of the Schuylkill and the Delaware were deeply absorbed in new varieties of love.

Imaginative, restless Theophilus R. Gates, emotionally intense and wrought to frenzy at the fear of spend-
ing his eternities with a scrawny, matter-of-fact wife,
preached a new gospel in the Philadelphia streets. One
might suppose that Philadelphia's strait and narrow
paths were ill-adapted for a shouting, ranting demon-
strator against the bonds of matrimony, but Gates
found willing listeners.

Especially he found pale Hannah Williamson,
high-strung, ill-balanced daughter of joy who hated
men who took their marriage vows too sadly. Hannah
was a fellow stroller of the streets and frequently could
hear Theophilus speak. She hated women too, for

Philadelphia ladies never saw pale Hannah as they passed, and they were spreading hateful gossip about her ways of life. Most of all she hated such females as the tight-lipped Mrs. Gates.

Theophilus, perhaps, was trapped. He knew full well that what the world required was violent religious revolution, tinged with what would now be termed red communism, but poor Theophilus had no designs on making war on marriage as a social institution. In his occasional magazine *Battle-Axe and Weapons of War* he argued for a new religious concept, one that might not bind him forever to his wife, but one which did not preach free love and promiscuity.

Hannah converted him to what she said were more delightful modes of living. The electric little lady aided him in an enrichment of his dogma. The creed of the Battle-Axes gained a new and heady doctrine: marriage was not intended to be permanent.

"Men and women," Gates declared as the result of a divine command, heard from the lips of Hannah, "had better change their partners twenty times over, under the best regulations they can make with each other, so as at length to have one with whom they can live in harmony, unity, and peace." The grammar was not perfect, but Theophilus, infatuated with his Hannah, was more concerned with ideas than with rhetoric. Probably he would have fervently denied that he was smitten, for Theophilus was well convinced that "love is an enchantment of the devil," but he left his wife to go adventuring with the more exciting charmer.

No one knows how Hannah and Theophilus, wandering about the countryside, came to such a hidden nook as Free Love Valley, but, once arrived, they met a friendly welcome. William Stubblebine gave them food and lodging. As they talked together after supper, he listened eagerly to the new doctrines. His vague, blue eyes were fascinated as taut, feverish Hannah told him that marriage need not be permanent. "No two people ought to live together if they cannot live in good-will, peace and comfort with each other. Any promise they have made in their ignorance," she said, "is not binding in justice, equity or common sense." His calloused hands twitched nervously as he watched his wife sit stern and straight, with thin lips tightly pressed together. Six children, long since sent unexpectedly to bed, strained to listen from their room above, but could not understand the quick, excited flow of words. They did not know why Mother cried when William shouted "Hallelujah," nor what was meant when Hannah welcomed their father to the sect.

Magdalena Snyder, twenty years younger than the thin-lipped Mary Ann, heard the stirring message soon. She, too, was much impressed. There were few young men in the valley; none had wooed her. Hannah, an indefatigable missionary, taught the girl that "in a holy community, there is no more reason why sex intercourse should be restrained by law than eating and drinking should be." "There is," urged Hannah, "as little cause for shame in the one case as in the other."

A leading Battle-Axe commandment declared that, if one believer came into a house to demand the person of another, the third, unnecessary, person must give place. Magdalena acted on the knowledge. She walked in the Stubblebine door as the family sat at supper. She asked that William obey the dictate of his conscience. As Hannah and Theophilus looked on approvingly, Stubblebine dismissed his wife and children. They might stay, he said, within the house, but Magdalena was to be spouse. Jacob, the oldest boy, protested, but William's answer was convincing.

"I have no cause to leave my wife," he said, "but the Bible tells me that I must not live with her if I see a woman that I think more of."

Two preachers in the valley failed to find the text on which Battle-Axes based their message, but the deposed Mary Ann was helpless against the combined force of Magdalena, Hannah, William, and Theophilus. Rather than stay with William's new mate, Mary Ann withdrew, taking with her all six children. William, to show that he bore her no ill will, made her a present of all his worldly goods except the house in which he and Magdalena were to live. Not long after, Mary Ann suffered a second disappointment when Jacob, soon after adolescence, embraced the Battle-Axe beliefs. Following the precedent he had seen, he stalked into his old home while Hannah was entertaining her younger sister Lydia and demanded that the slim girl obey the Battle-Axe commands and follow him.

William lived happily with Magdalena. For twenty years they prospered, by Free Love Valley standards. Other converts joined their faith. Each week the growing band, testifying to their steadfastness, walked down to a small pool in the center of the valley. There they disrobed, walked solemnly in single file through the shallow water, turned about, carefully averting their eyes from those who had not yet emerged, returned, and dressed. Nonbelievers were shocked, but when a pastor ventured to protest, he found his Sunday meeting interrupted. Battle-Axes, entering the building while the services were at their height, marched naked up the aisle, straight to the pulpit where the speechless clergyman stood open-mouthed, wheeled about, and silently departed.

Stubblebine died before Magdalena. As legal widow, Mary Ann demanded all his property. Magdalena indignantly protested that William had already given Mary all that she deserved and that his new estate belonged to her. But Mary Ann proved to the courts that she was William's lawful widow and that Magdalena was no legal wife. To add to Magdalena's anguish, Mary Ann arranged that William should be buried in her family's cemetery lot. And as a crowning insult to lonely Magdalena, when Mary died a few months later she was laid to rest beside her errant husband. For almost thirty years Magdalena saw the tombstones of her lover and the woman he had deserted side by side in Free Love Valley's little burial ground. When she, in time, was dead, the unforgiving Stubblebines placed her grave as far as possible from that of William.

Stubblebine hatred for Magdalena lasted long beyond her death. Her tombstone lacks the sculptured roses which local custom grants to every other grave, and the marker has been defaced. After the burial an unknown vandal, entering the tiny cemetery after dark, broke the tablet with a heavy sledge. Battle-Axes, loyal to their leader, mended the stone, but again an enemy destroyed the slab. This time the vandal carried off the upper piece of marble, so that today the grave of Magdalena Snyder, isolated in a corner of the churchyard, bears but a broken monument.

25

When Life Was Cheap

THE old era died in the decades just before the
Civil War. The Industrial Revolution, sweeping into
the valley of the Delaware, and transforming a peaceful
plantation country into what now came to be called the
workshop of the world, brought social evils in its train.
The same sad consequences that everywhere accompanied the coming of early laborsaving machinery disturbed the cities of the Delaware.

Fighting, tight-minded industrialists, struggling
the hard way from small beginnings into mastery of
manufacturing, had not the slightest sympathy for
Quaker gentleness. They viewed the Quaker toleration
as a sign of weakness and saw in Quaker calm only a
confession of defeat. Secure in their belief that the
laissez-faire philosophy of mid-Victorian times, together
with the Quaker quietude, would assure no interference
from the state, they doubled their aggressiveness. Employers whose greed was greater than their social-
mindedness swaggered triumphantly as bosses of the
valley.

Indeed, the placid Friends knew little of what was
really going on. Most of them were removed from
actual participation in the world of industry; few
worked in unsanitary mills; none were sweatshop labor-
ers. No Quaker families had to live in tiny "bandbox"
houses, where a crude ladder was the only means of

climbing from the small one-room lower floor to the single room above. The Friends were wholly unfamiliar with squalid slums where low-paid labor crowded. Therefore such protests as they made were merely academic, and were ignored by the intensely practical men who ruled the rising industries.

English, Welsh, and German labor was less placid; Scotch-Irishmen had lost nothing of their ancient zest for quarrel. When working hours grew and wages fell, these men protested angrily. Poorer sections of the cities seethed with discontent; violent agitation flamed against long working days, against wage cuts, against the vicious practice of keeping small children in the mills for endless hours. Had one dynamic labor leader, capable of recognizing the true cause of this unrest, appeared, the anger would have flared into a bloody social war.

But labor itself misunderstood the reasons for its suffering. Ignorant of economic history, unable to compare its plight with that of workmen of other lands where the Industrial Revolution had caused social dislocation, it sought a scapegoat. Demagogues traced the cause of all the evil to the coming of new immigrants who in race and creed and color were unlike the folk settled in the basin of the Delaware. These, it was said, were transported criminals and paupers, scourings of workhouses, beaten men of beaten peoples, come to take away the jobs of honest Americans. Since many of them came from southern Ireland, and were of the Catholic faith, Philadelphia became vigorously bigoted against the Roman Catholic Church. A growing group of Negroes, freed by their southern masters, had settled in the city and they, too, were singled out for persecution by low-grade whites who hated black competition.

The city government of Philadelphia, where the worst manifestations of mob spirit were arising, was much too weak to put effective brakes on the growing violence. The city had far outgrown the ancient boundaries laid down by William Penn; ugly slums sprawled far beyond the mile-wide area which Penn had set. The administrative frontier, beyond which Philadelphia police could exercise no jurisdiction, ran down the center of a crowded street in the built-up northern section of the city; the adjoining "suburb" of Northern Liberties was wholly indistinguishable from the city proper. On the south side, Moyamensing "suburb," itself a populous community, pressed just as close to Philadelphia. Other independent towns were separated from each other and from the metropolis by nothing more than an imaginary line.

Police were helpless. A fugitive from Philadelphia, escaping to the north side of Callowhill Street, could thumb his nose with impunity at the fuming officer; a Moyamensing culprit, dashing over South Street, found refuge in Philadelphia. Twenty-nine wholly independent cities, districts, boroughs, and townships governed the one region now included in the city of Philadelphia. None of the twenty-nine was rich enough, or strong enough, to guarantee itself a reign of law and order.

The Blood Tubs

Gangsterism wins where legal methods fail. Where legitimate authority is split too many ways, where official red tape tangles law enforcement, the racketeer may profit. In pre-Civil War Philadelphia, when authorized policemen could not keep the peace, lawless

gangsters blustered arrogantly. For more than a generation the calm city of brotherly love was a turbulent
hellhole where arson, riot, and murder were unchecked.

The gangs were petty chiselers whose pickings were
meager, but they insisted on their privileges. Modern
racketeering methods of "protection" or of muscling in
on business were unknown, but gangsters looked to
private citizens to make small contributions to picnic
funds, for "socials," and at stated intervals for promotion of goodwill. Each gang possessed its territory and
at the frontiers of the province chalked its name defi-
antly on the red-brick walls. The sign of Schuylkill
Ranger or Kensington Blood-tub, of Rats or Killers or
Swampoodle Terriers warned rivals against encroach-
ment.

But mere frontier signs were not enough to keep
off bold invaders. A growing gang, made confident
by numbers or past prowess, seeking to acquire new
lands or to annex a district for some ambitious young
lieutenant, might move into another gang's preserves.
Some restless spirits, fired by the fighting fever, might
stir up trouble, after some particularly joyous round of
free lunches at the bars, for pure love of battle. In
such event bricks, stones, and loaded clubs wrought
heavy havoc; brass-knuckled warriors jumped with
spiked boots upon their fallen foes. Gun fighting was
not common; the code of gangsterism much preferred
the hand-to-hand encounter.

Gangsters held a healthy hatred for each other,
but they were at one in their contempt for cops. The
poor policemen armed only with long billies of hardwood—officials were yet loath to arm their men with
pistols—faced a hopeless task in trying to put down
the riots. When wars were raging, a Bouncer or a
Ranger stood sentry to give warning. If officers were

numerous, gangsters hid their weapons quickly; only an unusual throng of peaceful corner loungers slouched idly by the cigar-store corner. But if a lone patrolman strolled by on his rounds, warring gangsters called a truce to pile on the common enemy. A bluecoat would be lucky to escape with any portion of his uniform, for the mob delighted wrenching away his shield or stealing his helmet. One famous gangster-girl, sweetheart of the Schuylkill Rangers, wore with proper pride a necklace of policemen's teeth, knocked out by her adoring swains.

Not all the riots were wars between the gangs. Almost any cause was good enough to stir hot blood into action. Once a restless Southwark crowd, promised the sight of a balloon ascension, got out of hand because the gasbag was not ready soon enough. Breaking through the fence that stood between them and the big balloon, the disappointed spectators ripped the great silk bag to ribbons. Then, rushing to the bar, they broke the bottles, smashed the glassware, stole the money in the till, and finished up the afternoon by tearing down the building. The police force, realizing the hopelessness of interfering, had hastily moved off to patrol the most distant section of their district.

A Moyamensing mob, righteously indignant that reformers had seen fit to start a temperance society, descended on a peaceful meeting, drove off a score of women who had gathered to plead with each other for prohibition, broke all the windows, smashed the doors, threw out and wrecked the furniture, and finally set fire to the ruins. The Moyamensing cops, fewer in numbers than their Southwark colleagues, saw nothing of the riot and, they later swore, had heard no sounds of rioting. Freed Negroes were a special target. Gangsters, cornered by the authorities, invariably insisted that Negroes had begun each riot and that all unfortunate events were due to their instigation. Almost every mob dispute ended in a combined assault on the blacks. This Moyamensing antitemperance riot developed into a race war lasting two days. Not even the sheriff with a sixty-man posse could quell the violence until he called for state troops to haul up enough artillery to command each street in the territory.

Kensington's "Fish-town Blood-tubs" followed the Moyamensing example. Angered because a Negro boy tried to steal a ride on the private Blood-tub merry-go-round, the gangsters marched on the Negro district. The terrified blacks fled into their houses, bolted their doors, slammed the shutters tight, and turned out all their lights. The Blood-tubs came into a peaceful block where not a soul was visible. They dragged logs from a near-by lumber yard, battered down doors, pulled cowering Negroes into the streets, beat them unmercifully, and burned the houses.

Volunteer firemen, rushing to put out the flames, found themselves in a Blood-tub ambush. Volleys of brickbats, torn up from the pavements, kept the firemen at a distance. Hoses were cut; fire carts were overturned. Two battalions of police, headed by the mayor, accomplished nothing, for the brickbat artillery kept them at bay. After two days and nights of constant warfare, the mayor capitulated; the Blood-tubs walked off unmolested on their solemn promise not to repeat the attack.

The truce was short-lived. Some Negroes, escaping from the terror, had huddled in a small frame meetinghouse. The Blood-tubs detoured from their direct homeward course, insisting that the frightened refugees were arming for attack. They ringed themselves about the building, while some of them hurried off to bring up wooden handcarts loaded with oil-soaked kindling to push up to the church walls. Then the building was fired, and Negroes were driven back into the flames until the City Troop, mobilized after too long delay, rescued the survivors. No punishment for these offenses was ever inflicted upon any member of the Blood-tub gang.

Such instances were not isolated cases. Time and time again during the 1830's and 1840's gangsters terrorized the town. Rivalries between volunteer fire companies, disputes over elections, jealousies between races, labor unrest, arguments over spheres of gang influence, all ended in wholesale rioting. Then when the State House bell was rung to call out troops order would be restored, but the troops seldom found rioters to punish, since the clanging of the bell served also as a warning to the gangs.

Indeed, the gangsters moved to take possession of the state militia, the one agency which could suppress mobs. By long-established custom, dating long before the Revolution, militiamen chose their own chiefs. Gangster members of the "Bloody Eighty-fourth" set up their own man, John Pluck, a hostler, as a candidate for colonel and by threatening to beat up anyone who failed to vote for him carried his election. More than ninety per cent of the regiment voted in his favor. The state authorities, however, refused to certify his victory and the city fathers took away the Bloody Eighty-fourth's drill ground because of the "drinking, tippling, cursing, swearing, etc., that went on there day and night." The regiment was never called upon for riot duty during the year of Pluck's disputed colonelcy.

26

Anti-Irish Riots

For a girl to wear a man's silk hat may be aesthetically indefensible, but it is certainly no crime; to teach street kids how to pray should merit a reward. Honora Power thought as much, but she was wrong: her silk hat incited riot and her piety led straight to open war. When gangsters saw her showing little children how to say their rosaries, they smelled a popish plot to turn the Delaware over to the Vatican.

Most of the gangsters were of native American origin and, as such, were highly susceptible to the wave of nationalism that swept the nation in the forties. Convinced that low wages and long hours were entirely due to willingness of Irish immigrants to work for less than good Americans, they heartily approved the resolution adopted in Germantown by the Know-Nothing party, demanding that immigrants be refused the right to vote or even to be naturalized. The mobsters shouted loudly that "bloody Irish transports" hated good free government, and that their Catholic churches were armed forts. In January, 1844, a meeting at the State House warned each patriotic citizen to protect the nation against seditious Irishmen. Nothing, of course, was said about the greater peril from lawless groups masquerading in the guise of superpatriots.

"Crazy Norah" Power, a familiar figure on the streets for almost two decades, was no spy. Her job was bill collecting, a service which she rendered well because delinquent debtors hated to see the queerly clothed, silk-hatted eccentric sitting on their steps. They paid their bills to get her out of sight. But demagogues had bellowed that all the Irish were suspect, even a silly woman at the turn of life who taught the children prayers.

A gangster threw a brick at Crazy Norah, and the poor girl screamed and ran. Hoodlums followed, yelling wildly, and a crowd collected. Excited mobs, not knowing what had happened but seeing only that poor Crazy Norah was hysterical, milled angrily about her, calling her bad names, threatening to do her harm if she persisted in her popish tricks. Then, tiring of the sport, they rushed off to wreck the Irish section, beating back the firemen with brick and stone bombardments. Again militiamen were summoned, but the mob, relying on the friendliness of guardsmen, stood their ground, mocking the commanders and daring the troops to fire.

Six Catholics were caught and murdered, one for the ostensible crime of "looking over a fence"; another, suspected of owning a gun, was dragged out of jail and hanged to a lamppost. Mobs burned the Catholic churches, wrecked parochial schools, destroyed convent hospitals, and put to flight the small-boy inmates of an orphanage. A theological library that contained books not elsewhere to be found in the United States was ransacked; its books were torn apart and burned. Every Catholic church in Philadelphia was attacked.

Amid the wild terrors poor Crazy Norah fled to safety in the Friends' Almshouse, where she remained for nearly twenty years, too frightened to stir out again upon the streets.

Philadelphia went under martial law. A large detachment of marines, landed from the warship *Princeton*, patrolled the streets, cutlasses in hand, accompanied by such militiamen as could be relied upon to stand firm against the gangsters. Ten thousand volunteers, formed into a "peace police," with white muslin badges to identify themselves, kept guard against new outbreaks. The city police, summoning its courage, ventured to arrest several of the chief offenders.

But the grand jury would not find true bills against the rioters, though overwhelming evidence piled up against them. Instead, the jury reported that the men arrested had been the sufferers, for, according to the jury, the Irish had provoked attack by breaking into Native American meetings and firing upon the speakers. The blame for the disturbance, the grand jury solemnly asserted, was due to "lawless, irresponsible men, some of whom had resided in the country only for a short period." Its presentment was a smashing victory for the Native American agitators.

The Irish were dismayed. A fiery young lawyer, William Dunn, expecting new attack, enrolled a hundred and fifty volunteers to protect church property and applied to Governor David Rittenhouse Porter for assistance; he was granted muskets from the state arsenal. His little army then retreated, on the Fourth of July, within the walls of St. Philip de Neri church in Southwark.

Word spread rapidly that the Catholics meant to fight. Mobs gathered round the church; the small police force appealed for aid. The sheriff brought a posse; an army, composed of Washington Blues, Cadwalader Grays, Montgomery Hibernia Greens, two rifle companies, and an artillery detachment armed with field pieces took post to protect the church.

Someone threw a stone at Brigadier General George

Cadwalader and he, jittery and hotheaded, ordered the troops to load their guns. Charles Naylor, former congressman and member of the sheriff's posse, stepped out in front of the field pieces and made a speech urging Cadwalader to hold his fire. Cadwalader, angered at civilian interference, arrested Naylor and sent him prisoner into the church to be guarded by Dunn's volunteers. During the altercation several "Church Burners," scooping water from the gutters and carrying hatfuls of water from the near-by pumps, drenched the priming of the guns and made them useless. Cadwalader, now thoroughly alarmed, withdrew his whole force within the church for safety.

Naylor's arrest infuriated the Know-Nothings. Angry rumors spread that the defender of the people was kept jailed by the Montgomery Hibernia Greens, an Irish Catholic command. The mob, vowing vengeance, pressed close up to the church and dared both Dunn and General Cadwalader to fire. They found two ancient cannon, loaded them with slugs and nails and scrap, and fired on the church. No harm was done to the thick stone walls by the bombardment, so the mob prepared a heavy battering ram and broke through the door. Cadwalader screamed to his troops to fire upon the mob, but the militiamen refused. Then, to restore the peace, Cadwalader delivered Naylor to his friends outside and promised to withdraw the soldiers if the mob would move away.

All went well until the Greens marched out. Then from every angle of the street came a shower of stones. They dove back into the church, but ventured out again under the protection of their fellow soldiers. Brickbats looped over the heads of the escort into the ranks of the Greens. They broke and fled, leaving their protecting riflemen. Several were captured by the

crowd and beaten. None of the escort moved to protect the badgered Irishmen.

Continued clanging of the State House bell called
more militia into action. Marching with fixed bayonets, with flags flying and bands playing, they marched
from Independence Hall to the beleaguered church.
Large crowds, attracted by the unusual spectacle of a
military parade on Sunday afternoon, jammed the narrow sidewalks and pushed into the streets. Thousands
of people pressed upon the troops from flanks and rear;
the soldiers were hopelessly engulfed. A new brickbat
barrage commenced; daring Know-Nothings grappled
with the bewildered soldiers, wrenched away their bayonets, twisted the swords from the hands of officers, and
stole the standards. The soldiers could not get room
enough to level their rifles.

Closer to the church, gunfire was exchanged between the soldiers and civilians. Native Americans
brought cannon, loaded with scrap iron, and fired them
at the advancing reinforcements; the militia, now recovered from confusion, answered with field pieces.
Sharp cannonading lasted through the night until cavalry charges cleared the streets. Many men were killed
and hundreds were seriously wounded. Five thousand
soldiers patrolled the Philadelphia streets for three
weeks after the disturbance had been suppressed.

These Anti-Catholic riots convinced both state and
city that reforms were desperately needed in the scheme
of law enforcement. A thousand uniformed city troopers were assigned to serve the sheriff; police forces were
greatly increased, and officers at last granted permission
to cross local boundary lines. The demonstration that
no single district of the twenty-nine component parts
of Philadelphia County could guarantee the peace

proved ample warrant for a movement to consolidate
the small communities into one major government.
Philadelphia city, in 1854, became coterminous with the
county.

27

The Copperhead Peril

GLOOM lay deep on the Delaware in 1862. Half the population denounced the Civil War as futile, pointing to the utter failure of the Federals to crush down the Confederacy; hundreds of prosperous businessmen, grown rich by trading with the South, regarded Lincoln as a menace; many men demanded that Pennsylvania secede or at least follow the Delaware example and send unofficial delegates to Richmond.

The Pennsylvania Germans were particularly restless. For years they had been stanchly Democratic; their representatives at Harrisburg and Washington had always worked well with the southern statesmen. Now that the dreaded "Brothers' War" was ranging, Confederate agents actively encouraged unrest among the German counties, pointing out that Pennsylvania in the past had not been properly appreciative of the German wishes and that the South was anxious to do full justice to them.

There was much reason for these complaints. For years this large minority of German-speaking people had fought discrimination. State laws ignored their loud demands that German-language schools be founded in the Pennsylvania German counties and that official records be maintained in German and in English. When the state passed laws providing universal public education, these counties rolled up huge majorities against the measure, only to find, when all the votes were counted, that their wishes had been overridden and their children were to be taught a wholly foreign tongue. More than 32,000 Pennsylvania Germans signed petitions for repeal of the compulsory school laws, but the legislature answered only by a scathing and contemptuous rebuke. Court proceedings were unfair, the Pennsylvania Germans said, because all testimony had to be in English, of which the juries in the German counties understood little.

Southern agents fanned the discontent, promising that Pennsylvania Germans would be granted preferred status if they brought the state into the Confederacy. Cleverly they invented a legend—since come to be widely accepted in circles which ought to know better —that German might have been the official language of the nation had not a Pennsylvanian, Speaker Frederick A. Muhlenberg, cast his deciding vote against the plan. Appealing to the Germans' love of freedom, the Southerners insisted that the North had insolently denied the rights that such a large minority had reason to expect.

Even slavery was no stumbling block to sympathy for the Confederacy. Pennsylvania Germans hated slavery, believing it unchristian and immoral, but to abolish slavery, many of them feared, would introduce a race equality in which few of them believed. Though hating southern arrogance, they were in no mood to kill their brothers in a war to free the Negroes, especially under leadership of Republican "radicals." There was a further fear that civil war might mean successful foreign intervention, perhaps a further heavy Irish immigration, quite possibly a clamping down on the state of control by secret orders such as the Masons.

According to the Pennsylvania German press, therefore, the Brothers' War was senseless, inhumane, unnecessary, and absurd. Upcountry editors demanded that the war be stopped, that prompt steps be taken for a peaceful arbitration of the quarrel, and that conscription be abolished. It is a proud feather in the Pennsylvania cap that the authorities allowed such sentiments without attempts to stop the freedom of the press.

Even among Unionists there was discontent, partly because Lincoln had not freed the slaves as soon as war began, more because the local military idol, Philadelphia-born George B. McClellan, had been removed from command. Some complained that the Federals were not aggressive, that Lincoln was too hesitant, and that troops should rush at once to Richmond; others were equally insistent that the northern generals were headstrong and would plunge the country into dire disaster.

Perhaps the key to the confusion lay in the geographic fact that Pennsylvania, Southern Jersey, and Delaware lay on the borderline between North and South. Plantation farming in southeastern Pennsylvania bred a character not too unlike that of the leisured South; people of the Delaware had never been close friends with "eastern states" nor with New York, but had close ties, socially and economically, with those who now were formal enemies. Delawareans and Jerseymen could not be moved by northern propaganda that the South was vicious, corrupt, and treacherous. Yet folk in Jersey, Delaware, and Pennsylvania were no friends of slavery, and they loved the Union. It was extremely difficult to make a final choice, and ofttimes families split badly in deciding, but the weight of popular opinion lay finally on the northern side.

Many, however, feared invasion, anticipating that when gray-clad troops arrived too many waverers would join Lee's men. When he moved up to Gettysburg, southeastern Pennsylvania trembled. Long lines of frightened refugees, driving carts, pushing barrows, or carrying their goods on their backs, crowded the dusty roads, hurrying to safety on the Jersey side of the river. Lancaster Pike was jammed with one-way traffic. Troops ordered west to reinforce the Union army met difficulty in getting through the throngs.

Indeed, the soldiers narrowly escaped attack. Tramping through the dust, the troops found hasty barriers thrown up against them at Paoli Tavern, close by the scene of Wayne's disaster. Few civilian men were visible, though women cowered close to trees and fence posts by the road. The men, they said, had gone away, but they seemed frightened as they spoke and contradicted themselves when cross-questioned closely. Suddenly the truth came out. A frightened horseback rider, catching sight of the advancing soldiers, had rushed back to warn the refugees that the Confederates were approaching from the east as well as from the west. The men had disappeared, to form an ambush for the enemy and to sell their lives as dearly as possible. In the dim light of the early morning the heavy dust had softened Union blue into Confederate butternut uniforms.

Many of the people feared capture. Twelve thousand Confederates, shut up in prison at Fort Delaware, near Salem, were always a potential peril. Three states were terror-stricken lest these captives break from jail and, joining with the northern Copperheads, seize possession of the river and its cities. The *Palmetto Flag,* a Philadelphia newspaper with avowed Confederate leanings, had made veiled threats of such a move. Moreover, many timid citizens were convinced that certain high-placed officers would not shrink from such a step. They remembered the frank statement made by Justice Woodward of the Pennsylvania Supreme Court: "If the

Union is to be divided, I want the line of separation to run north of Pennsylvania."

Had the captives been sturdy, there might have been a basis for the fears, but the Confederates, crowded on a marshy island which would have been too jammed with a third their number, were sick and ineffective. S. Weir Mitchell, then a Union army surgeon, reported that "the living had more life upon them than in them" and that no more than a small handful were active men.

Talk of treason penetrated even into the sacred circles of the Wistar Parties, those famous Philadelphia social gatherings held in memory of the great physician Caspar Wistar. So heated were the arguments at these intellectual groups that, for the first time in their four decades of history, meetings had to be suspended.

Union sympathizers withdrew from Philadelphia's famous social clubs to form their own societies. Led by Judge John Inness Clark Hare and by the sophisticated playwright George H. Boker, the more intense northern partisans formed an antislavery, anti-Confederate group since known as the Union League. It was its aim, as Boker solemnly declared, "to take treason by the throat" and to this day its by-laws contain a provision that no member may ever introduce a traitor within the League's property.

Scores of hickory handles stood inside the doors of the Union League's first clubhouse, ready for use whenever rebels might invade. Meanwhile, pending actual assault upon the Union League, the members subsidized recruiting, organized spy service in the South, assisted in financing the war and in carrying on effective propaganda against southern sympathizers. Other Union Leagues, modeled after that of Philadelphia, were organized in New York, Boston, and Chicago.

After Gettysburg, when fear of the Confederacy

faded, Federal sympathizers turned to less dramatic, but possibly more practical, affairs. Munitions manufacturing, the supply of necessary goods, and the raising of funds for northern hospitals through "Sanitary Fairs" absorbed the energies of folk along the Delaware.

Quite possibly the effects of unrestricted industrial expansion such as that of the Delaware valley in the Civil War era were quite as far-reaching as those of the war itself. Disturbed social conditions, complicated by mechanical revolution, lead inevitably to disorder and unrest. The rise of war profiteering, whether in legitimate business or, as some alleged, through sale of shoddy for good wool and of cheap substitutes for first-class goods, is bound to cause unhappiness.

Wealth came suddenly in the sixties. Northern businessmen, ironmasters, textile manufacturers, munitions makers, coal operators, provision merchants, contractors of a hundred varied sorts, reaped great, and sometimes unexpected, gains. The Delaware, center of the woolen trade and of the heavy industries, prospered through army orders.

War profiteers, with rare exceptions, sprang from a class which hitherto had never been important socially. Some few Philadelphia families, owning ancestral acres in the coal fields, were exceptions; more often, the newly rich were sons of recent immigrant or had themselves arrived but lately. Many of them untrained in ways of wealth, knew no other enjoyment of riches than vulgar ostentation. The lucky millionaires spent lavishly. Jewelers reported that more precious stones were sold in a few war years than in whole preceding generation. Men wore huge diamond waistcoat buttons, heavy rings and sparkling shirt studs women dressed gaudily, wearing long glittering neck laces and having their hair powdered with gold and silver dust.

Society along the Delaware, still true to Quaker principles of simplicity and moderation, was dismayed. Newcomers, powerful in finance, demanded entrance to exclusive functions. Admission to Philadelphia's famous Assembly, traditionally an exclusive ball limited to descendants of those who had founded it two centuries ago, was a prize persistently sought. Membership in the Philadelphia Club, oldest of its kind in the United States, and to the Fishing Company of the State in Schuylkill, a small group of bon vivants, were other important goals. Cruder social climbers, conscious of financial power, used their wealth as levers to buy or force their way into the strongholds of aristocracy. Few were successful, though some, more mighty than the rest or more acceptable, gained the charmed circle. Their descendants are today starchily unbending in defense of conservative traditions.

Rise of a rich new element drove the older fashionable leaders into self-imposed seclusion. Unable to keep pace with elaborate, expensive entertaining, influential families retired from open competition.

28

Mollie Maguires

Red-haired Jim McKenna rubbed his right eye, coughed, and asked the stranger if the night was dark. The man turned quickly, played nervously with his vest lapel, and grumbled that the times must mend. Something in the stranger's tone, perhaps, seemed ominous to Jim McKenna, for he asked softly and politely if the man was angry, and seemed relieved to hear that there was reason for the stranger's temper. John Kehoe, too, felt better, for a smile spread slowly over his broad Irish face; the two or three other miners in the shabby bar seemed to relax a bit.

McKenna sipped his drink a moment wondering, then spoke again inquiring, if he might be so bold, if the new arrival had been brooding on the troubles overseas. For McKenna felt, he said, that peace could not be long delayed now that the Frenchmen and the Spaniards were allied to stand up for the pope.

John Kehoe tightened, as though he did not hold with Red McKenna's politics, and Frank McHugh set down his bottle with such force that everyone in the saloon looked up to see if fights were starting. But the stranger put them at their ease. His mind, he said, was not on Europe, though he was, he hoped, a devout Catholic, but on poor Ireland's difficulties. He'd been thinking that it was a pity that the tenant farmers there could not unite against the landlords and that there never could be any happiness till Gladstone was put down.

McKenna grinned at the answer; Kehoe smiled again. McHugh, who had been glowering, red-faced, and belligerent, poured out a drink and pushed it toward the stranger. The little group of rough coal miners drank to Gladstone's fall. Then, since closing time was drawing near, Kehoe bought another bottle and suggested that they go over to his shack to finish up the whisky. They wandered off, still talking loudly of the Irish troubles.

Once safely out of sight and hearing of the miners left behind, McHugh slapped the stranger on the back. "Who sent you?" he asked quietly.

"I'm Mickey Doyle, from Mt. Laffee; Chris Donnelly, the bodymaster, told me to come here. I've got to talk to Jim McKenna."

Doyle had met the proper people; he had passed the formal tests and made correct responses. McKenna's sign in rubbing the right eye was capped when Mickey fingered his lapel; the curious questions, so foreign to the interests of coal miners of the upper Schuylkill, were challenges to which young Doyle had given the prescribed replies. The group of miners, whom he now knew to be fellow members of the great Irish secret brotherhood, the Mollie Maguires, gave him his instructions.

There is much room for doubt, even at this late date, concerning those instructions. Upstate coal regions, near the headwaters of the Lehigh and the Schuylkill, flamed with angry hatred against the city capitalists who owned the mines and who had given orders for a heavy cut in wages. To thousands of the Irish miners, newcome from overseas, the absentee ownership of coal seemed criminally similar to the absentee landlordism they had known in Ireland. To show their hatred of the system, lawless miners had been wrecking property, murdering the unhappy superintendents who had to do the dirty work for owners whom the miners never saw. Doyle, perhaps, was an imported killer, sent in from a distant mine field by his bodymaster, head of the local units of the Mollie Maguires, to kill unpopular John Jones, a mining boss.

For the state was terror-stricken; depression had hit a smashing blow. Soon after Appomattox, the war boom collapsed; busy mills, dependent wholly on the needs of Union armies, clanged their iron gates shut. Such industries as could survive at all worked half time only. Pay envelopes grew thin and missed a week or two each month. In place of feverish activity came unemployment, poverty, and deep despair. Labor troubles flamed angrily.

The truth is that people lost their nerve. Big businessmen, faced with economic setback, had no guide for conduct. Geared to rising markets, accustomed to prosperity, they stood by helpless when flush times faded. When panic cut the bottom out of business, the economic structure crashed, credit disappeared, and paper dollars lost their buying power. The bosses decreed that wages should be cut, heedless in their terror of the awful consequences to the men who worked for daily pay. Then came the great Long Strike of 1875 that ran for half a year, wrecking the unions and leaving the Mollies as the only force that kept the miners from complete despair.

By their own accounts, the Mollies were a friendly, law-abiding people. Proudly they pointed out that, during the thirty years of their existence, there had been little crime in regions where they had dominated. In eight years there had been no murder, no assault, no felonies of any sort in Schuylkill County, where the band was strongest.

Yet popular report ran differently. Those outside the Mollie ranks declared that the Mollie Maguires ruled the hard-coal counties with a bloody dictatorship, that thirty thousand sworn allies were masters of the state. Judges, sheriffs, and policemen trembled when they heard the war song, a ballad brought from Ireland:

> In Cavan town, where we sat down,
> Our Irish hearts to inspire,
> There's bould recruits, and undaunted yout's,
> An' they're led by Mollie Maguire.

Mickey Doyle appeared just at the moment when the skies were blackest for the Mollies. A dozen foremen had been killed, some in the open sight of hundreds of spectators none of whom had ever seen the murderers before. When Jones was killed, two mornings after Mickey met his fellow Mollies in the tavern, a vigilante group arrested Mickey Doyle, the hard-faced stranger, on the charge of murder.

Jim McKenna, Mickey's friend, was the chief witness against him. Carefully, and by reference to sheaves of voluminous notes, the red-haired Jim gave testimony that Mickey was a gunman and that Kehoe and McHugh were his accomplices in murder.

For Jim McKenna was a labor spy, a Pinkerton detective planted within the Mollie membership to learn their secrets. For three years he had sat, in coarse brown clothes and red yarn comforter, puffing a dirty cutty pipe, listening to Mollie Maguire conspiracies; prodding them to action when they seemed reluctant, but always conveniently ill when there was murder to be done.

No one is proud today of the results that followed.

In no portion of America was the decade following the Civil War an age of glory, but it was surely not in keeping with the great tradition of the Delaware, where tolerance and kindliness had flourished, that agents provocateurs and labor spies should thus find their first important use in labor troubles. Jim Mc-Kenna, who in reality was James McParland, Ulster-born soldier of fortune, pioneered a dirty trade.

McParland gets the glory, but the motivating brain was that of Franklin Gowen, president of the Philadelphia and Reading Railway, who was both financier and lawyer. Gowen was the man who, Mollies said, had decreed wage reductions; he was the big boss of anthracite who had monopolized the mines in order to provide a steady flow of freight for Reading trains; as a former Schuylkill County district attorney he was well acquainted with the Mollie tactics and, according to contemporary testimony, was the man who super-vised the drawing of the jury list which tried the Mollie cases. Gowen steered the Reading into bankruptcy, but his conduct of the murder trials resulted in the death of Mickey Doyle and eleven other Mollies and in the jailing as conspirators of twenty-eight other members of the secret brotherhood. The power of the Mollie Maguires was completely shattered.

Gowen did not live long to celebrate his triumph. Resigning from the Reading after the road had fallen into bankruptcy, Gowen fired a bullet into his head, for reasons no one has satisfactorily explained. Mollie Maguire apologists asserted loudly, without a shadow of authority, that he had been driven by remorse.

The Reading, one should here remark, has not invariably been happy in its leaders. Major George F. Baer, once a successful prosecutor of cases against the road, was taken by the railroad into its own employ and later became president. The little bearded financier, almond-eyed and thin-lipped, a close associate of J. P. Morgan, was the Reading chief at the time of the great mine strike of 1902. He gained a nation-wide attention by declining outside mediation.

"The rights and interests of the laboring man," he was credited with writing, "will be protected and cared for, not by the labor agitators, but by the Christian men to whom God in His infinite wisdom has given the control of the property interests of the country."

As "Divine-Right" Baer, the Reading president was caricatured in thousands of publications throughout the United States. Some contemporary commentators thought that his unfortunate remarks were largely responsible for Theodore Roosevelt's sensational threat to take over the anthracite mines as a national duty if the operators and the men did not immediately come to terms.

29

The Gang's All Here

THE Prophet Nehemiah was a war horse of reform. Last of the Romans, a political descendant of Gaius Gracchus, his white beard waved, like the plumes of Henry of Navarre, in the forefront of every battle. He was Patrick Henry in his oratory, Lincoln in his zeal for equality of man, a Lee in leadership.

Those metaphors are mixed designedly, for they all refer to the same hero, uncompromising Rudolph Blankenburg, leader during forty years for civic betterment. Invariably a lone dissenter, sneered at for futility, hated for his reforming zeal, yet always feared by those he termed "the powers that prey," he emerged as victor in his final struggle. And this, too, was typical, for Rudolph Blankenburg was all his life a living paradox.

Stanchly Republican in politics, he fought a constant bitter battle against the leaders of his party; in the most American of all the major cities he was a German immigrant; a wealthy man, he championed consistently the underdog; a hardheaded, practical man of business, he came to the United States on a Quixotic mission to free the Negroes from the servitude of which he'd read in *Uncle Tom's Cabin;* an intense believer in individualism, he organized the greatest movements for community co-operation ever seen in the history of public charity. Political and banking leaders used to answer pleas for contributions to relieve the sufferers of the Johnstown flood, the Russian famines, and the Charlestown earthquake by the promise "I will contribute if you will join me in a movement to suppress that interminable, pestiferous nuisance, Rudolph Blankenburg," but they liked the man for his after-dinner wit, his cheerfulness, his joking, and his zest for life. He was no long-nosed Puritan.

Blankenburg found a region steeped in graft and crooked politics, dominated by a group of professionally friendly politicians who proudly called themselves the "Gang." Cynical, unprincipled, boldly unscrupulous, the little leaders who ruled wards as their private satrapies took dirty money from petty grafts and from the keepers of brothels, gambling dives, and cheap saloons. The more important leaders blackmailed public utilities into giving campaign contributions under threat of hampering regulations, assessed public employees a portion of their pay, took cuts from favored contractors, and some accepted open bribes. From the time of Jim McManes, boss of the Gas House Ring in 1880, down to contemporary times Philadelphia has seldom been free of political bondage; other sections of the river valley have been almost as subservient to party bosses.

The so-called "better classes" had long since retreated from the field. Conservative aristocrats, feeling slight sympathy for the uncouth immigrants flooding in from Europe, fled from the arena; new-rich millionaires looked upon the foreigners as merely raw material for industry. John Christian Bullitt, coming from Kentucky and thus ignorant of local proprieties, might be concerned with making better city charters; a Biddle or two, belonging to a rebellious clan that felt itself above mere hampering conventionalities, might take a fleeting interest in civic matters, but the rest of the well-born stood contemptuously aloof. Blankenburg plunged deep into the midst of practical politics.

There was much for him to do. Jim McManes, once a boy worker in the cotton mills, had modernized the well-tried principles of Tom McKean. Brooking no argument, accepting no advice, the fighting Ulsterman dominated Philadelphia as his own. The great historian, Henry C. Lea, seeking a fit word to call the master, found no better name than "boss." Wherever in America political autocracy has spread, the title "boss" has stuck to the leader of the machine.

McManes maced the streetcar companies, the gasworks, and the railroads, demanding that they swell his war chest and hire their unskilled labor through the Gang's ward leaders. In this way he gained financial backing and added to the patronage that his "band of brothers" needed and clamped his hold on the city. Reformers voiced a meek protest, but McManes handled them with skill. To some he gave good jobs, thus silencing their cries; others he "framed" by catching them in compromising circumstances; still others he ignored or made ridiculous.

But Blankenburg was proof against such methods. The lithe, active German, devoutly Quaker in belief, was free from thought of sin and, comfortably rich by clever trading, was unbribable. Cartoonists lampooned him, making fun of his squat figure and of the bushy beard that framed the bullethead above the sturdy shoulders, but Blankenburg was undismayed. He carried war into the McManes camp, went eagerly on the stump, and acted out dramatic scenes in which he carried on imaginary conversations between Gang leaders. The public was convulsed with laughter, but the Gang was much too well entrenched to be defeated by such measures.

For greedy Gangsters the period was rich with opportunity. Peter A. B. Widener, investing his profits from Civil War meat contracts in street railway transportation, needed political assistance and was generous to those who served him well. Bill Elkins, an early partner in Standard Oil, land speculator and a pioneer in gas, joined ruthless Thomas Dolan in taking over a monopoly of city lighting. Their United Gas Improvement Company—invariably known as the UGI—proved properly appreciative of those who did it favors. Blankenburg and others shouted that the Gang was grafting and that McManes and his band of brothers were receiving bribes, and proof of certain nasty deals seemed past all doubt, but the traction people and the gas crowd had their way.

The Greeks came bearing gifts to Blankenburg. Matthew Stanley Quay, state boss and sly manipulator, made oily overtures, promising to help Blankenburg defeat the Gas House Ring if, in return, the war horse would lend a helping hand to Quay. It was, perhaps, the only time that Blankenburg had offers of assistance from a politician, but the German was not seduced. He knew that Quay was gunning for the Philadelphia graft and that the squint-eyed, semi-Indian state boss was hoping for election to the Senate. He turned down Quay's offer and saw his suspicion verified when Quay joined up with disgruntled Gang ward leaders in a so-called "Hog Combine" that toppled Jim McManes from his throne. Quay, proudly calling himself the "Republican Tilden," aimed thereafter at the presidential nomination of his party. A noisy group of hard-palmed claquers applauded lustily when Pennsylvania offered Matt Quay's name to the 1896 convention.

Then new leaders, largely contractors, came into control. By Pennsylvania practice, cities cleaned their streets, removed their ashes, and disposed of garbage by letting bids. A new triumvirate gloried in its opportunity. An ex-police magistrate, a favored public contractor, and a former saloonkeeper, banding together, distributed the contract plums in Philadelphia.

Jim McNichol built a boulevard from northeast Philadelphia to the county line, a splendid avenue that turned at times to run through land on which politicians held options; he built gigantic filtration plants that netted millions in profit. The cold-blooded Vare brothers of South Philadelphia, even in the early days eying eagerly the chances of becoming the supreme masters of the town, took double pay for hauling garbage and ashes from the streets and for dumping those same ashes on the marshes by the river. Asphalt magnates and oil companies shared the spoils that came from contracts.

Blankenburg was helpless to prevent the looting. The Gang controlled the mayor, owned ninety per cent of the City Council membership, bossed the police, managed all but three magistrates, and even, through the local school boards, ran the schools. The only thing he could do to halt the contract scandals was to carry on intensive public agitation.

The Old Warhorse of Reform was a spectacular campaigner. Each year, a week or so before election, Blankenburg was certain to spring a new sensation, buttressed with affidavits and so timed that it was difficult to draw up a convincing answer. One year he clamored violently against a mayor who had sold out to the Gang, after having been elected with reform support; at another time, he brought up detailed proof that the state was paying $545 each for desks and that public buildings supposedly trimmed with good mahogany were tricked out in painted putty. He made

detailed charges that the new state capitol was a graft-
ers' paradise where more than half the thirteen million
dollars spent had been stolen from the treasury.   At
yet another time he called the roll of those unfortunates
whom the Gang had driven into suicide or who had gone
to prison for their crimes.

His crowning achievement, however, was his capture of a regular Republican meeting, where Gang candidates were gathered to assert their confidence in the
party leadership.   It was an exploit which for strategy
and efficient planning has seldom seen its match, and
it was particularly effective because everything had been
cut and dried for an old-fashioned Gang jubilation.

Never in its history had so many Philadelphians
turned out at a mass meeting.   Long before the speeches
were to start, the hall was packed with men; ten thousand others, unable to jam themselves into the audi-
torium, blocked traffic in the streets.   It was a cheering
sight for politicians, particularly in this crucial 1905
campaign when reformers were insisting that the Gang
was on the run.

A strange crowd, too, some thought, for caps were
rare and derby hats, the hallmark of professionals, were
missing.   Few smoked cigars and none were chewing
gum; there was no whispering from the corner of the
mouth as men sat waiting for the speeches to begin.
The crowd lacked all the features of a conventional
mass meeting in election time, but that was all the more
assuring, so the leaders thought, for it meant that the
silent vote, the unpredictables, had been won over to
the Gang.

Happily the chairman banged his gavel, calling for
the invocation; then, when all had listened reverently,
he invited them to join in singing "My Country, 'Tis
of Thee," the anthem which, by old tradition, starts off

every rally. They sang it well, too well perhaps, for there was vibrancy and spirit in the music, not at all in keeping with the perfunctory noises usually heard at politicians' gatherings. The men were singing with devotion, as though it were a hymn. The chairman, vaguely worried because things were moving much too smoothly, turned to introduce his speaker, first of the three hand-picked candidates whom the bosses had selected.

"Yea, City Party," roared a voice and from a thousand others came a yell. Blue and gold City Party badges jumped from a thousand pockets to brighten coat lapels. "We want Blankenburg," another shouted. Rhythmically the audience fell into a chant, "We want Rudy . . . We want Rudy . . . We want Rudy . . ."

The Gang chairman was aghast. Nothing like this had ever been heard before; his meeting was entirely out of hand. He pounded angrily with his gavel, so hard that the handle snapped; he waved his hands, shouting for silence in a voice that could not reach the middle of the hall. City Party workers, handling the crowd with the efficiency of college cheerleaders, kept the chant alive. A stocky, white-bearded German jumped onto the stage. It was Rudolph Blankenburg, inventor of the plot to pack the meeting with church-member sympathizers.

The three Gang candidates were prisoners, and their helpless chairman, flanked now by stalwart City Party men, was nothing but a silent witness. Blankenburg held up his hand for quiet; when the chant subsided, he told the meeting that the time had come to put the question straight to the candidates whether they were honest men or tools of the Machine.

"Personally you are very likable fellows," Blankenburg continued, speaking to the captured candidates, "but politically you represent a system that I think damnable. Under this boss rule, everyone connected with this city government is a slave, no matter whether he is mayor or whether he holds the smallest, worst paid city post. Are you going to be free if you are chosen to your office? Will you give us a city clean, a city honest, a city healthful, a city moral and a city orderly? We have been governed by a generation of misrule, alternately corrupt and incompetent, sometimes both. Do you have the vision of clean, pure, honest government, and will you work to make that vision into fact?"

The candidates were stunned. At any other time they might have risen to their feet to talk in platitudes and to assure the voters of their zeal for public service. But Blankenburg had, just a week or two before, caught one of their own leaders in a most unfortunate remark, when the leader, thinking he was wholly among friends, had tried to be facetious and said that he was sick of talk of civic righteousness. Blankenburg's newspaper had been hammering every day, in small cartoons on each page of the paper, against the Gang flag of the Jolly Roger which was lettered with the politician's unfelicitous remark. The candidates were only too aware that they must be specific in their statements.

Seldom have politicians been at such a disadvantage. Blankenburg fired point-blank questions, asking them about the six million dollars graft in a filtration plant; he asked about the fraud in Philadelphia's smallpox hospital affair where patients had been killed by inefficiency of care; he probed their knowledge of stuffed ballot boxes and of bribery, of crooked district attorneys and of straw-bail cases; he wanted to know their views about padded payrolls and concerning violent assaults by Gang politicians against reformers; and then, when they had weakly cut themselves away from

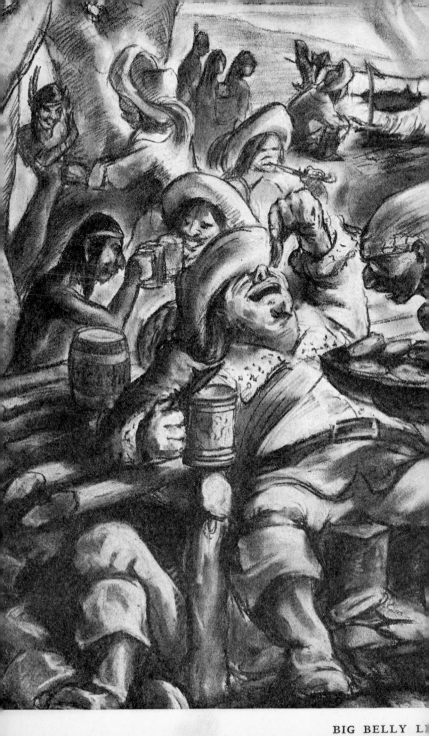

BIG BELLY LI

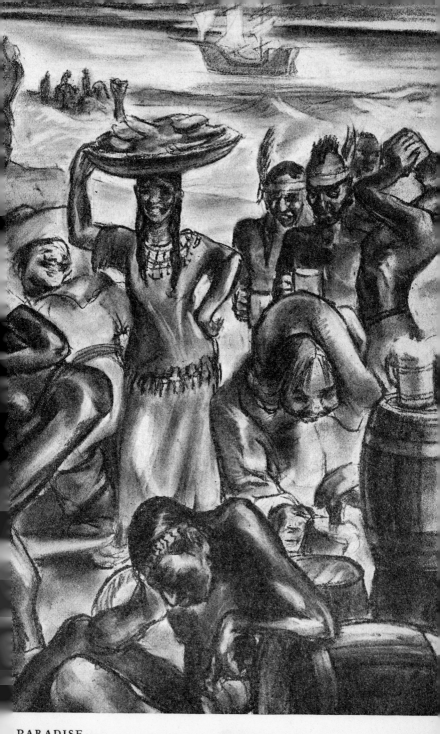

PARADISE

Gang support by denying their own leaders, Blankenburg opened fire on them for their own offenses.

"You have called me, in your public speeches, a Russian Jew, and you have also said that I am anti-Semite; you say that I am drunk each night and that I am a prohibitionist; you say I am self-seeking. Why have you spoken lies like these about myself and all my fellow reform leaders?"

It was a hopeless rout, and the reform newspapers made startling headlines of the meeting. Gang journals had no mention of the affair. It is a sad commentary on the voters of the city that the election, two weeks later, triumphantly returned the Gang to power.

The band of brothers rolled in wealth. Allies in city offices drew specifications in such fashion that favored contractors were sure to win; they slipped to politicians advance information concerning rival bids. Blankenburg exposed the practices, but the public paid no heed; he demanded that Gang-appointed inspectors be more zealous in their duties, but found no popular support even when he showed that the public paid for marble buildings but got cement instead. He fought a lone game, for the Gang bought off his associates by jobs and cash. The three Vare brothers, George, Ed, and Bill, made fortunes in garbage contracts; "Strawberry Jim" McNichol, who specialized in paving and street cleaning, built up a large-sized fortune; Iz Durham, the "peerless leader," lived in luxury on his profits.

All worked in close co-operation. When John Wanamaker, temporarily allied with Blankenburg, offered to give Philadelphia a million dollars for the right to run streetcars, the politicians stood firm to give the exclusive rights away for nothing to their Philadelphia Rapid Transit Company friends and, to prevent all future competition, made the franchise run for nine hundred and ninety-nine years. The Widener-Elkins-Dolan group, together with Charles T. Yerkes, whose career is thinly disguised in Theodore Dreiser's trilogy, found the politicians extremely helpful. When UGI wanted to reduce the yearly rental it was paying to the city the Gang whipped its henchmen into line to rush the revision through the Councils.

Blankenburg roared a protest and this time, favored by a split within Gang ranks, he finally aroused popular opinion. An outraged mob marched on City Hall, armed with ropes, threatening to hang to the nearest lamppost anyone who voted for revision. A reform party leaped into existence, elected a reform mayor, chose Blankenburg as county commissioner, and caused the scheme to be sidetracked. But, after clamor died away, the bill was quietly put through the Councils. The Gang emerged as strong as ever.

As county commissioner, Blankenburg pried deep into the secrets of the Gang. He found that ballot-box stuffing had been developed to a science, that groups of "repeaters" moved from ward to ward "voting the tombstones," casting ballots in the names of honest citizens who were late in coming to the polls, "voting the pet cats and dogs." Blankenburg revealed more than a hundred thousand false names on the registration lists, but when he tried to get allies to help him create a new party of reformers, his friends too often turned out to be self-seekers, false helpers, or venal timeservers acting in the interest of the Gang. Against his will, for there was literally no one else to do the job, Blankenburg was compelled to run for mayor.

He was elected in 1911. Gang-ruled councilmen blocked his efforts at reform and, though Old Dutch Cleanser made some healthful innovations, particularly in the conduct of the public works department under

Morris Llewellyn Cooke and in purifying the police department, the Blankenburg mayoralty fell short of expectation. At the end of his term Philadelphia slipped back into its comfortable delinquency for, happily for the Gang, the constitution of the state forbids a mayor to succeed himself. The bosses were again triumphant.

Of all the bosses, Boies Penrose was unquestionably the most dramatic and colorful. One of the few Pennsylvania blue bloods to mix in politics, he frankly disdained the masses and the leaders whom they tolerated. Clever and quick-minded, a master of popular psychology, he thoroughly enjoyed the sport of running intellectual rings around his slower-witted foes. Devastatingly honest in his cynicism, he scorned pretense and abhorred shams; he despised the stuffed shirts of society and, though he could converse on terms of ease with intellectuals, he openly preferred the company of coarser, more earthy people. Brought up to salons and parlors, he enjoyed saloons and was not above a hearty interest in brothels; he gloried in shocking the gentlemanly set and, on summer trips in his yacht *Betty*, he liked to stand naked on the deck in full sight of fashionable beaches.

Pennsylvania did not love him, nor did its voters choose him for his statesmanship. Penrose bulled his way into importance, using every method known to machine politicians. Not suave and sly like his first patron, Matthew Stanley Quay, not hypocritical like some of the alleged reformers with whom Blankenburg tried to work, not coldly heartless like the Vares, Penrose won mastery by his money, his intelligence, and his political craft.

Penrose scorned the petty grafts. Knowing that the business leaders worshiped the protective tariff, Penrose made himself the tariff spokesman. His spellbinders talked of nothing else, warning that low duties were synonymous with free trade and that free trade inevitably meant soup kitchens for the workingman. Few voters understood the economic argument, but the speeches sounded well and business leaders underscored the fears by promising that, if ever Democrats should win, the mills and factories would shut their doors. In return for this support, and for the campaign contributions which the manufacturers chipped in, Penrose guaranteed that there would be no hostile legislation.

That Gang rule was inefficient and corrupt, that political offices were overstaffed with useless "drones" whose sole function was to roll up Gang majorities, and that Pennsylvania lagged in social legislation were minor prices to be paid for guarantees that tariffs would stay high. Both state and cities were, in Lincoln Steffens's words, "corrupt and contented"; citizens cared not that Elihu Root had called the dominant party "a corrupt and criminal organization masquerading under the name of Republican."

Not until long after the World War was it fashionable to profess other than standpat Republican ideas. On each election night, while party leaders feasted at the Union League, organization henchmen marched downtown, transparent banners boasting the size of the majority rolled up by their wards, singing "Hail, hail, the Gang's all here; what the hell do we care?" Probably no other politicians in the world have ever strode forward to a Gilbert and Sullivan tune, and it is worthy of note that this one was borrowed from a most appropriate source, *The Pirates of Penzance*. On the roof of Republican headquarters a cannon boomed triumphant salutes to Penrose and his Gang.

30

The Bosses Strut

Pennsylvania's neighbors could point no finger of shame at its thralldom. Its fellow states were equally subjected. New Jersey had no freedom. For years the state was so controlled that it was dubbed the State of the Camden and Amboy Railroad.

Indeed, the Jerseymen were proud to be politically the railroad's private property. The corporation was a Jersey enterprise, manned by Jerseymen, financed by Jersey capital, operating for promotion of New Jersey interests. It seemed but natural that, to guarantee the welfare of the line, no candidate should dare to run for office without the railroad's open approval. An independent who aspired to be governor, or even to go to Trenton as a legislator, seemed a traitor to his state. A politician who might venture to suggest a bill for legislative passage knew that he had no hope of victory if the Camden and Amboy turned thumbs down on it. It was a stunning blow to Jersey pride when, without a moment's advance warning, the Camden and Amboy owners sold their railway to the alien Pennsylvania Railroad.

Sale of the Amboy to "foreigners" led to violent conflicts in the capitol at Trenton. "Reformers," pledged to force the railroad to pay its proper share of taxes, were chosen by several of the counties; a slight majority of legislators were, however, loyal to the company. When the antirailway men arrived to take their seats, Amboy partisans refused to let them enter on their duties. Locking themselves behind barricaded doors, corporation agents assumed political control. Reformers, climbing into the Senate chamber through the windows, fought fist-fights with railway men on the Senate floor. When their right to take part in lawmaking was eventually recognized, the reformers tried to name an antirailway man as New Jersey's United States senator, but the angry Amboy men nominated and elected a railroad superintendent to that office.

A second lockout, a few years later, created a situation in which New Jersey had two bodies, each claiming to be the rightful Senate. One group was recognized by the Assembly, but repudiated by the governor; a second, accepted by the governor, was turned down by the lower house. The antigovernor and antirailroad faction stormed the Senate chamber in the night. They burst open a light door leading to the gallery; a more agile statesman jumped from the gallery balustrade to a gas fixture, and swung himself to the floor. Quickly unlocking the doors, he let his colleagues into the chamber, where they held a midnight session. The governor called out the militia to expel them from the room. Eventually, when the case was taken into court, the raiding party won the right to take their seats.

Race-track gambling introduced new complications into Jersey politics. A Philadelphia bartender, William J. Thompson, keen, shrewd, with mustache and beard like Napoleon III, took over a tract of water front at Gloucester, just across the Delaware from Philadelphia, near the old Dutch fort. The so-called "Duke of Gloucester" started a wide-open town, where liquor, vice, and gambling were unchecked. Similar communities were established near New York and on the seashore.

Gloucester and the other race-track towns were not easily reformed. Swarms of illegal voters crossed the river on election day to help pile up tremendous machine majorities; on several occasions, when the polls opened, citizens found the boxes already stuffed with votes. Arrests were futile, for the gamblers owned the government. Police were hesitant to make arrests; when proved "floaters" or ballot-box stuffers were taken before magistrates, the latter freed the prisoners, often severely reprimanding the policeman for unnecessary arrests. In the rare event that a culprit was convicted, a venal pardon board canceled the sentence and set the floater free. And as a final recourse, if by any remarkable chance reformers cast more votes than the machine deposited, corrupt election officers could be relied upon to "count out" the antiorganization candidate.

The Duke of Gloucester and his fellows then looked about for wider fields. Thompson had himself elected to the legislature; other gamblers went to Trenton as lawmakers from their districts. The Gloucester race-track starter was named speaker of the House; through his biased rulings, no opposition member was allowed to take the floor. State laws were passed, giving to every town the right to set up race tracks and to license gambling houses; though the governor vetoed the measures, at the behest, according to the race-track speaker, of "old women and dominies," they were repassed over the veto.

These were the legislatures which made New Jersey a haven for corporations. During the time when small business was being integrated into large monopolies, some states endeavored to restrict the growth of trusts. New Jersey, seeking revenue that would come from corporation fees, welcomed the monopolies. If, the Jersey laws provided, a company would keep a representative in the state and pay the tiny fees demanded, all business might be transacted elsewhere. Attorneys in Trenton, Camden, and other Jersey towns fastened long notice boards to their office walls announcing that they were the "head officer" of a score or more corporations. The plan worked well until Delaware bid for corporation business by requiring even less than Jersey and by setting lower fees.

Corruption was open and unchecked. Elections for United States senatorships, then chosen by joint ballot of both legislative branches, went regularly to the highest bidder. Pennsylvania was particularly flagrant; in 1897, the machine, forthright and cynical, dumped a quarter of a million dollars cash into the pockets of legislators to bribe them away from their support of John Wanamaker, the Philadelphia merchant.

Delaware, however, was the scene of the most spectacular attempts to buy elections. For seventeen years John Edward Addicks, copper promoter, speculator, and "Napoleon of Gas," poured money into politics. Learning that by Delaware law no delinquent taxpayer had the right to vote, he built up a following by paying the back taxes of hundreds of citizens. On election day his agents manned the polls, handing out two-dollar bills to any voters who would promise to support an Addick's candidate. Anti-Addicks legislators were offered unlimited drawing accounts if they would shift to his support.

Addicks was not able to buy the state, though he spent upward of three million dollars in the effort. He did, however, prevent the election of a rival. During two complete Congressional sessions, Delaware had but one senator, since Addicks, unable to win the election, refused to permit another candidate to win; in one Congress, from 1903 to 1905, Delaware had no senators whatever at Washington. Financial reverses, caused by the collapse of copper prices, destroyed the Addicks fortune and caused him to withdraw from competition.

Overt bribery of legislators has nothing commendable to offer, but crude corruption served one useful purpose. Delaware had developed a habit of choosing senators for family reasons rather than for statesmanship; senatorial dynasties were being established. In Pennsylvania, Simon Cameron served three terms as senator and handed his toga to his son, James Donald Cameron, who stayed in office twenty years. Matthew Quay virtually threw the nomination to Penrose. New Jersey chose three generations of Frelinghuysens for the senatorship; Delaware sent four Bayards to Washington for a total of forty-five years' service and three Saulsburys whose combined terms covered fifty-eight years. For eighteen years two Saulsbury brothers sat together as the senators from Delaware. Nearly all these men, it must be admitted, were excellent administrators; some were brilliant, but the hereditary principle seemed in contravention of democracy. Vote buying, never defensible, elected fewer good men, but it did destroy the dynasties.

31

Custom Is King

TRADITION rules the river. Old customs, ancient habits, well-tried folkways are preferred. Small stores, not yet absorbed into all-conquering chains, throw in the thirteenth bun for steady customers who buy a dozen; tradesmen, totting up a bill that totals a few cents above the even dollar, knock off the extra pennies, but expect that customers draw checks that are as generous when bills run high into the nineties. Music lovers mightily resent suggestions that a cleanup program rid the old Academy of Music of the famous bat that, once or twice a season, throws the opera or the Philadelphia Orchestra into mild confusion. Such things have always had their place along the Delaware River.

For, though the business enterprises of the stream have changed, the people are not different. They still prefer their Sunday dinner in the middle of the day; they still, with quiet superiority, refer to "the university" as though Pennsylvania were the only institution of its rank; they still go forth in spring to seek arbutus on the wooded hills of Wissahickon as in the days when that fragrant early blossom was as plentiful as buttercups. Candid and outspoken, sublimely certain of their well-established social position, the folk along the Delaware seem often not to know that times have changed and that the river is no longer the one great waterway that leads from rural America to the foreigners beyond.

Convention is king in staider social circles. No institution that was ever valuable is allowed to wither on the vine. Associations for the catching of horse thieves, once essential in the slow days of the eighteenth century, meet solemnly each spring to reassure themselves that they are still alive, though none of the wide-waisted members has moved to snare a thief in nearly half a century. Ceremoniously the president of the Historical Society of Pennsylvania dons the sacred ring that contains a hair of William Penn as a symbol that the founder is still present, in substance as well as spiritually. Carefully the city fathers refrain from trespassing upon the tiny tract of ground that Penn set apart in central Philadelphia as a camping place for Indians. With heavy ritual convivial members of the Clover Club rise cumbrously to sing the famous "Darby Ram," and former students of the Academy of Fine Arts romp through the rowdy old Academy Fling.

University of Pennsylvania men rise loyally to wave their hats in unison while their band plays "The Red and Blue"; Bryn Mawr girls wake early in the morning of May Day, once each four years, to play medieval English morality dramas on the college lawn; Princeton lads in white beer suits stage deadly strife each decade against the eating clubs which disturb the true foundations of their democracy.

Such observances are required by ancient custom, as are snapper soup on Thursday evening, fish and chips on Friday, salt mackerel for Sunday morning breakfast and British kippers on ordinary days. They must not be disturbed, lest the social heavens fall. The socially correct are as hidebound in such matters as are the poor unfortunates of Lombard Street who put their trust in "Hy John" houses where voodoo doctors treat the ailing poor with rattlesnake concoctions and tinctures of white mice and herbs.

Nowhere is conservatism more pronounced than in the kitchen, where Delaware delicacies are unsurpassed. Succulent diamond-back terrapin, stewed with sherry or Madeira, planked shad, dainty grilled reedbirds, fresh shot in the marshes of the river, fiery pepper-pot soup, well cooked with tripe, and rich oyster stews, complete with hard-water Trenton crackers and with pepper hash, are the closest earthly equivalent of ambrosia. But they must be made in close conformity to ancient custom; the recipes must not be varied. Etiquette is strict about such matters, and the host who tries a new invention of his own gets talked about in a fashion that can never be lived down.

So, too, is rich, wholesome ice cream, smooth and soft and irresistibly enticing, a dainty to be tasted for its own seductive self. No well-brought-up Philadelphian would insult it with a chocolate smothering, with chopped nut garnishing, with a syrupy flavor. Those poor unfortunates who know it only as a factory product, made by commercial formula, have tasted hokey-pokey, not the true ice cream from Philadelphia freezers.

Cinnamon bun, made by little German bakers in out-of-the-way establishments, merits medals for its delicacy if made with spice and sugar, with wholesome butter and molasses, not too sticky, and free from nuts and raisins. Delaware valley bakeries sell jelly-roll, rich and satisfying pies, mince and honest pumpkin, with none of your sweet potato or squash mixture, deep-dish apple pie, served with thick slabs of York State cheese, and cheesecake too, a happy, charming food if properly prepared but sad, indeed, if not made by the proper recipes.

More difficult to come upon, but worthy of the search, is beaten biscuit, made of dough laboriously hammered with an ax on a chopping block until the proper blisters are created, but these round dainties must be eaten fresh and hot, for, once cooled, the biscuit is too floury and hard. Marylanders from the Eastern Shore are adept at making beaten biscuit, just as well-made fruitcake, rich and heavy, kept fresh by careful wrappings and by wine libations through the winter, is the pride of Delaware. A proper hostess brings out the fruitcake on state occasions, served paper-thin on the finest of porcelain.

Pennsylvania Germans also boast their specialties, though few of them are dainty. Spicy scrapple, made of odds and ends of pork, with corn meal and fragrant herbs, was once a special dish for slaughtertime in late November, but it is today a year-round dish, supplanting in many homes the salt mackerel and waffles which were once the Sunday breakfasts. Corn-meal mush, fried in thin slices and served with blackstrap molasses, wins no culinary prizes but is a stand-by for thousands. The Pennsylvania Germans can work miracles with pork and beef; their pies are famous.

Farther down the Delaware, particularly on the New Jersey shore, come oyster pies, baked with a quarter pound of butter and a pint of whole, rich milk, boiled tripe with oysters, and a savory composed of oysters, mushrooms, and Madeira that is worth a trip across a continent. On the west shore of the river, in Sussex, fried chicken, cooked without an armor plate of batter, is as irresistible as the appetizing fried peach, cooked in butter, of the whole roast suckling pig, served with an apple in its mouth. Folk along the Delaware know how to eat.

They drink well too. Small children sip rich raspberry vinegar, made of apple cider that has stood all night on ripe, sugared berries, or root beer which, invented by a Salemite, has spread throughout a nation, but in manhood they graduate to nobler beverages. Outside the ranks of New Orleans magicians, no one has ever matched the famous Fish House punch of Philadelphia, an insidious, authoritative drink, built on a brandy base, but with so many grand ingredients blended so expertly that the drinker cannot possibly identify the formula. This, and the smooth, deceptive eggnog, of milk and spice and egg and rum, traditionally served at New Year's and Easter, are masterpieces of bartending art.

Yet folk along the Delaware do not claim preeminence as a culinary center; instead, in this, as in all other forms of culture, the valley people deprecate their merits. Modestly they give credit to their rivals in more pushing sections, but themselves stay sedulously in retirement. People of the Delaware seem often, therefore, to be stricken with nostalgia, to look backward toward a golden age long distant, they seem defensive.

The trait is deep-rooted on the Delaware. None of the great local universities offer courses in the history of the river; the schools pay slight attention to the great events that have occurred in Delaware, in Pennsylvania, or in New Jersey. High school curricula ignore the story of the local past: the books give only a brief nod to Washington's crossing of the Delaware, ignore Brandywine and even Valley Forge; no author of a text used in the schools gives even a line to the Paoli Massacre, or mentions Rodney's Ride. Heroes of other sections receive warm welcome in school and college teaching, but the local lads who built the nation are forgotten. To hear the people talk, you might think they hated their homeland, that, in the words of one disappointed New York editor, Philadelphia really is the city of brotherly hate.

This does not mean that towns along the Delaware lack pride; it only testifies to the retiring spirit of the people. Each individual settlement along the river prides itself on its uniqueness and calmly knows its own achievements, but in a gentle, unobtrusive way that is quite free from brashness or from boasting. Salem and New Castle, for example, each considers that it is the only true repository of the authentic colonial spirit and each disdains the other's claim. Philadelphia and Camden, separated only by the river, look scornfully across the stream and each wonders how the other can be happy in its sordidness.

Strangers newly come into the valley find themselves baffled by what seems a stiff aloofness; they cannot understand the Delaware's reluctance to experiment. A new idea finds slow acceptance, for, according to the sages of the Delaware, "the plan might work in other places, where conditions are entirely different, but circumstances are peculiar here. What goes in Boston or New York would never be accepted by our people." But it would be wrong to think this attitude a blind conservatism.

To speak of cities in the valley of the Delaware is, after all, something of a misnomer. A city is an integrated unit, having a common spirit and communal pride, boasting a special individuality; its residents while not wholly standardized, bear at least remote resemblance to each other. Little of this is true on the Delaware; cities of that stream are groups of neighbor hoods, often only a collection of villages loosely bound into municipalities.

Philadelphia, the metropolis, best illustrates the incoherence of Delaware river towns. For years the socially elite were bound by ironclad custom to reside within a narrow area, eight blocks long by three blocks wide, centering on sacrosanct Rittenhouse Square. No "gentleman," it was well understood, could live across the Schuylkill in West Philadelphia or, under any conceivable circumstance, over the Delaware in Camden. Gentle folk dealt only at the proper stores, dined only at a few approved restaurants, attended certain colleges (among which, in recent years, the University of Pennsylvania was not invariably numbered), consulted the properly endorsed physicians, and finally were buried by the right undertaker in the especially select cemeteries.

Other sections of the city were veritable foreign settlements. Since no gentleman lived north of Market Street and since his engagements, short of death itself, narrowed his movements within a square mile or two of central city ground, outlying regions were almost as much cut off as though they were in foreign lands. Middle-class English monopolized Kensington, Germans ruled the vague area toward the northwest known popularly as Brewerytown, and beyond them were the Irish. Nestling close to Rittenhouse Square itself was the Black Belt, and farther to the south a large and growing Italian settlement.

These regions were, however, not so static as was Rittenhouse Square; while the latter long continued to be the aristocratic social center, population shifts, owing to immigrant migrations and intracity movements, brought important changes. In many sections of the town newcome Irish and Germans replaced English, later arrivals of Russian and Polish Jews displaced the Germans and the Irish, Negroes from the South took over areas abandoned by their predecessors. But of all this Rittenhouse Square was unaware.

The first breach in the conservative tradition that nothing of importance happened north of Market Street came with the construction of the new Academy of Fine Arts building, in 1872, a block and a half north of the dead line. The Academy, always a pet of social Philadelphia, thus defied convention, but, as a resort of unpredictable and not invariably responsible artists, it was able to survive. The Rittenhouse Square elite trekked north once a year to the private viewing of the Academy's excellent exhibition, but ventured no farther into the great unknown.

Years later, soon after the turn of the century, Oscar Hammerstein, seeking a site for a new opera house where his troupe might compete with the Philadelphia performances of New York's Metropolitan company, built a garish, crimson-and-gold theater more than a mile above the sacred Market Street line. His showmanship, his admirable publicity devices, above all his outstanding corps of artists, brought him a temporary victory over conservatism, but, after peace was made between Hammerstein and the Metropolitan forces, opera returned to the old Academy of Music, south of Market Street. Hammerstein's house decayed, fell to lower uses, and eventually ceased to be used for either opera or theater.

Far to the north, however, in Germantown and Chestnut Hill, on high land once used for country homes for Philadelphia citizens, well-established families, noted rather for ancestry than for wealth, are seated. They scornfully look down on those nouveaux riches who have built larger houses just beyond them in the Whitemarsh country. Germantown affects, also, a superiority over the much wealthier Main Line, northwest of Philadelphia, and over the folk who dwell northeast in the lovely, rolling Huntingdon Valley.

Though each group dwells in what appears, at superficial glance, to be isolation, the castes are cut across by intellectual interests. The Delaware is by no means a land of social snobbery, nor is it unduly self-contained. Silas Weir Mitchell's Saturday Nights, where was heard the best talk in Philadelphia until the physician's death in 1914, were attended by a cross section of the city. Horace Howard Furness's Sunday Afternoons at Wallingford were popular with the keenest intellects. These were, to be sure, exceptional affairs, for men flocked to hear the caustic, biting criticisms by Weir Mitchell as they later crowded to hear Joe Pennell's acid devastations of his brother artists or his lightning thrusts at the evils of prohibition, and an afternoon at the Furness mansion was so unpredictable that no man dared omit a call. The great Sumatra orangutan, which had the freedom of the house until it grew so vicious that it had to be sent off to the zoo, the four-foot lizard, which Furness affectionately called "my God-damned iguana," the seemingly countless kittens, which played about the folio-lined Furness study, lent excitement to the Sunday Afternoons. If these were sluggish, there was always a good chance that young Bill Furness, tattooed from pate to toe, might give an exhibition or that the disillusioned sister, so deaf that she missed most of the conversation, would start a soiree on her independent own. There was, in such company, no need to imagine the merry uncertainties of *You Can't Take It With You*.

More recently, Henry Drinker's Sunday musicales at Merion, where guests unite in chorale singing and impromptu melody, cut through narrow geographic boundaries. The witty Franklin Inn, lineal descendant of the Mitchell salon, where writers, artists, and publishers lunch together amid brilliant, and often savage, argument, the fashionable Contemporary Club, whose two hundred members hear excellent discussions, and the convivial Clover Club, of politicians and newspapermen, recruit their membership from every section.

32

Modest Self-Restraint

Twice a year, the transfer agent at the old Academy of Music, Philadelphia's temple of the arts, looks forward to a job. Two days after Christmas, a quiet, ancient grande dame will arrive to sell her share of stock; in March, as buds begin to swell, she will arrive to buy it back. Year after year, this same transaction is the only transfer, short of death bequest, in the Academy's stock ownership.

The ancient lady is a thrifty soul who knows her rights. Stockholders in the old Academy are highly privileged; their special perquisites include a front-row seat at any function held within the building: since the opera, the Philadelphia Forum, the Orchestra, and all other large-scale cultural functions must, by local custom, take place in the Academy, stockholders have free entree to whatever is afoot.

They cannot, however, trade their rights to any other person. Two hundred and fifty of the best seats in the house are set aside in case stockholders come to claim admission, but the owner must appear in person. Not even the wife of a stockholder can crash the gate unless the lady owns a share in her own name.

The quiet, ancient lady lives in the true spirit of the Delaware. Gentle but persistent, innocent though shrewd and businesslike, calm and sedate but unbreakable in her determination, she molds rules to her own purposes. Now that her blood is thinning, she goes south each year to Florida, but, just before she takes the train, she calls at the Academy, and "sells" her stock to her best friend in order that the perquisites shall not be wasted. Then, when summer birds return, she comes back home and "buys" her stock again. The transfer books at the Academy contain a lengthy list of these wash sales.

For the Delaware breeds canniness and, some say, parsimony. Not the calculating closeness, it should be understood, of cold New England, where a living must be wrested from the rocks, for the Delaware is generous by nature and it drains a gracious land. Its spreading meadows thick with grass, its lush grainfields, and its rolling, fertile hills preclude the thought of stinginess. There never can be mean, tightfisted misers in a land that blooms each spring with cream-white dogwood, wild pink azalea, golden daffodils, and the varied blues of violet and quaker-lady. Though the climate swings sometimes to extremes, the region is a smiling land.

But the people have been trained in simple, unpretentious ways. Sprung from the Friends, who scorned luxury as they scorned sin, and from the prudent Pennsylvania Germans, who sought only peace, cleanliness and a full barn, the Delaware folk developed a cult of moderation, cautiousness, and toleration. They were pleasant people, well-mannered and polite, kindly to their neighbors, moved by sympathy for the afflicted— it was no accident that the almshouses, asylums for insane, hospitals, and such social institutions appeared first along the Delaware—but they kept both feet firmly planted on the ground. Seldom were they swept away by strange enthusiasms or by eccentric cults. Certain of their economic security in a river valley that was fertile beyond all expectation, the people of the Delaware lived quietly and well.

Culture fashioned in the Quaker pattern will not flower quickly, nor will it dare strike out in unconventional direction. Quaker self-repression, modesty, and shy retirement fitted well with the calm spirit of the placid stream. The Delaware has never claimed to be a land where poets sang, where brilliant repartee flashed bright, or where originality was ever highly prized. True it is that the region was a temporary home for Poe, Whittier, and Whitman and that Charles Brockden Brown, America's first professional man of letters, lived along the river; Louisa May Alcott was Pennsylvania-born and so were other writers, but the poet and the novelist were strange phenomena in a land where many earnest people frowned on self-expression. Poe was never truly in the stream of Pennsylvania life; Whittier, the Quaker poet, felt at home among his spiritual kinsmen but wrote few masterpieces on the Delaware; poor Walt Whitman was outside the pale.

Lounging, frowsy and unkempt, in his straight unpainted chair propped against the ferryhouse, munching peanuts cadged from friendly vendors, shouting lusty "howdys" to all and sundry as they passed, Whitman seemed anything but a proper poet. Gently reared Philadelphians, devoted to their Whittier and Tennyson, saw no merit in his loud, unpolished verses; they deplored his lack of self-restraint. Many were shocked to hear that he lived in a tiny house, cooking all his food on a smoky, coal-oil stove, eating his meals from thick china plates from the top of a dry-goods box, sleeping on a bed that was unmade from one Sunday to the next. The "good, gray poet," riding back and forth on the limitless ferry pass provided for him by one of his more astute friends, leaning over the rail in coldest wintry weather for the sheer joy of watching the ice crunch beneath the flat bow of the ferryboat, standing on the open platform of the trolley cars, his long beard streaming, was surely not in tune with the late-Victorian Delaware. Good form ruled the river then, propriety was king, but Whitman scorned them both. Quiet Quakers thought he might be great, but they failed to absorb him within their fellowship.

It would be an error to assume that Quaker minds, like Quaker garb, were wholly buff and gray. Though Delaware folk showed slight imagination in the arts and though they failed signally to appreciate such unique geniuses as Poe and Whitman, they were adept at dealing with culture of a more traditional type. Just as the Delaware developed no great innovator in jurisprudence, but is nationally famous for the innumerable skilled lawyers who could use the law as a tool, just as the educational institutions turned out few theoreticians, but thousands of surgeons, physicians, and men of practical scholarship, so the Delaware is noted for the editors who channeled and directed thought.

They were, for the most part, concerned with politics, particularly in the early days when Philadelphia was the nation's capital and when polemic writing was pungent, violent, and virulent or, in more recent times, when a more mature America, convinced at last that convention was king, was striving to learn etiquette and culture. The cult of the gentleman was largely a Philadelphia product; more women learned how to be a lady from the Philadelphia fashion magazines than from any other single source.

Louis Antoine Godey, who flourished from 1830 until the decade of the seventies, began the process and, in his *Lady's Book*, a magazine, "entirely the production of lady writers," set the tone for good society. It was a crystallizing influence, devoted rather to pointing out those "pure virtues and moral influences which constitute woman's mission" than a trail-blazing publication, but the Delaware has always approved conservatism, and *Godey's Lady's Book* was exactly in the tradition of the river. Though neither the owner nor his editor, Sarah Josepha Hale, author of "Mary's Lamb," was of Quaker origin and though neither had been brought up on the river, both were so thoroughly steeped in the Delaware's conservatism, self-effacement, and simplicity as to make the magazine a perfect medium for the river's special character. Thousands of women throughout the land consciously molded themselves into the style which the Delaware River folk thought proper for themselves.

Even more effective was the more recently established *Ladies' Home Journal,* which, under the dual direction of Cyrus H. K. Curtis, publisher, and Edward W. Bok, editor, dominated the cultural ideas of a later time. Bok, a tall, handsome, Dutch immigrant, sublimely confident of his opinions, deliberately set out to raise the living standards of the nation. Not content to follow slavishly the Godey precedent, he undertook determined "crusades" against false standards and ugliness. His unrelenting journalistic wars against billboards and patent medicines, his emphasis on artistry in decoration and, above all, his sage counsel, under the pseudonym "Ruth Ashmore," to young girls on matters of good form and etiquette probably did more to bring beauty, sound taste, and healthfulness to American communities than has ever been accomplished by any other editor in history. It is, of course, sophisticated fashion to decry the *Ladies' Home Journal* and its sister magazine, the *Saturday Evening Post,* as bourgeois, philistine, and materialistic, but no more important mass publications have ever been issued in our land. In their soundness, their philosophy, their conventionality, even in their stodginess, these magazines, though, like the *Lady's Book*, conducted and edited by men originally foreign to the Delaware tradition, are typical of the character preferred along the river.

Though Bok retired in 1930, after forty years of editorship, his stamp still lies upon the river people. By various foundations, Bok perpetuates the search for high ideals. An annual Philadelphia Award of $10,000, paid to that person who has contributed most during the preceding year to the cultural development of the community, the establishment of special prizes for firemen and policemen, an American Peace Award of $100,000 for the best plan for American co-operation toward permanent peace, all testify to Bok's continuing influence in the community. His autobiography, *The Americanization of Edward Bok*, won the Pulitzer prize in 1921.

Tuck Your Neck In

Those who know the river best are well aware that the beauty of its landscape lies in its simplicity, its harmony, its classic moderation of proportion. There are no jutting peaks, no wide-ranging plains, no tangled and majestic forests. The Delaware is placid, civilized, serene.

So with the people, too. Public opinion frowns on individual brilliance, preferring that greater genius who submerges self in common welfare. The man who seeks to make himself a personage attains less happiness along the Delaware than the public servant who perfects a rounded, co-operative group.

James Huneker learned the lesson to his cost when, trying to hurry the staid community toward modern art of the Bohemian stamp, he dashed himself against the rock of disapproval. Richard Harding Davis learned to his astonishment that Philadelphians preferred reporting that was plain and factual to writing that was feverish and sparkling. Not even Leopold Stokowski, wizard of the Philadelphia Orchestra, could break the Delaware tradition, for though his orchestra was triumphantly successful and though devoted debutantes watched breathlessly the conscious artistry of Stokowski's gestures, subscribers clamored for the well-worn classics when the maestro wanted to perform modern music.

John Frederick Wolle, master of musicianship, knew his public better. Annually at Bethlehem he led his famous choir in a two-day festival that interpreted Bach's oratorios in a spirit that came close to reverence. His singers, forgetful of themselves, "sang out of worshipping hearts to the greater glory of God" and, under Wolle's clever leadership, they "accomplished miracles." The slender, vibrant Wolle, a martinet in discipline, gave music that was in perfect keeping with the self-repressing spirit of the Delaware.

The passion for effacement finds expression in the architecture. Rows of red-brick, three-story houses, white trimmed and green shuttered, with flights of glistening white marble steps leading to polished oak doors, were long typical of the area. The community remains today one of small, private homes—eighty-five per cent of Philadelphia's 433,000 residences are single-family houses, mostly of from five to seven rooms—though, as elsewhere in America, apartments are replacing single dwellings and brownstone takes the place of brick. Footscrapers standing at the bottom of the steps to clean mud off the boots of visitors, "busybody" mirrors at the upper windows to give timely warning as to who is walking down the street or is waiting at the door, were necessary adjuncts to a well-kept home. Even in the more pretentious suburban building of to-day, whether on the swank Main Line or in more modest Jersey settlements, houses are almost indistinguishable from one another.

There are, to be sure, remarkable exceptions to the standard. Such gems of architecture as Bryn Athyn Cathedral and Valley Forge Memorial Chapel, with their Gothic triumphs and their stained-glass artistry, prove that building skill has not been wholly lost, for these are show places of fine art.

It is essential that the beauties of these newer structures be stressed lest casual visitors imagine that the awful monstrosity known as Philadelphia's City Hall be taken as representative of the region's architectural taste. A squat, square structure, topped by a five-hundred-foot tower on which stands a twenty-six-ton statue of William Penn, the City Hall is definitely bad. Begun in 1871, after a referendum vote in which the citizens wisely refused to let the building be placed in Independence Square, the structure was half a century in building at a cost staggeringly above the estimates.

Much of the twenty-four million dollars expended went into elaborate and almost unbelievable carving. Statues of Swedes and Indians, each twenty-four feet high, of caryatides bearing armloads of all the food grains grown in the Americas, half-length figures of every nationality represented in the population, busts of long-forgotten minor politicians, ornament the crowded public building. At one entrance a frieze of sculptured playful kittens greets the passerby; at another, naked Negroes and Chinese sweat as they support the vaulted ceiling. No other city office in America is so ornately carved; few are so unattractive in appearance.

Artistic gems are visible in the country regions. Numberless covered bridges once spanned the Delaware and the smaller streams, and though many of these were washed away by floods or declared too obsolete to handle modern traffic, many still remain. At Valley Forge, in Chester County, among the Pennsylvania German people, and at other isolated points in the interior, the long, red-colored covered bridge, built, in all probability, after the style of Switzerland, still carries traffic.

So, too, in the hinterland, are unique costumes to be found. Near Lancaster, broad brims of the bearded Amish testify to the persistence of a stubborn people who believe that motorcars are sinful and buttons are against the will of God. Quaker garb is less plentiful than heretofore, even at the quarterly meetings, but gray bonnets and plain dress have not disappeared. The folk of the Delaware are conservatives who do not willingly let custom die. They pride themselves upon their martyrdom, and boast of it.

33

Communal Friendship

THERE's comradeship along the Delaware. Its pleasant, happy people, serene in spirit, moderate in tone, easy in manner, work well together and play well too. Blessed by rich resource of stream and field and mine and forest, economically secure, their leisure time was well invested in co-operative recreation.

The fun is communal; professional amusements have never won a high regard. Connie Mack, major league baseball pilot for more than forty years, won a Bok Award for service to the community in developing eight pennant winning teams, and great ballplayers from the almost prehistoric times when Ed Delahanty led his league in batting and Billy Hamilton was a base-running sensation, down through the days of screwball Rube Waddell, have had their following of wide-eyed admirers, but the Delaware is not a stronghold for professional athletes. Its loyalty is to the amateur, and to the local institution. Princeton, Pennsylvania, Lehigh, Villanova, Lafayette, and Temple have their earnest partisans in football; Haverford and Swarthmore are followed closely, though the former prefers cricket and the latter holds that its lacrosse is better sport.

There is no season when the river is deserted. In dead of winter, when the upper Delaware is frozen tight from shore to shore and the only signs that nature is alive consist of shiny laurel bushes and dark-green rhododendron glimpsed through the violet shadows of the wooded hills, skaters skim along the stream. Ice-boating, swiftest of terrestrial travel, holds its thrill and, all too infrequently, great ox-roasts may be held on mid-river ice, or elaborate frost-fairs, with booths selling a thousand different commodities, are set up in tents on the frozen stream. South of Trenton, constant traffic on the river breaks the ice and makes these festivals impossible, but in particularly cold winters of the past frost-fairs and ox-roasts have been held off Philadelphia.

Graybeards may grieve that these old pastimes are no more, but few will mourn the death of one Delaware peculiarity. December ice piles up against the shore, heaved by the tides into a jumbled mass of huge, irregular ice cakes. In early January comes a thaw, setting the ice adrift in bergs which to small-boy eyes seem arctic in immensity. Against the strict injunctions of their elders, adolescents once played "Kidney Benders," a follow-my-leader game of iceberg jumping that had all the thrill of log riding and Alpine climbing. Few players, inexplicably enough, were drowned in Kidney Bending, though many a boy was drenched in icy water and the incidence of colds, perhaps even of pneumonia, must have been appalling. For some reason, known only to youthful sense of propriety in timing, Kidney Benders was a January game; when the same opportunities returned at the great spring thaws, Kidney Benders was completely out of season. Quite possibly the sound of ball on bat was too alluring.

Spring sees new life on the streams. Rowing clubs, banded into a Schuylkill Navy, prepare for their regattas, training oarsmen who have won a wide renown. Forty years ago a famous Vesper crew swept the Thames at Henley; more recently Joe Burk, from the Rancocas, and Jack Kelly, a Falls of Schuylkill boy, won both the Diamond Sculls and the Olympic prizes.

Rowing is only one of the spring interests. The river, bordered by its bright gold forsythia, edged by delicately green willows standing with their feet buried in the intensely green early grass, comes quickly into vigorous activity. On week ends after daylight-saving time begins, when cherry trees are foaming and dogwood is about to flower, bungalows fill up with city fugitives who come to fix their boats for summer use. From primitive launches, whose owners twist energetically at always recalcitrant flywheels, come sounds of starting, even from the engines which forever need adjustment and repair; from lordly cabin cruisers equipped with every luxury that imagination can desire come cloying smells of fresh spar varnish. Small sailboats in their sheltered dry docks are calked and painted; old sails are spread on the grass to be inspected for mold and to be stitched tight; long lists are made of new supplies to be bought during the interminable days before the week end comes again. The swimming partisans dip tentative toes into the water; canoeists, sweatered heavily, paddle happily, calling greetings to each bungalow they pass.

Not all the sportsmen are on the riverbank, to be sure. Golfers are in force, led by an astonishing number of girl linksmen who, leagued in a gigantic tournament of more than a hundred teams, compete for club championships. Tennis players limber up on overcrowded park courts to which the wise repair at daybreak in order to secure a reservation for the day. Vacant lot ballplayers, adepts at bocce, the bowls game beloved by all Italians, roller-skated shinny players find release for energies in springtime. Almost every telephone pole in crowded downtown districts bears a bottomless peach basket for impromptu outdoor basketball.

People love to play along the Delaware, even if that play is merely passive. Horse shows are a serious, engrossing interest, as befits a land so similar to England in appearance. At Devon in the end of May, at Bryn Mawr and at Wilmington, formal exhibitions, carefully steeped in etiquette and ceremony, become virtually compulsory functions at which the Social Register must appear. The horses, possibly, are secondary in importance to fashion, and of late the horse shows have become a more sophisticated version of the country fair, but there exists an authentic love of horseflesh. Small, but intensely loyal, groups of devotees pass from estate to estate, week after week in springtime, to admire the same selected local horses. In recent years dog shows have become a favored diversion, but the horse is still king along the Delaware, nor has the sport been ruined by professional admixture. Despite the Duke of Gloucester's track, or the race course latterly set up in Delaware, the region has never been particularly addicted to gambling on the races.

Fox hunting flourishes; indeed, in southeastern Pennsylvania the sport has passed into a cult. Nor is membership in one of the great clubs, Radnor, Rose Tree, or Pickering, merely a nominal gesture; twice a week throughout the hunting season, pink-coated riders scour the countryside before they go into town to work at daily tasks. At other times informal bands, who carefully do not wear club livery unless in actual pursuit of foxes, exercise the hounds in cubbing or follow the pack on an aniseed trail. Each spring a magnificent fox hunt, combining the seven most important packs of hounds, commemorates the anniversary of the fictional hunt described by Bayard Taylor in the Pennsylvania classic novel, *The Story of Kennett*.

The same strong British bent explains the interest in cricket. Soon after the Civil War, Lancashire weavers, moving into Kensington to man the textile mills, brought the game with them as an almost year-round sport. Cricket gained an instant popularity; scores of teams, notably at Merion, Germantown, and Philadelphia, played lengthy schedules, interrupted only when a visiting British ship came into port and offered outside competition. Local colleges accepted cricket eagerly; at Haverford, and for a time at Pennsylvania, the game was ranked among the major sports; at the former institution it surpassed football in popularity. On a dozen occasions all-Philadelphia cricketeers competed successfully with major clubs of the British Isles; visiting teams from Bermuda, the West Indies, or England arrived almost every year.

Summer sees the river at its best. A hot spell comes in late May or early June, another brackets the Fourth of July; except for these few days when the mercury is in the nineties, the weather is most often balmy, with soft south winds blowing, not too hot for comfort in the middle of the day, delightful in the evenings.

People of the Delaware revel in the open air. Shaded from the sun by lawn umbrellas, suburbanites enjoy their gardens, for the flowers of the valley are superb. Only the estates of tidewater Virginia match the gardens of the Delaware in loveliness, and, of the two, the Delaware valley has a wider range of color and variety. The garden is the leisure center. At breakfasttime and luncheon, at tea and oftentimes at dinner, it is the preferred spot for small tables to be set; in early morning and at dusk, when winds are cooler and the sun shines with less fire, the garden is irresistible.

City dwellers also live outdoors, for the open porch, typical of standard architecture in one-family houses, becomes an extra room. Screened and lighted, fitted up with swinging couches and with taborets, it is the living space for countless thousands. Close to the sidewalk, closer still to next-door neighbors, the open porch invites hospitality and friendliness. Men and women, rocking comfortably, exchange neighborhood gossip, discuss the news or listen to the muffled sounds of radios transferred for the summer to the porches. People of the Delaware are comrades; the porch brings them closer to each other and makes for better understanding. Snobbishness is at a discount; tolerance and love of fellow man are favored. The early Quakers did not bring the porch with them from England, nor was it favored in the early days when houses were more distant from each other, but the Friends of Penn's time would have given it a hearty welcome and their blessing. It is thoroughly in harmony with the spirit of the Delaware.

On gala nights, the front porch widens. To aid a local church, to help some neighborhood improvement, or just to satisfy the craving for extending friendships, neighbors string yards of colored bunting, hang lines of colored lights, fasten up innumerable flags and tack hand-lettered streamers to their houses. As in the old-time country fair, these neighborhood "block parties" sell cakes and jellies, pies and pickles, knickknacks and odds and ends; they hold foot races for the small fry; a brass band plays while adolescents dance on porches or on the sidewalks, refreshing themselves with lemonade, root beer, and coffee. On elaborate occasions, local statesmen give talks that are more noted for their gaiety and local quip than for weighty comment on affairs of national importance.

Block parties rarely attract outsiders, for their appeal is frankly neighborly. Few formalities are observed, whether the party is held on the street or, as often happens in the summer, in the wider expanse of the public parks, but through its influence the residents of the district come to know each other closely and to feel the thrill of common interest. The block party is invaluable as a socializing influence.

More intimately connected with the river is the "moonlight," a favored summer diversion for the sentimental. The great days of the river steamers are no more, for speedy transportation took away their need, but the steamship has not vanished from the river. Dancing clubs, known locally as "socials," cannot bear to stay indoors in summer, nor do they wish to break up their good-fellowship by disbanding for half a year. Many of them, therefore, hire a riverboat to sail on moonlit nights, while they dance on the deck or sit hand in hand enjoying cool evening breezes.

Upstream the moonlights ply from Philadelphia to the head of navigation just below the stony rifts at Trenton, stopping at Andalusia to view the gardens or at the mouth of the Rancocas to put ashore those few who would prefer canoeing for the evening. At Beverley, on the Jersey side, the well-taught captain whistles politely to the huge iron dog that stands on the sloping lawn, and tells his trusting passengers that on his last trip up the dog responded with a courteous bark; at Edgewater Park he points out that in the old days the bank was famous for its floral butterflies, now withered to oblivion; at Bordentown, opposite the restored manor at Pennsbury, he speaks of romantic, tree-shaded Point Breeze, where Joseph Bonaparte, eldest brother of Napoleon, lived with Quakeress Annette Savage, his American bride. At Bordentown, however, he will say, that Joseph showed but little of the glory that had once been his; neighbors knew him not as ex-king of Naples and of Spain, but only as the alien Count de Survilliers. And so the moonlight goes on to Trenton, where the steamer, coming within the shadow of the gold-domed State House, close by the Hessian Barracks whose inmates Washington so completely surprised, turns about for a more leisured downstream course. And now the captain, wise in many a moonlight, speaks no more of history, but lets his passengers sit quietly on the benches, whispering softly to each other, or lets the dance be unrestrained.

More moonlights take the southern voyage, because it is a longer trip and has a more romantic history. For seven decades the river trip was popular, on the beloved *Major Reybold*, named for the innovator who first made Delaware peaches a successful crop, or on the "mammoth, three-deck iron steamer *Republic*," which plied for years on the Delaware. The former had devoted patrons who believed that its bell tones were sweet because, when the ship's bell was cast, the Reybold family tossed its silver into the crucible. Many a *Major Reybold* passenger grieved at the loss of a personal friend when the steamer burned and sank one night at its dock; the more credulous are certain that on moonlight nights the bell still rings from beneath the waters. But the old *Republic* had its partisans as well; more than one happy couple, whose romance had flowered on a river trip, took passage on the old ship for old times' sake when, visiting New York, they found the *Republic*, under a new name, sailing the Coney Island run.

The southern trip has other goals than merely moonlight sailing. Starting in the early morning, when passengers can see the sights of Camden, where victrolas and soups are made, past the Duke of Gloucester's track and past the Navy Yard at League Island, the merrymakers have a full day's cruise. Those who know their history can speak of Dutch and Swedish settlements, of Big Belly Printz at what is now called Essington, where nowadays the great steam yachts are moored, of New Castle, whose huge gray icebreaker stones are favored haunts for fishermen, of the strange duPont dynasty that owns the river front at Carney's Point and along the Brandywine, and of Salem where the Albion Knights once planned a paradise. They speak, too, of the Whorekill and of the gallant fight at Lewes against the British in the War of 1812 and then, arriving at Cape May, they tell of early voyagers who nosed their little ships into the stream.

But the vast majority of passengers on a moonlight are not keen for history; they are living in the present, and, if their minds stray far from their companions on the deck, they think of active pleasures, of the fine fishing to be found at Fortescue and Bower's Beach, of the luscious oysters to be had at Maurice River, of adventure to be tasted on the freighters that steam slowly out to sea. More than any of these joys, each young man's attention is riveted on the lady by his side, which is why the understanding captains of a moonlight flash their searchlights on the shore to pick out objects that may be of interest, but carefully refrain from casting too much light on the couples seated on the decks or leaning on the rails.

34

New Year's Shooters

Summer lingers long on the Delaware, to compensate perhaps for short, untimely springs which come too late and jump much too precipitately into torrid weather. All through September, summer lasts, and often well into October, and then, retiring slowly from the scene, gives way to golden autumn. This, too, is a time of glory. Maples mellow into soft-toned amber or blush scarlet in the swamps. Hickories and tulip poplars are a bronze and saffron hue; the gums blaze brilliant red and gold. Far up the stream the valley flames in beauty.

It is a pity that few strangers know the river at this time of loveliness. New York intellectuals who spend their summers in Bucks County must go home to work before the valley reaches its triumphant peak of loveliness; painters of the New Hope group are all too often at their posts of duty in the art schools of Philadelphia or New York to revel in the sheer delight of autumn along the stream. Summer residents of the Water Gap, sojourners at the summer camps from Stroudsburg north to Milford, trout fishermen along the upper Delaware miss much of beauty, for the river's boldest, wildest color comes in late October and November. The clear blue light of summer becomes a gold and purple mistiness; soon it will fade into the winter's violet.

But winter also has its blessings. Late in November, and again close to the Christmas season, comes a cold snap that makes false threats of arctic blizzards, but, for those who can survive the threat, winters on the Delaware are not severe. December is a pleasant month, except for that false week of fear, and January is more usually mild than bitter. February is a month of worries, but the month is short and there are promises of bud and blossom.

Much may be forgiven a season that has brought such joy to mortals, for, from the Germans of the Delaware and Schuylkill valleys has come much of our traditional Christmas charm. The tinseled, decorated tree that now is indispensable for all America first gained its popularity among these Pennsylvania Germans; the close connection between Christmas and Santa Claus—a German saint—was first established by the people of the Delaware. New Netherlanders knew their own St. Nicholas, patron of December 6th, but Pennsylvania Germans swore by their Kriss Kringle who loved little children even more than had St. Nicholas. When the friendly struggle for supremacy was over, Kriss Kringle was triumphant; he had pulled St. Nicholas over to the German date, though losing, perhaps, his own identity when the Hollander took over Christmas as his own. No celebrant in all America had thought to honor Christmas by a lighted Norway spruce until the Pennsylvania Germans of the Delaware and Schuylkill valleys taught us how to glorify the day.

But New Year's is the day traditional along the Delaware, for then the sherry waits in every parlor and eggnog flows from every bowl. By ancient custom, neighbors exchange visits to renew their friendliness and comradeship. On New Year's Day the Quaker reticence breaks down; the Pennsylvania German doffs his quiet mantle. It is the Delaware's great day of mimicry and pageant.

Promptly at eight o'clock in the morning the strains of "Oh, dem golden slippers," traditional song of jubilee, sound from the horns of the Silver Crown New Year's Club, oldest of the famous Mummers. Then, for four full hours of the wintry morning, thousands of gaily dressed masqueraders march on Broad Street, re-enacting in exaggerated caricature those local happenings which have caught popular attention in the year just past. Lampooning the stuffed shirts, mimicking the pompous, the paraders satirically advise the city officials how to carry on their duties. They would, with all goodwill, perform such service for a wider field had not Councils, fearing international repercussion, forbade the Mummers to take off the worthies of other lands.

The license thus allowed on New Year's Day might easily develop into libel; the freedom of expression might be turned to bitterness and hate, but civic pride is powerful; though the Mummers gaily tread on eggshell subjects with a heavy boot, there is no malice or vindictiveness in their impersonations. The great parade is full of satire and derision, but it is never cynical and never vicious.

Learned commentators, unwilling to accept such jubilation at its gay face value, have often sought to trace the origin of the unique parade. Some find its inspiration in the ancient Swedish custom of merrymaking from Christmas till the old year dies; others are convinced that the Mummers are survivals of the medieval English players who at Christmastime showed how St. George slew the dragon; a third group sees them as modern Lords of Misrule; a few, delving deep into forgotten history, think they are cultural descendants of those early Christians who once ran about in masks to ridicule the pagan superstitions. The truth is less glamorous; the Mummers, more certainly, are the outgrowth of the former custom on the Delaware whereby the irrepressibles "shot the New Year in" by fusillades of guns.

The Mummers—or, to give them their old-fashioned and more proper name, the Shooters—are formed for New Year's larking. Named either for their political patrons or for some generous merchant who donated heavily to the club treasury, the clubs work steadily throughout the year arranging floats, designing and creating rich satin costumes, planning new features for display. Their labor culminates in a festive New Year's Eve dance which lasts all night and from which the members go forth to their street parade. The fact that every celebrant has been up all night, welcoming the New Year's coming, explains what, to many, has seemed incomprehensible, the singularly early starting time for the parade.

Certain features are traditional. Club captains wear "capes" of incredible magnificence. Great trains of richly embroidered silk, hanging from their shoulders, trail far behind, kept clear of the ground by swarms of costumed page boys. Huge feathered headdresses tower high above the captains' heads. So heavy are the costumes that the wearers are literally bowed down by their burdens; they stagger, rather than walk, along the four-mile course. Lieutenants wear costumes of less elegance, but they, too, require a corps of page boys on their journey. A well-equipped fancy-dress club will have as many as a score of such elaborate capes.

Clowns and female impersonators—no woman may take part in the parade—dudes, acrobats, and all the

personages dear to burlesque stages, comprise the special contribution of the so-called "comic clubs" which
are the larger, and more appreciated, portion of the
long parade. The humor here is broad and, some say,
vulgar, but the spirit robs the Shooter of intentional
offense. In recent years the gay-clad string bands have
proved immensely popular.

Until the opening of the present century, the
Shooters paraded independently, competing for cash
prizes offered by merchants of the various neighbor-
hoods; but in 1901 Philadelphia City Councils organized
the scattered showings into one parade. The Silver
Crown Club leads the march by its seniority; other
positions are awarded by lot. Invariably both the drawings and the prize awards cause prolonged bickerings,
and lead to loose charges of favoritism against the
judges; yearly disappointed Shooters shout that they
never will march again, but, after a month or two of
angry accusation, tempers cool and work begins on next
year's celebration. Indeed, if truth be told, they were
active on the coming costumes even while they were
protesting that they never would take part again. "The
Neck," that portion of South Philadelphia close to the
confluence of the rivers, sometimes seems to live only
for the sake of New Year's Day parading.

So, with the dawn of a New Year on the Delaware,
a cycle closes, to begin again in merrier, more pleasant
form. The year of jollity is over; friendliness, neigh-
borliness, and service to mankind have prevailed, but
with characteristic modesty, with trained restraint, the
people of the Delaware renew their ancient mission, now
three centuries old. The river flows placidly to the
sea, gentling those who dwell along its banks, soothing
them to harmony, softening their parochial ideas. If it
has not always been successful in attaining peace and

bringing brotherhood to man, it certainly has mollified his passions; often it has brought a quiet happiness out of what seemed hopelessly discordant elements. The Delaware has molded men; it has helped to make a nation.

Acknowledgments and Bibliography

MATERIAL for *The Delaware* has been drawn from a wide variety of sources, ranging from the material to be found in contemporary manuscripts to the folk tales of the people living in the region. Old diaries and journals, many of them reproduced in the sixty-four volumes of the *Pennsylvania Magazine of History and Biography*, the eight volumes of *Sketches* of the Montgomery County Historical Society, the publications of the Gloucester, Salem, Chester, Bucks, Berks, Northampton, and Delaware county groups, others dug from the dusty attics of the Delaware valley, have been most productive. The *State Archives* of New Jersey, Delaware, and Pennsylvania, the last named of which, in nine series, is peculiarly important, have also been drawn upon, as have the invaluable numbers of *Hazard's Annals* and his *Registers*.

Newspapers have proved helpful though they, like the folk tales of the neighborhood, have required extensive checking. The files of the *Honey Brook Herald*, edited by Martin L. Andes, are rich in historical lore. Herman L. Collins's column, signed "Girard," in the Philadelphia *Inquirer*, Harrison Fry's special articles in the Philadelphia *Evening Bulletin* and "stories" by Edward Robins and others, including the late William Perrine, in the *Bulletin's* famous *Men and Things* department, have frequently contained interesting reminiscence. Edward Hocker's frequent "Norris" articles in the Norristown *Times-Herald*, the helpful items in the Wilmington *Every Evening*, the Salem *Standard*, the Easton *Express*, the Trenton *Times*, and half a dozen other Delaware valley papers encourage further research into the past files of the press. The author has, it is safe to say, dug deep into Delaware valley journalism from pre-Revolutionary times down to the present.

Far too many individuals have helped in gathering material for them all to be listed here individually. The writer has endeavored to thank them in person and by correspondence, and, though their names are omitted here, he has no thought of slighting their valuable assistance. The same gratitude ought also to be expressed to those great scholars of the past—men like Ellis Paxson Oberholtzer, Francis M. Brooke, Jones Detweiler, S. Gordon Smyth, Julius Sachse, Anthony Higgins, Henry C. Conrad, Judge Charles B. Lore, Alexander B. Cooper, and Samuel Whitaker Pennypacker—who left their collected notes for later inspection and to T. Lane Bean, General W. W. H. Davis, Judge J. Smith Futhey, and Gilbert Cope whose county histories are of such importance. To editors, librarians, and curators of historical societies from Walton down to Lewes, on both shores of the river, the author wishes to extend a particularly hearty appreciation.

Above all others, the writer is overwhelmingly indebted, both for assistance and for unfailing inspiration, to the brilliant and tireless person to whom *The Delaware* is dedicated. Her modest self-deprecation, so typical of the river people, forbids the use of her full name.

ACRELIUS, ISRAEL, *A History of New Sweden,* translated by William M. Reynolds. Philadelphia, 1874.
Politics, economics and sociology of the colony until 1748.
ANBUREY, THOMAS, *Travels Through the Interior Parts of America, 1797-1811,* 2 vols. London, 1789.
Much of this, especially the famous paragraphs describing bundling and the passages concerning the Delaware area, is borrowed without credit from Burnaby, *q.v.*
BALDWIN, WILLIAM C., "The Story of Elizabeth Montgomery," *New Delawarean,* November, 1938.
A "profile" of an early Victorian snooper after historical gossip.

BANNING, MRS. HENRY G., "Miss Vining, a Revolutionary Belle," in *American Historical Register*, July, 1895.

The same story of Wayne's Delaware love is reprinted, with a few additions, in the Wilmington *Every Evening*, August 18, 1928.

BARBE-MARBOIS, FRANÇOIS, MARQUIS DE, *Our Revolutionary Forefathers*. New York, 1929.

Philadelphia diary, 1779-1785, of the secretary of the French legation. He liked the Delaware, but deplored the modesty of American ladies.

BARTON, THOMAS, *The Conduct of the Paxton Men Impartially Represented*. Philadelphia, 1764.

The title is a misnomer. Barton takes sides in the Paxtang matter.

BECK, HENRY C., *Fare to Midlands*. New York, 1939.

——— *Forgotten Towns of Southern New Jersey*. New York, 1936.

——— *More Forgotten Towns*. New York, 1937.

A Camden *Courier* editor explores the ghost towns of southern and central New Jersey.

BERNARD, JOHN, *Retrospections of America* (1797-1811). New York, 1887.

A famous London actor found Philadelphia attractive, though the people seemed fidgety.

BINING, ARTHUR CECIL, *Forges and Furnaces of Pennsylvania*. Philadelphia, 1914.

The best account of the flourishing eighteenth century iron industry.

——— *Pennsylvania Iron Manufacture in the 18th Century*. Harrisburg, 1938.

Condensed and less definite account than the above, but correcting a few minor errors.

BOLLES, A. S., *Pennsylvania, Province and State*, 2 vols. Philadelphia, 1899.

BOUDINOT, ELIAS, *Life and Letters*, edited by Jane Boudinot. Philadelphia, 1896.

An imperfect collection, but noteworthy for its reference to the famous Lydia Darragh episode.

BOWDEN, ROBERT DOUGLAS, *Boies Penrose*. New York, 1937.

A good biography of the Big Grizzly is still needed.

BRISSOT DE WARVILLE, J. P., *New Travels in the United States of America, 1788*. London, 1792.

Written to praise "the prodigious effects of liberty on morals, on industry and on the amelioration of man." He loves the Delaware. "A glass of cider . . . appeared to me superior to the most exquisite wines."

BROWNING, CHARLES H., *The Welsh Settlements of Pennsylvania*. Philadelphia, 1912.

The leading authority on a still too unfamiliar subject.

BUCK, WILLIAM J., *The History of the Indian Walk*. Philadelphia, 1886.

The story of the infamous Walking Purchase.

BURNABY, REV. THOMAS, *Travels Through the Middle Settlements of America, 1759-1760*. London, 1798.

"Pennsylvanians . . . are frugal and industrious . . . not remarkably courteous . . . by far the most enterprising people upon the continent. . . . The women are exceedingly handsome . . . since their intercourse with the English officers, they are greatly improved . . ." Burnaby wrote the classic account of bundling.

BURNHAM, SMITH, *The Battle of Brandywine*, Second Report, Pennsylvania Historical Commission. Harrisburg, 1918.

CHASTELLUX, MARQUIS DE, *Travels in North America, 1780-1782*, 2 vols. Dublin, 1787.

One of the Forty Immortals, an aide to Rochambeau, the author was highly pleased with the Delaware, but saddened to find but two pretty women. He disliked the Quakers, and disapproved of "Miss Viny," for which he gained Brissot's violent hatred.

CONRAD, HENRY C., *A History of Delaware*, 3 vols. Philadelphia, 1908.

COOPER, THOMAS, *Some Information Respecting America.* London, 1794.

"I know of very few objections that can be made to the State of Pennsylvania . . . Book societies are everywhere . . . I know of only one professed 'gentleman' . . ."

DAY, SHERMAN, *Historical Collections of Pennsylvania.* Philadelphia, 1843.

A voluminous collection of anecdote, event, and statistical detail.

DRAKE, SAMUEL ADAMS, *The Campaign of Trenton, 1776-1777.* Boston, 1895.

DUNAWAY, WAYLAND FULLER, *A History of Pennsylvania.* New York, 1935.

EGLE, WILLIAM H., *A History of the Commonwealth of Pennsylvania.* Philadelphia, 1883.

Largely a rewriting and a continuation of Sherman Day's *Collections.*

ELLET, ELIZABETH F., *The Court Circles of the Republic.* Hartford, 1869.

The beauties, chivalries, and fashions of Philadelphia, capital of the U. S. A.

FARIS, JOHN T., *Old Churches and Meeting-Houses In and Around Philadelphia.* Philadelphia, 1926.

——— *Old Roads Out of Philadelphia.* Philadelphia, 1917.

FERRIS, BENJAMIN, *A History of the Original Settlements on the Delaware.* Wilmington, 1846.

FISHER, SYDNEY GEORGE, *The Making of Pennsylvania.* Philadelphia, 1916.

Particularly good for the Pennamite Wars and the Welshmen.

——— *Pennsylvania, Colony and Commonwealth.* Philadelphia, 1897.

Sketchy, impressionistic, and not always accurate.

——— *The Quaker Colonies.* New Haven, 1919.

——— *The True William Penn.* Philadelphia, 1900.

GARBER, JOHN PALMER, *The Valley of the Delaware.* Philadelphia, 1934.

GATES, THEOPHILUS R., *Battle-Axes and the Weapons of War*. July, August and December, 1837.

The pamphlets that touched off the Free-Love Valley craze.

GLENN, THOMAS ALLEN, *Merion in the Welsh Tract*. Norristown, 1896.

Particularly valuable for genealogists.

GODFREY, CARLOS E., *When Boston Was New Jersey's Capital*. New Jersey Historical Society, *Proceedings,* January, 1933.

GORDON, T. F., *History of Pennsylvania from Its Discovery Until 1776*. Philadelphia, 1829.

GRAYDON, ALEXANDER, *Memoirs of a Life Chiefly Spent in Pennsylvania*. Harrisburg, 1811.

Invaluable for manners and customs of his time.

HARLAND, MARIAN, *More Colonial Homesteads*. New York, 1899.

Contains reference to the Mary Vining story.

HAZARD, SAMUEL, *Pennsylvania, Its History*. Philadelphia, 1850.

Based on the famous Hazard's *Annals,* which are unmatched for importance.

HECKEWELDER, REV. JOHN, *History, Manners and Customs of the Indian Nations*. Philadelphia, 1819.

This famous missionary still remains the great authority on the Lenni-Lenape. His Indian vocabulary, though certainly unministerial, was probably of the highest usefulness to wandering white gentlemen.

HILTZHEIMER, JACOB, *Extracts from Diary*, edited by Jacob Cox Parsons. Philadelphia, 1893.

Memoirs of a merchant and sportsman who knew everybody in town.

HOCKER, EDWARD W., *Germantown, 1683-1933*. Germantown, 1933.

In this book, as in his famous "Norris" papers contributed to the Norristown *Times-Herald,* Hocker shows himself a master of historical lore.

JAMES, REESE D., *Old Drury of Philadelphia, 1800-1835*. Philadelphia, 1932.

Theatrical history, supplementing the Pollock volume.

JENKINS, HOWARD M., *Historical Collections of Gwynned*. Philadelphia, 1897.

The Welsh Tract on the eastern bank of the Schuylkill.

——— *Pennsylvania, Colonial and Federal*, 3 vols. Philadelphia, 1903.

Almost entirely political and not too inspiriting.

JOHNSON, AMANDUS, *The Swedish Settlements on the Delaware*, 2 vols. Philadelphia, 1911.

A definitive, but alas! costly account of the Swedes.

JOHNSON, ROBERT G., *Historical Account of the First Settlement in Salem*. Philadelphia, 1839.

LEWIS, JOSEPH J., *History of Chester County*, Letters in West Chester *Village Record*, 1824.

The source for several much more pretentious histories of the county, by the man originally selected to be Anthony Wayne's biographer.

LINCOLN, ANNA T., *Three Centuries Under Four Flags*. Rutland, Vt., 1937.

A sketchy, and unhappily not always authoritative, history of Wilmington.

LIPPARD, GEORGE, *The Legends of the American Revolution*. Philadelphia, 1876.

Wholly unreliable, but quite readable, anecdotes which once were accepted as authentic fact.

LIPPINCOTT, HORACE MATHER, *Colonial Homes of Philadelphia and its Neighborhood*. Philadelphia, 1912.

——— *Early Philadelphia, its People, Life, and Progress*. Philadelphia, 1917.

LOSSING, B. J., *Field Book of the Revolution*, 2 vols. New York, 1852.

A pictorial account of the various camps and battlefields.

MARSHALL, CHRISTOPHER, *Extracts from Diary*, edited by William Duane. Albany, 1877.

Firsthand narration of the stirring events from 1774 to 1781.

MARTIN, JOHN HILL, *History of Chester*. Philadelphia, 1877.

MONTGOMERY, ELIZABETH, *Reminiscences of Wilmington*. Philadelphia, 1851.

Virtually the entire Mary Vining story stems from this source. Miss Betsy seems to have been an indefatigable gossip columnist.

NOLAN, J. BENNETT, *Annals of the Penn Square*. Philadelphia, 1933.

———— *George Washington and the Town of Reading*. Reading, 1931.

Rich stores of breezy and original material concerning the upper Schuylkill.

OBERHOLTZER, ELLIS PAXSON, *The Literary History of Philadelphia*. Philadelphia, 1906.

Complete as far as it goes, but no writers who were living at the time of publication are included.

PARKINSON, RICHARD, *A Tour In America, 1798-1800*, 2 vols. London, 1805.

"Generally speaking, as a body of people, the Americans are bad . . . few of them will become rich . . . even the fair sex seemed to want softness of temper."

PENNYPACKER, SAMUEL W., *Pennsylvania in American History*. Philadelphia, 1910.

A battling defense of the state against New England's presumptions, by an antiquarian, and a former governor.

PINKERTON, ALLAN, *The Molly Maguires and the Detectives*. New York, 1877.

Rather too smug and righteous, but a stirring story none the less.

POLLOCK, THOMAS C., *The Philadelphia Theater in the Eighteenth Century*. Philadelphia, 1932.

PONTGIBAUD, CHEVALIER, *A French Volunteer in the War of Independence*, translated by Robert B. Douglas. New York, 1898.

He was astonished by the simplicity and democracy of American officials.

POWELL, WALTER A., *A History of Delaware*. Boston, 1928. Conrad's is far superior.

RAUM, JOHN O., *A History of New Jersey*, 2 vols. Philadelphia, 1877.

―――― *History of the City of Trenton*. Trenton, 1871. Arid, but complete, recitals of political and economic matters.

REED, WILLIAM B., *Life and Correspondence of Joseph Reed*, 2 vols. Philadelphia, 1847. A mine of information dealing with a statesman who has never received his just tributes.

REPPLIER, AGNES, *Philadelphia: The Place and the People*. New York, 1898. Belatedly, the Delaware valley will appreciate what shrewd appraisals this acidulous essayist has been writing for half a century.

ROBIN, ABBÉ CLAUDE, *New Travels Through North America, 1781*. Philadelphia, 1783. "Pennsylvania soon became the most virtuous and happy colony that history has ever recorded."

ROBINS, EDWARD, *Romances of Early America*. Philadelphia, 1902. The Mary Vining story by a member of the family who is now president of the Historical Society of Pennsylvania.

SACHSE, JULIUS F., *The German Pietists of Pennsylvania*. Philadelphia, 1895.

―――― *The Wayside Inns of Lancaster Pike*. Lancaster, 1912. Uncritical, but exciting legends of the countryside are interspersed with much excellent historical material. Much of the data first appeared in the West Chester (Pa.) *Village Record*, 1877 to 1887.

SACKETT, WILLIAM EDGAR, *Modern Battles of Trenton*, 2 vols. Trenton, 1895.

Inside story of political machinations of New Jersey statesmen.

SCHARF, J. THOMAS, *History of Delaware, 1609-1888.* Philadelphia, 1888.

SCHARF, J. THOMAS, and WESTCOTT, THOMPSON, *History of Philadelphia,* 3 vols. Philadelphia, 1884.

The latter remains the best local history of the city. The early chapters of the Scharf book are almost identical with those of Scharf and Westcott.

SCHOEPF, JOHANN DAVID, *Travels in the Confederation, 1783-1784,* edited by Alfred J. Morrison, 2 vols. Philadelphia, 1911.

An excellent account of America by a skilled reporter, though somewhat unkind to his German kinsmen. He liked America, and especially he liked the Delaware. "Gallant adventures are little known and still less practiced in this last refuge of virtue."

SÉGUR, PHILIPPE PAUL, COUNT DE, *Memoirs and Recollections,* 2 vols. London, 1825.

"The whole town of Philadelphia is one noble temple raised to the spirit of toleration."

SELLERS, CHARLES COLEMAN, *Theophilus the Battle-Axe.* Philadelphia, 1930.

An all-too-brief biography of Theophilus Gates.

SELSAM, J. PAUL, *The Pennsylvania Constitution of 1776.* Philadelphia, 1936.

Inner workings of the radical movement during the Revolution.

SICKLER, JOSEPH S., *The History of Salem.* Salem, N. J., 1937.

The town's postmaster digs deep into the foibles of his historic settlement.

SIPE, C. HALE, *The Indian Chiefs of Pennsylvania.* Butler, Pa., 1927.

—— *The Indian Wars of Pennsylvania.* Harrisburg, 1929.

The two books overlap considerably, but they are complete accounts, by a Pennsylvania lawyer and state senator.

SMITH, SAMUEL, *History of New Caesaria, or New Jersey.* Burlington, N. J., 1765.

Surprisingly modern-type history, replete with interesting detail.

SMITH, WILLIAM, *A Brief State of the Province of Pennsylvania.* London, 1755.

STEWART, FRANK, "Major John Fenwick," Salem (N. J.) *Standard and Jerseyman*, 1939.

Prolix and ill-arranged but detailed and authoritative.

STILLE, CHARLES J., *Major-General Anthony Wayne and the Pennsylvania Line.* Philadelphia, 1893.

Purely military biography by a former president of the Historical Society of Pennsylvania.

STONE, FREDERICK D., *The Battle of Brandywine.* Philadelphia, 1895.

STOUDT, REV. JOHN BAER, *The Liberty Bells of Pennsylvania.* Philadelphia, 1930.

STRYKER, WILLIAM S., *The Battle of Monmouth*, Princeton, 1927.

———*The Battles of Trenton and Princeton*, Trenton, 1895.

THOMAS, GABRIEL, *Historical and Geographical Account of Pennsylvania and West New Jersey.* London, 1698.

TRAUBEL, HORACE, *With Walt Whitman in Camden*, 3 vols. Philadelphia, 1906-1914.

Boswellian reports of the poet's every utterance by the former editor of the *Conservator*, which accents the third syllable, please.

TWINING, THOMAS, *Travels in America a Hundred Years Ago.* New York, 1900.

An East Indian nabob is astonished that Penn was forgotten by 1795. "It is possible that Penn's name is held in respect . . . but I never heard it mentioned in general society, nor observed that it was common."

UPLAND (PA.), *Record of the Court, 1676-1681.* Philadelphia, 1860.

WANSEY, HENRY, *Journal of an Excursion to the United States, 1794.* Salisbury, England.

A Wiltshire clothier went to breakfast with Washington and reports on the social life of the American capital.

WARD, CHRISTOPHER, *The Dutch and Swedes on the Delaware*. Philadelphia, 1930.

—— *New Sweden on the Delaware*. Philadephia, 1938.

—— *Jonathan Drew*. New York, 1932.

New Sweden is a reprinting of the early chapters of *Dutch and Swedes; Jonathan Drew*, a novel, gives vivid pictures of the period about 1820.

WATSON, ELKANAH, *Men and Times of the Revolution*. New York, 1856.

He found too much treating, too much drinking, and too cold manners.

WATSON, JOHN FANNING, *Annals of Philadelphia*, 3 vols. Philadelphia, 1857.

Men, manners, and *curiosa* of the Delaware valley. An invaluable book, though its items require verification before acceptance.

WEYGANDT, CORNELIUS, *Philadelphia Folks*. New York, 1938.

—— *The Dutch Country*. New York, 1939.

—— *The Red Hills*. Philadelphia, 1929.

—— *The Wissahickon Hills*. Philadelphia, 1930.

—— *Down Jersey Way*. New York, 1940.

Familiar essays concerning ways and institutions.

WHARTON, ANNE HOLLINGSWORTH, *Salons, Colonial and Republican*. Philadelphia, 1900.

A modernized version of the Ellet books.

WILDES, HARRY EMERSON, *Valley Forge*. New York, 1938.

The story of the Revolution in the Middle States, with the background and subsequent history of the encampment site.

WISTAR, SALLY, *Journal*, edited by Albert Cook Myers. Philadelphia, 1902.

Excerpts are also to be found in Watson and in Jenkins.

WOOD, LESLIE C., *Rafting on the Delaware*. Livingstone Manor, N. Y., 1934.

Exceptionally good account of the lumbering industry and its people.

Fiction writers have been concerned chiefly with the Revolutionary War period and with the clash of social codes in more modern times. As early as 1800, Charles Brockden Brown wrote a novel, *Arthur Mervyn*, dealing with the yellow fever epidemic of 1793, and, in the mid-forties George Lippard put forth an exciting story, originally entitled *The Monks of Monk Hall*, and later renamed *The Quaker City*, but these were exceptional topics.

Toward the close of the nineteenth century, when interest in the Revolution revived, Joseph Altsheler wrote *In Hostile Red*, a tale of the British campaigns in the Delaware valley, but Dr. S. Weir Mitchell's *Hugh Wynne, Free Quaker*, a story of the Revolution, was vastly more popular. In *The Red City*, published in 1908, Mitchell gained renewed popularity for a novel dealing with the second Washington administration. He had already, in *Hephzibah Guinness*, written of the Quaker life along the Delaware. A similar Revolutionary vein was tapped by Gertrude Crownfield, in 1934, with her *Where Glory Waits*, a fictionalized account of the love affair between Mary Vining and Anthony Wayne. Emma Raynor's *In Castle and Colony* took the quarrel between Big Belly Printz and Peg-leg Stuyvesant as its central theme.

Deeper social import is to be found in Cyrus Townsend Brady's novel of 1903, *A Doctor of Philosophy*, wherein he discusses the plight of a highly educated Negro girl who falls in love with a son of one of the old Philadelphia families. Dr. Brady had not, however, pioneered in the novel of social significance, for, as early as 1885, Ellen Kirk, in *A Midsummer Madness*, had written of the country-house life along the banks of the Delaware in much the same vein as was later to be followed by Francis Biddle in *The Llanfair Pattern* and William C. Bullitt in *It's Not Done*, a searing story that ran through twenty-four printings. The most recent of the Philadelphia novels is Christopher Morley's admirable *Kitty Foyle*.

Index